Estimated Minimum Sodium, Chloride, and Potassium Requirements for Healthy Persons

Age	Weight (kg)	Sodium (mg)*†	Chloride (mg)*†	Potassium (mg)‡
MONTHS				
0-5	4.5	120	180	500
6-11	8.9	200	300	700
YEARS				
1	11	225	350	1000
2-5	16	300	500	1400
6-9	25	400	600	1600
10-18	50	500	750	2000
>18§	70	500	750	2000

*No allowance has been included for large, prolonged losses from the skin through sweat.
†There is no evidence that higher intakes confer any additional health benefit.
‡Desirable intakes of potassium may considerably exceed these values (~3500 mg for adults).
§No allowance has been included for growth. Values given for people under 18 years of age assume a growth rate corresponding to the 50th percentile reported by the National Center for Health Statistics and averaged for males and females.

Estimated Safe and Adequate Daily Dietary Intakes (ESADDIs) of Selected Vitamins and Minerals*

Category	Age (years)	Vitamins		Trace Elements†				
		Biotin (µg)	Pantothenic acid (mg)	Copper (mg)	Manganese (mg)	Fluoride (mg)	Chromium (µg)	Molybdenum (µg)
Infants	0-0.5	10	2	0.4-0.6	0.3-0.6	0.1-0.5	10-40	15-30
	0.5-1	15	3	0.6-0.7	0.6-1	0.2-1	20-60	20-40
Children and adolescents	1-3	20	3	0.7-1	1-1.5	0.5-1.5	20-80	25-50
	4-6	25	3-4	1-1.5	1.5-2	1-2.5	30-120	30-75
	7-10	30	4-5	1-2	2-3	1.5-2.5	50-200	50-150
	11+	30-100	4-7	1.5-2.5	2-5	1.5-2.5	50-200	75-250
Adults		30-100	4-7	1.5-3	2-5	1.5-4	50-200	75-250

*Because there is less information on which to base recommendations for allowances of minerals, these figures are not given in the main table of RDAs and are provided here in the form of ranges of recommended intakes.
†Since toxic levels for many trace elements may be reached with only several times usual intakes, the upper levels for the trace elements given in this table should not be habitually exceeded.

CONTEMPORARY NUTRITION

Third Edition

GORDON M. WARDLAW, Ph.D., R.D., L.D.

School of Allied Medical Professions
Division of Medical Dietetics
The Ohio State University

with 318 illustrations

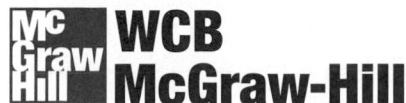

WCB McGraw-Hill

Boston, Massachusetts   Burr Ridge, Illinois   Dubuque, Iowa
Madison, Wisconsin   New York, New York   San Francisco, California   St. Louis, Missouri

WCB/McGraw-Hill

A Division of The McGraw·Hill Companies

Publisher **James Smith**
Senior Acquisitions Editor **Vicki Malinee**
Managing Editor **Janet Russell**
Project Manager **Linda McKinley**
Production Editor **René Spencer**
Designer **Elizabeth Fett**
Manufacturing Manager **Theresa Fuchs**

Third Edition

Printed in the United States of America

Composition by Graphic World, Inc.
Color separation by Color Associates
Printing/binding by Von Hoffmann Press

ISBN 0-8151-9050-6

97 98 99 00 / 9 8 7 6 5 4 3 2

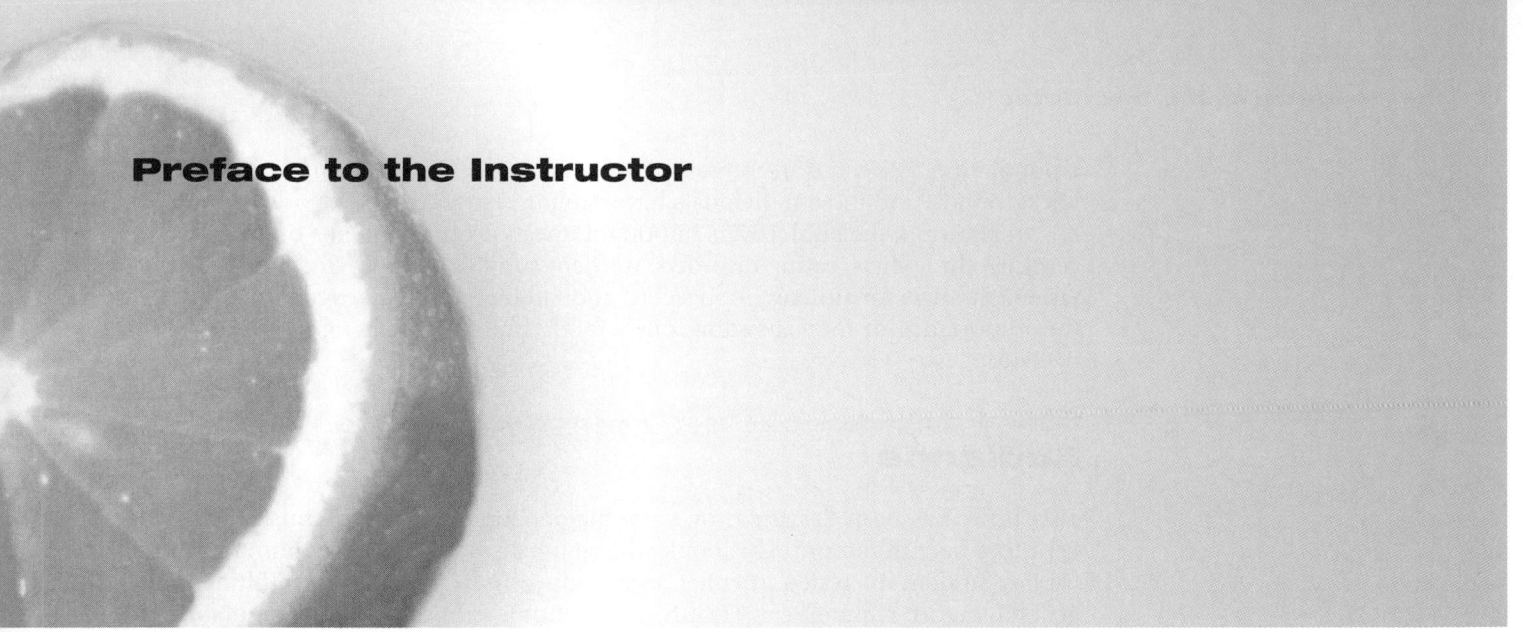

Preface to the Instructor

If you teach nutrition, you undoubtedly already find it a fascinating topic. However, nutrition can also be quite frustrating to teach. Claims and counter-claims abound regarding the need for certain constituents in our diets. Sodium is a good example. One group of researchers promotes a low-sodium diet for the general population as an effective preventive measure for high blood pressure. Other groups believe that normal blood pressure values can often be maintained despite the excess intakes of sodium common among Americans.

As an author, I too am aware of conflicting opinions in our field and thus draw on as many sources as possible in the continual updating of this textbook, now in its third edition. I have incorporated much new material, especially from recently published articles in major nutrition and medical journals, supplements to the *American Journal of Clinical Nutrition*, and the latest edition of *Modern Nutrition in Health and Disease*, edited by Shils, Olson, and Shike.

This textbook continues to differ significantly from all others in the field. Like other textbooks, it focuses on the latest research in nutrition, but it goes further by documenting important research studies throughout the chapters and listing those references at the end of each chapter. In all, the book strives to present many perspectives in current nutrition research so that you and your students can better understand and participate in debates about current nutrition issues.

Personalizing Nutrition

One prominent theme in nutrition research today is *individuality*. Not all of us, for example, find that saturated fat in our diets raises our blood cholesterol values above recommended standards. Each person responds individually, often idiosyncratically, to nutrients, and that is something I continually point out in this textbook.

Moreover, even at this basic level the book discussions do not assume that all nutrition students are alike. Chapter content repeatedly asks students to learn more about themselves and their health status and to use this new knowledge to improve their health. After reading this textbook, students will understand much more clearly how the nutrition information given on the evening news, on cereal-box labels, in popular magazines, and by government agencies applies to them. They will become sophisticated consumers of both nutrients and nutrition information. They will understand that their knowledge of nutrition allows them to personalize information, rather than follow every guideline issued for an entire population. After all, a population by definition consists of individuals with varying genetic and cultural backgrounds, and these individuals have varying responses to diet.

In addition, the book covers important questions that students often raise concerning ethnic diets, eating disorders, nutrient supplements, phytochemicals, vegetarianism, diets for athletes, food safety, and fad diets, with an overall emphasis on the importance of understanding one's food choices and changing one's diet as needed.

Audience

This book has been designed for a nonmajors audience. The chemistry has been kept to a bare minimum. This book will be most suitable as a beginning textbook for any student interested in either an introduction to nutrition or fulfillment of a general-science requirement. Health majors, home economics majors, nursing students, physical education students, and students in other health-related areas will also find this text appropriate. Because of the flexible chapter organization and content, this book can be adapted for students of diverse educational backgrounds.

Although the book is most suitable for a semester-length course, it can also be used in a quarter-length course by omitting chapters or multiple sections within chapters. An important feature of this text is that it is presented in five segments:

PART I   NUTRITION: A Key to Health
PART II   NUTRIENTS: The Heart of Nutrition
PART III   ENERGY: Balance and Imbalance
PART IV   NUTRITION: A Focus on Life Stages
PART V   NUTRITION: Beyond the Nutrients

This organization facilitates tailoring the text to your specific course needs.

New to This Edition

The third edition of *Contemporary Nutrition: Issues and Insights* incorporates several new features designed to enhance student learning and understanding:

Key Chapter Concepts

Each chapter opens with a list of key points the chapter will make. This piques student interest and focuses attention on important chapter ideas.

New Critical Thinking Questions

Each chapter presents two scenarios that allow students to apply information they have learned to practical situations. These questions will help students put the information in the chapter into the context of daily life and, by doing so, will enhance learning. Answers appear in the back of the book so that students can compare their thinking with that of the author.

Expanded Coverage of Nutrition Labeling

Constance J. Geiger, Ph.D., R.D., a noted authority on food-labeling issues and a consultant to the food industry, contributed to the Nutrition Issue in Chapter 2. This up-to-date essay reviews food labeling in detail. Then, in the remaining chapters of the book, sample labels are shown to reinforce the value of reading food labels and help the student practice obtaining important information from this nutrition tool.

Expanded Coverage of Ethnic Diets

The Nutrition Issue in Chapter 12 takes a broad look at ethnic influences on the American Diet. Chapter 6 covers the recently proposed Mediterranean diet pyramid.

New Nutrition Insight Boxes

Phytochemicals and other breaking topics are discussed in these new sections in each chapter.

Over 100 New Full-Color Illustrations

New figures provide a more colorful look at nutrition and effectively convey important nutrition concepts.

Food Guide Pyramid Illustrations

Sixteen colorful variations on the USDA Food Guide Pyramid illustrate the nutrient density of the various food groups.

Additional Features

This text is organized in response to the needs of instructors and students:

General Content and Controversial Topics Are Well Referenced

More than 80% of the references material is from sources published since the last edition of this text, published in 1994. As instructors, we demand the latest information to present to our students. Providing this up-to-date research not only gives students the most accurate picture of nutrition today but also directs them to current materials for further study.

Separate Chapters on Weight Control and Eating Disorders

These very controversial and current topics are discussed thoroughly.

Emphasis on Nutrient Density

Discussions of nutrients concentrate on the most nutrient-dense sources of foods. Leading food sources in the U.S. diet are identified for each nutrient when those data are available.

Application of the Exchange System

An outline of the 1995 version of the Exchange System is presented in Chapter 2 and can be used or omitted at your discretion. The use of the Exchange System is covered in detail in Appendix D and reinforced in the Student Study Guide.

Emphasis on Behavior-Change Strategies

Behavior-change strategies are introduced in Chapter 10, Weight Control, and then developed in detail in Chapter 12, Charting a Course for Change. The book encourages students to plan diets that will enhance health maintenance. The strategies allow students to apply the foundations of the course to daily life. Once students are able to put the main nutrition concepts into perspective, they can set nutritional goals and change their diets accordingly.

Summary Tables

Some chapters contain large summary tables detailing the major points. These tables are convenient capsules for reference.

Design

Choosing the illustrations for this textbook was quite exciting. This textbook is far ahead of any in the field in depicting important biological and physiological phenomena, such as transport across cell membranes, blood glucose regulation, digestion and absorption, cancer progression, and fetal development. The extensive three-dimensional graphic presentations in this book make nutrition principles come alive for students.

In addition, many sources are used to provide what is likely to be the best photographic program in any nutrition text. The many full-color photographs in this text were researched and selected to reflect a modern view of food presentation and food consumption.

Humor has been used throughout the text to aid the learning process. *Contemporary Nutrition: Issues and Insights* includes some of the best work of our nation's leading cartoonists. The cartoons make important nutrition points in a way that students will remember.

Pedagogy

The following pedagogical features were designed not only to interest the student but also to continually reinforce the learning process:

Assess Yourself

This exercise at the beginning of each chapter helps students explore their food habits and piques their interest in the nutritional information in the chapter. For example, the assessment in Chapter 6 focuses on saturated fat and cholesterol intake, which is a key discussion point in the chapter.

Key Chapter Concepts

Chapters open with key points to stimulate student interest and focus attention on important chapter content.

Another Bite

These are short paragraphs spaced throughout the book that apply the information in the chapter to various situations or provide another vantage point from which to view, and perhaps better appreciate, the text material.

Margin Notes

Margin notes throughout the book provide clinical examples, references to other chapters, clarification of ideas, and further details about key concepts.

Margin Definitions

Important terms are set in boldface type at first mention. More difficult terms are defined in the text's margins. All boldface terms appear in the glossary.

Concept Check Boxes

Concept Checks summarize chapter content every few pages, reinforcing students' understanding of the material.

Nutrition Insight Boxes

Each chapter contains short essays, often on controversial topics in nutrition, such as the role of fat replacements in our diets.

Rate Your Plate Boxes

These activity boxes at the end of each chapter let students put theory into practice. The suggested assignments are usually proactive and at times ask students to carefully analyze part of their current diet or nutrition-related lifestyle.

Critical Thinking Questions

Each chapter contains two scenarios that ask students to apply information they have learned to practical situations. Answers are provided at the end of the book.

Chapter Summary Points

The content of each chapter is summarized in seven to ten major points. This feature, together with the Key Chapter Concepts and Concept Checks, will help students review for examinations.

Study Questions

About ten questions at the end of each chapter encourage students to probe deeper into the chapter content, making connections and gaining new insights.

Up-To-Date References

Each chapter contains about 30 current references, most published since 1994.

Nutrition Issue Boxes

These essays at the end of each chapter extend the chapter content by adding more detailed and controversial material.

Glossary

A comprehensive glossary of more than 500 key terms is included for the student's reference. The glossary contains pronunciation keys for many unfamiliar words.

Supplementary Materials

The latest supplementary materials are provided to both the student and the instructor to make better use of the text and the concepts presented in the course:

Instructor's Manual and Test Bank

Prepared by Sandra Walz, Ph.D., R.D., this comprehensive teaching aid is available to adopters of the book and includes chapter summaries with suggestions for teaching difficult material: activities; suggested readings; activities to use with Mosby's NutriTrac software, source lists of supplementary materials; and a "survival" section, addressed to the novice instructor, that discusses class organization, scheduling, and problem areas such as cheating.

Extensively reviewed for clarity and accuracy, the test bank features approximately 1500 test items (multiple choice, short answer, and matching questions) coded for level of difficulty and type of knowledge being tested.

Student Study Guide

Prepared by Gordon M. Wardlaw, this student aid has been thoroughly reviewed by experienced instructors and developed in consultation with a learning-theory expert. This comprehensive guide reinforces concepts presented in the text and integrates them with study activities, such as flash cards, to emphasize key concepts. It features vocabulary review and sample examinations structured to reflect the actual examinations students will face in the classroom.

Computerized Test Bank

Instructors who adopt the text may receive EsaTest, a computerized test bank package compatible with IBM and Macintosh microcomputers. This test-generation software combines a number of user-friendly aids, enabling the instructor to select, edit, delete, and add questions and construct and print tests and answer keys. EsaTest also offers EsaGrade, a convenient electronic gradebook.

Transparency Acetates

Text adopters may receive full-color transparency acetates. They feature key illustrations from the text, with large, easy-to-read labels.

Mosby's NutriTrac Software

Available for Windows and Macintosh, this nutrient-analysis software allows you and your students to analyze diets easily, using an icon-based interface and on-screen help features. Foods for breakfast, lunch, dinner, and snacks may be selected from more than 2250 items in the database. Records may be kept for any number of days. The program can provide intake analyses for individual foods, meals, and days, or for an entire intake period. Intake analyses can compare nutrient values to RDA or RNI values and to the USDA Food Guide Pyramid and provide breakdowns of fat and calorie sources. Further activities for students to use with NutriTrac can be found in the Instructor's Manual.

ViewStudy™ Presentation Software

Available to qualified adopters, this CD-ROM, compatible with either Windows or Macintosh, contains key illustrations from the text. Images are arranged by chapter, and a slide-show tool allows selection of prearranged images. Illustrations can also be printed full size for use as acetates and may be exported for use with other programs and applications, such as the computerized testbank.

Special Acknowledgments

I would like to thank Janet Russell, who supported and assisted me through every step of the revision. Vicki Malinee and Jim Smith facilitated the difficult decisions that frequently arose. René Spencer did excellent and careful production work and copyediting. Sally Smith, R.D., proofread the entire manuscript.

Reviewers

As with the earlier editions, the goal is to provide the most accurate, up-to-date, and useful introductory nutrition text available. I, along with my publisher, would like to recognize and thank those people whose direction and insight guided the latest and first and second editions.

For the Third Edition:

John S. Avens, Ph.D.
Colorado State University

Hattie M. Middleton, Ph.D., R.D., L.D., C.H.E.
University of Northern Iowa

Susan G. Munroe, Ph.D.
University of Tennessee

Debra L. Ohlfs, R.D.
College of the Desert

Kaye L. Stanek, Ph.D.
University of Nebraska

Allison Stephen
University of Saskatchewan

Susan S. Yaple, M.Ed., R.D.
Spalding University

For the Second Edition:

Sandra L. Andrews, Ph.D.
Michigan State University

Liz Applegate, Ph.D.
University of California–Davis

Brenda Breeding, M.S.
Oklahoma City Community College

Faye C. Stucy Johnson, Ed.D., R.D., C.H.E.
California State University–Chico

Michael K. McIntosh Ph.D., R.D., L.D.N.
University of North Carolina–Greensboro

Dorice M. Narins, Ph.D.
Texas Woman's University

Marcia Nahikian-Nelms, M.Ed., R.D.
Southeast Missouri State University

Samuel C. Smith, Ph.D.
University of New Hampshire

Shirley Snarr, Ph.D.
Eastern Kentucky University

Wendy M. Stephens, M.S.
Luther College

Maureen C. Zimmerman, M.P.H.
Mesa Community College

For the First Edition:

Sara Anderson, Ph.D., R.D.
Southern Illinois University–Carbondale

Joan Benson, M.S., R.D.
University of Utah

Effie Creamer, Ph.D.
Eastern Kentucky University

Julie Ray Friedman, Ph.D.
State University of New York–Farmingdale

Deloy Hendricks, Ph.D.
Utah State University

Michael Hudecki, Ph.D.
State University of New York–Buffalo

Wendy Hunt, M.S., R.D.
American River College

Gladys Jennings, M.S., R.D.
Washington State University

Nelda Loper, M.S., R.D.
Seminole Community College

Margaret Ann McCarthy, M.P.H., R.D.
Eastern Kentucky University

Marsha Read, Ph.D.
University of Nevada

Joanne Spaide, Ph.D.
University of Northern Iowa

Diana Spillman, Ph.D., R.D.
Miami University

Kaye Stanek, Ph.D., R.D.
University of Nebraska

Ann Stasch, Ph.D.
California State University–Northridge

This book began with a dream. Each new edition is fostered by the excitement that improvements bring and ends with the revision of an innovative textbook that continues to set a standard for introductory nutrition textbooks.

Gordon M. Wardlaw

About the Author

GORDON M. WARDLAW, Ph.D., R.D., L.D., teaches nutrition to students in the Division of Medical Dietetics, School of Allied Medical Professions, The Ohio State University. Dr. Wardlaw is the author of many articles that have appeared in prominent nutrition, biology, physiology, and biochemistry journals and was the 1985 recipient of the American Dietetic Association's Mary P. Huddleson award. Dr. Wardlaw is a full member of the prestigious American Society for Nutritional Sciences and is certified as a Specialist in Human Nutrition by the American Board of Nutrition.

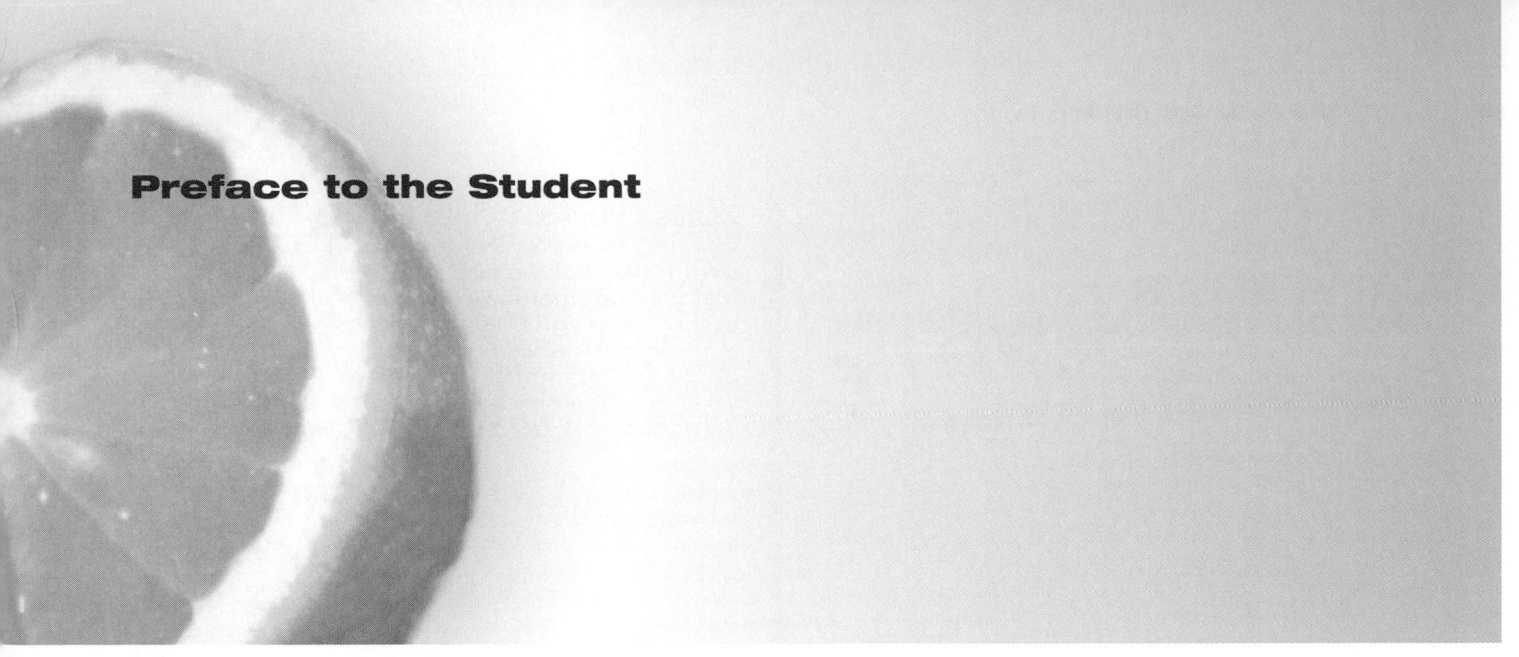

Preface to the Student

Cholesterol, sports drinks, food labeling, bulimia nervosa, alternative sweeteners, vegetarianism, and *Salmonella* food-borne illness—you have probably heard about the topics. Which of them are important considerations in your life or that of someone you know?

Americans pride themselves on their individuality. Nutritional advice should be given accordingly. For example, not all of us have high blood cholesterol and thus don't have this significant risk factor for premature development of heart disease. The need to tailor dietary advice to each person's individual nature is the basic approach of this book. First you are briefly introduced to the study of nutrition and ways to be a knowledgeable consumer. With so much information floating around—both accurate and inaccurate—you should know how to make informed decisions about your nutritional well-being. Then you will learn the basic principles of nutrition and discover how to apply the concepts in this book that pertain specifically to you.

The text discusses some of the most interesting and important elements of nutrition and food consumption to help you understand both how your body works and how your food choices affect your health.

Features
Planning a New Way of Eating

Many of the basic guidelines for planning a healthy diet are presented early in the text, including a description of the USDA Food Guide Pyramid in Chapter 2. Later, in Chapter 12, you learn the steps involved in setting nutritional goals and designing a diet plan to attain those goals.

Understanding the World Around Us

In a college environment, it is often difficult to envision how real the problem of world hunger is. Chapter 18 examines the problem of undernutrition and the conditions that create it. The chapter allows you to explore possible solutions that offer hope for the future of our world.

Pedagogy

Contemporary Nutrition: Issues and Insights incorporates some important tools (called *pedagogy*) to help you learn nutrition. The next few pages graphically point out how to use these study aids to your best advantage.

ASSESS yourself

How Does Your Diet Rate for Variety?

Directions: Check the box that best describes your eating habits.

How often do you eat:	Seldom or never	1 or 2 times a week	3 to 4 times a week	Almost daily
1. At least six servings of bread, cereals, rice, crackers, pasta, or other foods made from grains (a serving is one slice of bread or about ½ cup of cereal, rice, etc.) per day?	☐	☐	☐	☐
2. Foods made from whole grains?	☐	☐	☐	☐
3. Three different kinds of vegetables—about ½ cup each—per day?	☐	☐	☐	☐
4. A dark green leafy vegetable, such as spinach or broccoli?	☐	☐	☐	☐
5. Two kinds of fruit (whole piece) or fruit juice (¾ cup) per day?	☐	☐	☐	☐
6. Two servings of 2-3 ounces of lean meat, poultry, fish, eggs, dry beans, or nuts per day?	☐	☐	☐	☐
7. Two servings (three if teenager, pregnant, or breast-feeding) of a combination of milk (1 cup), yogurt (1 cup), or cheese (1½ ounce) per day?	☐	☐	☐	☐

SCORING: Compare your behaviors with the preferred practices.

Question 1: Almost Daily

Eating breads and cereals will not make you fat. Excess energy generally comes from the fat and/or sugar you may eat with them. Both whole-grained and enriched breads and cereals provide starch and essential nutrients.

Question 2: Almost Daily

Whole-grained breads and cereals contain vitamins, minerals, and dietary fiber that are lacking in the diets of some Americans. Select whole-grain cereals and bakery products, or make your own and use whole-wheat flour.

Question 3: Almost Daily

Vegetables vary in the amounts of vitamins and minerals they contain, so it's important to include several kinds every day.

Question 4: 3 to 4 Times a Week

Spinach and other dark green leafy vegetables are excellent sources of some nutrients and are lacking in many

Question 5: Almost Daily

Fruits taste good and are good for you. Choose several different kinds each day.

Question 6: Almost Daily

Most Americans include some meat, poultry, or fish in their diets regularly. Dry beans and peas, peanut cluding peanut butter), nuts and seeds, and eggs can be used as alternatives.

Question 7: Almost Daily

Adults as well as children need the calcium and other nutrients found in milk, cheese, and yogurt.

Each chapter begins with an **ASSESS YOURSELF.** This exercise will help you assess your own food choices and health history and habits. Review this again when you finish the chapter and think about how you will apply the chapter's content to your individual situation.

Key Chapter Concepts set the stage for learning at the start of chapter content and will focus your attention on important chapter ideas.

Key Chapter Concepts

- The scientific method of carefully examining hypotheses is a step-by-step, deliberate process, but no quicker method of testing ideas is as reliable.
- We tend to believe what we hear often or what close acquaintances tell us. When it comes to health practices, this well-meaning advice does not substitute for scientific verification of safety and effectiveness.
- The federal government provides minimal regulation of nutrient supplements and herbal remedies. "Let the buyer beware" is prudent advice to follow when using these products. Knowl-

- edge and professional guidance are important.
- Fraudulent claims for dietary and health-related remedies have always been part of our culture. Quacks prey primarily on older people and people with incurable diseases, such as AIDS.
- Consumers should carefully scrutinize the credentials and motives of anyone providing medical or health advice. Bogus practitioners with phony credentials are widespread.
- If it sounds too good to be true, it probably is. The medical community would gain nothing by holding back an effective cure from the public, despite what the quacks contend.

The Nature and Costs of Quackery

Quack
A person who does not have the medical skills or knowledge that he or she claims to have.

Health fraud
FDA defines health fraud as the promotion, advertisement, distribution, or sale of articles, intended for human or animal use, that are represented as being effective to diagnose, prevent, cure, treat, or mitigate disease (or other conditions) or provide a beneficial effect on health, but which have not been scientifically proven safe and effective for such purposes. Such practices may be deliberately deceptive or done without adequate knowledge or understanding of the article.

Fad is a shortened version of fiddle-faddle, which means to "play with" and then "cast aside."

Dictionaries define *quack* as "a pretender of medical skill; a charlatan" and "one who talks pretentiously without sound knowledge of the subject discussed." Quackery encompasses fraudulent actions, claims, and practices promoted by quacks, usually for their own profit.[1] In effect, quackery is a form of **health fraud**. Quacks argue that their alternative therapies and dietary regimens are the best road to health, and they decry more credible, science-based approaches as conspiracies perpetrated by a blind, money-mad medical-care industry. Many quacks lack any conscience or feeling for others; they selfishly take what they want and do as they please, leaving a trail of broken promises.[1,2] Deliberate deception is a hallmark of quacks. In contrast, other advocates of ineffective and unproven remedies sincerely believe in their products. They may be victims of quackery themselves or may merely wish to believe in something they hope will make them better. In their naivete and enthusiasm they pass on misinformation.[3]

Americans spend billions of dollars every year on quackery, often in search of a "quick fix" and sometimes in a desperate attempt to cure themselves of illness. Over $30 billion is spent on health fraud, including unnecessary vitamin and mineral supplements; substances such as bee pollen, ginseng root, and dried algae; and a wide range of herbal products. These items are taken in hopes of curing everything from the common cold, AIDS, and cancer to chronic diseases such as diabetes, heart disease, arthritis, Alzheimer's disease, and chronic fatigue syndrome.[7,10,13]

The Victims of Quackery

Can you say you were never a victim of quackery? Health fraud and quackery fool many people who are neither gullible nor ignorant. Quacks also prey on the unsuspecting, people who do not imagine that others are capable of doing such underhanded things. Until something bad happens, we usually don't recognize dishonest treatment. When we get "burned" by "hot" health frauds and other fads, a wiser skepticism results (Table 3-1).[3]

In many cases, people who follow the fraudulent health advice proffered by quacks lose only money. For others, however, quack practices can be dangerous. For example, dietary restrictions can be very hazardous to individuals who are ill or recovering from disease, pregnant women, infants, and growing children.[12] Moreover, if trying a quack remedy delays needed medical treatment, patients may suffer needless physical harm. Cancer patients, for instance, sometimes waste money on useless and unproved remedies instead of effective treatment and consequently risk dying

Throughout each chapter are **bold-faced key terms.** These are terms you will need to be familiar with throughout your study. The more difficult terms include a definition in the text's margins. All boldfaced terms appear with their definitions and pronunciations in the **glossary** at the end of the text.

You'll find that the numerous full-color, 3-dimensional **illustrations** almost jump off the page and will help nutrition "come alive" for you.

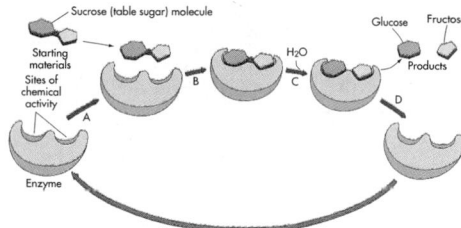

Figure 4-7 *A model of enzyme action. Enzymes act as catalysts to speed chemical reactions, including those that contribute to the digestion of foodstuffs. In this example an enzyme is contributing to the breakdown of sucrose (From A to D)into the smaller sugar forms glucose and fructose. Only these smaller sugar forms are absorbed from the small intestine to enter the bloodstream. Note that with some enzymes the reaction can go both ways. In addition, sometimes energy input is needed to allow the enzyme to push the reaction along.*

Each type of enzyme can speed only one specific type of chemical process. For example, enzymes that recognize and digest table sugar ignore milk sugar (lactose). The body can even increase the synthesis of certain digestive enzymes in response to the type of diet consumed—for example, producing more fat-digesting enzymes in response to a high-fat diet.[17]

Enzyme actions occur only under rather specific conditions. Besides working only on particular types of chemicals, enzymes are sensitive to acid and alkaline conditions, temperature, and the types of vitamins (acting as **coenzymes**) and minerals they require. Digestive enzymes that work in the acid environment of the stomach do not work well in the alkaline (basic) environment of the small intestine.

Again, the pancreas is a major site of production for digestive enzymes. In **cystic fibrosis**—an inherited disease of infants, children, and sometimes adults—the pancreas is often affected. It develops thick mucus that blocks its ducts, and active cells then die.[19] As a result, the pancreas is not able to effectively deliver its digestive enzymes into the small intestine. Digestion of carbohydrate, protein, and—most notably—fat is impaired because the needed enzymes are not released in adequate amounts. Often these enzymes must be ingested in capsule form with meals to aid in digestion.

Coenzyme
The active form of many vitamins; the coenzyme aids enzyme function.

Cystic fibrosis
A disease that often leads to overproduction of mucus, among other effects. Mucus can invade the pancreas, decreasing enzyme output. The lack of enzyme output then contributes to fat malabsorption.

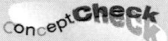

Concept **Check**

The gastrointestinal (GI) tract consists of the mouth, esophagus, stomach, small intestine, large intestine (colon), rectum, and anus. Organs associated with the GI tract are the liver, gallbladder, and pancreas. Together these organs perform the digestion needed to extract nutrients from food and funnel them into the bloodstream. In the GI tract, peristalsis propels food from the esophagus to the anus. During this journey, digestion is aided by enzymes produced by the mouth, stomach, pancreas, and small intestine cells. The transit time between eating food and eventually eliminating the indigestible remains is usually about 1 to 3 days.

The **CONCEPT CHECKS** appear every few pages and summarize content. If you don't understand what the Concept Check says, you should reread the preceding section in the textbook.

TABLE 1-2

Essential Nutrients in the Human Diet and Their Classes*

ENERGY-YIELDING NUTRIENTS

Carbohydrate	Fat (lipids)†	Protein (amino acids)	Water
Glucose‡ (or a carbohydrate that yields glucose)	Linoleic acid (omega-6)	Histidine	Water
	α-Linolenic acid (omega-3)	Isoleucine	
		Leucine	
		Lysine	
		Methionine	
		Phenylalanine	
		Threonine	
		Tryptophan	
		Valine	

VITAMINS

Water-soluble	Fat-soluble
Thiamin	A
Riboflavin	D§
Niacin	E
Pantothenic acid	K
Biotin	
B-6	
B-12	
Folate	
C	

MINERALS

Major	Trace	Questionable
Calcium	Chromium	Arsenic
Chloride	Copper	Boron
Magnesium	Fluoride ‖	Cadmium
Phosphorus	Iodide	Cobalt
Potassium	Iron	Lithium
Sodium	Manganese	Nickel
Sulfur	Molybdenum	Silicon
	Selenium	Tin
	Zinc	

*This table includes nutrients that the current RDA publication lists for humans. Some disagreement exists over the questionable and other minerals not listed. Dietary fiber could be added to the list of essential substances, but it is not a nutrient (see Chapter 5).
†The lipids listed are needed only in slight amounts, about 2% of total energy needs (see Chapter 6).
‡In order to prevent ketosis and thus the muscle loss that would occur if protein was used to synthesize carbohydrate (see Chapter 5).
§Sunshine on the skin also allows the body to make vitamin D for itself (see Chapter 8).
‖Primarily for dental health (see Chapter 9).

Below, nutrients are shown sorted into three groups: (1) those that primarily provide us with energy, (2) those that are important for growth and maintenance, and (3) those that act to keep body functions running smoothly. Some overlap exists between these groupings. The energy-yielding nutrients make up a major portion of most foods.

1. Provide energy	2. Promote growth and development	3. Regulate body processes
carbohydrates		
proteins	proteins	proteins
lipids	lipids	lipids
(fats and oils)	vitamins	vitamins
	minerals	minerals
	water	water

Carbohydrates. Carbohydrates provide a major source of fuel for the body, specifically 4 **kilocalories (kcal)** per gram. Small carbohydrate forms are called *sugars* or

Believing that a vitamin supplement provides the nutrition her body needs, Janice regularly takes such supplements while skimping on normal meals. How would you explain to her that the foods in a well-balanced diet are a more reliable source of essential nutrients than such supplements?

(For suggested answers to the Critical Thinking Questions in this and every chapter, turn to the back of the book.)

Kilocalorie (kcal)
The heat needed to raise the temperature of 1000 grams (1 liter) of water 1° Celsius. This is the same as raising the temperature of about 4 cups of water to 2° F.

The numerous **tables** throughout the text provide convenient capsules of information for your reference.

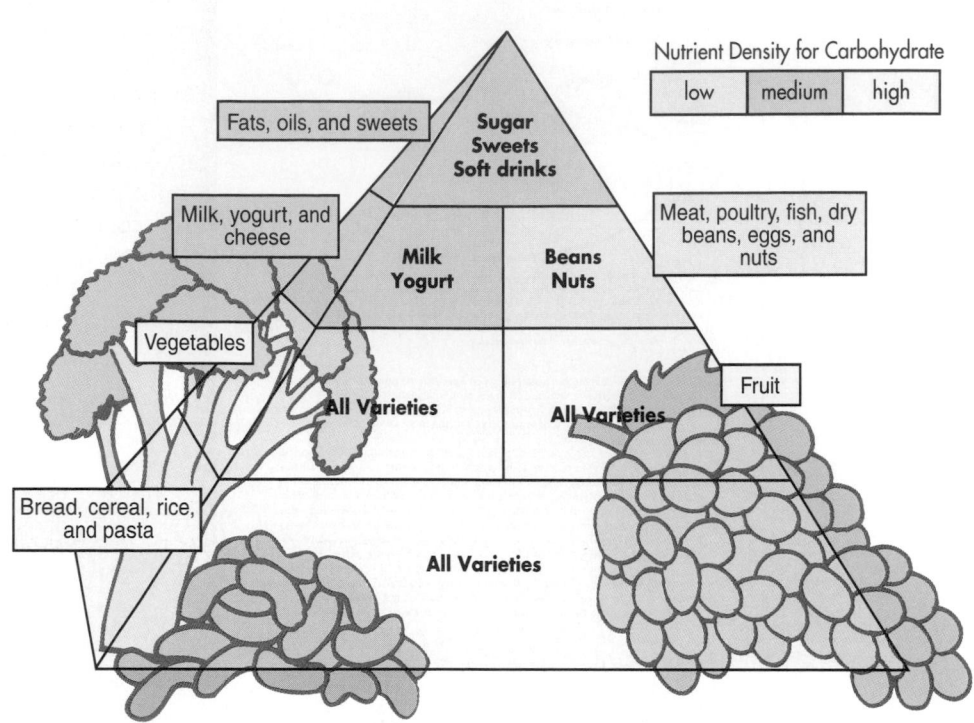

Nutrient Density for Carbohydrate

low	medium	high

Fats, oils, and sweets

**Sugar
Sweets
Soft drinks**

Milk, yogurt, and cheese

**Milk
Yogurt**

**Beans
Nuts**

Meat, poultry, fish, dry beans, eggs, and nuts

Vegetables

All Varieties

All Varieties

Fruit

Bread, cereal, rice, and pasta

All Varieties

Leading food sources for major nutrients are identified in **16 colorful variations** of the USDA Food Guide Pyramid. These illustrations will enable you to gain a further understanding of the distribution of nutrients among food groups.

Figure 5-10 *Sources of carbohydrates from the Food Guide Pyramid. The bread, cereal, rice, and pasta group, fruit group, vegetable group, and milk, yogurt, and cheese group contain many foods rich in carbohydrate. The background color of each group indicates the average nutrient density for carbohydrate in that group.*

ANOTHER BITE boxes are short paragraphs within the text designed to provide you with a different perspective on chapter material or more detail. You'll discover new and different ways to apply information.

Chapter 4   The Human Body: A Nutrition Perspective   123

A Closer Look at the Digestive Process

Even before we eat a morsel of many foods, the work of digestion—the breakdown of foods into usable forms we can absorb—is often already partially accomplished. Cooking or other preparations, such as marinating, pounding, or dicing, have probably begun the process. Starch granules in foods swell as they soak up water during cooking, making them much easier to digest. Cooking also softens the tough connective tissues in meats and the fibrous tissue of plants, such as is found in broccoli stalks. As a result, the food is easier to chew, swallow, and break down during later digestion. As you will see in Chapter 17, cooking also makes many foods, such as eggs, meats, fish, and poultry, much safer to eat.

Key Digestive Processes in the Stomach

The stomach secretes a major enzyme used for protein digestion. The release is controlled by a hormone. Just thinking about or chewing food stimulates nerves in the brain that control special hormone-producing cells in the base of the stomach. The hormone's release signals cells in the stomach to produce enzymes and acid.

You might wonder how the stomach protects itself from the acid and enzymes it produces. First the stomach has a thick layer of mucus that lines and insulates it from the acid and enzymes produced for digestion. The production of acid and enzymes is also tied to the release of a specific hormone, and this release happens primarily when we are thinking about eating or actually in the process of eating. Lastly, as the concentration of acid in the stomach increases, acid production tapers off, also because of hormonal control.[5]

Key Digestive Processes in the Small Intestine

All liquids consumed with a meal combine with stomach acid to form a very watery food mixture called *chyme*. As chyme squirts into the upper small intestine (called the *duodenum*), the acid in the chyme triggers the release of another hormone that stimulates the pancreas to release bicarbonate. This neutralizes the acid. If the chyme is not neutralized, it corrodes the wall of the duodenum, and could quickly lead to an *ulcer*, because, unlike the stomach, the small intestine lacks a protective layer of mucus. This form of protection is not possible because it would impede nutrient absorption. A second hormone causes the pancreas and gallbladder to release their products—enzymes from the pancreas and bile from the gallbladder.

Chyme
A mixture of stomach secretions and partially digested food.

Ulcer
Erosion of the tissue lining in either the stomach or upper small intestine; generally referred to as a peptic ulcer.

In part because of hormonal fine-tuning, the digestive tract responds to the nutritional makeup and amount of the food consumed. Foods generally contain a mixture of macronutrients and vitamins and minerals; therefore a multiple enzymatic attack on the contents of the small intestine is the rule. The contention of the authors of some fad diet books that ingestion of certain combinations of foods, such as meats and fruits together, hinders the digestive process does not make sense in light of both our knowledge about gastrointestinal physiology and our collective experience.

Small Intestine: Site for Most Nutrient Absorption

Most nutrient absorption—that is, the transfer of nutrients from the intestine and to the bloodstream—occurs in the small intestine; little occurs in the stomach and large intestine.[6] The small intestine can absorb about 95% of the energy it receives

To briefly clarify and expand concepts presented, **margin notes** are provided for you. These help reinforce concepts you'll learn in every chapter. Critical thinking questions also appear in the margins to give you the opportunity to apply chapter content to real-life situations. Answers are in the back of the book.

Fad is a shortened version of fiddle-faddle, which means to "play with" and then "cast aside."

The Victims

Can you say you we
many people who a
pecting, people who
handed things. Unti
treatment. When we
skepticism results (T

In many cases,
quacks lose only mo
example, dietary res
covering from diseas
if trying a quack rem
less physical harm. C
and unproved remed

72

NUTRITION INSIGHTS are boxes within the text that allow you to learn more about timely topics that should be of interest to you.

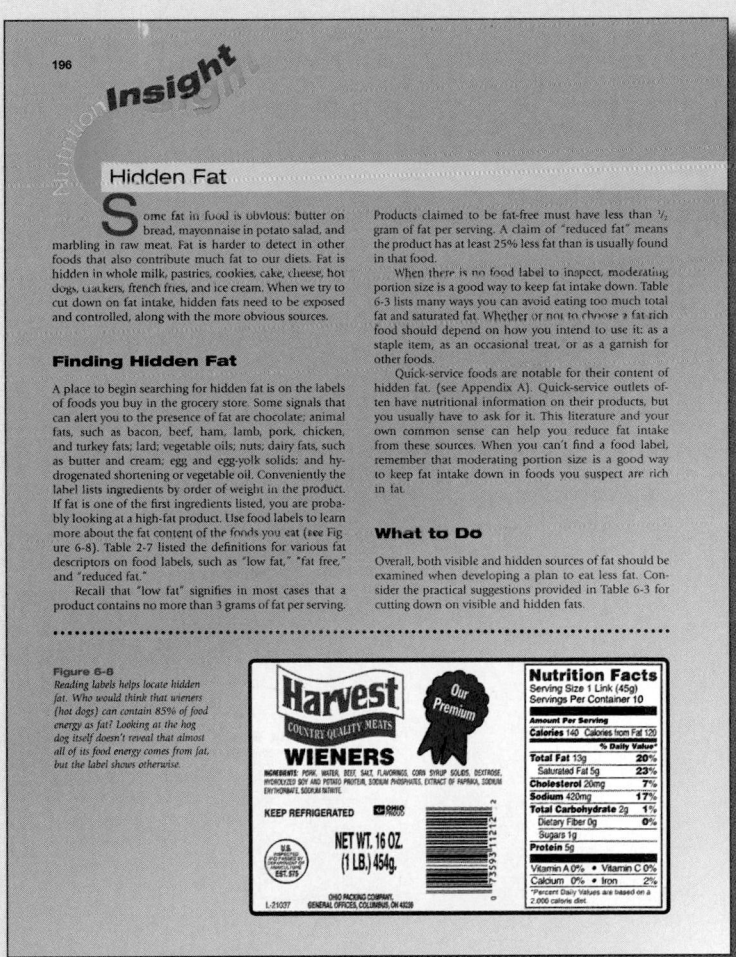

196

Insight

Hidden Fat

Some fat in food is obvious: butter on bread, mayonnaise in potato salad, and marbling in raw meat. Fat is harder to detect in other foods that also contribute much fat to our diets. Fat is hidden in whole milk, pastries, cookies, cake, cheese, hot dogs, crackers, french fries, and ice cream. When we try to cut down on fat intake, hidden fats need to be exposed and controlled, along with the more obvious sources.

Finding Hidden Fat

A place to begin searching for hidden fat is on the labels of foods you buy in the grocery store. Some signals that can alert you to the presence of fat are chocolate; animal fats, such as bacon, beef, ham, lamb, pork, chicken, and turkey fats; lard; vegetable oils; nuts; dairy fats, such as butter and cream; egg and egg-yolk solids; and hydrogenated shortening or vegetable oil. Conveniently the label lists ingredients by order of weight in the product. If fat is one of the first ingredients listed, you are probably looking at a high-fat product. Use food labels to learn more about the fat content of the foods you eat (see Figure 6-8). Table 2-7 listed the definitions for various fat descriptors on food labels, such as "low fat," "fat free," and "reduced fat."

Recall that "low fat" signifies in most cases that a product contains no more than 3 grams of fat per serving.

Products claimed to be fat-free must have less than $1/2$ gram of fat per serving. A claim of "reduced fat" means the product has at least 25% less fat than is usually found in that food.

When there is no food label to inspect, moderating portion size is a good way to keep fat intake down. Table 6-3 lists many ways you can avoid eating too much total fat and saturated fat. Whether or not to choose a fat-rich food should depend on how you intend to use it: as a staple item, as an occasional treat, or as a garnish for other foods.

Quick-service foods are notable for their content of hidden fat. (see Appendix A). Quick-service outlets often have nutritional information on their products, but you usually have to ask for it. This literature and your own common sense can help you reduce fat intake from these sources. When you can't find a food label, remember that moderating portion size is a good way to keep fat intake down in foods you suspect are rich in fat.

What to Do

Overall, both visible and hidden sources of fat should be examined when developing a plan to eat less fat. Consider the practical suggestions provided in Table 6-3 for cutting down on visible and hidden fats.

Figure 6-8
Reading labels helps locate hidden fat. Who would think that wieners (hot dogs) can contain 85% of food energy as fat? Looking at the hog dog itself doesn't reveal that almost all of its food energy comes from fat, but the label shows otherwise.

To reinforce the value of reading food labels, **sample labels** are illustrated throughout the text. These samples will help you practice obtaining important information from this nutrition tool.

RATE *your* Plate

What Is Your Fat and Cholesterol Intake?

How do your food practices compare with general guidelines suggested for fat, saturated fat, and cholesterol intake? Refer to the nutritional assessment you completed at the end of Chapter 2, and compare it with the guidelines listed below, issued by the American Heart Association and the National Cholesterol Education Program:

• Limit or reduce total fat intake to 30% or less of total energy intake.
• Reduce saturated fat intake to 7% to 10% of energy intake or less.
• Limit cholesterol to 200 to 300 milligrams per day.

To compare your nutritional assessment with these guidelines, first fill in the values for your intakes of the following:

TOTAL ENERGY: _____   TOTAL FAT: _____   SATURATED FAT: _____   CHOLESTEROL: _____

Now complete the following steps:

1. Multiply your total grams of fat by 9 (kcal per gram of fat). Then divide the result by your total energy intake. Next multiply this number by 100. This will give you the percentage of energy you consumed from fat.

   % OF ENERGY FROM FAT _____   IS IT 30% OR LESS OF TOTAL ENERGY?   YES _____   NO _____

2. Multiply your grams of saturated fat by 9 (kcal per gram of fat). Divide the result by your total energy intake. Now multiply this number by 100. This will give you the percentage of energy you consumed from saturated fat.

   % OF ENERGY FROM SATURATED FAT _____

   IS IT 10% OF ENERGY OR LESS?   YES _____   NO _____

3. Look at your milligrams of cholesterol.

   IS YOUR INTAKE LESS THAN 300 milligrams?   YES _____   NO _____

4. Look back at the foods you ate and notice the foods that contributed the most fat, saturated fat, and cholesterol. If you didn't meet one or more of the guidelines and had elevated LDL, how could you change what you ate that day to improve your diet?

5. Now take the next step. Do you know your HDL and LDL values? If not, have them checked soon. All adults should know whether these values are in the abnormal ranges.

6. Finally, fill in the following assessment of your risk for developing premature heart disease. Decide today how you could modify your diet and lifestyle, if necessary, to reduce your risk.

Do you have . . .	YES	NO		YES	NO
a history of smoking?	___	___	diabetes?	___	___
high blood pressure?	___	___	a history of physical inactivity?	___	___
high LDL?	___	___	a family history of premature heart disease?	___	___
low HDL?	___	___	a history of obesity?	___	___
			a diet that lacks sufficient B vitamins, such as B-6, folate, and B-12?	___	___

Other factors also could be considered, as discussed in the Nutrition Issue, but this provides a good start for assessing your risk.

At the end of each chapter is a **RATE YOUR PLATE** section that will help you apply a major concept in each chapter to your own life. The activity encourages you to look more carefully at your diet, examine your family history, or apply information to help other people you know.

NUTRITION ISSUES are boxes at the end of chapters that develop current topics in nutrition in greater detail than can be done in the chapter. Topics include nutrition and alcohol, heart disease, cancer, fad diets, and food labeling.

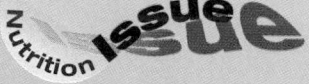

Nutrition Issue

Vegetarianism

Vegetarianism has evolved over the centuries from a necessity into an option (Figure 7-10). Historically, vegetarianism was linked with specific philosophies and religions or with science.[24] In the sixth century BC, Pythagoras advocated a meatless diet for its physical health, ecological, religious, and philosophical benefits.

Today there are about 12 million vegetarians in the United States, about double the number in 1985. Vegetarianism is popular among college students. Fifteen percent of college students in one survey said they select vegetarian options at lunch or dinner on any given day. In response, dining services offer vegetarian options at every meal, the most common being pastas with meatless sauce and pizza. A recent survey by the National Restaurant Association found that 20% of customers want a vegetarian option when they eat out. As nutrition science

has grown, new information has enabled the design of adequate vegetarian diets. It is important for vegetarians to take advantage of this information because a diet of only plants can lead to various nutrient deficiencies and to substantial growth retardation in infants and children.[1, 4, 7, 10] People who choose a vegetarian diet can meet their nutritional needs by following a few basic rules and knowledgeably planning their diets.

Recent studies show that death rates from some chronic diseases are lower for vegetarians than for nonvegetarians. Healthful lifestyles (not smoking, abstinence from alcohol and drugs, and increased physical activity) and social class bias probably partially account for these findings.[4] As noted in the last chapter, one study showed that a totally vegetarian diet coupled with physical activity, meditation, and smoking cessation led to regression of atherosclerosis.

WHY DO PEOPLE PRACTICE VEGETARIANISM?

People choose vegetarianism for a variety of reasons. Some believe that killing animals for food is unethical. Hindus and Trappist monks eat vegetarian meals as a practice of their religion. In the United States, many Seventh Day Adventists base their practice of vegetarianism on biblical texts and believe it is a more healthful way to live. Some people might pursue vegetarianism because meat is expensive.

People might choose vegetarianism after realizing that animals are not efficient protein factories. Animals actually use much of the protein they eat just to maintain themselves rather than to synthesize new muscle tissue. Animals that humans eat sometimes eat grasses that humans cannot digest. Many, however, also eat grains humans can eat.

People might also practice vegetarianism because it encourages a high intake of carbohydrates, vitamins A, E, and C, carotenoids, magnesium, and dietary fiber, while limiting saturated fat and cholesterol intake. This produces a diet closely resembling that suggested in the Dietary Guidelines for Americans covered in Chapter 2. Studies confirm that many vegetarians actually do eat nutritious, low-fat diets.[4]

FOOD PLANNING FOR VEGETARIANS

There are a variety of vegetarian styles. **Vegans** eat only plant foods. **Fruitarians** eat fruits, nuts, honey, and vegetable oils. This plan is not recommended because it can lead to nutrient deficiencies in people of all ages. **Lacto-vegetarians** modify vegetarianism a bit—they include dairy products

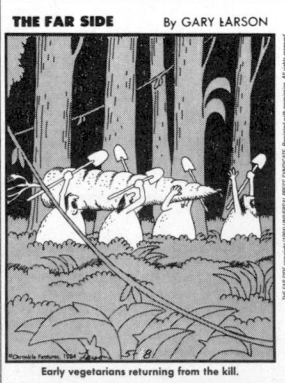

Figure 7-10 *The Far Side.*

Summary

➤ Nutrition is the study of what foods are vital for health and how your body uses nutrients to promote and support growth, maintenance, and reproduction of cells.

➤ The metric system is used throughout science. Lengths are expressed in meters, weights are expressed in grams, and volumes are expressed in liters. A meter equals about 39 inches, a kilogram is about 2.2 pounds, and a liter is about 1 quart.

➤ There are six classes of nutrients found in foods: (1) carbohydrates, (2) lipids (fats and oils), (3) proteins, (4) vitamins, (5) minerals, and (6) water. Carbohydrates, lipids, and proteins provide energy (kilocalories) for the body to use.

➤ A basic plan for health promotion and disease prevention includes eating a varied diet, performing regular physical activity, not smoking, getting adequate fluid and sleep, limiting alcohol intake, and limiting or coping with stress.

➤ Good nutrition should be based on eating the right foods rather than mostly relying on nutrient supplements. Getting necessary nutrients from foods minimizes nutrient imbalances and prevents most chances of toxicity from the resulting overnutrition.

➤ As nutritional health diminishes, nutrient stores in the body are depleted first. As stores are exhausted, the state of undernutrition causes biochemical reactions in the body to eventually slow down. Finally, clinical evidence of deficiency is apparent.

➤ Results from large nutrition surveys in the United States suggest that some of us need to concentrate on consuming foods that supply more vitamin A, certain B vitamins, calcium, iron, zinc, and dietary fiber.

➤ The taste and texture of foods primarily influence our food choices. Several other factors also help determine food habits and choices: our upbringing, various social and cultural factors, our self-image and the image we want to project to others, economics, and concerns about health.

➤ There are no true "junk" or "bad" foods. The focus should be on balancing a total diet by choosing many nutritious foods.

Study Questions

1 Name three chronic diseases associated with nutrition and a few corresponding risk factors.

2 Identify a nutrition-related disease that develops over many years before clinical symptoms are evident. Why is there such a long lag time?

3 List the energy values for a gram of carbohydrate, fat, protein, and alcohol.

4 Wendy's Big Bacon Classic contains 44 grams carbohydrate, 36 grams fat, and 37 grams protein. Calculate the percentage of energy derived from fat.

5 Outline the ABCDs of a nutritional assessment; that is, the activities performed to assess an individual's nutritional status.

6 According to national nutrition surveys, which nutrients tend to be underconsumed by many adult Americans. Why is this the case?

7 Over the next week, keep an eye out for subliminal cues in the media—TV, radio, magazines, etc.—for eating. What pattern do you see? (Hint: pizza delivery advertised during a sports show.)

Each chapter ends with a **SUMMARY.** These summary points convey the major ideas of each chapter.

There are approximately ten **STUDY QUESTIONS** per chapter. These provide an excellent review for studying for examinations.

Study Aids

A Student Study Guide and Mosby's NUTRITRAC software are available for use with *Contemporary Nutrition: Issues and Insights, third edition.* These instructional aids are designed to help you apply the major concepts developed in each chapter and prepare for classroom examinations.

Student Study Guide

Reviewed by instructors and developed in consultation with a learning theory expert, this valuable Study Guide by Gordon M. Wardlaw reinforces concepts presented in the text and integrates them with activities to facilitate learning.

• Sample examinations reflect the actual tests you will face in the classroom.
• Vocabulary review exercises increase your knowledge of terminology.
• Flash cards help you practice explaining the major concepts in the chapter to yourself and in turn test your understanding of these important concepts.
• Activities include fill-in tables, labeling, and matching terms. These activities follow the text discussion and are anchored with quotations and page citations from the text. An ongoing dietary analysis highlights the content of many chapters.

Mosby's NUTRITRAC

This nutrient-analysis software for Windows or Macintosh is accurate, up-to-date, and very easy to use. It lets you analyze food intakes with the click of a button. This unique program allows you to add foods from the food database for breakfast, lunch, dinner, and snacks for any number of days. The program then provides an intake analysis for an individual food, meal, day, or entire intake period. This software is powerful and very user-friendly:

- It's easy to use, with a visual design and on-screen help features.
- It's powerful, featuring a Food/Nutrient Database with more than 2250 foods and 33 nutrient values based on household measures from the USDA's Food Guide Pyramid for each food.
- It's up-to-date and compares the user's nutrient values to the USDA Food Guide Pyramid.
- It's thorough and authoritative—the food-intake analysis includes comparison of nutrient values to RDA or RNI values, calorie sources, and fat breakdowns.
- It's convenient and easily customized and maintains personal user profile(s), including height, weight, RDA category, activity level, and estimates of daily calorie needs.
- It's versatile and contemporary—quick-service and ethnic foods are contained in the Food/Nutrient Database.

A Request to Professors and Students Who Use This Book

As you might imagine, it is difficult to range across the vast areas of nutrition science, following all of the various controversies and new developments. I try my best but realize that sometimes I miss a side of an argument that deserves attention. If as you read this book you find content that you question or believe warrants a more detailed or broader look, feel free to contact me by mail, fax, or e-mail.

Gordon M. Wardlaw, Ph.D., R.D.
The Ohio State University
516H School of Allied Medical Professions
1583 Perry Street
Columbus, OH 43210
Fax: 614-292-0210
E-mail: wardlaw.1@osu.edu

Brief Contents

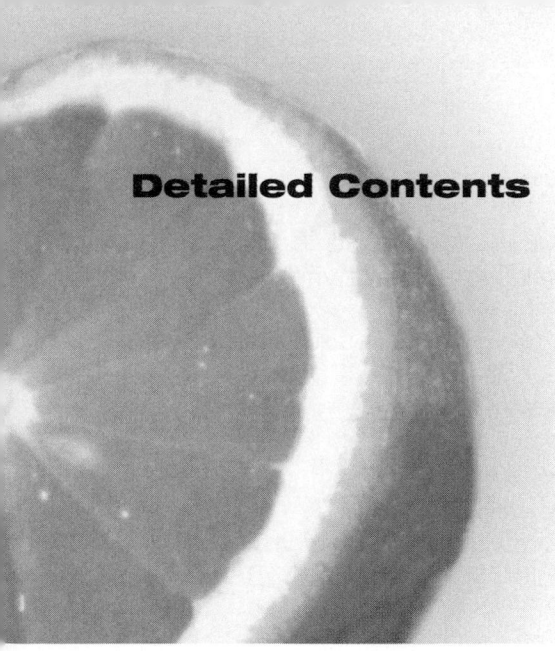

Detailed Contents

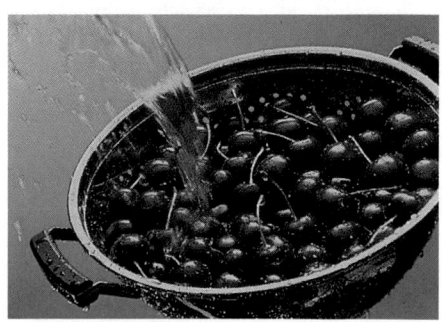

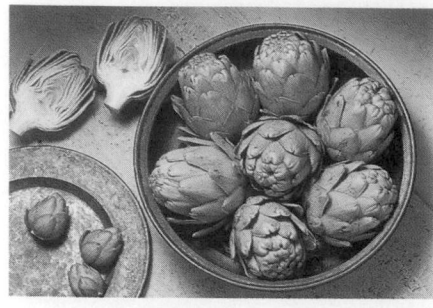

PART 3
ENERGY
Balance and
Imbalance

10 Weight Control, 350

11 NUTRITION: Athletics and Fitness, 400

12 Charting a Course for Change, 434

13 Anorexia Nervosa and Bulimia Nervosa, 458

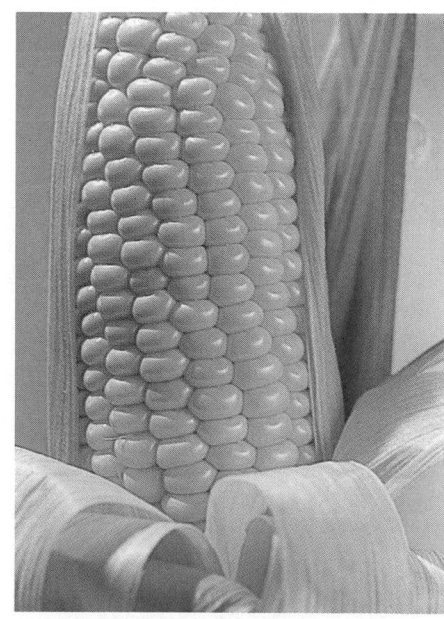

PART 4

NUTRITION
A Focus on Life Stages

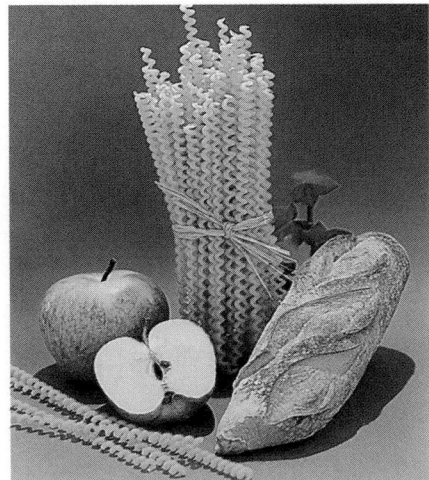

PART 5

NUTRITION
Beyond the Nutrients

NUTRITION

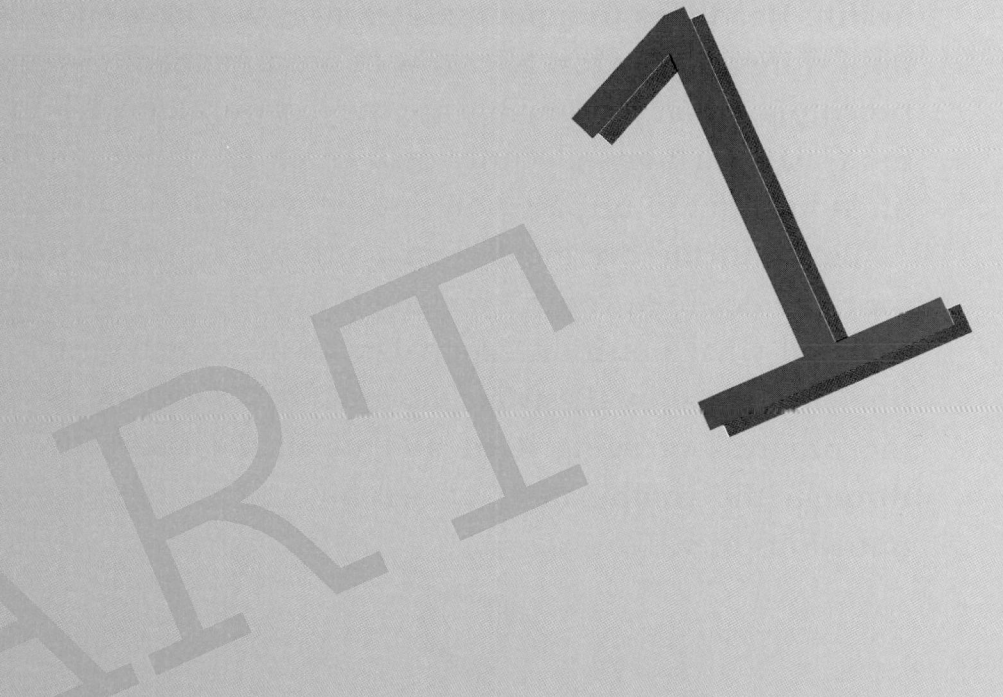

A Key to Health

PART 1

What You Eat and Why

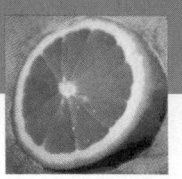

Do you need vitamin and mineral supplements? Are you getting too much fat and cholesterol? Is much of what you eat unsafe? Are some foods actually *junk foods*? Should you become a vegetarian? If you're confused about what you should eat, welcome to what is probably the fastest-growing club in the country. This chapter will help you sort out some of these issues as you are introduced to the science of nutrition.

For some time the media have been blasting us with information about nutrition and health. Headlines trumpet *breakthroughs* that frequently break down after further study. Bookstores display row after row of nutrition books—some excellent, some so-so, some ridiculous—that presumably are the last word on what to eat and what to avoid.[5] Some food manufacturers gleefully cash in on the latest nutritional marvel (whose wonders often turn out to be based on limited research).

But both the overrated claims and the sensible information spring from the same root: the desire to control our quality of life. As you begin this study of nutrition, keep in mind what nutrition expert Dr. Irwin Rosenberg recently provided as his "bottom line" for a healthy lifestyle: "Research has shown no better way to slow or even reverse the progress of aging itself and of all the age-related degenerative conditions than through the combination of aerobic and strength-building exercise and a balanced, nutritious diet."[16]

What Factors Determine Your Food Choices?

What are your favorite foods? Why do you like them? If only one's taste buds determined food preferences, you probably wouldn't try strong tasting or spicy foods. Which foods do most of the members of your family enjoy together? Which foods are consistently excluded, if any? Use the following survey to discover how significantly the factors listed determine why you eat the way you do. Circle the number reflecting the most appropriate answer.

		Not significant at all				Very significant	
1.	Weight control	0	1	2	3	4	5
2.	Health	0	1	2	3	4	5
3.	Food costs	0	1	2	3	4	5
4.	Convenience/Time	0	1	2	3	4	5
5.	Family background	0	1	2	3	4	5
6.	Advertisements (TV or radio)	0	1	2	3	4	5
7.	Emotions	0	1	2	3	4	5
8.	Peers (friends, co-workers)	0	1	2	3	4	5
9.	Customs/Ethnic background	0	1	2	3	4	5
10.	Physical activity habits	0	1	2	3	4	5

INTERPRETATION

Take note of the factors that scored 4 or 5. These are your most significant influences. Then, next to these put a PLUS (+) or MINUS (−) sign to indicate whether you feel they have been a positive or negative influence on your health.

This chapter asks you to examine what you eat and why, so you understand the origins of your eating habits. It includes a general discussion of why we eat what we do. Later you will also complete an activity that focuses on your reasons for choosing certain foods in a day's menu.

Key Chapter Concepts

- Poor nutrition contributes to much of the disease Americans experience.
- A varied diet coupled with regular physical activity is a goal for health.
- Nutrients are classed as carbohydrates, lipids (fats and oils), proteins, vitamins, minerals, and water. The lipids are especially rich in energy.
- Foods, rather than nutrient supplements, deserve the major focus in diet planning. Most

experts advocate increasing fruit and vegetable intake, rather than relying on nutrient supplements.
- Taste and texture primarily influence food choice. Health deserves a greater emphasis.
- There are no "junk" or "bad" foods per se. Focusing on the total diet is the best approach.
- Because genetic background influences health, family history for disease is important to consider.

Your Introduction to Nutrition

Although the science of **nutrition** is relatively young, we already know much about what nutrients are needed for an adequate diet and what foods provide them. In your lifetime you will eat about 70,000 meals and 60 tons of food. In this opening chapter you will take a close look at your eating habits and discover the underlying reasons for them. This is an important first step. People with nutritional lifestyles out of balance with their physiology are likely to have or eventually develop health problems. Ironically, people often have good intuitions about healthy food choices but fail to act on them. However, if you make even small changes in your behavior toward food, you can increase your chances for enjoying a long and vigorous life.[16] The more you know about nutrition and your health risks, the better you can plan diets to meet your nutritional needs.

Recent evidence points to poor diet as a **risk factor** for **chronic** diseases that are the leading causes of adult deaths: **heart disease, stroke, high blood pressure (hypertension), diabetes**, and some forms of **cancer**. Together, these disorders account for two thirds of all deaths in North America (Table 1-1). Not consuming enough **nutrients** also makes us more likely to suffer consequences of poor nutrition habits in later years, such as bone fractures from the disease **osteoporosis**. Iron-deficiency **anemia** is another possibility. At the same time, taking too much of a nutrient supplement—such as vitamin A, vitamin B-6, or copper—can be harmful. Another dietary problem, drinking too much alcohol, is associated with **cirrhosis** of the liver, some forms of cancer, accidents, and suicides. All of these consequences of modern living are partly an "affliction of affluence."[16]

The great tragedy is that these diseases are often preventable. Government scientists have calculated that a poor diet combined with a lack of sufficient physical activity accounted for 300,000 fatal cases of heart disease, cancer, and diabetes in 1990. Thus, the combination of poor diet and lack of physical activity is indirectly the second leading cause of death. As you gain understanding about your nutritional habits and increase your knowledge about nutrition, you have the opportunity to dramatically cut your risk for many of these problems.[18]

As you begin to study nutrition in this chapter, you will first learn the names of the nutrients you need. Then you will discover what those nutrients do in your body. Later you will learn how to evaluate a person's nutritional health, as well as evaluate how healthful the current American diet is. Finally, you will discover why people eat the things they do and the powerful influence of genetic background on your overall health.

Risk factor

A term used frequently when discussing diseases and factors contributing to their development. A risk factor is an aspect of our lives—such as heredity, lifestyle choices (i.e., smoking), or nutritional habits—that may make us more likely to develop a disease.

Chronic

Long-standing, developing over time; slow to develop or resolve. When referring to disease, this term indicates that the disease process, once developed, is slow and tends to remain; a good example is heart disease.

Heart disease

A disease characterized by the deposition of fatty material in the blood vessels that serve the heart. These deposits restrict blood flow through the heart, which in turn can lead to heart damage and death.

TABLE 1-2

Essential Nutrients in the Human Diet and Their Classes*

ENERGY-YIELDING NUTRIENTS

Carbohydrate	Fat (lipids)†	Protein (amino acids)	Water
Glucose‡ (or a carbohydrate that yields glucose)	Linoleic acid (omega-6)	Histidine	Water
	α-Linolenic acid (omega-3)	Isoleucine	
		Leucine	
		Lysine	
		Methionine	
		Phenylalanine	
		Threonine	
		Tryptophan	
		Valine	

VITAMINS

Water-soluble	Fat-soluble
Thiamin	A
Riboflavin	D§
Niacin	E
Pantothenic acid	K
Biotin	
B-6	
B-12	
Folate	
C	

MINERALS

Major	Trace	Questionable
Calcium	Chromium	Arsenic
Chloride	Copper	Boron
Magnesium	Fluoride ‖	Cadmium
Phosphorus	Iodide	Cobalt
Potassium	Iron	Lithium
Sodium	Manganese	Nickel
Sulfur	Molybdenum	Silicon
	Selenium	Tin
	Zinc	

*This table includes nutrients that the current RDA publication lists for humans. Some disagreement exists over the questionable and other minerals not listed. Dietary fiber could be added to the list of essential substances, but it is not a nutrient (see Chapter 5).
†The lipids listed are needed only in slight amounts, about 2% of total energy needs (see Chapter 6).
‡In order to prevent ketosis and thus the muscle loss that would occur if protein was used to synthesize carbohydrate (see Chapter 5).
§Sunshine on the skin also allows the body to make vitamin D for itself (see Chapter 8).
‖Primarily for dental health (see Chapter 9).

(For suggested answers to the Critical Thinking Questions in this and every chapter, turn to the back of the book.)

Critical Thinking

Believing that a vitamin supplement provides the nutrition her body needs, Janice regularly takes such supplements while skimping on normal meals. How would you explain to her that the foods in a well-balanced diet are a more reliable source of essential nutrients than such supplements?

Below, nutrients are shown sorted into three groups: (1) those that primarily provide us with energy, (2) those that are important for growth and maintenance, and (3) those that act to keep body functions running smoothly. Some overlap exists between these groupings. The energy-yielding nutrients make up a major portion of most foods.

1. Provide energy	2. Promote growth and development	3. Regulate body processes
carbohydrates	proteins	proteins
proteins	lipids	lipids
lipids (fats and oils)	vitamins	vitamins
	minerals	minerals
	water	water

Kilocalorie (kcal)
The heat needed to raise the temperature of 1000 grams (1 liter) of water 1° Celsius. This is the same as raising the temperature of about 4 cups of water to 2° F.

Carbohydrates. Carbohydrates provide a major source of fuel for the body, specifically 4 **kilocalories (kcal)** per gram. Small carbohydrate forms are called *sugars* or

TABLE 1-1		
Ten Leading Causes of Death in the United States		
Rank	**Cause of death**	**Percent of total deaths**
	All causes	100.0
1	Heart disease (primarily **heart attacks**)*	29
2	Cancer*	26
3	Cerebrovascular diseases (stroke)*	5
4	Chronic obstructive pulmonary diseases and allied conditions (lung diseases)	4
5	Accidents and adverse effects†	
	Motor vehicle accidents	3
	All other accidents and adverse effects	3
6	Pneumonia and influenza	3
7	Diabetes*	2
8	Acquired immunodeficiency syndrome (AIDS)	2
9	Suicide†	2
10	Homicide and legal intervention†	2

From Centers for Disease Control and Prevention, *Morbidity and Mortality Weekly Report*, December 16, 1994. Data are age-adjusted to the 1990 population.
*Causes of death in which diet plays a part.
†Causes of death in which excessive alcohol consumption plays a part.

What Is Nutrition?

The Council on Food and Nutrition of the American Medical Association defines *nutrition* as "The science of food, the nutrients and the substances therein, their action, interaction, and balance in relation to health and disease, and the process by which the organism ingests, digests, absorbs, transports, utilizes, and excretes food substances."

Nutrients Come From Food

What is the difference between food, nutrients, and nutrition? Food provides both the energy and the materials needed to build and maintain all body cells. Nutrients are the nourishing substances we must obtain from food. These essential substances are vital for growth from infancy to adulthood and the maintenance of body functions that keep us alive. For a nutrient to be considered essential, its omission from the diet must lead to a decline in certain aspects of human health, such as function of the nervous system. If the omitted nutrient is restored to the diet before permanent damage occurs, those aspects of human health hampered by its absence should regain normal function. In other words, the lost aspects of health are recovered when the body receives the essential nutrient.

Classes of Nutrients

You have probably heard the terms *carbohydrates, proteins, lipids* (fats and oils), *vitamins,* and *minerals.* These, plus **water,** make up the six classes of nutrients found in food (Table 1-2). Today we know that the minimum diet for human growth and development must contain about 45 essential nutrients.

Heart at
*Rapid fall in he
caused by reduc
through the hear
sels. Often part o
in the process (see*

Nutrients
Chemical substances in food that are essential parts of a diet. Nutrients nourish us by providing energy, materials for building body parts, and factors to regulate necessary chemical processes in the body. The body either can't make these nutrients or can't make them fast enough for its needs.

Some nutrients that perform life-sustaining functions can be produced by the body if they are missing from the diet. The essential nature of such nutrients sometimes is not clear cut. For example, the body requires a daily source of vitamin D, but the skin is capable of synthesizing its own vitamin D upon receiving sunlight. This reduces the daily need from dietary sources.

simple sugars. Table sugar is an example. Simple sugars, such as **glucose,** can chemically link together to form large storage carbohydrates called complex carbohydrates. One example is **starch** in potatoes.

Sugars impart sweetness to many foods. Aside from an enjoyable taste, sugars and other carbohydrates in our diets are primarily necessary to satisfy the energy needs of body **cells.** When you do not eat enough carbohydrate to supply one particular sugar (glucose) to your cells, your body will be forced to take what it can from storage and also make this sugar from other important body structures. However, because we generally eat plenty of carbohydrate each day, the latter rarely happens.

We begin digesting some of the starches in our diets as soon as we put them into our mouths. The process continues until starches and large sugars break down into single sugar **molecules** (like glucose) for absorption into the bloodstream. The chemical links between the sugar molecules in certain complex carbohydrates cannot be broken down by human digestive processes. These carbohydrates are part of what is called *dietary fiber.* These fibers then pass down the intestinal tract to provide bulk for the stool (feces) formed in the large intestine (colon). Chapter 5 focuses on the family of carbohydrates.

Lipids. Lipids are a second general class of nutrients that contain the familiar fats and oils. This book primarily uses the more familiar term, fat. Most lipids supply fuel for the body in a very concentrated form, specifically 9 kcal per gram. By common definition, fats are solid at room temperature and oils are liquid. The fatty acid is the basic structural unit of most lipids, just as sugars make up most carbohydrates. Another key characteristic of lipids as a class is their inability to dissolve in water.

There are two basic types of fatty acids found in lipids: saturated and unsaturated. (These chemical definitions are discussed in greater detail in Chapter 6.) Fats and oils in foods are always a combination of both saturated and unsaturated fatty acids. The dominant type of fatty acid determines the lipid's characteristics, such as whether it's solid or liquid at room temperature. Saturated fatty acids, such as those found in high amounts in animal fats, generally form lipids that are solid or semi-solid at room temperature. Unsaturated fatty acids, such as those found in high amounts in plant oils, form lipids that are liquid at room temperature.

Unsaturated fatty acids are essential nutrients in a diet, in part because they help regulate some important body functions, such as blood pressure. They are also needed for brain development in infancy and the synthesis and repair of vital cell parts. You need only about 1 tablespoon of a common vegetable oil (like those found in supermarkets) per day to supply your body with essential fatty acids. The average American diet supplies about 3 times the amount needed. Chapter 6 focuses on lipids, especially their connection to heart disease.

Proteins. Proteins are a third class of nutrients. These form a major part of the body structure. Muscles contain much protein. A major part of bones is also protein. Important parts of blood, most **enzymes,** some **hormones, cell membranes,** and components of the immune system come from proteins.

Proteins can also provide energy for the body, specifically 4 kcal per gram. Typically, little protein is used for that purpose in terms of daily energy use. The basic unit of protein structure is the **amino acid.** Amino acids join together to form proteins. Twenty or so common amino acids are found in food; nine of these are essential parts of an adult's diet.

Most of us eat about one and a half to two times more protein than the body needs to maintain health. In a healthy person this amount of extra protein in the diet is generally not harmful—it simply reflects the standard of living and the dietary habits that most Americans enjoy. The excess is mostly

---

Cell
The basic structural unit of all living organisms. Cells living and working together compose our bodies. Each body cell metabolizes nutrients in order to stay alive. Surrounding the cell is a cell membrane made mostly of lipids and protein. Inside each cell, tiny structures known as "organelles" are individually responsible for different cell processes, such as reproduction.

Molecule
A group of like or unlike atoms chemically linked together. It is similar to a compound, which is a group of different types of atoms bonded together in definite proportion.

Enzyme
A compound that speeds the rate of a chemical process but is not altered by the process. Almost all enzymes are proteins (see Chapters 4 and 7).

Hormone
A compound secreted into the bloodstream that acts to control the function of distant cells.

used for fuel; some may be made into fat or carbohydrate. Chapter 7 focuses on proteins.

The fourth and fifth classes of nutrients are vitamins and minerals. These nutrients form key regulators and structural parts in the body. While vitamins and minerals are vital to good health, they are needed only in small amounts in our diet. In fact, large amounts of some can cause harmful effects. This is one reason why foods rather than nutrient supplements deserve the primary focus for meeting nutrient needs. Any use of supplements needs to be done with care and knowledge because nutrient imbalances and toxicity are both distinct possibilities. This is discussed in more detail in Chapter 3.

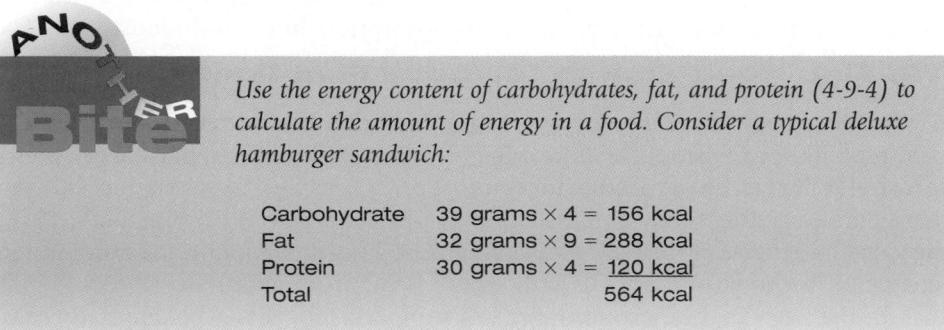

Use the energy content of carbohydrates, fat, and protein (4-9-4) to calculate the amount of energy in a food. Consider a typical deluxe hamburger sandwich:

Carbohydrate	39 grams × 4 =	156 kcal
Fat	32 grams × 9 =	288 kcal
Protein	30 grams × 4 =	<u>120 kcal</u>
Total		564 kcal

Chemical reaction

An interaction between two chemicals that changes them both.

Vitamins. Vitamins are carbon-containing compounds that enable many **chemical reactions** to occur in the body, some of which release the energy stored in carbohydrates, fats, and proteins. The vitamins themselves provide no energy to the body. We need 13 different vitamins; 4 are fat soluble (they dissolve in fat) and 9 are water soluble (they dissolve in water). The two groups of vitamins often act quite differently. For example, cooking destroys water-soluble vitamins much more readily than it does fat-soluble vitamins. Water-soluble vitamins are also excreted from the body much more readily than fat-soluble vitamins. Thus, the fat-soluble vitamins, especially vitamins A and D, are much more likely to build up in excessive amounts in the body and can then cause illness. Vitamins, with a focus on their role in the fight against cancer, are discussed in Chapter 8.

Metabolism

Chemical processes in the body that allow for life.

Minerals. Minerals also play an important role in the body's **metabolism,** such as magnesium for carbohydrate use. In addition, minerals help make up the body's structure and form key components of the bloodstream. Minerals by themselves provide no energy to the body. We know of about 16 essential minerals. Because of their simple structure, minerals are not destroyed during cooking but can still be lost if they leak into the water used for cooking and then that water is not consumed. Minerals are the focus of Chapter 9, especially their relation to bone health and blood pressure.

Water. Water is the sixth and last class of nutrients. It nourishes us in many ways. It is vital in the body because it dissolves substances, lubricates structures such as joints, and provides a way to transport nutrients and waste. Our body cells are composed of mostly water. The body itself is about 60% water. The body even makes water as a by-product of chemical reactions in cells. The bulk of our daily fluid need of about 8 cups (2 liters) comes from a combination of foods, fluids, and water itself. Compare 8 cups of water with our daily needs of 9 tablespoons of protein, $1/4$ teaspoon of calcium, and $1/1000$ teaspoon (a 2-microgram speck) of vitamin B-12 each day. Water is examined in detail in Chapter 9.

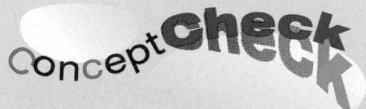

Concept**Check**

The food you eat contains six vital classes of nutrients: carbohydrates, lipids (fats and oils), proteins, vitamins, minerals, and water. The energy (kcal) you use comes mainly from carbohydrates and lipids. Growth and replacement of body cells require both proteins and lipids. Vitamins and minerals have many functions, including aiding in the chemical processes of energy metabolism. Water is the medium of life—a liquid that transports the substances in the body.

We Also Need Energy for Body Functions

We get the energy to perform body functions and do work from carbohydrates, fats, and proteins (see Table 1-2). Foods generally provide more than one energy source. **Alcohol** is also an energy source for some of us, supplying 7 kcal per gram. It is not considered a nutrient, however, because it has no required function. Still, alcoholic beverages—generally also rich in carbohydrate—are the third leading contributor of energy to the American diet.

The energy that our cells use actually comes from carbon-hydrogen chemical bonds found in carbohydrate, fat, protein, and alcohol. This energy is originally put in those bonds during photosynthesis, when plants use solar energy to make glucose and other carbon-containing compounds. In doing so, plants trap the sun's energy in the form of chemical bonds (see Chapter 5 for details).

The body then transforms the energy trapped in these compounds into other forms of energy to help do the following:

- build other compounds
- perform muscular movements
- promote nerve transmissions
- maintain **ion** balance within cells

As noted earlier, the energy in food is often measured in terms of calories. Technically, a calorie is the amount of heat it takes to raise the temperature of 1 gram of water 1 degree **Celsius** (1° C, centigrade scale). Because a calorie is such a tiny measure of heat, food energy is more often expressed in terms of the kilocalorie, or kcal, which equals 1000 calories. A kcal is the amount of heat it takes to raise the temperature of 1000 grams (1 L) of water 1° C. The term *kilocalorie* and its abbreviation *kcal* are used throughout this book. In everyday life the word *calorie* is often used loosely to mean *kilocalorie*. The values given on food labels in calories are actually in kilocalories. A suggested intake of 2000 calories on a food label is really 2000 kcal, or enough energy to raise the temperature of 2 million grams of water 1° C.

Carbohydrates, proteins, lipids, and alcohol provide the body with differing amounts of energy. Use of the 4-9-4 rule for carbohydrate, fat, and protein to determine energy content of a food was shown earlier. You can also use the 4-9-4 rule to determine what portion of total energy intake is contributed by the various energy-yielding nutrients. Assume that one day you consume 290 grams of carbohydrates, 60 grams of fat, and 70 grams of protein. This consumption yields a total of 1980 kcal ([290 × 4] + [60 × 9] + [70 × 4] = 1980). The percentage of your total energy intake derived from each nutrient can then be determined:

% of kcal as carbohydrate = (290 × 4) ÷ 1980 = 0.586 or 59%
% of kcal as fat = (60 × 9) ÷ 1980 = 0.273 or 27%
% of kcal as protein = (70 × 4) ÷ 1980 = 0.141 or 14%

Ion
An atom with an unequal number of electrons and protons. Negative ions have more electrons than protons; positive ions have more protons than electrons.

Nutrition Insight

Math Tools for Nutrition

You will use a few mathematical concepts in studying nutrition. Besides performing addition, subtraction, multiplication, and division, you need to know how to calculate percentages and convert English units of measurement to metric units.

Percentages

The term *percent* (%) refers to a part of the total when the total represents 100 parts. For example, if you earn 80% on your first nutrition examination, you will have answered the equivalent of 80 out of 100 questions correctly. This equivalent could be 8 correct answers out of 10; 80% also describes 16 of 20 (16/20 = 0.80 or 80%). The best way to master this concept is to calculate some percentages. Some examples are given below:

Question	Answer
What is 6% of 45?	$0.06 \times 45 = 2.7$
What is 32% of 8?	$0.32 \times 8 = 2.6$
What percent of 16 is 6?	$\frac{6}{16} = 0.375$ or 37.5%
What percent of 99 is 3?	$\frac{3}{99} = 0.03$ or 3%

Joe ate 15% of the adult Recommended Dietary Allowance (RDA) for vitamin C at lunch. How many milligrams did he eat? (RDA = 60 milligrams)

0.15×60 milligrams = 9 milligrams

It is difficult to succeed in a nutrition course unless you know what a percentage means and how to calculate one. Percentages are used frequently when referring to menus and nutrient composition.

The Metric System

The basic units of the metric system are the meter, which indicates length; the gram, which indicates weight; and the liter, which indicates volume. The inside cover of this textbook lists conversions from the metric system to the English system (pounds, feet, cups) and vice versa. Here is a brief summary:

One meter is 39.4 inches long, or about 3 inches longer than 1 yard (3 feet).
    A meter can be divided into 100 units of centimeters, or into 1000 units of millimeters.
    A millimeter is about the thickness of a dime.
    There are 2.54 centimeters in 1 inch and about 30 centimeters in 1 foot.
A person 6 feet tall is equivalent to 183 centimeters tall.
A gram is about 1/30 of an ounce (28 grams to the ounce).
Five grams of sugar or salt is about 1 teaspoon.
    A pound weighs 454 grams.
A kilogram is 1000 grams, equivalent to 2.2 pounds. To convert your weight to kilograms, divide it by 2.2 A 154-pound man weighs 70 kilograms (154/2.2 = 70).
    A gram can be divided into 1000 milligrams or 1,000,000 micrograms.
    15 milligrams of zinc (approximately the adult RDA) would be a few grains of zinc oxide.
Liters are divided into 1000 units called milliliters.
    One teaspoon equals about 5 milliliters, 1 cup is about 240 milliliters, and 1 quart (4 cups) equals almost 1 liter (0.946 liter to be exact).

If you plan to work in any scientific field, you will need to learn the metric system. **For now, remember that a kilogram equals 2.2 pounds, an ounce weighs 28 grams, 2.54 centimeters equals 1 inch, and a liter is almost the same as a quart.** In addition, know what the prefixes micro (1/1,000,000), milli (1/1000), centi (1/100), and kilo (1000) represent.

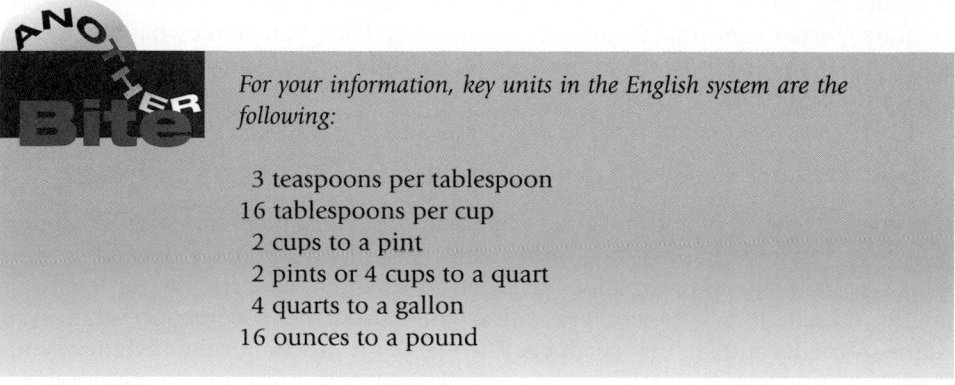

For your information, key units in the English system are the following:

3 teaspoons per tablespoon
16 tablespoons per cup
2 cups to a pint
2 pints or 4 cups to a quart
4 quarts to a gallon
16 ounces to a pound

Are You What You Eat?

The amounts of nutrients that your body needs vary widely from one nutrient to another. Nutrient quantities also vary from food to food. Each day we need about 1 pound (500 grams) of energy-yielding substances in the food we eat. Add to this about 5 pounds of water. We need to take in vitamins regularly but in very small amounts—100 milligrams or less. Although we should eat about 1 gram of some minerals—such as calcium and phosphorus—each day, many minerals are needed in quantities of only milligrams or less. For example, you need about 10 to 15 milligrams of iron each day, which is just a few grains of iron oxide.

Figure 1-1 shows the proportion of nutrients in a human body, compared with the proportions of the same nutrients in cooked steak and a cooked stalk of broccoli. Note how the nutrient composition of the body differs from the nutritional profiles of the foods we eat. This is because growth, development, and later maintenance of the human body are directed by the genetic material inside the cell. This genetic blueprint determines how each cell uses the nutrients to perform body functions. These nutrients can come from a variety of sources. Cells are not affected by

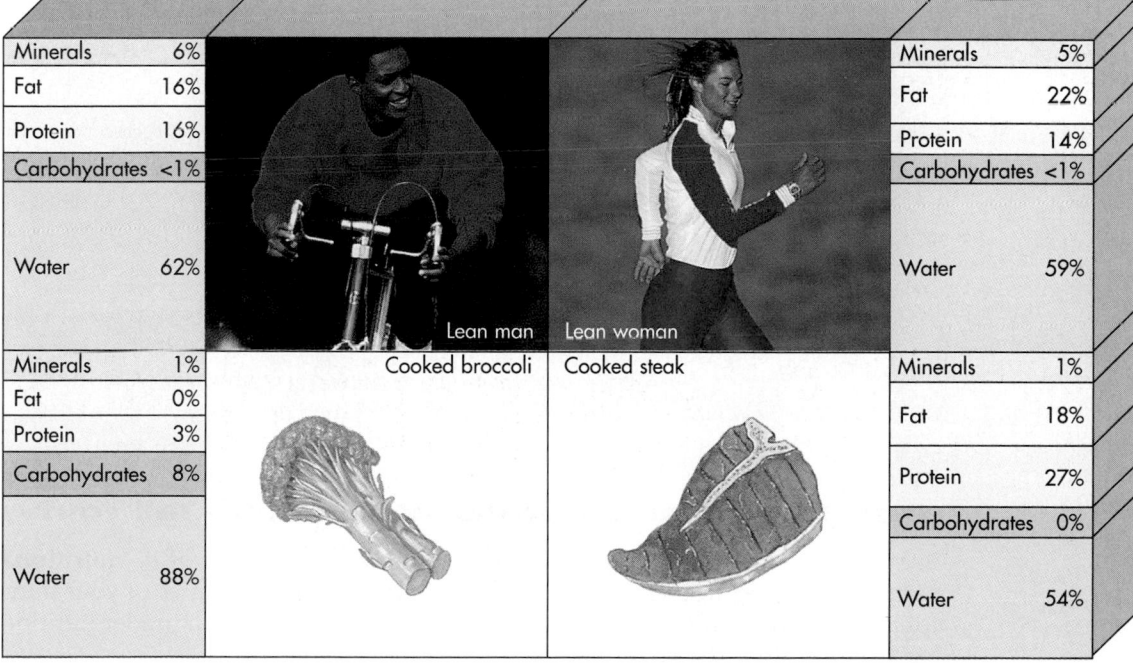

Minerals	6%	Lean man	Lean woman	Minerals	5%
Fat	16%			Fat	22%
Protein	16%			Protein	14%
Carbohydrates	<1%			Carbohydrates	<1%
Water	62%			Water	59%
Minerals	1%	Cooked broccoli	Cooked steak	Minerals	1%
Fat	0%			Fat	18%
Protein	3%			Protein	27%
Carbohydrates	8%			Carbohydrates	0%
Water	88%			Water	54%

Figure 1-1 *The properties of nutrients in the human body don't necessarily match those found in foods.*

Genes

The hereditary material on chromosomes that makes up DNA. Genes provide the blueprints for the production of cell proteins.

Anthropometry

Pertaining to the measurement of body weight and the lengths, circumferences, and thicknesses of parts of the body.

Biochemical deficiency symptoms

Nutrition deficiency symptoms observed in the blood or urine, such as low amounts of nutrient by-products or low enzyme activities. These indicate reduced biochemical functioning in the body.

Clinical deficiency symptoms

Generally, a change in health status noted by the individual (such as stomach pain) or noticed by a clinician during physical examination (the latter is technically called a clinical deficiency sign).

Nutritional status

The nutritional health of a person as determined by anthropometric measurements (height, weight, circumferences, and so on), biochemical measurements of nutrients or their by-products in blood and urine, a clinical (physical) examination, and a dietary analysis.

whether the amino acids available come from animal or plant sources. The carbohydrate glucose can come from sugars or starches. Thus, you aren't what you eat. Instead, what you eat provides your cells with the ability to function as directed by the **genes** housed in these cells.[17]

How Could Your Nutritional State Be Measured?

The measurements of your height, weight, and body circumference—called *anthropometry*—can reveal something about your current nutritional state (Table 1–3). This type of evaluation, explained in detail in Chapter 10, is simple but less informative than a full biochemical evaluation, which measures blood concentrations of some nutrients and their by-products. The search for **biochemical deficiency symptoms** relies on an expensive procedure, and most of the tests can be done only in specialized laboratories. Another way to find out about your nutritional state is to get a thorough physical **(clinical)** examination and undergo a detailed evaluation of your diet. Together these activities form the **ABCDs** of nutritional assessment: **a**nthropometric measurements, **b**iochemical assessment, **c**linical examination, and **d**iet history. Furthermore, because family history plays an important role in determining nutritional and health status, it also must be carefully recorded and critically analyzed as part of a nutritional assessment. Additional related background components could include (1) a medical history, especially for any disease states or treatments that could impede nutrient absorptive processes or ultimate use; and (2) socioeconomic history, to determine the ability to purchase and prepare appropriate foods needed to maintain health.

TABLE 1-3

Components of a Nutritional Assessment

Component	Example
Background histories	Medical history, including current diseases and past surgeries
	Medications history
	Social history (marital status, cooking facilities)
	Family history
	Economic status
Nutrition parameters	**A**nthropometric assessment: height, weight, skinfold thickness, arm muscle circumference, and other parameters
	Biochemical (laboratory) assessment of blood and urine: enzyme activities, concentrations of nutrients or their by-products
	Clinical assessment (physical examination): general appearance of skin, eyes, and tongue; rapid hair loss; sense of touch; ability to walk
	Diet history: usual intake or record of previous days' meals

What Could Such a Nutritional Check-Up Tell You?

Overall, the body's nutritional health is determined by the sum of its **nutritional status** with respect to each needed nutrient. Three general categories of your nutritional status for each nutrient are recognized—desirable nutrition, undernutrition, and overnutrition—based on the ABCD evaluation (Table 1-4).

Desirable nutrition. The nutritional status for a particular nutrient is desirable when body cells have enough of the nutrient to support normal metabolism as well as surplus stores that can be mobilized in times of increased need. A desirable nutritional state can be achieved by obtaining essential nutrients from a variety of foods. This then contributes to maintenance of a healthy body.

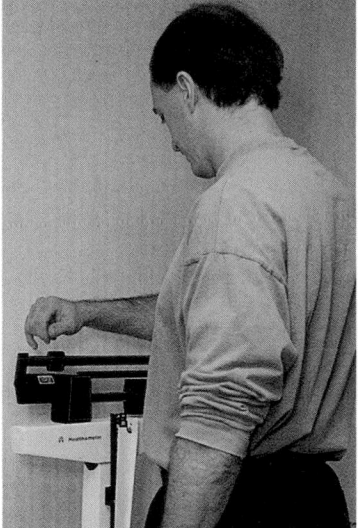

Body weight is a key component of a nutrition assessment.

TABLE 1-4

Categories of Nutritional Status with Respect to Iron*

General conditions	Conditions with respect to iron
Overnutrition: nutrients consumed in excess of body needs (degree of toxicity varies for each nutrient)	Results in toxic damage to liver cells; may contribute to heart disease
Desirable nutrition: nutrients consumed to support body functions and stores of nutrients for times of increased need	Adequate liver stores of iron, adequate blood values for iron-related compounds
Undernutrition: nutrient intake does not meet nutrient needs	Many changes in body functions are associated with a decline in iron status
Depleted tissue stores	Ferritin, an iron-containing protein in the blood, drops below normal values
Reduced biochemical function	Hemoglobin, an iron-containing pigment in the red blood cells, drops below normal values
Clinical evidence of deficiency	Pale complexion; greatly increased heart rate during activity; "spooning" of the nails in a severe deficiency; poor body temperature regulation

*This general scheme can apply to all nutrients. Iron was chosen because you are likely to be familiar with this nutrient.

Undernutrition. When nutrient intake does not meet nutrient needs, stores of nutrients soon become depleted by ongoing body use, some sooner than others. This results in **undernutrition**. Now the body slides into a state in which it cannot function appropriately. Although body stores of nutrients can make up for a poor diet over a short time, they do not last indefinitely. Once stores are depleted, the body attempts to obtain essential nutrients from itself. This continues to drain nutrients from vital tissues.

The demand for these nutrients exists partly because the body is in a constant state of turnover. Cells lining the intestinal tract, for example, are replaced every 2-5 days, and red blood cells live only about 120 days. To support this turnover, body stores may be sufficient to compensate for an inadequate diet for a brief period of time, but serious problems can arise from an inadequate diet in the long run. Some women in the United States, for example, do not consume sufficient iron and eventually deplete their iron stores. Reduced biochemical and, ultimately, body functions, such as reduced red blood cell production, develop. Eventually clinical evidence, such as pale skin and poor body temperature regulation, of an iron deficiency can develop.

Just not feeling well, let alone the long-term effects of poor nutrition, is unpleasant. It's wise for you to begin understanding how diet relates to health now—

Undernutrition
Failing health that results from a long-standing dietary intake that does not meet nutritional needs.

sound nutrition practices will move you toward your goal of good health for the rest of your life. Now that you know that foods supply you with the essential nutrients needed to help achieve and maintain good health, you are urged to take a closer look at your diet.

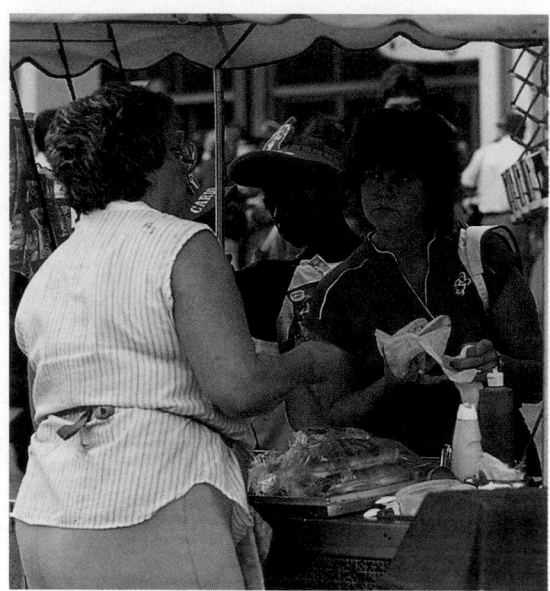

The major nutritional problems in the United States are primarily caused by overindulgence, especially of fat and total energy intake.

Overnutrition

A state in which nutritional intake exceeds the body's needs.

Overnutrition. Prolonged consumption of more nutrients than the body needs can lead to **overnutrition.** In the short run, for instance a week or two, overnutrition may cause no problems. Over time, however, some nutrients may eventually increase to toxic amounts, which can lead to serious disease. Iron overload, for example, can result in liver failure, and too much vitamin A can lead to many negative effects. The most common type of overnutrition—excess intake of energy-yielding nutrients—is the principal cause of obesity. Note that the average adult gains 15 to 20 pounds from ages 18 to 54 years. In the long run, an overweight condition can lead to serious diseases, such as certain forms of diabetes and cancer.

For most vitamins and minerals, the gap between desirable intake and overnutrition is wide. Therefore, even if people take a typical multiple vitamin and mineral supplement daily, they probably won't receive a harmful amount of any nutrient. The gap between optimal intake and overnutrition is narrowest for vitamin A and vitamin D, as well as calcium, iron, and other minerals. In very high doses, vitamin B-6 and the vitamin niacin can cause health problems. It is important to remember that high doses of some vitamins and minerals are toxic to the body. If you take nutrient supplements, keep a close eye on your total vitamin and mineral intake both from food and from supplements (again, see Chapter 3 for further advice on use of nutrient supplements).

At the beginning of the twentieth century, undernutrition was the main concern of nutrition scientists. Now, as we approach the end of the century, our attention needs to be directed toward both undernutrition and overnutrition in the United States and throughout the world.

Recognizing the Limitations of Nutritional Assessment

A long time may elapse between the initial development of poor nutritional health and the first clinical evidence of a problem. For example, a diet high in animal fat often increases blood **cholesterol** concentration without producing any clinical symptoms for years. However, when the blood vessels become sufficiently blocked by cholesterol and other materials, chest pain during physical activity may develop. This buildup of fatty substances also may eventually provoke a heart attack. Thus, a person may be on the road to developing a serious disease, but because it progresses slowly, its effects won't be obvious until quite late—perhaps too late.[16] A lot of current nutrition research aims to develop better methods for early detection of nutritional problems.

One example of a delay in symptoms causing serious consequences occurs with calcium deficiency, a particularly relevant issue for adolescent females. A goal should be to build dense bones, especially during the years of adolescent growth and development, by consuming adequate calcium. Still, many young women consume well below the recommended amount of calcium[1] but often suffer no ill effects in their younger years. However, women whose bone-density values do not reach full potential during the years of growth are likely to face an increased risk for osteoporosis later in life. This example highlights the idea that prolonged inadequate intake of certain nutrients can result in an eventual decline in health and performance that will initially be unnoticed.[4]

Furthermore, clinical signs and symptoms of nutritional deficiencies are often not very specific. Typical evidence to look for—diarrhea, an irregular walk, facial sores—have many different causes. It is often hard to decide whether the problem is caused by faulty nutrition or some other medical disorder. Long lag times and vague symptoms often make it difficult to establish a link between an individual's current diet and nutritional state.

As you study nutrition and learn the importance of nutrients in foods, you may notice people who have very poor diets but show no outward clinical symptoms of poor health. Nonetheless, their health is probably declining in subtle ways. A good example is the role of calcium in bone development just described. In addition, a chronically insufficient intake of vitamin C likely encourages development of cataracts in the eyes.[20] Heart disease also is related to low intakes of vitamin B-6, folate, and vitamin B-12. An insufficient intake of these vitamins leads to elevated blood concentrations of the substance homocysteine, which in turn promotes the development of heart disease.[3]

Often it is not possible to separate the best nutritional state from one that is slightly jeopardized. We can usually distinguish between distinct **malnutrition** and good nutrition, but the gray area—the gradual slide from a "good" to a malnourished state caused by earlier significant undernutrition or overnutrition—is hard to detect. For example, a very sophisticated test is needed to detect elevated blood homocysteine. In the case of cataracts, clinical evidence of the disease is the first warning sign. This observation is not intended as a scare tactic, but rather to provide reasons why a careful evaluation of the adequacy of *your* diet is worth the effort.

Table 1-5 shows the close relationship of nutrition and health. Chapter 2 helps you plan your diet to maximize health and minimize the development of nutrition-related diseases. For now, keep in mind that poor nutrition habits often catch up with us, bringing in turn ill health.[4]

Throughout this book practical tests that can tell you much about your current nutritional state will be discussed. Consider setting a goal to learn as much as you can about your nutritional status and total health as you study nutrition. You should also learn as much as you can about your family history for nutrition-related illnesses and other diseases (see the Nutrition Issue at the end of the chapter).

Cholesterol
A waxy lipid found in all body cells. It has a structure containing multiple chemical rings that is found only in foods that contain animal products (see Chapter 6).

Malnutrition
Failing health that results from long-standing dietary practices that do not coincide with nutritional needs.

Critical Thinking

Tom loves to eat hamburgers, fries, and lots of pizza with double amounts of cheese. He rarely eats any vegetables and fruits, but instead snacks on cookies and ice cream. He insists that he has no problems with his health, is rarely ill, and doesn't see how his diet could cause him any health risks. How would you explain to Tom that despite his current good health, his diet could predispose him to future health problems?

TABLE 1-5

What To Expect from Adequate Nutrition and Good Health Habits

DIET

Eating enough essential nutrients and meeting energy needs help prevent
  Birth defects and low birth weight in pregnancy
  Stunted growth and poor resistance to disease in infancy and childhood
  Poor resistance to disease in adulthood
  Deficiency diseases, such as cretinism (lack of iodide), scurvy (lack of vitamin C), and anemia (lack of iron, folate, or other nutrients)

Eating enough calcium helps
  Build bone mass in childhood and adolescence
  Prevent some adult bone loss, especially among older individuals

Obtaining adequate intake of fluoride and minimizing sugar intake helps prevent
  Dental caries

Eating enough dietary fiber helps prevent
  Digestive problems such as constipation and probaly some forms of intestinal cancer

Eating enough vitamin A and carotenoids may help reduce
  Susceptibility to some cancers
  Degeneration of the retina (intake of carotenoids specifically)

Moderating energy intake helps prevent
  Obesity and related diseases, such as diabetes, high blood pressure, cancer, and premature heart disease

Limiting intake of sodium helps prevent
  High blood pressure and related diseases of the heart and kidney in susceptible people

Moderating intake of saturated fat helps prevent
  Premature heart disease

Moderating intake of essential nutrients by using vitamin and mineral supplements wisely, if at all, prevents
  Most chances for nutrient toxicities

PHYSICAL ACTIVITY

Adequate, regular physical activity helps prevent
  Obesity
  The major form of diabetes
  Premature heart disease
  Some adult bone loss
  Loss of muscle tone

LIFESTYLE

Minimizing alcohol intake helps prevent
  Liver disease
  Fetal alcohol syndrome
  Accidents

Not smoking helps prevent
  Lung cancer, other lung disease, and heart disease

In addition, minimum use of medication, no illicit drug use, adequate sleep, adequate fluid intake and a reduction in stress provide a more complete approach to good nutrition and health

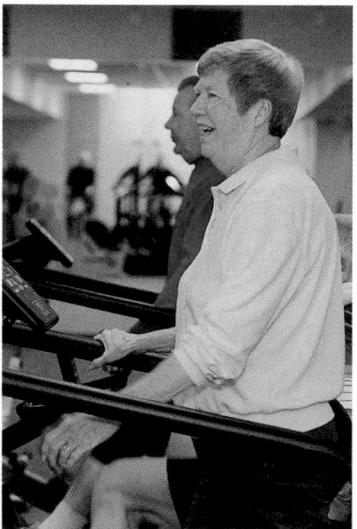

The need for regular physical activity continues through adult life.

Nutrition Insight

A Fountain of Youth?

Although most of us wish for a long life, we do not like to think of ourselves as suffering poor health when we are older. And rightly so! We can truly enjoy a long life only if we are productive and free of illness. Rather than suffer the ravages of heart disease, stroke, diabetes, osteoporosis, and other chronic diseases from the age of 50 or 60 years until death, we should strive to be as free from disease as possible and enjoy vitality even in the last years of life. Greater physical well-being contributes to our mental and social well-being.

Aging is a natural process: your body cells age no matter what health practices you follow. To a considerable extent, however, you can determine how quickly you age throughout your adult years. As we discuss in the Nutrition Issue at the end of this chapter, genetic background is very important in determining your risk of nutrition-related diseases; nonetheless, you also have some control over it. How you act now is important to your later health. Successful aging is a result of wise choices. Age quickly or age slowly—you have some choice in the matter.

The best way to promote your health and prevent chronic diseases in the future is to observe the following guidelines:

- Eat a healthful diet—a varied diet that helps avoid obesity should be a priority. The Food Guide Pyramid discussed in Chapter 2 is a great place to start. Choose moderate portion sizes and pay particular attention to serving sizes of high-fat foods. In addition, do not abuse nutrient supplements.
- Drink plenty of fluids—because the body is composed mostly of water, which is lost in perspiration and urine, water should continually be replaced. Aim to drink 6 to 8 glasses of water and other beverages daily.
- Physical activity—spend at least 30 minutes a day in a combination of brisk walking, jogging, swimming, stair climbing, and other activities that stimulate the cardiovascular system. Add to that some resistance exercise: situps, push-ups, presses, and curls with dumbbells, etc. See Chapter 11 for other options. But by all means, become and remain physically active.[14]
- Don't smoke—lung cancer, caused primarily by smoking cigarettes, is the only form of cancer for which yearly rates still increase. About half of regular cigarette smokers die as a direct result of smoking. In addition, a recent British study showed that smokers eat fewer fruits and vegetables and more saturated fat and sugar than nonsmokers. Currently, about 25% of adults smoke,

with low-income people more inclined to smoke than those with higher incomes. Slightly more men smoke than women. Moreover, many people find that once they begin smoking, they find it very hard to stop. Nicotine from tobacco is a very addictive substance.[8]
- Limit alcohol intake—don't drink more than 1 oz of alcohol per day on a regular basis. Women are cautioned to cut even that amount in half because they are more likely than men to develop cirrhosis of the liver with the same intake of alcohol. One 12-oz beer, a 5-oz glass of wine, or a mixed drink supplies about $\frac{1}{2}$ oz (15 grams) of alcohol. African-Americans are especially sensitive to the effects of alcohol on blood pressure. Furthermore, all women must avoid alcohol during pregnancy because it can harm the fetus, causing fetal alcohol syndrome (see Chapter 14 for a discussion of this disease).
- Get adequate sleep—establish a regular schedule to allow for an average of 7 to 8 hours of sleep a night. If you have difficulty sleeping, look for factors that may be interfering, such as noise, stress, caffeine-containing products, lack of physical activity, and late-night eating.
- Limit stress or adjust to the causes of stress—practice better time management, relax, listen to music, have a massage, and stay physically active. Do what works for you. In addition, maintaining self-esteem, interpersonal relationships, and a positive outlook contributes to limiting stress and reinforces wellness.
- Consult health-care professionals on a regular basis—early diagnosis is especially important for controlling the damaging effects of many diseases.

Your key to optimal health is to discover how to maintain your best physical, mental, psychological, and social states. There is no general formula for achieving this ideal. Each of us must juggle and balance personal goals with the opportunities and obstacles we encounter. Proper diet is not the only thing to consider. As just discussed, other behavior is also critical. Taking responsibility for yourself is central to achieving long-term health. As individuals, we can do a lot to improve our health by establishing good health behavior. This is a goal of Chapters 1 and 2.

Focusing on disease prevention may not allow you to live longer—because heredity, accidents, and other things are outside your control—but you'll probably live a healthier life.[16]

Health Objectives for the United States for the Year 2000

Health promotion and disease prevention have been public health strategies in the United States since the late 1970s. One part of this strategy is *Healthy People 2000*, a report issued in 1990 by the U.S. Department of Health and Human Services' Public Health Service. This report consists of national health promotion and disease prevention objectives for the nation for the year 2000 and assigns each of the objectives to appropriate federal agencies to address.

Healthy People 2000's nutrition-related challenges address the following:

Obesity

A condition characterized by excess body fat, often defined in clinical settings as 20% above healthy (also called desirable) body weight. See Chapter 10 for more details.

- Iron-deficiency anemia (degree of progress currently unclear)
- Stunted growth in infants and children (progress is being made)
- High fat intake (progress is being made, especially by women)
- **Obesity** (we are currently losing this battle)
- Elevated blood cholesterol (progress is being made)
- High sodium intake (degree of progress currently unclear)
- Low calcium intake (mixed findings on progress to date)
- Low complex carbohydrate and dietary fiber intakes (no data on progress to date)
- The need for more home-delivered meals for elderly people (no data on progress to date)
- A relative lack of breastfeeding, poor general nutrition knowledge, and the lack of nutrition education (mixed findings on progress to date)

The main objective of *Healthy People 2000* is to promote healthful lifestyles and reduce preventable death and disability in all Americans.

The American Diet

For most of us living in America, our main dietary sources of energy are carbohydrates, fats, and proteins. If we ignore alcohol, adults consume about 16% of their kcal as proteins, 50% as carbohydrates, and 34% as fats.[12] These percentages are estimates and vary slightly from year to year and from person to person.

Animal sources supply about two thirds of protein intake for most Americans; plant sources supply only about one third. In many other parts of the world, it is just the opposite: plant proteins—from rice, beans, corn, and other vegetables—dominate protein intake. About half the carbohydrate in American diets comes from simple sugars; the other half comes from starches (such as in pastas, breads, and potatoes). About 60% of our dietary fat comes from animal sources, and 40% from vegetable sources.

Profiling the American Diet

Salt

Generally refers to a compound of sodium and chloride in a 40:60 ratio.

Our information about the American diet comes from large surveys designed to find out what and when people eat. Results from these surveys and other studies show that we eat a wide variety of foods. Many people are meeting their nutrient needs; others are not. Chapter 2 will look at this situation in more detail. For now, note that studies show that some of us should choose more foods that are rich in iron, calcium, vitamin A, various B vitamins, vitamin C, zinc, and dietary fiber.[1] Many experts recommend that we eat less fat. Chapter 2 gives specific suggestions on how to do just that. In addition, we should match energy intake with need. Overnutrition is usually tied to an overindulgence in fat and alcoholic beverages. African-Americans may need to pay special attention to the amount of sodium (**salt** is a mixture of sodium and chloride) and alcohol in their diets because they have a greater chance of developing high blood pressure than other ethnic groups in America, and these substances are linked to that health problem. Actually, a careful look at sodium and alcohol intake—along with saturated and total fat intake—is a useful task for everyone.[23]

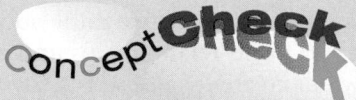

The energy to fuel our bodies comes mostly from carbohydrates, fats, and proteins. A desirable nutritional state results when the body has enough nutrients to function fully and contains stores to use in times of increased needs. When nutrient intake fails to meet body needs, undernutrition develops. Poor body functioning and physical evidence of a nutrient deficiency eventually can develop. Overloading the body with nutrients, leading to overnutrition, is another potential problem to avoid. Surveys in the United States show that we generally have a variety of food available to us. However, some of us could improve our diets by focusing on good food sources of iron, calcium, vitamin A, various B vitamins, Vitamin C, zinc, and dietary fiber. In addition, some of us should use more moderation when consuming energy, fat, sodium, and alcoholic beverages. These recommendations are consistent with an overall goal to attain and maintain good health.

How Aware Are We of Our Nutritional Health?

Judging from the responses of over half of the people in several large surveys, Americans are concerned about good nutrition and have a general awareness of possible health hazards from overeating, especially the dangers of too much fat, sodium, and energy in a diet. Many people aren't willing to critically examine their own food habits, however. Although they may be concerned, they don't make changes to improve their diets.[13] Most people enjoy eating and cooking, but unfortunately don't think of or use the principles of nutritional science.

A recent telephone survey of the dietary habits and attitudes of 1000 adult Americans representative of the U.S. population showed that 26% of the respondents felt that nutrition was important, they were careful about what they ate, and they were doing things right. Another 36% knew that they were not doing much to manage their diets but were not interested in changing because it would mean giving up their favorite foods and take too much time. The remaining 38% believed that diet was fairly important, but only about half of them were doing as much as they thought they should do because most did not want to give up the foods they like and they thought that making changes would take too much time. Thus, the unwillingness of some people to significantly change many of their nutritional practices is probably the major impediment to improving their diets.

Currently, many Americans are concerned about excessive consumption of several dietary components. About 60% are concerned about fat and cholesterol in their diets; 40%, about sodium; and 30%, about caffeine. Energy intake, sugar, and additives are of less concern.[11] In another survey, 44% of adults said they heard far more about what not to eat than what they should eat.

On a per-person basis, Americans consumed roughly 18 pounds of butter and 270 pounds of whole milk per year in the 1920s and 1930s, whereas today they consume less than 5 pounds of butter and 111 pounds of whole milk, often substituting margarine and low-fat or nonfat milk. Therefore progress is being made in reducing key sources of fat and cholesterol in our diets.[22] Nevertheless, many of us need to do more to improve our diets, as discussed further in Chapter 2.

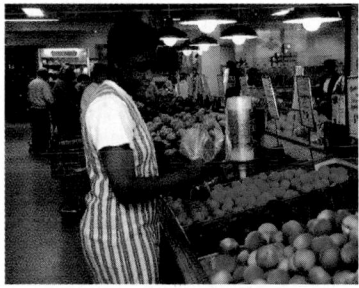

Most Americans enjoy a wide bounty of foods from which to choose.

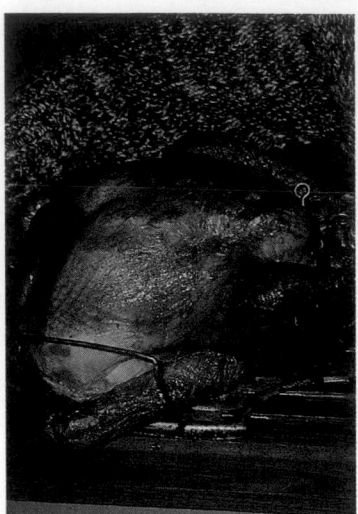

Holiday traditions help mold our food choices.

What Influences Our Food Choices?

Does what you eat say something about you? Our daily food choices have a lot to do with our age, gender, genetic makeup, occupation, and lifestyle; where we live; and our family and cultural background. We eat primarily for nourishment, but food means far more to us than that. Food symbolizes much of what we think about ourselves. We can use it to project a desired image. We bond relationships and express friendships around the dinner table. We show our creativity and sensitivity by what we serve to others in our homes. The common use of food as a gift is evidence that food signifies friendliness. We cope with stress and tension by eating or not eating. Food can be used as a reward—a dinner out to celebrate a new job or an ice cream cone for an A on a test. Some of us make special foods and elaborate preparations to observe national holidays and religious feast days.

Throughout our lives we spend 13 to 15 years of our waking hours eating. Taste and texture are the most important things that influence our choice of food. After that we consider the cost and convenience of food. What we eat ends up revealing much about who we are—politically, religiously, and socially. Behavior, perception, and environment influence food habits (Figure 1-2). While some people have no concern for nutrition, others will agonize endlessly over the taste, energy and fat content, and general nutritional value of everything they eat. Where do you fit into the food and nutrition picture?

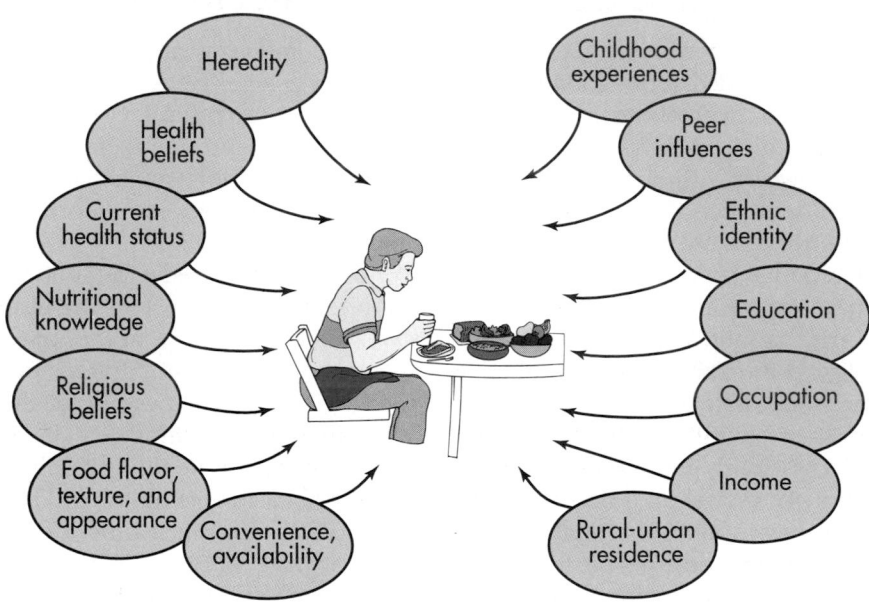

Figure 1-2 *Food behavior is influenced by many sources. Which are important in your life?*

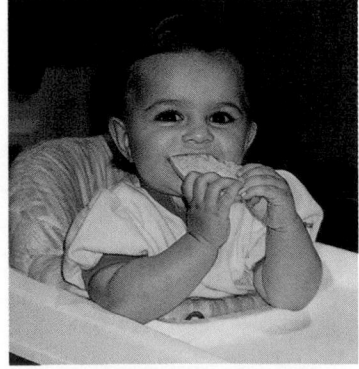

Food likes and dislikes are shaped by early experiences, among other factors.

Our Early Experiences with Food

Our food preferences begin early in life and then change as we interact with parents, friends, and peers.[15] Exposure to people, places, and situations often leads us to expand and change our food patterns. Our earliest food memories may include pancakes on Saturday mornings or hot cocoa on cold winter days. Unfortunately, as young children our food experiences may have been severely limited by parents or other adults responsible for us. Adults may have introduced us to only a small subset of available foods because some excellent foods are often considered inappropriate for children. For example, at what age did you discover lentils, spinach salad, or salmon?

Just being exposed to a variety of foods can help make us less resistant to try new foods. Young children prefer foods that are sweet or familiar. Preschoolers are usually quite willing to try new things. During school years, children are often strongly influenced by their peers. Adults need to give children under their care a variety of foods to try. It may take time, but children usually come to accept new foods (see Chapter 15).[15]

Some inborn reactions to foods include universal enjoyment of sweet and salty foods and dislike of bitter and sometimes spicy, burning ones. Sweet foods are usually safe to eat. We need to eat *salt* in foods (both the sodium and the chloride in table salt are essential nutrients), although the amount needed is only about $1/4$ teaspoon a day. Some bitter-tasting foods are poisonous. However, our inborn responses to some foods can change once we know a food is safe, allowing us to enjoy foods such as jalapeño peppers and fiery curries.

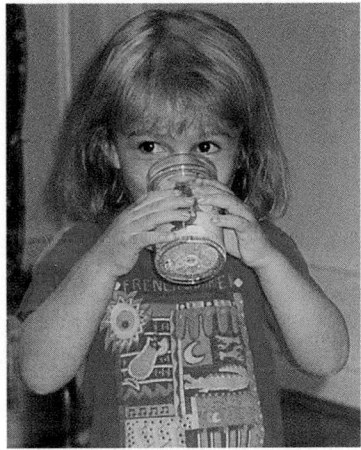

Healthy eating habits, such as often drinking milk with meals, ideally start early in life.

Habit

Some food choices are tied to our routines and habits. The ease with which we can obtain certain foods influences our choices. Most of us eat from a core group of foods. Only about 100 basic items account for 75% of an individual's total food intake. Narrowing our food choices provides us with security. In this context eating quick-service food (often called "fast food") at a restaurant such as McDonald's provides common expectations, experiences, and behaviors.

People often agree that their cooking habits are very similar to those of their mothers. How closely do your habits reflect what your mother taught you? Have you considered taking a cooking class to expand your food choices?

Health

About half of us consider nutrition, or what we think are good food habits, an important influence on our food purchases. Those Americans who tend to make better food choices are often well-educated, middle-class professionals. These are the same people who often are health oriented and who have an active lifestyle. Still, all of us should pay attention to nutritional health. In fact, increased health awareness among minority peoples is a major goal of current federal government health strategies.

Sugar used to be the main diet monster; now fat and cholesterol have the limelight.[22] As a result, manufacturers are racing to the market with reduced-fat or nonfat items (many also are lower in cholesterol and sodium), including mayonnaise, salad dressings, cheese, dairy spreads, frozen desserts, luncheon meats, sausage, and butter sprinkles.[7]

Some of us are concerned enough about our health that we want to change our diets. Even so, food tastes and habits still strongly influence us. When people are asked why they don't include foods they know to be healthful in their diets—for instance, yellow vegetables, low-fat milk, margarine, and whole-wheat bread—they say they don't like them. Similarly, people don't want to give up foods such as whole milk, rich cheeses, and fatty meat because they like them too much. This even is the case if they think they should limit fat intake and lower-fat varieties are available.

The modern supermarket is responding to our health concerns by providing fresh, frozen, ready-to-eat, international, gourmet, ethnic, **vegetarian,** and even not-so-healthful foods. Salad bars in supermarkets have become a big hit, especially for single people. Stores are stocking more foods lower in fat, salt, and sugar. They are carrying low-fat varieties of cheeses, yogurts, and peanuts; pure fruit juices; high-fiber cereals; whole-grain breads; fruits canned in natural juices; low-sodium soups

Vegetarian
A person who avoids eating animal products to a varying degree ranging from consuming no animal products to simply not consuming four-footed animal products (see Chapter 7).

and sauces; low-fat turkey and chicken franks; and many kinds of fish. We can select from a variety of bulk foods sold in bins, including beans, rice, flours, dried fruits, nuts, and grains. Most foods provide information on the nutritional content. There are many options for us as we head down the road to good nutrition. We just have to follow the right directions.

Advertising

To capture consumers' interest, the food industry spends well over $6 billion annually on advertising and another $26 billion on packaging (another form of advertising)—a total of more than $32 billion. Some of this advertising is helpful, as when it promotes the importance of calcium and fiber in our diets and encourages us to consume more low-fat and nonfat milk products, fruits, vegetables, and lean meats.[6] The food industry, however, does not promote all foods equally: sellers tend to emphasize brand-name foods, especially highly sweetened cereals, cookies, cakes, and pastries, because they bring higher profits. Food manufacturers often pay for the best place in the supermarkets: at the end of the aisle and, depending on the product, at the child's or adult's eye level.

Restaurants and Eating Out

Restaurants have long been a growth industry in America.[24] Nowadays about 45% of all food dollars are spent on meals outside the home. On weekdays, lunch is eaten out by 30% of all adults and dinner by 24%. Restaurant excursions are no longer a splurge but a real convenience for many people. Traveling sales representatives, students, truck drivers, and others regularly stop at quick-service restaurants. Drive-through restaurants are now a part of our culture, whereas 40 years ago they were much less common. Today, people drive through, wolf down 1200 kcal (about half their daily energy needs) via a burger, fries, and shake, and are on their way. Indeed, 8% of all food purchased in restaurants is consumed in the car.

Many restaurants, including quick-service restaurants, offer healthful alternatives to their energy-dense and high-salt foods. Yogurt has replaced ice cream in shakes, and low-fat hamburgers are offered in many restaurants. Salad bars are everywhere. Grilled chicken, fresh fruit, whole-grain muffins, and low-fat milk are widely available as well. Consumers must support this healthier fare by buying it if it is to succeed in a marketplace driven by profit.[10]

Still, the temptation to consume foods rich in fat and high in salt is often hard to resist when we eat out. The reality is that a cheeseburger, french fries, and a milk shake are more appealing than a well-stocked salad bar for many of us (Figure 1-3). Thus food chosen in a restaurant is generally poorer in nutritional quality than food eaten at or brought from home. Regular visitors to quick-service restaurants must be especially careful about the food choices they make if they want to have a healthy diet.

Social Factors

Many social changes in recent years have strongly affected the food marketplace, especially the large increases in the number of working women and single parents, both young and old. As a result of these and other factors, a general "time-famine" is emerging. Many people now turn to quick-service restaurants for meals on the run. Supermarkets are also competing for these restaurant customers, with already-prepared foods, microwavable entrees, and various other frozen foods being especially popular. Quick to meet the demand, food producers have increased the number of foods that require little or no preparation.[19] Almost 1000 new microwavable products were introduced in a recent year. Surveys show that one third

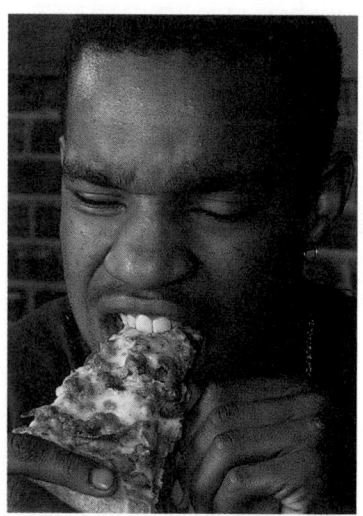

Recently a market research firm surveyed the eating habits of people in 2000 American households. The top meal choice was pizza, followed by ham sandwich, hot dog, peanut butter and jelly sandwich, steak, macaroni and cheese, turkey sandwich, cheese sandwich, hamburger on a bun, and spaghetti.

FOR BETTER OR FOR WORSE / By Lynn Johnston

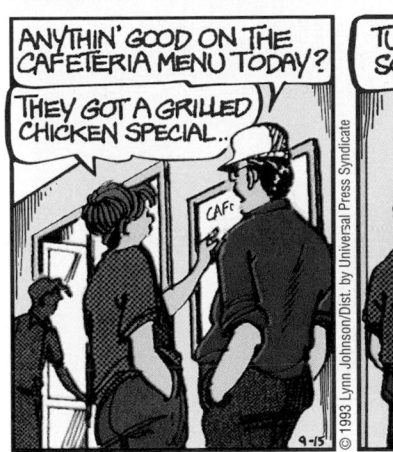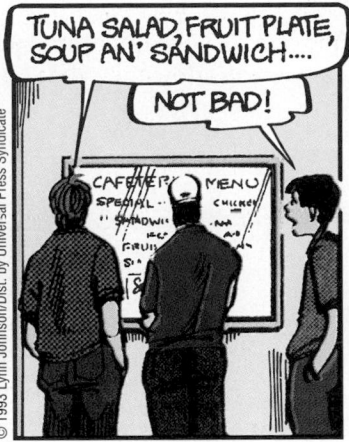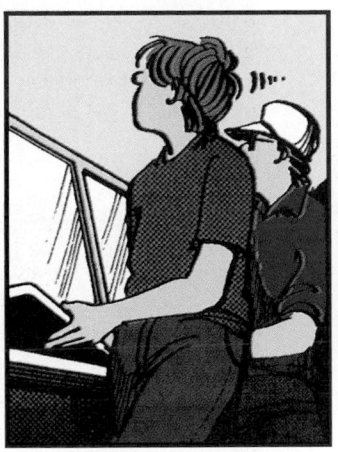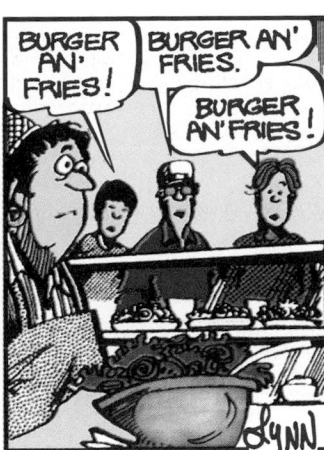

Figure 1-3 *For Better Or For Worse.*

to one half of consumers eat such foods regularly in order to save time. Sales of ready-to-eat and microwavable products marketed directly to children and weight-conscious adults are among the fastest-growing product segments.

As the age of the U.S. population has increased, so has the consumption of certain foods, such as shellfish, fresh vegetables, and alcoholic beverages. For older adults, new health and nutrition problems often arise and compel changes in food habits (see Chapter 16).

Overall, in today's fast-paced world, many people are looking for ways to save time. Current surveys show that women want to spend only 30 minutes or less each day selecting and cooking food, and men want to spend only 15 minutes on such activities.[10] Not only do many people eat away from home, they also skip meals. In a recent survey of college students, more than half reported that they ate only two meals a day, eating many snacks to make up the difference. In families, approximately 30% of adults skip breakfast, which is the appropriate meal to replace the carbohydrate stores used during the night's sleep. Although skipping breakfast

ANOTHER Bite

You eat because you see it, you hear it cooking, you smell it, or it's time to eat. All of these stimuli are concentrated in a mall: the food is there, it smells good, and there's so much to choose from. In addition, food may be the most affordable temptation at the mall. After a few hours of trekking through a mall, you would swear you had walked miles. But you would have to walk almost twice around the average mall to chalk up a mile—and that's only 100 kcal worth of physical activity.

The source of shopper's fatigue is psychological—styles, prices, lines, crowds . . .
Tired and frustrated,
the next step is hungry!

Think about that the next time you go shopping. Eat before you go, take a healthful snack, or be on your guard as you sample the smells.

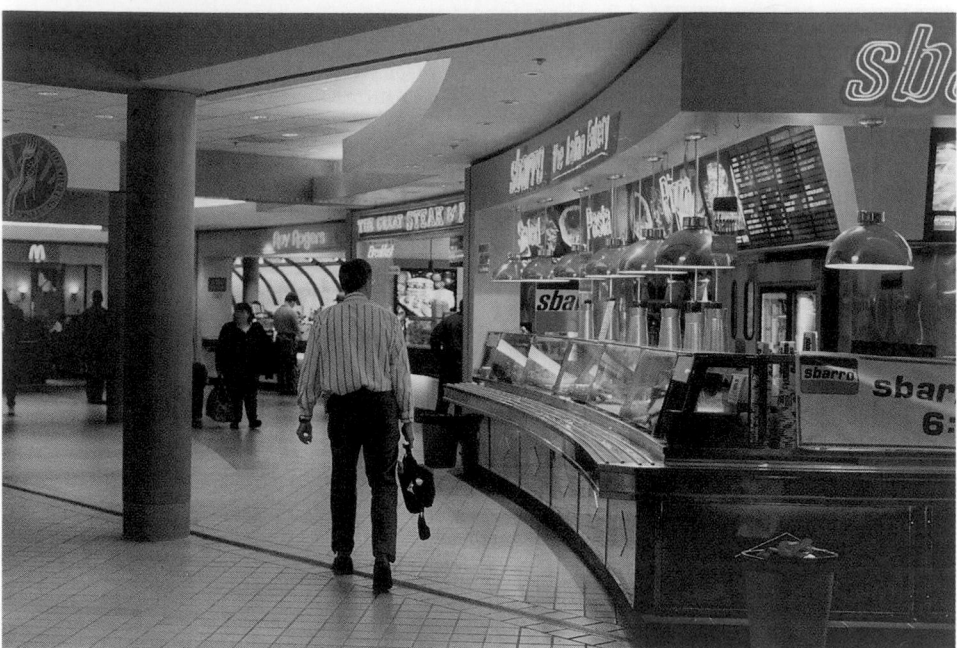

Mall munching can be convenient but costly in terms of the amount of energy consumed.

might save you a few minutes, you are likely to be less alert and less efficient than if you had eaten this meal. Thus you will most likely get much more accomplished during the day if you just take 20 minutes to relax and enjoy a nutritious breakfast.

It is also desirable to try to eat with others often. Meal time is a key social time of the day. The Japanese are ahead of us in recognizing that food's powers go beyond the realm of nutrition. Their national dietary guidelines, which like ours stress the importance of eating a variety of foods, maintaining healthy weight, and limiting fat in the diet, also advise people to make all activities pertaining to food and eating pleasurable.

Economics

Food habits are also influenced by the amount of money an individual or family has available for food purchases. As income increases, so do meals eaten away from home. More affluent people also tend to consume more vegetables, fruit, cheese, meat, fish, poultry, and fat, while eating fewer dried beans and less rice. However, the relationship between income and overall food consumption is not as strong as you might expect, probably because food is relatively inexpensive in the United States. The average American spends only 11% of after-tax income for food: 6% for food at home and 5% for food away from home. Compare this to about 50% of income spent on food in China or India. Nevertheless, high meat prices have led to the use of beef as an ingredient rather than as a centerpiece in some households; chicken, turkey, and fish are used as alternatives.[19]

Improving Our Diets

Our cultural diversity, varied cuisines, and generally high nutritional status should be points of pride for Americans.[5] Today we can choose from a tremendous variety of food products, the result of continual innovation by food manufacturers.

TABLE 1-6

Years When Common American Foods Were Introduced

1875—Chocolate milk	1941—Cheerios
1876—Heinz ketchup	1944—Hawaiian Punch
1891—Fig Newtons	1946—Minute Rice, frozen orange
1896—Tootsie Roll	juice, instant coffee
1897—Jell-O	1950—Sugar Corn Pops
1897—Grape-Nuts	1952—Kellogg's Sugar Frosted Flakes
1898—Graham crackers	1953—Sugar Smacks, frozen pizza
1907—Hershey's Kisses	1956—Duncan Hines brownie mix
1912—Life Savers	1956—Jif peanut butter
1912—Oreos	1958—Tang
1916—All-Bran	1960—Instant potatoes
1921—Mounds, Wonder bread	1963—Tab
1923—Milky Way	1965—Shake 'n Bake
1923—Reese's Peanut Butter Cup	1966—Cool Whip
1927—Kool-Aid	1968—Pringles, Care Free sugarless
1928—Rice Krispies	gum
1930—Birds Eye frozen foods	1976—Country Time lemonade
1930—Snickers	1981—TCBY frozen yogurt
1932—3 Musketeers, Fritos corn chips	1984—Diet Coke (with aspartame)
1934—Ritz crackers, Bisquick	1986—Pop Secret microwave popcorn

Modified from Staten V: *Can you trust a tomato in January?* New York, 1993, Simon & Schuster, and from other sources.

In 1994 alone, some 15,000 new food products were introduced in the United States.

The American food supply does not stand still but is in a constant state of evolution. During the last hundred years, the United States has led the world in creating new food products (Table 1-6). From toaster pastries to microwave popcorn, the variety of food products in a typical supermarket is nearly limitless. Even astronauts in space have their unique food product: a plastic bag containing the nutritional equivalent of an entree, two side dishes, and a beverage, which is kneaded for several minutes and then squeezed into the mouth.

Today we are eating more breakfast cereals, pizza, pasta entrees, stir-fried meat and vegetables served on rice, salads, tacos, burritos, and fajitas than ever before. Sales of whole milk are down, while in the same time period sales of nonfat and 1% low-fat milk have increased.[19] Consumption of frozen vegetables, rather than canned vegetables, is also on the rise.

More than half the shoppers in a recent survey said they are eating more fruits and vegetables to contribute to healthful diets. Shoppers said they are also eating less meat (34%), fewer fats and oils (25%), and less sugar (19%) and more chicken (16%), dietary fiber (16%), and fish (14%).[11] Still, soft drinks are more popular than milk, although not as beneficial to the diet. Overall many of these recent diet changes are advantageous; some are not.[9]

Today, Americans live longer than ever before and enjoy better general health. Many also have more money, more diverse food and lifestyle choices to consider, and more time to relax and enjoy life. The nutritional consequences of these trends are not fully known. Deaths from heart disease and strokes, for example, have dropped dramatically since the late 1960s, partly because of better medical care and diets. Still, if affluence leads to sedentary lifestyles and high intakes of fat, sodium, and alcohol, it can be a villain.[4] Because of better technology and greater choices, we can have a much better diet today than ever before—if we know what choices to make.

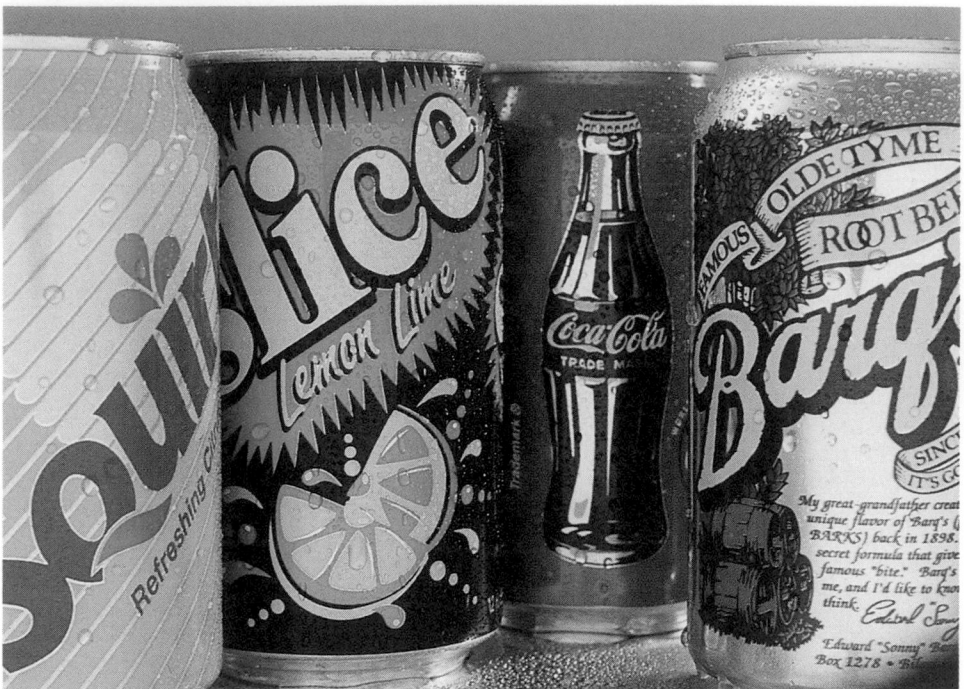

Today, soft drinks are more popular than milk, although not as beneficial to the diet.

Confusing and conflicting health messages also hinder diet change. Nutrition science does not have all the answers, but enough is known to (1) help you set a path to good health and (2) put diet-related recommendations you hear in the future into perspective. See Chapter 2 for details.

The goal of this book is to help you find the best path to good nutrition. There are no "junk" or bad foods, but some foods provide relatively few nutrients in comparison to energy content and thus contribute to less nutritious food behaviors. One's overall diet is the proper focus in a nutritional evaluation. Chapter 2 will emphasize this point and show you how to balance your diet. As you move toward your nutritional goals, remember your health is partly your responsibility. Your body has a natural ability to heal itself. Offer it what it needs, and it will serve you well.[16]

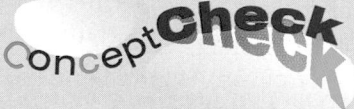

Food choices are influenced mainly by taste and texture. Recently, factors such as health concerns, economics, convenience, and social structure are also becoming important dietary determinants. Good food habits developed and strengthened early in life can provide many benefits in later years.

Summary

➤ Nutrition is the study of what foods are vital for health and how your body uses nutrients to promote and support growth, maintenance, and reproduction of cells.

➤ The metric system is used throughout science. Lengths are expressed in meters, weights are expressed in grams, and volumes are expressed in liters. A meter equals about 39 inches, a kilogram is about 2.2 pounds, and a liter is about 1 quart.

➤ There are six classes of nutrients found in foods: (1) carbohydrates, (2) lipids (fats and oils), (3) proteins, (4) vitamins, (5) minerals, and (6) water. Carbohydrates, lipids, and proteins provide energy (kilocalories) for the body to use.

➤ A basic plan for health promotion and disease prevention includes eating a varied diet, performing regular physical activity, not smoking, getting adequate fluid and sleep, limiting alcohol intake, and limiting or coping with stress.

➤ Good nutrition should be based on eating the right foods rather than mostly relying on nutrient supplements. Getting necessary nutrients from foods minimizes nutrient imbalances and prevents most chances of toxicity from the resulting overnutrition.

➤ As nutritional health diminishes, nutrient stores in the body are depleted first. As stores are exhausted, the state of undernutrition causes biochemical reactions in the body to eventually slow down. Finally, clinical evidence of deficiency is apparent.

➤ Results from large nutrition surveys in the United States suggest that some of us need to concentrate on consuming foods that supply more vitamin A, certain B vitamins, calcium, iron, zinc, and dietary fiber.

➤ The taste and texture of foods primarily influence our food choices. Several other factors also help determine food habits and choices: our upbringing, various social and cultural factors, our self-image and the image we want to project to others, economics, and concerns about health.

➤ There are no true "junk" or "bad" foods. The focus should be on balancing a total diet by choosing many nutritious foods.

Study Questions

1 Name three chronic diseases associated with nutrition and a few corresponding risk factors.

2 Identify a nutrition-related disease that develops over many years before clinical symptoms are evident. Why is there such a long lag time?

3 List the energy values for a gram of carbohydrate, fat, protein, and alcohol.

4 Wendy's Big Bacon Classic contains 44 grams carbohydrate, 36 grams fat, and 37 grams protein. Calculate the percentage of energy derived from fat.

5 Outline the ABCDs of a nutritional assessment; that is, the activities performed to assess an individual's nutritional status.

6 According to national nutrition surveys, which nutrients tend to be undercon- sumed by many adult Americans. Why is this the case?

7 Over the next week, keep an eye out for subliminal cues in the media—TV, ra- dio, magazines, etc.—for eating. What pattern do you see? (Hint: pizza delivery advertised during a sports show.)

References

1 Alaimo K and others: Dietary intake of vitamins, minerals, and fiber of persons ages 2 months and over in the United States: Third National Health and Nutrition Examination Survey, Phase 1, 1988-91, *Advance Data* 258(Nov 14):1, 1994.

2 Blau HM, Springer ML: Gene therapy—a novel form of drug delivery, *New England Journal of Medicine* 333:1204, 1995.

3 Boushey CJ and others: A quantitative assessment of plasma homocysteine as a risk factor for valvular disease, *Journal of the American Medical Association* 224:1049, 1995.

4 Diet, nutrition, and prevention of chronic diseases—a report of the WHO study group on diet, nutrition, and prevention of noncommunicable diseases, *Nutrition Review* 49:291, 1991.

5 Harper AE: The 1990 Atwater lecture: the science and the practice of nutrition: reflections and directions, *American Journal of Clinical Nutrition* 53:413, 1991.

6 Heimendinger J, Van Duyn MAS: Dietary behavior change: the challenge of recasting the role of fruits and vegetables in the American diet, *American Journal of Clinical Nutrition* 61(suppl):1397S, 1995.

7 Hollingsworth P: Lean times for U.S. food companies, *Food Technology*, p. 22, July 1995.

8 Kessler DA: Teens talk with FDA Commissioner about smoking, *FDA Consumer*, p. 23, January-February 1996.

9 Liebman B: The changing American diet, Nutrition Action Health Letter, p. 8, June 1995.

10 Lofgren PA and others: Eating in America today, *Food and Nutrition News* 66:9, 1994.

11 McBean LD: Consumer attitudes and behavior regarding diet, nutrition, and health, *Dairy Council Digest* 65:31, 1994.

12 McDowell MA and others: Energy and macronutrient intakes of persons ages 2 months and over in the United States, *Advance Data*, number 225, October 24, 1994, Centers for Disease Control, USDHS.

13 Morreale SJ, Schwartz WE: Helping Americans eat right, *Journal of the American Dietetic Association*, 95:305, 1995.

14 Pate RR and others: Physical activity and public health: a recommendation from the Centers for Disease Control and Prevention and the American College of Sports Medicine, *Journal of the American Medical Association* 273:402, 1995.

15 Pipes PL, Trahms CM: *Nutrition in infancy and childhood*, ed 5, St Louis, 1993, Mosby.

16 Rosenberg IH: Keys to a longer, healthier, more vital life, *Nutrition Reviews* 52:S50, 1994.

17 Simopoulos AP: Genetic variation and nutrition, part I and part II, *Nutrition Today* 30:157 (part I) and 194 (part II), 1995.

18 Siwek J: Ten steps to healthier patients in 1995, *American Family Physician* 51:33, 1995.

19 Stillings BR: Trends in foods, *Nutrition Today* 29:6, 1994.

20 Taylor A and others: Relations among aging, antioxidant status, and cataract, *American Journal of Clinical Nutrition* 62 (Suppl):1439S, 1995.

21 Thomas PR, Earl R: Creating the future of nutrition and food sciences, *Journal of the American Medical Association* 94:257, 1994.

22 Trends study examines food shoppers concerns, *Community Nutrition Institute Nutrition Week* p 4, June 23, 1995.

23 U.S. Public Health Service: Nutrition in adults, *American Family Physician* p 1485, May 1, 1995.

24 Warshaw HS: America eats out: nutrition in the chain and family restaurant industry, *Journal of the American Dietetic Association* 93:17, 1993.

25 Whittaker L: Clinical applications of genetic testing: implications for the family physician, *American Family Physician* S3:2077, 1996.

26 Williams RR: *Diet, genes, early heart attacks, and high blood pressure.* In Kotsonis FN, Mackey MA, editors: *Nutrition in the '90s,* New York, 1994, Dekker.

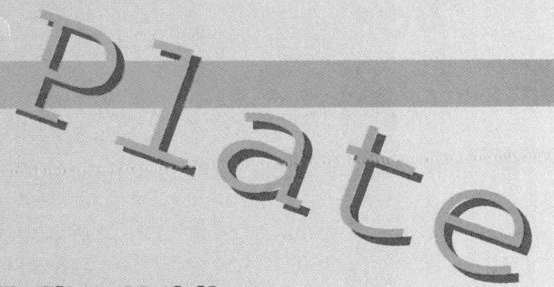

RATE Your Plate

Examine the Factors that Affect Your Eating Habits

Choose one day of the week that is typical of your eating pattern. In the table below, list all foods and drinks you consumed for 1 day. In addition, write down the approximate amounts you ate in units like cups, ounces, teaspoons, and tablespoons. Check the food composition table in Appendix A for examples of appropriate serving units for different types of foods, such as meat, vegetables, etc. Figure 12-4 in Chapter 12 shows an example of a completed form. Appendix C contains a blank form. After completing this activity, you will use this list of foods for future activities.

After you record each food, drink, and serving size, indicate in the table why you chose to consume each item. Use the following symbols to indicate your reasons. Place the corresponding abbreviation in the space provided, indicating why you picked that particular food or drink. Use additional sheets of paper as needed.

TAST	Taste/texture	**HUNG**	Hunger
CONV	Convenience	**FAM**	Family/cultural
EMO	Emotions	**PEER**	Peers
AVA	Availability	**NUTR**	Nutritive value
ADV	Advertisement	**$**	Cost
WTCL	Weight Control	**HLTH**	Health

There can be more than one reason for choosing a particular food or drink.

Time	Minutes spent eating	M or S*	H†	Activity while eating	Place of eating	Food and quantity	Others present	Reason for food choice

*M or S: Meal or snack
†H: Degree of hunger (0 = none; 3 = maximum)

APPLICATION

Now ask yourself what your most frequent reason is for eating or drinking. To what degree is health a reason for your food choices? Should you make it a higher priority?

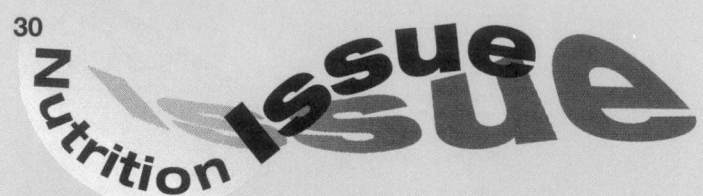

Genetics and Nutrition

The growth, development, and maintenance of cells, and ultimately of the entire organism, are directed by genes present in the cells. The genes contain the codes that control expression of individual traits, such as height, eye color, and susceptibility to many diseases (Figure 1-4). An individual's genetic risk for a given disease is an important factor, although often not the only factor, in determining whether he or she develops that disease.[25]

NUTRITIONAL DISEASES WITH A GENETIC LINK

Most chronic diseases in which nutrition plays a role are also influenced by genetics. The risks of developing heart disease, high blood pressure (hypertension), obesity, diabetes, cancer, and osteoporosis are influenced by interactions between genetic and nutritional factors. Studies of families, including those with twins and adoptees, provide strong support for the effect of genetics in these disorders. In fact, family history is considered to be one of the important factors in the development of many serious diseases (Figure 1-5).

Heart disease

About one of every 500 people in the American population has a defective gene that greatly delays cholesterol removal from the bloodstream.[26] As you will learn in Chapter 6, this and other genetic effects leads to an increased risk of developing heart disease at a young age. Diet changes can help these people, but medications and possibly surgery may be needed to address these problems.

Hypertension

An estimated 10% to 15% of the American population is very sensitive to salt intake. When these salt-sensitive individuals consume too much salt, their blood pressure climbs above the desirable range. The fact that more of these people are African-American than White suggests a genetic component.[17] At present, the only way to determine whether individuals with hypertension are salt sensitive is to place them on a salt-restricted diet and see if their blood pressure falls. Note also that many cases of hypertension are unrelated to salt sensitivity and are caused by other factors (see Chapter 9).

Obesity

Most obese Americans have at least one parent who is also obese. Findings from many human studies suggest that a variety of genes are involved in the regulation of body weight. Little is known, however, about the specific nature of these genes in humans or how the actual changes in body metabolism (such as lower energy use in general or fat use in particular) are produced. A protein produced by one of these genes, called *leptin*, has recently been isolated. The place at which leptin acts in the brain has also been identified. The relevance of this research is discussed in Chapter 10. For now, note that finding the genes that may increase the risk for obesity is a area of intense scientific research.

Still, although some individuals may be genetically predisposed to store body fat, whether they actually do so depends on how much excess energy—above energy

PEANUTS

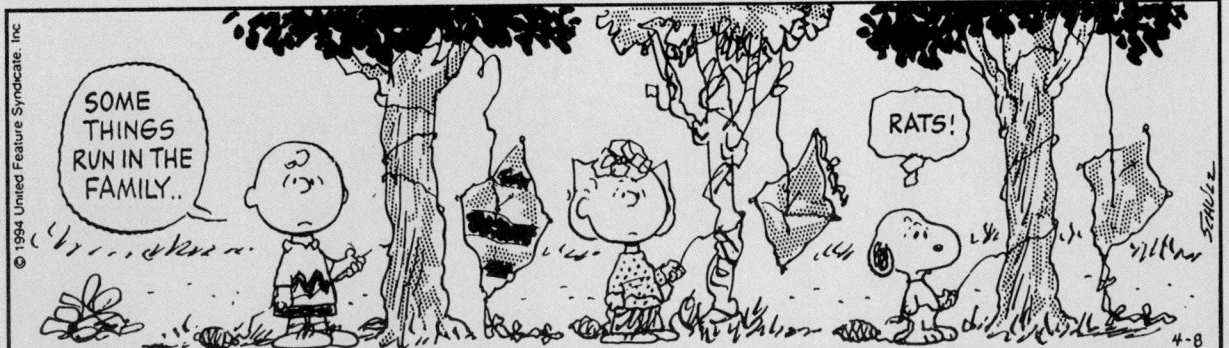

Figure 1-4 *Peanuts.*

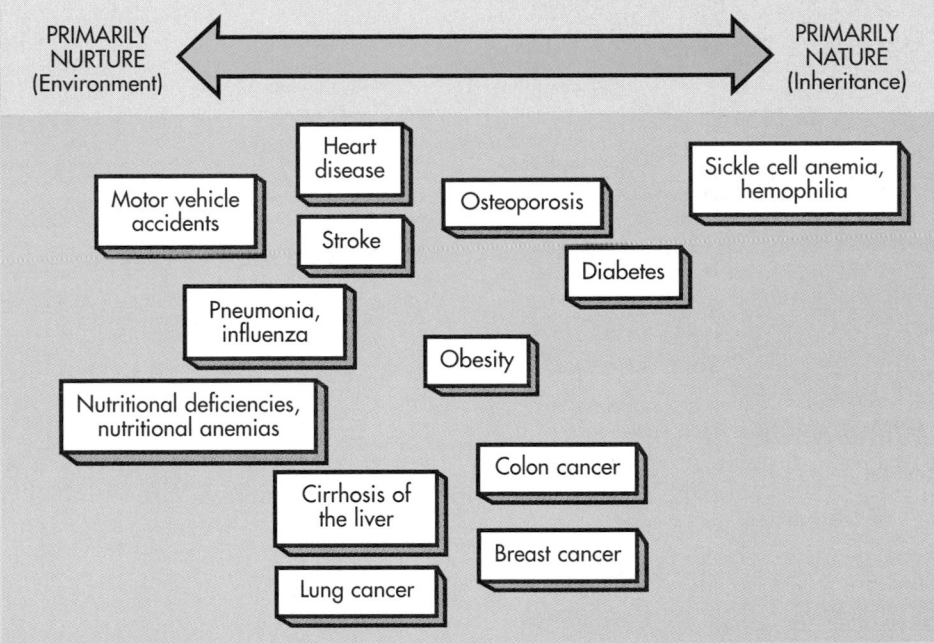

Figure 1-5 *Common causes of death and illness in our population vary in their links to genetic and environmental influences. We must consider both nature and nurture influences as we study each disease.*

needs—they ultimately consume. A common concept in nutrition is that *nurture*—how people live and the environmental factors that influence them—allows *nature*—each person's genetic potential—to be expressed. Although not everyone with a genetic tendency toward obesity develops this condition, they do have a higher lifetime risk than individuals without a genetic predisposition to obesity.

Diabetes

Both of the two common types of diabetes have genetic links, as revealed by family and twin studies.[17] Only sensitive and expensive testing can determine who is at risk. The form of diabetes involved in 90% of all cases also has a strong link to obesity. A genetic tendency for this major form of diabetes will be expressed once a person becomes obese but often not before, again illustrating that nurture affects nature.

Cancer

A few types of cancer (e.g., colon and breast cancer) have a strong genetic link, and genetics may play a role in others.[17] Still, nutritional and other environmental factors are also important. Because obesity increases the risk of many forms of cancer, a diet high in energy and fat is also a risk factor. And one third of all cancers result from smoking. Again, genetics is often not enough—environment also contributes to the risk profile.

Osteoporosis

Bone mineral content, and in turn bone strength, is similar in twins as well as in mothers and their daughters. The exact relative importance of genetic versus dietary factors is unknown, but a number of genes have been shown to contribute to a person's overall risk. In any case, children and adolescents need to consume sufficient calcium to build strong, dense bones, thus reducing the risk of problems, particularly osteoporosis in women, later in life. Adults should then continue that practice. The porous bones that are a result of osteoporosis greatly increase the risk of fractures, especially in the wrist, spine, and hip. As discussed in Chapter 9, the risk of osteoporosis can be greatly reduced by a combination of medical and nutritional means if therapy is started at least by midlife.

YOUR GENETIC PROFILE

From this discussion you can see that a family history of certain diseases raises your risk of developing those diseases. By recognizing your potential for developing a particular disease, you can avoid behavior that contributes to it. In general, the more of your relatives who had a genetically transmitted disease and the closer they are related to you, the greater your risk. One way to assess your risk is to put together a family tree of illnesses and deaths by compiling a few key facts on your primary relatives: siblings, parents, aunts and uncles, and grandparents.

Continued.

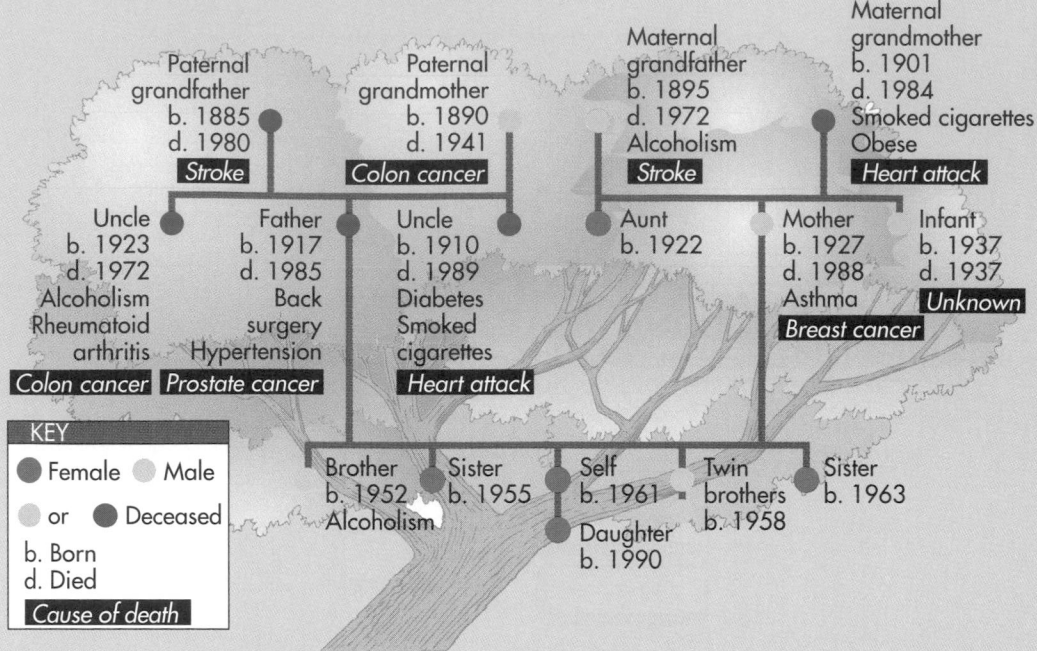

Figure 1-6 *Example of a family tree. Create your family tree of frequent diseases, age, and cause of death, using the example here as a guide. Then show your tree to your physician to get a full picture of what the information means for your health.*

Figure 1-6 shows an example of a family tree (also called a genogram). In this family, prostate cancer killed the man's father. This means that the son should be tested regularly for prostate cancer. His sisters should consider frequent mammograms because the mother died of breast cancer. Because heart disease and stroke are also common in the family, all the children should adopt a lifestyle that minimizes the risk of developing these diseases. Colon cancer is also evident in the family, so careful screening throughout life is important. Finally, alcoholism seems to run in the family, which is true of many American families. Whether nature or nuture is more important in the development of alcoholism is unclear. This is discussed further in Chapter 16.

GENE THERAPY

Scientists are currently developing therapies to correct some genetic disorders, such as a form of muscular dystrophy and a rare immune system disorder. Another example is **cystic fibrosis,** which affects one of every 2500 newborns and also illustrates a main approach to gene therapy. The genetic defect in cystic fibrosis, which must be inherited from both parents to cause the disease, typically leads to a buildup of sticky mucus in the lungs and respiratory tract, among other health problems. The accumulated mucus sets the stage for respiratory infections; generally, death from respiratory complications occurs before the age of 30.

Recently, scientists have inserted the correct gene into inactivated **viruses** and had patients inhale the viruses. Some of the inserted genes appear to enter the patients' lung cells and reduce the severity of the disease. Although this work is in its preliminary phase, experts believe that gene therapy will one day become a practical treatment for many people with cystic fibrosis.[2]

For other genetic diseases the correct genes are inserted into previously extracted body cells, and then the cells are injected back into the body. As the genes involved with more diseases are identified, gene therapy will likely become more common, but much more research is needed for that to happen.[2]

NUTRITIONAL IMPLICATIONS OF GENETIC RISK

Today in the United States, newborns are routinely tested for **phenylketonuria,** an inherited metabolic disease that leads to mental retardation and other problems if appropriate treatment is not given. Infants found to have this disorder are put on a special diet that reduces development of the disease (see Chapter 7 for details).

In contrast to infants with phenylketonuria, individuals with genetic predispositions for many other diseases do not always develop disease. In addition, because genetic background does influence disease risk, certain dietary guidelines are more beneficial for some people than for others.[21] For example, people prone to osteoporosis, as we mentioned earlier, need to be more aware of calcium intake; salt intake is a more important focus for people especially susceptible to high blood pressure.

It is not possible, given the resources presently allocated to medical care in America, to identify all people at genetic risk for the major chronic diseases and other health problems.[25] Thus many health authorities feel it is reasonable to give a general nutrition message to everyone, noting that some people will benefit from the advice much more than others. Throughout this book discussions will point out how you can personalize nutrition advice based on your genetic background. In this way, you can identify and avoid the "controllable" risk factors that would contribute to development of genetically linked diseases present in your family.

Tools for Diet Design

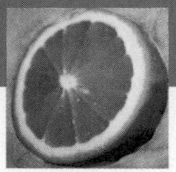

Have you felt bombarded

and confused by wild claims about the health benefits of certain foods? As consumers focus more and more on diet and disease, food manufacturers are churning out products that claim all sorts of health benefits.[13] Supermarket shelves resemble an 1800s medicine show: "Take fish oil capsules to avoid a heart attack." "Eat more olive oil and oat bran to lower blood cholesterol." "Strengthen your bones with calcium-fortified orange juice." What's behind these claims?

Advertising aside, poor eating habits are linked to many leading causes of death in America—high blood pressure, heart disease, cancer, liver disease, and diabetes.[2] Today, eating too much—specifically, eating excessive proportions of energy, fat, sodium, sugar, and alcohol—is increasingly common. How should we respond to all this information? The good news is that a variety of well-chosen foods can supply enough of the six essential classes of nutrients needed for health.[8]

In this chapter you will explore the healthful diet that nutrition scientists recommend—one that minimizes the risks for developing various chronic diseases. You will also acquire the practical tools required for evaluating and planning a healthful diet.

How Does Your Diet Rate for Variety?

Directions: Check the box that best describes your eating habits.

How often do you eat:	Seldom or never	1 or 2 times a week	3 to 4 times a week	Almost daily
1. At least six servings of bread, cereals, rice, crackers, pasta, or other foods made from grains (a serving is one slice of bread or about ½ cup of cereal, rice, etc.) per day?	☐	☐	☐	☐
2. Foods made from whole grains?	☐	☐	☐	☐
3. Three different kinds of vegetables—about ½ cup each—per day?	☐	☐	☐	☐
4. A dark green leafy vegetable, such as spinach or broccoli?	☐	☐	☐	☐
5. Two kinds of fruit (whole piece) or fruit juice (¾ cup) per day?	☐	☐	☐	☐
6. Two servings of 2-3 ounces of lean meat, poultry, fish, eggs, dry beans, or nuts per day?	☐	☐	☐	☐
7. Two servings (three if teenager, pregnant, or breast-feeding) of a combination of milk (1 cup), yogurt (1 cup), or cheese (1½ ounce) per day?	☐	☐	☐	☐

SCORING: Compare your behaviors with the preferred practices.

Question 1: Almost Daily

Eating breads and cereals will not make you fat. Excess energy generally comes from the fat and/or sugar you may eat with them. Both whole-grained and enriched breads and cereals provide starch and essential nutrients.

Question 2: Almost Daily

Whole-grained breads and cereals contain vitamins, minerals, and dietary fiber that are lacking in the diets of some Americans. Select whole-grain cereals and bakery products, or make your own and use whole-wheat flour.

Question 3: Almost Daily

Vegetables vary in the amounts of vitamins and minerals they contain, so it's important to include several kinds every day.

Question 4: 3 to 4 Times a Week

Spinach and other dark green leafy vegetables are excellent sources of some nutrients and are lacking in many diets.

Question 5: Almost Daily

Fruits taste good and are good for you. Choose several different kinds each day.

Question 6: Almost Daily

Most Americans include some meat, poultry, or fish in their diets regularly. Dry beans and peas, peanuts (including peanut butter), nuts and seeds, and eggs can be used as alternatives.

Question 7: Almost Daily

Adults as well as children need the calcium and other nutrients found in milk, cheese, and yogurt.

Key Chapter Concepts

- The watchwords of nutrition are *variety, balance,* and *moderation* when it comes to designing a diet.
- The Food Guide Pyramid provides a blueprint for a healthful diet and is a great place to begin when evaluating daily food intake.
- Dietary Guidelines issued by the federal government encourage a varied diet; daily physical activity; plenty of fruits, vegetables, and grains; and moderation in fat, cholesterol, sugar, and sodium intake. Moderation in alcohol intake, if not complete abstinence, is also advised.
- Recommended Dietary Allowances provide a benchmark for evaluating nutrient intake by groups of healthy people. These allowances should be met by consuming a variety of nutrient-rich foods—not relying on mostly nutrient supplements.
- The Nutrition Facts label on foods provides important information that helps consumers evaluate individual food choices.

A Food Philosophy That Works

You may be surprised to learn that what you should eat to minimize the risk of developing the common nutrition-related diseases seen in the United States is exactly what you've heard many times before: **consume a variety of foods balanced by a moderate intake of each food.** A variety of foods is best because no one food meets all your nutrient needs. Human milk comes close to meeting all of an infant's needs, except that it provides only limited amounts of iron, vitamin D, and fluoride. Cow's milk contains very little iron; neither form of milk provides dietary fiber. Meat provides protein but little calcium. Eggs have no vitamin C and provide little calcium because the calcium is mostly in the shell. Thus, you need variety in your diet because the required nutrients are scattered among many different foods.[10]

Health professionals have recommended the same basic diet and health plan for the past 30 years: watch how much you eat, focus on the major food groups, and stay physically active.[9] Whole grains, fruits, and vegetables have always been among the "good guys" in our diet.

It is disappointing, however, that according to a recent survey conducted by the American Dietetic Association, two of five people in the United States believe that following a healthful diet means giving up foods they enjoy. To the contrary, a healthful diet requires only some simple planning and doesn't have to mean deprivation and misery. Besides, eliminating favorite foods typically doesn't work for "dieters" in the long run. The best plan consists of learning the basics of a healthful diet—a variety and balance of foods from all food groups and moderate consumption of all foods. These aspects of a healthful diet—variety, balance, and moderation—will be continually stressed throughout this book. Let's now fine-tune this advice.

Some people would like to live on pizza alone. What are pizza's nutrient strengths and inadequacies? Check the food composition table in Appendix A for the vitamin C content of cheese pizza. How many slices would you need to eat to yield the vitamin C RDA of 60 milligrams? (Answer: 25 slices)

Variety

For variety in your diet, choose a number of different foods within any given food group rather than the "same old thing" day after day. Variety makes meals more interesting and helps ensure that a diet contains sufficient nutrients. For example, carrots may be your favorite vegetable, but if you choose carrots every day as your only vegetable source, you may miss out on the vitamin folate. Other vegetables, such as broccoli and asparagus, are rich sources of this nutrient. This concept is true of all classes of foods: fruits, vegetables, grains, etc. Different foods within each class vary somewhat in the nutrients they contain, but they generally provide similar types of nutrients.[23]

A varied diet can make eating fun too—no one ever said that we have to eat the same foods and meals that we've eaten since childhood.

Balance

One way to balance your diet as you consume a variety of foods is to select foods from the five major food groups every day:

- Milk, yogurt, and cheese
- Meat, poultry, fish, dry beans, eggs, and nuts
- Vegetable
- Fruit
- Bread, cereal, rice, and pasta

A lunch consisting of a bean burrito with tomatoes accompanied by a glass of milk and an apple covers all groups. Fats, oils, and sweets can also be added to your diet to increase its flavor and help deliver certain nutrients, such as vitamin E and essential fatty acids.

Moderation

Eating moderately requires planning your entire day's diet so that you juggle nutrient sources. For example, if you eat something relatively high in fat, sugar, salt, or energy, such as a bacon cheeseburger with a regular soft drink at a quick-service restaurant, you should eat other foods that are less concentrated sources of the same nutrients, such as fruits and salad greens, the same day. If you choose salty ham for dinner, opt for fresh or frozen vegetables prepared without salt to accompany it. If you prefer whole milk to low-fat or nonfat milk, cut the fat elsewhere in your meals. Try low-fat salad dressings, or use jam rather than butter or margarine on toast. Overall, strive to simply moderate—rather than eliminate—intake of some foods.[11]

In this country, the food supply is abundant and generally safe, most of us can afford a healthy diet, and a huge variety of food products is available. With intelligent planning, you can have a healthful diet that includes foods you like and is compatible with your family and cultural traditions, lifestyle, and budget (Figure 2-1). Although there are no "good" or "bad" foods as such, many Americans have

> **Variety**—Choose different types of foods within each food group.
>
> **Balance**—Choose foods from all five food groups.
>
> **Moderation**—Control portion size so that balance and variety are possible in your diet.

FRANK & ERNEST ® by Bob Thaves

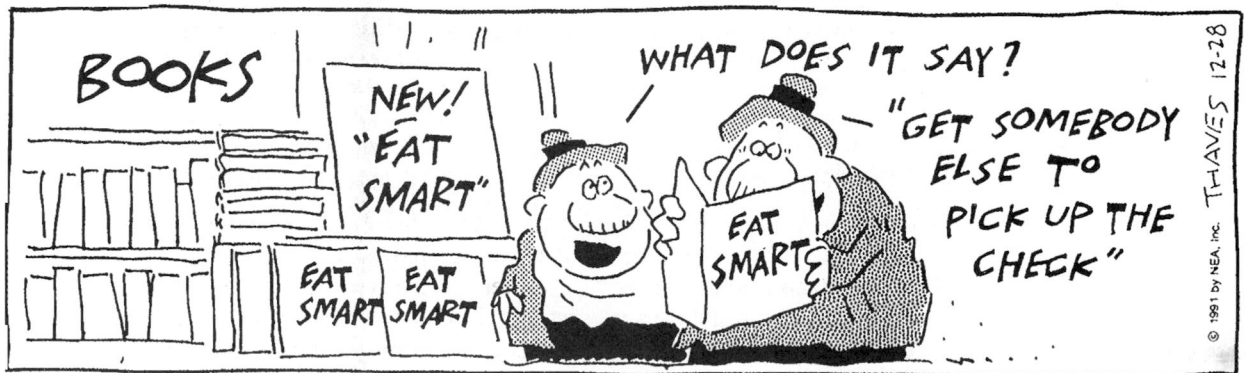

Figure 2-1 *Frank and Ernest.*

diets overloaded with high-fat foods (e.g., whole milk, doughnuts, french fries, hot dogs, meatloaf), white bread, and sugared soft drinks. Such diets lack the foundations of a healthy food plan—variety, balance, and moderation—and pose substantial risks for nutrition-related diseases.[24] The following sections describe various tools and nutrient guidelines for planning healthy diets.

The Food Guide Pyramid— A Menu-Planning Tool

Since the early twentieth century, researchers have worked to clarify the science of nutrition by using practical terms so that people with no special training could estimate whether their nutritional needs were being met. A seven–food-group plan, based on foods traditionally eaten by Americans, was one of the first formats. Daily food choices had to include items from each group. This plan was simplified by the mid-1950s to a four–food-group plan: a milk group, a meat group, a fruit and vegetable group, and a breads and cereals group. The entire plan was designed to provide a minimum foundation for a diet and represented about 1200 to 1400 kcal per day. Other food choices were to be added to meet daily energy needs.

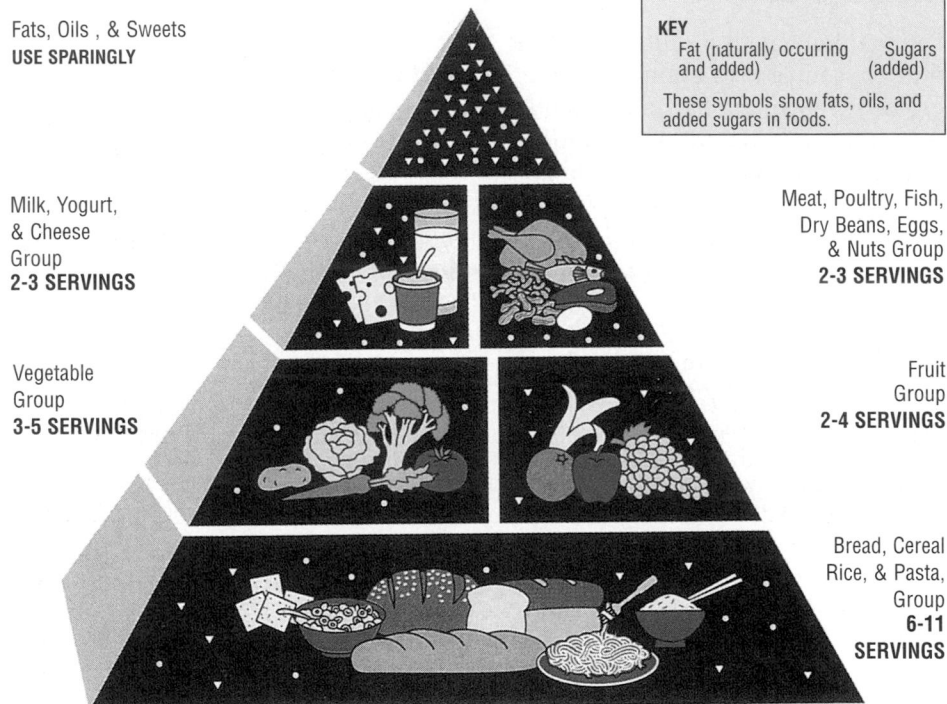

Figure 2-2 *USDA's Food Guide Pyramid. This guide lists the food groups and the number of servings to consume from each group. Note that for children, teenagers, and adults under age 25, 3 servings should be chosen from the milk, yogurt, and cheese group. Once you have estimated your energy needs, recommended servings from the other groups with wider ranges are as follows:*

Energy intake	1600 kcal	2200 kcal	2800 kcal
Bread group	6	9	11
Vegetable group	3	4	5
Fruit group	2	3	4
Meat group	2, for a total of 5 oz	2, for a total of 6 oz	3, for a total of 7 oz

In recent years the Food Guide Pyramid, which is designed to represent a total diet providing sufficient protein, vitamins, and minerals, has been introduced (Figure 2-2). This plan goes beyond earlier guides to suggest a pattern of food choices for the entire day, rather than simply a foundation diet.[23] The major changes from earlier food guides include an increase in total fruit and vegetable servings from 4 per day to 5 to 9 per day and an increase in bread and cereal servings from 4 per day to 6 to 11 per day. One goal of these changes is to provide the bulk of dietary energy intake from carbohydrates while moderating fat intake.[1]

Components of the Food Guide Pyramid

The number of servings to consume from each food group in the current Food Guide Pyramid depends on a person's age and energy needs. Serving size is also adjusted downward for young children (see Chapter 15). Table 2-1 lists serving sizes and amounts for adults of various ages. The table also lists the major nutrients each food group supplies. Note the similarities and differences among the groups. The plan for an adult over 24 essentially consists of the following:

- 2 servings from the milk, yogurt, and cheese group
- 2 to 3 servings from the meat, poultry, fish, dry beans, eggs, and nuts group (5 to 7 ounces total)
- 3 to 5 servings from the vegetable group
- 2 to 4 servings from the fruit group
- 6 to 11 servings from the bread, cereals, rice, and pasta group

For some population groups—children, teenagers, adults under age 25, and pregnant or breast-feeding women—3 servings of the milk, yogurt, and cheese group are recommended.

Foods from a final category, which is not a group per se, include fats, oils, and sweets. These can be eaten to help meet individual energy needs but should not replace foods from other groups.

Planning Menus with the Food Guide Pyramid

Table 2-2 illustrates a 1-day menu based on the Food Guide Pyramid. Remember the following points when using the Food Guide Pyramid to plan daily menus:

1. The Guide does not apply to infants or children under 2 years of age.
2. No one food is absolutely essential to good nutrition. Each food is deficient in at least one essential nutrient.
3. No one food group provides all essential nutrients in adequate amounts. Each food group makes an important, distinctive contribution to nutritional intake.
4. Variety is the key to success of the guide and is first guaranteed by choosing foods from all the groups. Furthermore, one should consume a variety of foods within each group.
5. The foods within a group may vary widely with respect to nutrient and energy content. For example, the energy content of 3 ounces of baked potato is 98 kcal, whereas that of 3 ounces of potato chips is 470 kcal. Compare an orange and an apple with respect to vitamin C, using the food composition table in Appendix A.

Overall, the Food Guide Pyramid incorporates the foundations of a healthy diet: variety, balance, and moderation. The nutritional adequacy of diets planned using this tool, however, depends on selection of a variety of foods. In addition, to ensure enough vitamin E, vitamin B-6, magnesium, and zinc—nutrients sometimes low in diets based on this plan—consider the following advice:

TABLE 2-1

The Food Guide Pyramid—A Summary

Food group

Milk, yogurt, and cheese

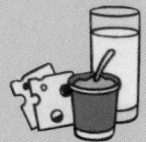

Meat, poultry, fish, dry beans, eggs, and nuts

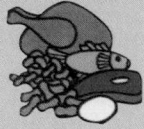

Fruits

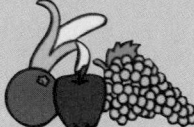

Vegetables

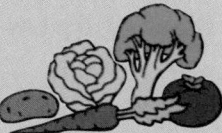

Bread, cereal, rice, and pasta

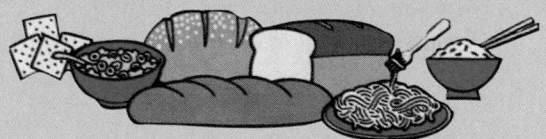

Fats, oils, and sweets

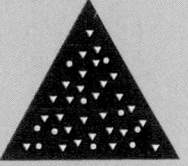

*Consuming the minimum number of servings from each food group provides about 1600 to 1800 kcal. Most adults must consume at least this much energy to meet their RDAs for nutrients, depending on use of nutrient-fortified foods and nutrient supplements.
†May be reduced for child servings.
‡≥25 years of age.
§Primarily in plant protein sources.
‖Only in animal foods.

Number of servings*	Major contributions	Foods and individual serving sizes†
2 (adult‡) 3 (children, teens, young adults, and pregnant or lactating women)	Calcium Phosphorus Carbohydrate Protein Riboflavin Vitamin D Magnesium Zinc	1 cup milk 1½ oz cheese 2 oz processed cheese 1 cup yogurt 2 cups cottage cheese 1 cup custard/pudding 1½ cups ice cream
2-3	Protein Thiamin Riboflavin Niacin Vitamin B-6 Folate§ Vitamin B-12‖ Phosphorus Magnesium§ Iron Zinc	2-3 oz cooked meat, poultry, or fish 1-1½ cups cooked dry beans 4 tbsp peanut butter 2 eggs ½-1 cup nuts
2-4	Carbohydrate Vitamin C Folate Magnesium Potassium Dietary fiber	¼ cup dried fruit ½ cup cooked or canned fruit ¾ cup juice 1 whole piece of fruit 1 melon wedge
3-5	Carbohydrate Vitamin A Vitamin C Folate Magnesium Potassium Dietary fiber	½ cup raw or cooked vegetables 1 cup raw leafy vegetables ¾ cup vegetable juice
6-11	Carbohydrate Thiamin Riboflavin¶ Niacin Folate# Magnesium# Iron¶# Zinc# Dietary fiber#	1 slice of bread 1 oz ready-to-eat cereal ½ cup cooked cereal, rice, or pasta ½ hamburger roll, bagel, or English muffin 3-4 plain crackers

Food from this category should not replace any from the other groups. Amounts consumed should be determined by individual energy needs.

¶If enriched.
#Whole grains especially.
To quickly estimate serving sizes, use the following equivalents:
A thumb = 1 oz of cheese   A fist = 1 cup
A thumb tip = 1 tsp   A handful = 1 or 2 oz of a snack food
Palm of a hand = 3 oz

TABLE 2-2

Putting the Food Guide Pyramid into Practice

Meal	Servings/food group*
BREAKFAST	
1 peeled orange	1 fruit
1½ cups Cheerios	2 bread
with ½ cup 1% milk	½ milk
1 slice raisin toast	1 bread
with 1 tsp margarine	1 fat/sweet
Optional: coffee or tea	
LUNCH	
Ham sandwich	
2 slices whole-wheat bread	2 bread
2 oz ham	1 meat
2 tsp mustard	
1 apple	1 fruit
2 oatmeal-raisin cookies (small)	2 fat/sweet
Optional: diet soda	
3 PM STUDY BREAK	
1 whole bagel	2 bread
1 tbsp peanut butter	¼ meat
½ cup 1% milk	½ milk
DINNER	
Lettuce salad	
1 cup romaine lettuce	1 vegetable
½ cup sliced tomatoes	1 vegetable
1 tbsp Thousand Island dressing	1 fat/sweet
½ grated carrot	½ vegetable
3 oz broiled salmon	1 meat
½ cup rice	1 bread
¾ cup green beans	1 vegetable
with 1 tsp margarine	1 fat/sweet
Optional: coffee or tea	
LATE-NIGHT SNACK	
1 cup low-fat fruit yogurt	1 milk
NUTRIENT BREAKDOWN	

1800 kcal

Carbohydrate	55% of kcal
Protein	20% of kcal
Fat	25% of kcal

Meets RDA/ESADDI values for all vitamins and minerals for a 25-year-old adult. For adolescents and adults under age 25, add one additional serving from the milk, yogurt, and cheese group.
*Names of food groups abbreviated as follows: milk = milk, yogurt, and cheese group; meat = meat, poultry, fish, dry beans, eggs, and nuts group; bread = bread, cereal, rice, and pasta group; fat/sweet = fats, oils, and sweets category.

1. Choose low-fat and nonfat items from the milk, yogurt, and cheese group. By reducing energy intake in this way, you can select more items from other food groups.
2. Include vegetables that are good sources of proteins, such as beans, at least several times a week because these are rich in minerals and dietary fiber.
3. For vegetables and fruits, try to include a dark green vegetable for vitamin A and a vitamin C–rich fruit, such as an orange, every day. Surveys show that only 25% of adults eat a green vegetable on any given day. Increased consumption

TABLE 2-3

Tips for Including More Fruits and Vegetables in Your Diet

- Include vegetables in main and side dishes. Add these to rice, omelets, potato salad, tuna salad, and pasta. Try broccoli or cauliflower florets, mushrooms, peas, carrots, corn, or peppers.
- Choose fruit-filled cookies, such as fig bars.
- Use fresh or canned fruit as a topping for puddings, hot or cold cereal, pancakes, and frozen desserts.
- Put raisins, grapes, apple chunks, pineapple, grated carrots, zucchini, or cucumber into coleslaw, chicken salad, or tuna salad.
- Be creative at the salad bar: try fresh spinach, leaf lettuce, red cabbage, sprouts, zucchini, yellow squash, cauliflower, peas, mushrooms, or red or yellow peppers.
- Pack fresh or dried fruit for snacks away from home instead of grabbing a candy bar or going hungry.
- On sandwiches, lettuce and tomato are just the beginning. Add slices of cucumber or zucchini, bean sprouts, spinach, carrot slivers, or snow peas.
- Try one or two vegetarian meals per week, such as beans and rice or pasta, or spaghetti, squash, and tomato sauce.
- When daily protein intake more than meets required amounts, reduce the meat, fish, or poultry in casseroles, stews, and soups by one third to one half and add more vegetables (and legumes).
- In the refrigerator, keep a bowl of fresh vegetables handy for snacks.
- Choose 100% fruit or vegetable juices instead of soft drinks.
- Have a bowl of fruit on hand.
- Switch from iceberg lettuce to leaf lettuce, such as romaine.
- Use salsa as a dip for chips.

of these foods is important because they contribute vitamins, minerals, and dietary fiber. (Table 2-3).

4. Choose whole-grain varieties of breads, cereals, rice, and pasta often, because they contribute dietary fiber. A daily serving of a whole-grain breakfast cereal is an excellent choice because the vitamins and minerals typically added to it, along with dietary fiber, help fill in the potential gaps listed above.

Following the Food Guide Pyramid makes it possible to create daily diets containing as few as 1600 to 1800 kcal (see Table 2-2), sufficient for a sedentary adult or an older person. Not following this advice can leave a diet of 1600 to 1800 kcal short on the nutrients just mentioned. Recall that excessive consumption of any one food—even ones considered "healthy"—is also not desirable and possibly risky. Overall, our diets must continue to be balanced, though with less consumption of high-fat meat and high-fat dairy products—which are staples of the American diet—to moderate fat intake.[24]

If 1600 to 1800 kcal represents too much food energy for you, you should first consider becoming more physically active rather than eating less. Obtaining enough nutrients from a diet that supplies fewer than 1600 kcal per day is very difficult. If you can't increase your energy output, you could make a special attempt to choose regularly some nutrient-fortified foods (e.g., breakfast cereals). As discussed in Chapter 3, the average person does not usually need nutrient supplements, but certain people may benefit from this practice, such as pregnant women and older people with limited energy intakes. In addition, for those whose diets do not include meat or other animal products, the Nutrition Perspective on vegetarianism

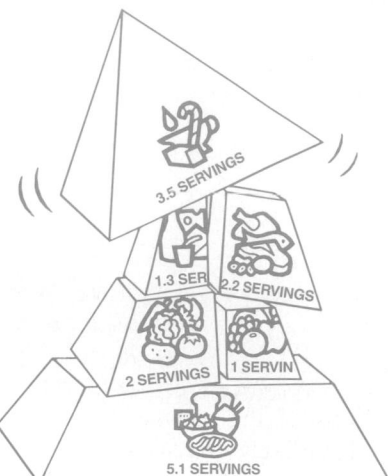

Current U.S. diet in terms of the Food Guide Pyramid.[21]

in Chapter 7 provides advice on adapting the Food Guide Pyramid to that dietary practice.

Evaluating the Current American Diet Using the Food Guide Pyramid

The average American diet, based on a recent survey of 2000 households, failed to meet the serving recommendations in the Food Guide Pyramid for all food groups. For example, the average diet included only 1 fruit serving (rather than the recommended 2 to 4 servings) and only 2 vegetable servings (rather than 3 to 5 servings). These were the most underrepresented groups. In contrast, the fats, oils, and sweets were well represented.[21]

How Does Your Current Diet Rate?

Regularly comparing your daily food intake with the Food Guide Pyramid recommendations is a relatively simple way to evaluate your overall diet. Strive to meet the recommendations. If that is not possible, identify the nutrients that are low in your diet based on the nutrients found in each food group (see Table 2-1). For example, if you do not consume enough from the milk, yogurt, and cheese group, your calcium intake is most likely too low. After completing the Rate Your Plate activity at the end of this chapter, you will be able to determine more accurately which nutrients are too low in your current diet and by how much. Armed with this knowledge, find foods that you enjoy that supply those nutrients, such as calcium-fortified orange juice. Customizing the Food Guide Pyramid to accommodate your own food habits may seem a daunting task now, but it is not difficult once you gain some additional nutrition knowledge.

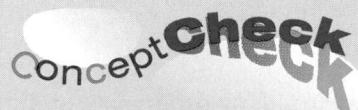

Concept Check

Variety, balance, and moderation are the foundations of a healthy diet. The Food Guide Pyramid translates these foundations and general needs for carbohydrate, protein, fat, vitamins, and minerals into the recommended number of daily servings from each of five major food groups and is a convenient and valuable tool for planning daily menus.

Critical Thinking

Devan has grown up eating the typical American diet. Having recently read and heard many news items about the relationship between nutrition and health, he is beginning to look critically at his diet and is considering making changes. However, he doesn't know where to begin. What advice would you give him?

Dietary Guidelines—Another Tool for Menu Planning

The Food Guide Pyramid was designed to help meet nutritional needs for carbohydrate, protein, fat, vitamins, and minerals. However, most of the major chronic "killer" diseases in America, such as heart disease, cancer, and alcoholism, are not primarily associated with deficiencies of these nutrients.[17] Nor are deficiency diseases, such as scurvy (vitamin C deficiency) and pellagra (niacin deficiency), still common. For many Americans, the primary dietary culprit is an overconsumption of one or more of the following: energy, saturated and total fat, cholesterol, alcohol, and sodium (salt). Underconsumption of calcium, iron, folate and other B vitamins, zinc, or dietary fiber is also a problem for some people.

Nutrition **Insight**

Phytochemicals

Foods of plant origin contain a variety of substances that, unlike the vitamins and essential minerals, are not absolutely required parts of the diet. Still, many of these substances probably provide significant health benefits. Considerable research attention is now focused on the role of these substances, often called *phytochemicals* (*phyto* means "plant"), in reducing the risks for certain diseases.[3] Because current vitamin and mineral supplements contain few or none of these potentially beneficial substances, they must be obtained from the diet.

Numerous epidemiological studies show reduced cancer risk among people who regularly consume fruits and vegetables.[6] This is true for cancer of the gastrointestinal tract, breast, lung, and bladder. Researchers surmise that some phytochemicals present in the fruits and vegetables block the cancer process. The cancer process is described in the Nutrition Issue in Chapter 8. For now, realize that cancer develops over many years via a multistep process. If an agent such as a phytochemical can block any one of the steps in this process, the chances that cancer will ultimately appear in the body are reduced. Other phytochemicals have been linked to a reduced risk of the major form of heart disease.[6] Could it be that because man evolved on a plant-based diet, the body developed with a need for these phytochemicals to maintain optimal health?

Currently, the pharmaceutical industry is experimenting with various phytochemicals in supplement form to be used in the prevention and treatment of disease. However, this work will involve only a few of the many potentially beneficial phytochemicals present in a diet that follows the Food Guide Pyramid recommendation of a total of at least 5 servings of fruits and vegetables a day. It will likely take many years for scientists to unravel the important effects of the myriad of phytochemicals in foods, and it is unlikely that all will ever be available in supplement form.[16] For this reason, leading cancer researchers suggest that a diet rich in fruits and vegetables is the most reliable way to obtain the potential benefits of phytochemicals.[22]

Table 2-4 lists a variety of phytochemicals under study with their common food sources. Table 2-3, featured earlier in the chapter, provided a number of suggestions for including more phytochemicals—essentially more fruits and vegetables, as well as more whole grains and legumes—in a diet. Currently, many researchers are studying phytochemicals, but you don't have to wait to take advantage of what are likely to be their major findings.

Note that only one in ten Americans consumes a combination of 5 servings of fruits and vegetables each day. Furthermore, a vitamin and mineral supplement won't make up for the potential health benefits forfeited by skimping on phytochemical-rich foods. Some nutrition experts are discussing the possibility of enriching certain foods with phytochemicals, analogous to the addition of thiamin, niacin, riboflavin, and iron to enrich flour. You can watch for this as you purchase foods over the coming years. This practice, however, will probably not outweigh the benefits of a diet that emphasizes the bottom half of the Food Guide Pyramid.[22]

TABLE 2-4

Some Phytochemicals Currently under Study

Phytochemical	Food source
Polyphenols (flavonoids; e.g., quercetin)	Onions, garlic, red wine, tea (especially green)
Indoles	Cruciferous vegetables*
Isothiocyanates (e.g., sulforaphane)	Cruciferous vegetables, especially broccoli
Carotenoids	Orange, yellow, and green vegetables; some fruits
Allyl sulfides	Onions, garlic, leeks, chives
Isoflavones (e.g., genistein)	Legumes (e.g., soybeans)
Monoterpenes (e.g., limonene)	Oils from citrus fruits; nuts, seeds
Phytic acid	Whole grains, legumes
Lignan	Seeds; some fruits and vegetables
Ellagic acid	Grapes
Caffeic acid, ferulic acid	Fruits
p-Coumaric acid, chlorogenic acid	Fruits and vegetables
Glutathione	Fruits and vegetables (also freshly prepared meats)

*Cruciferous vegetables include bok choy, broccoli, brussels sprouts, cabbage, cauliflower, collards, kale, kohlrabi, mustard greens, rutabaga, turnip greens, and turnips.

Dietary guidelines
General goals for nutrient intakes and diet composition set by the USDA and the Department of Health and Human Services (DHHS).

In response to concerns regarding disease patterns in the United States, since 1980 the USDA and Department of Health and Human Services (DHHS) have published **Dietary Guidelines** to aid diet planning. The latest version of these guidelines is summarized as follows[17]:

- Eat a variety of foods.
- Balance your food intake with physical activity; maintain or improve your weight.
- Choose a diet with plenty of grain products, vegetables, and fruits.
- Choose a diet low in fat, saturated fat, and cholesterol.
- Choose a diet moderate in sugars.
- Choose a diet moderate in salt and sodium.
- If you drink alcoholic beverages, do so in moderation.

A Closer Look at the Dietary Guidelines

The Dietary Guidelines refer to a total intake over a day or week, not to a single meal or certain foods. To further interpret these general guidelines, consider the following points covered in the Dietary Guidelines pamphlet *Nutrition and Your Health: Dietary Guidelines for Americans.*

Eat a variety of foods. Consume the recommended number of daily servings from the Food Guide Pyramid. Choose a variety of foods within each group. Grain products, along with fruits and vegetables, are the basis of healthful diets. Limit fats and sugars added in food preparation and at the table. Many women and adolescent girls need to eat more calcium-rich and iron-rich foods. Supplements are generally not needed and do not substitute for proper food choices. Vegetarian diets are consistent with the Dietary Guidelines but must be planned with care (see Chapter 7).

Balance the food you eat with physical activity—maintain or improve your weight. Try to do 30 minutes or more of moderate physical activity daily. Devote less time to sedentary activities, such as sitting; spend more time in activities such as walking. High-fat foods contain more energy per serving than other foods and may increase the likelihood of weight gain. Unless nutritious snacks are part of the daily meal plan, snacking may also lead to weight gain. Most adults should not gain weight. Generally, a gain of more than 10 to 16 pounds after age 21 is not recommended. The more you surpass the healthy weight range for your height, the higher the weight-related risk (see Chapter 8 for tables describing healthy weight). Excess fat in the abdominal (stomach) area poses a greater health risk than excess fat in the hips and thighs. Slow weight loss is recommended, when needed. Extreme approaches to weight loss, such as self-induced vomiting, are not appropriate and can be dangerous to your health.

Choose a diet with plenty of grain products, vegetables, and fruits. Most fruits and vegetables are naturally low in fat and provide many essential nutrients. Eat more of these, along with more grain products (breads, cereals, pasta, and rice).

Choose a diet low in fat, saturated fat, and cholesterol. Fats and oils and some types of desserts and snack foods that contain fat provide a great deal of energy but few nutrients. It is important to choose lower-fat options among these foods to leave room for the recommended servings from the five groups in the Food Guide Pyramid. The fats from meat, milk, and milk products are the main sources of saturated fats in most diets. Dietary cholesterol comes from animal sources; many of these foods are also high in saturated fat.

Choose a diet moderate in sugars. Because maintaining a nutritious diet and a healthy weight is crucial, sugars should be used in moderation by most healthy people and sparingly by people with low energy needs. Both sugars and starches can also promote tooth decay. The more you consume them and the longer they reside in the mouth, the greater your risk for tooth decay.

Choose a diet moderate in salt and sodium. Salt and other sodium-containing ingredients are often used in food processing. Most Americans consume more sodium than they need. Many dietary and lifestyle choices influence blood pressure. There is no way at present to tell who might develop high blood pressure from eating too much sodium. However, consuming less salt or sodium is not harmful and can be recommended for the healthy normal adult.

If you drink alcoholic beverages, do so in moderation. Alcoholic beverages supply energy but few or no nutrients. Although moderate drinking is associated with a reduced risk of certain forms of heart disease, high amounts of alcohol raise the risk for high blood pressure, stroke, heart disease, certain cancers, liver and pancreas disease, accidents, violence, suicides, birth defects, and death by other causes. Those who should not drink are children and adolescents, pregnant women, people who plan to take part in activities that require attention or skill (e.g., driving), and people taking certain medications. A moderate alcohol intake consists of two or fewer servings of 12 ounces of beer, 5 ounces of wine, or 1½ ounces of distilled spirits (80 proof) per day. Women should generally limit alcohol to one serving per day (see the Nutrition Insight in Chapter 1). Any use should be with meals.

A shortcut method for healthy weight gives 100 pounds for the first 60 inches for women and an extra 5 pounds for every inch thereafter. The corresponding values for males are 106 pounds to start and 6 additional pounds per inch over 60 inches.

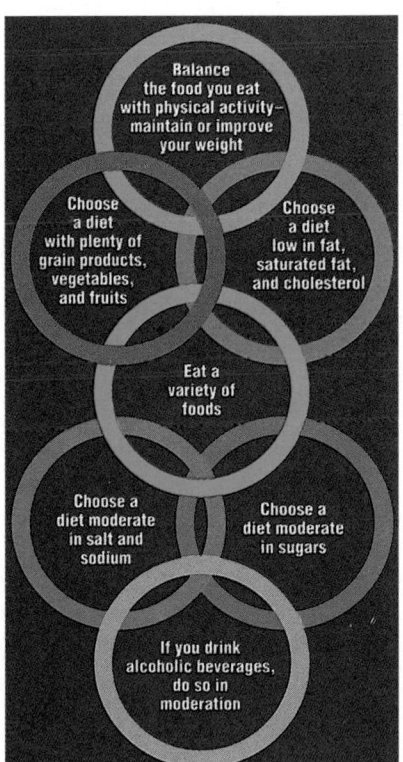

Practical Use of the Dietary Guidelines

The Dietary Guidelines are designed to promote adequate vitamin and mineral intake with the first guideline: Eat a variety of foods. Then the Guidelines emphasize changes that will reduce the risk of obesity, high blood pressure, heart disease, diabetes, and alcoholism.

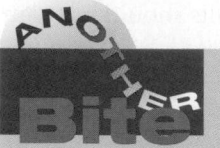

Do you know your blood cholesterol value? Blood pressure values? Although you may feel you are not susceptible to the problems listed previously, it is still a good idea to have your blood cholesterol and blood pressure measured every few years to verify you are right.

The Dietary Guidelines are not difficult to implement (Table 2-5). In addition, this overall diet approach is not especially expensive, as some people suspect. Fruits, vegetables, and low-fat and nonfat milk are no more costly than the chips, cookies, and soft drinks they should in part replace.

Chapter 16 will discuss diet recommendations for adults issued by other scientific groups. In essence, the current recommendations of the American Heart Association, U.S. Surgeon General, National Academy of Sciences, American Cancer Society, Canadian Ministries of Health (see Appendix F), and World Health Organization are consistent with the spirit of the Dietary Guidelines. All of these groups encourage people to modify their eating behavior in ways that are both healthful and pleasurable.[17]

The Dietary Guidelines and You

When using the Dietary Guidelines, you should consider your own state of health. Make specific changes and see whether they are effective. Note that results are some-

TABLE 2-5

Advice for Applying the Dietary Guidelines to Practical Situations

You usually eat this:	Reconsider and eat this:
White bread	Whole-wheat bread (less nutrients lost in refinement/processing)
Sugared breakfast cereal	Low-sugar cereal (use the kilocalories you save for a side dish of fruit)
Cheeseburger and french fries	Hamburger (hold the mayonnaise) and baked beans (for less fat and cholesterol, and the benefits of plant proteins)
Potato salad at the salad bar	Three-bean salad
Doughnut, chips, salty snack foods	Bran muffin or bagel (little or no cream cheese)
Soft drinks	Diet soft drinks (save the kilocalories for more nutritious foods)
Boiled vegetables	Steamed vegetables (for more nutrient retention)
Canned vegetables	Frozen vegetables (less nutrients lost in processing)
Fried meats	Broiled meats (watch the fat drain away)
Fatty meats, like ribs	Lean meats, like ground round (also, eat chicken and fish often)
Whole milk and ice cream	1% or nonfat milk and sherbert or frozen yogurt (to reduce saturated fat intake)
Mayonnaise or sour cream salad dressing	Oil and vinegar dressings or diet varieties (to save kilocalories)
Cookies for a snack	Popcorn (air popped with minimal margarine)
Heavily salted foods	Foods flavored primarily with herbs, spices, and lemon juice

times disappointing, even when you are following a diet change very closely. Some people can eat a lot of saturated fats and still keep blood cholesterol under control. Other people, unfortunately, have high blood cholesterol even if they eat a diet low in saturated fats. Such people don't benefit from the same diet that helps other people. Differences in genetic background are a key cause, as emphasized in Chapter 1.

Most nutrition and health researchers agree with the guidelines set by our major health and science institutions. Varying your food choices; controlling body weight; performing regular physical activity; watching total fat intake; eating plenty of grains, fruits, and vegetables; moderating salt and sugar use; and moderating alcohol intake are generally advised. Although everyone has individual nutritional needs and risks of developing certain diseases, tailoring a unique nutrition program for every American citizen is unrealistic. The Food Guide Pyramid and the Dietary Guidelines provide adults with simple advice that can be actively practiced by anyone willing to take a step toward good health. In effect, the Guidelines promise our nation a healthy future at minimal cost (sacrifice) to society.[5] Reaping the many benefits of good health requires only a small effort and a little knowledge—you are urged to continue the challenge of understanding more about how nutrition relates to you. In later chapters, you will see how to tailor diet planning for individuals with various specific needs and characteristics. There is no "optimal" diet. Instead, there are numerous healthful diets.[11]

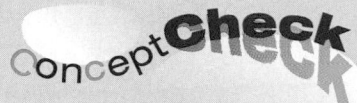

Dietary guidelines have been set by a variety of private and government organizations. These guidelines are designed to reduce the risk of developing obesity, high blood pressure, diabetes, heart disease, and alcoholism. To do so, they first recommend eating a variety of foods, ideally by following the Food Guide Pyramid. They also recommend performing regular physical activity, limiting energy intake to match energy output, and moderating total fat, saturated fat, salt, sugar, and alcohol intake, while focusing more on fruits, vegetables, and grain products in daily menu planning.

Recommended Dietary Allowances

Before designing a diet plan, such as the Food Guide Pyramid, we must determine what frequency and amount of each nutrient are needed. People have puzzled over this question for centuries. During World War II, when many men were rejected from military service because of the effects of poor nutrition on their health, the need for official dietary recommendations was recognized. In 1941 a group of 25 scientists formed the first Food and Nutrition Board. They established dietary standards for evaluating the nutritional intakes of large populations and for planning agricultural production. This Board developed the first **Recommended Dietary Allowances (RDAs).** They left open the option to revise the RDAs as better scientific evidence became available. Every 4 or 5 years the RDAs are revised using the following guidelines[8]:

1. Estimate how much of each essential nutrient the average healthy person requires to maintain that health and how those requirements vary among people.
2. Increase the average **requirement** to cover the needs of almost all members of the population. This usually means increasing the average requirement by approximately 30% to 50%. Thus, if the average requirement for a vitamin is 20

Recommended dietary allowances (RDAs)
Recommended intakes of nutrients that meet the needs of almost all healthy people of similar age and gender. RDAs are established by the Food and Nutrition Board of the National Academy of Sciences.

Requirement
The amount of a nutrient required by one person to maintain health. This varies among individuals. No one knows his or her true requirements for various nutrients.

Nutrition **Insight**

Health Claims on Foods—
What Is Currently Allowed and What Isn't

As noted at the beginning of the chapter, consumers have begun to focus more on diet and disease, and at the same time food manufacturers are asserting that their products have all sorts of health benefits. This campaign began in earnest in 1984, when the Kellogg Company, in conjunction with The National Cancer Institute, printed a health claim on its "high fiber" cereals stating that fiber may help prevent certain forms of cancer. This type of label message was not allowed at the time and caused a heated debate among nutrition scientists. After reviewing hundreds of comments on the proposed rule allowing health claims, the Food and Drug Administration (FDA), which has legal oversight over most food products, decided to permit this and other health claims with certain restrictions.

Currently, FDA limits the use of health messages to specific diseases in which there is significant scientific agreement concerning the relationship between a nutrient, food, or food constituent and the disease. The currently allowed claims may show a link between the following:[14]

- A diet with enough calcium and a reduced risk of osteoporosis
- A diet low in total fat and a reduced risk of some cancers
- A diet low in saturated fat and cholesterol and a reduced risk of heart disease
- A diet rich in dietary fiber–containing grain products, fruits, and vegetables and a reduced risk of some cancers
- A diet rich in fruits, vegetables, and grain products that contain fiber and a reduced risk of heart disease
- A diet low in sodium and a reduced risk of high blood pressure
- A diet rich in fruits and vegetables and a reduced risk of some cancers
- A diet adequate in folate and a reduced risk of neural tube defects (a type of birth defect)

A "may" or "might" qualifier must be used in the statement. In addition, before a health claim can be made for a food product, it must meet two general requirements. First, the food must be a "good source" (before fortification) of dietary fiber, protein, vitamin A, vitamin C, calcium, or iron. The legal definition of "good source" appears in Table 2-7 (in the Nutrition Issue). Second, a single serving of the food product cannot contain more than 13 grams of fat, 4 grams of saturated fat, 60 milligrams of cholesterol, or 480 milligrams of sodium. If a food exceeds any one of these amounts, no health claim can be made for it despite its other nutritional qualities. For example, even though whole milk is high in calcium, its label can't make the health claim about calcium and osteoporosis because whole milk contains 5 grams of saturated fat per serving.

In addition, the product must meet criteria specific to the health claim being made. For example, a health claim regarding fat and cancer can be made only if the product contains 3 grams or less of fat per serving, which is the standard for low-fat foods.

The primary danger with health claims is that not all the facts may be presented in some cases. For example, claims about dietary fiber often omit negative information, such as the fact that too much wheat-bran fiber can lead to decreased absorption of iron, zinc, and calcium, as well as to intestinal problems, such as gas. A more complete statement is that too much—as well as too little—dietary fiber can be harmful.

Some food manufacturers have asked the FDA to amend the regulations governing health and nutrient-content claims to allow greater flexibility in the language of these claims.[18] One request involves changing the "jelly bean" rule, which establishes a minimum nutrient content for any food with a health claim on its label. As it stands now, a manufacturer could not add the calcium equivalent of a glass of milk to a jelly bean and then make a nutrient claim on the package label about calcium and a reduced risk of osteoporosis. Some manufacturers are also lobbying for the right to make health claims based on the findings of an "objective panel" of qualified experts rather than exclusively on the conclusions of FDA. These efforts could effectively thwart the original intent of FDA rules, which are designed to restrict health claims to truly healthful foods—foods with no nutritional drawbacks that increase health risks.

The bottom line for health claims is honesty. FDA is vigilant in controlling the claims made about foods on supermarket shelves. We will have to see to what extent FDA regulation is reduced as private interest groups promote their own agendas.

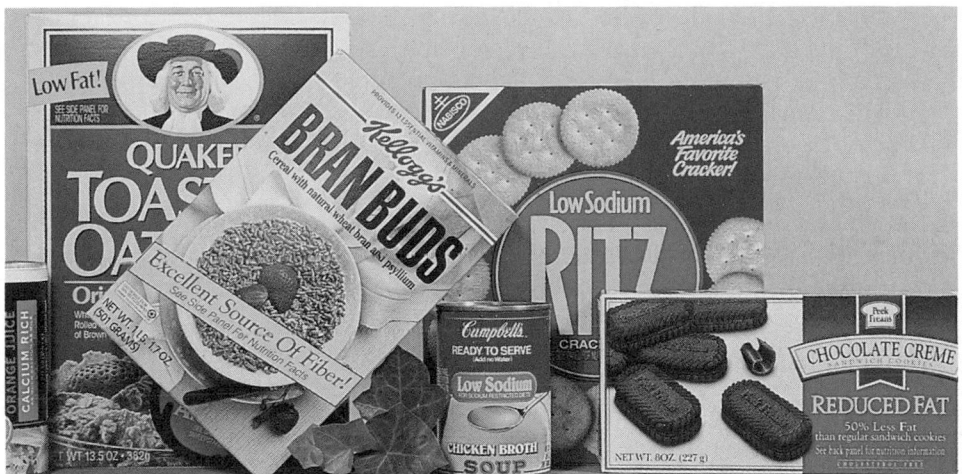

Many food packages prominently feature health claims.

milligrams, the RDA may be 28 milligrams per day, or 40% higher than the average value.

3. Increase the RDA again to make up for cooking losses and inefficient use by the body, as well as for cases in which greater nutrient needs are placed on the body, such as in pregnancy.

4. Use scientific judgment to establish allowances when specific data are limited.

Using this process, the Food and Nutrition Board determines RDAs for healthy males and females of various age-groups. See the inside cover of this book for the specific recommendations.

The RDAs are your guide for estimating your nutritional needs. Strive to obtain these nutrients from foods, rather than relying mainly on vitamin and mineral supplements. Using foods is important because as a whole they contain all essential nutrients. Only 19 of approximately 45 necessary nutrients—not counting certain essential amino acids that make up food protein—have an RDA. Not enough is known about many nutrients for the Food and Nutrition Board to establish an RDA. However, all essential nutrients should be part of your diet.

The RDAs Are Not for Amateurs

One common misconception about the abbreviation RDA is that the "D" stands for "daily." It stands instead for "dietary." We don't need to eat the RDA for each nutrient every day because our bodies store nutrients for later use. Think instead of averaging the RDA for vitamins and minerals over a week's time: some days you eat more, and some days you eat less, but the average for 3 to 7 days should meet the RDA. That can be extended to months for vitamin A and vitamin B-12 because they are not readily excreted by the body.

Notice also that the "R" does not stand for "required," but "recommended." Furthermore, because of the way they are set, RDAs are most relevant to nutritional activities involving population groups, not individuals. Activities in which the RDAs are valuable and correctly used include the following:

- Planning and obtaining food supplies for population groups, such as schools, college dormitories, hospitals, and health-care facilities
- Establishing standards for food assistance programs, such as food stamps
- Evaluating dietary survey data, such as those collected by the federal government
- Developing food and nutrition information and education programs, such as those provided by federal food assistance programs

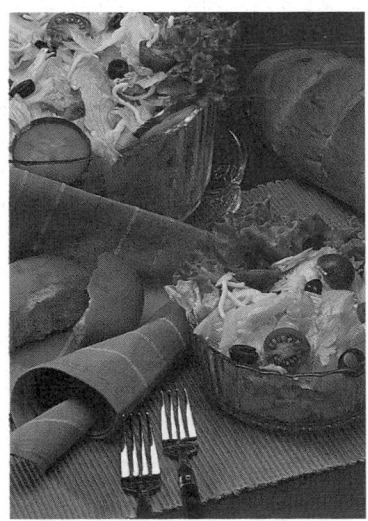

Focus on nutrient-rich foods as you strive to meet the Recommended Dietary Allowances.

- Establishing food-labeling standards, such as the Daily Values that appear as part of the Nutrition Facts panel on food labels
- Regulating food fortification, such as setting standard fortification policies for enriched bread, milk, and infant formulas
- Developing new or modified food products, such as rations used by soldiers in military combat and astronauts in space

The RDAs are not to be interpreted as specific personal nutritional requirements for individuals. Those values can be scientifically determined only in a laboratory. Because the allowances are set quite high, healthy people should not expect their health to improve if they eat more than the RDA levels of various nutrients.[12] The Food and Nutrition Board's goal in establishing RDAs is to prevent Americans from getting either too much or too little of the needed nutrients.

Potential positive effects from nutrient intakes well above what can be obtained from food are medical or pharmacological in nature. The RDAs do not address these uses of nutrients, although intakes much above RDA amounts show efficacy in clinical practice in a limited number of diseases. This topic will be discussed in more detail later. Keep in mind, however, that many people believe if a little of something is good, a lot must be better. This can lead to trouble with some nutrients, as you will see in Chapters 8 and 9. The Rate Your Plate activity at the end of this chapter will help you evaluate how well you are meeting the RDAs set for your age and gender.

In sum, the RDAs are estimates of the amount of each nutrient that should be consumed by groups of healthy people to meet their nutritional needs. The word *healthy* needs emphasis. The RDAs apply only to people who are not taking medications or suffering from diseases that increase nutrient needs, are not experiencing temperature extremes, and do not participate in long, strenuous physical activity.[8]

A Close Look at One RDA: Protein

Eating protein regularly is critical to maintaining your health. The RDA for protein is 0.8 gram per kilogram of healthy body weight (or about 0.35 gram per pound) for an adult.[8] That amount allows daily protein intake to balance the body's normal protein losses from hair, skin, stool, and so on and allows the body to maintain protein **equilibrium** (Figure 2-3). (Chapter 7 contains more details on proteins in the body.) The recommendation also allows for some extra protein to stock the body's protein stores. In this way, protein status of the body should stay about the same each day.

When setting the RDA for children, scientists add extra protein to create the **positive balance** necessary to accommodate daily growth needs in new cells. For children it is not enough to balance daily protein losses and store a little extra; to provide for growth, children must regularly take in more protein than they lose. The RDA is adjusted to account for this. The same is true for pregnant women.

If you total the amount of protein you eat in 1 week and divide by seven, you will have your average daily protein consumption. If that value is close to the RDA, you are most likely eating enough protein. Even if you eat less protein than the RDA, you might not suffer ill effects because your needs are most likely less than the RDA. As a general rule, however, the further you stray below the RDA—particularly as you approach less than half the recommendation—the greater your risk of a nutritional deficiency from the resulting **negative balance** that will follow.

Symptoms of nutritional deficiencies may be subtle and develop slowly. It takes a long time to detect problems such as a weakened immune system, reduced chemical processing in body cells, or an impaired ability to carry oxygen in the blood. If you suspect that your diet is not nutritious enough, don't wait for warning signs to develop. Start eating a diet that meets the RDAs set for all listed nutrients for your age and gender rather than risking the development of health problems from poor nutrition.

Equilibrium

A state in which nutrient intake equals nutrient losses so that the body maintains a stable condition.

Positive balance

A state in which nutrient intake exceeds losses. This causes a net gain of the nutrient in the body, such as when tissue protein is gained during growth.

Negative balance

The state in which nutrient losses from the body exceed intake, as in cases of starvation.

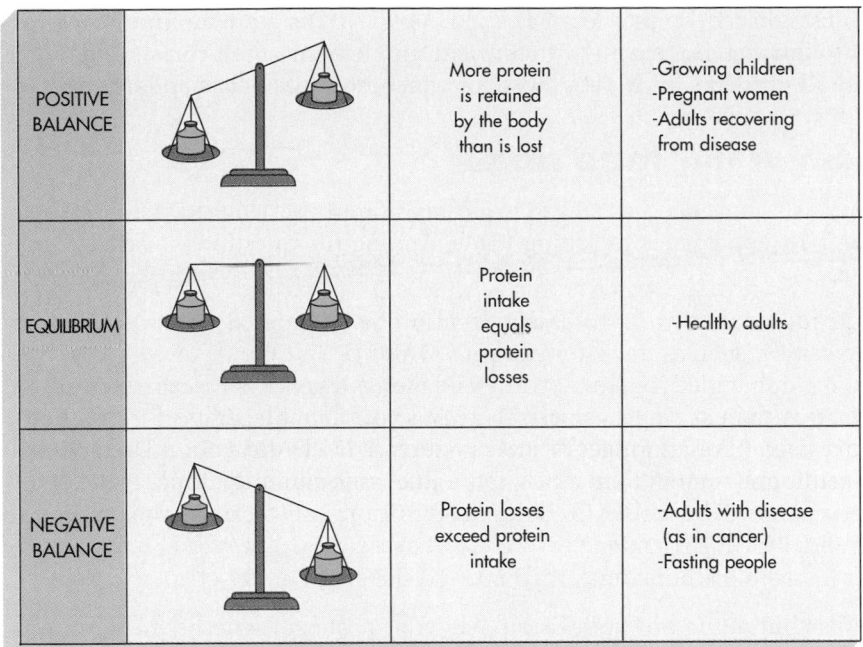

POSITIVE BALANCE		More protein is retained by the body than is lost	-Growing children -Pregnant women -Adults recovering from disease
EQUILIBRIUM		Protein intake equals protein losses	-Healthy adults
NEGATIVE BALANCE		Protein losses exceed protein intake	-Adults with disease (as in cancer) -Fasting people

Figure 2-3 *Nutrient balance using protein as an example. The concept of positive balance, equilibrium, and negative balance applied to the health status of a person with respect to all nutrients.*

RDAs for Energy Needs

RDAs for nutrients are set high enough to meet the needs of almost all healthy people. In contrast, the Food and Nutrition Board sets the RDAs for energy at the average needs for various age groups (see inside cover). Note that no extra amount is added for human variability, as is done for nutrient RDAs.[8] Unlike most vitamins and minerals, excess energy consumed (above energy needs) is not excreted. Thus, to promote weight maintenance, a more conservative standard must be set for energy needs than for nutrient needs. The Board also warns that the energy RDA is only a rough estimate, because energy needs depend on energy use. For most adults, the ability to obtain and maintain a healthy weight is the best yardstick of energy balance—energy intake matching energy output.

Other Nutrient Standards Set by the Food and Nutrition Board

In addition to the RDAs, the Food and Nutrition Board sets two other types of numerical standards for certain nutrients.

Estimated safe and adequate daily dietary intakes (ESADDIs). *ESADDIs* have been established for several nutrients, including copper, biotin, and chromium (see inside cover). The Board determined that insufficient data were available to set RDAs for these nutrients but that enough data were available to suggest a range for a reasonable intake for groups.[8]

Minimum requirement. Minimum requirements, the third type of numerical standard, have been set for sodium, potassium, and chloride (see inside cover). These values represent minimum nutrient needs. Note that these amounts are much less than typical intakes of sodium or chloride but are about equal to Americans' typical intake of potassium.[8]

To date, the Food and Nutrition Board has set no numerical standards for carbohydrates, fats, and some other essential nutrients. Nonetheless, if you meet all the

Estimated safe and adequate daily dietary intakes (ESADDIs) *Nutrient-intake recommendations made by the Food and Nutrition Board for certain nutrients when not enough information is available to establish RDAs. The recommendations specify an intake range rather than a single value for each nutrient.*

standards established by the Board (i.e., RDAs, ESADDIs, and minimum requirements) through diet, not mostly with nutrient supplements, then you should obtain enough of all nutrients, including those for which no numerical standards exist.

Revision of the 1989 RDAs

When scientists convened in 1993 to begin revision of the 1989 RDAs, they began discussing new approaches to setting RDAs. Among the questions raised were the following:[4,15]

- Should concepts of chronic disease prevention be considered when developing the allowances, such as those for vitamins C and E?
- Should recommended intakes for different ages and genders be expressed as ranges rather than as single values? There was considerable support for presenting the revised RDAs as ranges of intake—such as likely deficient, RDA, and upper safe amount—rather than as a single value, as is currently done.
- Should separate RDAs be set for older people? Currently a category exists for age 51 and older for each gender.
- Should RDAs for carbohydrate, total fat, and dietary fiber be set?

Work is continuing on the revision. Ask your professor whether new information is available.

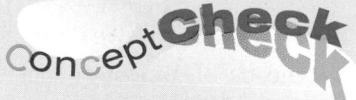

Concept**Check**

Recommended Dietary Allowances represent the nutrient needs for groups of healthy people, not of individuals per se. RDAs are established for specific age and gender categories. No one knows his or her own nutritional requirements; the best general rule is that the further you stray from the RDAs set for your age and gender, the greater your chance of having a nutritional deficiency.

Daily Values: The Standards Used for Food Labeling

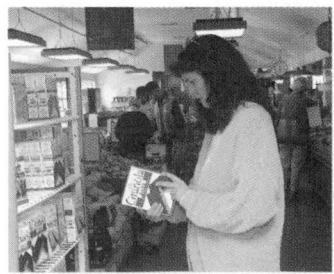

Nutrient content in foods is expressed on the nutrition label in terms of Daily Values.

The RDAs are not used in food labeling because they are age and gender specific. We can't have different packages for men and women or for teens and adults. The Food and Drug Administration (FDA) has developed a set of generic standards, called *Daily Values,* that are used to express the nutrient content of foods for the Nutrition Facts panel on food labels. The content of a particular nutrient is listed on labels as a percentage of the Daily Value. These percentages serve as a bench mark for evaluating the nutrient content of foods. They do not, however, represent a set of tailor-made recommendations for an adult. You will see why once the method for setting Daily Values is described.

The Daily Values are based on two sets of dietary standards. The first, **Reference Daily Intakes (RDIs),** are for vitamins and minerals. The second, **Daily Reference Values (DRVs),** are standards for protein and various dietary components that have no RDA (e.g., total fat, cholesterol, and dietary fiber). These two terms—*Reference Daily Intakes* and *Daily Reference Values*—do not appear on labels. To make reading labels less confusing for consumers, the term *Daily Value* is used to represent the combination of these two sets of dietary standards.[14]

Standards set for nutrients
that have RDAs, called
RDIs

Standards set for many
nutrients that do not have
RDAs, called DRVs

Daily Values consist of RDI and DRV standards for use in the Nutrition Facts panel of food labels

Reference Daily Intakes (RDIs)

Reference Daily Intakes (RDIs) make up the majority of the Daily Values. The RDIs were determined by the FDA using a compilation of the RDA values published in 1968. Essentially, RDIs were set as the highest RDA values within specific age categories. For example, consider iron: in 1968 the RDA for adult men was 10 milligrams per day and that for adult women and adolescents was 18 milligrams per day. The iron RDI for adults is the higher value: 18 milligrams per day. Appendix C lists the RDIs used for various age groups. Typically the RDI for people over 4 years of age is used to set the Daily Values on most food packages.

The RDI values currently in use, which are based on the 1968 RDAs, are generally slightly higher than 1989 RDAs. Therefore when you read a cereal label that claims a serving provides 25% of the Daily Value for a vitamin or mineral, you can generally be sure that it will provide at least 25% of the RDA for your age and gender if the nutrient has an RDA. This is especially true for vitamin E, vitamin B-12, and folate because current RDAs are lower than those of 1968. Your individual need, if it is different from the Daily Value, will probably be lower. An exception is calcium for the age group 11 to 24 years; the RDI and, hence, the Daily Value are 200 milligrams lower than the current RDA.

Many scientists support revision of the RDIs based on the 1989 RDAs.[19] However, some scientists and the vitamin industry in general oppose this revision because it would reduce many RDIs. Some opponents believe that the public generally underconsumes some of the nutrients covered (e.g., vitamin E). Because the amounts of nutrients added to "fortified" foods, such as breakfast cereals, are related to the RDI values, reduction of these values might have health consequences for some consumers. Revision of the RDIs would also reduce the market for the vitamins and minerals used in fortification, with unfavorable economic consequences for supplement manufacturers. It is unclear which group's interests and opinion will prevail.

Daily Reference Values (DRVs)

The Daily Values for some food constituents are based on Daily Reference Values (DRVs) rather than RDIs. Except for the protein DRV, which is based on RDA values, the other DRVs cover certain dietary components that have no true RDA: total fat, saturated fatty acids, cholesterol, carbohydrate, fiber, sodium, and potassium. The DRVs are intended to help consumers evaluate their food choices by comparing their actual intakes of these food constituents with desirable (or maximum) intakes.[20] Appendix C lists the DRVs. The amounts for energy-yielding nutrients are based on 30% of total kcal from fat, 60% from carbohydrate, and 10% from protein.

Note that many of the DRVs, such as those for saturated fat, total fat, and dietary fiber, are related to total energy intake. By accounting for this, you can evaluate your diet even if your energy intake is more or less than the standard energy intake, 2000 kcal, used on the label. For example, if you consume only 1600 kcal per day, the total percentage of Daily Value for each of these dietary components should add up to no more than 80%, because $1600 \div 2000 = 0.8$, or 80%. If you eat 2800

Daily values
A set of standard nutrient-intake values developed by FDA and used as a reference for expressing nutrient content on nutrition labels. The Daily Values include two types of standards—RDIs and DRVs.

Reference daily intakes (RDIs)
Nutrient-intake standards set by FDA based on the 1968 RDAs for various vitamins and minerals. RDIs have been set for four categories of people: infants, toddlers, people over 4 years of age, and pregnant or lactating women. Generally the highest RDA value in each category is used as the RDI. The RDIs constitute part of the Daily Values used in food labeling.

Daily reference values (DRVs)
Nutrient-intake standards established for protein and some other dietary components lacking an RDA, including fat, saturated fat, cholesterol, carbohydrate, dietary fiber, sodium, and potassium. The DRVs for cholesterol, sodium, and potassium are constant; those for the other nutrients increase as energy intake increases. The DRVs constitute part of the Daily Values used in food labeling.

kcal, your total percentage of Daily Value for each of these components in all the foods you eat in one day can add up to 140%, because 2800 ÷ 2000 = 1.4, or 140%. However, the % Daily Values for some dietary constituents, such as cholesterol and sodium, are not adjusted for differences in energy intake.

Daily Values in Perspective

The Nutrition Facts panel on the label of a food product lists various components of the food as a percentage of their Daily Values. Use this information to learn more about your food choices. For example, suppose that one serving of a macaroni and cheese product contains 15% of the Daily Value for iron. Since the Daily Value for iron is 18 milligrams, this product contains about 3 milligrams of iron per serving (18 × 0.15 = 2.7 milligrams). The Nutrition Issue at the end of this chapter describes nutrition labels on foods in detail.

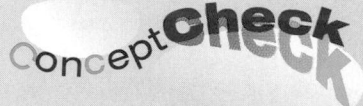

Daily Values are currently used as a bench mark for representing the nutrient content of foods on nutrition labels. Nutrient content is expressed as percentages of the Daily Values, which in turn are based on Reference Daily Intakes (RDIs) or Daily Reference Values (DRVs). The RDIs for vitamins and minerals constitute the majority of Daily Values and are based on the 1968 RDAs. The DRVs have been set for protein and some nutrients that don't have an RDA, such as fat, cholesterol, and dietary fiber. To decrease confusion, the Daily Value is the only term that appears on food labels.

Nutrient Density Can Help Guide Food Choice

Nutrient density

The ratio formed by dividing a food's contribution to nutrient needs by its contribution to energy needs. When its contribution to nutrient needs exceeds its energy contribution, the food is considered to have a favorable nutrient density.

As you've seen already, the RDAs are used for planning and evaluating complete diets of groups of individuals. However, these nutrient standards aren't useful for assessing the nutritional quality of an individual food. For this purpose the concept of **nutrient density** has gained acceptance in recent years.

To determine the nutrient density of a food, simply compare its vitamin or mineral content with the amount of energy it provides. The higher a food's nutrient density, the better it is as a nutrient source. Comparing the nutrient density of different foods is an easy way to estimate their relative nutritional quality. Generally, nutrient density is assessed with respect to individual nutrients. For example, many fruits and vegetables have a high content of vitamin C compared with their modest energy content: that is, they are nutrient-dense foods for vitamin C. Moreover, as Figure 2-4 shows, nonfat milk is much more nutrient dense than sugared soft drinks for many nutrients.

Menu planning focuses mainly on the total diet—not on selection of one critical food as key to an adequate diet. Nonetheless, nutrient-dense foods—such as nonfat and low-fat milk, lean meats, beans, oranges, carrots, broccoli, whole-wheat bread, and whole-grain breakfast cereals—do help balance less nutrient-dense foods—such as cookies and potato chips—that many people like to eat. The latter are often called empty-calorie foods because they tend to supply much energy as sugar and/or fat but few other nutrients.

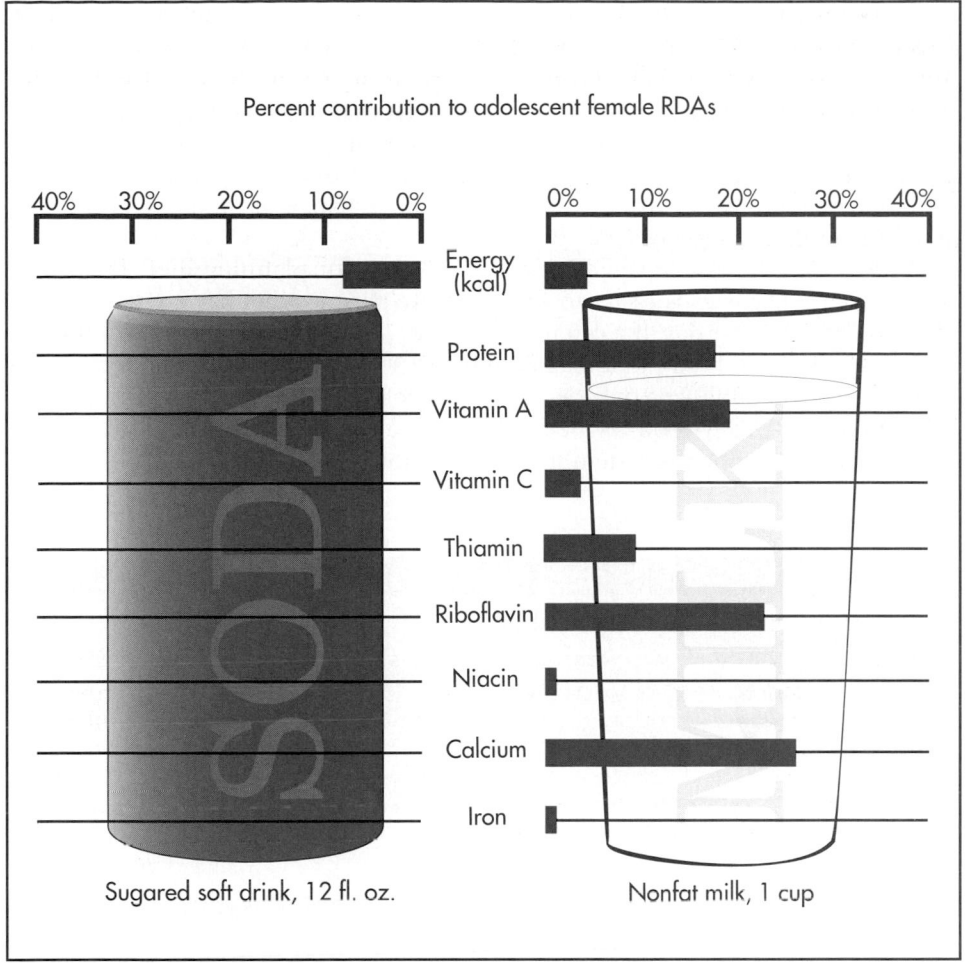

Percent contribution to adolescent female RDAs

| 40% | 30% | 20% | 10% | 0% | | 0% | 10% | 20% | 30% | 40% |

Energy (kcal)

Protein

Vitamin A

Vitamin C

Thiamin

Riboflavin

Niacin

Calcium

Iron

Sugared soft drink, 12 fl. oz.   Nonfat milk, 1 cup

Figure 2-4 *Comparison of the nutrient density of a sugared soft drink with that of nonfat milk. Choosing a glass of nonfat milk makes a significantly greater contribution to nutrient intake in comparison with a sugared soft drink. An easy way to determine nutrient density is to see how many of the nutrient bars are longer than the kcal bar. The soft drink has no longer nutrient bars. Nonfat milk has longer nutrient bars for protein, vitamin A, thiamin, riboflavin, and calcium. Including many nutrient-dense foods in your diet aids in meeting nutrient needs.*

Critical Thinking

Your classmate John is having trouble understanding the concept of nutrient density. How could you demonstrate to him that nonfat (skim) milk is a more "nutrient-dense" source of calcium than whole milk?

Searching for nutrient-dense foods is important in some cases. For example, this strategy can aid diet planning for people who tend to consume little food energy, including some older people and those following weight-loss diets.

The Exchange System: a Final Menu-Planning Tool

The **Exchange System** is a valuable tool for quickly estimating the energy, protein, carbohydrate, and fat content of a food or meal. Although learning to use the Exchange System is a bit tedious, it greatly simplifies menu planning. The Exchange System organizes many details of the nutrient composition of foods into a manageable framework, allowing you to plan daily menus without having to look up or memorize the nutrient values of numerous foods. Thus, the time you spend now becoming familiar with the Exchange System can pay dividends in the future.

Exchange system
A system for classifying foods into numerous lists based on their macronutrient composition and establishing serving sizes so that one serving of each food on a list contains the same amount of carbohydrate, protein, fat, and energy content.

In the Exchange System, individual foods are placed into three broad groups: carbohydrate, meat and meat substitutes, and fat. Within these groups are lists that contain foods of similar macronutrient composition: various types of milk; fruit; vegetables; starch; other carbohydrates; various types of meat and meat substitutes; and fat. These lists are designed so that when the proper serving size is observed, each food on a list provides about the same amount of carbohydrate, protein, fat, and energy (Table 2-6). This equality allows the exchange of foods on each list—hence the term *Exchange System.*

The Exchange System was originally developed for planning diets for people with diabetes. Diabetes is easier to control if the person's diet has about the same composition day after day. If a certain number of "exchanges" from each of the various lists is eaten each day, that regularity is easier to achieve. However, because the Exchange System provides a quick way to estimate the energy, carbohydrate, protein, and fat content in any food or meal, it is a valuable menu-planning tool. Appendixes D and E describe the system fully and demonstrate how to use it.

TABLE 2-6

Nutrient Composition of Exchange System Lists (1995 Edition)

Groups/lists	Household measures*	Carbohydrate (gram)	Protein (gram)	Fat (gram)	Energy (kcal)
CARBOHYDRATE GROUP					
Starch	1 slice, ¾ cup raw, or ½ cup cooked	15	3	1 or less†	80
Fruit	1 small/medium piece	15	—	—	60
Milk	1 cup				
Skim/very low-fat		12	8	0-3†	90
Low-fat		12	8	5	120
Whole		12	8	8	150
Other carbohydrates	Varies	15	Varies	Varies	Varies
Vegetables	1 cup raw or ½ cup cooked	5	2	—	25
MEAT AND MEAT SUBSTITUTES GROUP	1 oz				
Very lean		—	7	0-1	35
Lean		—	7	3	55
Medium-fat		—	7	5	75
High-fat		—	7	8	100
FAT GROUP	1 tsp	—	—	5	45

From American Diabetes Association and American Dietetic Association: *Exchange lists for meal planning,* 1995.
*Just an estimate. See exchange lists for actual amounts.
†Calculated as 1 gram for purposes of energy contribution.

Epilogue

The tools discussed in this chapter greatly aid in menu planning. Menu planning can start with the Food Guide Pyramid. The totality of choices made within the groups can then be evaluated using the Dietary Guidelines. Individual foods that make up a diet can be examined more closely using the comparison to the Daily Values listed on the Nutrition Facts panel of the product. For the most part, these Daily Values are in line with the Recommended Dietary Allowances. The Nutrition Facts panel is especially useful in identifying nutrient-dense foods—foods that are high in a specific nutrient, such as the vitamin folate, but low in comparison to the relative amount of energy provided. Once mastered, the Exchange System is helpful for formulating a menu plan that meets specific carbohydrate, fat, and protein goals. Generally speaking, the more you learn about and use these tools, the more they will benefit your diet.

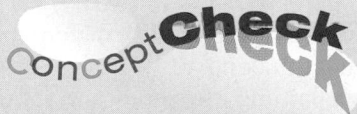

Nutrient density is a measure of the nutrient contributions made by each food compared with its total energy content. Nutrient-dense foods supply much of one or many nutrients while providing a relatively modest energy content.

The Exchange System makes it possible to design and follow a precise diet that yields desired ratios of carbohydrate, fat, and protein, while accounting for total energy intake. When the set serving sizes are observed, all the foods within each of the various Exchange System lists yield similar contributions of carbohydrate, fat, protein, and energy. Because of their similar nutrient profiles, the foods in each group can be "exchanged" for one another.

Summary

➤ The Food Guide Pyramid is designed to translate nutrient recommendations into a food plan that exhibits variety, balance, and moderation. The best results are obtained by using low-fat or nonfat dairy products; including some vegetable proteins in addition to animal-protein foods; including citrus fruits and dark green vegetables; and emphasizing whole-grain breads and cereals.

➤ Dietary Guidelines have been issued to help reduce chronic diseases in our population. The Guidelines emphasize eating a variety of foods; performing regular physical activity; maintaining or improving weight; moderating consumption of fats, cholesterol, sugar, salt, and alcohol; and eating plenty of grain products, fruits, and vegetables.

➤ Recommended Dietary Allowances (RDAs) are set for many nutrients. These amounts yield enough of each nutrient to meet the needs of groups of healthy people within specific gender and age categories. The current RDAs, published in 1989, are in the process of being revised.

➤ Daily Values are used as a basis for expressing the nutrient content of foods on the Nutrition Facts panel. Reference Daily Intakes (RDIs), which are derived from the 1968 RDA values, constitute the majority of the Daily Values. Daily Reference Values (DRVs) have been set for some nutrients with no RDA, such as fat and dietary fiber; they compose the rest of the Daily Values.

➤ Nutrient density reflects the nutrient content of a food in relation to its energy (kcal) content. Nutrient-dense foods are relatively rich in nutrients, in comparison with energy content.

➤ The Exchange System provides a valuable tool for estimating the carbohydrate, fat, protein, and energy content of a food or meal and for planning a diet to correspond to specific goals for carbohydrate, fat, protein, and energy consumption.

Study Questions

1 Describe the philosophy underlying the creation of the Food Guide Pyramid. What dietary changes would you need to make to meet the Pyramid guidelines on a regular basis?

2 Describe the intent of the Dietary Guidelines. Point out one criticism for its general application to all American adults.

3 Based on surveys of current food patterns of adults, suggest two key dietary changes the typical American adult should consider making.

4 What three key points should you make when explaining the significance of the RDAs to a friend?

5 How do RDAs differ from Daily Values (made up of RDIs and DRVs) in intention and application?

6 How would you explain the concept of nutrient density to a fourth-grade class?

7 Describe how the Exchange System can be used to help design a diet, based on what the system can predict and monitor.

Read the Nutrition Issue before answering the last question.

8 Nutritionists encourage all people to read labels on food packages to learn more about what they eat. What four nutrients could easily be tracked in your diet if you regularly read the Nutrition Facts panels on food products?

References

1 Achterberg C and others: How to put the Food Guide Pyramid into practice, *Journal of the American Dietetic Association* 94:1030, 1994.

2 ADA Reports: Position of the American Dietetic Association and Canadian Dietetic Association: women's nutrition and health, *Journal of the American Dietetic Association* 95:362, 1995.

3 ADA Reports: Position of The American Dietetic Association: Phytochemicals and functional foods, *Journal of the American Dietetic Association* 95:493, 1995.

4 Anonymous: How should the Recommened Dietary Allowances be revised? A concept paper from the Food and Nutrition Board, *Nutrition Reviews* 52:216, 1994.

5 Blackburn H: Strategies for reducing dietary risk factors: the high risk individual versus population-wide interventions, *Nutrition* 10:636, 1994.

6 Block G, Langseth L: Antioxidant vitamins and disease prevention, *Food Technology* July 1994.

7 FDA's final regulations on health claims for foods, *Nutrition Reviews* 51:90, 1993.

8 Food and Nutrition Board, National Academy of Sciences–National Research Council: *Recommended Dietary Allowances,* revised, Washington, DC, 1989.

9 Goldberg JP: Nutrition and health communication: the message and the media over half a century, *Nutrition Reviews* 50:71, 1992.

10 Hahn NJ: Variety is still the spice of a healthful diet, *Journal of the American Dietetic Association* 95:1096, 1995.

11 Harper AE: Nutrient standards for today—another view, *Nutrition Today* July/August 1993.

12 Hegsted DM: Nutrition standards for today, *Nutrition Today,* March/April 1993.

13 Herbert V, Kasdan TS: Misleading nutrition claims and their gurus, *Nutrition Today* May/June 1994.

14 Kurtzweil P: Food label makes good eating easier, *FDA Consumer* September 1995.

15 Lachance P, Langseth L: The RDA concept: time for a change? *Nutrition Reviews* 52:266, 1994.

16 Marwick C: Learning how phytochemicals help fight disease, *Journal of the American Medical Association* 274:1328, 1995.

17 McBean L: The Dietary Guidelines: change and implications, *Dairy Council Digest* 67:7, 1996.

18 Mermelstein NH: A regulatory look back at 1995, *Food Technology* December 1995.

19 Rosenberg IH: The new Reference Daily Intakes: for better or for worse? *Nutrition Reviews* 50:119, 1992.

20 Saltos E and others: The new food label as a tool for healthy eating, *Nutrition Today,* May/June 1994.

21 Schweitzer CM and others: How do Americans eat (and think they eat) today? *Food & Nutrition News* 67 (2):11, 1995.

22 Voelker R: Ames agrees with mom's advice: eat your fruits and vegetables, *Journal of the American Medical Association* 273:1077, 1995.

23 Welsh S and others: Development of the Food Guide Pyramid, *Nutrition Today* Nov/Dec 1992.

24 Wynder EL and others: Nutrition: the need to define optimal intake as a basis for policy decisions, *American Journal of Public Health* 82:346, 1992.

RATE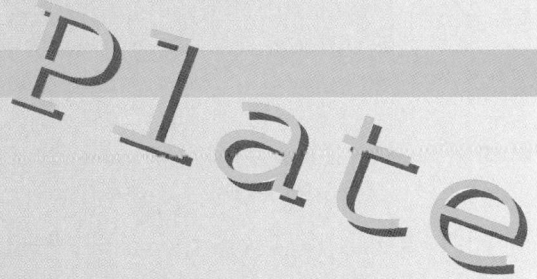

Does Your Diet Meet the RDAs and Food Guide Pyramid Recommendations?

Complete either Part I or Part II. Then complete Parts III, IV, and V. (For help in following the instructions for this activity, see the sample assessment in Appendix B.)

PART I

Manual RDA analysis

A. Take the information from the 1-day food-intake record you completed in Chapter 1 and record it on the blank form provided in Appendix B or by your instructor. Be sure to record the food or drink ingested and the amount (e.g., weight) consumed. NOTE: Your instructor may require you to keep the food record for more than 1 day.

B. Review the 1989 RDAs on the inside cover of this book and choose the appropriate recommendations for your gender and age. Write the appropriate value for each nutrient on the line on the form labeled "Your RDA." NOTE: The values for sodium and potassium from the table on the inside cover of the book are labeled "Estimated Sodium, Chloride, and Potassium Requirements of Healthy Persons."

C. Look up the foods and drinks that you listed on the form in the food composition table, Appendix A. Record on the form the amounts of each nutrient and the kcal present in them, based on the serving size and the number of servings you ate. For example, if you drank 2 cups of milk and the serving size listed in Appendix A is 1 cup, double all nutrient values as you record them. If the food is not listed, choose a substitute, such as cola for rootbeer.

D. For each food and drink, add the amounts in each column and record the results on the line labeled "Totals."

E. Compare the totals to your RDAs. Divide the total for each nutrient by the specific RDA or minimum requirement and multiply that by 100. Record the result on the line labeled "% of Your RDA."

F. Keep this assessment for use in subsequent activities in other chapters.

PART II

Computer RDA analysis

A. Obtain copies of the computer software from your instructor. Load the software into the computer.

B. Choose RDAs based on your age and gender.

C. Enter the information from the 1-day food intake record you kept in Chapter 1. Be sure to enter each food and drink and the specific amount you ate.

D. This software program will give you the following results:

1. The appropriate 1989 RDA value for each nutrient

Continued.

2. The total amount of each nutrient and the kcal consumed for the day

3. The percentage of the 1989 RDA for each nutrient that you consumed

E. Keep this assessment for use in subsequent activities in other chapters.

PART III

Evaluation of nutrient intakes as a percentage of RDAs

Remember that you don't necessarily need to consume 100% of the 1989 RDA values. A general standard is at least 70% averaged over 5 to 8 days. It is best not to exceed 500% to avoid potential toxic effects.

A. For which nutrients did your intakes fall below 70% of the 1989 RDAs?

B. Did you exceed the minimum requirements for sodium? To what degree?

C. For which nutrients did you exceed the RDA by greater than 500% (5 times greater)?

D. What dietary changes could you make to correct or improve your dietary profile? If you're not sure, future chapters will help guide your decisions.

PART IV

Food Guide Pyramid

Using the same food-intake record used in Part I or II, place each food item in the appropriate group of the Food Guide Pyramid in the chart below. That is, for each food item indicate how many servings it contributes to each group based on the amount you ate (see Table 2-1 for serving sizes). Note that many of your food choices may contribute to more than one group. For example, toast with margarine contributes to two categories: (1) the breads, cereals, rice, and pasta group; and (2) fats, oils, and sweets. After entering all the values, add the number of servings consumed in each group. Finally, compare your total in each food group with the recommended number of servings shown in Figure 2-2. Enter a minus sign (−) if your total falls below the recommendation or a plus sign (+) if it equals or exceeds the recommendation.

PART V

Further diet evaluation

Do the weaknesses, if any, suggested in your nutrient analysis (see Part III) correspond to missing servings in the Food Guide Pyramid chart? If so, consider changing your food choices based on the Food Guide Pyramid to help improve your nutrient profile. Finally, indicate whether your day's diet did or did not conform to the following items in the Dietary Guidelines:

	Yes	No
• Eat a variety of foods.	_____	_____
• Choose a diet with plenty of grain products, vegetables, and fruits.	_____	_____
• Choose a diet low in fat, saturated fat, and cholesterol.	_____	_____
• Choose a diet moderate in sugars.	_____	_____
• Choose a diet moderate in salt and sodium.	_____	_____
• Drink alcoholic beverages in moderation, if at all.	_____	_____

If your diet comes up short on any of these evaluations, take appropriate action to improve your eating patterns.

INDICATE THE NUMBER OF SERVINGS THAT EACH FOOD REPRESENTS							
Food or beverage	Amount eaten	Milk, yogurt, and cheese	Meat, poultry, fish, dry beans, eggs, and nuts	Fruit	Vegetable	Bread, cereal, rice, and pasta	Fats, oils, and sweets

Nutrition Issue

What's On The Label?

Constance J. Geiger, PhD, RD

People today are very interested in nutrition and health. Increased consumer interest in health has resulted in the greater availability of foods lower in energy content, sodium, and fat and higher in dietary fiber. Consumers also have more nutrition information than ever before, thanks to expanded food labeling mandated by the federal government. What can a food label tell you, and how can it help you learn about nutrition?

For the most part, foods packaged and sold in any U.S. supermarket are labeled with the product name, name and address of the manufacturer, amount of product in the package, and ingredients, which are listed in descending order by weight if the food contains more than one ingredient. With the exceptions of fresh fruits, vegetables, fish, meats, and poultry, almost all other foods are labeled in this manner (Figure 2-5).

- The % Daily Values listed on the label show consumers how a particular food fits into their daily nutrition needs.
- Serving sizes are more realistic, are expressed in common household and metric units of measure, and are more consistent across product lines.
- Important information (e.g., fat, saturated fat, cholesterol, and sodium content) is highlighted.
- Descriptive terms for nutrient content, such as "low fat" and "light," can be used only if the product meets strict definitions set by FDA.
- Health claims must be supported by scientific findings approved by FDA, as discussed in the Nutrition Insight. An example is the claim that calcium may help prevent osteoporosis.
- Ingredient labeling is now required on all foods hav-

THE MIDDLETONS

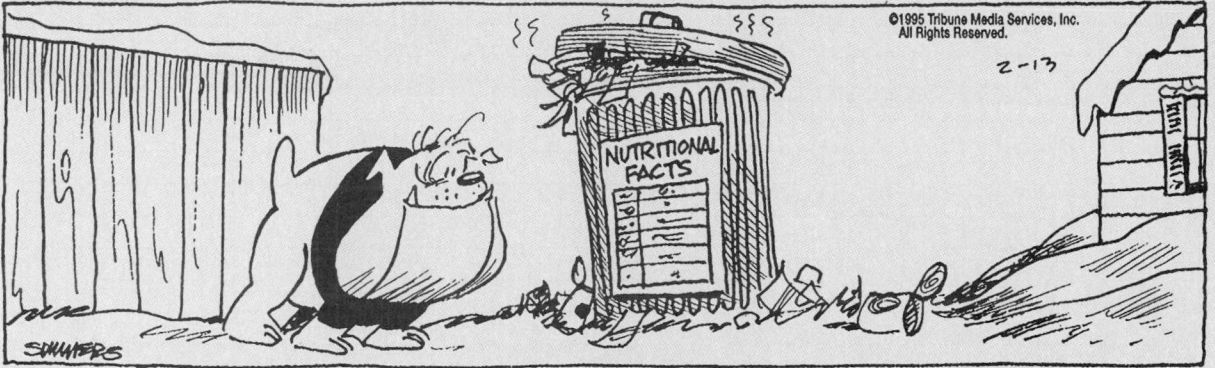

Figure 2-5 *The Middletons.*

In the United States, FDA regulates labeling of processed foods. USDA regulates the labeling of processed meat and poultry products (e.g., sausage pizza) and meat and poultry. Alcoholic beverages are regulated by the Bureau of Alcohol, Tobacco, and Firearms.

In 1990 FDA began a three-step approach for updating the nutrition label, and in November 1990 the Nutrition Labeling and Education Act (NLEA) became law. This law mandated nutrition labeling of almost all processed foods and affected the entire nutrition label. The advantages of the new label are many:

- Consumers can easily determine which foods are healthful because almost all labels now include a Nutrition Facts panel.

ing more than one ingredient. Fuller disclosure of ingredients is required, such as the specific food coloring agents used.

Because of the new regulations, consumers can learn more about the foods they eat and have more confidence in what they read on the label. Let's look at these specific changes in more detail.

NUTRITION LABELS ARE REQUIRED ON MOST FOOD PRODUCTS

Nutrition labels are mandatory on nearly all packaged foods and processed meat products (e.g., chili, hot dogs). Supermarkets may voluntarily provide information on raw, single-ingredient meat, poultry, fish, fruit, and vegetable products. This information often appears as large posters in the appropriate sections of a store. Nutrition information may also be provided in brochures and videos and on the fresh product itself.

LABELS PROVIDE DETAILED NUTRITION INFORMATION

A typical food label is shown in Figure 2-6. Mandatory food components must be listed on the Nutrition Facts panel, whereas listing of other (voluntary) components is optional. The order in which components must appear on the label is shown below, with mandatory components underlined:

- Total kcal (listed as calories)
- kcal from fat
- kcal from saturated fat
- Total fat
- Saturated fat
- Polyunsaturated fat
- Monounsaturated fat
- Cholesterol
- Sodium
- Potassium
- Total carbohydrate
- Dietary fiber
- Soluble fiber
- Insoluble fiber
- Sugars (includes both added and naturally occurring sugars)
- Sugar alcohols (e.g., the sugar substitutes xylitol, mannitol, and sorbitol)
- Protein
- Vitamin A
- Percentage of vitamin A present as beta-carotene
- Vitamin C
- Calcium
- Iron
- Other essential vitamins and minerals. (Thiamin, riboflavin, and niacin are not mandatory items, because deficiencies of these nutrients are rarely seen. They may, however, be listed voluntarily, such as is typical for breakfast cereals.)

If a claim is made about any of the optional components, or if a food is fortified or enriched with any of them, nutrition information for the specific components becomes mandatory.

An optional footnote for packages of any size is the number of kcal per gram of fat (9), carbohydrate (4), and protein (4).

SERVING SIZE IS UNIFORM WITHIN A FOOD CLASS

Serving sizes are defined by regulation and required for nutrition labeling, and they must be translated into a statement using common household measures, such as cups, items, and ounces, on labels. This uniformity

The nutrition label uses the term *calorie* for energy values, but *kilocalorie* values are actually listed. The term *kilocalories* (kcal) will be used in discussing labeling to be consistent throughout the book. Note that by convention the capitalized term *Calorie* is equivalent to kilocalorie when used to express energy content.

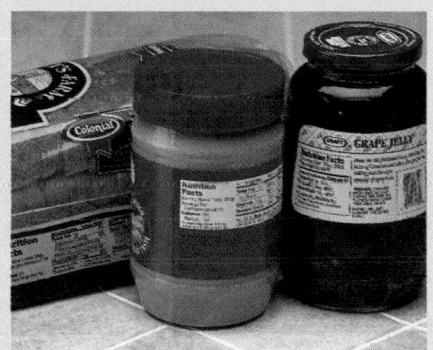

The food labels on these three products can be combined to indicate nutrient intake for a meal—a peanut butter and jelly sandwich.

Key Label Tips
- You can believe the claims on the package.
- You can easily compare products because serving sizes are comparable for similar foods.
- The % Daily Value shows if a product is high or low in a nutrient.
- By consulting the Daily Values, you can determine how much (or how little) of the major nutrients you should eat daily.

Continued.

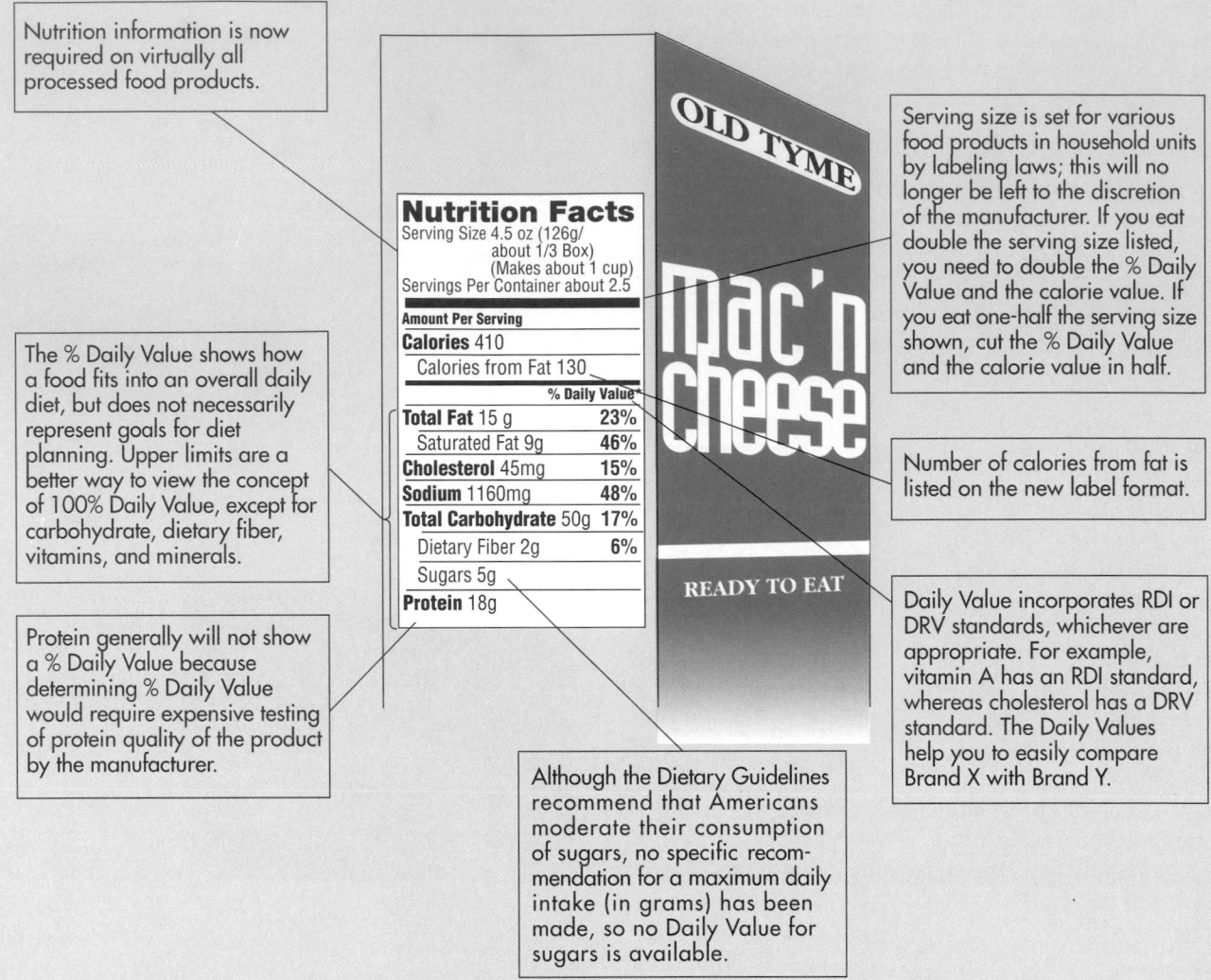

Nutrition information is now required on virtually all processed food products.

Serving size is set for various food products in household units by labeling laws; this will no longer be left to the discretion of the manufacturer. If you eat double the serving size listed, you need to double the % Daily Value and the calorie value. If you eat one-half the serving size shown, cut the % Daily Value and the calorie value in half.

The % Daily Value shows how a food fits into an overall daily diet, but does not necessarily represent goals for diet planning. Upper limits are a better way to view the concept of 100% Daily Value, except for carbohydrate, dietary fiber, vitamins, and minerals.

Number of calories from fat is listed on the new label format.

Protein generally will not show a % Daily Value because determining % Daily Value would require expensive testing of protein quality of the product by the manufacturer.

Daily Value incorporates RDI or DRV standards, whichever are appropriate. For example, vitamin A has an RDI standard, whereas cholesterol has a DRV standard. The Daily Values help you to easily compare Brand X with Brand Y.

Although the Dietary Guidelines recommend that Americans moderate their consumption of sugars, no specific recommendation for a maximum daily intake (in grams) has been made, so no Daily Value for sugars is available.

Nutrition Facts
Serving Size 4.5 oz (126g/ about 1/3 Box) (Makes about 1 cup)
Servings Per Container about 2.5

Amount Per Serving

Calories 410

Calories from Fat 130

	% Daily Value*
Total Fat 15 g	23%
Saturated Fat 9g	46%
Cholesterol 45mg	15%
Sodium 1160mg	48%
Total Carbohydrate 50g	17%
Dietary Fiber 2g	6%
Sugars 5g	
Protein 18g	

OLD TYME
Mac'n cheese
READY TO EAT

Figure 2-6 *The Nutrition Facts panel on a current food label. The box is broken into two parts: A is the top, and B is the bottom. The % Daily Value listed on the label is the percentage of the generally accepted amount of a nutrient needed daily that is present in 1 serving of the product. You can use the % Daily Values to compare your diet with current nutrition recommendations for certain diet components. Let's consider dietary fiber. Assume that you consume 2000 kcal per day, which is the energy intake corresponding to the % Daily Values listed on labels. If the total % Daily Value for dietary fiber in all the foods you eat in one day adds up to 100%, your diet meets the recommendations for dietary fiber.*

makes it easier for consumers to interpret serving-size information.[14]

MOST NUTRIENT AMOUNTS ARE EXPRESSED AS % DAILY VALUES

The actual amount of each listed component present in a serving size is indicated on the label. The amounts of most components also are expressed as percentages of their Daily Value (% Daily Value), as explained earlier in the chapter.

On many labels, the bottom portion of the Nutrition Facts panel lists the Daily Values for selected di-

etary components, such as fat, cholesterol, and total carbohydrate. The values for both a 2000 and 2500 kcal diet are given. However, the % Daily Values listed in the top portion are based on an intake of 2000 kcal per day.

You can use the Daily Values to help monitor your intake of certain nutrients. For example, the label for the macaroni and cheese product shown in Figure 2-7 indicates that 1 serving (1 cup) of this product provides 23% of the Daily Value for fat (65 grams), or 15 grams of fat (0.23 × 65 = 15). The Daily Value for fat of 65 grams was set to provide 30% of the energy content of a 2000

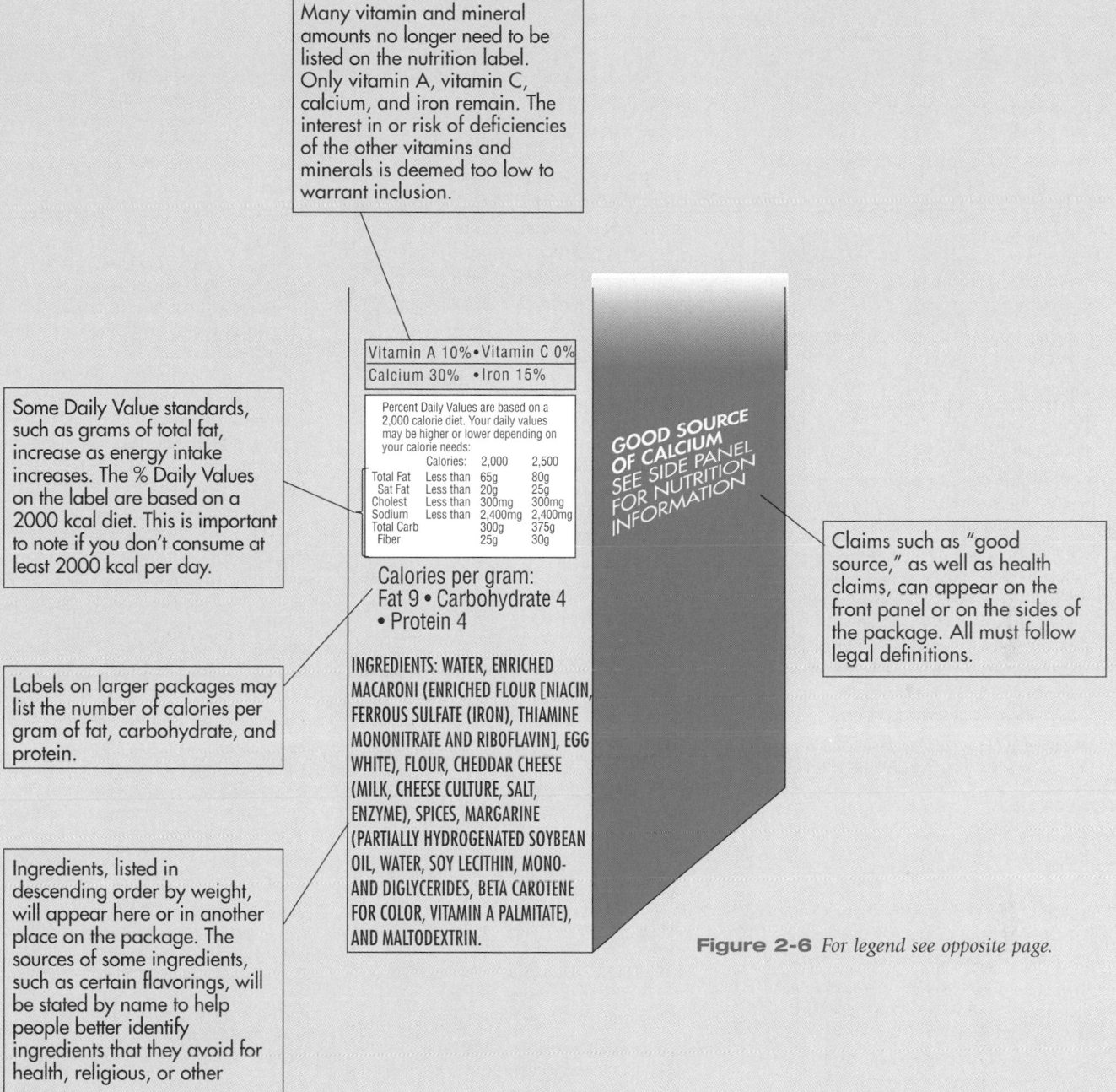

Many vitamin and mineral amounts no longer need to be listed on the nutrition label. Only vitamin A, vitamin C, calcium, and iron remain. The interest in or risk of deficiencies of the other vitamins and minerals is deemed too low to warrant inclusion.

Some Daily Value standards, such as grams of total fat, increase as energy intake increases. The % Daily Values on the label are based on a 2000 kcal diet. This is important to note if you don't consume at least 2000 kcal per day.

Labels on larger packages may list the number of calories per gram of fat, carbohydrate, and protein.

Ingredients, listed in descending order by weight, will appear here or in another place on the package. The sources of some ingredients, such as certain flavorings, will be stated by name to help people better identify ingredients that they avoid for health, religious, or other reasons.

Claims such as "good source," as well as health claims, can appear on the front panel or on the sides of the package. All must follow legal definitions.

Figure 2-6 *For legend see opposite page.*

kcal diet, the maximum recommended contribution from fat:

$$\frac{(0.30 \times 2000 \text{ kcal})}{9 \text{ kcal/gram of fat}} = 67 \text{ grams}$$

The calculated value of 67 is rounded to 65 for simplicity. Now, suppose that the first fat-containing food you eat one day is 1 serving of this macaroni and cheese product. You then would have 50 grams of fat (65 − 15) to use for other food choices during the rest of the day, or 77% of the Daily Value allotment (50 ÷ 65 = 0.77 or 77%).

Because the Daily Value for fat is related to total energy intake, this calculation yields a different result for an energy intake of 2500 kcal. At that energy intake the fat allotment is 80 grams. Thus, the total fat in 1 serving of the macaroni and cheese would provide 19% of the Daily Value, leaving 81% of the daily allotment for other food choices during the rest of the day.

NUTRIENT-CONTENT CLAIMS MUST FOLLOW STRICT LEGAL GUIDELINES

Food companies may use descriptive terms such as "low fat" or "sugar free" to help guide food choices, but such

Continued.

TABLE 2-7

Definitions for Nutrient Claims on Food Labels

SUGAR

- *Sugar free:* less than 0.5 grams per serving.

- *No added sugar; without added sugar; no sugar added:*
  - No sugars are added during processing or packing, including ingredients that contain sugars (for example, fruit juices, applesauce, or jam).
  - Processing does not increase the sugar content above the amount naturally present in the ingredients (A functionally insignificant increase in sugars is acceptable for processes used for purposes other than increasing sugar content.)
  - The food that it resembles and for which it substitutes normally contains added sugars.
  - If the food doesn't meet the requirements for a low- or reduced-calorie food, the product bears a statement that the food is not low-calorie or calorie-reduced and directs consumers' attention to the nutrition panel for further information on sugars and calorie content.

- *Reduced sugar:* At least 25% less sugar per serving than usual food.

CALORIES

- *Calorie free:* Fewer than 5 kcal per serving.

- *Low calorie:* 40 kcal or less per serving and, if the serving is 30 grams or less (or 2 tablespoons or less) per 50 grams of the food.

- *Reduced or fewer calories:* At least 25% fewer kcal per serving than usual food.

FIBER

- *High fiber:* 5 grams or more per serving. (Foods making high-fiber claims must meet the definition for low fat, or the level of total fat must appear next to the high-fiber claim.)

- *Food source of fiber:* 2.5 to 4.9 grams per serving.

- *More or added fiber:* At least 2.5 grams more per serving than usual food.

FAT

- *Fat free:* Less than 0.5 gram of fat per serving.

- *Saturated fat free:* Less than 0.5 gram per serving, and the level of trans fatty acids not exceeding 0.5 gram per serving (Chapter 6 describes trans fatty acids).

- *Low fat:* 3 grams or less per serving and, if the serving is 30 grams or less (or 2 tablespoons or less) per 50 grams of the food.

- *Low saturated fat:* 1 gram or less per serving and not more than 15% of kcal from saturated fatty acids.

- *Reduced or less fat:* At least 25% less per serving than usual food.

- *Reduced or less saturated fat:* At least 25% less per serving than usual food.

CHOLESTEROL

- *Cholesterol free:* Less than 2 milligrams of cholesterol and 2 grams or less of saturated fat per serving.

- *Low cholesterol:* 20 milligrams or less cholesterol and 2 grams or less of saturated fat per serving, and if the serving is 30 grams or less, or 2 tablespoons or less, per 50 grams of the food.

- *Reduced or less cholesterol:* At least 25% less cholesterol and 2 grams or less of saturated fat per serving than usual food.

SODIUM

- *Sodium free:* Less than 5 milligrams per serving.

- *Very low sodium:* 35 milligrams or less per serving and, if the serving is 30 grams or less, or 2 tablespoons or less, per 50 grams of the food.

- *Low sodium:* 140 milligrams or less per serving and, if the serving is 30 grams or less (or 2 tablespoons or less) per 50 grams of the food.

- *Light in sodium:* At least 50% less per serving than usual food.

- *Reduced or less sodium:* At least 25% less per serving than usual food.

OTHER TERMS:

- *Fortified/Enriched:* Vitamins and/or minerals have been added to the product in amounts in excess of at least 10% of that normally present in usual product.

- *Healthy:* An individual food that is low fat and low saturated fat and has no more than 360 to 480 milligrams of sodium or 60 milligrams of cholesterol per serving can be labeled "healthy" if it provides at least 10% of vitamin A, vitamin C, protein, calcium, iron, or dietary fiber.

- *Light or Lite:* The descriptor "light" or "lite" can mean two things: first, that a nutritionally altered product contains one-third fewer kcal or half the fat of the usual food (if the food derives 50% or more of its energy from fat, the reduction must be 50% of the fat); and second, that the sodium content of a low-calorie, low-fat food has been reduced by 50%.

  In addition, "light in sodium" may be used for foods in which the sodium content has been reduced by at least 50%. The term "light" may still be used to describe such properties as texture and color as long as the label explains the intent; for example, "light brown sugar" and "light and fluffy."

- *Diet:* A food may be labeled with terms such as "diet," "dietetic," "artificially sweetened," or "sweetened with nonnutritive sweetener" only if the claim is not false or misleading. The food can also be labeled "low calorie" or "reduced calorie."

- *Good source:* "Good source" means that a food contains 10% to 19% of the Daily Value for a particular nutrient.

- *High:* "High" means that a food contains 20% or more of the Daily Value for a particular nutrient.

- *Natural:* The food must be free of food colors, synthetic flavors, or any other synthetic substance.

TERMS APPLYING ONLY TO MEAT AND POULTRY PRODUCTS REGULATED BY USDA

- *Extra lean:* The product has less than 5 grams of fat, 2 grams of saturated fat, and 95 milligrams of cholesterol per serving (or 100 grams of an individual food).

- *Lean:* The product contains less than 10 grams of fat, 4.5 grams of saturated fat, and 95 milligrams of cholesterol per serving (or 100 grams of an individual food).

Many definitions are from FDA's *Dictionary of Terms,* as established in conjunction with the 1990 NLEA.

terms must meet strictly defined government standards. For example, if a food is labeled as "low calorie," the product must contain 40 kcal or less per the official serving size. In the past the nutrient-content claims on labels did not have legal definitions. For example, the term "light" or "lite" could mean light in color, weight, or energy. Now there are uniform definitions for all such terms used (Table 2-7).

Nutrient-content claims include terms such as "free," "low," "good source," "high," as well as "reduced," "light" or "lite," "less," "fewer," "more," "lean," and "extra lean." These terms or their allowed synonyms usually appear on the front label, although manufacturers may place them on other parts of the label, too.

SOME FOODS DON'T HAVE TO BE LABELED

Several categories of food are exempt from mandatory labeling, although they can carry voluntary nutrition information. However, if one of these foods carries a health or nutrient-content claim, it must also have a label meeting all current requirements. Among the foods exempt from nutrition labeling are the following:

- Foods served for immediate consumption, such as those served in hospital cafeterias and on airplanes and those sold by food service vendors (e.g., mall cookie counters, sidewalk vendors, vending machines)
- Ready-to-eat foods that are not for immediate consumption but are prepared primarily on site (e.g., bakery, deli, candy store items)
- Foods shipped in bulk, as long as they are for sale in that form to consumers
- Plain coffee and tea, some spices, and other foods that contain no significant amounts of any nutrients
- Foods produced by small businesses or packaged in small containers

SPECIAL REGULATIONS APPLY TO PROTEIN LABELING

Because protein deficiency is not a public health concern in the United States, declaration of the % Daily Value for protein is not mandatory on foods for people over 4 years of age. If the % Daily Value is given on a label, FDA requires that the product be analyzed for protein quality. Because this procedure is expensive and time consuming, many companies opt not to list a % Daily Value for protein. However, labels or foods for infants or children under 4 years of age must include the % Daily Value for protein, as must the labels on any food carrying a claim about protein content (see Chapter 15).

YOU CAN USE FOOD LABELS TO IMPROVE YOUR DIET

The new food labels, which are found on almost all processed food products (and voluntarily placed on many fresh foods) allow you to make informed food choices that are part of a healthy diet. Now a quick glance can tell you the nutrient content of your frozen dessert, candy bar, cookie, or other foods whose labels provided no nutrition information in the past. You can use the % Daily Value to compare food products and see if a food has a little or a lot of a nutrient. The % Daily Values let you gauge the approximate amount you should consume each day. You can now rely on nutrient-content claims such as "fat-free" because there are strict definitions for use of such claims. Use claims such as "high" and "good source" as signals to include foods with dietary fiber and vitamins and minerals. "Free" and "low" claims help you moderate your intake of fat, saturated fat, and cholesterol. Health claims provide general dietary guidance about diet and prevention of chronic diseases. Use them to make wise choices among foods. Overall, the food label is an important tool in choosing a healthful diet that supports the Food Guide Pyramid and the Dietary Guidelines.

Dr. Geiger is president of Geiger & Associates and is an adjunct research assistant professor at the University of Utah, both in Salt Lake City, Utah. Her company specializes in food labeling, health communications, and government affairs consulting for the food industry, health profession associations, and food trade organizations.

Nutritional Advice

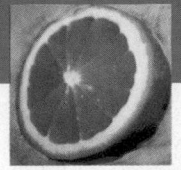

Facts and Fallacies

ADVICE ABOUT FOODS TO EAT AND AVOID IS OVERWHELMING:

- Eat organic produce to avoid pesticides.
- Don't eat processed foods that contain preservatives.
- Take large doses of vitamin C to cure colds.
- Herbal remedies are natural and therefore safe.
- Choose baked goods made with honey instead of sugar.
- Shark cartilage is a reliable cure for cancer.
- Death begins in the colon.

Sound convincing? Have you heard these statements argued both ways? Contradictory advice can be confusing. How do you distinguish food fact from fiction? Many food products and legitimate businesses ride a nutritional bandwagon. Unfortunately, so do quacks.[21] This chapter presents popular nutrition myths and misconceptions. Familiarity with the claims and methods of quackery can help you distinguish between sound and unsound nutritional advice. If you can spot a myth, you can protect yourself from pretentious health claims and fraudulent food promotions and practices.[12] More information on fad diets can be found in Chapter 10. For now, let's distinguish the credible advice from common fallacies about nutrition and other health-related areas.

Can You Spot a Quack?

Quacks are people who exaggerate health claims. Every day, people fall prey to quackery. By following quack advice, you can lose considerable money. You can also damage your health. Americans spend at least $30 billion a year on quackery and related health fraud. Protect yourself by knowing what to look for.

Put a "Q" in blanks preceding statements that describe quacks. Write "E" before statements that describe reliable nutrition experts.

_____ 1. They use anecdotes and testimonials to support their claims. They refer to stories of people being cured of cancer or arthritis by using product X as proof of the effectiveness of the product.

_____ 2. They promise quick, dramatic, miraculous cures.

_____ 3. They hold credentials recognized by responsible scientists or educators.

_____ 4. They say that most disease is caused by faulty diet and can be treated with "nutritional" methods.

_____ 5. They support the pros and cons of a claim with scientific studies and evidence.

_____ 6. In literature they use or write, they cite few if any scientific studies to support the product or claims.

_____ 7. They claim that most food additives and preservatives are safe; however, some still require further testing and study.

_____ 8. They claim that "natural" vitamins are better than synthetic ones.

_____ 9. They say you can get all nutrients necessary for a healthful diet from the supermarket.

_____ 10. They tell you not to trust the medical community.

_____ 11. They tell you that no food is really good or bad, but that all foods provide some nutritional value—some more than others.

_____ 12. They claim that modern food processing methods and storage remove all or almost all nutritive value from food.

_____ 13. They say that organically grown foods are not necessarily superior to plants cultivated using chemical fertilizers.

_____ 14. They claim that they are being persecuted by orthodox medicine and that their work is being suppressed because it is controversial.

_____ 15. They recommend that everybody take vitamins, eat health foods, or do both because diet alone does not supply enough nutrients.

Interpretation

Characteristics of a quack: 1, 2, 4, 6, 8, 10, 12, 14, 15

Characteristics of an expert: 3, 5, 7, 9, 11, 13

Put the total number you answered correctly in this blank _____

Were you able to tell the difference between a quack and a reliable expert? _____
_____

From Herbert V, Barrett S: Twenty-one ways to spot a quack, *Nutrition Forum*, p. 65, September 1986.

Key Chapter Concepts

- The scientific method of carefully examining hypotheses is a step-by-step, deliberate process, but no quicker method of testing ideas is as reliable.
- We tend to believe what we hear often or what close acquaintances tell us. When it comes to health practices, this well-meaning advice does not substitute for scientific verification of safety and effectiveness.
- The federal government provides minimal regulation of nutrient supplements and herbal remedies. "Let the buyer beware" is prudent advice to follow when using these products. Knowl-
edge and professional guidance are important.
- Fraudulent claims for dietary and health-related remedies have always been part of our culture. Quacks prey primarily on older people and people with incurable diseases, such as AIDS.
- Consumers should carefully scrutinize the credentials and motives of anyone providing medical or health advice. Bogus practitioners with phony credentials are widespread.
- If it sounds too good to be true, it probably is. The medical community would gain nothing by holding back an effective cure from the public, despite what the quacks contend.

The Nature and Costs of Quackery

Quack

A person who does not have the medical skills or knowledge that he or she claims to have.

Health fraud

FDA defines health fraud as the promotion, advertisement, distribution, or sale of articles, intended for human or animal use, that are represented as being effective to diagnose, prevent, cure, treat, or mitigate disease (or other conditions) or provide a beneficial effect on health, but which have not been scientifically proven safe and effective for such purposes. Such practices may be deliberately deceptive or done without adequate knowledge or understanding of the article.

Dictionaries define *quack* as "a pretender of medical skill; a charlatan" and "one who talks pretentiously without sound knowledge of the subject discussed." Quackery encompasses fraudulent actions, claims, and practices promoted by quacks, usually for their own profit.[1] In effect, quackery is a form of **health fraud.** Quacks argue that their alternative therapies and dietary regimens are the best road to health, and they decry more credible, science-based approaches as conspiracies perpetrated by a blind, money-mad medical-care industry. Many quacks lack any conscience or feeling for others; they selfishly take what they want and do as they please, leaving a trail of broken promises.[12] Deliberate deception is a hallmark of quacks. In contrast, other advocates of ineffective and unproven remedies sincerely believe in their products. They may be victims of quackery themselves or may merely wish to believe in something they hope will make them better. In their naivete and enthusiasm they pass on misinformation.[3]

Americans spend billions of dollars every year on quackery, often in search of a "quick fix" and sometimes in a desperate attempt to cure themselves of illness. Over $30 billion is spent on health fraud, including unnecessary vitamin and mineral supplements; substances such as bee pollen, ginseng root, and dried algae; and a wide range of herbal products. These items are taken in hopes of curing everything from the common cold, AIDS, and cancer to chronic diseases such as diabetes, heart disease, arthritis, Alzheimer's disease, and chronic fatigue syndrome.[7,10,13]

The Victims of Quackery

Fad is a shortened version of fiddle-faddle, which means to "play with" and then "cast aside."

Can you say you were never a victim of quackery? Health fraud and quackery fool many people who are neither gullible nor ignorant. Quacks also prey on the unsuspecting, people who do not imagine that others are capable of doing such underhanded things. Until something bad happens, we usually don't recognize dishonest treatment. When we get "burned" by "hot" health frauds and other fads, a wiser skepticism results (Table 3-1).[21]

In many cases, people who follow the fraudulent health advice proffered by quacks lose only money. For others, however, quack practices can be dangerous. For example, dietary restrictions can be very hazardous to individuals who are ill or recovering from disease, pregnant women, infants, and growing children.[12] Moreover, if trying a quack remedy delays needed medical treatment, patients may suffer needless physical harm. Cancer patients, for instance, sometimes waste money on useless and unproved remedies instead of effective treatment and consequently risk dying

---

TABLE 3-1

Advertising Claims Used to Promote Quack Products and Services and Rebuttals

"Our product has FDA approval."
Manufacturers are prohibited by law from claiming to have FDA approval.

"Our case histories and testimonials are reliable and useful."
Such testimonials may come from people with chronic ailments who (1) have had a symptom-free period, (2) have had a spontaneous remission, (3) have experienced a placebo effect, or (4) have been misdiagnosed. Celebrities and sports heroes often give testimonials in exchange for payment.

"The medical profession's attempts to persecute our company hide the truth."
The medical/scientific community uses the scientific method when testing validity of health claims. Double-blind studies prevent the results from being biased. The medical profession seeks truth; it does not bear grudges.

"Words like *wondrous, breakthrough, ancient, secret,* and *revolutionary* herald a reevaluation we should all consider."
True medical breakthroughs are never secret. They are reported in medical journals and the general media, not in the back sections of magazines and in leaflets.

"Our product cures many ailments overnight."
No single product can be effective for a wide variety of ailments; any claim for a quick and painless cure is usually too good to be true.

---

from a curable form of the disease.[15] A good example is the craze surrounding shark cartilage, which has not been shown to be effective. Even if it were effective, it would have to be injected in the body rather than ingested, because digestion in the stomach and intestine would dismantle it.

Older people are particularly vulnerable to quackery. Many of them have several chronic diseases, some of which have no effective cure, such as certain forms of arthritis. The resulting pain and disability lead people to seek alternative approaches. Their wish to heal their failing bodies can be a powerful force.[10] Access is easy; invitations to be healed are everywhere. It's even cheaper than seeing a physician.[5] The naive hope of such relief sells many useless, expensive cures to frightened and weary older people.

Some experts theorize that a new fringe group of people has emerged recently, called the "worried well." These are people seeking what they believe might be a deeper sense of well-being. This drives them to seek alternative methods of health care. Other people may be nostalgic for the simplicity of bygone days that herbs and other "natural" products seem to represent (Figure 3-1).

Usually you first need a physician's diagnosis for conditions requiring detailed nutrition advice. An exception to this might be losing weight when you are otherwise healthy. An accurate diagnosis by a physician is needed because you could have a condition that actually results from another disease. A physician needs to evaluate your total health to properly diagnose problems.

CALVIN & HOBBES

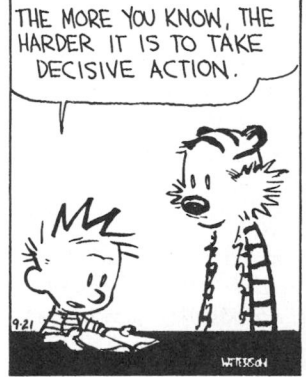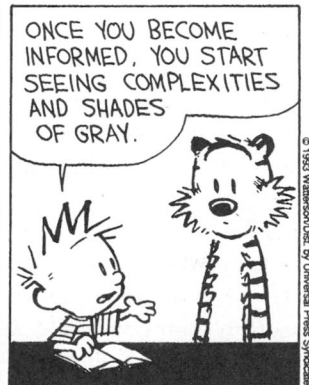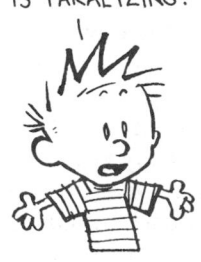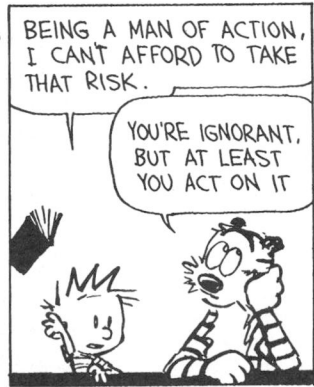

Figure 3-1 *Calvin and Hobbes.*

The Media's Role in Fostering Quackery

People tend to believe what they hear repeatedly. As with any type of brainwashing, a repeated claim can seem real even when it has no basis in fact. Unsound nutritional claims flood the media, food shelves, and conversations of those seeking good health. Fringe health groups are not the only sources for this false information. A well-meaning but poorly informed medical reporter on the nightly news may unknowingly mislead you. Because a sliver of truth underlies many claims, separating fact from fiction can stump even health professionals. For instance, a product promoted as a treatment for multiple ailments may be effective in relieving one complaint but totally worthless for the others. Comprehensive knowledge is often needed to distinguish fact from food fad.[2]

Today, especially, the popular media often publicize preliminary research information in an effort to enhance audience ratings. Adding to the problem, promoters may quickly turn preliminary research findings into sales pitches, products, and services. The purveyors of such misleading information are favored as guests on talk shows and sources for magazines and newspapers. Quack ideas are everywhere, but repetition does not make them valid.[12]

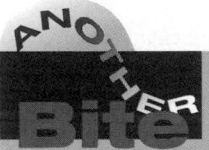

Despite its broad powers, the government often fails to protect consumers from false advertising and misleading health claims. However, with some basic knowledge you can protect yourself from quackery. The following pages will alert you to a truer picture of reality: Let the buyer beware.

Most medical advances are discovered in steps over long periods—rarely in a miraculous flash. Promising preliminary results often are not supported by additional research.[18] By and large, "miracle" cures are found only in tabloids and paid advertisements, not in reputable scientific journals. You need not rely on sensational media accounts, slick "infomercials," and talk shows to learn about important new developments. Any credible new finding will be familiar to most physicians and reported in a responsible manner by the mainstream media.[3]

This chapter begins with a look at the methods by which scientific evidence is obtained. Then it describes some common fraudulent concepts and the ways quacks typically operate. Finally, you will learn how to avoid becoming a victim and what you can do to help put a stop to quackery.

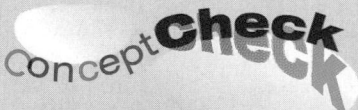

Quackery is at work whenever the promises for a food or medical regimen go beyond its scientifically established benefits. The victim pays not only in dollars and cents but sometimes in physical harm. Quack ideas are everywhere, but repetition does not make them valid. Miracle cures are myths. If a cure has not been reported in a scientific journal and physicians are not familiar with it, the cure is no miracle.

Applying Logic to Nutrition

Like other sciences the study of nutrition has developed through the use of the scientific method, a procedure for testing designed to detect and eliminate error. The first step is observation of a natural phenomenon. Scientists then suggest possible explanations, called *hypotheses,* about its cause. Distinguishing a true cause-and-effect relationship from mere coincidence can be difficult. For instance, earlier in this century many patients in mental hospitals suffered from *pellagra,* which suggested a possible relationship between mental illness and this disease. In time it became clear that this supposed connection was simply coincidental; the real culprit was the poor diet common in mental institutions at that time.

To test hypotheses and eliminate coincidental explanations, scientists perform controlled, scientific **experiments.** The data gathered from these experiments may either support or refute each hypothesis (Figure 3-2). If the results of many experi-

Hypothesis
An "educated guess" by a scientist to explain a phenomenon.

Pellagra
A disease characterized by inflammation of the skin, diarrhea, and eventual mental incapacity caused by a dietary deficiency of the vitamin niacin.

Experiment
A test made to examine the validity of a hypothesis.

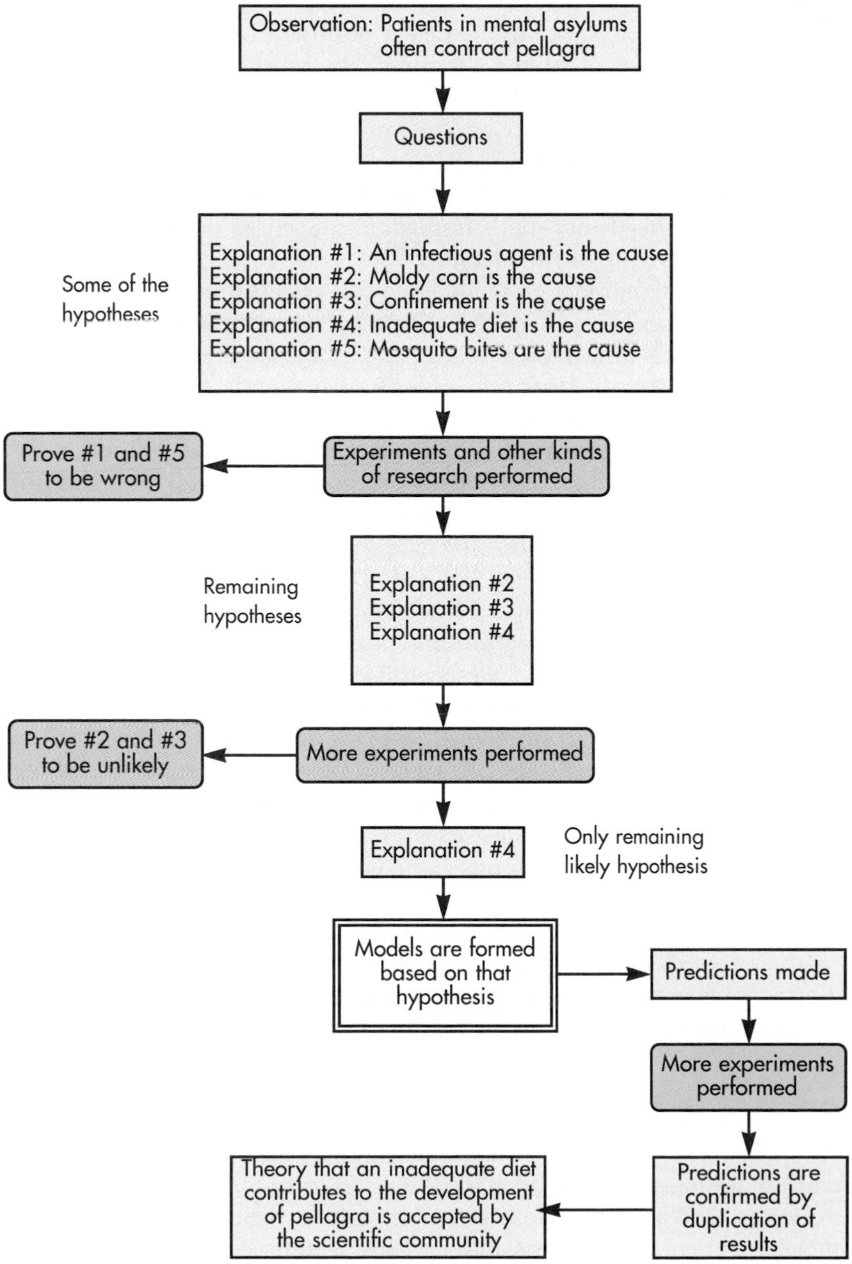

Figure 3-2
From question to theory—the process of science applied to nutrition. Only after careful and thorough analysis and repeated experimentation should a research finding influence our food choices, such as consuming the vitamin niacin to prevent development of pellagra.

Theory

An explanation for a phenomenon that has numerous lines of evidence to support it.

Scurvy

The deficiency disease that results after a few months of consuming a diet essentially free of vitamin C.

Mortality

A population's death rate. The term morbidity *refers to the number of sick persons in a population.*

Epidemiology

The study of how disease rates vary among different population groups. For example, the rate of stomach cancer in Japan could be compared with that in Germany.

Infectious disease

Any disease caused by invasion of the body by microorganisms, such as bacteria, fungi, or viruses.

ments support a hypothesis, the hypothesis becomes generally accepted by scientists and can be called a *theory* (such as the theory of gravity). Very often, the results from one experiment suggest a new set of questions to be answered.

The scientific method requires a skeptical attitude. Scientists must not accept proposed hypotheses and theories until they are supported by considerable evidence, and they must reject those that fail to pass critical analyses. Likewise, students should adopt a healthy skepticism and be critical of many current ideas about nutrition.[21]

Generating Hypotheses

Historical events have provided clues to important relationships in nutrition science. In the fifteenth and sixteenth centuries, for example, many European sailors on the long voyages to the Americas developed the disease **scurvy.** The sailors ate few fruits and vegetables, and eventually British scientists discovered that lime juice prevented or cured the scurvy. After this, sailors were given a ration of lime juice, earning them the nickname "limeys." This simple practice ensured a healthy workforce for the British navy and helped it dominate the seas worldwide. About 300 years later, scientists identified vitamin C, the nutrient present in fruits and vegetables that prevents scurvy.

During World War II the German army blockaded the Russian city of Leningrad, causing widespread semistarvation. Noting that lack of food was associated with increased infant **mortality,** scientists in North America extended the finding and eventually demonstrated that food supplements given to poor women improved their chances of delivering healthy babies.

In a related approach to using historical observation, scientists establish nutritional hypotheses by studying the different dietary and disease patterns among various populations in today's world. If one group tends to develop a certain disease whereas another group does not, scientists can speculate about the role diet plays in this difference. The study of diseases in populations is called *epidemiology.*

An example of this approach occurred in the 1920s, when Dr. Joseph Goldberger noticed that prisoners in jail—but not their jailers—suffered from pellagra. He reasoned that if pellagra was an **infectious disease,** both populations would suffer from it. Since this was not the case, he concluded that pellagra was probably caused by a dietary deficiency. Likewise, Dr. Denis Burkitt noted in the 1970s that Africans, who had lower rates of intestinal problems, consumed more dietary fiber than Englishmen. These observations suggested that dietary fiber contributes to intestinal health.

Historical and epidemiological findings can suggest hypotheses about the role of diet in various health problems. To prove the role of particular dietary components, however, requires controlled experiments. For instance, once the high incidence of pellagra in mental institutions during the 1920s was linked to poor diet, various foods were given to patients who had the disease. These experiments showed that yeast and high-protein foods could cure these patients if the disease was not in its final stage, indicating that pellagra results from a deficiency of some nutrient present in these foods. Eventually this nutrient was found to be niacin. Similarly, experiments in the 1970s showed that when people who consumed low amounts of dietary fiber increased their fiber intake, their intestinal health improved. These results established the importance of dietary fiber in intestinal health.

Animal Experiments

When scientists cannot test their hypotheses by experiments with humans, they often use animals. Much of what we know about human nutritional needs and functions has been generated from animal experiments. Still, human experiments are the most convincing to scientists. In the 1930s, scientists showed that a pellagra-like disease seen in dogs, called *blacktongue*, was cured by nicotinic acid. Only when nicotinic acid actually cured the disease in humans were scientists convinced that nicotinic acid, later identified as the vitamin niacin, was the critical dietary factor.

Today, we know that low doses of the mineral fluoride can stimulate growth in rats. However, we still do not know whether this is true for humans, because it is not practical to control the fluoride intake of humans accurately enough to answer the question. Thus, fluoride might stimulate growth in humans, but real proof is lacking.

In addition, use of humans in certain types of experiments is considered unethical. Although some people argue that animal experiments are also unethical, most people believe that the careful, humane use of animals is an acceptable alternative to using human subjects. For example, most people think it is reasonable to feed rats a low-copper diet to study the importance of this mineral in the formation of blood vessels. Almost universally, however, people would object to a similar study in infants.

The use of animal experiments to study the role of nutrition in certain human diseases depends on the availability of an **animal model**—a disease in laboratory animals that closely mimics a particular human disease. If no animal model is available and human experiments are ruled out, scientific knowledge often cannot advance beyond what can be learned from epidemiological studies.

Human Experiments

Various experimental approaches are used to test research hypotheses in humans, including case-control and double-blind studies.

Case-control study. In a case-control study, individuals who have the condition in question, such as lung cancer, are compared with individuals who do not have the condition. Comparisons are made only between groups that are matched for other major characteristics (e.g., age and gender) not under study. This type of study is in effect a microscopic epidemiological study. It may identify factors other than the disease in question, such as fruit and vegetable intake, that differ between the two groups, thus providing researchers with clues about the cause, progression, and prevention of the disease.

Double-blind study. An important approach for more definitive testing of hypotheses is the *double-blind study*, in which a group of subjects—the experimental group—follows a specific protocol (e.g., consuming a certain food or nutrient), and participants in a corresponding **control group** conform to their normal habits. People are randomly assigned to each group, as by the flip of a coin. Scientists then observe the experimental group over time to see if there is any effect that is not found in the control group. Sometimes subjects are used as their own control: first they are observed for a period of time, and then they are treated and their responses noted.

Two features of a double-blind study help reduce the introduction of bias (prejudice), which can easily affect the outcome of an experiment. First, neither the subjects nor the researchers know which subjects are in the experimental group and which are in the control group. Second, the expected effects of the experimental protocol are not disclosed to the subjects or researchers until after the entire study is completed. This approach reduces the possibility that researchers may see the change they want to see in the subjects to prove a certain "pet" hypothesis, even though such a change did not actually occur. This approach also reduces the chance that the subjects may begin to feel better simply because they are participating in a research study or receiving a new treatment, a phenomenon called the *placebo effect*.

Derived from the Latin word *placebo*, meaning "I shall please," the placebo effect cannot be explained by pharmacological or other direct physical action. It may

Before researchers conduct any research process using humans (or laboratory animals), they must first obtain approval from the Human Use (or Animal Use) Committee at their universities or companies. The committee determines if the experimental protocol is valid and assesses the risks and benefits of the potential therapy to the subject and, when appropriate, society at large. In human studies the committee insists that a document depicting the risks and benefits of the study be developed, which the subjects must receive and sign. The process is called *informed consent*, meaning the subject knows what he or she is expected to do in the research study and the associated risks.

Double-blind study
An experimental design in which neither the subjects nor the researchers are aware of the subject's assigment (test or placebo) or the outcome of the study until it is completed. An independent third party holds the code and the data until the study has been completed.

Control group
Participants in an experiment who are not given the treatment being tested.

Placebo
A fake medicine used to disguise the roles of participants in an experiment; if fake surgery is performed, it is called a sham operation.

instead be linked to a simple reduction in stress and anxiety.[19] At least one third of all patients will show improvement after receiving a placebo (fake medicine)—no matter what the illness.[24] Thus, it is critical to make allowances for the placebo effect in research studies.

In a double-blind experiment, the control group often receives a sugar pill or other placebo to camouflage who is in which group and thereby eliminate the bias introduced by the placebo effect. During the course of the experiment, neither the researchers nor the participants know who is getting the real treatment and who is getting a placebo. Sometimes only a single-blind protocol is possible, in which either the subjects or the researchers are kept in the dark. Now it is up to the experimental treatment—not just the practice of both groups taking a pill—to show an effect, if one is possible.

Drug studies lend themselves to double-blind protocols because it is often easy to substitute a placebo for the drug. However, food studies often cannot be placebo controlled. For example, disguising a diet high in fruits and vegetables from one devoid of them is difficult. In such a study the experimenters should try to ensure that the results from blood assays or other measurements are not revealed until the end of the study. In addition, the results should be kept from the subjects until the end of the study. These precautions can eliminate much potential bias. The more bias that is controlled in an experiment, the more confidence we can have in the results.

A recent example illustrates the need to test hypotheses based on epidemiological observations in double-blind studies. Epidemiologists using primarily case-control studies found that smokers who regularly consumed fruits and vegetables had a lower risk for lung cancer than smokers who ate few fruits and vegetables. Some scientisits proposed that beta carotene, a pigment present in many fruits and vegetables, could reduce the damage that tobacco smoke created in the lungs. This hypothesis helped fuel sales of beta carotene worth $100 million in 1995.

However, in double-blind studies involving heavy smokers, the risk of lung cancer was found to be higher for those who took beta carotene than for those who did not. Some investigators criticized this research, arguing that the beta carotene was given too late in the smokers' lives to be of much use, but even these critics did not suspect that the substance would increase cancer risk. After these results were reported, the federal agency supporting two large ongoing studies that employed beta carotene supplements called a halt to the research, stating that these supplements were ineffective in preventing both lung cancer and heart disease.[18]

Overall, health and nutrition advice provided by grandparents, parents, friends, and other well-meaning individuals can't be verified unless it is put to the ultimate scientific test—the double-blind study. Until that is done, we can't be sure that the substance or procedure in question is truly effective.[20] One reason for this is the power of the placebo effect. In addition, many common symptoms, such as sneezing, lower back pain, and headache, are short-lived and go away within a month or so without any treatment, reflecting the natural course of the underlying diseases. When people say "I get fewer colds now that I take vitamin C," they overlook the fact that many cold symptoms disappear quickly with no treatment; the apparent curative effective of vitamin C or any other remedy is often coincidental rather than causal to the natural healing process.[12]

The double-blind trial accounts for all these potential problems; no other approach does so. The only way of knowing if a treatment produces improvement in a particular condition is to compare individuals who get the treatment with those who don't. That's the comparison that quacks avoid at all costs. Medical practitioners must accept science as the ultimate arbiter of therapeutic efficacy and the source of new ideas, and so should you. Just because a product has been in use for a long time doesn't mean that it is better than nothing.[17]

All consumers need to become more sophisticated about science, its accepted standards of evidence, and its current limitations. Failure to do so leads many to a frantic pursuit of quack remedies. To ignore science is to follow an inferior path—

When you read accounts of scientific experiments, ask yourself: "Was a double-blind study protocol used? If a placebo could have been used, was it? During the experiment, were the researchers "blinded" as much as possible as to who received the experimental treatment and the effects of that treatment?"

the road of hard knocks. Those who follow this road learn about the dangers of various health practices primarily from the experiences of those harmed by them. A later discussion of herbal therapies provides numerous examples of this. Medical science does not ignore novel approaches to disease prevention and cure. Anecdotes and personal experiences are important clues to fruitful experimentation, but they are not credible evidence.[20]

Peer Review of Experimental Results

Once an experiment is complete, scientists summarize the findings and publish the results in a scientific journal. At the end of each chapter in this book, many reports are listed describing important experiments that have been published in scientific journals. Generally, before articles are published in scientific journals, they are critically reviewed by other scientists familiar with the subject. The objective of this peer review is to ensure that only high-quality research findings are published. This is an important step because most scientific research in this country is funded by the federal government, nonprofit foundations, drug companies, and other private industries. All these funding sources can have strong expectations about the research outcomes. In theory the scientists conducting these research studies will be fair in evaluating their results and will not be influenced by the funding agency. Peer review helps ensure that the researchers are as objective as possible. Results published in peer-reviewed journals, such as the *American Journal of Clinical Nutrition*, the *New England Journal of Medicine*, and the *Journal of the American Dietetic Association*, are much more reliable than those found in popular magazines or promoted on television talk shows. Unfortunately, reputable journals are not the main sources for the information presented in the popular media, and claims are seldom scrutinized by competent researchers for accuracy and scientific validity.[21]

Follow-Up Studies

Finally, even if an acceptable protocol has been followed and the results of a study accepted by the scientific community, one experiment is never enough to prove a particular hypothesis or provide a basis for nutritional recommendations. Rather, the results obtained in one laboratory must be confirmed by experiments conducted in other laboratories. Only then can we really trust and use the results. The more lines of evidence available to support an idea, the more likely it is to be true. It is important to avoid rushing to accept new ideas as fact or incorporating them into your health habits until they are proved by several lines of evidence (Figure 3-3). The best goal is to have a varied diet and consume all foods in moderation.[3]

Critical Thinking

For thousands of years, early man consumed a diet rich in vegetable products and low in animal products. These diets were generally lower in fat and higher in dietary fiber than modern diets. Do these differences in human diets throughout history necessarily tell us which diet is better—that of early man or modern man? If not, what is a more reliable way to pursue this question of potential diet superiority?

The American Dietetic Association has a toll-free hotline, staffed by registered dietitians, to answer consumers' food-related questions. Call (800) 366-1655, weekdays from 9 a.m. until 9 p.m. EST.

CATHY

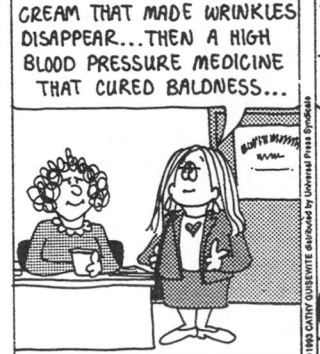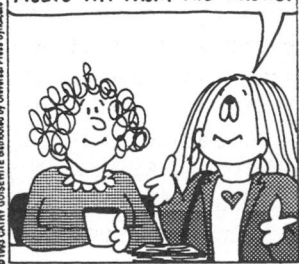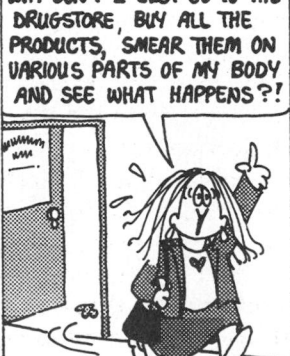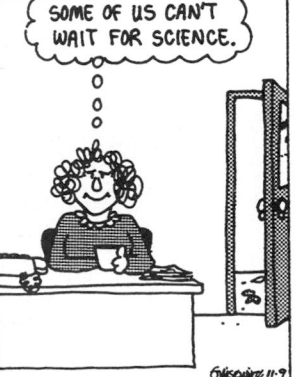

Figure 3-3 *Cathy.*

Nutrition **Insight**

How to Spot Front-Page Fallacies

By Anthony Schmitz

1. Study: Eating Citrus Can Help Against Cholesterol

Associated Press

MIAMI—Eating citrus can reduce cholesterol plaque in clogged arteries and help reverse atherosclerosis, a leading cause of heart attacks and strokes, researchers said Wednesday.

2. A two-year experiment with pigs found that citrus pectin—the sticky substance that's used to make jelly—reduces the formation of fatty plaque in coronary arteries, said D. Sigurd Normann of the University of Florida.

3. "The practical impact of our investigation is that we can tell a patient with severe atherosclerosis all is not lost," said fellow researcher Dr. James Cerda. "Based on this research, I would advise my patients with high cholesterol levels to eat a low-fat diet, get some exercise, and eat at least one grapefruit or several fresh oranges every day."

4. The researchers emphasized that citrus juice doesn't have the same beneficial effects because pectin is found only in the rind and in the pulp.

5. Normann, chief of cardiac pathology at the university's college of medicine, presented the study Thursday to the Federation of American Societies of Experimental Biology in Atlanta.

6. The primary grant for the research came from the Florida Citrus Commission, a state-appointed, industry-funded panel, but the commission played no role in reviewing the results, university officials said.

Normann said the study used pigs because their arteries and susceptibility to atherosclerosis are similar to humans'.

7. Dr. Margo Denke, a specialist with the Center for Human Nutrition at the University of Texas's Southwestern Medical Center in Dallas, said she was impressed with the research. The findings fit in with previous studies showing pectin, a type of soluble fiber, can reduce cholesterol levels.

"They saw the change in a very short period of time, which is quite dramatic," she said. "But I think that more research is going to need to be done, and we might not expect such a dramatic effect in humans."

The study indicated as little as one grapefruit a day was enough to show results, but Denke said some other research has suggested that higher amounts might be necessary.

Dr. George Lumb, a scholar in residence at Duke Medical School who has conducted research on heart disease for 30 years, questioned whether people would be willing to eat that much fresh citrus fruit every day. He said his research team is conducting studies on 24 volunteers with high cholesterol levels to test the effects of pectin-enriched fruit punch.

YOUR NEWSPAPER probably prints some type of food news every day. It may be important; it may be meaningless. Don't count on the editors' knowing the difference. You can defend yourself against half-baked findings and wild advice—if you read carefully. Here's how to skeptically evaluate the food news piece that you just read.

1. The bold, beckoning words at a newspaper story's top are usually cranked out by a special headline writer whose familiarity with the subject can be measured in minutes. If eating citrus can help against cholesterol, your first questions should be "How much citrus? Whom does it help?"

2. Now you know they're talking about pigs. Even if you have four legs and a snout, you shouldn't go for the pectin quite yet. The writer left out the study size—seven control pigs, seven pigs on pectin—which is too small to make the results widely applicable *even for pigs*. For humans, the conclusions are shakier still. That's not to say the research is irrelevant. Human arteries harden about the same way pigs' do. But the story doesn't say what else the pigs ate. Pigs are more sensitive to food's cholesterol content; we're more sensitive to saturated fat. Animal studies alone can't prove anything about human nutrition and health.

3. Did the pigs eat an amount of pectin that a reasonable pig, or a reasonable person, might eat? The answer (not that it's here) is no. Researchers fed 60-pound Yucatan micropigs half an ounce of pure pectin a day. Chances are you weigh two or three times more than a micropig. To have any hope of a cholesterol drop like that of the pigs, you'd have to eat at least *two dozen* grapefruits a day.

4. Great news if you eat grapefruit *rind*. Most people don't.

5. There's a big difference between papers delivered at a conference, such as this one, and papers published in the *Journal of the American Medical Association*, the *New England Journal of Medicine, Science, Nature,* and the like. Journal articles are usually reviewed by experts who help editors toss out the scientific chaff. Presentations at conferences aren't as carefully winnowed and shouldn't be taken as seriously.

6. If the bills are paid by the citrus industry, wouldn't the researchers inevitably find something good to say about grapefruits and oranges? Maybe; maybe not. "You can't jump to conclusions about bias," warns *Washington Post* science writer Victor Cohn. Some crooked researchers do get money from corporations, he notes. "But the peddler of a biased point of view is as likely to be an antiestablishment crusader or an academic ladder-climber as a corporate darling." You have to judge each study on its own merits.

7. The last paragraphs are often more helpful than the first. This is usually where outside experts comment, putting the finding in perspective. In this case Margo Denke, a member of the American Heart Association's nutrition committee, makes three good points: This study confirms others showing that soluble fiber lowers cholesterol. Humans, however, aren't the same as pigs. And there ought to be more research done before anyone climbs on the citrus bandwagon.

Anthony Schmitz is a contributing editor to *Health* magazine.

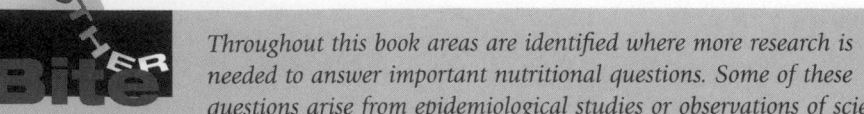

Throughout this book areas are identified where more research is needed to answer important nutritional questions. Some of these questions arise from epidemiological studies or observations of scientists and await testing in an experimental setting (either in an animal model or, even better, in a human clinical study). Until overwhelming evidence supports a hypothesis, it should not be considered a nutrition "fact."

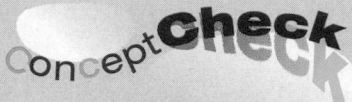

The scientific method is a procedure for testing designed to detect and eliminate error. Scientists suggest hypotheses to explain the causes of various observed phenomena and then test these hypotheses in controlled scientific experiments. If evidence from many experiments supports a hypothesis, it becomes generally accepted by scientists. An important approach for more definitive testing of hypotheses is the double-blind study, in which a group of subjects—the experimental group—follows a specific protocol and a corresponding control group takes a placebo. (This approach eliminates the bias introduced by the placebo effect.) Anecdotes and personal experiences, the trademarks of quacks, are not credible evidence for the beneficial effect of a dietary practice or supplement.

How to Evaluate Nutrition Claims and Advice

Based on what has been covered so far, the following suggestions should help you make healthful and economical nutrition decisions[2,3,12]:

1. Apply the basic principles of nutrition as outlined in Chapters 1 and 2 to any nutrition claim. Do you note any inconsistencies? Do reliable references support the claims? When evaluating a new diet in your favorite magazine, evaluate the advice using tools described in this book, including the Food Guide Pyramid, the Dietary Guidelines, and the principles of variety, balance, and moderation. Beware of the following:

   • Testimonials about personal experience
   • Disreputable publication sources
   • Dramatic results (rarely true)
   • Lack of evidence from supporting studies made by other scientists
   • Lists of good and bad foods
   • Statements that particular foods can cure specific diseases or that many harmful foods should be eliminated from your diet
   • Claims that only natural foods should be eaten because modern processing methods strip the nutritional value from foods
   • Assertions that sugar is a deadly poison
   • Warnings that stress greatly increases your need for nutrients

2. Examine the background and scientific credentials of the individual, organization, or publication making the nutritional claim. Usually a reputable author is one whose educational background or present affiliation is with a nationally recognized university or medical center that offers programs or courses in the field of nutrition, medicine, or a closely allied specialty.

A

35 Pounds of Fat.

DR. EDISON'S OBESITY PILLS AND REDUCING TAB- LETS CURED MRS. MANNING.

No Other Remedies But Dr. Edison's Reduce Obesity— Take No Others.

SAMPLES FREE—USE COUPON.

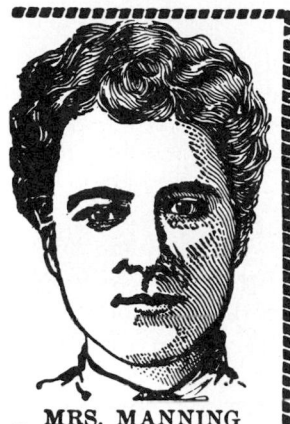

MRS. MANNING

Mary Hyde Manning, one of the best known of Troy's, New York, society women, grew too fleshy, and used Dr. Edison's Obesity Remedies. Read the letter telling of her reduction and restoration to health:—"In six weeks I was reduced 35 pounds, from 171 to 136, by Dr. Edison's Obesity Pills and Re- ducing Tablets. I recommend these remedies to all fat and sick men and women."

The following well-known men and women have been reduced by DR. EDISON'S OBESITY REME- DIES:

Mrs. H. Mershon, 156 South Jackson St., Lima, O., 148 lbs.

Mrs. Josephine McPherson, 7916 Wright St., Chi- cago, 42 lbs.

Rev. Edward R. Pierce, 410 Alma St., Chicago, 42 lbs.

C. C. Nichols, 145 Clark St., Aurora, Ill., 36 lbs.

Mrs. W. Davlin, Whitemore, O., 149 lbs.

W. H. Webster, 618 2d Ave., Troy, N. Y., 26 lbs.

J. M. McKinney, 4504 State St., Chicago, 30 lbs.

Mrs. J. M. McKinney, 4504 State St., Chicago, 33 lbs.

Mrs. A. Walker, 1104 Milton Place, Chicago, 20 lbs.

B

22% LESS BODY FAT IN SIX WEEKS

University studies have identified CHROMIUM PICOLINATE as a "trig- ger" for fat loss and lean muscle en- hancement. 200 micrograms taken daily caused a 22% fat loss in only 6 weeks.

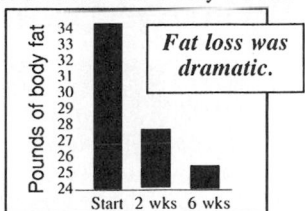

Fat loss was dramatic.

Men and women of every age are talking about the amazing benefits of this safe, es- sential nutrient:

WEIGHT LOSS • FAT LOSS MORE ENDURANCE AND STAMINA MORE LEAN MUSCLE

BODY GOLD is made to the exact specifications of the capsules used in the studies cited above. Each bottle of 60 cap- sules is a 2-month supply.

SATISFACTION GUARANTEED

(Check or money order only. Canada: U.S. $ m.o.)

Please rush ____ bottles of BODY GOLD @ $10.95 each + $2.50 total delivery.

Name_____

Address_____

City_____ State_____ Zip_____

BODY GOLD, 5930 La Jolla Hermosa, Dept. NH-123, La Jolla, CA 92037

Figure 3-4 *Quackery has been with us for ages. (A) Even at the turn of the century, people wanted to believe that fat could be lost without changing habits or without much effort, and (B) they still do.*

3. Be wary if the answer is "Yes" to any of the following questions about a health-related nutrition claim:
   - Are only advantages discussed and possible disadvantages ignored?
   - Are claims made about "curing" disease? Do they sound too good to be true?
   - Is extreme bias against the medical community or traditional medical treatments evident?
   - Are dire warnings and other fear-arousing techniques used?
   - Is a cure heralded as quick and painless?
   - Is the product promoted to combat a wide variety of diseases and conditions?
   - Is the claim touted as a new or secret scientific breakthrough (Figure 3-4)?

4. Note the size and duration of any study cited in support of a nutrition claim. The larger it is and the longer it went on, the more dependable its findings. Also consider the type of study. The results of clinical research comparing one carefully selected group with another, for example, are generally more signifi- cant than those that simply observe a large population for trends. Check out the group studied; a study of men or women in Sweden may be less relevant than one of men or women of Southern European, African, or Hispanic de- scent, for example. Keep in mind that "contributes to," "is linked to," or "is associated with" does not mean "causes."

5. Beware of press conferences and other hype. Nutrition scientists normally report their studies in reputable scientific journals. Top-notch research journals require that every article be reviewed by other scientists. Follow-up studies are

How to Find Reliable Nutrition Information

By Susan Calvert Finn, Ph.D., R.D.

Here in America, as we prepare to enter the twenty-first century, you can roam the information highway on your computer. You can scan a dazzling variety of CD-ROMs. You can receive information via fax or, of course, on television, on the radio, and through the "old-fashioned" channels of communication—newspapers, magazines, books, and conversation.

But proliferation of information doesn't mean increased accuracy or consistency, particularly in nutrition. Almost daily, Americans are asked to judge the reliability of reports, studies, and news releases that often seem contradictory. We are told that our diets should contain low fat, no fat, some fat. We've been advised to drink wine and to avoid wine. The virtues of antioxidants, vitamins, and minerals are extolled and refuted. We've witnessed the Great Olive Oil and the Great Oat Bran debates. "Experts" advise gimmicks and gadgets, pills and potions. As the traveling medicine men of the nineteenth century liked to say, whatever is being sold is good for what ails you.

Unreliable Nutrition Information

The reason for the explosion of nutrition information is relatively simple: everyone wants to be healthy and have a long, productive life. Consequently, health and nutrition are a multibillion dollar business—and where the dollar stakes are high, there are always unscrupulous players.

A recent Gallup survey revealed that 56% of Americans get their nutrition information from the media, 32% from physicians, and 31% from family or friends. These numbers indicate that more than two thirds of us are getting nutrition information from sources who may be untrained or unqualified. No wonder there is confusion.

Still another recent survey found that in 32 states "consumers had less than a fifty-fifty chance of finding a reliable 'nutritionist'" through the yellow pages of the phone book. The study further stated that "of the 618 entrants listed under the heading 'Nutritionists,' 358 (58%) [had] either spurious or suspicious [qualifications]. Sixty-three percent of the ads and boxed listings under this heading were for bogus nutritionists. . . . " These "experts" had degrees from correspondence schools or diploma mills or were using invalid regimens and diagnostic methods.

Sound Nutrition Information

With all of these pitfalls, where and how do you find legitimate experts—true professionals who offer valid diagnoses and prescribe safe and effective nutrition programs? A number of avenues are available. If you have access to an accredited university, you may be able to obtain current and authoritative information from faculty members, particularly those who teach nutrition, dietetics, health, and medicine. Similarly, many hospital dietetics departments can be valuable references.

Most public, private, and school libraries stock nutrition books by experts on topics you are researching. Be aware, however, that appearing in print does not necessarily make information credible. With all sources, it is essential to authenticate the background and training of the practitioner before accepting the material. If you have questions or doubts you can't resolve, check with recognized authorities or organizations such as the American Dietetic Association (ADA) and the National Council Against Health Fraud (Table 3-2)

The Registered Dietitian

The most dependable source for up-to-date, accurate nutrition data is a registered dietitian (R.D.). Registered dietitians are health-care professionals who are rigorously trained in a single specialty—nutrition science. Their goal is to promote health and fight illness by fostering the practice of proper nutrition. Through the ADA, R.D.s are the most reliable disseminators of educational and informational material on food and nutrition.

An R.D. analyzes each patient's situation, taking into account such factors as medical history, lifestyle, and eating habits, and tailors specific regimens to meet those unique needs. Because R.D.s do not make medical diagnoses, the patient is encouraged to consult a physician regularly.

What is it about registered dietitians that makes them so qualified? A registered dietitian has a bachelor's degree in food and nutrition from an accredited university, has had thorough and extensive professional practice under expert supervision, and has passed a comprehensive examination. There are over 65,000 registered dietitians in the United States, and they can be identified by the letters *R.D.* after their names.

More than half of all states license dietitians. Unfortunately, in the other states people with no training, experience, license, or specific qualifications can call themselves dietitians and nutritionists. Only a person who meets the qualifications listed above can use the designation "registered dietitian," which indicates that the practitioner is a trained, reputable expert who is educated in nutrition science and has both practical and theoretical experience.

As you seek nutrition information, you would do well to follow these guidelines. Keep in mind that availability doesn't mean accuracy, and abundance doesn't mean reliability. A good measure of common sense, sound research, and thorough verification of references and credentials will ensure that you have chosen an accurate and reliable source of information. Most health-care professionals are readily available and willing to answer questions or provide information. The benefits you will receive are well worth the extra effort required to secure their advice.

Dr. Finn is the Director of Nutrition Services for Ross Laboratories, a leading research facility and manufacturer of scientifically formulated nutritional products. She is past president of the American Dietetic Association and coauthor of *The Real Life Nutrition Book* (Penguin Books, 1992).

TABLE 3-2

Sources of Reliable Nutrition Information to Keep You Informed about the Latest Developments in the Field

NEWSLETTERS

American Institute for Cancer Research
1759 R St. N.W.
Washington, DC 20009

Center for Science in the Public Interest (CSPI)
1875 Connecticut Ave. N.W.
Suite 100
Washington, DC 20009

CNI Nutrition Week
Community Nutrition Institute
910 17th St. N.W., Suite 413
Washington, DC 20006

Dairy Council Digest
National Dairy Council
10255 West Higgins Road, Suite 900
Rosemont, IL 60018
(inexpensive)

Dietetic Currents
Ross Laboratories
Director of Professional Services
625 Cleveland Ave.
Columbus, OH 43216
(free)

Egg Nutrition Center
1819 H St. N.W., No. 510
Washington, DC 20009
(free)

Environmental Nutrition
52 Riverside Dr.
New York, NY 10024

Food and Nutrition News
National Livestock and Meat Board
444 Michigan Ave.
Chicago, IL 60611
(free)

Harvard Medical School Health Letter
Department of Continuing Education
25 Shattuck St.
Boston, MA 02115

Healthline
830 Menlo Ave. #100
Menlo Park, CA 94025

Healthy Weight Journal
402 South 14th Street
Hettinger, ND 58639

National Council Against Health Fraud Newsletter (NCAHF)
P.O. Box 1276
Loma Linda, CA 92354

National Heart, Lung, and Blood Institute
9000 Rockville Pike, Building 31, Room 4A21
Bethesda, MD 20892

Nutrition Forum
JB Lippincott Company
East Washington Sqaure
Philadelphia, PA 19105

Nutrition & the M.D.
Raven Press
1185 Avenue of the Americas
New York, NY 10036

Nutrition Research Newsletter
P.O. Box 700
Pallisades, NY 10964

Tufts University Diet & Nutrition Letter
P.O. Box 10948
Des Moines, IA 50940

University of California at Berkeley
Wellness Letter
P.O. Box 420148
Palm Coast, FL 32142

INTERNET SITES

American Dietetic Association http://www.eatright.org

International Food Information Council (IFIC)
　http://ificinfo.health.org/homepage.htm

National Council Against Health Fraud (NCAHF)
　http://www.primenet.com/~ncahf/

Vegetarian Resource Group (VRG)
　http://envirolink.org/arrs/VRG/home/html

US Dept of Agriculture http://www.usda.gov

National Agricultural Policy and Promotion
　http://www.usda.gov/fcs/cnpp.html

Food and Nutrition Information Center
　http://www.nalusda.gov/fnic/

Center for Food Safety and Applied Nutrition
　http://vm.cfsan.fda.gov/index.html

Center for Science in the Public Interest
　http://.cspinet.org

Consumer Information Center
　http://www.gsa.gov/staff/pa/cic/cic.html

National Food Safety Database
　http://www.agen.ufl.edu/~foodsaf.html

NCI International Cancer Information Center
　http://wwwicic.nci.nih.gov

NATIONAL PERIODICALS

American Health
Better Homes and Gardens
Consumer Reports
Good Housekeeping
Health
Parents

then demanded before hypotheses can be supported. One study may not prove anything, but a body of research, in which evidence accumulates bit by bit, can uncover the truth.

6. When you meet with a nutrition professional, you should expect that he or she will do the following:
   - Ask questions about your medical history, lifestyle, and current eating habits. The professional may ask you to keep a detailed diet diary to establish a baseline before making major diet changes or recommendations.
   - Formulate a diet plan tailored to your needs, as opposed to simply tearing a form from a tablet that could apply to almost anyone.
   - Schedule follow-up visits to track your progress, answer any questions, and help keep you motivated.
   - Involve family members in the diet plan, when appropriate.
   - Consult directly with your physician and readily refer you back to your physician for those health problems a nutrition professional is not trained to treat.

7. Avoid practitioners who prescribe vitamin and mineral supplements for everyone or sell them in connection with their practice.

8. Examine product labels carefully. Be skeptical of any product promotion not clearly stated on the label. A product is not likely to do something that is not specifically claimed on its label or package insert (legally part of the label).

One insidious ploy of quacks is to suggest that the medical establishment deliberately keeps important discoveries away from patients and inhibits the inquiry of unorthodox practitioners. With regard to therapies and medicine, nothing is further from the truth.[15] Physicians would like nothing more than to cure the common diseases that currently elude effective therapy. Keep in mind that family and friends of physicians, not to mention physicians themselves, may suffer from such diseases. However, these professionals know from experience the importance of protecting the public against unfounded and unproven remedies. If a new approach to therapy can be proved safe and effective, it will be endorsed and applied. Consider how quickly new drugs for the treatment of AIDS are employed once approved by FDA.

The Many Faces of Nutrition Quackery

As previously noted, we are all exposed daily to unsound nutrition claims through radio, television, newspapers, books, and magazines. Some dubious claims about a variety of nutrition products are listed in Table 3-3. In this section, the pros and cons of organically grown food, health foods, and food additives—the subjects of numerous myths—are discussed. Then you'll learn about several "alternative" nutritional therapies promoted as cures for many diseases. Medically supervised nutritional therapy is recommended for certain specific diseases, including nutrient-deficiency diseases. However, the cure-all claims of meganutrient therapies, macrobiotics, and herbal therapies amount to nothing more than quackery.

Organically Grown Produce

Pesticide scares crop up in the news as regularly as harvest season. One year we hear apples are unsafe; the next year it may be that grapes can kill. The public listens. To placate public fears, supermarkets now stock produce once found only in health food stores. Today, organic produce is a $330 million industry. Though large, it still represents only about 2% of the U.S. food production, partly because of its higher price.

Organic farmers usually avoid pesticides and use natural soil improvers, such as compost, instead of synthetic fertilizers. They rotate crops to enrich soil further and may control pests with biological methods. However, despite all the hoopla about

Pesticide
A general term for an agent that can destroy bacteria, fungi, insects, rodents, or other pests.

TABLE 3-3

Dubious Claims for Nutrition Products

Food	Claims	Facts
Acidophilus milk (contains bacteria that ferment milk sugar)	Aids digestion; promotes health of digestive tract	This may be of value to people who cannot readily digest milk sugar (lactose) or need to reestablish intestinal bacteria after long-term antibiotic therapy
Alfalfa sprouts	Have nutrients not available in other vegetables	They have less nutritional value than broccoli, carrots, and spinach; alfalfa tea can disturb digestion and respiration
Amino acid tablets	Help build muscle mass	Amino acids make up proteins; an abundant amount is supplied by diets following the Food Guide Pyramid
Bee pollen	A perfect food; can help athletic and sexual performance; prevents cancer, infection, and allergy; prolongs life; promotes both weight loss and gain	Its nutrients are found in conventional foods; no evidence shows that it helps athletes; people allergic to specific pollens can develop severe allergic reactions after ingestion
Bioflavonoids ("vitamin P")	Essential for good health; provides resistance to colds and flu	Bioflavonoids are not vitamins or essential nutrients
Blackstrap molasses (less refined form of molasses)	Wonder food that can restore hair and cure anemia	Although contributes to iron intake, it has no effect on hair color and does not cure anemia
Bone meal	A rich source of calcium	Calcium in bone meal is poorly absorbed and can contain high amounts of lead
Brewer's yeast	Excellent diet supplement	This is a good source of protein and several B vitamins, but adds nothing to a balanced diet and has an unsavory taste for some
Brown rice	Most perfect food; improves health even if eaten exclusively	Although nutritous, it lacks some needed nutrients and must be complemented by other foods to maintain health
Cider vinegar	Keeps body in balance; thins blood; aids digestion	No evidence exists to support these claims
Fertile eggs	Nutritionally superior to unfertilized eggs; have fewer unnatural hormones	Fertilization does not add to an egg's nutritional value
Fish oil capsules	Lowers blood cholesterol	They can be used to lower some blood lipids (only cholesterol when given in very high doses), but they can also make control of blood glucose in diabetes more difficult (see Chapter 6)
Garlic	Purifies blood; reduces high blood pressure; prevents diabetes and heart disease	Garlic and onion contain substances that help prevent blood cells from clumping into blood clots
Kelp (type of seaweed)	Good source of iodide; energy booster;	This is a good source of iodide but more expensive than iodized salt
Lecithin	Reduces heart disease risk	The body makes *all the* lecithin it needs
Oat bran	Superior food ingredient for lowering blood cholesterol	Only effective in very high doses; reducing saturated fat in the diet is a more reliable way to lower blood cholesterol (see Chapter 6)
Para-aminobenzoic benzoic acid (PABA)	Can prevent or reverse graying in hair when ingested orally	PABA is a vitamin for bacteria but not for humans; it is a useful ingredient in sunscreens
Spirulina (blue-green algae)	Aids in weight loss; helps people with diabetes, liver disease, and ulcers	It is a good source of protein, but more expensive than conventional foods; there is no evidence that it promotes weight loss or has medical value

organically grown food in recent years, no consistent definition of this term exists. Currently, some states require that no pesticide be used for 3 years before foods can be labeled as organic; other states require 1 year. Other states either have not specified the time or have no specific laws on this issue. The inconsistency or absence of state laws prompted Congress to call for federal standards defining organic farming methods in the Farm Bill passed in 1990. Once these standards are implemented, which is expected by October 1996, both USDA and FDA will enforce them. Until federal standards are in place, a "certified organic" label is the most reliable indicator that "organic" practices were followed in producing a particular food.

Organic
Anything that contains carbon linked to hydrogen in the chemical structure.

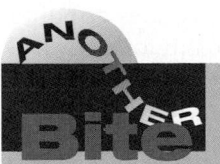

*In chemical terms, all substances containing carbon atoms plus hydrogen atoms are **organic** compounds. According to this definition, all carbohydrates, fats, and proteins are organic, regardless of how they are produced. **Inorganic** compounds, such as minerals and water, do not contain carbons attached to hydrogens. These terms, based on simple chemical concepts, are common in nutrition and have little to do with organic farming.*

Inorganic
Anything that is free of carbon linked to hydrogen in the chemical structure.

Advocates of organically grown foods claim that they are more nutritious and less hazardous to your health than conventionally grown foods. These purported advantages presumably justify the extra cost of organic produce. Let's examine the facts to see just how organic and nonorganic foods differ[2]:

1. Surveys have found that both organically and conventionally grown foods contain similar levels of pesticide residues. Cross-contamination from wind and groundwater partly accounts for this. Washing fruits and vegetables removes some external pesticide residue from foods. According to FDA, the tiny amounts of pesticides that may remain on foods pose no significant health risk for the average person (see Chapter 17 for a detailed discussion). Although proper handling of pesticides by producers is important, many of the most dangerous pesticides have been banned in this country. Those currently in use are regulated so that even if they are consumed over a lifetime, the risk that they will cause cancer in a typical consumer is less than one in a million.

2. The soil nutrients required by plants in the greatest amounts are nitrogen, potassium, and phosphorus. It makes no difference to plants whether these nutrients come from natural fertilizers, such as manure, or from those in chemical fertilizers made in factories. The key issue is whether sufficient amounts of the main soil nutrients are available to crops—not whether natural or manufactured fertilizer is used.

3. The genetic makeup of a plant largely determines its nutrient content and needs. Plants thrive when the soil is rich in nutrients. Long-term studies find no differences in the nutritional value of organically and conventionally grown crops.

4. The flavor of a plant food depends on its freshness, hereditary makeup, and harvest time. Organic food moves through its own separate distribution and marketing system to avoid any possibility of being commingled with nonorganic food. Compared with conventional foods, organic foods tend to be handled less efficiently and more slowly on the way to stores. Thus the organic produce available to consumers often has a poorer quality and more spoilage than conventionally grown and distributed produce.

Rather than wasting your money on organic produce, consider buying the freshest foods available. These will have the best taste and highest vitamin content. If you choose to spend the extra dollars for organic foods, try to find out your store's current standards for labeling foods "organic."

Health Foods: Much Ado about Nothing?

Today's health food stores often sell not only vitamins and other supplements but also breads, produce, pasta, juices, and a variety of other products. The proprietors promise that their products are minimally processed and have no additives or other artificial ingredients. Still, can a line be drawn between processed and unprocessed foods? For example, consider a cracker. Making a single cracker requires grinding, mixing, boiling, baking, and pressing—a lot of processing. Yet health food crackers get a "health food" label (and price tag) because they contain no artificial coloring or preservatives. Is this fair?

Actually the term *health food* is inherently misleading. All foods eaten in moderation can be healthful in the context of a balanced diet. All foods, even Popeye's spinach, can be unhealthful when eaten in excess. For example, some foods, whether bought in a health food store or a grocery store, can contain naturally occurring toxins: aflatoxins in grains, solanine in green parts of potatoes, goitrogens in some raw vegetables, and other poisons in mushrooms and herbs (see Chapter 17). Most of these naturally occurring toxins are harmless when eaten in small amounts in foods as part of a balanced diet.

Many foods found in health food stores serve important nutritional roles: whole-grain products, fruits and vegetables, juices, yogurt, tofu, and nut butters. However, these nutritious food products can be bought at most grocery stores, generally at lower cost. In addition, although some highly touted health food snacks may contain dietary fiber and other nutritious things, they are also high in fat.

Health food stores also sell many nonfood nutritional products of dubious value. For example, digestive enzymes, amino acid supplements, bee pollen, ginseng, protein supplements, and primrose oil play no important nutritional role in diet planning despite promotional claims to cure all kinds of ailments (see Table 3-2).

Let's look more closely at food processing and the use of additives, two practices health food proponents denounce. Then the problem of regulating nutritional products will be covered.

Food processing. Rice, wheat, and other grains—the seeds of grasses—have a germ (seed) surrounded by starch. The starch provides nourishment once the seed sprouts. A layer of bran and an outer, inedible hull protect the germ and starch. Edible whole grains, such as rice and whole wheat, contain everything but the hull. Most methods of grain processing strip away some nutrients. The valuable dietary fiber in the bran layer and the important nutrients in the germ are removed to produce the white rice and flour many desire. Food processors enrich some white rice and flour by adding the significant nutrients that were lost. However, **enriched** foods lack the dietary fiber and some nutrients contained in the corresponding whole-grain foods.

Thus the brown rice, whole-wheat flour, and other whole-grain products touted by health food advocates do offer more dietary fiber, protein, and certain vitamins and minerals than their more highly processed counterparts. Still, most grocery stores stock these staples at lower prices than health food stores normally charge.

However, not all food processing involves removal of healthful ingredients. Indeed, some nutrients are commonly added to such foods as breakfast cereals. This process, called *fortification,* makes foods more nutritious in some respects. In some cases, processing is critical to food safety. For example, unprocessed (raw) milk can contain microorganisms that cause disease. The **pasteurization** of milk (heating it

---

Be assured that if all the health food stores in the United States were closed, no one's health would necessarily suffer. The stores serve no essential function—grocery stores and supermarkets can supply all our nutrient needs.

Enriched

A term generally meaning that the vitamins thiamin, niacin, and riboflavin and the mineral iron have been added to a grain product to improve nutritional quality.

Pasteurization

The process of heating food products to kill pathogenic microorganisms. One method heats milk to 161°F for at least 20 seconds.

to high temperatures for a short time) kills microorganisms capable of causing disease, such as bacteria and viruses. Even when produced under high standards of cleanliness, raw milk may contain dangerous microorganisms, which can cause serious illness in children and other susceptible people.

Each type of processed food, then, deserves a separate evaluation. Overall, whole grains are more nutritious than refined grains, but fortified processed breakfast cereals are important in many children's diets. As stated in Chapter 2, you should focus on the quality of your total diet, not fixate on particular food choices.

Food additives. Food manufacturers add **preservatives** and other additives to many products. The controversy surrounding use of additives is largely groundless in view of their usefulness and safety. The three most widely used additives—sugar, salt, and corn syrup—are all found naturally. These three—plus citric acid (found naturally in oranges and lemons), baking soda, vegetable colors, mustard, and pepper—account for over 98% by weight of all food additives used in the United States.

Additives are used in food processing for several purposes:

- To retard the growth of microorganisms
- To prevent unpleasant flavors in fat by reducing the incidence of **rancidity**
- To improve flavor and appearance
- To keep mixtures from separating
- To retain food crispness

Some preservatives, such as vitamin C, are nutrients; others may prevent the formation of cancer-causing chemicals. The vitamins and minerals added to various products clearly raise the nutrient value of these foods. Moreover, many common additives contribute to the taste of foods.

As discussed in Chapter 17, the safety of food additives is monitored by FDA. Nonetheless, some people are still skeptical; health food advocates, in particular, often question the safety of and need for additives. Remember, though, that food additives not only contribute nutrients and enhance food safety but also prevent quick spoilage. By minimizing food spoilage and waste during distribution and in the home, additives ensure the year-round availability of many food products. For the consumer, insisting on additive-free foods can mean higher prices and less availability.

Even without additives, some unprocessed foods contain natural—yet potentially **toxic**—substances. Our body's defense mechanisms help guard against harm from additives and other foreign compounds. Liver enzyme systems and the constant shedding of the intestinal tract are two of the many means by which our bodies defend themselves.

Overall, scientific experts believe that the benefits of food additives—safer foods, improved nutritional quality, less waste, and lower prices—far outweigh the minimal or nonexistent health risks associated with their use.

Regulation of nutritional products. The health food industry, which generates a billion dollars per year, is subject to relatively little regulation. FDA works hard to investigate complaints of quackery and harm to individuals caused by fraudulent nutrition products, but it does not have enough time or money to investigate all leads. In addition, the Dietary Supplement Health and Education Act of 1994 classifies vitamins, minerals, amino acids, and herbal remedies as "foods" and effectively restrains FDA from regulating them as heavily as food additives and drugs. According to this act, rather than the manufacturer having to prove a nutritional product is safe, FDA must prove it is unsafe before preventing its sale. In contrast, the safety of food additives and drugs must be demonstrated to FDA's satisfaction before they are marketed.

Currently, a supplement or herbal product can be marketed without FDA approval if (1) there is a history of its use or other evidence that it is expected to be

Preservatives
Compounds that extend the shelf life of foods by inhibiting microbial growth or minimizing the destructive effect of oxygen and metals.

Rancid
Having a disagreeable odor or taste, usually caused by fat breakdown.

Toxic
Poisonous; caused by a poison.

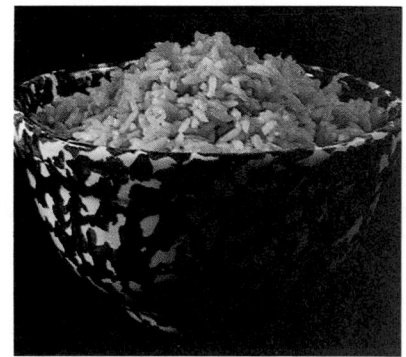

Rice is often given high status in health food circles.

reasonably safe when used under the conditions recommended or suggested in its labeling and (2) the product is labeled as a dietary supplement. It is permissible for the labels on such products to claim a benefit related to a classic nutrient-deficiency disease, describe how a nutrient affects human body structure or function, and claim that general well-being results from consumption of the ingredient(s).

Although their claims do not have to be approved by FDA, manufacturers must have evidence that their marketing statements are truthful and not misleading. There is no guarantee, however, that anyone will ever confirm this. In addition, the label of products bearing such claims must prominently display in boldface type the following disclaimer: "This statement has not been evaluated by the Food and Drug Administration. This product is not intended to diagnose, treat, cure, or prevent any disease." Despite this statement, when consumers find these products on the shelves of supermarkets, health food stores, and pharmacies, they may mistakenly assume FDA has carefully evaluated the products.

The fact remains that many Americans are willing to try bogus health food products and believe in their miraculous actions. Popular products claim to increase muscle growth, enhance sexuality, boost energy, reduce body fat, increase strength, supply missing nutrients, increase longevity, and even improve brain function. For example, "smart drugs" are a popular supplement of the 1990s that supposedly improve thinking. Some "smart drugs" are herbal mixtures and others are prescription drugs that are sold illegally by foreign mail-order distributors.

Clearly many nutritional products commonly found in health food stores are not strictly regulated in terms of safety or effectiveness. Few have been thoroughly evaluated by reputable scientists. If you embark on a self-cure by means of such products, you will probably waste money and possibly risk ill health.[3]

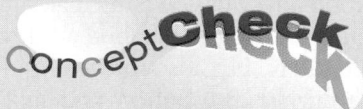

Choosing organically grown and natural foods to avoid pesticides, chemical fertilizers, additives, and artificial ingredients is expensive and offers no real benefit. The nutritional value of organic foods is no higher than that of similar foods produced by conventional methods. Food processing that includes the use of additives often increases the safety of foods, enhances their nutritional value, and improves their taste, appearance, and shelf life. FDA, the nation's federal food regulatory watchdog, requires testing of all food additives when safety is questioned. Many nutritional products typically found in health food stores are ineffective and possibly hazardous. The grocery store, not the health food store, is the place to seek the foods you need to nourish your body.

Meganutrient Therapies and Supplement Use

About 35 years ago a few physicians began treating schizophrenic patients with **megadoses** of vitamins (quantities of more than 10 times the RDA). Today this approach is used by a tiny minority of physicians, who call it *meganutrient, orthomolecular,* or *nutritional therapy.* Although chemical imbalances in the body contribute to many diseases, meganutrient therapies have not been accepted as remedies to these imbalances. The risk of such therapies outweighs their dubious benefits.[3]

In some specific cases, vitamin and mineral supplements may be advisable in smaller amounts. However, you should seek professional advice to evaluate whether supplementation is in your best interest. The reason for this cautious approach is that supplementation with some vitamins and minerals can counteract the effect of certain medications and also produce toxic effects. The Nutrition Issue discusses this topic in greater detail.

Megadose
Quantity of nutrient greater than 10 times one's RDA value listed in the 1989 publication.

Macrobiotics

Macrobiotics, a quasireligious/philosophical way of life founded by the late Japanese philosopher George Ohsawa, advocates a mainly vegetarian diet. Foods of animal origin are used as condiments rather than main dishes. Ohsawa outlined a 10-stage Zen macrobiotic diet, with each stage being more restrictive. In the highest stage, followers are to consume only brown rice and water. This eating plan was purported to overcome many illnesses attributed to dietary excesses. Though no scientific evidence supports the claims, proponents believe macrobiotics cures anemia, arthritis, appendicitis, cancer, cataracts, tuberculosis, diabetes, epilepsy, heart disease, hernia, leprosy, and schizophrenia.

Today, under the leadership of Michio Kushi, Ohsawa's followers promote macrobiotics as a cancer cure. In fact, this diet can interfere with legitimate cancer treatment because patients lose their appetite, as well as weight. Also, the diet may not meet the increased nutritional needs of some cancer patients.

Current macrobiotic diets are less restrictive than earlier versions. Proponents now recommend whole grains (50% to 60% of each meal), vegetables (25% to 30% of each meal), whole beans or soybean-based products (5% to 10% of daily food), nuts and seeds (small amounts as snacks), miso soup, herbal teas, and small amounts of white meat or seafood once or twice weekly. Do you see any important foods missing from this diet?

The American Academy of Pediatrics cautions that a macrobiotic diet is especially hazardous to children. Recently, some children following macrobiotic diets were diagnosed with **rickets.** This bone disease was linked in these cases to deficient vitamin D and calcium intake. Vitamin D–fortified milk in the diet would add these nutrients.[8] In addition, children may be unable to eat enough of the bulky foods composing macrobiotic diets to meet their needs for energy, protein, and many vitamins (see Chapter 15). Deficiencies of these nutrients can stunt growth.

Herbal Therapies

Throughout history, healers have gone to the garden, forest, and sea to seek herbal remedies. By definition, herbs are flowering plants that have nonwoody aboveground stems. Largely by trial and error, the leaves and seeds of various herbs, roots, and barks were found to possess medicinal properties. As early as the second century BC, the Egyptians used myrrh, cumin, peppermint, caraway, fennel, and clove oil for various ailments. In sixteenth-century Europe, physicians began experimenting with sarsaparilla, the dried root of the smilax plant, in an attempt to cure venereal disease. Later the root was used to treat chronic rheumatism and skin disease. When late-nineteenth-century physicians abandoned belief in its medicinal powers, sarsaparilla found new life as a syrup for soft drinks.[25]

Most plant substances, however, still remain in the forest. The National Cancer Institute is the world's leader in the search for medicinal compounds in plants. For example, the agency has tested extracts from 30,000 plant species for activity against cancer. This work identified five anticancer compounds from flowering plants that have been approved for use in cancer patients. Other plant-derived compounds are currently being tested for safety and effectiveness in clinical trials but haven't yet been approved. Traditional knowledge of the healing properties of plants provides leads for scientists to explore.[27] Any promising compounds they isolate are subjected to rigorous FDA-approved tests to determine safety, effectiveness, and side effects. This controlled testing provides a wealth of information far exceeding that available for herbal remedies.[11]

In 1993 Congress created an Office of Alternative Medicine within the National Institutes of Health. The primary purpose of this office is to evaluate the safety and efficacy of herbal and other alternative medical therapies, some of which include nutritional components.[16] Members of Congress with a personal interest in herbal therapies, as well as individuals in the herbal and alternative medicine field, pushed for

Macrobiotics
A food plan that emphasizes vegetable foods over animal foods, often with heavy use of brown rice.

Rickets
A disease characterized by softening of the bones because of poor calcium deposition. This deficiency disease arises from insufficient vitamin D activity in the body.

To compare this food plan with a recommended vegetarian diet, see Chapter 7.

creation of this office.[17] Opinions vary on the wisdom of this decision. Some practitioners argued that fair evaluation of alternative therapies was long overdue. Although not generally supported by the medical profession or taught in medical schools, such therapies are used in one form or another by an estimated one in three Americans. Conversely, many scientists warned that the Office of Alternative Medicine simply provides an air of respectability for quacks and charlatans and wastes money that would be better spent on more promising areas of scientific research.[20]

Little scientific data are available concerning the therapeutic value and safety of the 7000 or so herbs used in traditional medicine, which has been practiced and chronicled primarily by the Chinese.[14,26] Proponents of herbal medicine suggest that its safety and efficacy have been well established during its 4000-year history. These individuals also point to the widespread use of herbal therapies in Europe, especially Germany. Still, numerous reports have documented significant health risks associated with use of some herbal and alternative remedies, sometimes resulting in death. Studies especially implicate germander, comfrey, chaparral, yohimbe, lobelia, jin bu huan, products containing stephanie and magnolia, senna, hai gen fen, paraguay tea, kombucha tea, tung shueh (Chinese black balls), ma huang (Ephedra), and willow bark.[6,11,14,23,25]

There is also a distinct risk that an herbal product may be mislabeled, laced with prescription drugs, or subject to extreme variations in potency. Thus, herbal products should be used with great caution and only in consultation with a person's primary physician. Otherwise, potential side effects may go undiagnosed, or dangerous herb-medicine interactions may develop. Pregnant and nursing women and anyone with chronic and serious health problems should not take herbal supplements unless their physicians consent to the practice[11] and monitor them for potential complications. For example, abdominal pain, darkened urine, and jaundice can signal liver complications caused by an herb.[11]

FDA advises anyone who experiences adverse side effects from an herbal remedy to contact a physician. Physicians are encouraged to report such adverse effects to the agency's hotline for professionals. The agency also suggests contacting the state and local health departments and consumer protection agency.

Not all herbal remedies are ineffective, but in many cases too little information is available to guide their safe use or determine whether the benefits are worth the risks.[9] Remember that herbal remedies, unlike conventional drugs, are not regulated by FDA. Our knowledge about these products is based largely on folklore and tradition, not reliable scientific research. Moreover, although some herbs are clearly dangerous, no warning labels are required on herbal products.

Some herbalists claim that natural herbs cannot harm people. No evidence supports this claim. Indeed, if there's one thing experts agree on, it's this: An herb that has the ability to heal also has the ability, if misused, to harm. In addition, many conditions for which herbs are recommended (such as diabetes and arthritis) are not suitable for self-treatment.[11] For a balanced, thoughtful discussion of herbal remedies, consult *The Honest Herbal* by Verro Taylor, an expert in the medicinal use of plants.[25]

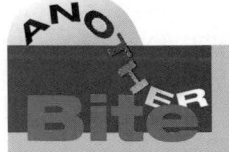

Today the American public can buy herbs in pill form. Nature's Sunshine Products markets more than 70 different individual herbs and about 60 herbal combinations, some containing as many as 18 different herbs. These herbal pills and capsules have the safe appearance of traditional medicines. A little pill seems more legitimate than a mixture of magic potions. The potions, however, are the same; only the packages are different. Estimated yearly sales of Nature's Sunshine Products exceed $60 million.

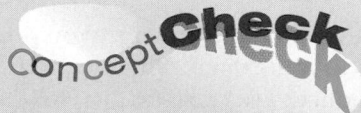

Therapies based on herbs or megadoses of vitamins and minerals lack scientific endorsement and may be dangerous. Likewise, macrobiotic diets do not cure disease. Such diets can even harm children through inadequate nutrient intake. Unlike prescription medicines, herbal remedies are not regulated by FDA. Most of the many herbs used today have not been rigorously tested for efficacy and safety. Moreover, numerous reports indicate that herbal remedies have caused significant adverse effects, even death in some cases. Any use of herbal products or alternative medical practices must be undertaken with caution and under the supervision of your primary physician.

How Nutrition Quackery Spreads

Quackery is easier to perpetuate than you might think. Again, the reality is "let the buyer beware." To avoid becoming a victim of quackery, you need to understand the tactics of quacks and recognize their promotional strategies.

Skirting the Law Is Easy

Our devotion to free speech can harm the consumer and protect the phony-food promoter. For example, those who make false claims for a product but do not actually sell it cannot be charged with fraud or other legal violations. Labeling a vitamin as a cure for cancer on the package itself or package insert is illegal. However, a TV talk show guest or magazine writer can make testimonials about wonder cures without facing prosecution. Retailers can then refer to the talk show or magazine article in their sales pitches, thereby passing along misinformation. They can refer customers to more misinformation in popular literature and materials distributed by supplement manufacturers. Storekeepers attending seminars sponsored by trade organizations can gather these illegal claims and pass them on in the privacy of health food stores. Individuals who use bogus products and practices are also free to spread such misinformation to their friends and neighbors.[2]

Some quacks are impostors who purchase bogus credentials from unaccredited diploma mills. These may look impressive, but they're not worth the paper on which they are printed. Dr. Victor Herbert, a noted "quack buster" and nutrition scientist, purchased two diplomas—one from the American Association of Nutrition and Dietary Consultants, the other from the equally "prestigious" International Academy of Nutritional Consultants—by submitting the name and address of the applicant, along with a check for $50. The first certificate was inscribed with the name of Dr. Herbert's pet poodle, Sassafras; the other belongs to his cat, Charlie (Figure 3-5).[3]

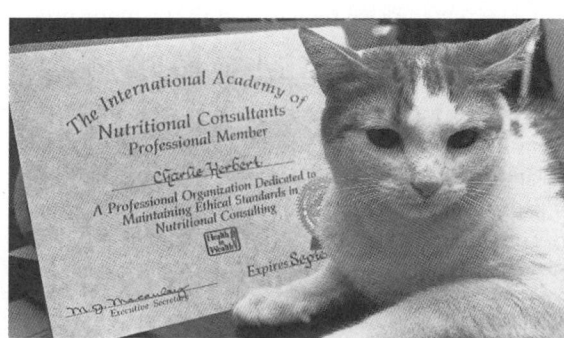

Figure 3-5 *Consumers need to be wary of people with credentials from "diploma mills." Charlie Herbert (the cat) is a nutrition consultant, according to the diploma purchased by his owner. Seek out a true nutrition professional for dietary advice—a registered dietitian (R.D.).*

Popular Books Promote Dubious Theories

The health food industry's well organized promotion machine capitalizes on popular books. Nutri-Books, the largest distributor, stocks more than 2000 titles, most of which promote questionable health ideas and products. *Life Extension*, a 1982-1983 best-seller, was based on a medically unacceptable premise; building on data taken from animal experiments, the authors generalized that underfed humans might live to 150 years of age. (Chapter 16 discusses the research behind this premise.) According to the publisher's promotions the authors appeared on national TV more than a dozen times. The magazine *Health Foods Business*, which reports industry trends, noted that sales of "antioxidants, moisturizers, and antiaging products" promoted by the book jumped after its publication. A number of companies even designed new products to take advantage of the book's popularity.[2]

Coinciding with public concern about AIDS, the 1985 publication of *Dr. Berger's Immune Power Diet* sparked the marketing of many health food products promising to boost the immune system. This book gives unreliable dietary advice.

Michio Kushi's books touting macrobiotics as a "nutritional cure" for cancer and heart disease continued to be best-sellers throughout the 1980s and 1990s. Books supporting herbal therapy instead of prescribed medicine—such as those by James Balch, M.D.—are commonplace on the health food store bookshelf, alongside numerous books on weight loss.[3]

Sales Pyramids Widen the Distribution Network

Many companies market food supplements, diet plans, and other health products using person-to-person sales. Anyone can become an independent distributor. Simply complete an application form, pay a small fee for a sales kit of product literature, and practice the pitch. Companies require no knowledge of nutrition or health care. Pitch the product with personal testimonials and persuade others to become distributors. This type of distribution system, known as a *sales pyramid*, is a typical get-rich-quick scam. When sales mount, distributors make money from a percentage of the sales of those below them in the pyramid. Like many such scams, promises of profits that continually multiply are rarely fulfilled.[2]

Health Food Stores and Pharmacies Provide Easy Outlets

Although it is illegal for storekeepers to diagnose or prescribe, they often do both. No special knowledge or training is required to become a salesperson at a health food store. Employees in these stores typically obtain information by reading books and magazines that promote supplement products for the treatment of virtually all health problems. Investigators from the American Council on Science and Health uncovered the following practices in a survey of health food stores in a three-state area[3]:

- When asked about eye symptoms characteristic of glaucoma, 17 of 24 storekeepers suggested a wide variety of products; none recognized that urgent medical care was needed.
- When asked over the telephone about a sudden, unexplained 15-pound weight loss in 1 month, 9 of 17 storekeepers recommended products sold in their store; only 7 suggested medical evaluation.
- Nine of 10 storekeeprs recommended bone meal and dolomite, products considered hazardous because they are often contaminated with lead.
- Nine stores made false claims about the effectiveness of bee pollen.
- Ten stores made false claims about RNA (ribonucleic acid, a part of almost all cells).

The investigators concluded that most clerks in health food store give advice that is irrational, unsafe, and illegal. As major purveyors of misinformation, these stores play no legitimate role in maintaining the health in Americans.

Although many consumers are wary of health food stores, they don't expect quackery in reputable pharmacies. Yet the typical pharmacy stocks hundreds of supplements, many completely useless. Colorful posters and brochures describing what vitamins do in the body are often prominently displayed. These tend to promote sales by encouraging customers to think that if a little is good, more is better. Most pharmacists know that "nutrition insurance" is not usually needed, that "stress" supplements are a scam, and that doses above the RDA are rarely appropriate. Yet pharmacists throughout the United States profit from public confusion by marketing supplements in their stores.[2]

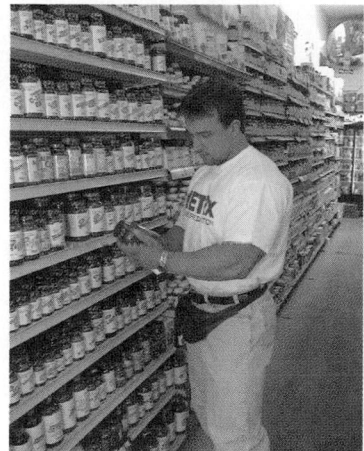

Health food stores and pharmacies sell billions of dollars in vitamin supplements each year.

Chiropractors and Homeopaths Peddle Bogus Remedies

Research supports the effectiveness of spinal manipulation, performed by trained chiropractors, as therapy to ease lower back pain and related ills. However, chiropractors are not medical doctors and have only a specialized expertise; for this reason, they may not recognize possible side effects from therapy or spot other medical problems a person may have. Moreover, many chiropractors sell vitamins and herbal remedies as part of their practice. They may use their analysis, muscle testing, inappropriate blood tests, and "electrodiagnostic" gadgets (fancy galvanometers) to determine the alleged need for supplements. Inappropriate tests are also used to diagnose nonexistent food allergies.[4] An individual contemplating chiropractic therapy should avoid any practitioner who sells nutritional products or offers unusual tests. A more conservative chiropractor who will discuss the proposed therapy with the person's primary physician is preferable. A safer approach is first to discuss the specific health concern with a physician.

Like chiropractors, homeopaths are nonphysicians who practice an alternative therapy. No reputable evidence supports the effectiveness of homeopathy. Introduced in the early 1800s, homeopathic therapy involves administration of minute doses of substances that create the symptoms associated with the disease being treated. For example, a person with influenza might be given a very weak herbal potion that induces fever.

As medical treatment became more scientific and effective, homeopathy declined in the United States to the point of being little more than a curiosity. It remained popular in Europe, however, and has recently been making a comeback here. The homeopathic principle that the activity of a substance increases as it is diluted is scientifically unfounded. The general approach, which amounts to little more than pure quackery, only survives because generations of charlatans periodically reintroduce it.[2] Any apparent benefits from homeopathic procedures can be explained by the tendency of most mild illnesses to naturally improve with time and/or by placebo effects. Furthermore, even if homeopathic portions are harmless, their use can keep patients from seeking effective medical care.

Phony Organizations Fool the Public

Some organizations with scientific-sounding names actually jeopardize public health with misleading nutritional information. The National Health Federation (NHF), for instance, promotes the gamut of alternative health methods with its theme of "freedom of choice" in health matters. Actually NHF just about locks out one choice—medically acceptable types of treatment. Its underlying message implies that anyone opposing NHF ideas is part of an anticonsumer conspiracy controlled by the government, organized medicine, and big business.[2]

NHF publications criticize such proven public health measures as pasteurizing milk, vaccinating for polio, and fluoridating water. This group, based in Monrovia, California, stretches its influence to Washington, D.C., filing lawsuits against government agencies and helping defend people prosecuted for selling questionable "health" products or services.

More than one slipshod organization, billing itself as a scientific "foundation" working for the public good, actually sells enticing cure-alls for common ailments. Often such pseudoprofessional organizations claim to have an impressive board of "scientific advisors" bearing PhD degrees or holding positions in universities and research centers around the world. In some cases, further investigation has shown that many members of the scientific advisory committees do not even exist.[3]

Telling the difference between a reputable and a bogus organization is not always easy, even for health care professionals. The following practices suggest that an organization may be in the business of duping the public and making a profit:

- It advertises a "comprehensive plan" or "health package" that cures such common ailments as arthritis or chronic diseases such as diabetes or cancer.
- It offers members "discount" prices for nutrition products.
- It relies on personal anecdotes rather than scientific studies published in peer-reviewed journals to support its message.

Be wary of any organization that engages in such practices or appears reluctant to provide full information about its staff, directors, and services at minimal cost.

Combatting Quackery

If you suspect false claims, seek answers from reputable sources:

- The local public health department
- Medical societies
- Other professional organizations (Table 3-4)
- Registered dietitians in hospitals and private practice
- The medical or nutrition departments of universities and colleges

FDA also responds to inquiries about product claims. A local FDA office may be listed in the telephone book under Health and Human Services in the U.S. Government listings. False or misleading advertising about nutrition products is handled by the Federal Trade Commission (FTC), not FDA. In addition, the Postal Service can take action against people making false claims for products sold through the mail. Postal prosecution has been fairly effective in curbing this type of quackery.

You can also fight quackery through the media. If you notice a newspaper article, radio or television broadcast, or advertisement that contains health misinformation, complain to the source. Call the station or paper. Consider enlisting the help of the National Council Against Health Fraud, Inc. (Box 1276, Loma Linda, Calif. 92354). Some people fear that speaking out against quackery will put them in legal jeopardy. It won't if they stick to the facts and avoid name calling. You need not label someone a "quack" to speak out against false claims for a product.[2]

When a friend, relative, or fellow student is buying into quackery, consider the following tactics:

1. Ask whether the claim or product has scientific studies to support its message. If it does, take the literature to a reputable source (such as those listed previously) for evaluation and share the professional's opinion with your friend.
2. If the product is a diet, evaluate it in terms of the Food Guide Pyramid. Does the diet stand on its own for balance, variety, and moderation?
3. Remember that people try new things for a number of reasons. The best you may do is provide an objective opinion and let your friend decide.

TABLE 3-4

Where to Complain About Quackery and Health Fraud

In matters of health there should be no tolerance for deception. A small effort in opposing quackery may save many people from being hurt—and may even save a life. If more than one agency seems appropriate for a problem, contact each one.

Problem	Agencies to contact
False advertising	FTC Bureau of Consumer Protection* Regional FTC office Editor or station manager of media outlet where ad appeared
Product marketed with false or misleading claims	FDA national or regional office* State attorney general State health department Local Better Business Bureau Congressional representatives
Bogus mail-order promotion	Chief Postal Inspector, U.S. Postal Service*
Improper treatment by licensed practitioner	Local or state professional society (if practitioner is a member) Local hospital (if practitioner is a staff member) State licensing board National Council Against Health Fraud Task Force on Victim Redress
Improper treatment by unlicensed individual	Local district attorney State attorney general National Council Against Health Fraud Task Force on Victim Redress

From Barrett S: Nutrition quackery—a brief look at the marketplace, Healthline, p. 2, October 1991.
*Federal agency addresses: FDA, 5600 Fishers Lane, Rockville, MD 20857 [800/332-1088]; FTC Bureau of Consumer Protection, 6th and Pennsylvania Ave N.W., Washington, DC 20580; Chief Postal Inspector, 475 L'Enfant Plaza S.W., Washington, DC. 20260-1100; regional offices are listed in the blue pages of telephone directories in the areas where they are located.

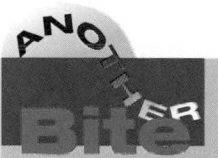

Quacks are experts at "bio babble." The use of pseudomedical terminology may sound legitimate to a person unfamiliar with genuine terms. The following buzzwords are warning flags for quackery: holistic, homeopath, naturopath, nutripath, clinical ecology, cytotoxic testing, and psychic surgeon. Worthless diagnostic methods and treatments include saliva tests, iridology (close examination of the eye), cellulite removal, applied kinesiology, metabolic therapy, hair analysis done by mail-order laboratories, coffee enemas, chelation therapy, and colonic irrigation/detoxification. Rigorous scientific testing has disproved the effectiveness of many of these.[2]

Hair analysis is an experimental research tool used in mineral research. It has little or no place in clinical practice, except in the diagnosis of late mercury or other metal poisoning.

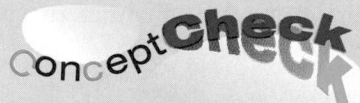

Quacks promote their ideas through fringe health practitioners, salespeople, and the mainstream media. As long as people seek eternal health and quick cures, disreputable health practitioners will thrive. Health food retailers often suggest remedies for illnesses best treated by a medical professional. Protect yourself by being an informed and skeptical consumer.

Summary

➤ The scientific method is a logical approach for determining the accuracy of hypotheses ("educated guesses"). A double-blind study is the gold standard for experimental work because it reduces the potential for bias introduced by the investigators, subjects, and especially the placebo effect.

➤ Though capable of causing bodily harm, quackery hits most people in the pocketbook. However, abandoning medical therapy for a quack remedy can also have serious physical consequences.

➤ Organically grown and so-called health foods provide alternatives to foods grown with chemical fertilizers and pesticides and processed foods containing artificial ingredients and additives. Although these alternate foods are rarely harmful, their nutritional benefits are few and they are often more expensive than conventional foods.

➤ Quacks often suggest that the average diet lacks vitamins and minerals and should be supplemented with their products. Better advice is to choose whole grains, fruits and vegetables, and other selections from the Food Guide Pyramid to provide excellent nutrition. An excess of certain vitamin and mineral supplements, such as vitamins A and D and the minerals iron and copper, can cause harm.

➤ Herbal remedies and megadose vitamin and mineral therapies are not necessarily reliable and may be dangerous.

➤ Consumers who feel shortchanged by orthodox health care provide a large and willing market for those promoting questionable and dangerous nutritional advice. Before accepting alternative health products or suggestions, check for supporting evidence and reputable credentials. If in doubt, check with a physician or registered dietitian.

Study Questions

1 Outline what a double-blind study protocol would contain. Why is this considered the "gold standard" for the assessment of possible health benefits of any substance?

2 What are five tipoffs to "junk science"?

3 What is the difference between a typical and an "organic" product? What do these products have in common?

4 What products are typically sold in health food stores? Which products are potentially harmful?

5 List three "alternative" therapies and provide a brief explanation of each therapy's approach. Why might these therapies be potentially dangerous?

6 What groups of people in the United States do you think may be more susceptible to nutrition fraud? Why? What products are frequently sold to such groups of people?

7 Briefly discuss the implications of the 1994 Dietary Supplements Act with respect to the use of herbal products.

Answer the next question after reading the Nutrition Issue.

8 List some common claims for vitamin and mineral supplements. Evaluate these claims—why are or why aren't such claims accurate? In what situations are vitamin or mineral supplements sometimes warranted? Unsafe?

References

1 ADA Reports: Position of the American Dietetic Association: Food and nutrition misinformation, *Journal of the American Dietetic Association* 95:707, 1995.

2 Barrett S: *Health schemes, scams, and frauds,* Mt. Vernon, N.Y., 1990, Consumer Reports Books.

3 Barrett S, Herbert V: *The vitamin pushers,* Amherst, N.Y., 1994, Prometheus Books.

4 Barrett S: Chiropractic: uncertain benefits, significant risks, *Healthline* January 1996.

5 Campion EW: Why unconventional medicine? *The New England Journal of Medicine* 283:282, 1993.

6 Centers for Disease Control: Unexplained severe illness possibly associated with consumption of kombucha tea—Iowa, 1995, *Journal of the American Medical Association* 275:96, 1996.

7 Colman LM and others: Use of unproven therapies by people with Alzheimer's disease, *Journal of the American Geriatric Society* 43:747, 1995.

8 Dagnelie PC, van Staveren WA: Macrobiotic nutrition and child health: results of a population-based, mixed-longitudinal cohort study in The Netherlands, *American Journal of Clinical Nutrition* 59(suppl):1187S, 1994.

9 Delbanco TL: Bitter herbs: mainstream, magic and menace, *Annals of Internal Medicine* 121:803, 1994.

10 Furnham A, Forey J: The attitudes, behaviors and beliefs of patients of conventional vs. complementary (alternative) medicine, *Journal of Clinical Psychology* 50:458, 1994.

11 Herbal roulette, *Consumer Reports* November 1995.

12 Herbert V, Kasdan TS: Misleading nutrition claims and their gurus, *Nutrition Today* 29:28, 1994.

13 Kassler WJ and others: The use of medicine herbs by human immunodeficiency virus–infected patients, *Archives of Internal Medicine* 151:2281, 1991.

14 Koff RS: Herbal hepatotoxicity, *Journal of the American Medical Association* 273:502, 1995.

15 Lowenthal RM: On eye of newt and bone of shark, *The Medical Journal of Australia* 160:323, 1994.

16 Marshall E: The politics of alternative medicine, *Science* 265:2000, 1994.

17 Marwick C: Growing use of medical botanicals forces assessment by drug regulators, *Journal of the American Medical Association* 273:607, 1995.

18 Marwick C: Trials reveal no benefit, possible harm of beta carotene and vitamin A for lung cancer prevention, *Journal of the American Medical Association* 275:422, 1996.

19 Spiro HM: The art and science of placebos, *Scientific American: Science and Medicine* March/April, 1996.

20 Stalker DF: Evidence and alternative medicine, *The Mount Sinai Journal of Medicine* 62:132, 1995.

21 Stare FJ: Combatting misinformation—a continuing challenge for nutrition professionals, *Nutrition Today* May/June 1992.

22 Thomas PR: Food for thought about dietary supplements, *Nutrition Today* 31:46, 1996.

23 Stehlin IB: An FDA guide to choosing medical treatments, *FDA Consumer* June 1995.

24 Turner JA: Placebo effects on pain, *Healthline* April, 1995.

25 Tyler VE: *The honest herbal,* ed 3, New York, 1993, Pharmaceutical Products Press (an imprint of the Haworth Press, Inc.).

26 Wu C: Yin and yang—Western science makes room for Chinese herbal medicine, *Science News* 148:172, 1995.

27 Xue T: Exploring chinese herbal medicine can foster discovery of drugs, *The Scientist* February 19, 1996.

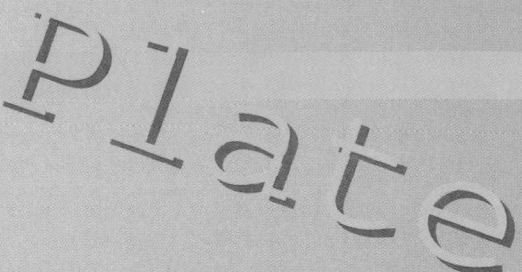

RATE *Your Plate*

Should I Bag the Brown Food?

Many articles in popular magazines have provocative titles. Finding truth amid this hype is a challenge. Your powers to evaluate such claims should have been sharpened with this chapter. These consumer skills will save money, disappointment, and wasted time. The following article simulates those found in popular health and fitness magazines. Using information from this chapter, critically evaluate the article's claims and air of authority.

Conquering the Blues with Brown Food

By Wilma Fuzzlenuts, N.D.C.

Do you often feel like you are living in slow motion? Are you always tired? Is fun the last thing on your mind? You might be suffering from what doctors now call Chronic Fatigue Syndrome—also called "Yuppie Flu." Many respectable scientists and doctors attribute the syndrome to a continual viral infection. Dr. Mickey Fibernugget, an endocrinologist, commented, "I was seeing so many tired patients in my practice that I knew it had to have some medical cause."

Would you like to have more energy? Feel sexier? Recapture that ambition to succeed in life? Well, a little known medical breakthrough may be the stroke of luck to lead you from your troubles. Recently discovered in a small laboratory and medical clinic in Bentenhausen,

Norway, this miracle diet has not yet reached the desks of most physicians, dietitians, and scientists.

When Dr. Val Hornwhipper, Ph.D., noted psychologist, fed his tired patients a diet of only brown food, their energy level and vigor vastly improved. Dr. Hornwhipper claims his Brown Food Empowerment Diet changes lives after only 2 weeks.

How does the brown food diet restore vigor? According to Dr. Nord Viplaugher, noted scientist of the Chocolate Guild in Norway, this exciting new diet speeds up your metabolic rate. You immediately feel energized. Viplaugher refers to this biochemical effect as "catalytic kinetics." In addition, brown food naturally causes your body's immune cells to destroy many different viruses.

By properly incorporating foods like brown rice, chocolate, brown bean soup, brown bread, and coffee, you can eliminate fatigue problems. Helen Howrowitz says, "After following the Brown Food Empowerment Diet for 1 week I felt like I could run a marathon." Vird Veerplank, world-class cross country skier, raved, "I've never performed like this in my sport." Over 20 psychologists and physicians now promote this exciting fatigue-buster.

Why feel tired for even 1 more day? Buy Dr. Hornwhipper's book, *The Brown Food Empowerment Diet* and begin waking up to high energy days. You have discovered a future your physician probably never dreamed of.

Wilma Fuzzlenuts is a National Dietary Consultant for the Wambaugh Holistic Eating Center. She has run five marathons and has worked in nutrition for 10 years. Much of her knowledge comes from personally experimenting with foods to improve her athletic performance.

EVALUATION

1. Evaluate this article using characteristics of food faddists (p. 71) and "How to Evaluate Claims" (pp. 82-83). In your critique, include aspects of the article that intrigued you and aspects that made you suspicious.

2. Consider doing the same type of evaluation on a health-related article from a magazine or newspaper. Are you surprised by the unfounded statements that appear? These are allowed by our laws, so we must stay vigilant in our evaluation of health messages.

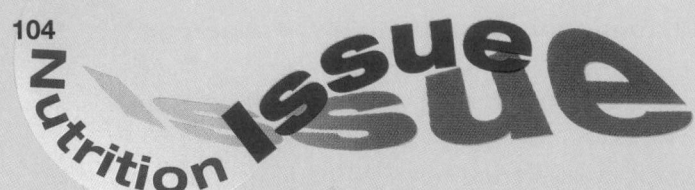

Nutrition Issue

Vitamin and Mineral Supplements—Who Needs Them?

Opinions about vitamins have changed since the turn of the century, when Casimir Funk coined the term. At first, vitamins were merely a curiosity. Later they became the subject of intense scientific scrutiny and research. Today, vitamins are promoted as cure-alls by many health food enthusiasts and consumed as supplements by about 50% of the American population on at least an occasional basis. Supplements are big business; in fact, their sales have nearly tripled since 1976, today exceeding $4 billion annually.

The grocery carts of health food shoppers often contain bottles of vitamin and mineral supplements tucked amid the breads and grains. The two most popular purchases are vitamin C and multiple vitamin and mineral products. People who buy these supplements often worry that their normal diets fail to provide sufficient nourishment. Table 3-5 analyzes common sales pitches for supplements. Do any look familiar?

When respondents in various surveys have been asked to state their most important reason for taking sup-

---

TABLE 3-5

Analysis of Scare Tactics Used to Promote Vitamins

Claim	Comment
"Remember that the health of your eyes, teeth, bones, and internal system depends on a sufficient intake of these vital nutrients."	Messages of this type, intended to make a person nutrient conscious, are true but misleading. They never say how to tell whether a person is getting enough.
"Of the approximately 45 nutrients that are considered essential in meeting daily body requirements, many cannot be manufactured or stored by the body. These nutrients must be ingested daily."	This claim subtly exaggerates the likelihood of deficiency. The body's storage of water-soluble vitamins is limited, but occasional low dietary intake poses no danger.
"How much of your vitamin C gets lost on the way to the table? Picking, packing, processing—all these plus transportation can lead to the destruction of part of the vitamin C in your foods."	The real issues are how much vitamin C remains in one's diet and whether it is enough. Following the Food Guide Pyramid ensures an adequate intake of vitamin C.
"No matter how hard you try, in our fast-paced society, it's often difficult to make sure you're getting enough essential vitamins and minerals in the food you eat."	This claim exaggerates the difficulty of balancing one's diet.
"Most packaged foods have many, if not all, of the natural nutrients removed during processing and replaced with chemicals."	This statement greatly exaggerates the amount of nutrients lost in processing and exploits public fear that our foods contain too many chemicals.
"Our soils are depleted."	This claim falsely suggests that adequate nutrition can be obtained only by ingesting food supplements or special foods.
"I take my vitamins every day. Just to be on the safe side." (Said by man pictured climbing a steep mountain.)	This is a misleading comparison of the dangers of mountain climbing and of not taking daily vitamin pills.

From Cornacchia HJ, Barrett S: *Consumer health,* St Louis, 1993, Mosby.
These vitamin-related issues are discussed in more detail in Chapter 8.

plements, the answers generally fall into the following categories:

- To supplement the diet (31%): "I don't get a balanced diet at all times"; "I don't eat right"; "I don't get enough vitamins during the day"; "I'm an irregular eater."
- Healthful/makes me feel better (30%): "To be healthy"; "As a health supplement"; "They're good for you"; "For general health reasons."
- For energy/strength (12%): "Give me pep"; "To keep going"; "I am run down"; "As a pick-me-up."
- Doctor recommended/prescribed (17%)
- Pregnant (5%)

Surveys also show that about 60% of the supplements sold in the United States consist of multiple vitamin and mineral preparations. Among single-nutrient supplements, iron, vitamin E, vitamin C, and calcium are the most popular.

Some vitamin manufacturers advertise that stress raises vitamin needs. For these hucksters, stress can mean physical demands, overwork, or mental burdens. A vitamin vendor might suggest you raise your intake

Do you take vitamin supplements? Why? If not, why not?

As discussed in this chapter, supplements and other nutritional products are not closely regulated like regular medications. FDA must have evidence that a supplement is inherently dangerous or marketed with illegal claims before it can take any action. Once again, the reality is *buyer beware*. Because of the inflated claims about many supplements and the possible dangers associated with overuse, consumers should seek guidance from professionals about the need for and proper use of supplements.

WHO NEEDS SUPPLEMENTS?

Nutrition scientists generally agree that most people can obtain the vitamins and minerals they need if they eat a healthy diet. If you eat a balanced, lowfat, varied diet that conforms to the Food Guide Pyramid and engage in regular physical activity, you probably don't need supplements.[22] If your diet doesn't meet the guidelines discussed in Chapter 2, first try improving your diet where needed. Only after that should you consider taking a supplement, such as additional calcium if your diet does not include many rich sources. Re-

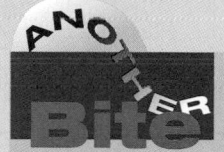

In 1990 Miles Laboratories (makers of One-A-Day products) signed a 3-year "assurance of discontinuance" order with the attorneys general of several states and agreed to pay $10,000 to each. Without admitting wrongdoing, the company pledged not to claim that (1) the average consumer needs a supplement to prevent mineral and vitamin loss, (2) vitamins can prevent or reverse lung damage caused by pollution, (3) routine daily stress depletes vitamins, and (4) routine physical exercise depletes essential minerals. More recently the Federal Trade Commission settled with the corporate parent of GNC, the largest health-food chain in the country, for payment of a $2.4 million civil penalty—without admitting any wrongdoing—based on several years' worth of charges. According to the Commission, GNC had failed to substantiate disease-treatment, weight-loss, muscle-building, and endurance claims for more than 40 products.

around examination time or before a big date. Other supplement companies target athletes, homemakers, and busy executives by plugging products for each group's special needs. Some companies make no health claims at all and rely on the product's name or fast-talking salespeople to sell it.

In fact, no scientific evidence demonstrates that we need more vitamins during emotional stress, mental activity, or routine exercise. Strenuous physical activity primarily increases the need for energy, carbohydrates, and water. The body's natural instinct to eat will ensure that these nutrients are replaced. As we discuss in Chapter 8, extra vitamins do not provide extra energy.

member that regularly eating fortified breakfast cereals can supply significant amounts of many vitamins and minerals (Figure 3-6). Before you begin supplementation, we advise you to discuss your plan with a physician, who may refer you to a registered dietitian.

Recently a panel of scientists from the American Institute of Nutrition and the American Society for Clinical Nutrition suggested a few cases in which vitamin and mineral supplementation should be considered. They are as follows:

- Women with excessive bleeding during menstruation may need extra iron.

Continued.

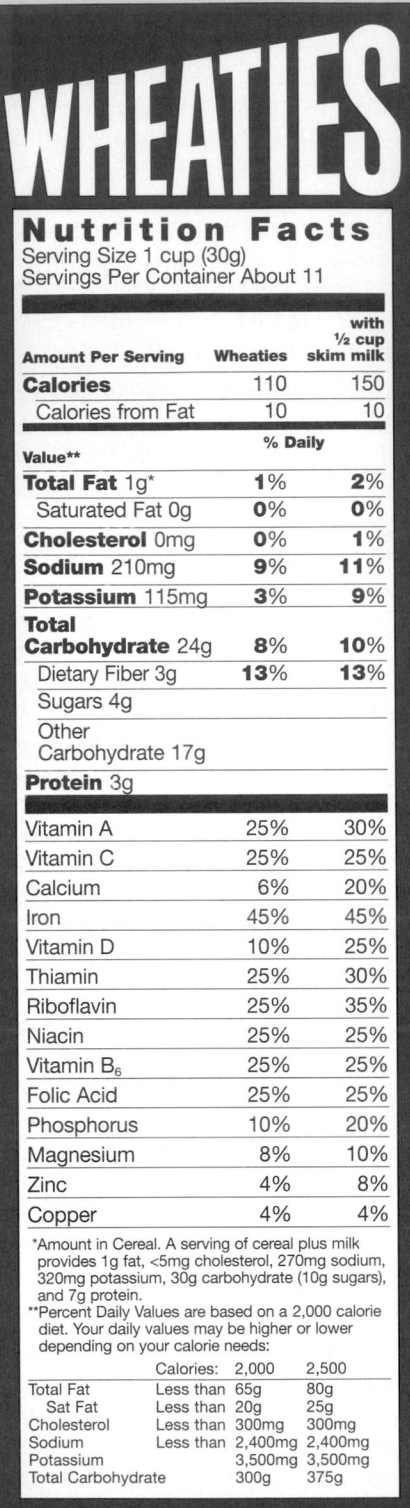

WHEATIES

Nutrition Facts
Serving Size 1 cup (30g)
Servings Per Container About 11

Amount Per Serving	Wheaties	with ½ cup skim milk
Calories	110	150
Calories from Fat	10	10
	% Daily Value**	
Total Fat 1g*	**1%**	**2%**
Saturated Fat 0g	**0%**	**0%**
Cholesterol 0mg	**0%**	**1%**
Sodium 210mg	**9%**	**11%**
Potassium 115mg	**3%**	**9%**
Total Carbohydrate 24g	**8%**	**10%**
Dietary Fiber 3g	**13%**	**13%**
Sugars 4g		
Other Carbohydrate 17g		
Protein 3g		
Vitamin A	25%	30%
Vitamin C	25%	25%
Calcium	6%	20%
Iron	45%	45%
Vitamin D	10%	25%
Thiamin	25%	30%
Riboflavin	25%	35%
Niacin	25%	25%
Vitamin B$_6$	25%	25%
Folic Acid	25%	25%
Phosphorus	10%	20%
Magnesium	8%	10%
Zinc	4%	8%
Copper	4%	4%

*Amount in Cereal. A serving of cereal plus milk provides 1g fat, <5mg cholesterol, 270mg sodium, 320mg potassium, 30g carbohydrate (10g sugars), and 7g protein.
**Percent Daily Values are based on a 2,000 calorie diet. Your daily values may be higher or lower depending on your calorie needs:

	Calories:	2,000	2,500
Total Fat	Less than	65g	80g
Sat Fat	Less than	20g	25g
Cholesterol	Less than	300mg	300mg
Sodium	Less than	2,400mg	2,400mg
Potassium		3,500mg	3,500mg
Total Carbohydrate		300g	375g

Figure 3-6 *The amount of vitamin and mineral fortification in a typical breakfast cereal. Note that two of the four fat-soluble vitamins are included.*

- Women who are pregnant or breast-feeding may need extra iron, folate, and calcium.
- People with very low energy intakes need a range of vitamins and minerals.
- Some vegetarians may need extra calcium, iron, zinc, and vitamin B-12.
- Newborns, under the direction of a physician, need a single dose of vitamin K.

Individuals with other illnesses or diseases and those who use certain medications may require supplementation with specific vitamins and minerals under the direction of a physician. For example, people taking some types of **diuretics** often require extra potassium. The treatment of osteoporosis may include vitamin D and calcium supplements. Women who are able to become pregnant may need folate supplements if their diets do not provide enough, as deficient folate status increases the risk of certain birth defects (see Chapter 8). Individuals with food allergies may need supplements if they avoid entire food groups, such as in severe milk allergy.

Supplementation during illness and drug therapy needs to be directed by a physician because some vitamin and mineral supplements can cause harm by themselves or counteract the actions of certain medications. For example, vitamin B-6 can offset the action of a medication used in treating Parkinson's disease. High intakes of vitamin E can inhibit vitamin K metabolism, thereby increasing the effect of some anticoagulants (e.g., warfarin). Conversely, high intakes of vitamin K reduce the action of some anticoagulants.

WHICH SUPPLEMENT SHOULD YOU CHOOSE?

If you decide to take a vitamin and mineral supplement, which one should you choose? The guidelines set forth by the Council on Scientific Affairs of the American Medical Association recommend that a supplement contain no more than 50% to 150% of the adult Daily Values (formally called U.S. RDAs) for vitamins A, D, E, and C, folate, thiamin, riboflavin, niacin, vitamin B-6, and vitamin B-12. The Council does not recommend that the supplement contain biotin or pantothenic acid (because deficiencies are so unlikely), or vitamin K (because it can disturb oral anticoagulant therapy). For minerals, consider using the same guideline: 50% to 150% of the Daily Value as an upper limit, or up to 100% of the estimated safe and adequate daily dietary intake (see the inside cover of this book). All of these guidelines are usually observed in a basic one-a-day type vitamin, but read the label to be sure. For example, many B-complex products are quite unbalanced, with one tablet providing 33% of the Daily Value for biotin and up to 6670% or more for thiamin.

A balanced supplement formulation conforming to the above guidelines minimizes the chance of vitamin and mineral competition, toxicity, and other undesirable effects. The following examples illustrate such problems:

- Excessive intake of vitamin C can cause overabsorption of iron and lead to iron toxicity in susceptible people. Consuming excessive amounts of vitamin C may also inhibit copper absorption and decrease the effectiveness of certain diagnostic tests for diabetes or cancer.

- Excessive zinc intake can inhibit iron and copper absorption.
- Excessive fluoride exposure during childhood may stain and even weaken the teeth (see Chapter 9).
- Large amounts of folate can mask signs and symptoms of a vitamin B-12 deficiency, thereby preventing the early diagnosis of a potentially life-threatening condition.
- Vitamins A and D, calcium, and selenium can produce toxic effects at intakes only two to five times above their Daily Values (see Chapters 8 and 9).

Critical Thinking

Many vitamin supplements supply nutrients in amounts that exceed the Daily values listed on the label. Miguel believes that "more is better." How can you explain to him that the supplement he is about to start taking is "worse," since it contains amounts that exceed the Daily Values by ten times for many nutrients, including vitamin A?

These examples highlight the reasons that you should consult with a physician and registered dietitian before beginning vitamin and mineral supplementation. Only then can you appropriately evaluate whether use of particular supplements is in your best interest.

In selecting a supplement, many consumers wonder if so-called natural vitamins are superior to synthetic ones. Natural vitamins are isolated from various food products, whereas synthetic vitamins are produced chemically. Although the chemical structures of a few synthetic vitamins differ slightly from their natural counterparts, the body does not distinguish between them. Thus the actions of the natural and synthetic forms of a vitamin in the body are identical. The only real difference between them is price: natural vitamins cost more.

Another consideration is whether the supplement contains superfluous ingredients, such as para-aminobenzoic acid (PABA), hesperidin complex, inositol, bee pollen, and lecithin. Either these substances are produced, in sufficient amounts by the body, such as with lecithin, or they are pure and simple quackery, as with bee pollen. These extraneous substances are frequently found in expensive supplements sold at health food stores and by mail.

CURRENT CONTROVERSIES ABOUT SUPPLEMENTS AND ADDITIONAL FORTIFICATION

Some nutrition experts recommend broadening the concept of the RDA to include two sets of recommended intakes. According to this proposal, lower RDA values would be designed to prevent known vitamin deficiency diseases (similar to the current RDAs), whereas higher RDA values would seek to optimize the potential disease-preventing properties of nutrients such as vitamins C and E. Many people would probably require supplements to meet the higher values for vitamin E (see Chapter 8). Scientists are still debating whether healthy people who eat a varied diet would benefit from taking vitamin and mineral supplements, as this proposal suggests. Currently, both FDA and the National Academy of Sciences state that recommending supplements to the general public is premature.[22]

Because the diets of many Americans do not follow the Food Guide Pyramid, some scientists suggest that further fortification of certain food products may be prudent. Limited fortification worked to improve health in the 1940s, when the government mandated the addition of thiamin, niacin, riboflavin, and iron to refined grains. Would the overall health of the nation be improved further if the government required additional fortification? Or would this lead to unbalanced nutrient composition and untoward effects? There is no consensus on this question. Consuming a healthy, balanced diet is still the prevailing advice—boring as it may sound to people seeking a simpler solution.

NUTRIENTS
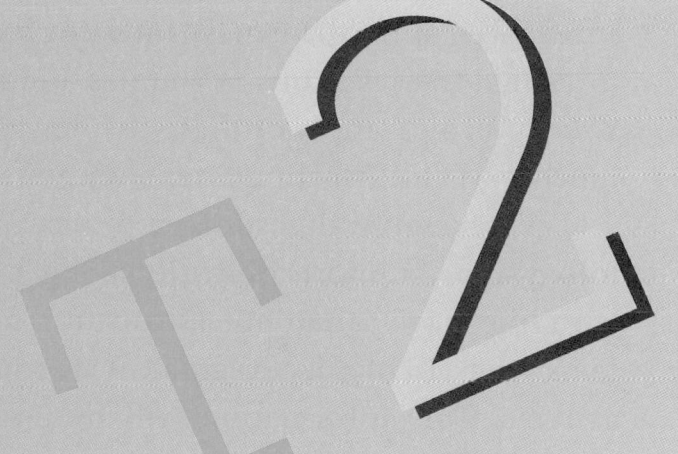
The Heart of Nutrition

PART 2

The Human Body: A Nutrition Perspective

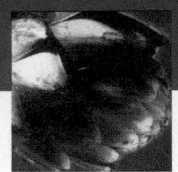

MERELY EATING FOOD WON'T nourish you. You must first digest the food—in other words, break it down into usable forms of the essential nutrients so they can be absorbed into the bloodstream. Once nutrients are taken up by the bloodstream, they can be distributed to body cells.

We rarely think about, let alone control, the digesting and absorbing of foods. Except for a few voluntary responses—such as deciding what and when to eat, how well to chew food, and when to eliminate the remains—most digestion and absorption processes control themselves. We don't consciously decide when the pancreas will secrete digestive substances into the small intestine or how quickly to propel foodstuffs down the intestinal tract. Various hormones and the nervous system help control these functions.[5] Your only awareness of these involuntary responses may be a hunger pang right before lunch or a "full" feeling after eating that last slice of pizza.

Let's examine digestion and absorption as part of the study of the human physiology that supports nutritional health. In the process you will become acquainted with the basic anatomy (structure) and physiology (function) of several body systems: the circulatory, regulatory (control), digestive, excretory, storage, and immune systems. This information will be used as you take a more detailed look at the six classes of nutrients in later chapters.

CHAPTER 4

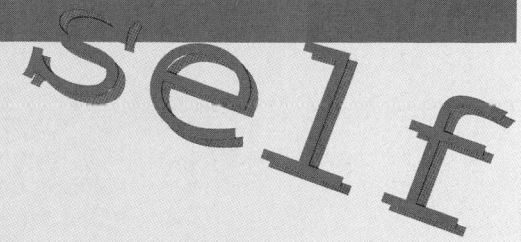

How Healthy Is Your Digestive Tract?

We rarely think about our digestive tract until we notice an unpleasant symptom. However, there are eating routines we can practice to keep this system functioning efficiently. The following assessment is designed to get you to examine your habits and symptoms associated with the health of your digestive tract. Put a "Y" in the blank to the right of the question to indicate a yes and an "N" to indicate a no.

1. Do you have a family history of digestive tract problems such as ulcers, hemorrhoids, diverticulosis, constipation, and lactose intolerance? _____

2. Do you feel pain in your stomach region about 2 hours after you eat? _____

3. Do you smoke cigarettes? _____

4. Do you take aspirin frequently? _____

5. Are you currently experiencing greater than normal stress and tension? _____

6. Do you feel the gnawing pain of heartburn in your upper chest at least once a week? _____

7. Do you frequently lie down immediately after eating? _____

8. Do you feel abdominal pain, bloating, and gas about 30 minutes to 2 hours after consuming milk products? _____

9. Do you often have to strain while having a bowel movement? _____

10. Do you drink less than 6 to 8 cups of fluids per day? _____

11. Are you physically active (jog, swim, walk briskly, row, stairclimb) for less than 30 minutes per day? _____

12. Do you eat a diet relatively low in dietary fiber? (A diet high in dietary fiber contains liberal quantities of whole fruits, vegetables, legumes, nuts and seeds, and whole-grain breads and cereals.) _____

13. Do you frequently experience diarrhea? _____

14. Do you frequently use laxatives or antacids? _____

INTERPRETATION

Add up the number of Ys and record the total in the blank to the right. _____

If you score between 8 and 14, your habits and symptoms suggest that digestive problems are present and/or you risk experiencing digestive tract problems in the future. This chapter examines the processes of digestion and absorption. How these normal processes can be disrupted will be discussed. Take particular note of the habits you can adopt to contribute to the health of your digestive tract.

Key Chapter Concepts

- The cell is the basic building block of body tissues. DNA in cells determines the cell type, its function and structure, and the kind of chemical produced.
- Blood travels the pulmonary circuit, picking up oxygen at the lungs. Then, via the systemic circuit, the blood delivers essential nutrients, energy, oxygen, and water to all body cells. Water-soluble compounds absorbed into the body enter the portal vein and travel to the liver before distribution to other organs. Fat-soluble compounds enter the lymphatic system, which eventually connects directly to the bloodstream.
- The kidneys, skin, and lungs all perform excretory functions for the body.
- The gastrointestinal (GI) tract is a hollow tube that consists of the mouth, esophagus, stomach, small intestine, large intestine (colon), rectum, and anus. The liver, gallbladder, and pancreas participate in digestion and absorption and play especially important roles in digesting protein, fat, and carbohydrate.
- Enzymes and hormones contribute to the digestive process. Most digestion and absorption occur in the small intestine. Little digestion and absorption occur in the stomach or large intestine, with the exception of some protein, which is digested in the stomach.
- Final water and mineral absorption takes place in the large intestine. Products from bacterial breakdown of some plant fibers and other substances are also absorbed here. Plant fibers and other materials that are not digested are eliminated in the feces.
- Nutrients are constantly present in the blood for immediate use and stored to a greater or lesser extent in body tissues for later use when a sufficient food source is unavailable.

Tissue

A group of cells designed to perform a specific function; muscle tissue is an example.

Organ

A group of tissues designed to perform a specific function—for example, the heart. It contains muscle tissue, nerve tissue, and so on.

Organism

A living thing. The human body is an organism consisting of many organs acting in a coordinated manner to support life.

Body Systems Used in Digestion and Absorption

Many aspects of human anatomy and physiology contribute to nutritional health. In this context the stomach and intestinal tract should quickly come to mind, but other systems, such as the circulatory system, excretory system, endocrine system, and nervous system, also play key roles. Use of carbohydrate, protein, fat, vitamins, minerals, and water requires input from all these systems[9] (Table 4-1).

From Cells to Organ Systems

The various body systems are composed of millions of cells. (See Appendix G for a review of the parts and structure of a cell if you do not recall this from previous course work.) Each cell is a self-contained, living entity. Cells represent the basic building blocks of the body and ultimately form all body structures.

When cells of the same type work together for a common purpose—bound together by intercellular substances—they form **tissues,** such as bone, cartilage, muscle, and nerve. Often two or more tissues combine in a particular way to form more complex **organs,** such as skin, kidneys, and liver. At still higher levels of coordination, several organs can cooperate to achieve a common purpose and form an organ system, such as the respiratory system or the digestive system. The human body is a coordinated unit of many such organ systems and is called an **organism**[5] (Figure 4-1).

Every cell in the human body performs a specialized job. A cell's master plan for its work and for generating the corresponding machinery necessary to do its work is encoded into the cell's genetic material, the **deoxyribonucleic acid (DNA).** The DNA acts as a blueprint for synthesizing specific proteins required to perform specific tasks in the body. Although most cells in our bodies contain the same DNA information, each cell is programmed to use only the parts of the DNA instructions that apply to its own tasks, depending on the type of tissue it is part of. For example, stomach cells and bone marrow cells receive the same master plan. However, stomach cells use only a subset of the DNA code to make **mucus,** while cells in the

TABLE 4-1

Organ Systems of the Body

System	Major components	Functions
Integumentary	Skin, hair, nails, and sweat glands	Protects, regulates temperature, prevents water loss, and produces a substance that converts to vitamin D
Skeletal	Bones, associated cartilage, and joints	Protects, supports, and allows body movement, produces blood cells, and stores minerals
Muscular	Muscles attached to the skeleton	Produces body movement, maintains posture, and produces body heat
Nervous	Brain, spinal cord, nerves, and sensory receptors	A major regulatory system: detects sensation, controls movements, controls physiological and intellectual functions
Endocrine	Endocrine glands such as the pituitary, thyroid, and adrenal glands	A major regulatory system: participates in the regulation of metabolism, reproduction, and many other functions
Cardiovascular	Heart, blood vessels, and blood	Transports nutrients, waste products, gases, and hormones throughout the body; plays a role in the immune response and the regulation of body temperature
Lymphatic	Lymph vessels, lymph nodes, and other lymph organs	Removes foreign substances from the blood and lymph, combats disease, maintains tissue fluid balance, and aids in fat absorption
Respiratory	Lungs and respiratory passages	Exchanges gases (oxygen and carbon dioxide) between the blood and the air and regulates blood acid-base balance.
Digestive	Mouth, esophagus, stomach, intestines, and accessory structures	Performs the mechanical and chemical processes of digestion, absorption of nutrients, and elimination of wastes
Urinary	Kidneys, urinary bladder, and the ducts that carry urine	Removes waste products from the circulatory system; regulates blood acid-base balance, overall chemical balance, and water balance
Reproductive	Gonads, accessory structures, and genitals of males and females	Performs the processes of reproduction and influences sexual functions and behaviors

(Modified from Seely RR and others: *Essentials of anatomy and physiology*, St Louis, 1991, Mosby.)

bone marrow that make the oxygen-carrying protein hemoglobin use a different subset of the DNA code.[5]

Chemical processes occur all the time in every living cell: the chemical synthesis of new substances is balanced by the chemical breakdown of other materials into smaller units. For these reactions to occur, the cell requires a continuous supply of energy and oxygen. Cells also need water, the medium in which they live. Furthermore, they need their own building blocks, especially the materials they can't make themselves—the essential nutrients supplied by food. These substances enable the tissues, composed of individual cells, to function properly.

Healthful nutrition can supply an adequate amount of nutrients to all body cells. Still, to ensure the best use of these nutrients by cells, the following organ systems must also be healthy and working efficiently.

Circulatory System

Blood travels two basic routes. In the first route it circulates from the right side of the heart, through the lungs, and then back to the heart (the pulmonary circuit). Then, in the second route the blood circulates between the left side of the heart and all other body parts, eventually returning back to the heart (the systemic circuit)

Deoxyribonucleic acid (DNA)
The site of hereditary information in cells; DNA directs the synthesis of cell proteins.

Mucus
A thick fluid secreted by glands throughout the body. It contains a compound that is both carbohydrate and protein in nature. Mucus acts as both a lubricant and protectant for cells.

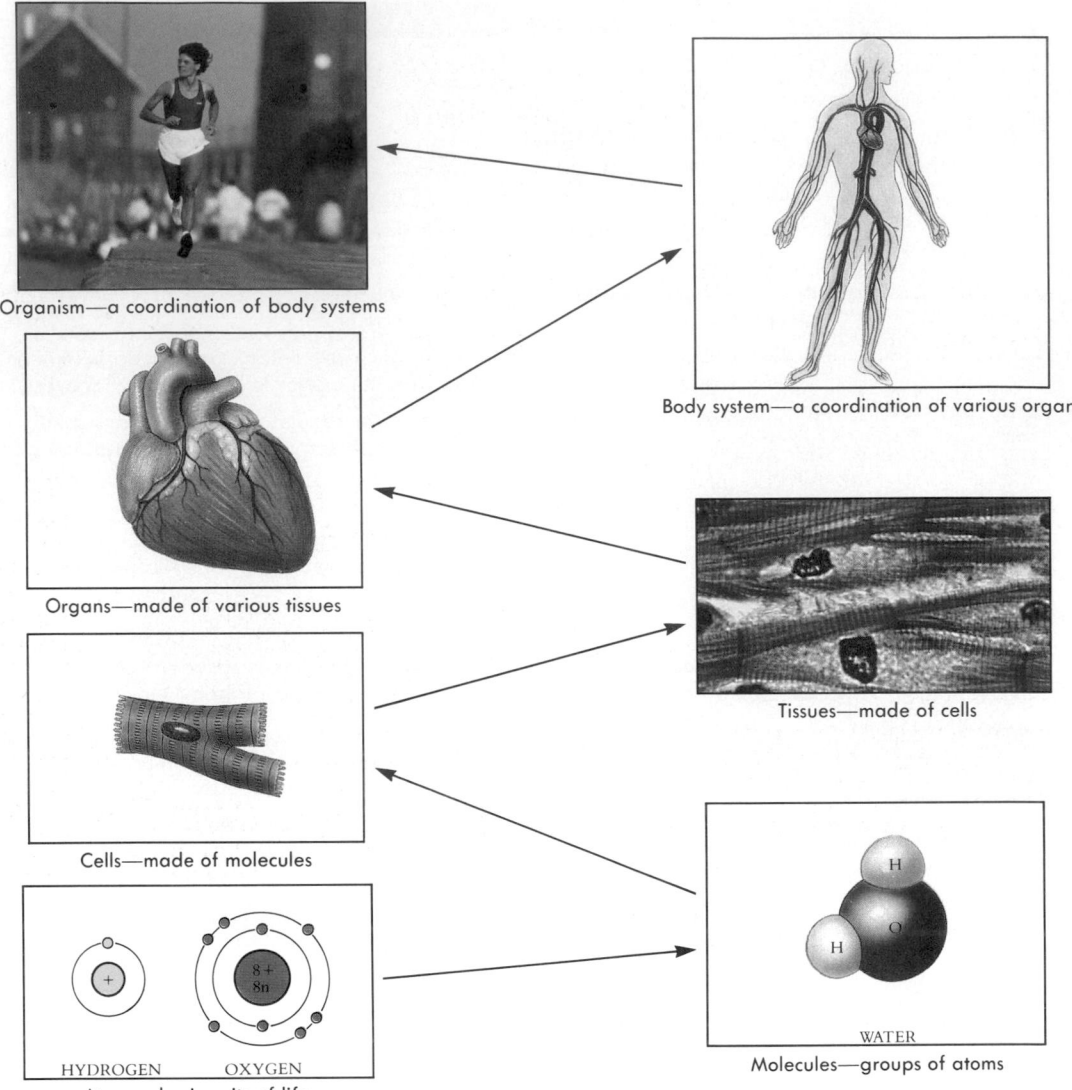

Organism—a coordination of body systems

Body system—a coordination of various organs

Organs—made of various tissues

Tissues—made of cells

Cells—made of molecules

HYDROGEN   OXYGEN

Atoms—basic units of life

WATER

Molecules—groups of atoms

Figure 4-1 *The levels of human biological organization. We are as simple as a collection of atoms and as complex as a whole organism.*

(Figure 4-2). The heart is a muscular pump that normally contracts and relaxes 50 to 90 times per minute while the body is at rest. This continuous pumping keeps blood moving through the circuits.[5]

The circulatory system distributes nutrients yielded from digestion and absorption, along with oxygen from the air, to all body cells. All blood goes to the lungs to pick up oxygen and release carbon dioxide. The oxygenated blood then returns to the heart to be pumped to all other body tissues. In the capillaries, cells exchange nutrients and wastes with the blood: cells empty their waste products into the blood and take nutrients from it. Capillaries, networks of tiny blood vessels, service every region of the body via individual capillary beds that are only one cell layer thick. Nutrients, gases, and other substances can pass through capillary cells to both enter into and exit out of other body cells. In this way, cells can take up needed nutrients and oxygen from the bloodstream and return waste products to the bloodstream for external excretion later.[5]

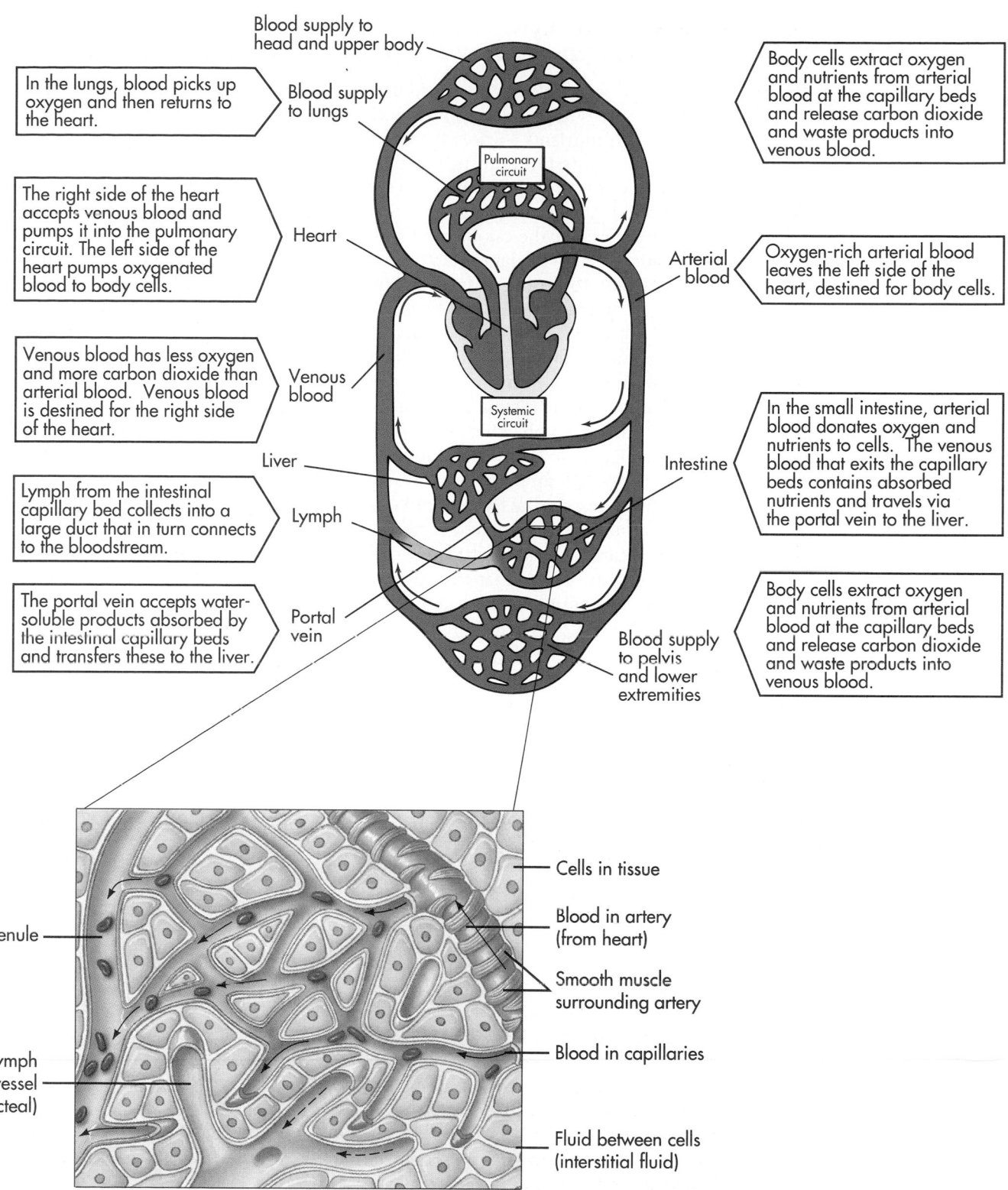

In the lungs, blood picks up oxygen and then returns to the heart.

The right side of the heart accepts venous blood and pumps it into the pulmonary circuit. The left side of the heart pumps oxygenated blood to body cells.

Venous blood has less oxygen and more carbon dioxide than arterial blood. Venous blood is destined for the right side of the heart.

Lymph from the intestinal capillary bed collects into a large duct that in turn connects to the bloodstream.

The portal vein accepts water-soluble products absorbed by the intestinal capillary beds and transfers these to the liver.

Blood supply to head and upper body

Blood supply to lungs

Pulmonary circuit

Heart

Venous blood

Systemic circuit

Liver

Lymph

Portal vein

Body cells extract oxygen and nutrients from arterial blood at the capillary beds and release carbon dioxide and waste products into venous blood.

Arterial blood

Oxygen-rich arterial blood leaves the left side of the heart, destined for body cells.

Intestine

In the small intestine, arterial blood donates oxygen and nutrients to cells. The venous blood that exits the capillary beds contains absorbed nutrients and travels via the portal vein to the liver.

Blood supply to pelvis and lower extremities

Body cells extract oxygen and nutrients from arterial blood at the capillary beds and release carbon dioxide and waste products into venous blood.

Venule

Lymph vessel (lacteal)

Cells in tissue

Blood in artery (from heart)

Smooth muscle surrounding artery

Blood in capillaries

Fluid between cells (interstitial fluid)

Figure 4-2 *Blood circulation throughout the body. This represents the route blood takes through the two circuits that begin and end at the heart. The red color indicates blood that is richer in oxygen; blue is for blood carrying more carbon dioxide. Oxygen and nutrients are exchanged for carbon dioxide and waste products in the capillaries, the points at which the arteries and veins merge. The bottom box shows a close up of a capillary bed in the small intestine, including the location of the lymphatic vessels. This second set of circulatory vessels—part of the lymphatic system—picks up fluid that builds up between cells (interstitial fluid) and large particles, such as some fats. This fluid and the particles become lymph, which travels through further lymph vessels to reach the bloodstream. Lymph vessels in the intestine are also called* lacteals.

Portal and Lymphatic Circulation Plays an Important Role in Nutrient Absorption

Fluids and particles, once absorbed through the intestinal wall, travel one of two different routes. One pathway is the bloodstream. As just noted, the blood—laden with oxygen and nutrients—leaves the heart and enters the arteries. Some of this blood travels to the intestine and ends up in capillary beds inside the intestine. From there, some nutrients are taken up by intestinal cells for nourishment, whereas much of the nutrients from recently eaten foods transfers into the bloodstream. The actual transfer points are the capillary beds. The blood then passes into veins and eventually collects in a very large vein, called the **portal vein** (see Figure 4-2). This vein leads directly to the liver. Most veins in the body double back directly to the heart. However, by going first to the liver, the portal vein enables the liver to process absorbed nutrients before they enter the general circulation of the bloodstream. Water-soluble nutrients—such as glucose and amino acids—enter the bloodstream through this portal vein.[5]

The **lymphatic system** is the other system of circulatory vessels that serves the body. It carries lymph, which is mostly composed of a clear fluid that forms between cells (see Figure 4-2). This fluid filters into tiny lymphatic vessels composing a one-way network that funnels lymph from all over the body into large lymphatic vessels. From these vessels, the lymph fluid empties into major veins returning to the heart. The lymphatic system thereby serves as a second route to return fluids that emanate from the capillaries and ultimately return to the circulatory system.

Lymphatic vessels that serve the small intestine play an important role in nutrition. These vessels pick up and transport the majority of products yielded from fat absorption. These products are too large to enter the bloodstream directly. The lymphatic vessels from the intestine drain into a large duct that connects with the bloodstream through a vein near the neck. Most of the absorbed fat products eventually enter the bloodstream in this way.[9] Other parts of the lymphatic system also serve critical functions in the immune system.[1]

Lymphatic system

A system of vessels that can accept fluid surrounding cells and large particles, such as products of fat absorption. This lymph fluid eventually passes into the bloodstream via the lymphatic system.

TABLE 4-2

Important Secretions and Products of the Digestive Tract

Secretion	Site of production	Purpose
Saliva	Mouth	Contributes to starch digestion, lubrication
Mucus	Mouth, stomach, small intestine, large intestine	Protects cells, lubricates
Enzymes	Mouth, stomach, small intestine, pancreas	Promote digestion of foodstuffs into particles small enough for absorption
Acid	Stomach	Promotes digestion of protein among other functions
Bile	Liver (stored in gallbladder)	Suspends fat in water to aid fat digestion in the small intestine
Bicarbonate	Pancreas	Neutralizes stomach acid when it reaches the small intestine
Hormones	Stomach, small intestine	Stimulate production and/or release of acid, enzymes, bile, and bicarbonate; help regulate peristalsis and overall GI tract flow

Regulatory (Control) Systems

The hormonal and nervous systems have regulatory functions that greatly influence nutrient use in the body. The term *hormone* comes from the Greek for "to stir or excite." To be a true hormone, a regulatory compound must have a specific synthesis site from which it enters the bloodstream to reach target cells.

The hormone insulin helps control the amount of glucose in the blood, and thyroid hormones help control the body's metabolic rate. Other hormones are especially important in regulating digestive processes, such as the hormone gastrin, which is produced in the stomach[9] (Table 4-2).

Many hormonelike compounds also control important aspects of GI function. These compounds diffuse from GI tract cells or nerve endings to act on nearby cells. Many of these hormonelike compounds are found in both the intestine and the brain. When a person thinks about eating or prepares to eat, the whole GI tract begins to prime itself for action. Hormonelike substances participate in this process.[5]

Nervous system input is also important for the GI tract. Nerves influence acid **secretion** in the stomach and regulate intestinal muscle action. The senses of sight, hearing, touch, smell, and taste all use nerve pathways to communicate information—such as the availability of food or the need for it—to the brain. Some nutrients are important in nerve functioning, especially the vitamins thiamin and niacin.

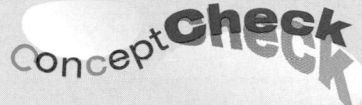

Digestion and absorption require the coordinated efforts of many body systems. These processes aid in supplying energy, oxygen, water, and essential nutrients to all body cells. The circulatory and lymphatic systems transport nutrients throughout the body. The hormonal and nervous systems have regulatory (control) functions that help direct nutrient use and the digestive process.

The Anatomy and Physiology of Digestion

The **gastrointestinal (GI) tract** is the site of nutrient **digestion** and later of absorption. This tract is a long, hollow tube stretching from the mouth to the anus (Figure 4-3). Nutrients from the food we eat must pass through the walls of this tube—from the inside to the outside—to be absorbed into the bloodstream. The GI tract promotes digestion and absorption through a variety of functions: it simultaneously moves and mixes foods (as part of a process called *motility*). The GI tract also secretes chemical substances to promote the breakdown of foods. Finally, the GI tract eliminates wastes. Adding to this, the GI tract promotes nutrient production; the bacteria living in the intestine make vitamin K, which we can then use.[16] Most of these processes are under autonomic control; that is, they are involuntary. Almost all functions involved in digestion and absorption are controlled by hormones, hormonelike compounds, and nerves.[9]

The Flow of Digestion

Let's review the major body parts of the GI tract, starting with the mouth. As you put food into your mouth, the typical response is a sudden rush of **saliva**. This saliva, secreted by special glands in the mouth, contains mucus that envelops and lubricates each morsel, easing its passage down the GI tract (see Table 4-2). Saliva also

Secrete
To produce and then release a substance, generally called a **se-cretion**, *from a cell into the body.*

Gastrointestinal (GI) tract
The main sites in the body used in nutrient digestion and absorption. It consists of the mouth, esophagus, stomach, small intestine, large intestine, rectum, and anus.

Digestion
The process whereby food is broken down into forms that can be taken up by the GI tract.

Saliva
A watery fluid produced by the salivary glands in the mouth; it contains lubricants, enzymes, and other substances.

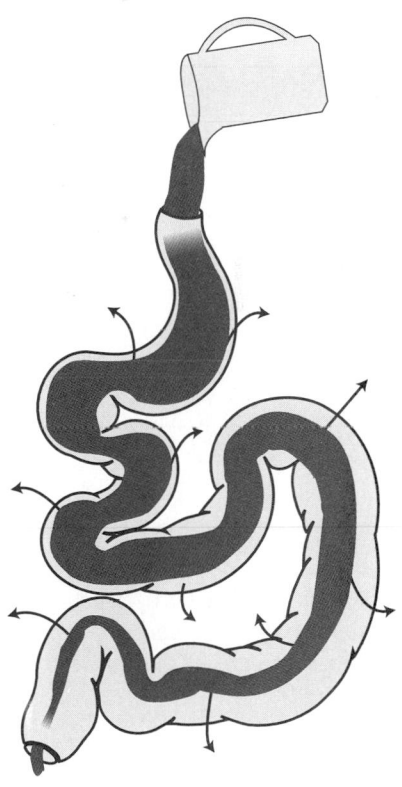

As the intestinal contents pass down the tract, nutrients are absorbed from the "hollow tube" into the body.

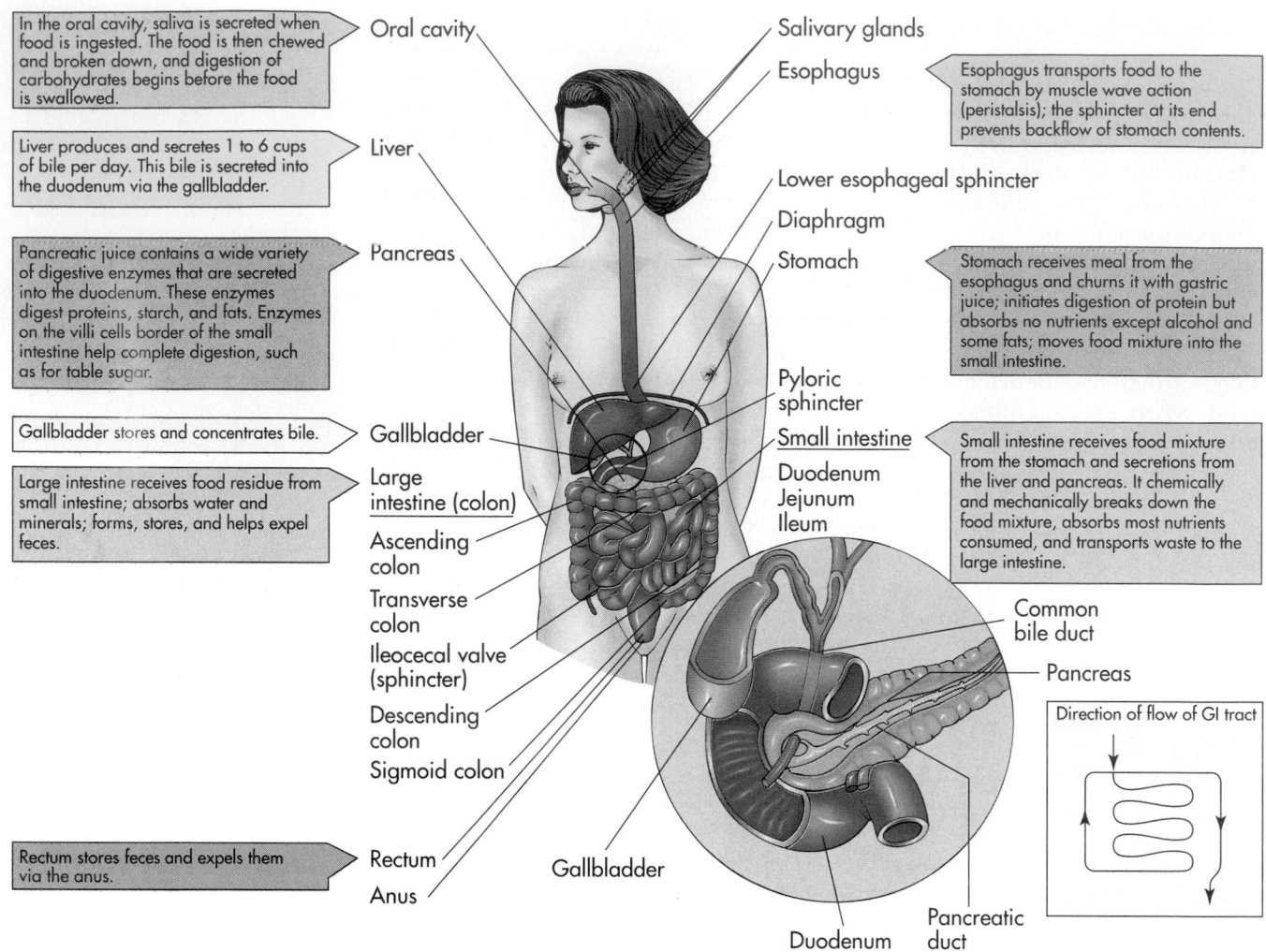

In the oral cavity, saliva is secreted when food is ingested. The food is then chewed and broken down, and digestion of carbohydrates begins before the food is swallowed.

Liver produces and secretes 1 to 6 cups of bile per day. This bile is secreted into the duodenum via the gallbladder.

Pancreatic juice contains a wide variety of digestive enzymes that are secreted into the duodenum. These enzymes digest proteins, starch, and fats. Enzymes on the villi cells border of the small intestine help complete digestion, such as for table sugar.

Gallbladder stores and concentrates bile.

Large intestine receives food residue from small intestine; absorbs water and minerals; forms, stores, and helps expel feces.

Rectum stores feces and expels them via the anus.

Oral cavity
Liver
Pancreas
Gallbladder
Large intestine (colon)
Ascending colon
Transverse colon
Ileocecal valve (sphincter)
Descending colon
Sigmoid colon
Rectum
Anus

Salivary glands
Esophagus
Lower esophageal sphincter
Diaphragm
Stomach
Pyloric sphincter
Small intestine
Duodenum
Jejunum
Ileum

Esophagus transports food to the stomach by muscle wave action (peristalsis); the sphincter at its end prevents backflow of stomach contents.

Stomach receives meal from the esophagus and churns it with gastric juice; initiates digestion of protein but absorbs no nutrients except alcohol and some fats; moves food mixture into the small intestine.

Small intestine receives food mixture from the stomach and secretions from the liver and pancreas. It chemically and mechanically breaks down the food mixture, absorbs most nutrients consumed, and transports waste to the large intestine.

Common bile duct
Pancreas
Gallbladder
Duodenum
Pancreatic duct

Direction of flow of GI tract

Figure 4-3 *Physiology of the GI tract. Many organs cooperate in a regulated fashion to allow digestion and subsequent absorption of nutrients in foods.*

contains specific **enzymes** that break down large carbohydrates into small units. Chewing then breaks food into small pieces, exposing more food surface to digestive action. The more surface exposed, the more efficient digestion is in the mouth and throughout the entire GI tract as well.[9]

The tongue aids chewing and also contains taste sensors for sweet, salt, sour, and bitter.[5] The sweet and salt sensors are near the tip of the tongue; the sour and bitter sensors are near the base. A fifth taste sensation called *umami* has been proposed. This taste sensation is elicited by monosodium glutamate. Brothy, meaty, and savory are examples of umami sensations. Monosodium glutamate is often added to Chinese and Japanese foods to enhance the umami flavor.

The sensation of flavor is aided by input from the approximately 6 million **cells** in the nose that can detect hundreds of thousands of different molecules.[2] Overall, flavor is a complex combination of taste, smell, physical sensations from certain chemicals in foods (such as in chili peppers), and textural sensations. Flavor is also affected by human genetic variability in both taste and nasal sensations.[2]

A variety of diseases and drugs, as well as the effects of aging, can alter the sense of taste. Adding spices and flavorings to foods can enhance the pleasure of eating in these cases.

Umami

A brothy, meaty, savory flavor in some foods. Monosodium glutamate enhances this flavor when added to foods.

The mouth and stomach are connected by a tube called the *esophagus*. At its top is a flap of tissue (called the *epiglottis*) that prevents food from being swallowed into the trachea (windpipe). During swallowing, food lands on the flap, folding it down to cover the opening of the trachea. Breathing also automatically stops. These responses ensure that swallowed food will only travel down the esophagus, helped along by the lubricating mucus, muscular contractions, and gravity (Figure 4-4).

The food then enters the stomach, which is basically a 4-cup (1-liter) holding tank. Only proteins are significantly digested in the stomach. This protein digestion proceeds as the stomach secretes acid and enzymes to help break down the food and slowly churns these into the food. (Later sections discuss the role of acid and enzymes in the digestive process in detail.) A meal usually leaves the stomach within 2 to 4 hours after eating. Solids take longer than liquids to leave the stomach, and a fatty meal usually leaves later than a meal containing mostly protein or carbohydrate.[9]

The stomach is connected to the 10 feet of small intestine, which is coiled inside the abdomen. The considerable length of the small intestine provides ample opportunity for digestion to occur. The small intestine is then divided into three sections: the first part, the duodenum, is about 10 inches long; the middle segment, the jejunum, is about 4 feet long; and the last section, the ileum, is about 5 feet long. The small intestine is considered small because of its narrow (1 inch) diameter. Most digestion is completed in the duodenum and upper jejunum, with the help of enzymes made by intestinal cells and the pancreas.[9]

GI tract flow

Mouth
↓
Esophagus
↓

Stomach—4-cup (1 L) capacity. Food remains about 2 to 3 hours. High-fat meals take the longest time to empty.
↓

Small intestine—duodenum (10 inches long), jejunum (4 feet long), ileum (5 feet long)—about 10 feet (3.1 meters) in total length; food remains about 3 to 10 hours.
↓

Large intestine (colon)—cecum, ascending colon, transverse colon, descending colon, sigmoid colon—3½ feet (1.1 meters) in total length; food can remain up to 72 hours.

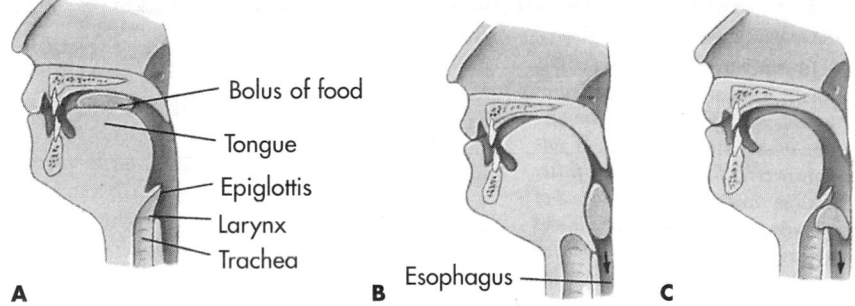

A **B** Esophagus **C**

Bolus of food
Tongue
Epiglottis
Larynx
Trachea

Figure 4-4 *The process of swallowing.* **A,** *During swallowing, food cannot normally enter the trachea because the epiglottis closes over the larynx.* **B,** *The arrow shows that this allows food to proceed down the esophagus.* **C,** *When a person chokes, food becomes lodged in the trachea, blocking air flow to the lungs. The food should have gone down the esophagus.*

Muscular contractions constantly mix the food in the small intestine. This churning enhances digestive action because it exposes more food surface to enzyme action. A meal remains in the small intestine about 3 to 10 hours. About 95% of a total meal has been digested by the time it leaves.[9]

From the small intestine, food moves into the large intestine, also called the *colon.* This organ is about 3½ feet long and is separated into five sections: the cecum, ascending colon, transverse colon, descending colon, and sigmoid colon. Bacteria in the large intestine digest mostly leftover plant fibers.[11] Little else remains to be digested. The food remnants and wastes stay in the large intestine for about 24 to 72 hours before being eliminated.

The large intestine ends in a cavity called the *rectum*, which connects to the anus, the end of the GI tube. These final sections work with the large intestine to prepare the feces for elimination.

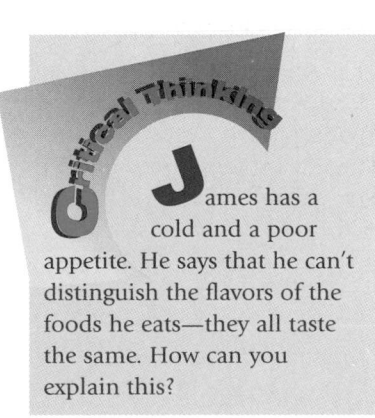

Critical Thinking

James has a cold and a poor appetite. He says that he can't distinguish the flavors of the foods he eats—they all taste the same. How can you explain this?

Bile

A substance secreted by the liver and stored in the gall-bladder; it is released into the small intestine to aid fat absorption by suspending fat in tiny droplets within a watery fluid.

Sphincter

A muscular valve; these vales help control flow of foodstuffs in the GI tract.

Heartburn

A pain emanating from the esophagus caused by stomach acid backing up into the esophagus and irritating its tissue.

As mentioned before, other organs associated with the GI tract aid digestion in the small intestine (see Figure 4-3 and Table 4-1). The liver secretes **bile** needed to digest fat. Bile helps suspend fat in the watery digestive mixture, making the fat more available to the digestive processes. This process is analogous to the way dishwashing liquid breaks up oil spots in dishwater. The body stores bile in the gall-bladder until it is needed.

The pancreas secretes enzymes that aid digestion and bicarbonate (the chemical in baking soda) to neutralize the acid produced earlier in the stomach. Ducts leading from the pancreas and gallbladder merge, allowing the pancreatic juices and bile to blend as they are released into the upper small intestine for digestion. In this way the liver, pancreas, and gallbladder work with the GI tract.

GI Tract Control Valves: Sphincters

A variety of ringlike muscles form valves, called *sphincters,* all along the GI tract (Figure 4-5). The mouth is one example. Sphincters retard or prevent backflow of partially digested food. These sphincters respond to various stimuli, such as signals from the nervous system, hormones, acid versus alkaline conditions, and the pressure that builds up around sphincters.[5] A sphincter in the lower esophagus (lower esophageal sphincter) is critical in preventing backflow of stomach contents up into the esophagus. If highly acidic stomach contents come in contact with the esophagus, they can cause pain, known as **heartburn**.[8] Another sphincter (pyloric sphincter), located at the base of the stomach, controls the flow of processed foodstuffs from the stomach into the small intestine. Only about a teaspoon (a few milliliters) at a time of acidic stomach contents squirt into the small intestine. Such small amounts enable bicarbonate from the pancreas to efficiently neutralize the acid coming from the stomach. The key controlling event is the sensation of acid on the intestinal side of the sphincter. When acid is sensed, the flow of stomach content stops. Once the acid is neutralized, flow from the stomach can begin again.[21]

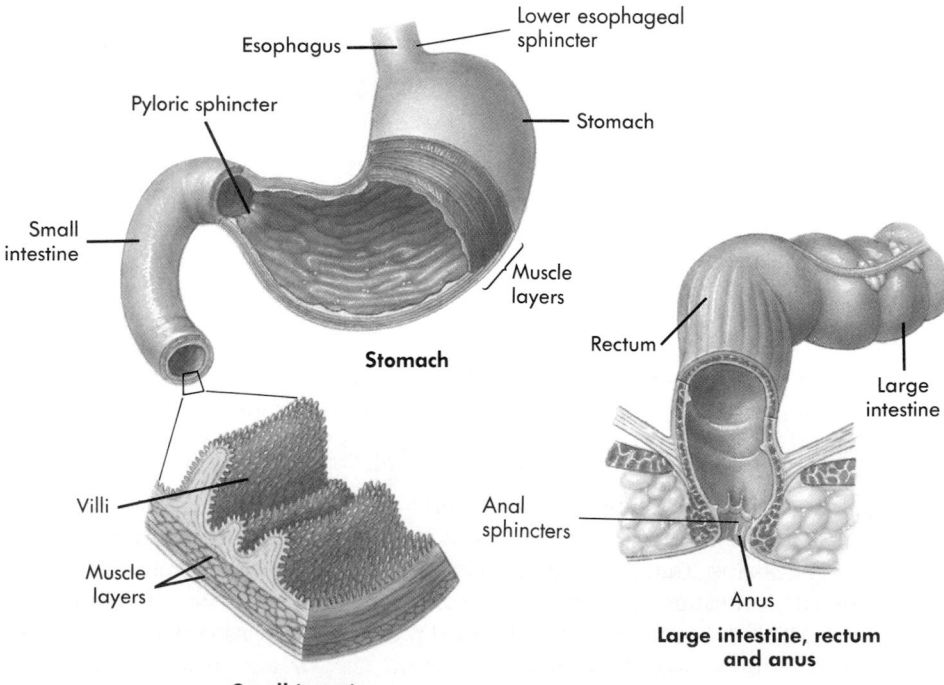

Figure 4-5 *A close-up view of the intestinal tract—muscles, sphincters, and villi. These features of the GI tract perform key roles in digestion, absorption, and elimination.*

At the end of the small intestine, another sphincter (typically called the *ileocecal sphincter*) prevents the contents of the large intestine from reentering the small intestine. At the end of the large intestine are two final anal sphincters, one of which is under voluntary control. Once children are toilet trained, they can generally determine when the outer anal sphincter will relax and when it will stay rigid, in turn affecting whether elimination occurs. Relaxation of the sphincter allows for elimination.

GI Tract Propulsion: Peristalsis

Food is propelled down the GI tract mainly by a wavelike process called *peristalsis.* A snake swallowing its prey illustrates the process. Groups of muscles encircle the GI tract, whereas other groups run along its length (see Figure 4-5). When food is swallowed, coordinated squeezing and shortening by the muscle groups in the esophagus create the first waves. In the stomach, the same muscle action creates a mixing and grinding motion. The most active peristaltic waves occur in the small intestine, about every 4 to 5 seconds (Figure 4-6). In contrast, the large intestine has very sluggish peristalsis, using occasional large contractions to help eliminate the feces.[5]

Peristalsis
A coordinated muscular contraction that serves to propel food down the GI tract.

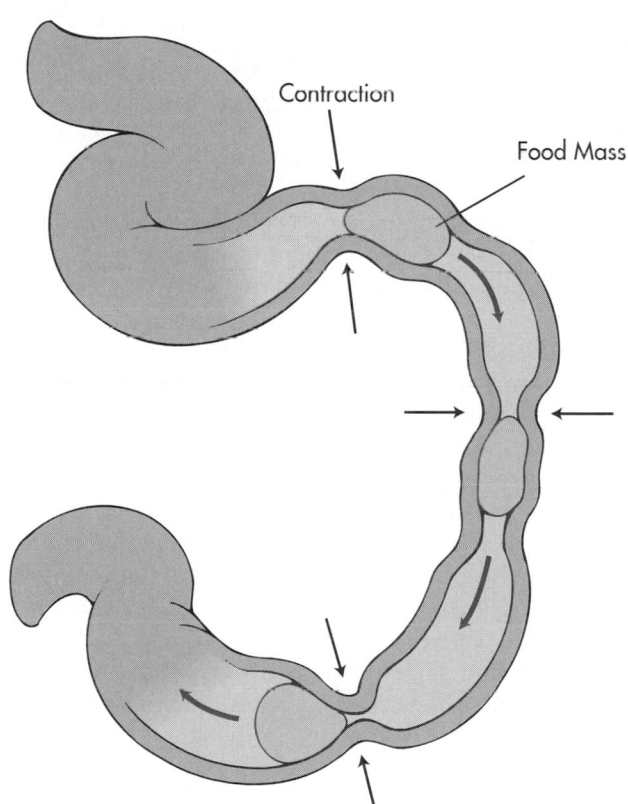

Contraction

Food Mass

Figure 4-6 *Peristalsis. Peristalsis is a progressive type of movement, propelling material from point to point along the GI tract. To begin this, a ring of contraction occurs where the GI wall is stretched, passing the food mass forward. The moving food mass triggers a ring of contraction in the next region, which pushes the food mass even farther along. The net result is a ring of contraction that moves like a wave along the GI tract, pushing the food mass forward.*

Enzymes Play a Vital Role in Digestion

As noted earlier, enzymes are critical to digestion. These substances essentially enhance digestion by making chemical breakdown more likely to happen. Enzymes bring specific chemicals close together and then create an environment that allows the chemicals to change in chemical structure (Figure 4-7). Almost every chemical process in the body, and especially digestive processes, requires an enzyme to hasten the event. Figure 4-7 shows how an enzyme contributes to the breakdown of table sugar (sucrose) into the smaller sugars glucose and fructose. Only the latter sugars are absorbed from the GI tract. The pancreas and small intestine produce most digestive enzymes. A few are secreted by the mouth and stomach.

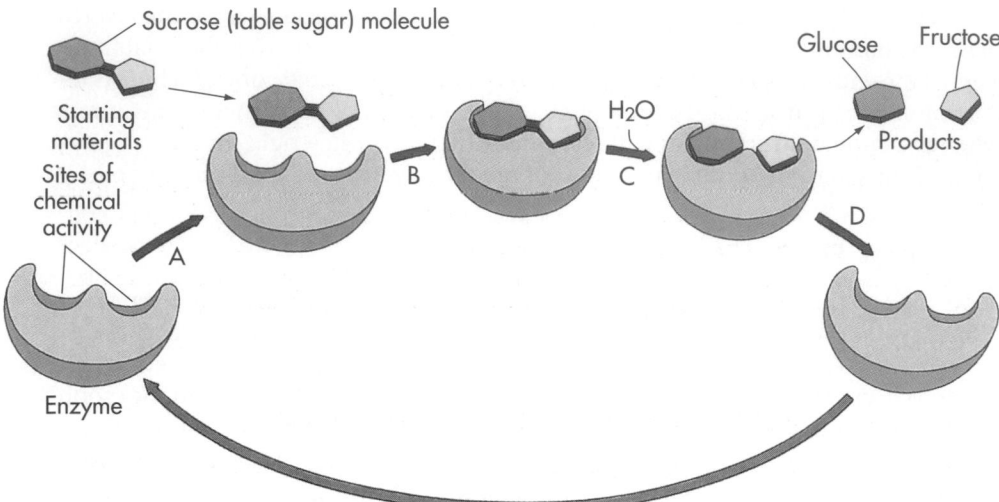

Figure 4-7 *A model of enzyme action. Enzymes act as catalysts to speed chemical reactions, including those that contribute to the digestion of foodstuffs. In this example an enzyme is contributing to the breakdown of sucrose (From **A** to **D**)into the smaller sugar forms glucose and fructose. Only these smaller sugar forms are absorbed from the small intestine to enter the bloodstream. Note that with some enzymes the reaction can go both ways. In addition, sometimes energy input is needed to allow the enzyme to push the reaction along.*

Each type of enzyme can speed only one specific type of chemical process. For example, enzymes that recognize and digest table sugar ignore milk sugar (lactose). The body can even increase the synthesis of certain digestive enzymes in response to the type of diet consumed—for example, producing more fat-digesting enzymes in response to a high-fat diet.[17]

Enzyme actions occur only under rather specific conditions. Besides working only on particular types of chemicals, enzymes are sensitive to acid and alkaline conditions, temperature, and the types of vitamins (acting as **coenzymes**) and minerals they require. Digestive enzymes that work in the acid environment of the stomach do not work well in the alkaline (basic) environment of the small intestine.

Again, the pancreas is a major site of production for digestive enzymes. In **cystic fibrosis**—an inherited disease of infants, children, and sometimes adults—the pancreas is often affected. It develops thick mucus that blocks its ducts, and active cells then die.[19] As a result, the pancreas is not able to effectively deliver its digestive enzymes into the small intestine. Digestion of carbohydrate, protein, and—most notably—fat is impaired because the needed enzymes are not released in adequate amounts. Often these enzymes must be ingested in capsule form with meals to aid in digestion.

Coenzyme

The active form of many vitamins; the coenzyme aids enzyme function.

Cystic fibrosis

A disease that often leads to overproduction of mucus, among other effects. Mucus can invade the pancreas, decreasing enzyme output. The lack of enzyme output then contributes to fat malabsorption.

Concept Check

The gastrointestinal (GI) tract consists of the mouth, esophagus, stomach, small intestine, large intestine (colon), rectum, and anus. Organs associated with the GI tract are the liver, gallbladder, and pancreas. Together these organs perform the digestion needed to extract nutrients from food and funnel them into the bloodstream. In the GI tract, peristalsis propels food from the esophagus to the anus. During this journey, digestion is aided by enzymes produced by the mouth, stomach, pancreas, and small intestine cells. The transit time between eating food and eventually eliminating the indigestible remains is usually about 1 to 3 days.

A Closer Look at the Digestive Process

Even before we eat a morsel of many foods, the work of digestion—the breakdown of foods into usable forms we can absorb—is often already partially accomplished. Cooking or other preparations, such as marinating, pounding, or dicing, have probably begun the process. Starch granules in foods swell as they soak up water during cooking, making them much easier to digest. Cooking also softens the tough connective tissues in meats and the fibrous tissue of plants, such as is found in broccoli stalks. As a result, the food is easier to chew, swallow, and break down during later digestion. As you will see in Chapter 17, cooking also makes many foods, such as eggs, meats, fish, and poultry, much safer to eat.

Key Digestive Processes in the Stomach

The stomach secretes a major enzyme used for protein digestion. The release is controlled by a hormone. Just thinking about or chewing food stimulates nerves in the brain that control special hormone-producing cells in the base of the stomach. The hormone's release signals cells in the stomach to produce enzymes and acid.

You might wonder how the stomach protects itself from the acid and enzymes it produces. First the stomach has a thick layer of mucus that lines and insulates it from the acid and enzymes produced for digestion. The production of acid and enzymes is also tied to the release of a specific hormone, and this release happens primarily when we are thinking about eating or actually in the process of eating. Lastly, as the concentration of acid in the stomach increases, acid production tapers off, also because of hormonal control.[5]

Key Digestive Processes in the Small Intestine

All liquids consumed with a meal combine with stomach acid to form a very watery food mixture called *chyme.* As chyme squirts into the upper small intestine (called the *duodenum*), the acid in the chyme triggers the release of another hormone that stimulates the pancreas to release bicarbonate. This neutralizes the acid. If the chyme is not neutralized, it corrodes the wall of the duodenum, and could quickly lead to an **ulcer,** because, unlike the stomach, the small intestine lacks a protective layer of mucus. This form of protection is not possible because it would impede nutrient absorption. A second hormone causes the pancreas and gallbladder to release their products—enzymes from the pancreas and bile from the gallbladder.

Chyme
A mixture of stomach secretions and partially digested food.

Ulcer
Erosion of the tissue lining in either the stomach or upper small intestine; generally referred to as a peptic ulcer.

In part because of hormonal fine-tuning, the digestive tract responds to the nutritional makeup and amount of the food consumed. Foods generally contain a mixture of macronutrients and vitamins and minerals; therefore a multiple enzymatic attack on the contents of the small intestine is the rule. The contention of the authors of some fad diet books that ingestion of certain combinations of foods, such as meats and fruits together, hinders the digestive process does not make sense in light of both our knowledge about gastrointestinal physiology and our collective experience.

Small Intestine: Site for Most Nutrient Absorption

Most nutrient absorption—that is, the transfer of nutrients from the intestine and to the bloodstream—occurs in the small intestine; little occurs in the stomach and large intestine.[6] The small intestine can absorb about 95% of the energy it receives

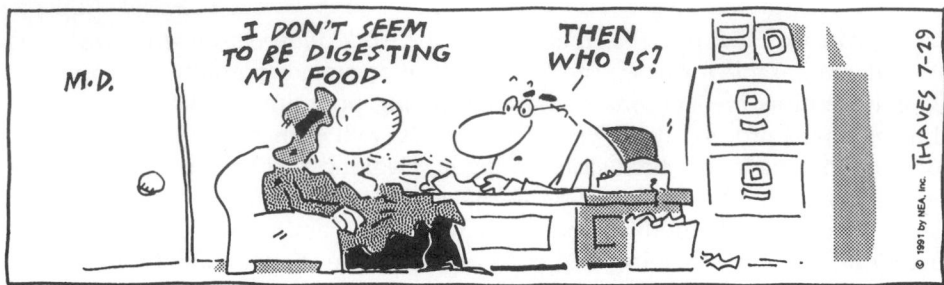

Figure 4-8 *Frank and Ernest. Reprinted by permission of NEA, Inc.*

in the form of protein, carbohydrate, fat, and alcohol (Figure 4-8). The mouth and stomach absorb only water, small amounts of alcohol, certain types of minor fats, and some glucose. The large intestine absorbs some minerals, water, and some fat and carbohydrate by–products (produced by bacterial action).[11]

The enormous surface area of the small intestine promotes efficient nutrient absorption. The wall of the small intestine is folded, and within the folds are fingerlike projections called *villi* (see Figure 4-5). These "fingers" are in constant movement, which helps trap foodstuffs between them to enhance absorption. Each villus "finger" is made up of numerous absorptive cells, and each of these cells has a highly folded cap. The combined folds, fingers, and folded caps in the small intestine increase its surface area 600 times beyond that of a simple tube.[5]

New absorptive cells are constantly produced and appear daily along the surface of each villus "finger," probably because absorptive cells are subjected to a harsh environment. This environment demands constant renewal of the intestinal lining as a biological necessity, and it leads to a high nutrient demand from the small intestine. The health of these cells is further enhanced by the various hormones and other substances that participate in or are produced as part of the digestive process.[17]

Villi

Fingerlike protrusions in the small intestine that participate in digestion and absorption of foodstuffs.

Absorptive cells

A class of cells that line the villi (fingerlike projections in the small intestine) and participate in nutrient absorption.

Passive absorption

Absorption that requires (1) ability of the substance to penetrate the absorptive surface and (2) a higher concentration of the substance in the intestinal lumen than in the absorptive cells. The higher concentration of the substance in the lumen of the intestine in comparison with that in the absorptive cells promotes the absorption of the nutrient.

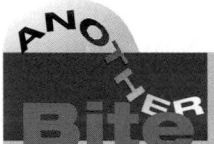

Cancer treatments often involve the use of medications (chemotherapy) to prevent rapid cell growth. Cancer cell growth is the intended target. However, although the medications can slow the growth of rapidly dividing cancer cells, they also affect other body cells that normally reproduce rapidly, such as the absorptive cells in the small intestine. This is the reason that diarrhea is a common side effect of chemotherapy.

Types and Means of Absorption

The small intestine absorbs nutrients into the intestinal cells through various means and processes. For nutrients such as fats the intestine is easily permeable. When the nutrient concentration is higher in the inside cavity (**lumen**) of the small intestine than in the **absorptive cells,** the difference in nutrient concentration drives absorption because nutrients naturally move from higher to lower concentrations. Fats and other nutrients now enter the absorptive cells from the lumen of the small intestine via this **passive absorption** route. Water and some minerals are also absorbed in this way[9] (Figure 4-9).

Another absorption mechanism uses both a carrier protein and energy input to actively pump nutrients from the lumen of the small intestine into the absorptive cells. This makes it possible for the body to take up nutrients even when they are not

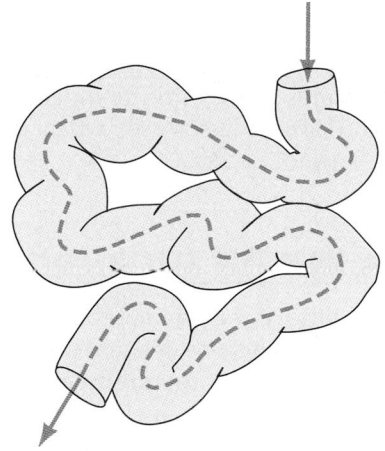

Lumen: The inside of a tube, such as the inside cavity of the GI tract.

Nutrient intake also directly influences nutrient absorption. For example, vitamin C in a meal modestly increases iron absorption in the same meal because it changes elemental iron into a more absorbable state (Fe^{2+}).

concentrated in the diet. Some sugars, for example, follow this route, called *active absorption.* The sugar glucose is much more concentrated in the absorptive cells than in the chyme in the small intestine because the absorptive cells are bathed by the glucose-rich bloodstream. To get glucose into the absorptive cells, given the high concentration already present (an uphill battle, so to speak), it must be pumped in using energy.[9] Still other sugars, such as fructose, follow **facilitated absorption.** A type of carrier protein is used, but no energy is expended in the transfer across the intestinal surface.[15]

Active absorption
Absorption using a carrier protein and expending energy. In this way the absorptive cell absorbs nutrients, such as glucose, when a high concentration of the nutrient is already present in the absorptive cells.

Facilitated absorption
Absorption in which a carrier protein shuttles substances into the absorptive cell but no energy input is needed. A concentration gradient higher in the intestinal contents than in the absorptive cell drives the absorption.

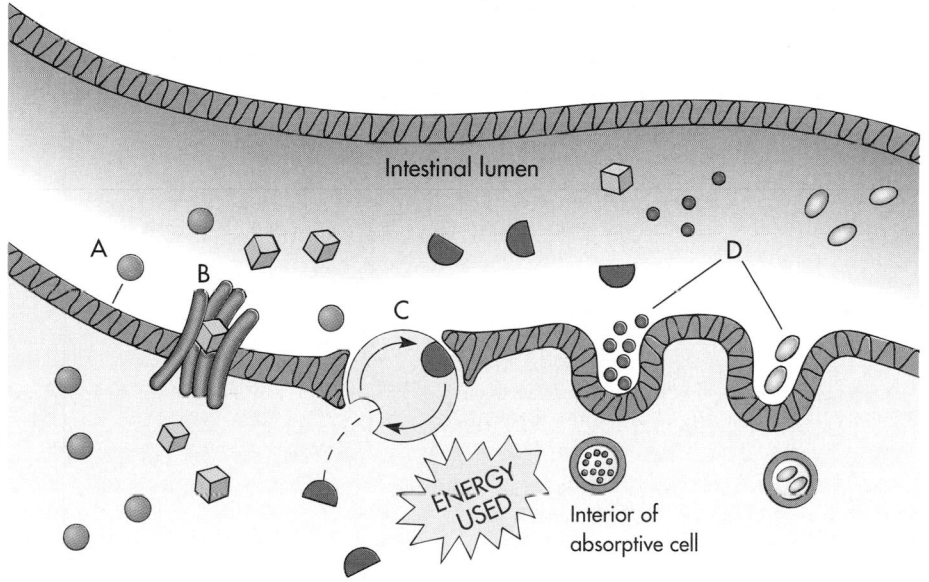

Intestinal lumen

A   B   C   D

ENERGY USED

Interior of absorptive cell

Figure 4-9 *Nutrient absorption relies on these major forms of absorptive processes.* **A,** *Passive absorption involves simple diffusion of substances across the cell membrane of absorptive cells. No energy is expended because the substances follow a favorable concentration gradient (from high to low concentrations). Water and fats are absorbed in this manner.* **B,** *Facilitated absorption uses a carrier protein or other process to aid in absorption of specific substances, such as fructose. No energy is expended; the process is simply aided by the carrier. Fructose undergoes facilitated absorption.* **C,** *Active absorption (transport) uses a carrier protein and expends energy in the process. The use of energy allows the absorptive cell to absorb nutrients against their concentration gradient (from low to high concentrations). Glucose undergoes active absorption.* **D,** *Phagocytosis—"cell eating" involves cells taking in substances, including whole particles, by forming an indentation in the cell membrane and then surrounding the particle, with eventual incorporation into the cell. This is an active form of transport of substances. Pinocytosis—"cell drinking" involves cellular uptake of liquids in a manner analogous to phagocytosis.*

Critical Thinking
The medical history of a young girl who is greatly underweight shows that she had three quarters of her small intestine removed after she was injured in a car accident. Explain how this accounts for her underweight condition, even though her medical chart shows that she eats well.

A further means of active absorption entails the absorptive cells' literally engulfing compounds (phagocytosis) or liquids (pinocytosis). A cell membrane can form an indentation itself so that when particles or fluids move into the indentation, the cell membrane surrounds and engulfs them. This process is used when an infant absorbs immune substances from human milk (see Chapter 13).

The Large Intestine Completes Absorption

When the intestinal contents enter the large intestine, little of the original foodstuff eaten still remains. Only a minor amount (5%) of carbohydrate, protein, and fat has escaped absorption (Figure 4-10). Some water is still present because the small intestine absorbs only 85% to 90% of the fluid it receives, which includes large amounts of GI-tract secretions produced during digestion. The remnants of the meal also include some minerals and food fibers.

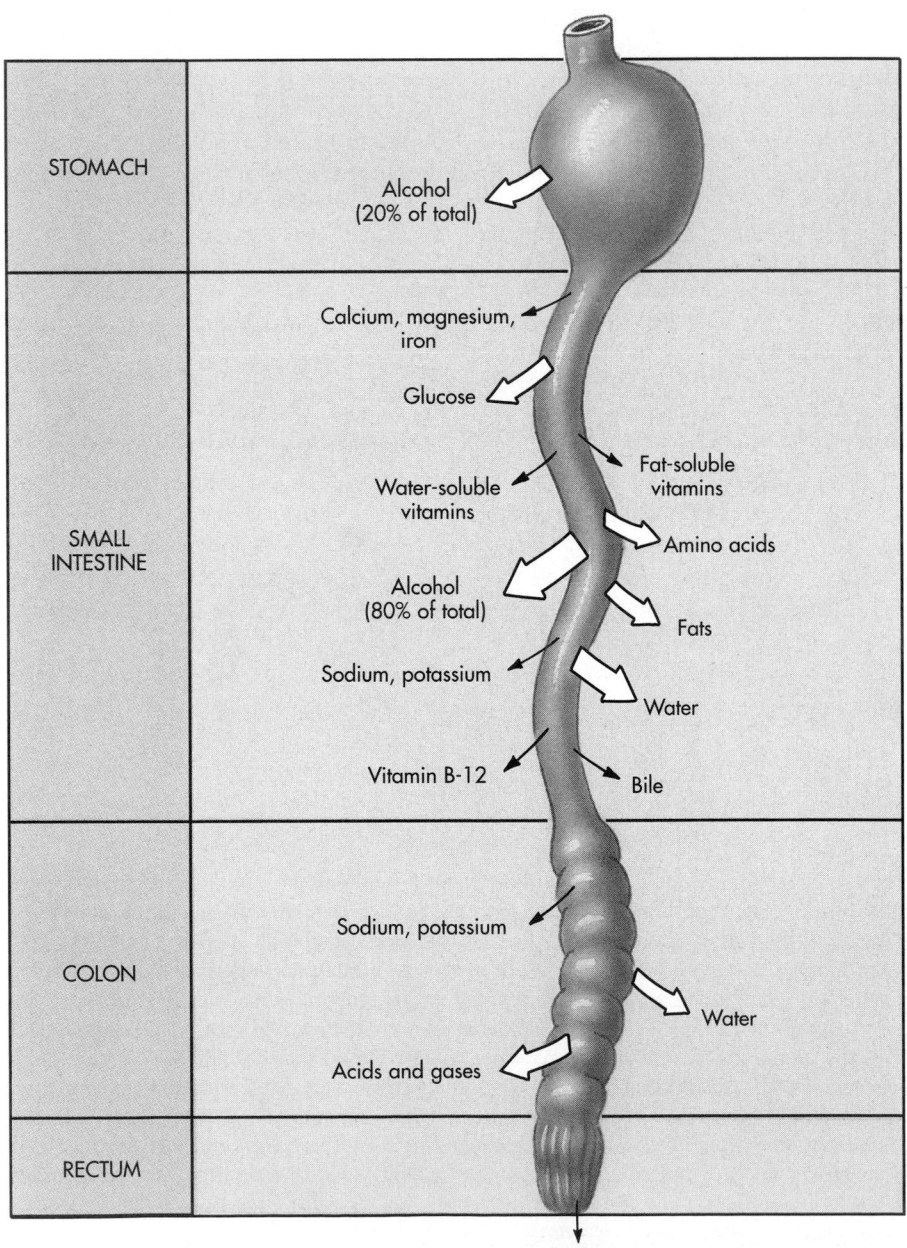

Figure 4-10

Major sites of absorption along the GI tract. The size of the arrow indicates the relative amount of absorption at that site.

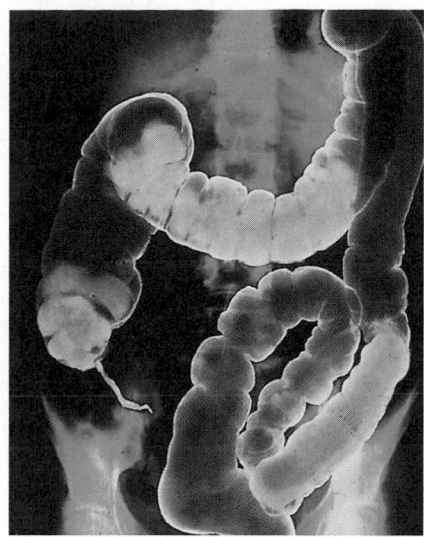

The colon has a large diameter and no villi.

In the upper half of the large intestine, much of the remaining water and the minerals—mostly sodium and potassium—are absorbed. The unabsorbed water now amounts to only a few ounces. Products from the metabolism of certain plant fibers and small amounts of undigested starches are also absorbed.[12] The contents of the large intestine are semisolid by the time they have passed through the first two thirds of it. The stool remains in the last third until muscular movements push it into the rectum to be eliminated. The presence of feces in the rectum stimulates elimination. What remains in the feces, besides water, are indigestible plant fibers, tough connective tissues (from animal foods), bacteria from the large intestine, and some body wastes, such as parts of dead intestinal cells.[5]

When either the small intestine or the pancreas is diseased, it may not produce enough of the important enzymes. People with cystic fibrosis may have this problem, as noted previously. A lack of enzymes can result in poor digestion and, consequently, very poor absorption of nutrients into the bloodstream. This condition accompanies many intestinal diseases. Any foodstuffs that enter the large intestine, rather than being absorbed mostly into the bloodstream from the small intestine, are metabolized by bacteria into acids and gas. A person with poor intestinal function often experiences severe abdominal discomfort caused by intestinal gas. Insufficient enzyme production or not enough time for complete enzyme action is often the source of these problems.[20]

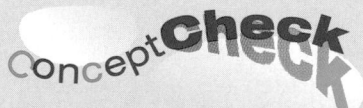

A variety of factors—such as hormones, nerves, muscles, and sphincters—help regulate the rate of digestion. Stomach acid and enzymes contribute to digestion of some foodstuffs. The small intestine is the major site for nutrient digestion and absorption, which are aided by enzymes and bile. Numerous folds and fingerlike projections in the small intestine create a large amount of absorptive surface for nutrient absorption. Because absorptive cells have a life span of only a few days, the lining of the small intestine is constantly renewed. Absorptive cells can perform passive types of absorption promoted by a concentration difference that is greater in the lumen of the intestine than in the absorptive cell. They also perform more active forms of absorption by either overcoming the resistance of high concentrations through the use of a carrier protein and energy input or physically engulfing compounds.

The Immune System—with a Nutrition Focus

Many types of body cells work in co-operation to maintain a defense against infection.[5] It is easy to show the importance of good nutrition for immune function. Early humans were plagued by famine, infections, and death. Today, because of better nutrition, many of us avoid that cycle. In striving to eat healthfully, however, we may easily go too far. Although a proper nutrient intake is needed to maintain immune function, excess quantities can in fact jeopardize it. In reviewing some major components of the immune system—the skin, intestinal cells, and white blood cells—let's also consider how nutrient intake affects each component (Figure 4-11).

Skin

The skin forms an almost continuous barrier surrounding the body. Invading microbes have difficulty penetrating the skin. However, if the skin is split by lesions, bacteria can easily penetrate this barrier. Skin health is hampered by deficiencies of such nutrients as essential fatty acids, vitamin A, niacin, and zinc.[4] Vitamin A deficiency also decreases gland secretions in the skin—necessary secretions that contain enzymes capable of killing bacteria. Bacterial eye infections in citizens of poorer countries are often due to vitamin A deficiency.

Intestinal Cells

The cells of the intestines form an important barrier to invading microbes. Not only are the cells closely packed together, but specialized cells that produce immune bodies—such as immunoglobulins—are also scattered throughout the intestinal tract.[1] These immune bodies bind to the invading microbes, preventing them from entering the bloodstream. This process is called "mucosal immunity." When either protein or vitamin A is deficient, the specialized cells produce fewer immune bodies.

For a person in a nutritionally deficient state, the intestinal cells break down so that microbes more easily enter the body and cause infections. Two common results of undernutrition are diarrhea and bacterial infections of the bloodstream. To protect the health of the intestinal tract, an adequate nutrient intake is necessary—especially of protein; vitamins A, B-6, B-12, and C; folate; zinc; and other nutrients needed for intestinal cell synthesis and maintenance.[4]

White Blood Cells

Once a microbe enters the bloodstream, white blood cells move in to attack it. A variety of types of white blood cells participate in this response and function in unique ways (see Figure 4-11). For example, a class called *phagocytes* circulates throughout the circulatory system, along with other immune system cells, and ingests and some-

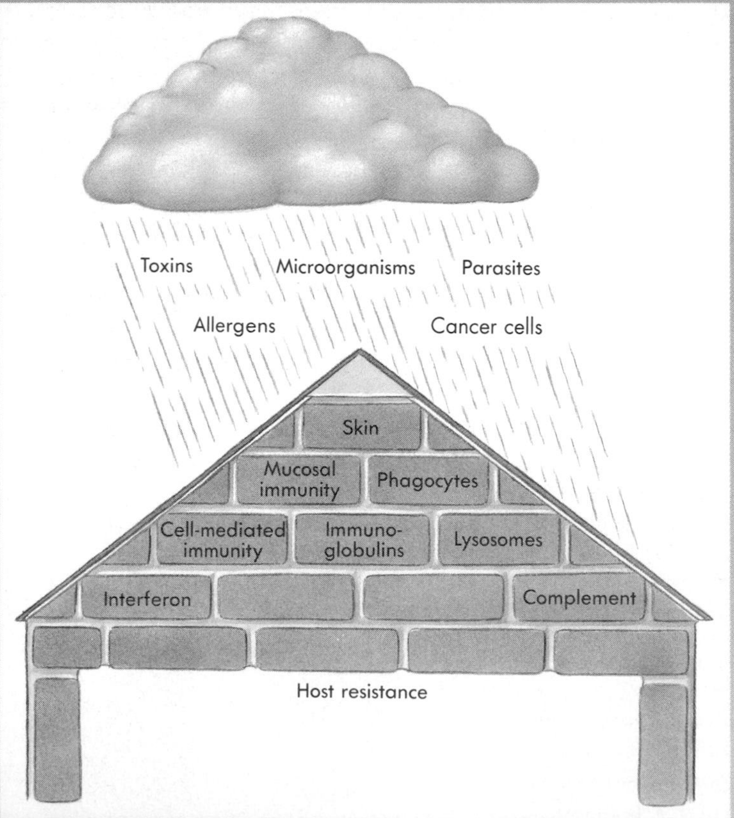

Figure 4-11 *Host protective factors. The immune system has many components, all of which are affected by nutrient intake.*

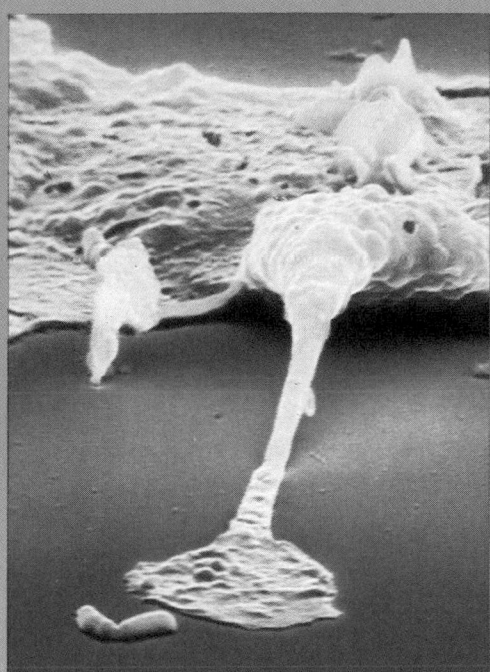

Proteins allow immune processes—like this white blood cell attacking a bacterium—to take place in the body.

One proof that nutrition is important to immune status is the body's response to microbes: microbes normally present in the body usually cause disease only in severely undernourished people. A good example is measles. Your parents probably had this viral infection and survived. (You were probably vaccinated against measles.) However, many undernourished children who contract it die. Thus the presence of a virus or microbe in the body does not guarantee its triumph over the immune system. However, if a person's health is already compromised through undernutrition, the chances that a destructive microbe will win are greater.

An infection that occurs primarily in undernourished people is called an ***opportunistic infection.*** Opportunistic infections are also characteristic of acquired immunodeficiency syndrome (AIDS), a disease in which one class of white blood cells becomes severely depleted. A type of pneumonia that rarely occurs in people with normal immune function is often able to take hold in people with AIDS.[20]

times digests microbes and foreign particles. Other white blood cells participate in cell-mediated immunity, achieved when certain immune cells recognize foreign cells and attack and destroy them. White blood cells, along with proteins in the blood called *immunoglobulins* and *complements,* contribute to an antibody response that binds microorganisms, engulfs and digests them, and then creates a template (memory) that allows future recognition of the microbe. Recognition allows more rapid attacks in the future.[1]

Your nutrient intake affects these white blood cells and protein factors. Some white blood cells live only a few days. Their constant resynthesis requires a steady nutrient input. The immune system needs (1) iron to produce an important killing factor that is used, (2) copper for the synthesis of a specific type of white blood cell, and (3) adequate amounts of protein; vitamins B-6, B-12, and C; and folate for general cell synthesis and, later, cell activity. Zinc and vitamin A are also needed for the overall growth and development of the immune cells.[4]

A Note of Caution

Many studies show that good nutritional status is associated with good immune status. However, other studies also show that an overabundance of certain nutrients can actually harm the immune system. Excess intake of total fat, polyunsaturated fatty acids, and vitamin E has been implicated in a decreased immune response. Taking too much zinc also appears to decrease immune function.[4] This decrease may be partially due to zinc's interference with copper absorption. The copper deficiency contributes to decreased synthesis of a specific class of white blood cells.

The message here is that eating a balanced diet will help us maintain the health of all components of our immune systems. Our bodies need this system to continuously defend us from harmful microbes in the environment. The diets of some older people are a concern in this context because their energy intakes may be too low to meet all nutrient needs. Careful nutrient supplementation, especially with vitamin C and vitamin B-6, then deserves consideration (see Chapter 16 for more details). However, keep in mind that consuming megadoses of nutrients is not going to boost the immune system to even higher abilities. In fact, it can harm certain aspects of immune function.[4]

Urea

Nitrogen-containing waste product found in urine. Most nitrogen excreted from the body leaves in this form.

Excretory System

The kidneys, digestive tract, skin, and lungs all remove wastes from the body. For example, as blood passes through the kidneys, body wastes such as **urea** are removed and shunted into the urine to be excreted (Figure 4-12). Excess intakes of water-soluble nutrients and other substances are also filtered and excreted in that manner. So, if the body already has enough vitamin C, for example, the kidneys screen the extra amount out of the blood and redirect it into the urine. The skin excretes body wastes, along with perspiration, through the pores. The lungs remove the carbon dioxide produced during the metabolism of energy-yielding nutrients, including carbohydrates, fats, and proteins. The carbon dioxide is then exhaled into the air.

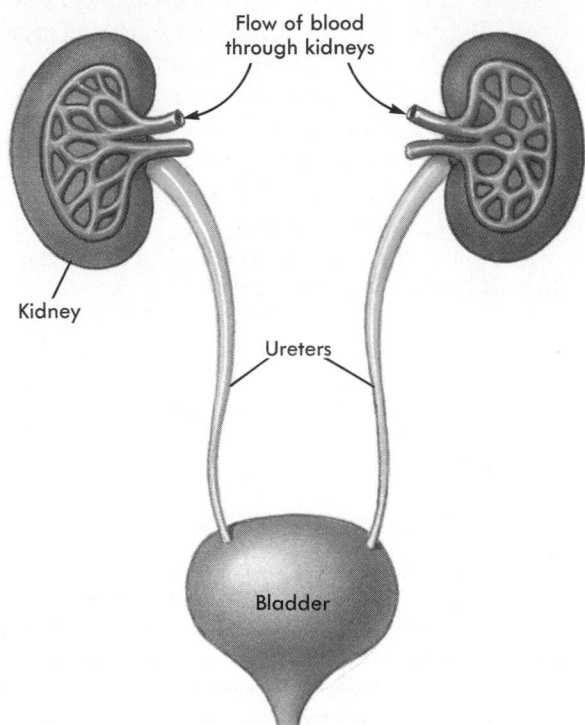

Figure 4-12 *The urinary tract. Blood enters the kidneys by way of the arteries. The kidney filters waste from the blood and sends it as urine to the bladder. The bladder then periodically eliminates the urine.*

Storage Systems

The human body must maintain reserves of nutrients. Otherwise, we would need to eat continuously. Storage capacity varies for each different nutrient. Most fat is stored at sites designed specifically for this—**adipose (fat) tissue.** Short-term storage of carbohydrate occurs in muscle and liver, and the blood maintains a small reserve of glucose and amino acids.[9] Many vitamins and minerals are stored in the liver. Other nutrient stores are found in individual cells.

When people do not meet their nutrient needs, some nutrients are obtained by breaking down a tissue that contains high concentrations of the nutrient. Calcium is taken from bone, and protein is taken from muscle. Neither bones nor muscles are meant to act as nutrient reserves, and nutrient losses in cases of deficiency harm these tissues.

Many people believe that if too much of a nutrient is obtained, for example from a vitamin or mineral supplement, only what is needed is stored and the rest is excreted by the body. Though partially true, as with vitamin C, the large dosages found frequently in supplements such as vitamins A and D can cause harmful side effects because these are not readily excreted. This is one reason that obtaining your nutrients from a balanced diet is the safest means to acquire the building blocks you need to maintain the good health of all body systems.

This review of human anatomy and physiology from a nutrition perspective sets the stage for developing a more detailed understanding of the nutrients. The next three chapters will build on this information.

Adipose (fat) tissue
A grouping of fat-storing cells.

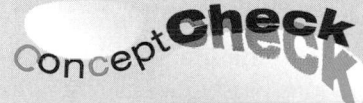

Concept**Check**

The kidneys, skin, and lungs all perform excretory functions of the body. The health of these organ systems depends on a sufficient and appropriate supply of nutrients. Nutrients are constantly present in the blood for immediate use and are stored to a greater or lesser extent in body tissues for later use when sufficient food is unavailable. However, when the body suffers a nutrient deficiency caused by an inadequate diet, it breaks down vital tissues for their nutrients, which can lead to ill health. Additionally, too much of any nutrient can be detrimental. It's best to focus on obtaining all essential nutrients from a balanced diet.

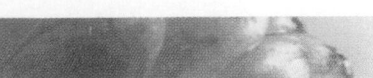

Summary

➤ The cell is the basic building block of body tissues. DNA is the blueprint found in all cells. This determines the cell type, its function and structure, and the kind of chemical each type of cell will produce.

➤ Blood travels the pulmonary circuit, picking up oxygen at the lungs. Then, via the systemic circuit, the blood delivers essential nutrients, energy, oxygen, and water to all body cells. Nutrients and wastes are exchanged between the blood and cells across the cell membrane.

➤ Water-soluble compounds in the villi enter the portal vein and travel to the liver. Fat-soluble compounds enter the lymphatic system, which eventually connects to the bloodstream.

➤ The gastrointestinal (GI) tract consists of the mouth, esophagus, stomach, small intestine, large intestine (colon), rectum, and anus. For the most part, digestion and absorption of nutrients occur in the small intestine.

➤ The liver, gallbladder, and pancreas participate in digestion and absorption. Products from these organs, such as enzymes and bile, enter the small intestine and play important roles in digesting protein, fat, and carbohydrate.

➤ Along the GI tract are ringlike valves (sphincters) that control the flow of food-stuffs. Muscular contractions, called *peristalsis,* propel the foodstuffs down the GI tract. A variety of nerves, hormones, and other substances control the activity of sphincters and peristaltic muscles.

➤ Digestive enzymes are secreted by the mouth, stomach, wall of the small intestine, and pancreas. The presence of food in the small intestine stimulates the release of pancreatic enzymes. Bile needed for fat digestion is synthesized by the liver, stored in the gallbladder, and released in digestion, as directed by hormonal action.

➤ The major absorptive sites consist of fingerlike projections called *villi,* located in the small intestine. Absorptive cells cover the villi. This intestinal lining is continually renewed. Absorptive cells can perform various passive and active forms of absorption and are able to absorb substances by physically engulfing them.

➤ Little digestion and absorption occur in the stomach or large intestine, but some protein is digested in the stomach. Some plant fibers and undigested starch are digested by bacteria in the large intestine; undigested plant fibers are eliminated in the feces.

➤ Final water and mineral absorption takes place in the large intestine. Products from bacterial breakdown of some plant fibers and other substances are also absorbed here. The presence of feces in the rectum provides a strong impetus for elimination.

➤ The kidneys, skin, and lungs all perform excretory functions for the body. Limited stores of nutrients are present in the blood for immediate use and stored to a greater or lesser extent in body tissues for later use when sufficient food is unavailable. When the body suffers a nutrient deficiency caused by a poor diet, it breaks down vital tissues for their nutrients, which can lead to ill health. Additionally, too much of any nutrient can be detrimental.

Study Questions

1 Provide examples of cells in the digestive system that carry out different tasks.

2 Explain how the nerves and hormones interact in "priming" the digestive tract.

3 Describe the physiological mechanisms by which the health and absorptive abilities of the cells of the small intestine are protected.

4 Outline the possible results of a highly diseased pancreas throughout the digestive process.

5 Explain why the small intestine is better suited than the other GI tract organs to carry out the absorptive process.

6 Explain where and how each of the following nutrients is absorbed:
  a Glucose
  b Fats
  c Amino acids
  d Water

7 Show where acid is secreted and how its production is controlled. What are its roles in digestion?

8 Describe the actions of the digestive hormones.

9 Indicate how blood is routed through the digestive system. Which nutrients enter the bloodstream directly? Which nutrients are first absorbed into the lymph?

References

1 Abbas AK, Lichtman AH, Pober JS: *Cellular and molecular immunology,* ed 2, Philadelphia, 1994, WB Saunders.

2 Axel R: The molecular logic of smell, *Scientific American,* p 154, October 1995.

3 Bonis PAL, Norton RA: The challenge of irritable bowel syndrome, *American Family Physician* 53:1229, 1996.

4 Chandra RK: Effects of nutrition on the immune system, *Nutrition* 10:207, 1994.

5 Ganong WF: *Review of medical physiology,* ed 15, Norwalk, Conn, 1995, Appleton & Lange.

6 Lentze MJ: Molecular and cellular aspects of hydrolysis and absorption, *American Journal of Clinical Nutrition* 61:946S, 1995.

7 Marshall BJ: Helicobacter pylori: The etiologic agent for peptic ulcer, *Journal of the American Medical Association* 274:1064, 1995.

8 Marshall JB: Severe gastroesophageal reflux disease, *Postgraduate Medicine* 97(5):98, 1995.

9 Mayes PA: Nutrition, digestion, and absorption. In Murray RK and others, editors: *Harper's Biochemistry,* Norwalk, Conn, 1993, Appleton & Lange.

10 Metcalf A: Anorectal disorders, *Postgraduate Medicine* 98:81, 1995.

11 Nordgaard I, Mortensen PB: Digestive processes in the colon, *Nutrition* 11:37, 1995.

12 Phillips J and others: Effect of resistant starch on fecal bulk and fermentation-dependent events in humans, *American Journal of Clinical Nutrition* 62:121, 1995.

13 Rao SSC: Functional colonic and anorectal disorders, *Postgraduate Medicine* 98:115, 1995.

14 Raymond KF: Gastroenterology and hepatology, *Journal of the American Medical Association* 273:1679, 1995.

15 Riby JE and others: Fructose absorption, *American Journal of Clinical Nutrition* 58:748S, 1993.

16 Roberfroid MB and others: Colonic microflora: nutrition and health, *Nutrition Reviews* 53:127, 1995.

17 Schneeman B: Nutrition and gastrointestinal function, *Nutrition Today,* p 20, Jan/Feb 1993.

18 Soll AH: Medical treatment of peptic ulcer disease, *Journal of the American Medical Association* 275:622, 1996.

19 Welsh MJ, Smith AE: Cystic fibrosis, *Scientific American,* p 52, December 1995.

20 Wilson JD and others: *Harrison's Principles of internal medicine,* ed 13, New York, 1994, McGraw-Hill.

21 Woodtli W, Owyang C: Duodenal pH governs interdigestive motility in humans, *American Journal of Physiology* 268:G146, 1995.

RATE

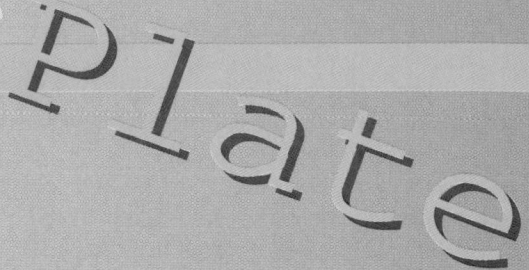

The Anatomy and Physiology of Digestion and Absorption

Label each organ shown in the figure below and note if (and if so, how) it participates in digesting, absorbing, and/or ultimately excreting the remains of what you ate for dinner last night. Later chapters cover the digestion and absorption of each nutrient in detail. Use this exercise to build your knowledge.

Pancreas	Epiglottis	Large intestine (colon)
Trachea	Pyloric sphincter	Rectum
Esophagus	Anus	Small intestine
Liver	Salivary glands	Gallbladder
Stomach	Mouth	Common bile duct

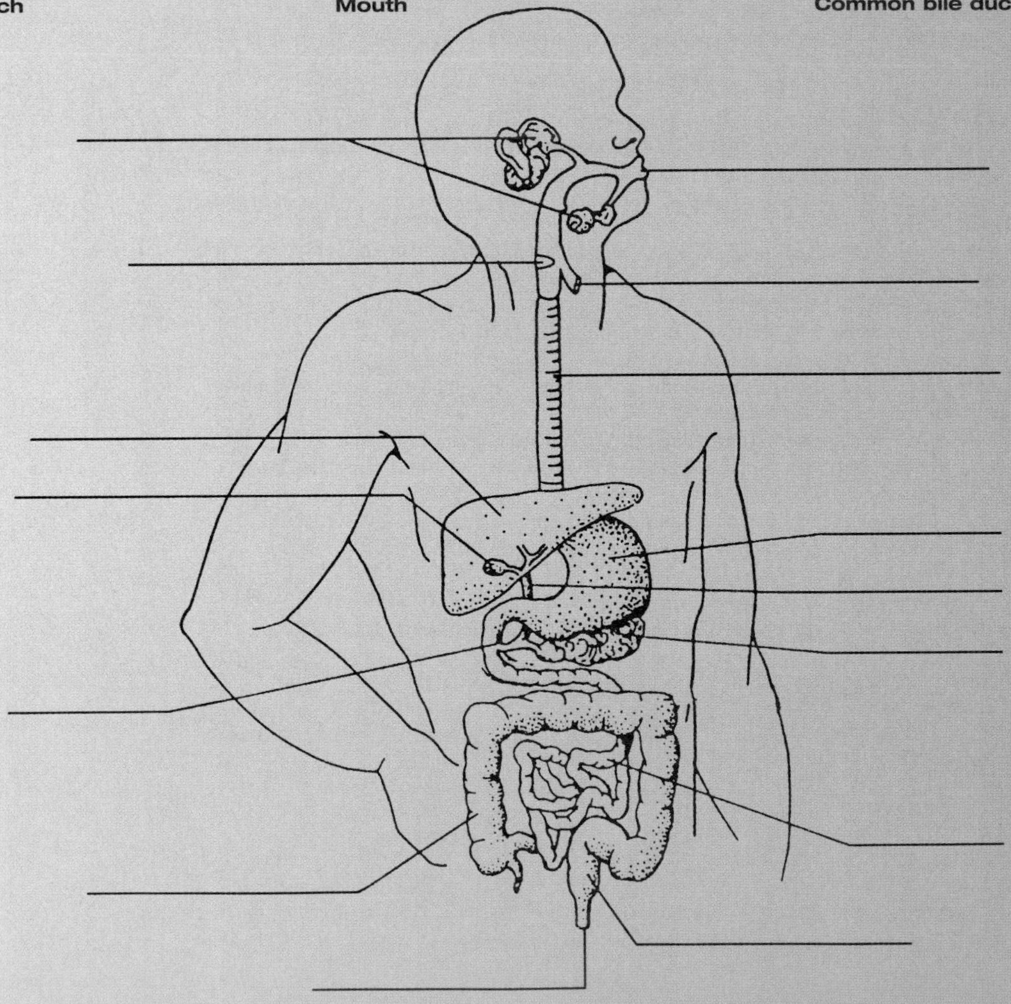

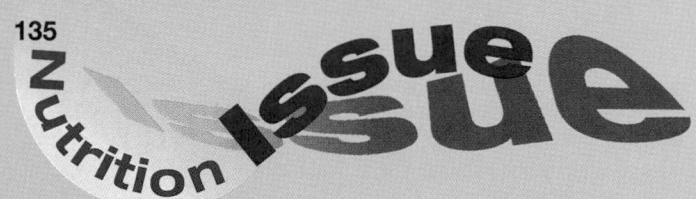

When the Digestive Processes Go Awry

The fine-tuned organ system we call the *GI tract* can develop problems. Knowing about these common problems can help you avoid them.

ULCERS

Many adults develop ulcers each year. The principal causes are a specific bacterial infection, use of aspirin and related medications, and disorders that cause excessive acid production in the stomach.[8] As the stomach lining deteriorates and loses its mucus layer protection, the acid erodes the stomach tissue. This specific chain of events will result in a gastric ulcer. Acid can also erode the tissue lining of the first part of the small intestine, the duodenum, and result in a duodenal ulcer. *Peptic ulcer* is the general term for both of these two cases.[20]

Some people are more susceptible to ulcers than others because their stomach and intestinal cells are less able to protect themselves from acid. In addition, recent research suggests that an infection by bacteria (specifically *Helicobacter pylori*) is an important cause of most ulcers.[14] Antibiotic and bismuth therapy directed at this bacterium, in combination with agents to decrease acid production by the stomach, is becoming part of routine care for ulcer patients who show evidence of a *Helicobacter pylori* infection.[18]

Most ulcers in young people occur in the duodenum; in older people they occur primarily in the stomach. The typical symptom of an ulcer is pain about 2 hours after eating. Digestive acids acting on a meal irritate the ulcer after most of the meal has moved to the jejunum area of the small intestine.

The primary risk associated with an ulcer is the possibility that it will eat entirely through (perforate) the stomach or intestinal wall. The GI contents could then spill into the body cavities, causing a massive infection, called *peritonitis*. In addition, an ulcer may erode a blood vessel, leading to massive blood loss (hemorrhage). For these reasons we should not ignore early warning signs of ulcer development.[20]

In the past, milk and cream therapy—the Sippy diet—was used to help cure ulcers. Clinicians now know that milk and cream are two of the worst foods for an ulcer. The calcium in these foods stimulates stomach acid secretion and actually inhibits ulcer healing.

Today a combination of approaches is used for ulcer therapy. As noted above, people infected with *Helicobacter pylori* are given medications to eradicate that agent. Antacid medications may also be part of ulcer

care. There is also a class of medicines called *H_2 blockers.* These include cimetidine (Tagamet), ranitidine (Zantac), and fa-motidine (Pepcid), all of which prevent histamine-related acid secretion in the stomach. The stomach cells produce histamine, and the diet supplies histamine from the breakdown of the amino acid histidine.

H_2 blockers
Medications such as cimetidine (Tagamet) that block the increase of stomach acid production caused by histamine.

Some of these medications are now available over the counter in nonprescription doses for cases of indigestion and heartburn (see next section). Medications that coat the ulcer, such as sucralfate (Carafate), are also commonly used today. Finally, medications that reduce acid production by the stomach, such as omeprazole (Prilosec), can be employed.[18]

People with ulcers should also refrain from smoking and minimize the use of aspirin and other related compounds. These practices reduce the mucus secreted by the stomach. Overall, this combination of medical and lifestyle therapies has so revolutionized ulcer therapy that dietary changes are of minor importance today (Table 4-3). Current diet-therapy approaches recommend simply avoiding foods that increase ulcer symptoms.

Stomach acid is not a problem for those not prone to or currently experiencing ulcers. The acid in the stomach enhances absorption of iron, calcium, and vitamin B-12. Acid also minimizes bacterial growth in the stomach; the stomach is essentially bacteria free because of its high acid content. Bacteria in food are quickly destroyed, which reduces the risk of these bacteria forming cancer-causing agents or leading to food-borne illness (see Chapter 17). Thus acid production by the stomach is an important part of the physiology of digestion and absorption.[9] This means that despite their usual presence alongside the breath mints in a convenience store, antacids should not be used excessively. If an antacid contains magnesium (and many do), magnesium toxicity is another possible result of antacid abuse.

HEARTBURN

Many adults regularly have heartburn. This gnawing pain in the upper chest is caused by the movement of acid from the stomach into the esophagus.[8] Unlike the stomach, the

Continued.

TABLE 4-3

Recommendations to Prevent Ulcers and Heartburn from Occurring or Recurring[20]

ULCERS

1. Stop smoking, if you are now a smoker.

2. Avoid aspirin, ibuprofen, and other aspirinlike compounds unless a physician advises otherwise.

3. Limit coffee, tea, and alcohol (especially wine), if this helps.

4. Limit pepper, chili powder, and other strong spices, if this helps.

5. Eat nutritious meals on a regular schedule.

6. Chew foods well.

7. Lose weight if you are currently overweight.

HEARTBURN

1. Wait about 3 hours after a meal before lying down.

2. Don't overeat at mealtime. Smaller meals that are low in fat are advised.

3. Observe the recommendations for ulcer prevention.

esophagus has no mucous lining to protect it, so acid quickly erodes the lining of the esophagus, causing pain.

An important dietary measure for avoiding heartburn is to eat smaller meals, especially meals that are low in fat (see Table 4-3). Fatty meals remain in the stomach longer than low-fat meals. The large volume of food and secretions that remains in the stomach creates pressure that can force the stomach contents up into the esophagus.

Several other steps may be taken to prevent heartburn. Cigarette smokers should quit smoking. In addition, it is best not to lie down after eating and to avoid foods and other substances that can specifically contribute to heartburn, such as chili powder, onions, garlic, peppermint, caffeine, alcohol, and chocolate. Individuals should discover irritants and tailor their diets accordingly.[20]

Certain physical conditions can lead to heartburn. For example, both pregnancy and obesity result in increased production of estrogen and progesterone. These hormones relax the lower esophageal (cardiac) sphincter, making heartburn more likely. A pregnant woman may find it helpful to eat smaller, more frequent meals. An obese person should slim down to a more healthy weight so that blood concentrations of these hormones decrease. Adipose (fat) tissue turns certain circulating hormones into estrogen; thus the more adipose tissue, the more estrogen is produced.

Occasional heartburn can be treated medically with antacids, over-the-counter H_2 blockers, and bismuth agents. Heartburn that recurs several times a week for at least a month should be investigated by a physician. Long-standing heartburn may require aggressive medical therapy because it can lead to alteration in the cells of the esophagus, which increases the risk of a rare form of cancer.[20]

CONSTIPATION AND LAXATIVES

Constipation, which is difficult or infrequent evacuation of the bowels, is commonly reported by adults. Slow movement of fecal material through the large intestine causes constipation. As fluid is increasingly absorbed during the extended time the feces stay in the large intestine, they become dry and hard.

Constipation
A condition characterized by infrequent bowel movements.

Constipation can result when people regularly inhibit their normal bowel reflexes for long periods.[13] People tend to ignore normal urges when it is inconvenient to interrupt occupational or social activities. Muscle spasms of an irritated large intestine can also slow the movement of feces and contribute to constipation. Medications such as antacids can also cause constipation.

Constipation is difficult to diagnose. The normal frequency of bowel movements is 3 to 12 times per week, varying from person to person. The best indication of constipation is unusually hard, dry feces at infrequent intervals, rather than failure to meet a general prescription of "once a day." Sudden, prolonged changes in the frequency of bowel movements should be evaluated by a physician. This may be a warning that a more serious intestinal disorder is developing.[13]

Eating foods with plenty of dietary fiber, such as whole-grain breads and cereals, is the best alternative for treating typical cases of constipation. Dietary fibers stimulate peristalsis by drawing water into the large intestine and helping form a bulky, soft fecal output. People with constipation should also drink more fluids. Eating dried fruits can help stimulate the bowel. In addition, people with constipation may need to develop more regular bowel habits; allowing the same time each day for a bowel movement can help train the large intestine to respond routinely. Finally, relaxation facilitates regular bowel movements, as does regular physical activity.[13]

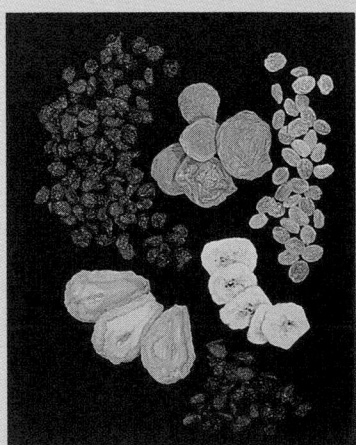

Eating dried fruit is another excellent way to increase your dietary fiber intake.

Laxative

A medication or other substance that stimulates evacuation of the intestinal tract.

Laxatives can also lessen constipation by irritating the intestinal nerve junctions to stimulate the peristaltic muscles or drawing water into the intestine to enlarge fecal output. The larger output stretches the peristaltic muscles, making them rebound and then constrict. Regular use of laxatives, especially irritating ones, can decrease muscle action in the large intestine, causing more constipation. The GI tract can in time actually become dependent on laxatives. Thus it is unwise for anyone to use laxatives routinely, although people in certain circumstances—for example, those who are bedridden or quite elderly—may need periodic help from laxatives to relieve constipation.[20]

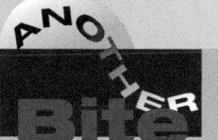

Perhaps you have heard that taking laxatives after overeating prevents deposition of body fat from the excess energy intake. This erroneous and dangerous premise has gained popularity among followers of numerous fad diets. You may temporarily feel less full after using a laxative because laxatives hasten emptying of the large intestine and increase fluid loss. Most laxatives, however, do not speed the passage of food through the small intestine, where digestion and most nutrient absorption take place. As a result, laxatives do not prevent fat gain from excess energy intake.

HEMORRHOIDS

Hemorrhoids, also called *piles,* are swollen veins of the rectum and anus. The blood vessels in this area are subject to intense pressure, especially during bowel movements. Added stress to the vessels from pregnancy, obesity, prolonged sitting, violent coughing or sneezing, or straining during bowel movements can lead to a hemorrhoid. Hemorrhoids can develop unnoticed until a strained bowel movement precipitates symptoms, which may include pain, itching, and bleeding.[10]

Itching, caused by moisture in the anal canal, swelling, or other irritation, is perhaps the most common symptom. Pain, if present, is usually aching and steady. Bleeding may result from a hemorrhoid and may appear in the toilet as a bright red streak in the feces. The sensation of a mass in the anal canal after a bowel movement is symptomatic of an internal hemorrhoid that protrudes through the anus.

Anyone can develop a hemorrhoid, and about half of adults over age 50 do. Pressure from prolonged sitting or exertion is often enough to bring on symptoms, although diet, lifestyle, and possibly heredity play a role. If you think you have a hemorrhoid, you should consult your physician. Rectal bleeding, although usually caused by hemorrhoids, may also indicate other problems, such as cancer.[20]

Hemorrhoids

Swollen veins of the rectum and anus, often protruding into the anus.

A physician may suggest a variety of self-care measures for hemorrhoids. Pain can be lessened by applying warm, soft compresses or sitting in a tub of warm water for 15 to 20 minutes. Dietary recommendations are the same as those for treating constipation, emphasizing the need to consume adequate dietary fiber and fluid.[10] Over-the-counter remedies can also offer relief of symptoms.

IRRITABLE BOWEL SYNDROME

Many adults have irritable bowel syndrome, a combination of cramps, gassiness, bloating, and irregular bowel function (diarrhea, constipation, or alternating episodes of both). It is more common in women than in men. A hallmark of the disease is pain relief after a bowel movement. The cause is thought to be altered intestinal peristalsis, coupled with a decreased pain threshold for abdominal distention. In other words, a minor amount of abdominal bloating causes pain that the average person would not sense.

Therapy is individualized and can include a trial of high-fiber foods; elimination diets that focus on avoiding dairy products and gas-forming foods, such as legumes and certain other vegetables; medications to treat the diarrhea or constipation; stress-reduction strategies; and psychological counseling.[3] Low-fat meals and smaller, more frequent meals may also help because large meals can trigger large intestine contractions. Although irritable bowel syndrome can be uncomfortable and upsetting, it is harmless; it carries no risk for cancer or other serious digestive problems.[20]

Carbohydrates

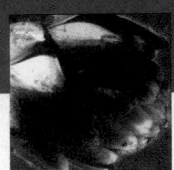

WHAT DID YOU EAT TO OBTAIN the energy you are using right now? The next three chapters will examine this question by focusing on the nutrients the human body uses for fuel. These energy-yielding nutrients are mainly carbohydrates (at 4 kcal per gram) and fats and oils (at 9 kcal per gram). Not much protein (at 4 kcal per gram) is used to fuel the body. Most people know that potatoes have carbohydrates and steak has fat and protein, but few people know what those terms signify. Knowing more about them helps you choose appropriate foods for your needs.

You have probably recently consumed fruits, vegetables, dairy products, cereals, breads, and pasta. All these foods supply you with carbohydrates. Unfortunately, the benefits of these foods are often misunderstood. Many people think carbohydrate-rich foods are necessarily fattening—they are not. In fact, they are much less fattening than fats and oils, pound for pound. Some people think sugars cause diabetes or hyperactivity—both highly unlikely. If you see carbohydrates as being unhealthful, it is unfortunate. In fact, carbohydrates, especially starch-rich foods, have been the class of nutrients most promoted by diet recommendations in the last 20 years and should constitute more than half your daily energy intake.[19,23] The link between fat—especially animal fat—and heart disease should prompt us all to switch our focus away from high-fat foods toward more high-carbohydrate foods. It is unfortunate that affluence tends to drive us the other way.

Examining Your Sugar Habits

One of the Dietary Guidelines for Americans you learned about in Chapter 2 says, "choose a diet moderate in sugars." In this chapter you will learn facts and fallacies about this recommendation. Complete this quiz about your sugar habits. Put a "Y" in the blank to the right of the questions to indicate yes and an "N" to indicate no. Don't answer the questions in the way you think they should be answered but according to what you generally do.

1. Do you read the ingredient labels to identify added sugars in a product? ____

2. Do you try to select items lower in sugar when possible? ____

3. Do you buy fresh fruits or fruits packed in water, juice, or light syrup, rather than those in heavy syrup? ____

4. Do you generally avoid or limit the serving size of foods high in sugar, such as prepared baked goods, candies, sweet desserts, soft drinks, and fruit-flavored punches? ____

5. Do you purposely try to reduce the sugar in foods you prepare at home? ____

6. Do you experiment with spices—such as cinnamon, nutmeg, and ginger—to enhance the flavor of foods, rather than using a lot of sugar? ____

7. Do you use home-prepared items (with less sugar) when possible instead of commercially prepared ones that are higher in sugar? ____

8. Do you try to use less of all sugars (white and brown sugar, honey, molasses, and syrups)? ____

9. Do you often reach for fresh fruit instead of sweets for dessert or when you want a snack? ____

10. Do you try to minimize the addition of sugar to foods, such as coffee, tea, cereal, and fruit? ____

INTERPRETATION

For every "Y" give yourself 0 points and for every "N" 1 point. Record your total points (from 0 to 10) in this blank. ____

The Dietary Guideline "Choose a diet moderate in sugars" encourages Americans to evaluate their total intake of sweetened foods and sugar. The higher your score on the quiz, the more you should reevaluate your sugar intake in an effort to comply with the Dietary Guideline. Although a current emphasis in diet planning is placed on increasing the total amount of carbohydrate in the diet, this should come mainly from grain, fruit, and vegetable sources. It's wise to keep an eye on carbohydrate intake from mainly sugar sources, such as regular soft drinks. Look through your answers and identify ways you could reduce your sugar intake. In the space below write one easy way.

_____
_____

As you read this chapter, you will find out how to and why you should examine your sugar intake, as well as reasons to examine whether you need to increase your starch and dietary fiber intake.

Key Chapter Concepts

- The simple sugars in our diets are made up primarily of monosaccharides and disaccharides.
- The monosaccharides include glucose, fructose, and galactose. Once absorbed via the small intestine and transported to the liver, much of the fructose and galactose is turned into glucose.
- The major disaccharides are sucrose (glucose plus fructose), maltose (glucose plus glucose), and lactose (glucose plus galactose). When digested, these yield monosaccharide forms.
- Starches are a more complex form of carbohydrate, containing multiple glucose units linked together. Glycogen is an animal form of starch that acts as a storage form of glucose in the liver and muscles.
- Dietary fibers include the indigestible forms of large carbohydrates—cellulose, hemicelluloses, pectins, gums, and mucilages—as well as the noncarbohydrate lignins. Dietary fiber, especially insoluble varieties, provides mass to the stool, thus easing elimination.
- Some starch digestion occurs in the mouth. Carbohydrate digestion is completed in the small intestine. Some plant fibers are digested by bacteria in the large intestine; undigested plant fibers end up in the feces.
- Lactose intolerance is a condition that results when cells of the intestine do not make sufficient lactase, the enzyme necessary to digest lactose. Undigested lactose travels to the large intestine, resulting in symptoms such as abdominal gas, pain, and diarrhea. Some people with lactose intolerance can tolerate cheeses and yogurt.
- Carbohydrates provide energy (4 kcal per gram), protect against needless metabolism of protein for energy, and provide flavor and sweetness to foods. Many carbohydrates can be metabolized to acids by bacteria on teeth. The acid can erode the tooth surface, leading to dental caries.
- A minimal intake of carbohydrate is 50 to 100 grams per day; 55% or more of total energy intake is good goal.
- Diets should be high in complex carbohydrates rather than fat. Starches such as potatoes, grains, pastas, fruits, and vegetables—essentially the bottom half of the Food Guide Pyramid—should be emphasized.
- The current advice for sugar intake is moderation. The use of alternative sweeteners such as aspartame can help in limiting sugar intake.

Forms of Simple Carbohydrates

Green plants create the carbohydrates in our foods. Leaves capture the sun's solar energy in special areas of their cells and transform it to chemical energy. This energy is then used to produce glucose from the carbon dioxide that leaves take from the air and the water that roots bring up from the soil. This complex process is called *photosynthesis*.

Photosynthesis

Process by which plants use solar energy from the sun to synthesize energy-yielding compounds, such as glucose.

Sugar

A simple carbohydrate with the chemical composition $(CH_2O)_n$.

$$\text{6 Carbon dioxide} + \text{6 Water} \rightarrow \text{The carbohydrate glucose} + \text{6 Oxygen}$$
$$(CO_2) \qquad\qquad (H_2O) \qquad\qquad (C_6H_{12}O_6) \qquad\qquad (O_2)$$

As the name suggests, most carbohydrate molecules are composed of carbon, hydrogen, and oxygen atoms. Simple forms of carbohydrates are called *sugars.* Larger, more complex forms are primarily called either *starches* or *dietary fibers,* depending on their digestibility by human GI tract enzymes. Starches are the digestible form.

Monosaccharides—Glucose, Fructose, and Galactose

Monosaccharide

A simple sugar, such as glucose, that is not broken down further during digestion.

Monosaccharides are the single sugar forms (*mono* means one) that serve as the basic unit of all sugar structures. Glucose is the major monosaccharide found in the body (Figure 5-1). Glucose is also known as *dextrose* or *blood sugar* because it is the major form of sugar found in the bloodstream. Glucose is a primary source of energy for human cells, although foods contain little in this form. Most glucose

Monosaccharides

Glucose

Fructose

Galactose

Disaccharides

Sucrose: glucose + fructose
Lactose: glucose + galactose
Maltose: glucose + glucose

Sucrose

Figure 5-1 *Some common sugars. Sucrose and fructose are the most common sugars in our diets.*

comes from sucrose (common table sugar), which is made up of the sugars glucose and fructose.[13] For the most part, sugars in foods are eventually converted to glucose in the liver and thus readily serve as a source of cellular energy.

Fructose, also called *levulose* or *fruit sugar,* is another common sugar. After it is consumed, fructose is absorbed by the small intestine and then transported to the liver, where it is quickly metabolized. Much is converted to glucose, and the rest goes on to form other compounds.[22] Most of the fructose as such in our diets comes from the use of **high-fructose corn syrup** in food production (see later discussion). Fructose also forms half of sucrose, as previously noted, and is found in fruits.

The sugar **galactose** has nearly the same structure as glucose. Large quantities of pure galactose do not exist in nature.[3] Instead, galactose is usually found attached to glucose in lactose, a sugar found in milk and other dairy products. After it is absorbed, galactose arrives in the liver. There it is either transformed into glucose per se or further metabolized. One product of this metabolism is glycogen, a special storage form of glucose found in liver and muscle.

Now is a good time to begin emphasizing a key concept in nutrition: the difference between *intake* of a substance and the body's *use* of that substance. The body often does not use all nutrients in their original states. Some of these substances are broken down and later reassembled into the same or a different substance when and where necessary. For example, much of the galactose in the diet is metabolized to glucose. When later required, as in the mammary gland of the lactating female, galactose is resynthesized by way of a wide variety of compounds.

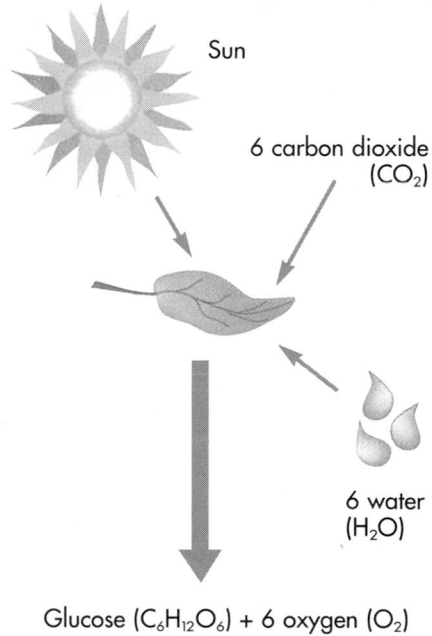

Sun

6 carbon dioxide
(CO_2)

6 water
(H_2O)

Glucose ($C_6H_{12}O_6$) + 6 oxygen (O_2)
Glucose is stored in the leaf, but can also undergo further metabolism

Disaccharides—Sucrose, Lactose, and Maltose

Disaccharides are formed when two monosaccharides combine (*di* means two). The most common disaccharides in food are sucrose, lactose, and maltose.

Sucrose—common table sugar—forms when the two sugars glucose and fructose join together. Sucrose is found in sugar cane, sugar beets, honey, and maple sugar. Animals do not produce it.

Disaccharides
Class of sugars formed by chemically linking two monosaccharides.

Lactose forms when glucose joins with galactose. Again, our major food source for lactose is milk products. A later Nutrition Insight discusses the problems that result when a person can't readily digest lactose.

Maltose forms when two glucose molecules combine. Maltose is of nutritional interest primarily because of its role in alcohol production in the beer and liquor industry. In the production of alcoholic beverages, starches in various cereal grains are first converted to simpler carbohydrates by enzymes present in the grains. The end products of this step—maltose, glucose, and other sugars—are then mixed with yeast cells in the absence of oxygen. The yeast cells convert most of the sugars to alcohol (ethanol) and carbon dioxide, a process termed *fermentation*. Little maltose remains in the final product. Few other food products and beverages contain maltose. In fact, most occurs during digestion of starch and in the mouth and small intestine.[22]

Monosaccharides and disaccharides are often referred to as *simple sugars* because they contain few sugar units. Food labels lump all these sugars under one category, listing them as "sugars."[19]

Fermentation

The conversion, without the use of oxygen, of carbohydrates to alcohols, acids, and carbon dioxide.

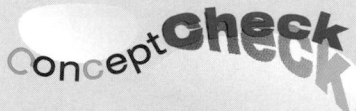

Important monosaccharides in nutrition are glucose, fructose, and galactose. Glucose is a primary energy source for body cells. Disaccharides form when two monosaccharides combine. Important disaccharides in nutrition are the table sugar sucrose (glucose joined with fructose), maltose (glucose joined with glucose), and the milk sugar lactose (glucose joined with galactose). Once digested into monosaccharide forms and absorbed, most carbohydrates are transformed into glucose in the liver.

Simple	*Monosaccharides* Glucose, fructose, galactose
	Disaccharides Sucrose, lactose, maltose
	Polysaccharides Starches (amylose), glycogen, most
Complex	dietary fiber

Forms of the More Complex Carbohydrates

The larger, more complex forms of carbohydrates are primarily called either *starches* or *dietary fibers*, depending on their digestibility by human GI tract enzymes. These more complex forms of carbohydrates are composed of many units of smaller, simpler carbohydrates and found primarily in grains, vegetables, and fruits. The Dietary Guidelines recommend that we consume a diet based on these foods as we attempt to moderate use of fat and simple sugars.[19]

Starches Are Digestible Polysaccharides

The scientific name for the large, complex carbohydrates is **polysaccharides.** Polysaccharides are very long carbohydrate chains composed of many monosaccharide units, mainly glucose (*poly* means many). Some polysaccharides have 3000 or more glucose units. These forms include **amylose** in plants, such as potato starch, and glycogen in animal tissues. When food labels list "Other Carbohydrates," this primarily refers to starch content.[19]

Amylose, a long, straight chain of glucoses (Figure 5-2), forms much of the starch found in vegetables, beans, breads, pasta, and rice. In corn, for example, glucose is converted to starch as the corn ages. This reflects the function of starch as a carbohydrate storage form in plants.

As noted before, glycogen (animal starch) is made by humans and is a storage form for glucose. This polysaccharide consists of a chain of glucoses with many branches. Enzymes that digest starches can start digestion only at the ends of the

Polysaccharides

Large carbohydrates containing from hundreds to 3000 or more glucose units; also known as complex carbohydrates.

Amylose

A straight-chain digestible polysaccharide made of glucose units; primary component of starch in foods.

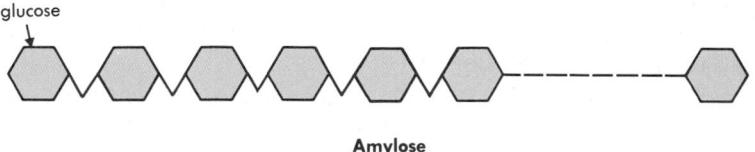

Amylose

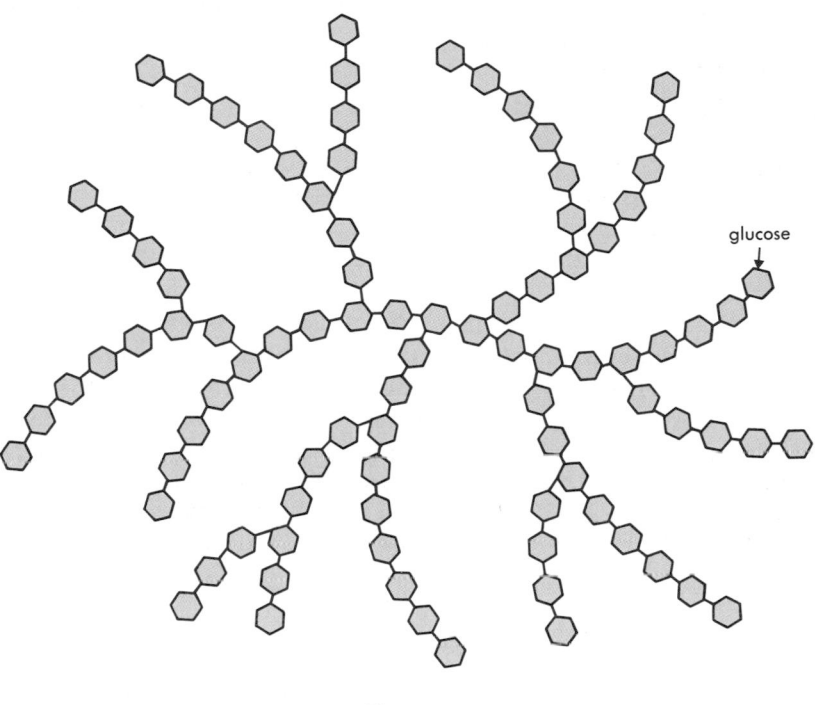

Glycogen

Figure 5-2 *Some common starches. We consume essentially no glycogen. All glycogen found in the body is made by our cells, primarily in the liver and muscles.*

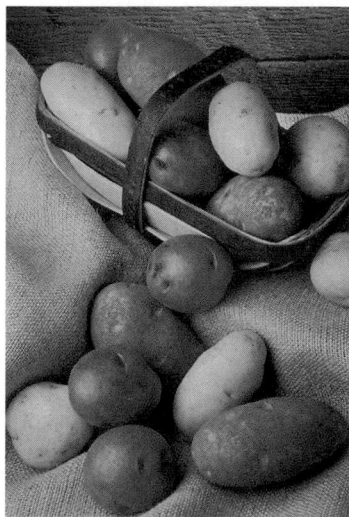

Potatoes are rich in plant starch.

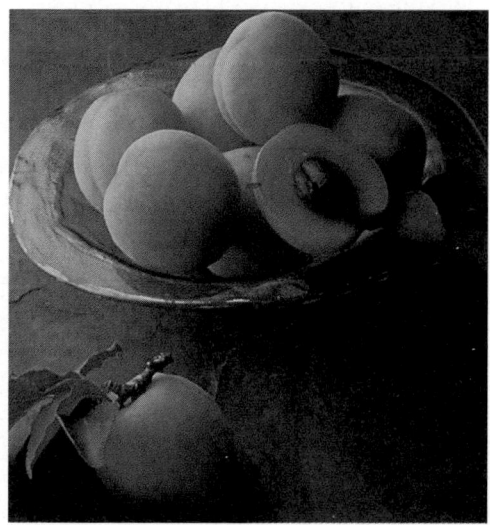

Fruits contain sugars, such as fructose.

molecule. The numerous branches of glycogen provide many sites (ends) for enzyme action. Glycogen is thus an ideal form for carbohydrate storage in the body because it can be quickly broken down.

The liver and muscles are the major storage sites for glycogen. Because only about 80 kcal of glucose are available from the blood, these storage sites for carbohydrate energy—amounting to about 1800 kcal—are extremely important. The 400 kcal of liver glycogen can be turned into blood glucose, but the 1400 kcal of muscle glycogen cannot. Still, glycogen in muscles can supply glucose for muscle use, especially during high-intensity and endurance exercise. (See Chapter 11 for a discussion of carbohydrate use in exercise.)

Dietary Fibers Are Primarily Indigestible Polysaccharides

Insoluble fibers

Fibers that mostly do not dissolve in water and are not metabolized by bacteria in the large intestine. These include cellulose, some hemicelluloses, and lignins.

Soluble fibers

Fibers that either dissolve or swell in water and are metabolized (fermented) by bacteria in the large intestine. These include pectins, gums, and mucilages.

Dietary fibers as a class are mostly made up of polysaccharides, but they differ from starches insofar as the chemical links that join individual sugar units cannot be digested by human enzymes in the GI tract.[3] This prevents the small intestine from absorbing the sugars that make up dietary fibers. Dietary fiber is not a single substance but a group of substances with similar characteristics (Table 5-1). The group comprises the carbohydrates cellulose, hemicelluloses, pectins, gums, and mucilages, as well as the noncarbohydrate lignins.

Cellulose, hemicelluloses, and lignins form the structural parts of plants. A cotton ball is pure cellulose. Bran fiber is rich in hemicelluloses. The woody fibers in broccoli are partly lignins. Because the majority of these compounds neither readily dissolve in water nor are metabolized by intestinal bacteria, they are called *insoluble fibers.*

Pectins, gums, and mucilages are contained around and inside plant cells. These compounds either dissolve or swell when put into water and are therefore called *soluble fibers.* These exist as gum arabic, guar gum, locust bean gum, and various pectin forms and are found in several foods, especially in salad dressings, some frozen desserts, jams, and jellies. Some forms of hemicelluloses also fall into the soluble category.

Most foods contain mixtures of soluble and insoluble fibers, but food labels do not distinguish between the two types. Still, if food is listed as a good source of one type of fiber, it usually contains some of the other type of dietary fiber as well. Therefore, when adding fiber-rich foods to your diet, you usually get both types.

TABLE 5-1

Classification of Dietary Fibers

Type	Component(s)	Examples	Physiological effects	Major food sources
INSOLUBLE				
Noncarbohydrate	Lignins	Wheat bran	Under study	All plants
Carbohydrate	Cellulose	Wheat products	Increases fecal bulk	All plants
	Hemicelluloses	Brown rice	Decreases intestinal transit time	Wheat, rye, rice, vegetables
SOLUBLE				
Carbohydrate	Pectins, gums, mucilages, some hemicelluloses	Apples Bananas Oranges Carrots Barley Oats Kidney beans	Delays gastric emptying; slows glucose absorption; can lower blood cholesterol	Citrus fruits, oat products, beans

Another term sometimes used for fiber is *crude fiber.* This term was coined in the 1800s to describe the amount of indigestible foodstuff present in animal feed. With the use of acids and then alkalis to chemically digest the animal feed, the amount of crude fiber was determined by measuring what remained "undigested"— mostly cellulose and lignins. Because other types of dietary fibers are destroyed by this type of treatment, substituting the term *crude fiber* for *dietary fiber* is misleading. If you see the term *crude fiber* on food composition tables, keep in mind that values reported often bear little resemblance to dietary fiber values. This point is important. When nutrition scientists talk about fiber, they are referring to dietary fiber. Other terms for fiber, such as *roughage* and *bulk,* are also no longer widely used.

We need much more data about the dietary fiber content of foods. In fact, researchers still disagree on the best means for determining dietary fiber content.[3] In all analyses used today, some dietary fiber is lost, which explains the occasional discrepancies between food tables and nutrition labels on foods.

You may think of wheat bran as pure fiber, but it is actually a mixture of several dietary fibers. It also contains some protein, fat, and trace minerals, as is true for all dietary fiber sources. The age of a plant may also influence its fiber composition; for example, young carrots contain very little lignin, whereas old carrots may contain 10% to 20% of this material.

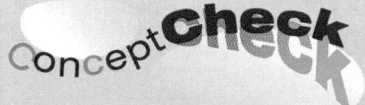

The major digestible polysaccharides—starches—contain multiple glucose units linked together. Glycogen is animal starch and acts as a storage form of glucose in the liver and muscles. Dietary fibers include the indigestible polysaccharides cellulose, hemicelluloses, pectins, gums, and mucilages, as well as the noncarbohydrate lignins. Diets based on starch-rich foods, particularly grains, pastas, fruits, and vegetables, are encouraged as replacements for diets based on mostly high-fat foods.

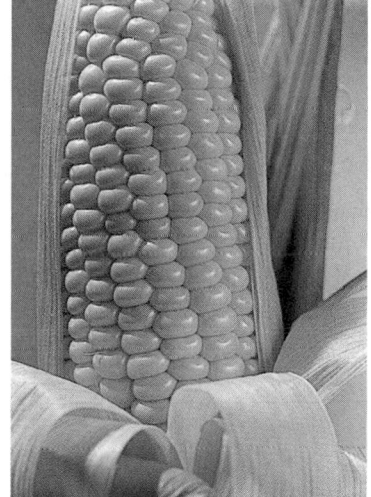

Making Carbohydrates Available for Body Use

As discussed in Chapter 4, simply eating a food does not supply nutrients to body cells. Digestion and absorption must occur first.

Carbohydrate Digestion

Carbohydrate digestion actually begins before we start eating. Preparing food can be viewed as the first step in digestion. Cooking softens tough connective tissues in the fibrous tissue of plants, such as broccoli stalks. When starches are heated, the starch granules swell as they soak up water, making them much easier to digest. All these effects of cooking generally make food easier to chew, swallow, and break down during digestion.

Digestion of the large carbohydrates—starches—begins as these mix with saliva during the chewing of food. Saliva contains an enzyme called *salivary amylase.* This enzyme breaks down starch into many smaller sugar units (disaccharides, such as maltose)[22] (Figure 5-3). You can observe this conversion while chewing a saltine cracker. Prolonged chewing of the cracker causes it to taste sweeter as some starch breaks down into the sweeter sugars.

Salivary amylase does not work in an acidic environment. Once food moves down the esophagus into the stomach, the stomach's acidity halts further salivary amylase action and subsequently any starch digestion. However, salivary amylase is not very important because the enzyme pancreatic amylase finishes in the small intestine what salivary amylase begins in the mouth.

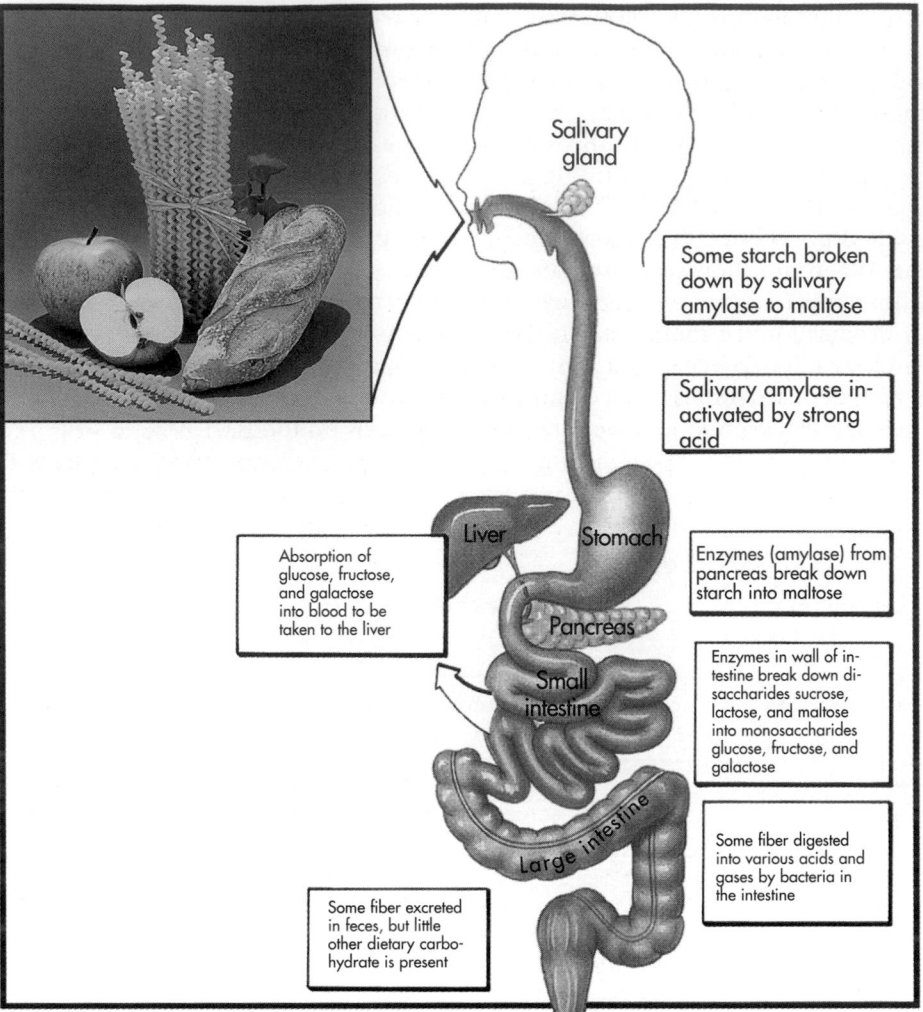

Figure 5-3 *Carbohydrate digestion and absorption. Enzymes made by the mouth, pancreas, and small intestine participate in the process of digestion. Most carbohydrate digestion and absorption take place in the small intestine.*

After the carbohydrates are in the intestine and pancreatic amylase has had time to act, the original carbohydrates in a food are now present as monosaccharides (mostly any glucose and fructose present as such in food), as well as disaccharides (maltose from starch breakdown, lactose mainly from dairy products, and sucrose from food preparation and that added at the table). Eventually all the disaccharide forms are digested to their monosaccharide forms by specialized enzymes attached to the cells of the small intestine. The enzyme maltase acts on maltose to produce two glucose molecules. Sucrase acts on sucrose to produce glucose and fructose. Lactase acts on lactose to produce glucose and galactose.[22]

When considering carbohydrate digestion, you should remember that key digestive enzymes come from both the pancreas and the cells of the intestinal wall. Intestinal diseases can interfere with the production of the intestinal wall enzymes. Such conditions may interfere with the efficient digestion of the sugars maltose, lactose, and sucrose. The portion of these carbohydrates that is not fully digested will not be absorbed. When these unabsorbed carbohydrates eventually end up in the large intestine, the bacteria there will use the sugars to produce acid and gas.[19] If produced in large amounts, these can cause abdominal discomfort. People recovering from intestinal disorders, such as diarrhea or bacterial infections, may need to avoid lactose for a few weeks if temporary lactose intolerance is experienced. Two weeks will be sufficient time for the small intestine to resume producing enough lactase enzyme to allow for lactose digestion.

Carbohydrate Absorption

Single sugars found naturally in foods and those formed as by-products of earlier starch digestion in the mouth and small intestine generally follow an active absorption process (one that requires energy input) when they are taken up by the absorptive cells in the small intestine.[22] Once glucose, galactose, and fructose enter the intestinal cells, they are transported via the portal vein to the liver. The liver then exercises its metabolic options—transforming monosaccharides into glucose and releasing them directly into the bloodstream, producing the storage form of the carbohydrate, glycogen, or producing fat. Of these three options, producing fat is the least likely.[15] Only a minor amount of starch (about 5%) escapes absorption. This travels down to the large intestine and is digested there by bacteria and then absorbed in the form of acids and gases, as with undigested lactose.[22]

Bacteria in the large intestine metabolize soluble fibers into such products as acids and gases. These can cause intestinal gas (flatulence). Gas is not harmful but can be inconvenient. However, the body tends to adapt over time and produce less gas.

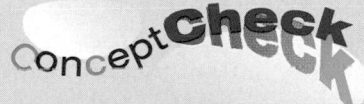

ConceptCheck

Carbohydrate digestion is the process of breaking down larger carbohydrates into their absorbable components. Digestion of starches begins in the mouth with salivary amylase. Enzymes made by the pancreas and small intestine complete the digestion of carbohydrates to single sugars in the small intestine. Primarily following an active absorption process, the single sugars—either resulting from the digestive process or present in the meal—are taken up by absorptive cells in the intestine and ultimately transported via the portal vein to the liver. Then the liver exercises its metabolic options, primarily producing glucose and glycogen.

Putting Simple Carbohydrates to Work in the Body

The functions of glucose in the body start with supplying energy, but that is only the beginning. Because the other sugars can generally be converted to glucose and starches are broken down to yield glucose, the functions described here apply to most carbohydrates.

Yielding Energy

The main function of glucose is to supply energy for the body: 1 gram of carbohydrate yields 4 kcal. Certain tissues in the body, such as red blood cells, can use only glucose and other simple carbohydrate forms for energy. Most parts of the brain also derive energy only from simple carbohydrates, unless the diet contains almost none. In that case, much of the brain can use partial breakdown products of fat—called *ketones*—for energy (see p. 152). Simple carbohydrates can also fuel muscle cells and other body cells, but many of these cells also use much fat for energy needs (see Chapter 11 for details).

In America, carbohydrates supply about 50% of our dietary energy; sugars and starches contribute about equal amounts. Worldwide, however, carbohydrates

Lactose Intolerance

The ability to digest lactose depends on the activity of the enzyme **lactase.** This enzyme, which is embedded within the surface of intestinal cells, splits lactose into glucose and galactose. These monosaccharides are absorbed from the small intestine into the bloodstream, but lactose is not. When lactase activity is low, lactose travels unaltered into the large intestine, where resident bacteria metabolize it into acids and gases, causing intestinal gas, bloating, cramping, and discomfort.[22]

Primary lactose intolerance is common in Asians, Hispanics, Native Americans, people of Mediterranean descent, African-Americans, and some other ethnic races. In this case, the loss of lactase activity is not due to another disease per se—hence its designation as a **primary disease.** Some individuals may be born with little or no lactase, but more commonly the lactase activity declines with age, starting at about 2 years of age. Even though lactose intolerance is more prevalent in some ethnic groups than others, between 30 and 60 million Americans and up to 75% of adults worldwide experience a large decrease in their ability to synthesize lactase as they age.[18] They are therefore unable to tolerate large amounts of milk products, since much of the lactose in these products tends to remain undigested.

Secondary lactose intolerance by definition develops as a result of another disease, as is true of **secondary diseases.** Most cases are caused by intestinal bacterial infections. The inability to digest lactose may also result from the use of certain medications, especially anticancer drugs. Both infection and some drugs can inhibit the growth of the rapidly reproducing cells that line the GI tract and produce lactase.

Clinically, lactose intolerance can be diagnosed from a history of gas and bloating after milk consumption. This history can then be confirmed by having the person consume lactose. If blood glucose does not rise much after consuming the lactose, lactose maldigestion is the likely cause. Other, more technical procedures are available to confirm the diagnosis of lactose intolerance.[24]

An individual who is sensitive to even small amounts of lactose must become an avid label reader in order to avoid products with ingredients such as milk, milk solids, casein, and whey. Some medications contain lactose as binders or fillers. Moderate lactose intolerance, however, is more common than nearly complete intolerance. Most people who are moderately intolerant quickly learn by trial and error how much lactose they can tolerate and easily adjust the amount of dairy products in their diet. Such people need not avoid all milk and milk products; nor is this recommended, because these foods are very good sources of calcium, riboflavin, potassium, and magnesium. Although these four nutrients are present in other food groups, many people don't eat much of these alternative sources. Obtaining enough of these nutrients is much easier if milk and milk products are included in the diet.

Several options are available to moderately lactose-intolerant individuals who prefer to continue using milk products. First, they can consume small portions of milk products and take them with other foods; this often works because they are able to digest some lactose but not large amounts at one time.[18] Also, fat in a meal slows digestion, leaving more time for lactase action. Secondly, they can eat cheese. Much lactose is lost when milk is made into cheese. Finally, they can consume yogurt. The bacteria that make yogurt provide their own lactase activity. Thus, if the yogurt contains active bacteria cultures, the lactose present is essentially digested by the yogurt. Freezing destroys the bacteria's activity, so frozen yogurt—as currently manufactured—may have little remaining lactase activity. In general, the foods tolerated best by lactose-intolerant individuals are hard cheeses and regular yogurt. However, sweetened yogurt typically may have as many as 240 kcal per serving, approximately three times more energy than a glass of nonfat milk, making it a high-calorie option. Supermarkets also sell low-fat, and nonfat aspartame-sweetened, fruit-flavored yogurts with as few as 120 kcal per serving (8 oz).

During the past few years, manufacturers have been producing low-lactose milk by treating regular milk with lactase isolated from yeast. The added lactase breaks down most of the lactose into glucose and galactose, yielding a milk that causes few symptoms in most moderately intolerant people. Compared with regular milk, low-lactose milk tastes sweeter because of its higher concentration of glucose, which is three to four times sweeter than lactose. Low-lactose milk can be made at home by adding a commercially available lactase preparation to regular milk. Lactase pills are also available and can be used at mealtimes. Few people actually need to use enzyme-treated milk or lactase pills, because their intolerance is moderate. Minor changes in diet suffice, even for people who feel they are quite sensitive to lactose.[24] For those who nevertheless wish to consume less lactose, these products allow greater versatility in the diet. Several options, then, are available to lactose-intolerant people, only one of which is abandoning milk products. People with severe lactase deficiency who avoid all dairy products should seek other sources of calcium (see Chapter 9).

account for about 70% of all energy consumed.[23] In North America and other industrialized areas where meat and overall fat intakes are high, carbohydrates end up supplying a lower percentage of total energy intake.

Regulating this energy source. Under normal circumstances a person's blood glucose concentration is regulated within a very narrow range. If blood glucose rises too high, the condition is called *hyperglycemia* (*hyper* means high, and *emia* means in the bloodstream). Excess glucose then spills over into the urine. This is what happens in people with poorly controlled or undiagnosed diabetes (see the Nutrition Issue in this chapter).[28] If blood glucose falls too low, a person feels nervous, irritable, and hungry, and may develop a headache. This is referred to as *hypoglycemia* (*hypo* means low). It is not too surprising that a headache results, because the brain is fueled almost entirely by glucose.[21]

Recall that when carbohydrates are digested and taken up by the absorptive cells of the small intestine, the portal vein then transports the resulting sugars to the liver. The liver is the first organ to screen the absorbed sugars. One of its roles is to guard against excess glucose entering the bloodstream after a meal.

The pancreas works with the liver to control blood glucose. As soon as eating begins, the pancreas releases small amounts of the hormone **insulin.** Once much glucose enters the bloodstream, the pancreas releases more insulin. This insulin stimulates the liver to synthesize glycogen—the storage form of glucose in the body—and stimulates muscle cells, adipose (fat) cells, and other cells to increase glucose uptake. By triggering both glucose storage in the liver and glucose movement out of the bloodstream into certain cells, insulin keeps glucose from rising too high in the blood (Figure 5-4).

Other hormones have the opposite effects of insulin. When a person has not eaten for a few hours and blood glucose begins to fall, the pancreas releases the hormone **glucagon.** This hormone prompts the breakdown of glycogen into glucose, which is then released from the liver into the bloodstream. In this way glucagon keeps blood glucose from falling too low (see Figure 5-4).

A different mechanism increases blood glucose during times of stress. **Epinephrine** (adrenaline) is the hormone responsible for the "flight or fight" reaction. Epinephrine and a related compound are released in large amounts from the adrenal gland (located on each kidney) and various nerve endings in response to a perceived threat, such as a car approaching head-on. These cause glycogen in the liver to break down into glucose. The resulting rapid flood of glucose from the liver into the bloodstream helps promote quick mental and physical reactions.

In essence, the actions of insulin on blood glucose are balanced by the actions of glucagon, epinephrine, and other hormones. If hormonal balance is not maintained, such as during over- or under-production of insulin or glucagon, major changes in blood glucose concentrations occur.

Before we move on, let's step back and look at one of the intricacies of our body's metabolism. To maintain blood glucose within an acceptable range, the body relies on a complex regulatory system. This provides a safeguard against extreme hyperglycemia or hypoglycemia if one control mechanism fails. Suppose instead there were only one mechanism for controlling blood glucose, such as a nerve connection between the brain and pancreas that when appropriately stimulated caused release of insulin. Damage to this nerve would prevent insulin release, causing extreme fluctuations in blood glucose, with dire physiological consequences. In fact, a disturbance in one of the body's control mechanisms—such as insulin release from the pancreas—can greatly influence blood glucose, but it doesn't knock out all of the other regulatory systems. The liver and adrenal glands still act to provide moderate regulation of blood glucose. This example of checks and balances is typical of how the body maintains blood and other tissue concentrations of its key constituents within fairly narrow ranges.

Hyperglycemia
High blood glucose; above 140 milligrams per 100 milliliters of blood.

Hypoglycemia
Low blood glucose; below 40 to 50 milligrams per 100 milliliters of blood.

Insulin
A hormone produced by the beta cells of the pancreas. Among other processes, insulin increases the synthesis of glycogen in the liver and the movement of glucose from the bloodstream into body cells.

Glucagon
A hormone made by the pancreas that stimulates the breakdown of glycogen in the liver into glucose; this ends up increasing blood glucose. Glucagon also performs other functions.

Epinephrine
A hormone also known as adrenaline; it is released by the adrenal gland (located on each kidney) and various nerve endings in the body. It acts to increase glycogen breakdown in the liver, among other functions.

quick mental + physical rxs

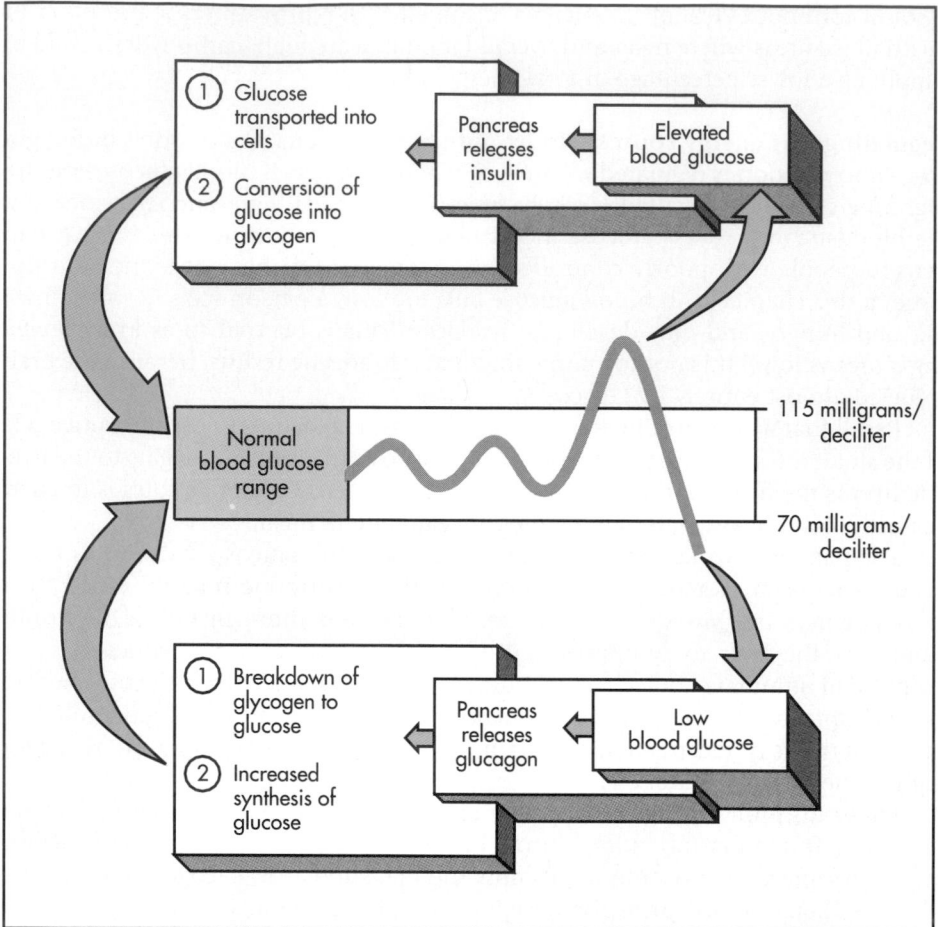

Figure 5-4 *Regulation of blood glucose. The hormones insulin and glucagon are key factors in controlling blood glucose. Other hormones, such as epinephrine, norepinephrine, cortisol, and growth hormone, also contribute to blood glucose regulation.*

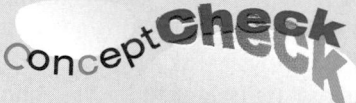

Blood glucose concentration is maintained within a very narrow range. When blood glucose rises after a meal, the hormone insulin is released in great amounts from the pancreas. Insulin acts to lower blood glucose by increasing glucose storage in the liver and glucose uptake by many body cells. If blood glucose falls during fasting, then glucagon and other hormones increase the liver's release of glucose into the bloodstream to restore normal blood glucose values. In a similar way the hormone epinephrine can make more glucose available in response to stress. This balance in hormone activity helps maintain blood glucose within a healthy range.

Flavoring and Sweetening Foods

Even a baby responds to sugars with a smile. On the tip of the tongue are sensors for tasting sweetness. The sensors recognize a variety of sugars and even some noncarbohydrate substances. Some sugars are sweeter than others; per gram, fructose is almost twice as sweet as sucrose under cold and acidic conditions, as found in soft drinks. Glucose and lactose are much less sweet than fructose (Table 5-2).

TABLE 5-2

The Sweetness of Sugars and Alternative Sweeteners

Type of sweetener	Relative sweetness* (sucrose = 1)	Typical sources
SUGARS		
Lactose	0.2	Dairy products
Maltose	0.4	Sprouted seeds
Glucose	0.7	Corn syrup
Sucrose	1	Table sugar, most sweets
Invert sugar†	1.3	Some candies, honey
Fructose	1.2-1.8	Fruit, honey, some soft drinks
SUGAR ALCOHOLS		
Sorbitol	0.6	Dietetic candies, sugarless gum
Mannitol	0.7	Dietetic candies
Xylitol	0.9	Sugarless gum
ALTERNATIVE SWEETENERS		
Cyclamate	30	Not currently in use in the United States
Aspartame	200	Diet soft drinks, diet fruit drinks, sugarless gum, powdered diet sweetener
Acesulfame-K	200	Sugarless gum, diet drink mixes, powdered diet sweeteners, puddings, gelatin desserts
Saccharin (sodium salt)	300	Diet soft drinks

From the American Dietetic Association, 1993.
*On a per gram basis.
†Sucrose broken down into glucose and fructose.

Sugars improve the palatability of many foods and thus enhance diets in general. For example, a small amount of sucrose on a grapefruit improves the taste of this sour fruit. Moderation in using sugars is recommended, but there is no need to believe that sugars are to be avoided altogether.[15]

Sparing Protein from Use as an Energy Source and Preventing Ketosis

The importance of carbohydrate fuel for the body cannot be overstated. As a fuel for the brain and red blood cells, carbohydrate is critical. If you don't eat enough carbohydrates, your body is forced to make glucose from other nutrients, mainly certain amino acids that make up proteins. When this occurs, some of the proteins from your diet can't be used to make body tissues and perform other vital functions. Under normal circumstances, sugars in the diet mostly end up as blood glucose to be used by the brain, red blood cells, and most other body cells for fuel. This allows proteins to be saved for their normal functions, like building and maintaining muscles. Therefore sugars are considered protein sparing.

During long-term starvation, proteins in the muscles, heart, liver, kidneys, and other vital organs break down into amino acids, and certain forms are turned into needed glucose. If the process occurs over weeks at a time, these organs become partially weakened. (See Chapters 7 and 18 for discussions of the specific effects of starvation.)

When you don't eat enough carbohydrates, an additional result is that fats don't break down completely in metabolism. In other words, without enough

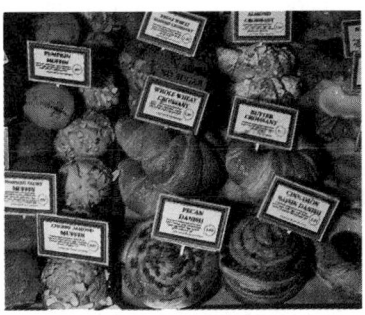

Many foods we enjoy are sweet and should be eaten only in moderation.

Ketone

Incomplete breakdown products of fat containing three or four carbons.

carbohydrate present, fat metabolism is hampered. Partial breakdown products of fats, called **ketones,** then form. This condition, known as **ketosis,** should be avoided because it disturbs the body's normal acid-base balance and leads to other health problems.[4]

For now, keep in mind that eating at least 50 to 100 grams of carbohydrates per day ensures complete metabolism of fats. It also prevents the body weakness that usually results from having to use protein to compensate for an insufficient carbohydrate intake. Still, typical adults in the United States need not worry. Our daily carbohydrate intakes usually exceed 100 grams, averaging closer to 200 to 300 grams per day.[23]

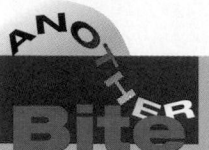

The life-threatening wasting of protein that occurs during long-term fasting has prompted companies that produce medical products for rapid weight loss to include 30 to 120 grams of carbohydrate in the formulation.* This significantly decreases protein breakdown and thereby helps protect vital tissues and organs, including the heart (see Chapter 10 for details).

*Most of these products are powders that can be mixed with different kinds of fluids, are consumed five or six times per day, and are very low in calories.

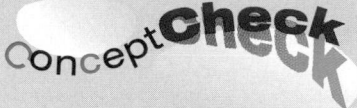

The major reason to consume carbohydrates is to provide glucose for the energy needs of red blood cells and parts of the brain. Eating less than 50 to 100 grams of carbohydrates per day forces the body to make glucose using primarily amino acids from proteins found in vital organs. A low glucose supply in cells also inhibits efficient metabolism of fats. Ketosis can then result.

Dietary Fiber Also Provides Health Benefits

Many types of dietary fiber absorb water and hold onto it in the intestine. When enough fiber is consumed, its water-retaining property helps enlarge and soften the stool, easing elimination. Basically the larger stool size stimulates the intestinal muscles that promote peristalsis (see Chapter 4). Consequently, less pressure is needed to expel the stool.[5] This link between dietary fiber and the health of the intestine has interested people for hundreds of years.

When too little dietary fiber is eaten, the opposite can occur: the stool may be small and hard. Constipation may result, requiring strong pressures to move the stool in the large intestine during elimination. Hemorrhoids may then result from excessive straining. Also, the high pressures can force parts of the large intestine wall to pop out from between the surrounding bands of muscle. This forms small pouches, called **diverticula,** leading to a condition called *diverticulosis.* About 50% of older people have many of these pouches (Figure 5-5). Diverticula rarely occur in people in developing countries, probably because of their high dietary fiber intakes. In contrast, people in Western countries often ingest much less dietary fiber in their diets.

Diverticulosis is normally not noticeable. But if the diverticula become filled with food particles, especially hulls or seeds, bacteria can metabolize them into acids

Diverticula

Pouches that protrude through the outside wall of the large intestine. Diverticulosis is the condition of having many diverticula in the large intestine.

and gases. This irritates the diverticula and may eventually cause inflammation, a condition known as *diverticulitis.* Treatment includes taking antibiotics to counter the bacterial action and eating a limited amount of dietary fiber to reduce the food source for bacterial activity. Once the inflammation subsides, a high dietary fiber intake (but free of seeds) is begun to ease elimination and reduce the risk of a future attack.

Insoluble fibers, particularly certain types of hemicelluloses, are the best fibers for increasing stool size. Again, bran—the fibrous covering of grain kernels—is rich in hemicelluloses. Because bran layers form the outer covering of all grains, whole grains are good sources of insoluble fiber. Increasing fluids is also important whenever a high fiber intake is instituted. Performing regular physical activity to stimulate peristalsis is also helpful for intestinal health.[5]

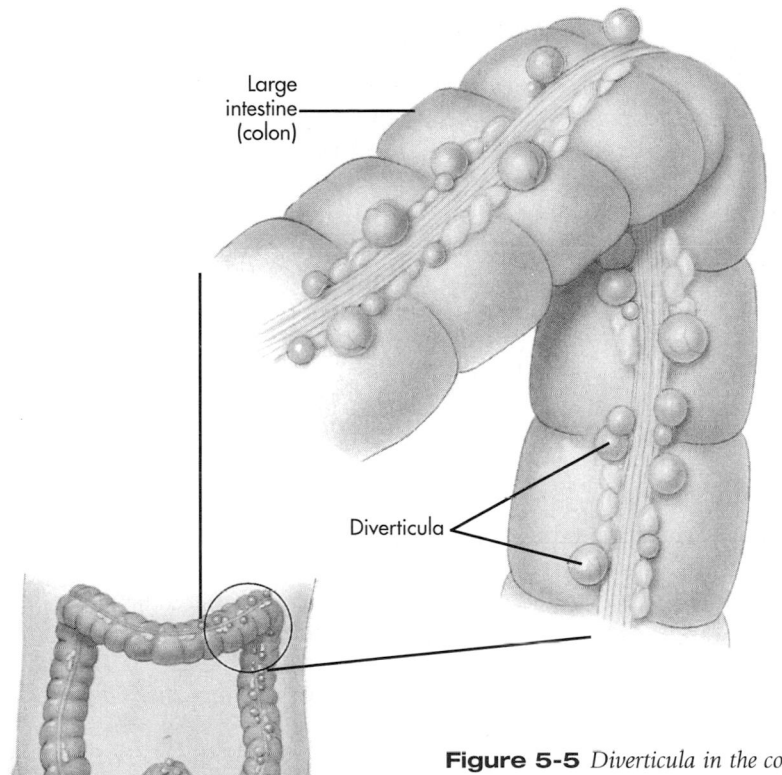

Large intestine (colon)

Diverticula

Figure 5-5 *Diverticula in the colon. A low-fiber diet increases the risk for their development.*

Diverticulitis
An inflammation of the diverticula caused by acids produced by bacterial metabolism inside the diverticula.

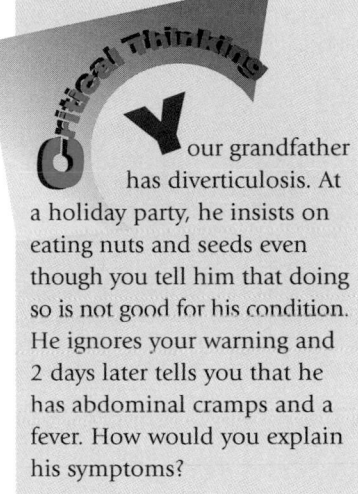

Critical Thinking

Your grandfather has diverticulosis. At a holiday party, he insists on eating nuts and seeds even though you tell him that doing so is not good for his condition. He ignores your warning and 2 days later tells you that he has abdominal cramps and a fever. How would you explain his symptoms?

Mortality
Synonymous with death; number of deaths.

Whole grains
Grains containing the entire seed of the plant, including the bran, germ, and endosperm (starchy interior). Examples include whole wheat and brown rice.

Can Dietary Fiber Play Other Roles in Preserving Health?

Dietary fiber may also play a key role in preventing colon cancer. Among the deadly cancers, colon cancer ranks second only to lung cancer in occurrence and **mortality** in the United States.[25] Dozens of epidemiological studies have linked its occurrence to diets low in **whole grains,** fruits, and vegetables—all good sources of dietary fiber—and high in fat, meat, and excess energy intake.[10] Many other factors, however, are also involved in the development of the disease, such as genetic background.[25] Weaker but intriguing evidence implicates obesity; smoking; a generous

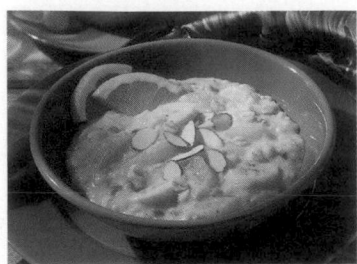

Oatmeal is a rich source of soluble fiber.

alcohol intake (more than two drinks per day); lack of regular physical activity; inadequate intakes of the vitamins C, D, and folate and the mineral calcium; and low starch intakes.[5,10,11,19,25] One study has also suggested long-term aspirin use might reduce the risk of colon cancer, but any use must be approved by a physician because of other health problems that may result, such as ulcers.[12]

Researchers are not sure how dietary fiber might reduce colon cancer development. However, they surmise that potential cancer-causing compounds in the intestinal contents are diluted by fluid attracted to the fibers, bound to the fibers, and more rapidly excreted as fibers speed passage of feces through the intestinal tract. Colon cancers have been prevented in laboratory animals by the use of dietary fiber. Preliminary evidence suggests that cellulose, hemicelluloses, and lignins serve major protective functions.

In human studies, dietary fiber from fruits and vegetables has tended to be most protective against colon cancer. This finding suggests that increased consumption of vitamin C and carotenoids from fruits and vegetables, or simply the reduction in meat and fat intake when a high-fiber diet is instituted, may exert the main protective effect, rather than dietary fiber alone.[10] Currently, foods, rather than nutritional supplements, are regarded as the best source of this preventive effect of dietary fiber. In a recent 4-year trial, consumption of vitamin E, vitamin C, and beta carotene supplements by people who had already had one occurrence of colon cancer was shown to be ineffective in reducing subsequent colon cancer risk.[14] Critics of the study suggest that 4 years is an insufficient treatment period to demonstrate the possible protective effects of supplements. Another supplement trial, extending over 10 years, will be completed soon; the results of this study should clarify the role, if any, of supplements in protecting against colon cancer.

Soluble fibers taken in high amounts in the diet can decrease blood cholesterol. The dose, if oat bran is used, needs to be about 80 to 100 grams (about $^3/_4$ of a cup uncooked) per day—not an easy feat. With cooked beans, about 150 grams ($1^1/_2$ cups) is needed. The effect is partly caused by inhibiting bile recycling in the intestinal tract. Bile, which is formed from cholesterol, is then pulled into the feces for elimination.[5] Additional mechanisms may be at work as well (see Chapter 6). Other rich sources of soluble fibers include fruits and vegetables in general, soybean fiber, rice bran, and **psyllium** seeds (found in many commercial fiber laxatives). Overall, a fiber-rich diet containing fruits, vegetables, beans, and whole grains (including whole-grain breakfast cereals) is advocated as part of a strategy to reduce heart disease risk.[29]

A diet high in fiber may also aid weight control and reduce the risk of developing obesity. The bulky nature of high-fiber foods fills us up without yielding much energy. High-fat foods tend to do just the opposite, contributing to obesity. Increasing intake of foods rich in dietary fiber is one strategy for remaining satisfied after a meal even if the fat content in a diet is low.[15]

Finally, when consumed in large amounts, soluble dietary fiber slows glucose absorption from the small intestine. This effect can be helpful in treatment of diabetes[2] (see the Nutrition Issue).

Psyllium

A mostly soluble type of dietary fiber found in the seeds of the plantain plant.

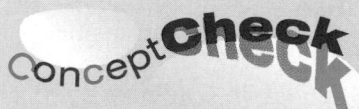

Make high-fiber food choices like vegetables a regular part of your diet.

Concept Check

Dietary fiber has been a subject of interest for centuries. Insoluble fiber forms are vital because they provide mass to the stool, which helps ease elimination and lessen the risk for developing diverticulosis. Fiber may also reduce the risk of colon cancer and obesity. Generous intakes of soluble fiber can help decrease blood cholesterol and moderate swings in blood glucose. Whole grains, vegetables, beans, and fruits are excellent sources of both types of dietary fiber.

History of Fiber in America

Folklore surrounding dietary fiber has been a part of American culture since the 1800s. Food faddism flourished during this time.

Sylvester Graham, a minister, traveled up and down the East Coast extolling the virtues of fiber in the 1820s and 1830s. Graham claimed that the true cause of disease was the removal of bran from flour during processing. The dark bread (brown bread) he recommended was later called Graham bread. Graham also believed that meat excited vile tempers and drove men to sexual excesses. He claimed that the bacterial infection cholera was the price for indulging in too much lewdness and chicken pie. He also claimed that people did not bathe enough and needed external applications of cold water at least weekly. Partly as a result of his advocacy, Saturday night baths and sitting-up exercises before open windows became common practices. His legacy to us is the Graham cracker. However, today's graham cracker bears little resemblance to the whole-grain product he promoted.

The next wave of fiber frenzy crested in the mid-1870s. Dr. John Harvey Kellogg was hired by the Seventh Day Adventist Church to manage their health sanitarium in Battle Creek, Michigan. Kellogg claimed that 90% of health ills centered in the stomach and bowels. He advocated ridding the digestive tract of "poisons" derived from meat-eating, drinking, and condiments. He believed that bowel eliminations should occur frequently. Tablespoons of sterilized bran were given to patients at every meal for laxative purposes. Lettuce and bran were commonly given at breakfast. Kellogg said, "Bran does not irritate, it titillates." Adherents, including many famous people, came from all over the United States to "take the cure" at the sanitarium. Dr. Kellogg became the first person to earn a million dollars from "health foods."

One man who came for a cure in 1891, Charles W. Post, decided he could do what Dr. Kellogg was doing. He created the Post Toasted Cornflakes Company, started producing Postum Cereal Food Coffee, and developed a hard-baked wheat cracker, which he broke into small pieces and called Grape Nuts. Sold as a health food in 1898, it was advocated as a food for the brain and a cure for appendicitis, loose teeth, consumption, and malaria. Post netted $1 million from his products in 1901 alone.

Not to be outdone, William Kellogg—John Harvey Kellogg's brother—began promoting the Kellogg Toasted Corn Flake Company in 1906. Today both companies are active in the breakfast cereal market. True to form, the Kellogg Company is still promoting fiber to Americans.

Fiber finally received its scientific letters in the early 1970s. Dr. Denis Burkitt, a noted British physician, observed that many "Western" diseases did not exist in Africa. These included diverticulitis, colon cancer, appendicitis, hemorrhoids, constipation, and other intestinal disorders. Burkitt surmised that the high-fiber intake of Africans was an important reason these diseases did not occur. He noticed that Africans had very large stools, almost twice the weight of stools from Westerners.

Many researchers followed Burkitt's lead. Soon studies showed that high-fiber intakes decreased the transit time of food through the GI tract—that is, the more fiber eaten, the less time needed to propel the undigested part through the intestinal tract to be eliminated. Researchers suggested that if the stool stayed in the colon for only a short time, less bacterial metabolism of the stool would occur. Thus probably fewer toxins and perhaps fewer **carcinogens** would form. This faster transit time is especially promoted by insoluble fibers.

As discussed in Chapter 2, the fiber argument sharpened in the mid-1980s when the Kellogg Company began promoting high-fiber cereals in the war against colon cancer. Actually, the company was following the lead of the National Cancer Institute. Scientists at the National Cancer Institute believed that a verifiable link existed between low-fiber diets and colon cancer and thought the public needed to be alerted.

The bold move by the Kellogg Company to promote fiber to Americans was criticized as premature by some scientists, who believed that if a low fiber intake was related to colon cancer, it was not a very strong association. Some scientists are still not convinced that a high-fiber diet will prevent enough colon cancer to justify giving fiber much publicity based on that health-related link. FDA does allow a fiber-related health claim on appropriate foods, stating a diet rich in dietary fiber–containing grain products, fruits, and vegetables *may* reduce the risk of some cancers and heart disease. Note that a "may" or "might" qualifier must be included in the claim. Overall, dietary fiber is important for regular bowel habits and may provide other health benefits as well.[5, 29]

Recommendations for Carbohydrate Intake

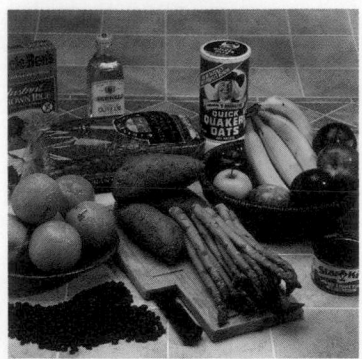

The fruits, vegetables, and grain products in this picture are all good sources of dietary fiber.

No RDA for carbohydrate intake has been established. As previously discussed, consuming at least 50 to 100 grams of carbohydrate per day is critical to prevent ketosis. The diet must also contain enough total energy to meet needs.

Consuming 50 grams of carbohydrate is easy. Just 3 pieces of fruit, 3 slices of bread, or a little more than 3 cups of milk suffice. In fact, eating so little carbohydrate that ketosis results is rare.

Beyond preventing ketosis, carbohydrates provide important fuel for the body. The average adult American eats more than 200 grams of a combination of all digestible carbohydrates—sugars and starches—per day. This adds up to about 50% of energy intake.[23] As noted in Chapter 2, many health authorities recommend boosting carbohydrate intake to 55% or more of energy intake and reducing fat intake, with an emphasis on grains, fruits, and vegetables[19] (Figure 5-6). As carbohydrate intake increases—by eating more foods from the bottom part of the Food Guide Pyramid—fat intake should automatically decrease, as long as added fat is kept to a minimum and foods are prepared and served without additional fat.

Keep in mind, however, that any nutrient can lead to health problems when consumed in excess, including carbohydrate and dietary fiber. High carbohydrate, high fiber, and low fat do not mean zero calories. Carbohydrates help moderate energy intake in comparison to fats, but the contribution of high-carbohydrate foods to total energy intake still needs to be watched. Generally speaking, though, Americans are becoming fatter not because they are eating too much bread and pasta but because they are physically inactive and their diets are high in fat.[15]

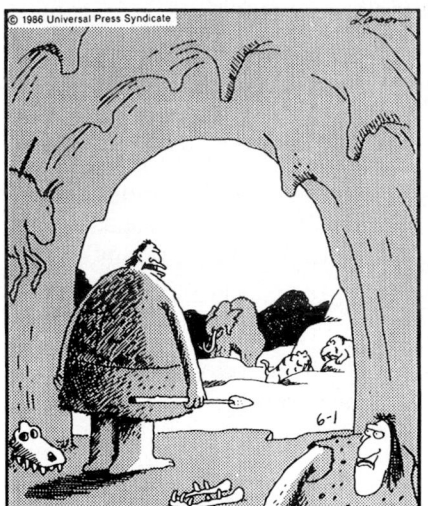

"Once in a while couldn't we just have some pasta?"

Figure 5-6 *The Far Side.*

Each day Americans eat about 70 to 100 grams of sugars, not including the lactose in dairy products. This 70 to 100 grams is made up of a combination of (1) sugars that naturally occur in foods, such as fruits, and (2) sugars that are added during food processing, such as in jam. This total sugar intake corresponds to about 18% of total energy intake.[9] Most of these sugars are added to foods and beverages during manufacturing. The rest occur naturally in foods or are added at the table. Overall consumption of sucrose has dropped in the last 10 years, but consumption of corn sweeteners has increased to make up for the decline. This is mostly because corn sweeteners are cheaper for food manufacturers to use than other forms of sugars.

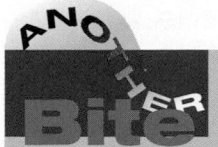

During food processing, the sugar content is often increased. Usually, the more processed the food, the higher the sugar content. An apple has 0 grams of added sugar, canned apples in heavy syrup have 10 to 15 grams, and one sixth of a 9-inch apple pie has 30 grams of added sugar. For comparison purposes, 1 teaspoon of sugar is 5 grams.

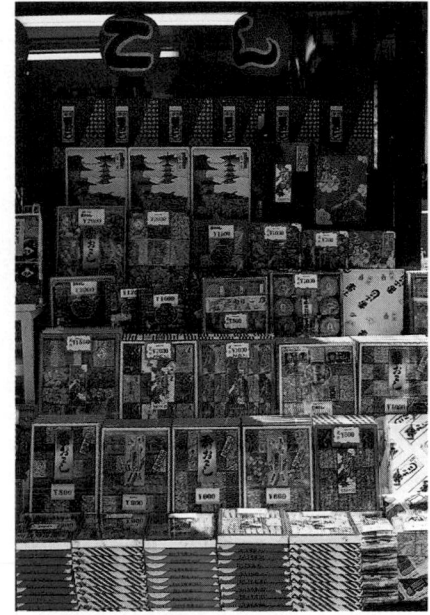

Candy and other sucrose-rich foods are part of diets worldwide, as shown in this photo from Japan.

Although a desirable amount of sugar intake has not yet been set, less than 10% to 15% of total energy intake is considered reasonable.[9] This allows for 10 to 15 teaspoons (50 to 75 grams) a day on a 2000-kcal diet, including what is added to foods, such as cookies and soft drinks. Table 5-3 shows some common sources of sugars in our diets. Are these foods major players in your diet?

Does This Mean Sugar Is Bad for You?

Some people think that all consumption of sugar is unhealthy. Certainly, foods high in simple sugars may supply few, if any, vitamins, minerals, or proteins compared with the number of calories they supply. However, if you can afford to consume some extra calories, moderate amounts of sugar are not harmful. Scientists think that sugar is mostly a problem when it is eaten at the expense of more nutritious foods. When this happens, a person could become deficient in vitamins and other important nutrients, especially if restricting energy intake from other sources.

Many reputable scientific groups have reviewed the current research concerning the health effects of the typical sugars in American diets. In general, these groups have given simple sugars a clean bill of health except for the tendency of many sugars to cause **dental caries**.[13] Caries are formed when sugars and other carbohydrates

TABLE 5-3

Some Sources of Sugars

Food	Serving	Teaspoons of sugar	Food	Serving	Teaspoons of sugar
BEVERAGES			**JELLIES AND JAMS**		
Cola drinks	1 (12 oz bottle or glass)	7	Apple butter	1 tbsp	1
			Jelly	1 tbsp	4-6
Ginger ale	1 (12 oz bottle)	10	Orange marmalade	1 tbsp	4-6
Orangeade	1 (8 oz glass)	5	Peach butter	1 tbsp	1
Root beer	1 (10 oz bottle)	4½	Strawberry jam	1 tbsp	4
Seven-Up	1 (12 oz bottle)	7½			
			CANDIES		
CAKES AND COOKIES			Average milk chocolate bar (e.g., Hershey's)	1 (1½ oz)	2½
Angelfood cake	1 (4 oz piece)	7	Chewing gum	1 stick	½
Applesauce cake	1 (4 oz piece)	5½	Fudge	1 oz square	4½
Banana bread	1 (2 oz piece)	2	Gum drop	1	2
Cheesecake	1 (4 oz piece)	2	Hard candy	4 oz	20
Chocolate cake (plain)	1 (4 oz piece)	6	Lifesavers	1	½
Chocolate cake (iced)	1 (4 oz piece)	10	Peanut brittle	1	3½
Coffee cake	1 (4 oz piece)	4½			
Cupcake (iced)	1	6	**CANNED FRUITS AND JUICES**		
Fruit cake	1 (4 oz piece)	5	Canned apricots	4 halves/1 tbsp syrup	3½
Jelly roll	1 (2 oz piece)	2½			
Orange cake	1 (4 oz piece)	4	Canned fruit juices, sweetened	½ cup	2
Pound cake	1 (4 oz piece)	5			
Sponge cake	1 (1 oz piece)	2	Canned peaches	2 halves/1 tbsp syrup	3½
Strawberry shortcake	1 serving	4			
Brownie (unfrosted)	1 (¾ oz)	3	Fruit salad	½ cup	3½
Chocolate cookie	1	1½	Fruit syrup	2 tbsp	2½
Fig newton	1	5	Stewed fruits	½ cup	2
DAIRY PRODUCTS			**BREAKFAST CEREALS***		
Ice cream	⅓ pint (3½ oz)	3½	Cheerios	1 oz	⅕
Ice cream bar	1	1-7 accord. to size	Special K	1 oz	⅔
			Total	1 oz	⅔
Ice cream cone	1	3½	Quaker 100% Natural	1 oz	2
Ice cream soda	1	5	Sugar Frosted Flakes	1 oz	2
Ice cream sundae	1	7	Sugar Smacks	1 oz	3
Malted milkshake	1 (10 oz glass)	5	Raisin Bran	1 oz	1½
Frozen yogurt	3 oz	3	Cracklin' Oat Bran	1 oz	1½
			Fruit Loops	1 oz	2½
			Cap'n Krunch	1 oz	2½
			Rice Krispies	1 oz	⅔

*As served; no sugar added by the consumer.

are metabolized into acids by bacteria that live in the mouth (Figure 5-7). The acid produced dissolves the tooth enamel and underlying structure. These bacteria lodge themselves in fissures in the teeth. Dentists now apply sealants to heavily fissured areas of certain teeth as a preventive measure. Bacteria also use the sugars to make plaque, a sticky substance that both adheres bacteria to teeth and diminishes the acid-neutralizing effect of saliva.

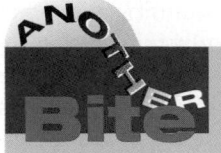

Certain foods—such as cheese, peanuts, and sugar-free chewing gum—can actually help reduce the amount of acid on teeth. Also, rinsing after meals and snacks reduces the acidity in the mouth.

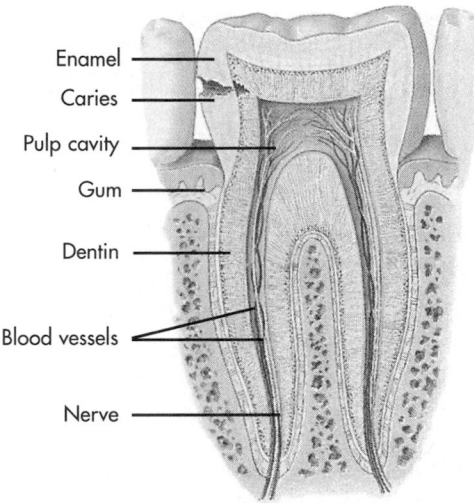

Enamel

Caries

Pulp cavity

Gum

Dentin

Blood vessels

Nerve

Figure 5-7 *Dental caries. Bacteria can collect in various areas on a tooth. Using simple sugars, bacteria then create acids that can dissolve tooth enamel, leading to caries. If the caries process progresses and enters the pulp cavity, damage to the nerve and resulting pain are likely. The bacteria also produce plaque whereby they adhere to the tooth surface.*

Overall, the frequency and amount of time that sugar is retained in the mouth play the greatest role in caries production from food. Sticky or gummy foods that are high in sugars—such as caramels and raisins—are the worst caries offenders, whereas liquid sugar sources—like fruit juices—are not nearly so bad.[1] Note also that sugar-containing foods are not the only foods that are turned to acid by the bacteria in the mouth. If held in the mouth for a long time, starch-containing foods (such as saltines and breads) may be acted on by enzymes in the mouth that break down the starch to sugar.[3] Frequent snacking on sugary foods especially affects dental health in the absence of good dental hygiene. Regular snacking allows the bacteria on the teeth continually to make acid. Limiting the intake of sweets or eating them with meals, instead of between meals or by themselves, is best. This way, other foods help dilute and neutralize the acid that is produced.

In the last 15 years, dental caries rates have decreased in the United States, even though simple-sugar consumption has remained about constant. This decline is primarily due to the addition of fluoride to water. When teeth develop in the presence of this mineral, they become much more resistant to acid (see Chapter 9). Partly because of this, the number of caries-free children increased from 37% in 1980 to 50% in 1988. Fluoride in toothpaste also contributes to dental health because it promotes remineralization of damaged teeth and inhibits the metabolism and growth of bacteria on the teeth.[1]

Are There Risks from Sugar Use Besides Dental Caries?

Some people claim that simple sugars cause heart disease, diabetes, hyperactivity, juvenile delinquency, obesity, and other problems. Little or no credible research supports these allegations. A cause-and-effect relationship between these conditions and consumption of sugars—specifically sucrose—has not been established. There is a widespread notion that high sugar intake by children causes hyperactivity, typically part of the syndrome called *attention deficit hyperactive disorder (ADHD)*. Some people claim that sucrose creates an excited—even antisocial—state, which may lead to violence and disruptive behavior. However, most research shows that sucrose itself is not the villain and indeed may have the opposite effect. A high-carbohydrate

Critical Thinking

John and Mike are identical twins who like the same games, sports, and foods. However, John likes to chew sugar-free gum and Mike doesn't. At their last dental visit, John had no dental caries, but Mike had two. Mike wants to know why John, who chews gum after eating, doesn't have cavities but he does. How would you explain this to him?

TABLE 5-4

Suggestions for Reducing Simple Sugar Intake

AT THE SUPERMARKET

- Read ingredient labels. Identify all the added sugars in a product. Select items lower in total sugar when possible.
- Buy fresh fruits or fruits packed in water, juice, or light syrup rather than those packed in heavy syrup.
- Buy fewer foods that are high in sugar, such as prepared baked goods, candies, sugared cereals, sweet desserts, soft drinks, and fruit-flavored punches. Substitute vanilla wafers, graham crackers, bagels, English muffins, and diet soft drinks, for example.
- Buy reduced-fat microwave popcorn to replace candy for snacks.

IN THE KITCHEN

- Reduce the sugar in foods prepared at home. Try new recipes or adjust your own. Start by reducing the sugar gradually until you've decreased it by one third or more.
- Experiment with spices such as cinnamon, cardamom, coriander, nutmeg, ginger, and mace to enhance the flavor of foods.
- Use home-prepared items (with less sugar) instead of commercially prepared ones that are higher in sugar.

AT THE TABLE

- Use less of all sugars. This includes white and brown sugars, honey, molasses, and syrups.
- Choose fewer foods high in sugar, such as prepared baked goods, candies, and sweet desserts.
- Reach for fresh fruit instead of a sweet for dessert or between-meal snacks.
- Add less sugar to foods—coffee, tea, cereal, and fruit. Get used to using half as much; then see if you can cut back even more.
- Cut back on the number of sugared soft drinks and punches you drink. Substitute water, fruit juice, and diet soft drinks.

Modified from USDA *Home and Garden Bulletin* No. 232-5, 1986.

It has been mentioned several times that milk and some dairy products contain the milk sugar lactose. This should in no way be construed to mean that milk is a food to avoid when limiting simple-sugar consumption. In fact, low-fat and nonfat dairy products have an overall high nutrient density and would be one of the last sources of sugars to limit.

meal, for example, calms many children and induces sleep; this effect may be linked to changes in the synthesis of certain neurotransmitters in the brain.[27] Negative behavioral changes probably result from the excitement or tension in situations in which high-sucrose foods are served, such as birthday parties and on Halloween. Any improvement in behavior observed in children on relatively sugar-free diets is probably due to the extra attention they receive, not the reduction in the intake of sugars.

In the final analysis, use of sugar should follow the same guideline given for many other food products—moderation. By regularly visiting the dentist, practicing good dental hygiene, and following the Food Guide Pyramid while keeping weight under control, you can consume sugar in reasonable amounts without risking your health. Table 5-4 lists ways to reduce sugar intake if you think you eat too much of it.

How Much Dietary Fiber Do We Need?

A reasonable goal for dietary fiber intake is 20 to 35 grams per day. The average intake for Americans is closer to 16 grams per day.[23] Men eat more dietary fiber on average than do women, partly because they eat more food. Increasing dietary fiber intake to 20 to 35 grams is not difficult to achieve (Table 5-5) and should prevent much of the diverticulosis that typically develops in Western countries. Eating a high-fiber cereal for breakfast is one easy way to increase dietary fiber intake. Whole-

TABLE 5-5

Sample 1750 Kcal Menu Containing 30 Grams of Dietary Fiber*†

Menu	Dietary fiber content (grams)
BREAKFAST	
1 cup orange juice	—
¾ cup Wheaties	3
½ cup 2% milk	—
1 slice whole-wheat toast	1.5
1 tsp margarine	—
Coffee	—
LUNCH	
2 oz lean ham	—
2 slices whole-wheat bread	3
2 tsp mayonnaise	—
¼ cup lettuce	0.2
⅓ cup baked beans	4.8
1 pear (with skin)	4
½ cup 1% milk	—
SNACK	
1 carrot (as carrot sticks)	2.2
DINNER	
3 oz broiled chicken (no skin)	—
1 baked potato (large, with skin)	4.8
1½ tsp margarine	—
1 cup cooked green beans	2.2
½ tsp margarine	—
1 cup 1% milk	—
1 apple (with peel)	3.7
SNACK	
1 raisin bagel	1.2
Total	30.6 grams

*The overall diet pattern is based on the Food Guide Pyramid
†Carbohydrate, 60% of kcal; protein, 20% of kcal; fat, 20% of kcal.

food sources such as cereals, not bran supplements, are preferable because foods provide a broader variety of nutrients, particularly many natural high-fiber foods—whole grains, fruits, vegetables, and beans. Note also that drinking fluids with fiber-containing foods is recommended because fibers tend to bind water. Recall from Chapter 2 that the Food Guide Pyramid suggests we consume 5 to 9 servings of fruits/vegetables and 6 to 11 servings of breads/cereals each day. All these food choices can provide dietary fiber (Figure 5-8).

Read the Label

To check for whole grains, read the label on the food package (Figure 5-9). Note that manufacturers often list enriched white flour as wheat flour on food labels. Many people think that if a product is labeled *wheat*, they are getting a whole-wheat product. However, if the label does not say whole-wheat flour in the ingredient list, it is not a whole-wheat product. Bread made from white (refined) flour lacks the bran that forms a protective coating around the wheat kernel. Bran makes flour coarser but contains important nutrients, including dietary fiber.

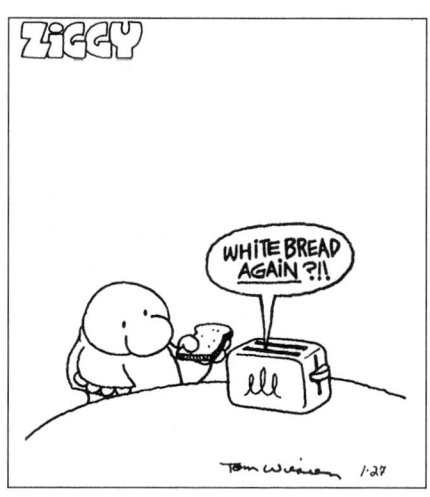

Figure 5-8
Ziggy.

Nutrition Facts

Serving Size 1 cup (55g/2.0 oz.)
Servings Per Container 10

Amount Per Serving	Cereal	Cereal with ½ Cup Vitamins A & D Skim Milk
Calories	170	210
Calories from Fat	10	10
	% Daily Value**	
Total Fat 1.0g*	**2%**	**2%**
Sat. Fat 0g	**0%**	**0%**
Cholesterol 0mg	**0%**	**0%**
Sodium 300mg	**13%**	**15%**
Potassium 340mg	**10%**	**16%**
Total Carbohydrate 43g	**14%**	**16%**
Dietary Fiber 7g	**28%**	**28%**
Sugars 17g		
Other Carbohydrate 19g		
Protein 4g		
Vitamin A	15%	20%
Vitamin C	0%	2%
Calcium	2%	15%
Iron	45%	45%
Vitamin D	10%	25%
Thiamin	25%	30%
Riboflavin	25%	35%
Niacin	25%	25%
Vitamin B_6	25%	25%
Folate	25%	25%
Vitamin B_{12}	25%	35%
Phosphorus	20%	30%
Magnesium	20%	25%
Zinc	25%	25%
Copper	15%	15%

*Amount in cereal. One half cup skim milk contributes an additional 40 calories, 65mg sodium, 6g total carbohydrate (6g sugars), and 4g protein.
**Percent Daily Values are based on a 2,000 calorie diet. Your daily values may be higher or lower depending on your calorie needs:

		Calories:	2,000	2,500
Total Fat	Less than		65g	80g
Sat Fat	Less than		20g	25g
Cholesterol	Less than		300mg	300mg
Sodium	Less than		2,400mg	2,400mg
Potassium			3,500mg	
Total Carbohydrate			300g	375g
Dietary Fiber			25g	30g

Calories per gram:
Fat 9 • Carbohydrate 4 • Protein 4

Ingredients: Wheat bran with other parts of wheat, raisins, sugar, corn syrup, salt, malt flavoring.

Vitamins and Minerals: iron, niacinamide, zinc oxide, pyridoxine hydrochloride (vitamin B_6), riboflavin (vitamin B_2), vitamin A palmitate, thiamin hydrochloride (vitamin B_1), folic acid, vitamin B_{12}, and vitamin D.

Nutrition Facts

Serving Size 1 cup (30g)
Servings Per Container about 13

Amount Per Serving	Cereal	with ½ cup skim Milk
Calories	120	160
Calories from Fat	10	15
	% Daily Value**	
Total Fat 1g*	**2%**	**2%**
Saturated Fat 0g	**0%**	**1%**
Cholesterol 0mg	**0%**	**1%**
Sodium 200mg	**8%**	**11%**
Potassium 55mg	**2%**	**7%**
Total Carbohydrate 25g	**8%**	**10%**
Dietary Fiber 1g	**6%**	**6%**
Sugars 13g		
Other Carbohydrate 11g		
Protein 2g		
Vitamin A	25%	30%
Vitamin C	25%	25%
Calcium	2%	15%
Iron	25%	25%
Vitamin D	10%	25%
Thiamin	25%	30%
Riboflavin	25%	35%
Niacin	25%	25%
Vitamin B_6	25%	25%
Folate	25%	25%

*Amount in Cereal. A serving of cereal plus skim milk provides 1.5g fat, <5mg cholesterol, 260mg sodium, 260mg potassium, 31g carbohydrate (19g sugar) and 6g protein.
**Percent Daily Values are based on a 2,000 calorie diet. Your daily values may be higher or lower depending on your calorie needs:

		Calories:	2,000	2,500
Total Fat	Less than		65g	80g
Sat Fat	Less than		20g	25g
Cholesterol	Less than		300mg	300mg
Sodium	Less than		2,400mg	2,400mg
Potassium			3,500mg	3,500mg
Total Carbohydrate			300g	375g
Dietary Fiber			25g	30g

INGREDIENTS: WHOLE OAT FLOUR (INCLUDES THE OAT BRAN), MARSHMALLOW BITS (SUGAR, MODIFIED CORN STARCH, CORN SYRUP, DEXTROSE, GELATIN; RED 40, YELLOW 5 & 6, BLUES 1 & 2 AND OTHER COLOR ADDED, ARTIFICIAL FLAVOR), SUGAR, CORN SYRUP, WHEAT STARCH, SALT, COLOR ADDED, CALCIUM CARBONATE, TRISODIUM PHOSPHATE, VITAMIN C (SODIUM ASCORBATE), A B VITAMIN (NIACIN), IRON (A MINERAL NUTRIENT), VITAMIN B_6 (PYRIDOXINE HYDROCHLORIDE), VITAMIN A (PALMITATE), VITAMIN B_2 (RIBOFLAVIN), VITAMIN B_1 (THIAMIN MONONITRATE), ARTIFICIAL FLAVOR, A B VITAMIN (FOLIC ACID), VITAMIN D, VITAMIN E (MIXED TOCOPHEROLS) ADDED TO PROTECT FRESHNESS.

Figure 5-9 *Reading The NUTRITION FACTS on food labels helps us choose more nutritious foods. Based on the information from these nutrition labels, which cereal is the better choice for breakfast? Consider the amount of dietary fiber in each cereal, based on the amount per 100 kcal. Did the ingredient lists give you any clues? (*NOTE: *Ingredients are always listed in descending order by weight on a label.) When choosing a breakfast cereal, it is generally wise to focus on ones that are rich sources of dietary fiber and low in fat. Simple sugar content can also be used for evaluation. However, sometimes this number does not reflect added sugar but simply the addition of fruits such as raisins, complicating the evaluation.*

TABLE 5-6

Increasing Dietary Fiber Intake Is Not Hard To Do

Try this:	Instead of this:	Dietary fiber bonus (grams)
Whole-wheat bread, 1 slice	White bread, 1 slice	1.5
Brown rice, $\frac{1}{2}$ cup	White rice, $\frac{1}{2}$ cup	2
Baked potato with skin, 1 medium	Mashed potatoes, $\frac{1}{2}$ cup	3
Unpeeled apple (or applesauce made with unpeeled apples), 1 medium	Regular applesauce, $\frac{1}{2}$ cup	1.5
Orange segments, 1 orange	Orange juice, 1 cup	2
Whole-grain cereal (hot or ready-to-eat), 1 cup	Sweetened cereal, 1 cup	2.5-5
Popcorn (lightly seasoned with butter or salt, if at all), 3 cups	Potato chips, 12	2
Bean dip, $\frac{1}{4}$ cup	Sour cream dip, $\frac{1}{4}$ cup	1.5
Kidney beans on salad, 2 tbsp	Bacon bits on salad, 2 tbsp	2
Salad, 2 cups	French fries, 12	1

In your search for dietary fiber, must you always avoid white bread, rolls, and fluffy, white pancakes? Must you always choose the whole-grain types? No. You don't have to give up favorite foods as long as you frequently choose whole-grain alternatives to refined breads and cereals. Again, the goal of 20 to 35 grams of dietary fiber a day is not that hard to attain (see Table 5-6).

Problems with High-Fiber Diets

Very high dietary fiber intakes—for example, 60 grams per day—can pose some health risks. Again, a high dietary fiber intake requires a high fluid intake. Not consuming enough fluid with the dietary fiber can leave the stool very hard, making elimination difficult and painful. Intestinal blockage has occurred in people who consume great amounts of wheat bran and oat bran. Large amounts of dietary fiber can also bind important minerals, especially calcium, zinc, and iron, making them less available to the body.[5] More studies are needed concerning the long-term effects of high-fiber diets on mineral status. High-fiber diets also contribute to intestinal gas. Finally, great amounts of dietary fiber can make children feel full before they eat enough food to meet energy needs. As with many practices, moderation with dietary fiber is the best approach.

Carbohydrates in Foods

The foods that yield the highest percentage of energy from carbohydrates are table sugar, honey, jam, jelly, fruit, and plain baked potatoes. These foods are nutrient dense for carbohydrate; that is, carbohydrates deliver much of their food energy. Corn flakes, rice, bread, and noodles all contain at least 75% of energy as carbohydrates. Foods with moderate amounts of carbohydrate energy are peas, broccoli, oatmeal, dry beans and other legumes, cream pies, french fries, and nonfat milk. In these foods the carbohydrate content is diluted either by protein, as in the case of nonfat milk, or by fat, as in the case of a cream pie.

Chocolate, potato chips, and whole milk contain 30% to 40% of energy as carbohydrates. Again, the energy supplied from the carbohydrate content of these foods is overwhelmed by either their fat content or their protein content. Foods with essentially no carbohydrates include beef, chicken, fish, vegetable oils, butter, and margarine.

Figure 5-10 shows that, in planning a high-carbohydrate diet, you need to emphasize potatoes, grains, pasta, fruits, and vegetables. You can't create a diet high in carbohydrate energy from chocolate, potato chips, and french fries because these foods contain too much fat. The percentage of energy from carbohydrate is more important than the total amount of carbohydrate in a food when planning a high-carbohydrate diet.

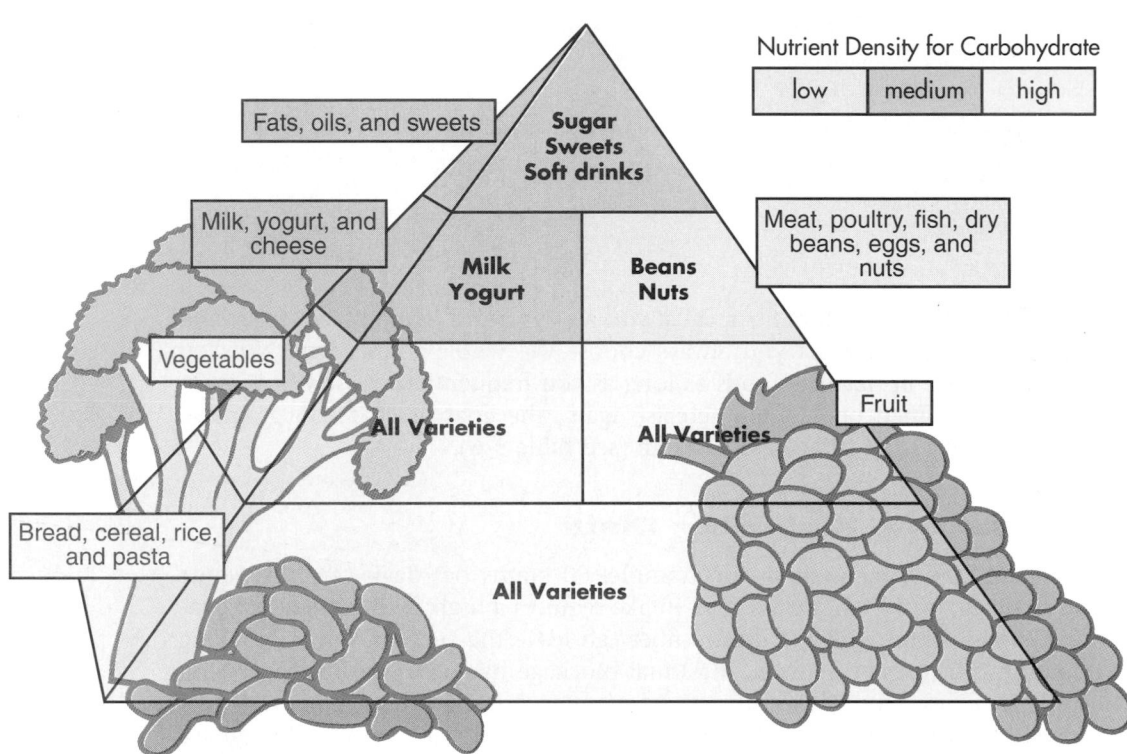

Figure 5-10 *Sources of carbohydrates from the Food Guide Pyramid. The bread, cereal, rice, and pasta group, fruit group, vegetable group, and milk, yogurt, and cheese group contain many foods rich in carbohydrate. The background color of each group indicates the average nutrient density for carbohydrate in that group.*

Nutritive Sweeteners in Foods

Sucrose is the tried-and-true sweetener. A relatively new sweetener in food is high-fructose corn syrup, which contains 40% to 90% fructose. It is made by treating corn starch with acid and enzymes. Much of the starch is broken down into glucose and then changed into fructose. The syrup is usually as sweet as sucrose. Its major advantage is that it is cheaper and can be shipped in a more concentrated form than sucrose. Also, it has better freezing properties because it doesn't encourage the formation of ice crystals. High-fructose corn syrups are used in soft drinks, candies, jams, jellies, other fruit products, and desserts.

In addition to sucrose and high-fructose corn syrup, brown sugar, turbinado sugar, honey, maple syrup, and other sugars are added to foods. Raw (unrefined) sugar is generally unavailable in the United States. FDA considers it unfit for human consumption. A partially refined version of raw sugar that can be sold is turbinado sugar. This has a slight molasses flavor. Brown sugar is basically sucrose containing some molasses; either the molasses is not totally removed from the sucrose during processing or it is added back to the sucrose crystals.

Maple syrup is made by boiling down the sap from sugar maple trees. Pancake syrup sold in supermarkets is sweetened mostly with corn syrup—not maple syrup.

To make honey, bees alter nectar from plants, breaking down the sucrose into fructose and glucose. Honey offers the same nutritional value as other simple sugar sources. A common misconception is that honey contains vitamins and minerals. It is a source of energy but little else (see Appendix A). Note that giving honey to infants is risky because it can contain spores of the bacterium *Clostridium botulinum*. These spores can develop into bacteria that cause fatal food-borne illness (see Chapter 17). Adults can safely consume honey because the acidic environment of an adult's stomach inhibits bacterial growth. An infant's stomach is not very acidic, leaving it susceptible to the risks this bacterium poses.

Only the sweetener black strap molasses, a by-product of sugar production, contains any appreciable amount of minerals. However, our consumption of molasses in foods is very low.

Alternative Sweeteners

People who want to limit sugar have two sets of alternative sweeteners to consider. One set is the sugar alcohols: **sorbitol,** mannitol, and xylitol. Today the one used in the greatest amounts in foods is sorbitol, which is found in some sugarless gum and some dietetic foods. Sugar alcohols yield energy (close to 3 kcal per gram) but are not readily metabolized by the bacteria in the mouth. Thus they do not promote dental caries. Nor do sugar alcohols cause as rapid a rise in blood glucose as do typical dietary monosaccharides—hence their use in dietetic foods. However, when taken in large amounts, sorbitol and mannitol can cause diarrhea because they are not readily absorbed from the small intestine. Products whose foreseeable consumption may result in a daily ingestion of 50 grams of sorbitol or mannitol must bear this labeling statement: "Excess consumption may have a laxative effect."

The other major class of alternative sweeteners currently available in the United States contains saccharin, aspartame, and acesulfame-K. Another sweetener, cyclamate, was banned in 1970 by FDA because of its link with cancer and birth defects. New research has introduced some questions about the necessity of such a ban. Depending on this reexamination, cyclamate could be back on the grocery shelves soon.

Saccharin. The sweetener **saccharin** was first produced in 1879. Although widely used in soft drinks and table sweeteners, it has been recently linked with cancer. Laboratory animals have developed bladder cancer when given high doses of saccharin, especially in the second generation after exposure. Arguments continue concerning the interpretation of data from these experiments, mostly because of saccharin's weak carcinogenic nature, if it is carcinogenic at all. In 1977 FDA attempted to ban saccharin because of this association with cancer. Many saccharin users protested a ban because it left them with no low-calorie sweetener (the others were not available in 1977). Public pressure persuaded Congress to prevent FDA from banning saccharin. In 1991 FDA withdrew its 1977 proposal to ban saccharin. However, products containing saccharin must contain a label of warning of the cancer risk.

Aspartame. In 1981 the alternative sweetener **aspartame** became available. Its trade name is NutraSweet when added to foods and Equal when sold as powder. Aspartame is composed of the amino acids phenylalanine and aspartic acid, with the

---

Names of sugars used in foods
  Sugar
  Sucrose
  Brown sugar
  Confectioners' sugar (powdered sugar)
  Fruit juice concentrate
  Syrup
  Turbinado sugar
  Invert sugar
  Glucose
  Levulose
  Polydextrose
  Lactose
  Honey
  Corn syrup or sweeteners
  High-fructose corn syrup
  Molasses
  Caramel
  Maple syrup
  Dextrose
  Fructose
  Maltose

Sorbitol
An alcohol derivative of glucose that yields about 3 kcal per gram but is slowly absorbed from the small intestine. It is used in some sugarless gums and dietetic foods.

Saccharin
An alternative sweetener that yields no energy to the body; it is 300 times sweeter than sucrose.

Aspartame
An alternative sweetener made of two amino acids (part of proteins) and methanol; it is about 200 times sweeter than sucrose.

CONTAINS: CARBONATED WATER, ORANGE JUICE, CITRIC ACID, NUTRASWEET* BRAND OF ASPARTAME**, POTASSIUM BENZOATE (A PRESERVATIVE), CITRUS PECTIN, POTASSIUM CITRATE, CAFFEINE, MALTODEXTRIN, GUM ARABIC, NATURAL FLAVORS, BROMINATED VEGETABLE OIL, YELLOW #5 AND ERYTHORBIC ACID (TO PROTECT FLAVOR).
*NUTRASWEET® AND THE NUTRASWEET SYMBOL ARE REGISTERED TRADEMARKS OF THE NUTRASWEET COMPANY.
PHENYLKETONURICS: CONTAINS PHENYLALANINE.

Note the warning for people with PKU that this diet soft drink with aspartame contains phenylalanine.

Phenylketonuria (PKU)

A disease in which the liver cannot readily metabolize the amino acid phenylalanine. Toxic by-products of phenylalanine can then build up in the body and lead to mental retardation.

Acesulfame-K

An alternative sweetener that yields no energy to the body; it is 200 times sweeter than sucrose.

addition of methanol. Because amino acids are the building blocks of proteins, aspartame belongs more in the protein class than in the carbohydrate class. Aspartame yields energy—4 kcal per gram—but is about 200 times sweeter than sucrose. This means that much less aspartame yields the same sweetening potency as sucrose. Today aspartame is used mostly in beverages, gelatin desserts, chewing gum, and other food items. FDA has recently expanded aspartame's uses to toppings and fillings for precooked bakery goods and cookies. Aspartame does not cause tooth decay. Like other proteins, however, aspartame is damaged when heated for a long time and thus cannot be widely used in products that require cooking.

In widespread use throughout the world, aspartame has been approved for use by more than 90 countries and endorsed by the World Health Organization, American Medical Association, American Diabetes Association, and American Academy of Pediatrics Committee on Nutrition. Although aspartame has never been linked with cancer, individuals have filed about 7000 complaints with FDA claiming adverse reactions to aspartame—headaches, dizziness, seizures, nausea, allergic reactions, and other side effects.

People who are sensitive to aspartame should avoid it. However, the percentage of sensitive people is extremely small. Considering its wide use, the relatively small number of complaints made against aspartame to date suggests most people can use it. In addition, careful research casts doubt on whether it causes headaches and mood swings or stimulates later food intake.[7]

Aspartame's phenylalanine content has concerned some people. Blood concentrations of this amino acid may increase significantly if aspartame is not consumed with the other amino acids normally found in protein foods. This problem can be easily avoided by consuming aspartame with protein foods. Some people are also concerned about the methanol content in asparatame. However, the amount of methanol in a soft drink sweetened with aspartame is not more than is found in a cup of many fruit or vegetable juices.

Overall the scientific community agrees that aspartame itself is safe; as previously noted, numerous scientific and medical groups support its use. An acceptable daily intake set by FDA is equivalent to about 14 cans of diet soft drinks a day for an adult or about 80 packets of Equal. Aspartame is safe for children and pregnant women to consume, but some scientists suggest cautious use by these groups.

One final note about aspartame: a rare disease called *phenylketonuria (PKU)* lessens a person's ability to metabolize phenylalanine. PKU is discussed in Chapter 7. For now, note that you were tested for this disease as an infant, probably before leaving the hospital. Labels on products containing aspartame warn people with PKU against using the product. Individuals carrying only one PKU gene in their DNA do not have the disease and can consume aspartame. Only a person with two PKU genes has inherited the disease and should not use aspartame.

Acesulfame-K. The newest sweetener in the United States, **acesulfame-K** (Sunette), was approved by FDA in July 1988. Acesulfame-K is 200 times sweeter than sucrose. Presently, it can be used in chewing gum, powdered drink mixes, gelatins, puddings, nondairy creamers, baked goods, yogurt, frozen desserts, syrups, and toppings. It contributes no energy to the diet because it is not broken down by the body. Acesulfame-K is used as a sweetener in foods and beverages in at least 60 countries including Canada. Acesulfame-K can be used in baking, whereas the current form of aspartame cannot because it breaks down when heated. Acesulfame-K may therefore become more widely used.

Other alternative sweeteners. Research continues on new forms of alternative sweeteners. Three are awaiting FDA approval:

- Alitame, which is formed from two amino acids and another small nitrogen group, is 2000 times sweeter than sucrose.

- Sucralose, which is made by substituting three chlorine atoms for three hydroxyl groups (−OH) on sucrose, is 400 to 800 times sweeter than sucrose and is approved for use in Canada, among other countries.
- D-Tagatose, a compound derived from lactose, has the same sweetness as sucrose but yields only half the energy.
- Thaumatins, proteins obtained from the fruit of the West African plant *Thaumatococcus danielii* that are 2000 times sweeter than sucrose.

Overall, alternative sweeteners enable people with diabetes to enjoy the flavor of sweetness while controlling sugars in their diets; they also provide noncaloric or very low-calorie sugar substitutes for persons trying to lose weight.[7] Thus alternative sweeteners provide people who want to reduce their intake of sugars with another flavorful option. In the future there will probably be more use of blends of the alternative sweeteners, such as aspartame and acesulfame. Improved flavor (more like sucrose) and greater sweetness from the various possible combinations can result. These blends are commonly used in Europe.

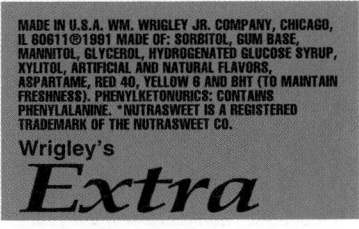

MADE IN U.S.A. WM. WRIGLEY JR. COMPANY, CHICAGO, IL 60611®1991 MADE OF: SORBITOL, GUM BASE, MANNITOL, GLYCEROL, HYDROGENATED GLUCOSE SYRUP, XYLITOL, ARTIFICIAL AND NATURAL FLAVORS, ASPARTAME, RED 40, YELLOW 6 AND BHT (TO MAINTAIN FRESHNESS). PHENYLKETONURICS: CONTAINS PHENYLALANINE. *NUTRASWEET IS A REGISTERED TRADEMARK OF THE NUTRASWEET CO.

Wrigley's
Extra

Sugar alcohols can be found in sugarless gum. Note that aspartame is also used to sweeten this product.

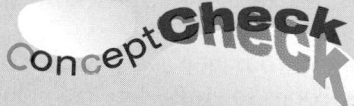

ConceptCheck

There is no RDA for carbohydrate; the best advice is an intake of more than 50 to 100 grams, emphasizing grains, vegetables, and fruits, to 55% or more of total energy intake. We should limit total consumption of simple sugars to about 10 to 15 teaspoons per day. Most simple sugars are added to foods and beverages during manufacturing or at the table. To reduce simple sugar consumption, one must eat fewer items that have had a lot of sugar added, such as some baked goods, certain beverages, and some breakfast cereals. Simple sugars contribute to dental caries and provide few vitamins and minerals, if any. There are three major alternative sweeteners available in America today—saccharin, aspartame, and acesulfame-K. These can aid in the goal of reducing simple sugar intake.

Summary

➤ The monosaccharides in our diet include glucose, fructose, and galactose (the latter as part of lactose). Once absorbed via the small intestine and transported through the portal vein into the liver, much of the fructose and galactose is turned into glucose.

➤ The major disaccharides are sucrose (glucose plus fructose), maltose (glucose plus glucose), and lactose (glucose plus galactose). When digested, these yield monosaccharide forms. Both monosaccharides and disaccharides are classified as simple sugars.

➤ Lactose is the sugar found in milk. Lactose intolerance is a condition that results when cells of the intestine wall do not make sufficient or any lactase, the enzyme necessary to digest lactose. Undigested lactose travels to the large intestine, resulting in such symptoms as abdominal gas, pain, and diarrhea. Most people with lactose intolerance can tolerate cheese and yogurt, although tolerance to dairy products as a whole varies among affected individuals.

➤ Some starch digestion occurs in the mouth. Carbohydrate digestion is finished in the small intestine. Some plant fibers are digested by the bacteria present in the large intestine; undigested plant fibers end up in the feces. Single sugars mostly follow an active absorption process in the small intestine. They are then transported to the liver.

➤ The major digestible polysaccharides—starches—contain multiple glucose units linked together. Glycogen is an animal starch that acts as a storage form of glucose in the liver and muscles.

➤ Carbohydrates provide energy (4 kcal per gram), protect against needless metabolism of protein for energy, and add flavor and sweetness to foods. They are not necessarily fattening. Many types of carbohydrates can be metabolized to acids by bacteria on teeth. The acid can erode the tooth surface, leading to dental caries.

➤ Dietary fibers include the indigestible polysaccharides cellulose, hemicelluloses, pectins, gums, and mucilages, as well as the noncarbohydrate lignins. Dietary fiber, especially insoluble varieties, provides mass to the stool, thus easing elimination. It may also decrease the risk for colon cancer. In high doses, soluble fibers can help control blood glucose in diabetic people and also lower blood cholesterol.

➤ There is no RDA for carbohydrate. A minimal intake of 50 to 100 grams is needed; 55% or more of total energy intake is recommended. If carbohydrate consumption is inadequate, the body can make what sugars it needs to support cell metabolism. However, if inadequate carbohydrate intake continues for weeks at a time, the price is a loss of body protein, ketosis, and a general weakening of the body.

➤ Diets high in complex forms of carbohydrates are encouraged as a replacement for high-fat diets, with an emphasis on starches. Foods to emphasize are potatoes, grains, pastas, fruits, and vegetables. Sugar intake should be limited to 10% to 15% of energy intake. Moderating sugar intake, especially between meals, reduces the risk of dental caries. Use of alternative sweeteners, such as aspartame, can help in limiting sugar intake.

Study Questions

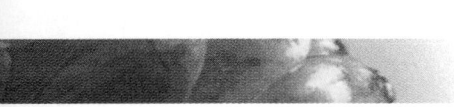

1 Outline the basic steps in blood glucose regulation, including the roles of insulin and glucagon.
2 What are the three major disaccharides? Describe how each plays a part in the human diet.
3 How do amylose and glycogen differ from one another? Why can this be important metabolically?
4 What are the important roles that dietary fiber plays in the diet?
5 What, if any, are the proven ill effects of sugars in the diet?
6 How is high-fructose corn syrup made? Why is its use in food products increasing?
7 Briefly describe the chemical structure, sweetness, and food uses of two alternative sweeteners.

After reading the Nutrition Issue, answer the following questions:

8 How does insulin-dependent diabetes differ from non–insulin-dependent diabetes in cause and treatment?
9 What dietary treatment is recommended for the common form of hypoglycemia?

References

1 American Dietetic Association Reports: Position of The American Dietetic Association: oral health and nutrition, *Journal of the American Dietetic Association* 96:184, 1996.

2 Anderson JW and others: Postprandial serum glucose, insulin, and lipoprotein responses to high- and low-fiber diets, *Metabolism* 44:848, 1995.

3 Asp NGL: Classification and methodology of food carbohydrates as related to nutritional effects, *American Journal of Clinical Nutrition* 61:930S, 1995.

4 Atkinson MA, Maclaren WK: The pathogenesis of insulin-dependent diabetes mellitus, *New England Journal of Medicine* 331:1428, 1994.

5 Bennett WG, Cerda JJ: Benefits of dietary fiber. *Postgraduate Medicine* 99(2):153, 1996.

6 Clark CM, Lee DA: Prevention and treatment of the complications of diabetes mellitus, *New England Journal of Medicine* 332:1210, 1995.

7 Drewnowski A: Intense sweeteners and the control of appetite, *Nutrition Reviews* 53:1, 1995.

8 Foster-Powell K, Miller JB: International tables of glycemic index, *American Journal of Clinical Nutrition* 62:871S, 1995.

9 Gibney M and others: Consumption of sugars, *American Journal of Clinical Nutrition* 62:178S, 1995.

10 Giovannucci E and others: Physical activity, obesity, and risk for colon cancer and adenoma in men, *Annals of Internal Medicine* 122:327, 1995.

11 Giovannucci E and others: Alcohol, low-methionine–low-folate diets, and risk of colon cancer in men, *Journal of the National Cancer Institute* 87:265, 1995.

12 Giovannucci E and others: Aspirin and the risk of colorectal cancer in women, *The New England Journal of Medicine* 333:609, 1995.

13 Glinsmann WH, Park YK: Perspective on the 1986 Food and Drug Administration assessment of the safety of carbohydrate sweeteners: uniform definitions and recommendations for future assessments, *American Journal of Clinical Nutrition* 62:161S, 1995.

14 Greenberg ER and others: A clinical trial of antioxidant vitamins to prevent colorectal adenoma, *New England Journal of Medicine* 331:141, 1994.

15 Hirsch J: Role and benefits of carbohydrate in the diet: key issues for future dietary guidelines, *American Journal of Clinical Nutrition* 61:996S, 1995.

16 Hollander PA: New oral agents for type II diabetes, *Postgraduate Medicine* 98(5):110, 1995.

17 Jaravi AE and others: The influence of food structure on postprandial metabolism in patients with non–insulin-dependent diabetes mellitus, *American Journal of Clinical Nutrition* 61:837, 1995.

18 Levine B: About lactose intolerance, *Nutrition Today* 31:79, 1996.

19 Lineback D, Dreher M: Complex carbohydrates: the science and the label, *Nutrition Reviews* 53:186, 1995.

20 Polonsky KS and others: Non–insulin-dependent diabetes mellitus—a genetically programmed failure of the beta cell to compensate for insulin resistance, *New England Journal of Medicine* 334:777, 1996.

21 Service FJ: Hypoglycemic disorders, *New England Journal of Medicine* 332:1144, 1995.

22 Southgate DAT: Digestion and metabolism of sugars, *American Journal of Clinical Nutrition* 62:203S, 1995.

23 Stephen AM and others: Intake of carbohydrate and its components—international comparisons, trends over time, and effects of changing to low-fat diets, *American Journal of Clinical Nutrition* 62:851S, 1995.

24 Suarez FL and others: A comparison of symptoms after the consumption of milk or lactose-hydrolyzed milk by people with self-reported severe lactose intolerance, *The New England Journal of Medicine* 333:1, 1995.

25 Truszkowski JA, Summers RW: Colorectal neoplasms, *Postgraduate Medicine* 98(5):97, 1995.

26 Wolever TMS, Miller JB: Sugars and blood glucose control, *American Journal of Clinical Nutrition* 62:212S, 1995.

27 Wolraich ML and others: Effects of diets high in sucrose or aspartame on the behavior and cognitive performance of children, *New England Journal of Medicine* 330:301, 1994.

28 Wylie-Rosett J, Mossavar-Rahmani Y: Diabetes and women's health, *Topics in Clinical Nutrition* 11:36, 1995.

29 Wynder EL and others: High fiber intake—indicator of a healthy lifestyle, *Journal of the American Medical Association* 275:486, 1996.

RATE 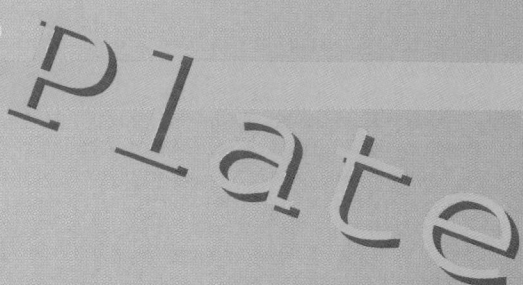 your Plate

How Does Your Diet Rate for Carbohydrate and Dietary Fiber?

Let's reevaluate the nutritional assessment you completed at the end of Chapter 2. Here are your tasks:

1. Look at your analysis and find the total number of grams of carbohydrate you ate.

   TOTAL GRAMS OF CARBOHYDRATE _____
   A. Did you consume more than the minimum amount to avoid ketosis, 50 to 100 grams?
   B. Now calculate the percentage of energy in your diet from carbohydrate. You will need the total grams of carbohydrate from your assessment as well as the total kcals you ate. Use this formula to calculate it:

   $$\frac{\text{Total grams of carbohydrate} \times 4}{\text{Total kcals consumed}} \times 100 = \text{\% of energy intake from carbohydrate}$$

   ANSWER: _____

   Was 55% or more of your total energy intake from carbohydrate? YES _____ NO _____
   If not, list several ways you could increase your carbohydrate intake.

   _____

   _____

   _____

2. Look again at the list of foods you ate, including the amounts, and determine the total amount of dietary fiber you consumed. If you have a computer analysis of your diet, your dietary fiber intake is listed in the printout. Otherwise, look up the dietary fiber content of each food you ate in the food composition table in Appendix A, then calculate your total intake, taking into account the amount of each food you ate.

   TOTAL AMOUNT OF DIETARY FIBER CONSUMED _____ grams
   A. Did you eat the 20 to 35 grams suggested in this chapter?
   B. If not, what could you do to increase your dietary fiber intake? What foods could you substitute for some of the foods you ate?

   _____

   _____

   _____

   _____

3. Finally, use Table 5-4 to see if you can reduce your intake of sugars, especially if you need to watch your total energy intake to maintain a healthy weight. What three foods might you limit in the future?

   _____

   _____

   _____

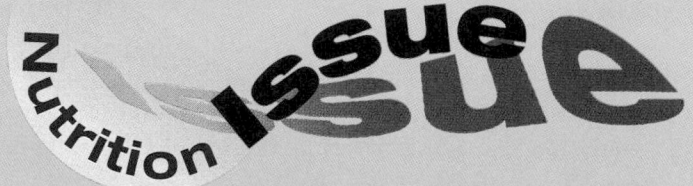

When Blood Glucose Regulation Fails

Improper regulation of blood glucose results in either hyperglycemia (high blood glucose) or hypoglycemia (low blood glucose). High blood glucose is most commonly associated with diabetes (technically *diabetes mellitus*), a disease that affects about 16 million Americans. Low blood glucose is a much rarer condition.

DIABETES MELLITUS

There are two major forms of diabetes: **insulin-dependent diabetes** (also called *type I* or *juvenile-onset diabetes*) and **non–insulin-dependent diabetes** (also called *type II* or *adult-onset diabetes*).

Insulin-dependent diabetes

The insulin-dependent form often begins in late childhood, around the age of 8 to 12 years, but can occur at any age. The disease runs in certain families, indicating a clear genetic link. The symptoms of the disease are abnormally high blood glucose after eating and the tendency to develop ketosis.[4]

The onset of insulin-dependent diabetes is generally associated with decreased release of insulin from the pancreas. As insulin in the blood declines, blood glucose increases, especially after eating. When blood glucose exceeds the kidney's capacity to recapture and return it to the bloodstream, excess glucose spills over into the urine. Figure 5-11 shows a typical glucose tolerance curve observed in a patient with this form of diabetes, following a test load of 50 grams (10 teaspoons) of glucose. Warning signs for diabetes are as follows: frequent urination and extreme thirst, constant hunger, fatigue, weakness, sudden weight loss, slowed healing of skin infections, and blurred vision.

An exciting new finding regarding the cause of insulin–dependent diabetes may help physicians treat this disease or even prevent its onset in the future. At least some cases of insulin-dependent diabetes begin with an immune system disorder that causes destruction of the insulin-producing cells in the pancreas. Most likely a virus or protein foreign to the body sets off the destruction.[4] Cow's milk is suspected of supplying such a protein, so its introduction before 1 year of age is not advised (see Chapter 15). In response to the destruction, the affected cells release other proteins that stimulate a more furious attack. Eventually the pancreas loses its ability to synthesize insulin, and the clinical stage of the disease begins. For this reason, early treatment to stop the immune-linked destruction may be important. Other researchers are attempting to extract insulin–producing cells from cadavers and infuse them into people with insulin-dependent diabetes. Both lines of research are continuing.

Currently, insulin-dependent diabetes is treated primarily by insulin therapy, either with injections one to six times a day or with an insulin pump. The pump dispenses insulin at a steady rate into the body, with

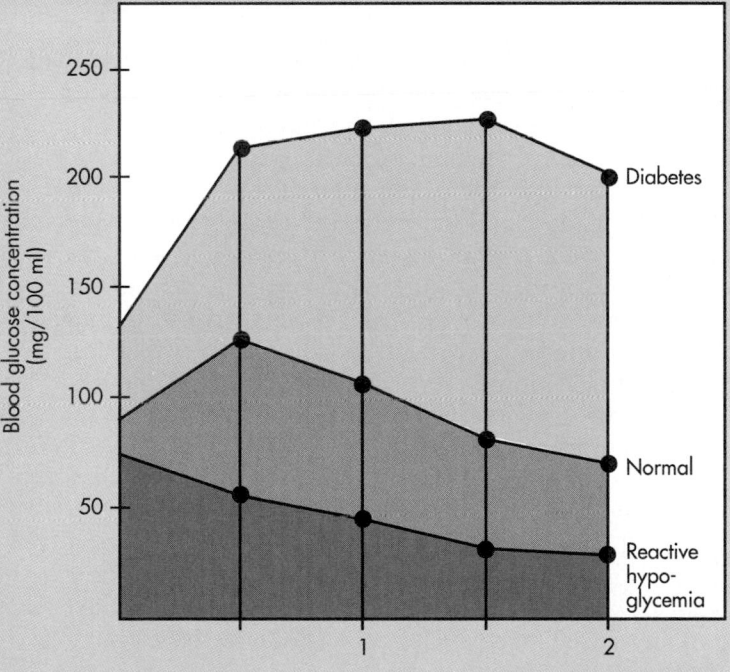

Figure 5-11 *Glucose tolerance test. These are typical responses seen after 50 grams (10 teaspoons) of glucose are ingested by a healthy person and by a person with uncontrolled diabetes mellitus or reactive hypoglycemia. Blood glucose concentration is determined during fasting and then at regular intervals after the person consumes the glucose load. The depiction of reactive hypoglycemia is theoretical; the actual existence of this syndrome is in question. In any case, true hypoglycemia is rare.*

Continued.

greater amounts delivered after each meal. Dietary measures include three regular meals and one or more snacks (including one at bedtime) having a regulated carbohydrate:protein:fat ratio to maximize insulin action and minimize swings in blood glucose concentrations. The diet should be rich in complex forms of carbohydrates, include ample dietary fiber, and supply an amount of energy in balance with energy needs.[28] If a high carbohydrate intake raises blood triglyceride and cholesterol concentrations beyond desired ranges, carbohydrate intake can be reduced and replaced with unsaturated fat. This change tends to reduce blood triglycerides and cholesterol.[28] Chapter 6 discusses how to implement such a diet. Moderate consumption of sugars with meals is fine as long as blood glucose regulation is preserved and the sugars replace other carbohydrates in the meal.[26] Overall the diet prescription needs to be individualized according to health status. Once sufficient protein is included in the diet, the rest of the energy is distributed between carbohydrate and fat, with minimal saturated fat intake.

In nondiabetic individuals, insulin output decreases as glucose is cleared from the bloodstream after a meal. Because this does not necessarily occur in diabetic people who are taking insulin, consumption of meals at regular intervals is especially important for them. If they skip meals, the injected insulin can cause severe hypoglycemia because it acts on whatever little glucose is available.

The hormone imbalances that occur in people with untreated diabetes lead to mobilization of body fat, which floods into liver cells. Ketosis results because the fat is mostly converted to ketones. Ketone concentration can rise excessively in the blood, eventually forcing ketones into the urine. These ketones pull sodium and potassium ions with them. This series of events can contribute to a chain reaction that eventually leads to dehydration, ion imbalance, coma, and even death, especially in people with poorly controlled insulin-dependent diabetes.[6]

Other complications of diabetes can be degenerative conditions, such as blindness, heart disease, kidney disease, and numbness from nerve damage; all are caused by long-term poor blood glucose regulation. These degenerative health problems arise in part from changes that occur in small blood vessels, namely the capillaries. Nerves can also deteriorate, resulting in many changes that decrease proper nerve stimulation. When this occurs in the intestinal tract, intermittent diarrhea and constipation result. Because of nerve deterioration in the extremities, many people with diabetes lose the sensation of pain associated with injuries or infections. Not having as much pain, they often delay treatment of hand or foot problems. This delay, combined with a rich environment for bacterial growth (bacteria thrive on glucose), sets the stage for complications in the extremities. High blood glucose also contributes to a rapid build-up of fats in blood vessel walls, which eventually chokes off the blood supply to nearby organs. See Chapter 6 for details on this latter process, called *atherosclerosis.*

Current research shows that the development of blood vessel and nerve complications of diabetes can be slowed with regular treatment directed at keeping blood glucose within the normal range.[6] The therapy poses some risks of its own, such as hypoglycemia, so it must be implemented under close supervision of a physician.

A person with diabetes generally must work closely with a physician to make the correct alterations in diet and medications and perform physical activity safely. Physical activity can enhance glucose uptake by muscles, which in turn can lower blood glucose. This outcome is beneficial, but people with diabetes need to be aware of their own blood glucose response to physical activity and compensate appropriately.

Non–insulin-dependent diabetes

Non–insulin-dependent diabetes usually begins after age 20 and more typically after age 40. This is the most common type of diabetes, accounting for about 90% of the cases diagnosed in the United States.[28] The number of people affected is on the rise, for the most part because of widespread inactivity and obesity and our ever-aging population. This type of diabetes is also genetically linked, but the initial problem often is not with the insulin-producing cells of the pancreas, but instead with the insulin receptors on the cell surfaces of certain body tissues, especially muscle tissues. Insulin needs to bind to these receptors if it is to promote glucose uptake in the tissues. If limited binding is instead the case, blood glucose is not readily transferred into cells, so the patient develops hyperglycemia as a result of the glucose's remaining in the bloodstream.[20] The pancreas attempts to increase insulin output to compensate, but its ability to do so is limited. Rather than insufficient insulin production, there is an abundance of insulin, particularly during the onset of the disease. As the disease develops, pancreatic function can fail, leading to reduced insulin output.[20]

Many cases of non–insulin-dependent diabetes are associated with obesity, especially when primarily abdominal in appearance, but the hyperglycemia is not directly caused by the obesity. In fact, some lean people also develop this type of diabetes. Obesity associated with oversized fat cells simply increases the risk for inefficient insulin binding to cells.

Non–insulin-dependent diabetes linked to obesity often disappears if the obesity is corrected. Achieving a more healthy weight should be a primary goal of treatment, but even limited weight loss can lead to better blood glucose regulation. Oral medications that increase the ability of the pancreas to produce insulin are often prescribed. New medications to slow starch digestion in the small intestine are also being employed.[16]

Sometimes it may be necessary to provide insulin injections because nothing else is able to control the disease. Regular physical activity also helps the muscles to take up more glucose. Regular meal patterns, with an emphasis on control of energy intake, consumption of complex forms of carbohydrates, and ample dietary fiber, is also important therapy. Moderate intake of sugars is fine with meals, but again these must be substituted for other carbohydrates, not simply added to the meal plan. Sugars should not be allowed to crowd out healthier food choices. Distributing carbohydrates throughout the day is also important because this helps minimize the high and low swings in blood glucose concentrations.

People with non–insulin-dependent diabetes who have high blood triglycerides should moderate their carbohydrate intake and increase their intake of unsaturated fat and dietary fiber, as noted earlier regarding people with insulin-dependent diabetes.[28]

Although many cases of non–insulin-dependent diabetes can be relieved by reducing excess fat stores, many people are not able to lose weight. They remain affected by diabetes and may experience the degenerative complications seen in the insulin-dependent form of the disease. Ketosis, however, is not usually seen in this form of diabetes.

The glycemic index: a tool for planning diabetic diets

Research concerning the body's response to various carbohydrates has led to development of a clinical tool known as the *glycemic index*. This index compares the total amount of glucose appearing in the blood after a specific food is eaten with the total amount of glucose appearing in the blood after the same amount of carbohydrate is eaten in the form of white bread or glucose.[8]

Several factors must be considered when predicting the glycemic index of a food, including its dietary fiber content, digestion rate, and total fat content. Whether the food is rich in sugar or starch is not as important.[17] Foods containing much soluble fiber (like oatmeal) are pro-cessed slowly and thus produce a slow increase in blood glucose after eating. In contrast, foods such as potatoes are broken down quickly, producing a rapid increase in blood glucose after eating. If a diabetic person eats many foods having low glycemic indices, such as whole fruits, milk, and beans, then each meal in the entire diet can contribute to blood glucose regulation.[2]

Hypoglycemia

As previously mentioned, diabetic people who are taking insulin sometimes have hypoglycemia if they don't eat frequently enough. Hypoglycemia can also develop in nondiabetic individuals. The two common forms of nondiabetic hypoglycemia are termed *reactive* and *fasting*. Al-though many people think they have hypoglycemia, few actually do.

Reactive hypoglycemia is described as irritability, nervousness, headache, sweating, and confusion 2 to 4 hours after eating a meal, especially a meal high in simple sugars. The cause of reactive hypoglycemia is unclear, but it may be overproduction of insulin by the pancreas in response to rising blood glucose. Some researchers are unwilling even to acknowledge the existence of reactive hypoglycemia, pointing out that the symptoms are more likely tied to recent intense exercise, psychological stress, medication use, or alcohol consumption.[21] **Fasting hypoglycemia** is usually caused by pancreatic cancer, which may lead to excessive insulin secretion. In this case, blood glucose falls to low concentrations after fasting for about 8 hours to 1 day. In some cases, both reactive and fasting hypoglycemia can be at work.

The diagnosis of hypoglycemia requires the simultaneous presence of low blood glucose and the typical hypoglycemic symptoms. Blood glucose of 40 to 50 milligrams per 100 milliliters is suggestive, but just having low blood glucose after eating is not enough evidence to make the diagnosis of hypoglycemia.

The popular press and television talk shows have popularized hypoglycemia, relating it to a variety of symptoms that most everyone has at one time or another. No clear evidence, however, has conclusively linked hypoglycemia to the difficulties popularly attributed to it: depression, chronic fatigue, allergies, nervous breakdowns, alcoholism, juvenile delinquency, childhood behavior problems, drug addiction, and inadequate sexual performance. Most people complaining of fatigue, shakiness, occasional heavy sweats, and emotional instability do not have documentable hypoglycemia. Furthermore, for most people in good health, eating simple sugars does not induce hypoglycemia. Unless a metabolic disorder is present, the body generally can respond adequately to an intake of simple sugars and starches.[21]

It is normal for healthy people to have some hypoglycemic symptoms, such as irritability, headache, and shakiness, if they have not eaten for a prolonged period of time. Although these symptoms don't necessarily indicate hypoglycemia, the standard nutrition therapy for them is one we all could follow. Eat regular meals, make sure you have some protein and fat in each meal, and eat complex forms of carbohydrates with ample soluble fiber. Avoid meals or snacks that contain little more than simple carbohydrates. If symptoms continue, try small protein-containing snacks between meals, such as half a turkey sandwich on whole wheat bread and half a glass of milk. Fat, protein, and soluble fiber in the diet tend to moderate swings in blood glucose. Lastly, moderate caffeine and alcohol intake.

Lipids

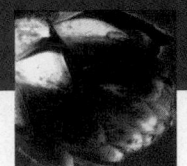

YOUR DOCTOR INFORMS YOU

that your "triglycerides are up." Your bill from a medical laboratory reads, "Blood lipid profile—$35." A health food advertisement suggests using omega-3 fatty acids from fish oils to lower blood cholesterol. Advertisers plug foods "lowest in saturated fat." All of these substances—triglycerides, omega-3 fatty acids, saturated fat, and cholesterol—are lipids, a collective term referring to fats and oils.

Lipids contain more than twice the energy per gram (9 kcal) as proteins and carbohydrates (4 kcal each). Consumption of certain saturated fatty acids also is linked to the risk of heart disease. For this reason, some concern about lipids is warranted, but lipids also play vital roles both in the body and in foods. Their presence in the diet is essential to good health.[30]

Let's look at lipids in detail—their forms, functions, metabolism, and food sources. This chapter will then conclude with a look at the link between lipid intake and the major "killer" disease in the United States, heart disease.

CHAPTER 6

Are You Eating A Diet That Includes Many Saturated-Fat Sources?

Instructions:

Check the food you would typically select from the two choices you are given.

1. ___ Bacon and eggs   ___ Ready-to-eat whole-grain breakfast cereal
2. ___ Doughnut or sweet roll   ___ White or whole-wheat roll, bagel, or bread, no margarine
3. ___ Breakfast sausage   ___ Fruit
4. ___ Whole milk   ___ Low-fat or nonfat milk
5. ___ Cheeseburger   ___ Turkey sandwich, no cheese
6. ___ French fries   ___ Plain baked potato or salad with low-cal or fat-free dressing
7. ___ Meal including fried hamburger or fatty beef   ___ Meal including broiled lean hamburger (ground round), chicken, or fish
8. ___ Creamed soup   ___ Clear soup (could have meat or vegetables in it)
9. ___ Potato salad   ___ Baked potato, plain
10. ___ Fruit/cream pie   ___ Graham crackers
11. ___ Ice cream   ___ Frozen yogurt, sherbet, or fat-reduced ice cream
12. ___ Butter or stick margarine   ___ Soft margarine in a tub

Interpretation

The foods listed on the left tend to be high in saturated fat, cholesterol, and total fat. Those on the right generally are low. If you want to reduce the risk of heart disease, choose the foods on the right more often than the foods on the left.

Key Chapter Concepts

- Lipids are a group of compounds that don't readily dissolve in water.
- Fatty acids are part of most lipids and can be grouped according to the type of bonds between the carbons: saturated fatty acids contain no double bonds, monounsaturated fatty acids contain one double bond, and polyunsaturated fatty acids contain two or more double bonds.
- Lipids composed of saturated fatty acids, such as in animal fat, tend to be solid at room temperature. Those with polyunsaturated fatty acids, such as in vegetable oils, are usually liquid at room temperature.
- Certain polyunsaturated fatty acids are essential parts of our diet because our bodies need them but don't produce them.
- Triglycerides are the major form of fat in food and in our bodies. Besides supplying certain essential polyunsaturated fatty acids to the body, triglycerides supply energy, allow efficient energy storage, insulate and protect the body, transport fat-soluble vitamins, and promote satiety. Fats also enhance the appeal and enjoyment of food by adding flavor and texture.
- Phospholipids are another class of lipids. They are derived from triglycerides. Phospholipids form important parts of cell membranes. Cholesterol is in the class of lipids called *sterols*. It forms part of vital compounds such as cell membranes, some hormones, and bile.
- Fats are carried in the bloodstream by various lipoproteins: chylomicrons, very low-density lipoproteins (VLDL), low-density lipoproteins (LDL), and high-density lipoproteins (HDL). Both elevated LDL and low HDL in the blood speed the development of heart disease.
- There is no RDA for fat. We need to eat at least the equivalent of about 1 tablespoon of plant oils daily in foods to get the specific polyunsaturated fatty acids our cells require. Our body cells make all the phospholipids and cholesterol we need.
- Major contributors of fat to our diets include animal foods, whole milk, and pastries.
- *Fat-free* does not mean *calorie-free*. As with other foods, the energy content of fat-free products must be considered when designing a diet.

Lipids in General

Lipids are a diverse group of chemical compounds, but they share one main characteristic: they do not readily dissolve in water.[18] Think of an oil and vinegar salad dressing. The oil is not soluble in the water-based vinegar; upon standing, the two separate into distinct layers, with oil on top and vinegar on the bottom.

The diversity of lipids is evident when you compare the structures of two of the many types: a fatty acid shown in Figure 6-1 and cholesterol on page 179.

As noted in Chapter 1, lipids that are solid at room temperature are called *fats*, and lipids that are liquid are called *oils*. Most people use the word *fat* to refer to all lipids because they don't know any differences exist. As already noted, however, *lipid* is a generic term that includes triglycerides and many other substances. To simplify our discussion, this chapter primarily uses the term *fat*; but as we will see later, not all the substances we call *fats* truly are fats. When necessary for clarity, the name of a specific lipid, such as cholesterol, will be used. This word usage is consistent with the way many people use these terms today.

Fatty Acids: The Simplest Form of Lipids

The **fatty acid** is common to most lipids, both in the body and in foods. It is basically a long chain of carbons linked together and flanked by hydrogen (see Figure 6-1). Fats in foods are not composed of a single type or category of fatty acid. Rather, each dietary fat is a complex mixture of different fatty acids. Butterfat, for example, contains numerous different fatty acids.

If all the links (technically referred to as *chemical bonds*) between the carbons are single connections and the carbons are filled with hydrogen, a fatty acid is said

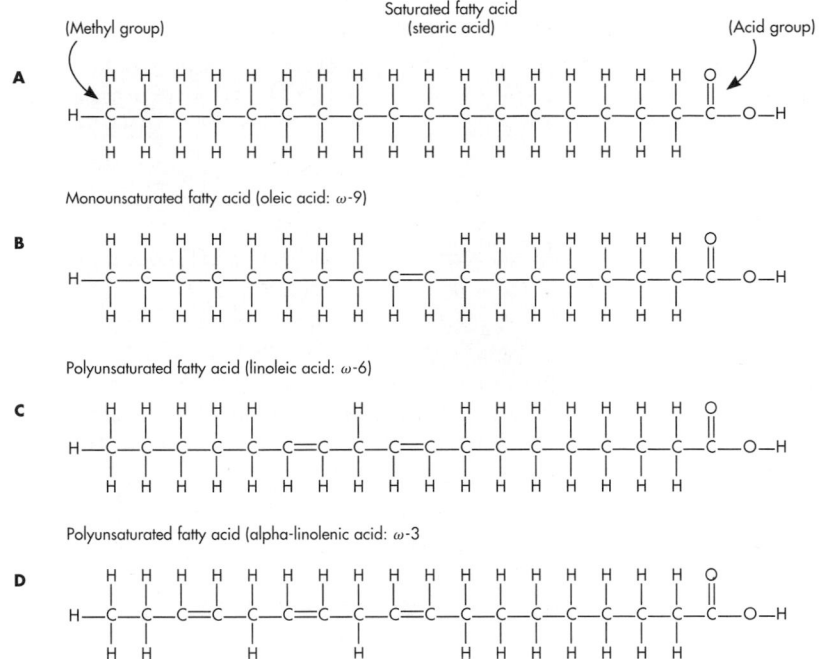

Figure 6-1 *Chemical forms of saturated, monounsaturated, and polyunsaturated fatty acids.*

to be **saturated** (see Figure 6-1, A). To understand this concept, picture a sponge saturated (full) with water.

As noted earlier, most fats high in saturated fatty acids, such as animal fats, remain solid at room temperature. A good example is the solid fat surrounding a piece of uncooked steak at room tempeature. Chicken fat, semisolid at room temperature, contains less saturated fat. In some foods, like whole milk, saturated fats are suspended in liquid, so the solid nature of these fats at room temperature is less apparent.

If a fatty acid is unsaturated, hydrogens are missing from the carbon chain, specifically at the area of the carbon-carbon double bonds (see Figure 6-1). If a fatty acid has one double bond between the carbons, it is **monounsaturated** (see Figure 6-1, B). Olive and canola oils contain a high percentage of monounsaturated fatty acids. If two or more bonds between the carbons are double bonds, the fatty acid is **polyunsaturated** and thus even less saturated with hydrogens (see Figure 6-1, C and D). Corn, soybean, and safflower oils are rich in polyunsaturated fatty acids.

Note, however, that dietary fats and oils contain a mixture of various saturated and unsaturated fatty acids (Figure 6-2). A fat or oil is classified as saturated, monounsaturated, or polyunsaturated based on the nature of the fatty acids present in the greatest concentration.

Chain length affects fatty acid characteristics. Fats in foods that contain primarily saturated fatty acids are solid at room temperature, especially if the fatty acids have a **long chain** (12 carbons or longer). **Medium-chain** saturated fatty acids (6 to 10 carbons long), such as those in coconut oil, produce liquid oils at room temperature. The shorter chain length overrides the effect of saturation. **Short-chain** saturated fatty acids (less than 6 carbons long) also form liquid oils at room temperature. Dairy fats are sources of these short-chain fatty acids. Fats containing primarily polyunsaturated or monounsaturated fatty acids are also usually liquid at room temperature. These are not affected by chain length.

Fatty acid
Acids found in fats. These are composed of a chain of carbons linked together. The chain is flanked by hydrogens and has an acidic chemical group at one end.

Saturated fatty acid
A fatty acid with no carbon-carbon double bonds.

Monounsaturated fatty acid
A fatty acid containing one carbon-carbon double bond.

Polyunsaturated fatty acid
A fatty acid containing two or more carbon-carbon double bonds.

Long-chain fatty acids
Fatty acids that contain 12 or more carbons.

Medium-chain fatty acids
Fatty acids that contain 8 to 10 carbons.

Short-chain fatty acids
Fatty acids that contain fewer than eight carbons.

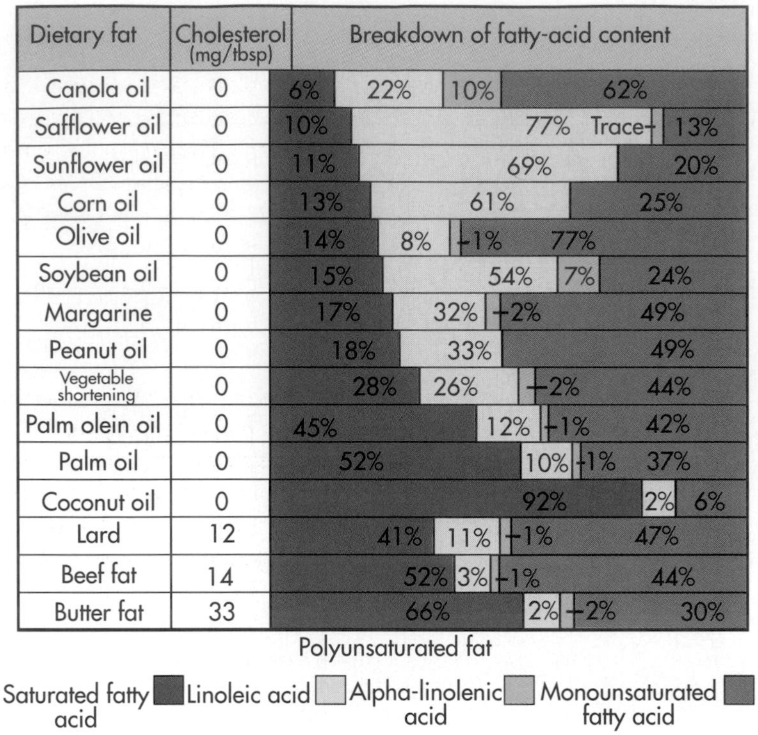
Dietary fat
Cholesterol (mg/tbsp)
Breakdown of fatty-acid content
Canola oil 0 6% 22% 10% 62%
Safflower oil 0 10% 77% Trace 13%
Sunflower oil 0 11% 69% 20%
Corn oil 0 13% 61% 25%
Olive oil 0 14% 8% 1% 77%
Soybean oil 0 15% 54% 7% 24%
Margarine 0 17% 32% 2% 49%
Peanut oil 0 18% 33% 49%
Vegetable shortening 0 28% 26% 2% 44%
Palm olein oil 0 45% 12% 1% 42%
Palm oil 0 52% 10% 1% 37%
Coconut oil 0 92% 2% 6%
Lard 12 41% 11% 1% 47%
Beef fat 14 52% 3% 1% 44%
Butter fat 33 66% 2% 2% 30%
Polyunsaturated fat
Saturated fatty acid
Linoleic acid
Alpha-linolenic acid
Monounsaturated fatty acid

Figure 6-2 *Comparison of dietary fats in terms of saturated fatty acids, the most common unsaturated fatty acids, and cholesterol content.*

Triglycerides

Fats and oils in foods are mostly in the form of triglycerides. The same is true for fats found in body structures. Some fatty acids are found attached to proteins in the bloodstream as they are being transported, but fatty acids usually do not exist in the body as such. Instead they form into triglycerides.[18]

Glycerol
A three-carbon alcohol used to form triglycerides.

Triglycerides contain a simple three-carbon alcohol, **glycerol,** which serves as a backbone for the three attached fatty acids. Removing one fatty acid from a triglyceride forms a diglyceride. Removing two fatty acids from a triglyceride forms a **monoglyceride.** Later we see that before most dietary fats are absorbed in the small intestine, the upper and lower fatty acids are typically removed from the triglyceride. This produces fatty acids and monoglycerides, which are absorbed into the intestinal cells. After absorption the fatty acids and monoglycerides are mostly re-formed into triglycerides.[18]

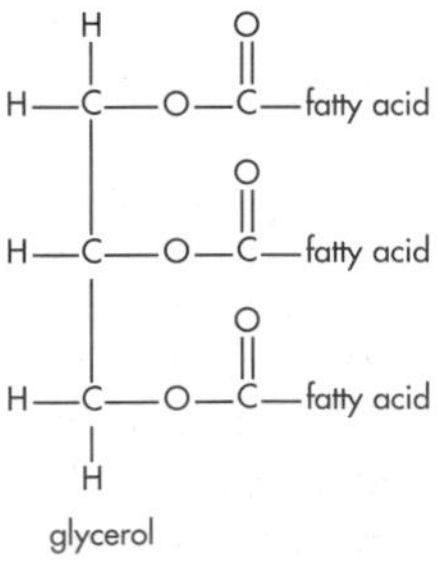
fatty acid
fatty acid
fatty acid
glycerol

Triglyceride.

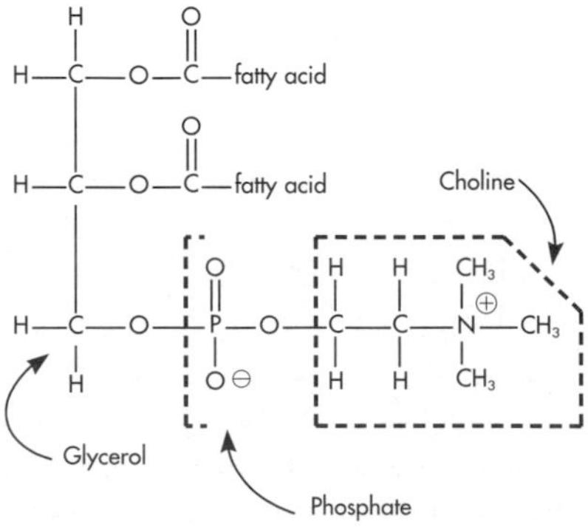
fatty acid
fatty acid
Choline
Glycerol
Phosphate

Lecithin.

Phospholipids

Phospholipids are another class of lipid. Like triglycerides, they are built on a backbone of glycerol. However, at least one fatty acid is replaced with a compound containing phosphorus (and often other chemicals, such as nitrogen). Many types of phospholipids exist in the body, especially in the brain. They form important parts of cell membranes.[18] The various forms of **lecithin** are common examples of phospholipids. These are found in body cells, where they participate in fat digestion in the intestine.

Sterols

Sterols are the last class of lipids this chapter covers. Their characteristic multi-ringed structure makes them different from the other lipids already discussed. Consider the important sterol cholesterol. This waxy substance doesn't look like a triglyceride—it doesn't have a glycerol backbone or any fatty acids. Still, because it doesn't readily dissolve in water, it is a lipid. Among other functions, cholesterol is used to form certain hormones and bile and is incorporated into cell membranes.[18]

Phospholipid
Any of a class of fat-related substances that contain phosphorus, fatty acids, and a nitrogen-containing base. Phospholipids are an essential part of every cell.

Lecithin
Phosopholipids that contain two fatty acids, a phosphate group, and a choline (vitamin-like) molecule.

Sterol
A compound containing a multi-ring (steroid) structure and a hydroxyl group (−OH).

Cholesterol.

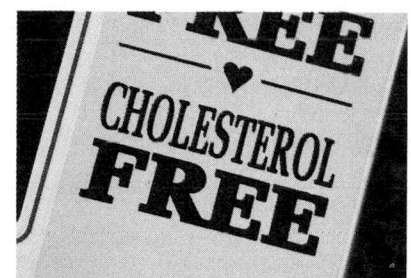

In choosing a diet lower in cholesterol, it's helpful to read food labels.

Concept**Check**

Lipids are a group of compounds that do not dissolve readily in water. They include fatty acids, triglycerides, phospholipids, and sterols. Fatty acids can differ from each other in the number of the double bonds between carbons in the carbon chain. Saturated fatty acids contain no carbon-carbon double bonds; that is, they are fully saturated with hydrogens. Monounsaturated fatty acids contain one carbon-carbon double bond, and polyunsaturated fatty acids contain two or more carbon-carbon double bonds.

Triglyceride is the major form of fat in the body and in food. It is formed by attaching three fatty acids to a glycerol backbone. Phospholipids differ from triglycerides: their glycerol backbone has fatty acids attached, but at least one fatty acid is replaced by another type of compound. Many phospholipids are present in cell membranes, and some act as emulsifiers. Sterols, another class of lipids, are constructed quite differently from either triglycerides or phospholipids. Cholesterol, a sterol, forms part of cell membranes, some hormones, and bile.

Functions of Lipids

The various classes of lipids have diverse functions in the body. All are necessary for health, but, as we will see, not all are needed in our diet. Of all the classes of lipids, only certain polyunsaturated fatty acids are essential parts of a diet.

Essential Fatty Acids

In the Greek alphabet, alpha is the first letter and omega is the last.

This essentiality of certain polyunsaturated fatty acids in the diet is based on the location of the carbon-carbon double bonds in the fatty acids. Greek letters are used to signify this location. For example, if the double bonds start after the third carbon (counting from the end with a -CH_3 group), the fatty acid is an **omega-3 (ω-3) fatty acid.** If these bonds start after the sixth carbon, it is an **omega-6 (ω-6) fatty acid,** and so on. **Alpha-linolenic acid** is the major omega-3 fatty acid found in food; **linoleic acid** is the major omega-6 fatty acid.

Humans can't produce omega-3 and omega-6 fatty acids; we get them only by ingesting them. That is why this structural uniqueness is important. These fatty acids are essential for us to eat because they participate in immune processes and vision, help form cell membranes, and aid in the production of hormonelike compounds.[18] Because we must get linoleic acid (omega-6) and alpha-linolenic acid (omega-3) from foods, they are called *essential fatty acids.*

We need to get about 1% to 2% of our total energy intake from linoleic acid. On a 2500-kcal diet, that corresponds to 1 tablespoon of plant oil each day. We easily get that much—via mayonnaise, salad dressings, margarine, and other foods—without even noticing. Barring these foods, regular consumption of whole grains and vegetables can also supply enough essential fatty acids.

Our diets should include a regular supply of either alpha-linolenic acid or its related omega-3 forms, such as **eicosapentaenoic acid (EPA).** To get this supply, we should eat fish—such as salmon, tuna, and sardines—about twice a week. Regular use of canola or soybean oil also supplies omega-3 fatty acids. However, the conversion of the omega-3 fatty acid present (alpha-linolenic acid) to EPA and related compounds appears to be relatively inefficient, especially in people who consume the usual amounts of linoleic acid, which slows the conversion process. Thus regular intake of fish is advised.[13]

This recommendation for consuming omega-3 fatty acids stems from the observation that compounds made from omega-3 fatty acids tend to decrease blood clotting and inflammatory processes in the body, whereas the omega-6 fatty acids generally increase these processes. Studies from Scandinavia, the Netherlands, and Japan show that people who eat fish about twice a week (total weekly intake: 8 ounces [240 grams]) run lower risks for heart attacks than do people who rarely eat fish. In these cases the omega-3 fatty acids in fish oil are probably acting to reduce blood clotting. Consequently the risk of heart attack decreases, especially for people already at high risk (see the Nutrition Issue at the end of this chapter to learn about the link between blood clots and heart attacks).

We need to remember, however, that blood clotting is a normal body process. Certain groups of people, such as Eskimos in Greenland, eat so much seafood that their blood-clotting ability can be impaired. An excess of omega-3 fatty acid intake can allow uncontrolled bleeding and may cause one type of **stroke.** Current studies also show that consuming large amounts of omega-3 fatty acids by using fish oil supplements can impede blood glucose regulation in people who have diabetes and can even raise blood cholesterol levels in some people. Excessive consumption of omega-3 fatty acids can be as problematic as inadequate consumption.

As a result, health experts recommend not using fish oil supplements—just stick to eating fish about two times a week.[13] Atlantic and Pacific herring, sardines, Atlantic halibut and salmon, lake trout, coho, pink and king salmon, bluefish, tuna,

Omega-3 (ω-3) **fatty acid**
An unsaturated fatty acid with its first double bond at the third carbon atom from the $-CH_3$ end.

Omega-6 (ω-6) fatty acid
An unsaturated fatty acid with its first double bond at the sixth carbon atom from the $-CH_3$ end.

Alpha-linolenic acid
An essential fatty acid with 18 carbons and three carbon-carbon double bonds (omega-3).

Linoleic acid
An essential fatty acid with 18 carbons and two carbon-carbon double bonds; omega-6.

and Atlantic mackerel are among the fish with the highest omega-3 fatty acid content. Oysters are also a source.

Effects of a Deficiency of Essential Fatty Acids

If you don't consume enough essential fatty acids, your skin will become flaky and itchy, and diarrhea and other symptoms eventually develop. However, because our bodies need the equivalent of only about 1 tablespoon of polyunsaturated plant oil a day, even a low-fat diet will provide enough EFAs if it follows the Food Guide Pyramid and includes some fish.

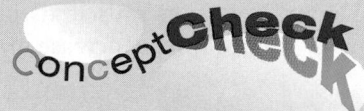

Because humans can't make either omega-3 or omega-6 fatty acids, which perform vital functions in the body, they are essential parts of a diet and therefore called essential fatty acids. Plant oils are generally rich in omega-6 fatty acids. Eating fish about twice a week is a good way to take in a healthful amount of omega-3 fatty acids.

Broader Roles for Fatty Acids and Triglycerides

Many key functions of fat in the body require the use of fatty acids in the form of triglycerides. Triglycerides are used for energy storage, insulation, transportation of fat-soluble vitamins, and the sensation of satiety (fullness) after eating.

Providing Energy for the Body

The fatty acids supplied by triglycerides both contained in the diet and stored in adipose (fat) tissue are the main fuel for muscles while at rest and during light activity. Only in endurance exercise, such as long-distance running and cycling, do muscles burn a lot of carbohydrate in addition to fatty acids. Other body tissues also use fatty acids for energy. Overall, about half of the energy used by the entire body at rest and during light activity comes from fatty acids. On a whole-body basis the use of fatty acids by muscles is balanced by the use of glucose by the brain and red blood cells. Recall from Chapter 5 that all cells also need carbohydrate to efficiently process fatty acids for fuel.[18]

Storing Energy

We store energy mainly in the form of triglycerides. The body's ability to store fat is essentially limitless. Its fat storage sites, adipose (fat) cells, can increase about 50 times in weight. If the amount of fat to be stored exceeds the ability of the cells to expand, the body can form new adipose cells. (This is discussed further in Chapter 10.)

An important advantage of using triglycerides to store energy in the body is that they are energy dense. Recall that these yield 9 kcal per gram, whereas proteins and carbohydrates yield only 4 kcal per gram. In addition, when we store triglycerides in

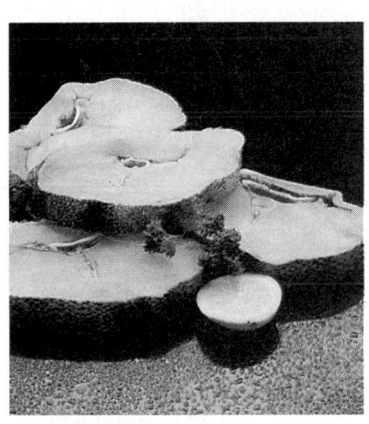

Eating fish about twice a week makes a healthy contribution to a diet.

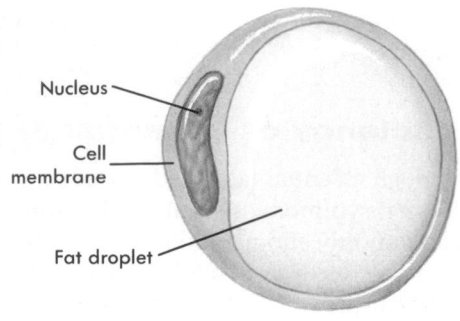

Nucleus

Cell
membrane

Fat droplet

Adipose cell.

adipose cells, we store little else; adipose cells contain about 80% lipid and only 20% water and protein. In contrast, imagine if we stored energy as muscle tissue, which is about 73% water. Body weight linked to energy storage would increase dramatically.

Insulating and Protecting the Body

The layer of fat just beneath our skin is made mostly of triglycerides. This fat tissue insulates and protects some organs—kidneys, for example—from injury. We usually don't notice the important insulating function of fat tissue, because we wear clothes and add more as needed. But a layer of insulating fat is quite apparent in animals, particularly in those cold climates. Polar bears, walruses, and whales all build a thick layer of fat tissue around themselves to insulate against cold-weather environments. The extra fat also provides energy storage for times when food is scarce.

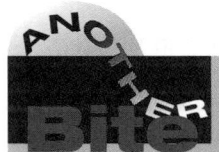

*We can never be totally fat free because fat is an essential part of all cells. However, people with **anorexia nervosa** often lose 25% or more of body weight and end up about as fat free as is biologically possible. This poses many health risks (see Chapter 13). In addition, in place of the layer of fat tissue under the skin, people with anorexia nervosa often develop downy hair called **lanugo** all over the body. These hairs insulate the body by standing up and trapping air.*

Transporting Fat-Soluble Vitamins

Triglycerides and other fats in foods carry fat-soluble vitamins to the small intestine and aid their absorption. If the small intestine is diseased, however, it may not be able to adequately digest and absorb fat from foods. When this happens, the unabsorbed fat carries the fat-soluble vitamins—A, D, E, and K—into the large intestine. From there they are eliminated with the feces, and the body loses the benefits of the vitamins. If the disease doesn't resolve quickly, medical attention is necessary.

People who absorb fat poorly, such as those with the disease cystic fibrosis, are also at risk for deficiencies of fat-soluble vitamins, especially vitamin K. A similar risk accrues from taking mineral oil as a laxative at mealtimes. Because the body cannot digest or absorb mineral oil, the undigested oil carries the fat-soluble vitamins from the meal into the large intestine, where they are eliminated.

Critical Thinking

In a class discussion, the topic of "diets" comes up. One of the most frustrating feelings dieters have, the students remark, is "being hungry all the time." Many dieters not only reduce their energy intake but also eliminate much of the fat from their diets. As a nutrition student, you suggest that some fat should be included in meals even on a weight-reduction diet. How would you justify this advice? What other diet changes could you suggest to help compensate for the reduced fat content in the meal?

Providing Satiety

If you are fond of cheesecake, you know that a little goes a long way. This is because triglycerides in foods help give us a full and contented feeling after a meal. The fat we eat triggers hormones that cause the stomach to retain foods longer than when we eat mostly carbohydrate or protein.[18] This is why a high-fat meal allows us to feel full longer.

Many people who want to lose weight cut much of the fat from their diet. However, if dieters cut too much fat, they lose its *satiety* value and get hungry more quickly. Thus reducing fat intake below about 20% of total energy intake can actually be self-defeating, unless high-fiber foods are added to contribute bulk, which also makes us feel full (see Chapter 10 for further discussion). Having some low-fat snacks around at times of intense hunger is also a good idea. Fruit is an excellent choice.

Phospholipids in the Body

Many types of phospholipids exist in the body, such as in the brain and other nerve tissue. Although phospholipids are necessary components of body tissues, however, we don't have to consume phospholipids as such because the body can make them when and where they are needed.

Some phospholipids, such as the family of compounds mentioned earlier called *lecithins*, function as **emulsifiers.** These allow fat and water to mix. By breaking fat globules into small droplets, emulsifiers enable a fat to be suspended in water. Here's how the process works: The fatty acid ends of lecithins attract fat. The phosphorus and nitrogen at the other end of lecithins form an area containing positive and negative charges. This area attracts water. When lecithins are added to an oil and water mixture, they act as bridges between the oil and water that in turn form tiny oil droplets surrounded by thin shells of water. In an emulsified solution, millions of tiny oil droplets are separated by shells of water (Figure 6-3).

Satiety
A state in which there is no longer a desire to eat; a feeling of satisfaction.

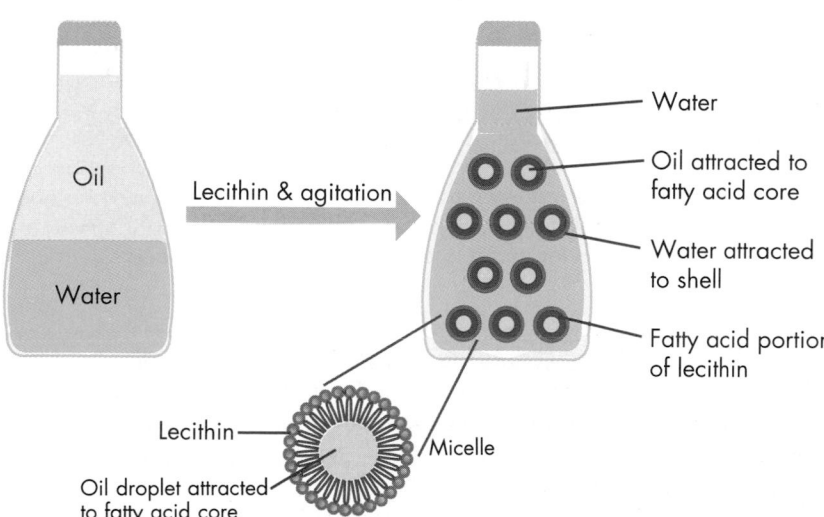

Figure 6-3 *Emulsifiers in action. Emulsifiers are what keep many brands of salad dressings and other condiments from separating into layers of water and fat. Emulsifiers like lecithins are ball-shaped molecules. They attract fatty acids inside, and have a water-attracting group on the outside. Add them to salad dressing, shake well, and they hold the oil in the dressing in the center of their molecules and keep the water on the outside, forming micelles. Emulsification is important in both food production and fat digestion/absorption.*

The body's main emulsifiers are the lecithins and **bile,** which are produced by the liver and released into the small intestine via the gallbladder during digestion. By breaking up the fat globules, the emulsifiers create more fat surface for fat-digesting enzymes to act on.[18]

Perhaps you've seen health food advertisements touting the importance of taking a lecithin supplement to maintain the health of body cells. This mistaken notion has also been promoted by some popular publications but has no scientific basis. Eating lecithin isn't even an efficient way to obtain it because the digestive system dismantles most of the lecithin before it enters the bloodstream. All the lecithin you need for digesting fat and other functions can be made by your body; in other words, lecithin is not an essential nutrient. What's more, large doses of lecithin can cause stomach upsets, sweating, salivation, and loss of appetite.

Cholesterol in the Body

Cholesterol forms part of some important hormones, such as estrogen, testosterone, and a form of the active vitamin D hormone. Cholesterol is also the building block of bile acids, which are needed for fat digestion. Finally, cholesterol is an essential structural component of cell membranes and the outer layer of particles that transport lipids in the blood, as discussed in the next section.[18] The cholesterol content of the heart, liver, kidney, and brain is quite high, reflecting its critical role in these organs.

Each day your liver makes about 1000 milligrams of cholesterol. About one third is made into bile; the rest circulates through the bloodstream to function as the body needs it.[18] In comparison, we eat about 200 to 400 milligrams of cholesterol per day. When a diet doesn't contain enough cholesterol, the liver makes what the body needs.

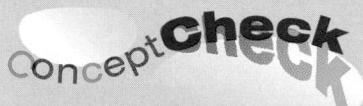

Triglycerides are the major form of fat in the body. Used for and stored as energy, they insulate and protect body organs, transport fat-soluble vitamins, and promote satiety. Many phospholipids act as emulsifiers, compounds that suspend fat as small droplets in water. Phospholipids also form parts of cell membranes and various compounds in the body. Cells produce all the phospholipids the body needs. Cholesterol, a sterol, forms part of cell membranes, hormones, and bile; it is essential to the body. Cholesterol is manufactured in the liver, and if sufficient amounts are not ingested, the body makes what it needs.

Making Fats Available for Body Use

Fat is digested and absorbed primarily in the small intestine.

Fat Digestion

In the first phase of fat digestion the stomach secretes an enzyme that acts primarily on triglycerides with fatty acids of short-chain and medium-chain lengths, such as those found in butterfat. The action of this enzyme, however, is usually dwarfed by that of an enzyme released from the pancreas and active in the small intestine. In addition, triglycerides and other lipids found in common vegetable oils and meats are generally not digested until they reach the small intestine (Figure 6-4).

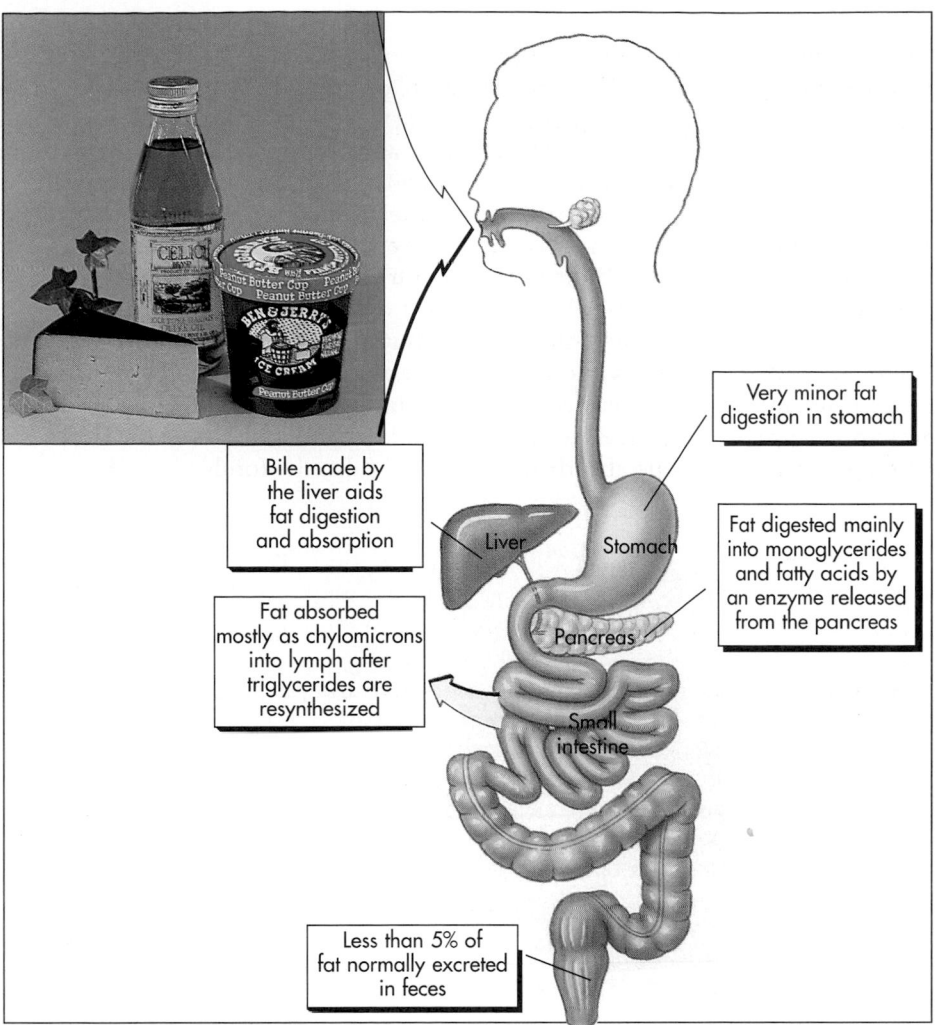

Bile made by
the liver aids
fat digestion
and absorption

Very minor fat
digestion in stomach

Liver   Stomach

Fat digested mainly
into monoglycerides
and fatty acids by
an enzyme released
from the pancreas

Fat absorbed
mostly as chylomicrons
into lymph after
triglycerides are
resynthesized

Pancreas

Small
intestine

Less than 5% of
fat normally excreted
in feces

Figure 6-4 *A summary of fat digestion and absorption. Chapter 4 covered general aspects of this process.*

In the small intestine, triglycerides break down into smaller products, namely monoglycerides (glycerol backbones with single fatty acids attached) and fatty acids. In the right circumstances, digestion is very rapid and thorough. The "right" circumstances include the presence of bile from the gallbladder.[18] Bile helps emulsify the digestive products of lipase action by forming water-soluble **micelles.** Bile, in effect, acts like dishwashing detergent when it breaks up oil spots in dishwater. Micelle formation improves digestion and absorption because as large fat globules are broken down into smaller ones, the total surface area for enzyme action increases.

During meals, bile circulates in a path that begins in the liver, goes on to the gallbladder, and then moves to the small intestine. After participating in fat digestion, the bile constituents are absorbed and end up back at the liver. This cycling of bile is called **enterohepatic circulation.** Approximately 98% of the bile is recycled. Only 1% to 2% ends up in the large intestine to be eliminated in the feces.[18] The Nutrition Issue explains that one common way to control very high blood cholesterol is to consume resins that bind bile constituents and draw them into the feces.[17] This treatment reduces bile's enterohepatic circulation. The liver is then forced to make new bile rather than use recycled bile. One building block for bile synthesis is cholesterol. The liver must take cholesterol out of the bloodstream to make new bile, thus lowering blood cholesterol.

Monoglyceride

A breakdown product of a triglyceride consisting of one fatty acid bonded to a glycerol backbone.

Micelle

An emulsification product in which individual emulsifiers organize with their fat-attracting parts to the center of the micelle and their water-attracting parts to the outside. Lipids are attracted to the center area, and water is attracted to the outside periphery. (See later section for details).

Enterohepatic circulation

Recycling of compounds between the small intestine and the liver over and over again, as happens with bile.

Lipoprotein

A compound found in the bloodstream containing a core of lipids with a shell of protein, phospholipid, and cholesterol.

Chylomicron

Lipoprotein made of dietary fats that are surrounded by a shell of cholesterol, phospholipids, and protein. Chylomicrons are made in the intestine after fat absorption and travel through the lymphatic system to the bloodstream.

Fat Absorption

Most products of fat digestion have by now been reduced to mere fatty acids and monoglycerides in the small intestine. These are passively absorbed as such into the absorptive cells of the small intestine. One key characteristic of fatty acids and monoglycerides affects their ultimate fate after absorption. If the chain length of a fatty acid is less than 12 carbon atoms (a short-chain or medium-chain variety), it is water soluble and will therefore probably travel as such through the portal vein to the liver. If the fatty acid is a long-chain variety (especially 14 or more carbon atoms), it must eventually be re-formed into a triglyceride and enter circulation via the lymphatic system.

To travel in the lymphatic system, the triglycerides are first combined with cholesterol and other substances and covered with a protein coat. The collective structure of lipid and protein is termed a **lipoprotein,** or, as in this specific case, a **chylomicron.** This chylomicron enters the lymphatic system and eventually the bloodstream to carry most of the absorbed fats yielded from the foods eaten.[18]

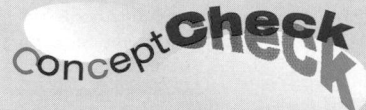

In the small intestine an enzyme released from the pancreas digests dietary triglycerides into smaller breakdown products, namely monoglycerides (glycerol backbones with single fatty acids attached) and fatty acids. The breakdown products are then passively absorbed into the absorptive cells of the small intestine. These products are mostly resynthesized into triglycerides and combined with cholesterol, protein, and other substances to yield a chylomicron. Chylomicrons enter the lymphatic system and eventually the bloodstream.

Carrying Fats in the Bloodstream

As noted earlier, fat and water don't easily mix. This incompatibility presents a challenge in transporting fats through the watery mediums of blood and lymph systems.

Carrying Dietary Fats

As just mentioned, once the various dietary fats are digested and absorbed into the small intestine cells, most of these fats are re-formed into triglycerides. These combine with phospholipids, protein, and cholesterol to form a chylomicron, one of many types of blood lipoproteins (see Figure 6-5). This lipoprotein structure allows fats to float freely in the water-based bloodstream.

Chylomicrons enter the lymphatic system and travel into the bloodstream. Once there the triglycerides in the chylomicrons are broken down into fatty acids and glycerol by an enzyme on the inside wall of the blood vessel. Muscle cells, adipose cells, and other cells in the vicinity then absorb most of the fatty acids. Cells can immediately use absorbed fatty acids for fuel, or they can re-form them into triglycerides and store them as such. Muscle cells tend to burn the fatty acids, whereas adipose cells tend to store them.

Transporting Various Fats Mostly Made by the Body

Note that in the clinical laboratory the amount of cholesterol in the HDL fraction of blood lipids is what is determined, rather than the amount of HDL itself. The same holds true for LDL. Thus it is more correct to refer to HDL cholesterol and LDL cholesterol. To simplify the discussion, generally the terms LDL and HDL will be used.

The liver produces more fat and cholesterol than does any other body organ. The source of the needed carbons, hydrogens, and energy to make such substances as triglycerides and cholesterol includes the carbohydrate and protein the liver takes up

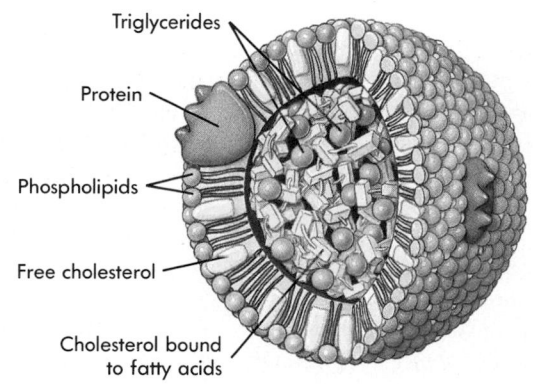

Triglycerides

Protein

Phospholipids

Free cholesterol

Cholesterol bound
to fatty acids

Figure 6-5 *The structure of a lipoprotein, namely an LDL. This structure allows fats to circulate in the water-based bloodstream. Various lipoproteins are found in the bloodstream. Chylomicrons carry fats absorbed from foods through the bloodstream to body cells. VLDLs do the same but mostly carry various lipids made by the liver. LDLs carry cholesterol to the body cells and result from metabolism of VLDLs. HDLs carry cholesterol primarily back to other lipoproteins that in turn are mostly taken up by the liver. Some HDLs also take their cholesterol load directly back to the liver.*

from the bloodstream. Any alcohol consumed can also be used as a source. The liver coats the cholesterol and triglycerides it makes with a shell of protein and lipids. This process produces what is called a **very low-density lipoprotein (VLDL)** (see Figure 6-5).

When the VLDLs leave the liver, the enzyme lipoprotein lipase on the blood vessels breaks down the triglyceride in the VLDLs into fatty acids and glycerol. Again fatty acids and glycerol are released into the bloodstream and are taken up by the body cells. Because fats are less dense than water, VLDLs become much heavier—proportionately denser—as triglyceride is released. Much of what eventually remains of these VLDLs becomes particles called **low-density lipoprotein (LDL).** LDL is composed primarily of cholesterol.[18]

LDL particles are absorbed from the bloodstream by cells and broken down. Most LDL is taken up by liver cells. Diets low in saturated fat and cholesterol encourage this process, whereas diets high in those lipids can reduce LDL uptake by the liver[31] (see the Nutrition Issue). The cholesterol and protein parts then are transported throughout the cell. In this way, liver and other body cells absorb the building blocks used to make bile, certain hormones, and other compounds.

If LDL is not rapidly taken up by this route, scavenger cells buried in blood vessels detect, alter **(oxidize),** engulf, and digest the extra circulating LDL. Once within the scavenger cells the oxidized LDL is prevented from reentering the bloodstream. Over time, cholesterol builds up in the scavenger cells, especially when the amount of LDL in the bloodstream is excessive.[24]

When scavenger cells have collected and deposited cholesterol for many years at a heavy pace, cholesterol builds up on the inner blood vessel walls—especially in arteries—and **plaque** develops (see Figure 6-11 in the Nutrition Issue). The plaque eventually mixes with protein and is then covered with a cap of muscle cells and calcium. Atherosclerosis, also referred to as *hardening of the arteries,* develops as plaque grows in the vessel. This eventually chokes off the blood supply to organs, setting the stage for a heart attack and other problems.[24] Plaque is probably first deposited to repair injuries in a vessel lining. The injuries that start plaque formation can be caused by smoking, diabetes, high blood pressure, and LDL itself. Viral and bacterial infections also are implicated.

A final critical participant in this extensive process of fat transport is the **high-density lipoprotein (HDL).** Its high proportion of protein makes it the heaviest

Very low-density lipoprotein (VLDL)
The lipoprotein that initially leaves the liver; it carries cholesterol and lipids newly synthesized by the liver.

Low-density lipoprotein (LDL)
The product of the VLDL metabolism that contains primarily cholesterol; elevated LDL is strongly linked to heart disease.

Oxidize
Specifically, to lose an electron or gain an oxygen atom.

Plaque
A cholesterol-rich substance deposited in the blood vessels; it contains various white blood cells, smooth muscle cells, cholesterol and other lipids, and eventually calcium.

High-density lipoprotein (HDL)
Lipoprotein, synthesized in part by the liver and intestine, that picks up cholesterol from dying cells and other sources and transfers it to the other lipoproteins in the bloodstream, as well as directly to the liver.

One type of compound that can cause oxidative damage to body constituents is free radicals. These are short-lived forms of compounds that exist with an unpaired electron. This causes an electron-seeking nature to complete the pair, which can be very destructive to electron-dense areas of a cell, such as DNA and cell membranes. Antioxidants can counter this destruction by stopping free radical reactions (see Chapter 8).

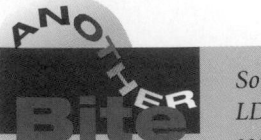

*Some nutrients have **antioxidant** properties. These likely reduce LDL oxidation in the bloodstream and thus slow LDL uptake into scavenger cells. Fruits and vegetables are rich in such antioxidants as **carotenoids** and vitamins C and E. Eating fruits and vegetables regularly is one positive step we can take to reduce cholesterol buildup and slow the progression of heart disease. Consuming megadoses of vitamins to do the same thing is controversial[8] (see Chapter 8). On the other hand, an excessive intake of iron probably speeds LDL oxidation, making it wise not to take an iron supplement unless a physician prescribes it. People who experience iron storage disease should pay special attention to this warning[9] (see Chapter 9).*

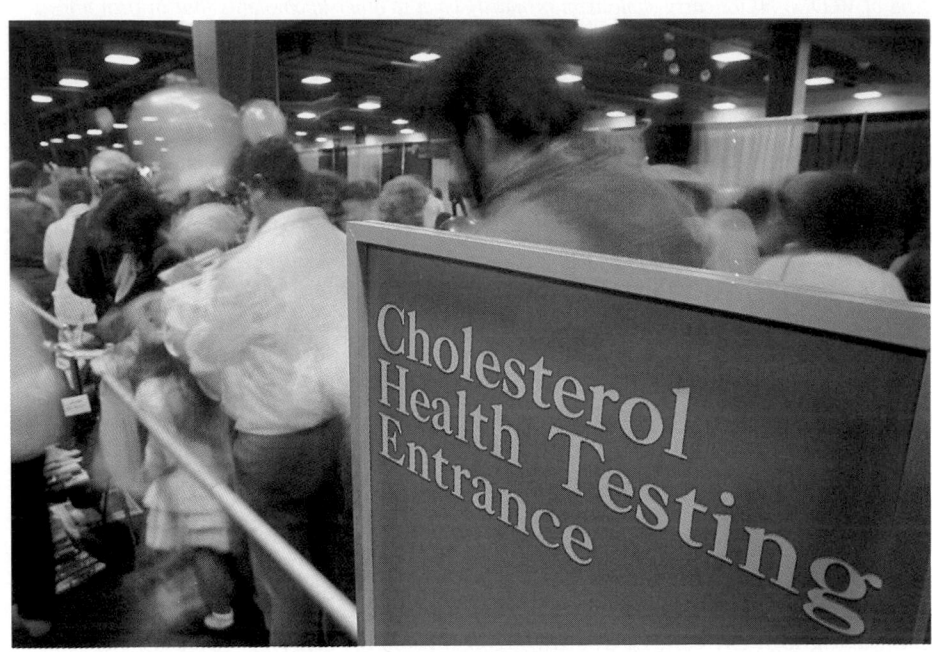

Every adult should know his or her blood lipoprotein status.

Antioxidant

Generally, a compound that can donate electrons to electron-seeking (oxidizing) compounds. This reduces the destructive nature of oxidizing compounds. Some compounds have antioxidant capabilities (that is, they stop oxidation) but are not electron donors per se.

Menopause

The cessation of menses in women, usually beginning at about age 50.

(densest) lipoprotein. The liver and intestine produce most of the HDL in the blood. It roams the bloodstream, picking up cholesterol from dying cells and other sources. HDL donates the cholesterol primarily to other lipoproteins for transport back to the liver to be excreted. Some HDL travels directly back to the liver.[18] Another beneficial function of HDL is that it may block oxidation of LDL.

Many studies demonstrate that the amount of HDL in the bloodstream can closely predict the risk for heart disease. The risk increases with low HDL because little blood cholesterol is transported back to the liver and excreted. Women tend to have high HDL, especially before **menopause,** whereas low values are more common in men.[23]

Because high HDL slows the development of heart disease, any cholesterol carried by HDL can be considered "good" cholesterol. By convention, then, cholesterol carried by LDL would be "bad" cholesterol because high LDL speeds the development of heart disease.

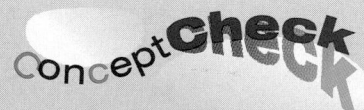

Exploring Another Dimension of Fat—Roles in Food

Various fats play important roles in foods. Much ingenuity must go into the production of fat-reduced products to preserve flavor and texture. In some cases, fat-free also means tasteless.

Fat Provides Flavor and Texture to Foods

Many flavorings dissolve in fat. Heating spices in oil intensifies the flavors of an Indian curry or Mexican dish far more than simply adding them at the table. The oil then carries these flavors to the sensory cells that discriminate taste and smell in the mouth. We quickly associate flavor with fatty foods.[4] Foods that have had too much fat removed often lack taste and may feel dry, as if they need something to bind them together.

If you've ever eaten a high-fat yellow cheese or cream cheese, you probably agree that fat melting on the tongue feels good. The fat in whole milk also gives body that nonfat milk lacks. This love of fat is universal. Western, Eskimo, and Mediterranean diets are all rich in fat. Immigrants to Western cultures, such as many Japanese, quickly embrace the high-fat diet found in the United States. A person who has been following a typical American diet will probably need some time to adjust to a lower-fat diet. It is possible that by emphasizing flavorful fruits, vegetables, and whole grains, we can reduce dietary fat, but the factors just reviewed usually tempt us to move toward the more familiar high-fat diet.[4]

Hydrogenation of Fatty Acids Is Needed for Some Types of Food Production

In some kinds of food production, such as pastry making, solid fats work better than liquid oils. In pie crust, for example, solid fats yield a flaky product, whereas crusts made with liquid oils tend to be greasy. The polyunsaturated fatty acids must become more saturated to solidify vegetable oils into shortenings and margarines for use in pastries and other products. In other words, more hydrogen must be added to turn double bonds between the carbons into single bonds. In the **hydrogenation** process the hydrogens are added by bubbling hydrogen gas into liquid vegetable oils (see Figure 6-6).

During hydrogenation, changes also occur in the fatty acid, casting it in a so-called trans shape from its more typical cis form. The resulting substance is called a **trans fatty acid.** This structural change also causes the fats to raise blood cholesterol,

Hydrogenation
Addition of hydrogen to a carbon-carbon double bond, producing a single bond. Because hydrogenation of unsaturated fatty acids in a vegetable oil increases its hardness, this process is used to convert liquid oils into more solid fats, which are used in making margarine and shortening. Trans fatty acids are a by-product of hydrogenation of vegetable oils.

Trans fatty acid
A form of an unsaturated fatty acid, usually a monounsaturated one when found in food, in which the hydrogens on both carbons forming the double bond lie on opposite sides of that bond. A cis fatty acid has the hydrogens lying on the same side of the carbon-carbon double bond.

Oleic acid   **Elaidic acid**

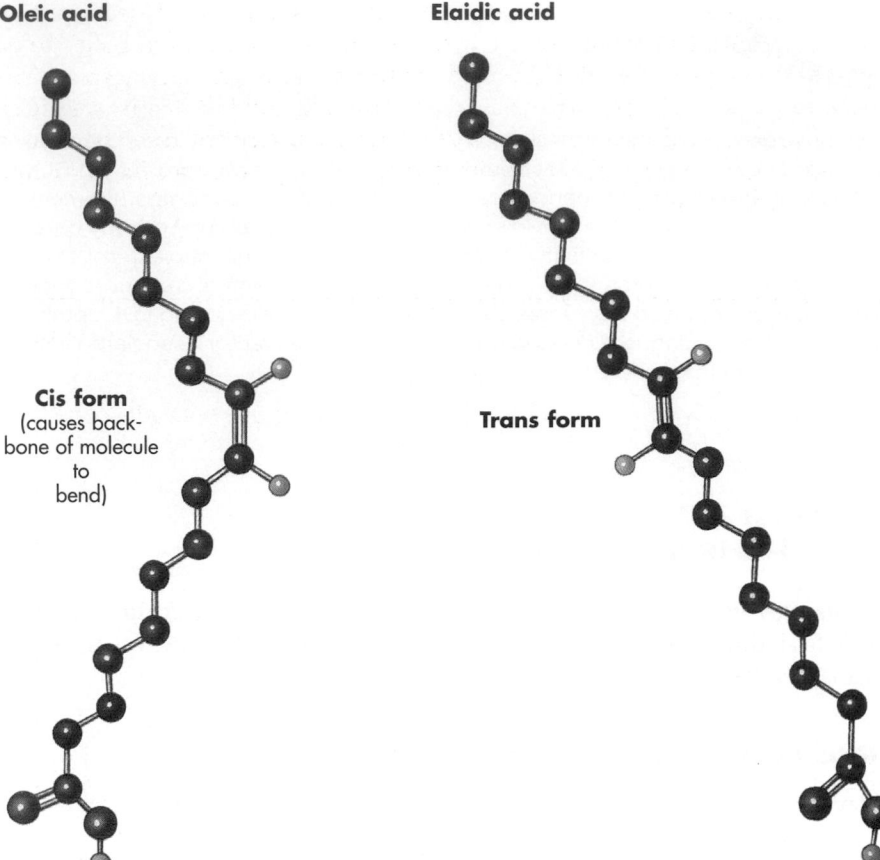

Cis form
(causes back-
bone of molecule
to
bend)

Trans form

*Cis form seen in double carbon-
carbon bonds in a fatty acid. The
hydrogens (in blue) lie on the same
side of the double bond. This causes
a "kink" at that point in the fatty
acid, which is typical of unsaturated
fatty acids in nature.*

*Trans form seen in double carbon-
carbon bonds in a fatty acid. The
hydrogens lie across from each other
at the double bond. This causes the
fatty acid to exist in a linear form,
like a saturated fatty acid.*

just as many saturated fats do. In particular, some experts suggest that people with elevated LDL should limit intake of hydrogenated fat[32] (see the Nutrition Issue). It is less clear that this is important for the average person, as long as total fat intake is not excessive.[1] Generally the more hydrogenation that occurs, the harder the product is; for example, stick margarine is more hydrogenated (saturated) than tub margarine. If a liquid oil is listed before any hydrogenated oil on food labels, the food probably contains a greater amount of unsaturated than saturated fat. Note that food labels don't currently list the amount of trans fatty acids present.

As public pressure has persuaded manufacturers to eliminate the tropical oils rich in saturated fat (palm, palm kernel, and coconut) from food processing, partially hydrogenated soybean oil has become the major replacement. During the next few days, study food labels and notice how many chips, snack products, and crackers contain a "partially hydrogenated vegetable oil."

It's easy to avoid eating much hydrogenated fat and in turn taking in high levels of trans fatty acids. First, use little or no stick margarine or shortening; instead, substitute softer, tub margarine (whose labels list vegetable oil or water as the first ingredient) and vegetable oils. Second, minimize consumption of deep fat-fried foods in restaurants, which tend to use hydrogenated fat in the fryer. Foods to eat sparingly include french fries, doughnuts, fried potato skins, and any deep fat-fried meat, fish, or poultry (Figure 6-7). As an alternative a typical hamburger sandwich, bowl of chili, and soft drink or milk in a quick-service restaurant contain minimal hydrogenated fat and still make a satisfying meal. Finally, limit intake of high-fat baked foods, such as pastries.

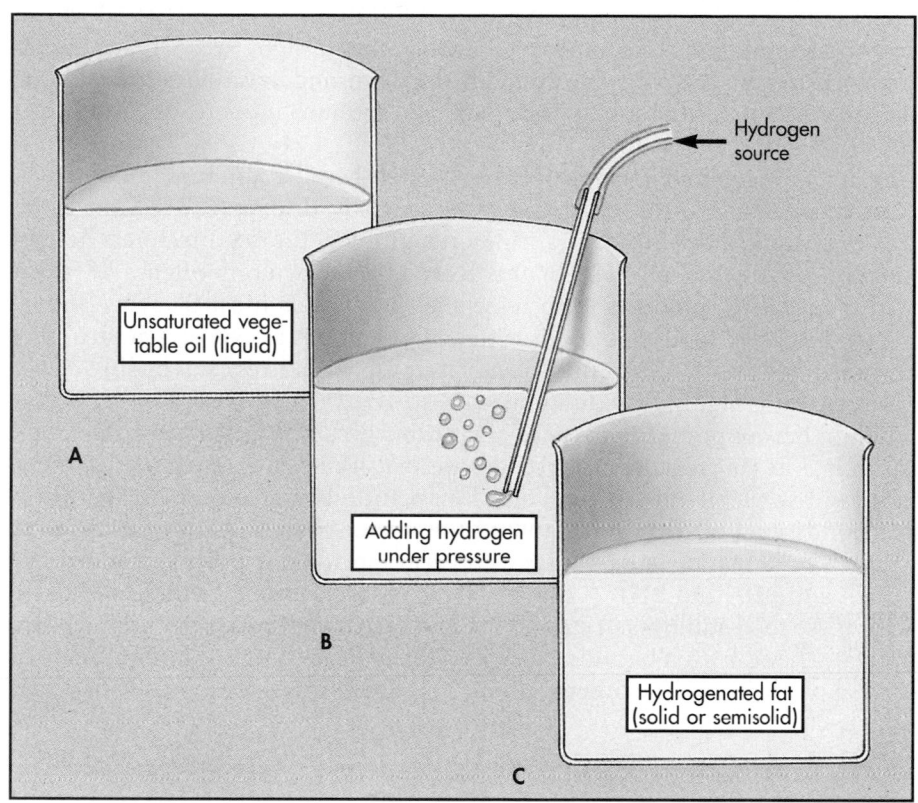

Figure 6-6 *How liquid oils become solid fats.* **A,** *Unsaturated fatty acids are present in liquid form.* **B,** *Hydrogens are added (hydrogenation), changing some carbon-carbon double bonds to single bonds and producing some trans fatty acids.* **C,** *The completed hydrogenated product, which is likely to be used in margarine, shortenings, or deep-fat frying.*

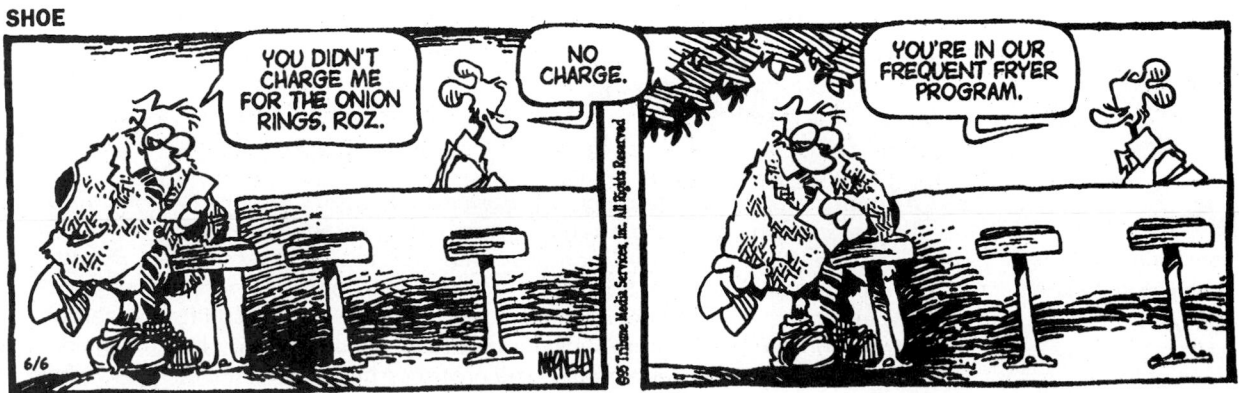

Figure 6-7 *Shoe.*

Rancid

Containing products of decomposed fatty acids; they yield unpleasant flavors and odors.

BHA and BHT

Butylated hydroxyanisol and butylated hydroxytoluene—two common synthetic antioxidants added to foods.

Emulsifier

A compound that can suspend fat in water by isolating individual fat droplets using a shell of water molecules or other substances to prevent the fat from coalescing.

An additional consideration is use of nondairy creamers. Initially these may appear to be a healthful substitute for cream, which is rich in saturated fatty acids. However, many nondairy creamers are rich in hydrogenated vegetable oils. Low-fat or nonfat milk is a better choice than liquid or dry nondairy creamer when you're trying to reduce hydrogenated fat intake.

Fat Rancidity Limits Shelf Life of Foods

Decomposing oils emit a disagreeable odor and also taste sour and stale. Stale potato chips are a good example. As double bonds in fatty acids break down, the by-products are said to be **rancid.** Ultraviolet rays of light, oxygen, and certain other procedures can break double bonds, break them, and in turn destroy the structure of polyunsaturated fatty acids. Saturated fats can much more readily resist these effects. Why?

Rancidity is not a major problem for consumers because although eating rancid oils can cause sickness, the odor and taste generally discourage us from eating enough to become sick. However, rancidity is a problem for manufacturers because it reduces a product's shelf life. For this reason, manufacturers often add hydrogenated plant oils to products to increase shelf life. Foods most likely to become rancid are deep-fried foods and foods with a large amount of exposed surface (such as powdered eggs or powdered milk). The fat in fish is also very susceptible to rancidity because it is highly polyunsaturated.

Vitamin E helps protect foods against rancidity because it acts as an antioxidant. It guards against fat breakdown caused by various agents, such as metals found as impurities in vegetable oils. The vitamin E in plant oils reduces the breakdown of double bonds in fatty acids. In Chapter 8 the role of vitamin E is explained more fully. When food manufacturers want to prevent rancidity in polyunsaturated fats, they often add **BHA** and **BHT.** (Chapter 17 discusses the safety of these additives.) Look for these food additives in salad dressings, cake mixes, and other products that contain fat. They can even be added to a food's paper packaging. Manufacturers also tightly seal products and use other methods to reduce oxygen levels inside packages.

Use of Emulsifiers Improves Many Food Products

Food manufacturers add emulsifiers in the preparation of many food products, primarily to improve texture. For example, lecithins, polysorbate 60, and other emulsifiers are added to salad dressings to keep the vegetable oil suspended in water. Eggs added to cake batters likewise emulsify the fat with the milk. Monoglycerides and related compounds are also good emulsifiers and for that reason are sometimes used in cake mixes and salad dressings. Over the next few days, examine the labels of salad dressings and cake mixes, and see how many emulsifiers are listed.

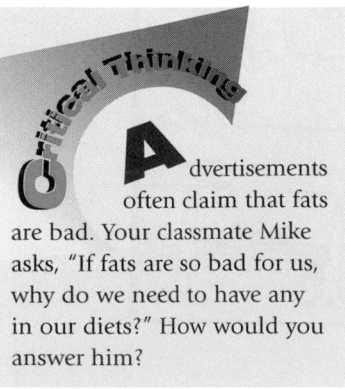

Critical Thinking

Advertisements often claim that fats are bad. Your classmate Mike asks, "If fats are so bad for us, why do we need to have any in our diets?" How would you answer him?

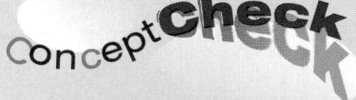

Concept Check

At room temperature, fats rich in saturated fatty acids tend to form solid fats, and fats rich in polyunsaturated and monounsaturated fatty acids tend to form liquid oils. During hydrogenation of unsaturated fatty acids, hydrogen is added to carbon-carbon double bonds to produce single bonds; some trans fatty acids are also created. Hydrogenation changes vegetable oil to solid fat. The carbon-carbon double bonds in polyunsaturated fatty acids are easily broken, yielding products responsible for rancidity. The presence of antioxidants, such as vitamin E in oils, naturally protects unsaturated fatty acids against oxidative destruction.

Continued.

Manufacturers can use hydrogenated fats and add synthetic antioxidants to reduce the likelihood of rancidity.

Commercial salad dressings find practical use for emulsification. Emulsifiers such as lecithins, polysorbate 60, and monoglycerides are added to salad dressings and other fat-rich products to keep the vegetable oils and other fats suspended in the water.

Recommendations for Fat Intake

There is no RDA for fat. To obtain the essential fatty acids, adults should consume about 4% of total energy intake from plant oils incorporated into foods and eat fish about twice a week. Recall that it takes only about 1 tablespoon of oil per day to meet linoleic acid needs. The typical American diet derives about 7% of energy content from polyunsaturated fatty acids. An upper limit of 10% of energy intake as polyunsaturated fatty acids is often recommended, in part because the breakdown (oxidation) of those present in lipoproteins is linked to increased cholesterol deposition in the arteries, as just discussed. This breakdown may also increase the risk of cancer. Depression of immune function is also suspected to be caused by an excessive intake of polyunsaturated fats.

Dietary fat supplies about 34% of Americans' total energy intake. Vegetable and animal foods each supply about half of the fat. Major sources of fat in the U.S. diet include animal flesh, whole milk, pastries, cheese, margarine, and mayonnaise.

Because many Americans are at risk for developing heart disease, the American Heart Association (AHA) promotes dietary changes aimed at reducing this risk (Table 6-1). Many health agencies agree with the AHA recommendation that total fat intake should not exceed 30% of total energy intake, with a ratio of about 10:10:10 for saturated to monounsaturated to polyunsaturated fatty acids.

TABLE 6-1

Dietary Guidelines for Healthy American Adults:
A Statement for Physicians and Health Professionals by
the Nutrition Committee, American Heart Association (AHA)*

1. Total fat intake should be less than 30% of energy intake.
2. Saturated fat intake should be less than 10% of energy intake.
3. Polyunsaturated fat intake should not exceed 10% of energy intake.
4. Cholesterol intake should not exceed 300 milligrams per day.
5. Carbohydrate intake should constitute 50% or more of energy intake, with emphasis on complex carbohydrates.
6. Protein intake should provide the remainder of the energy intake.
7. Sodium intake should not exceed 3 grams per day.
8. Alcohol consumption should not exceed about 1 ounce of ethanol per day. Two ounces of 100-proof whiskey, 10 oz of wine, and 24 oz of beer each contain about 1 oz of ethanol.
9. Total energy intake should be sufficient to maintain the individual's recommended body weight.
10. A wide variety of foods should be consumed.

From *Circulation* 77:721A, 1988.
*Chapter 2 listed the Dietary Guidelines for Americans. Chapter 16 reviews these guidelines in the context of adult health. "Moderate fat intake" is a common general health message for adults, regardless of who issues the report.

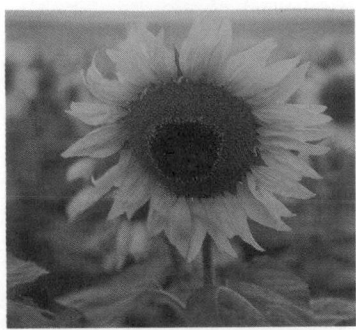

Plant oils should supply at least 4% of our total energy intake.

The intake of saturated fats currently averages about 12% of energy intake. The recommended reduction in saturated fat and cholesterol intake enhances the liver's ability to clear LDL from the bloodstream. Table 6-2 shows a diet that follows the basic AHA guidelines.

Current research shows that our palates adapt to a lower fat intake over time, so we miss it less. Reducing fat intake also allows us to include more healthful foods—fruits, vegetables, and whole grains—in our diets. A good start for this type of diet is a low-fat breakfast: one option is a high-fiber cereal, low-fat or nonfat milk, and fruit juice.[25]

For people who have elevated LDL even when following the guideline of 30% of energy intake from fat, the AHA recommends a more stringent diet that includes no more than 20% of total energy from fat. Some cancer researchers also advocate such a diet for adults in general (see Chapter 9). To achieve this goal, fat intake must be strictly limited (see Table 6-2). The advice and counsel of a registered dietitian are helpful in planning such diets.

The National Cholesterol Education Program, established in 1985, recommends reducing saturated fatty acids to 7% of total energy intake if elevated LDL does not respond to the reduction in saturated fat intake of 10% of energy intake. In other words, the lower the saturated fat intake, the better. Cholesterol intake in

TABLE 6-2

Daily Menus Containing 2000 Kcal and Various Percentages of Fat

30% OF ENERGY AS FAT	Teaspoons of fat	20% OF ENERGY AS FAT	Teaspoons of fat
Breakfast			
Orange juice, 1 cup	0	Same	0
Shredded wheat, ¾ cup	⅕	Same	⅕
Bagel, toasted	⅕	Same	⅕
Margarine, 2 tsp	1¾	Margarine, 1 tsp	⅞
1% milk, 1 cup	½	Nonfat milk, 1 cup	⅒
Lunch			
Whole-wheat bread, 2 slices	½	Same	½
Roast beef, lean, 2 oz	1	Ham, broiled, 2 oz	½
Mayonnaise, 2 tsp	1½	Mayonnaise, 1 tsp	¾
Lettuce	0	Same	0
Tomato, sliced	0	Same	0
Animal crackers, 8	⅕	Same	⅕
Snack			
Apple	⅙	Same	⅙
Dinner			
Pork chop, broiled, 3 oz	2⅓	Halibut, broiled, 3 oz	⅔
Pasta, 1½ cup	⅔	Pasta, 2½ cups	1
Margarine, 2 tsp	1¾	Margarine, 1 tsp	⅞
Broccoli, ½ cup	0	Same	0
1% milk, 1 cup	½	Nonfat milk, 1 cup	⅒
		Banana	⅒
Snack			
Raisins, 2 tbsp	0	Raisins, ¼ cup	0
Popcorn, air-popped, 6 cups	½	Same	½
With 2 tsp margarine	1¾	With 1 tsp margarine	⅞
TOTALS	14½		7½

this regard should be limited to 300 milligrams per day, with a reduction to 200 milligrams per day if LDL remains elevated when following a fat-restricted diet containing the higher amount of cholesterol. Recall that adults consume an average of about 200 to 400 milligrams of cholesterol per day, with men generally consuming the higher amount. By encouraging a reduction in total fat, saturated fat, and cholesterol intake, all of these suggestions are in line with the Dietary Guidelines discussed in Chapter 2. Keep in mind, however, that the latter two suggestions are most important for people with elevated LDL.

Unfortunately, exceeding 30% of energy intake of fat is all too easy. For example, a bologna and cheese sandwich with mayonnaise contains about 39 grams of fat, or about 60% of the fat allowance for a 2000-kcal diet. A half-cup serving of premium ice cream contains about 18 grams, and a slice of apple pie contains about 19 grams, almost all of which is in the crust. A large order of McDonald's fries has 22 grams. Do you still want to routinely order fries?

Most people probably have no idea how much of the energy in their diets comes from fat. You've already tracked your food intake for one day. The Rate Your Plate exercise asks you to compare your fat intake to current guidelines. Using the information on food labels and occasionally recording and analyzing daily food intake allow you to track your fat intake.

A final note: The advice to consume 20% to 30% of energy as fat does not apply to infants and toddlers below the age of 2 years.[30] These youngsters are forming much new tissue, especially in the brain, so their intake of fat and cholesterol should not be greatly restricted. After that age, children should gradually adopt a diet that contains no more than 30% of energy from fat and 300 milligrams of cholesterol per day (see Chapter 15 for details). As children begin to consume less fat, they should replace the missing energy with more grain products, fruits, vegetables, and low-fat milk products.

Recommendations for fat intake are stated as a percentage of total energy intake—usually 20% or 30%. This chart shows how many grams of fat per day are allowed with diets ranging from 1000 to 3900 kcal.

Energy intake (kcal)	Fat intake grams	
	30% of energy	20% of energy
1000	33	22
1200	40	27
1500	50	33
1800	60	40
2100	70	47
2400	80	53
2700	90	60
3000	100	67
3600	120	80
3900	130	87

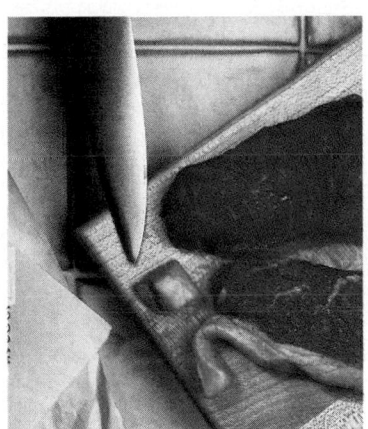

Trim meats before cooking to help reduce your fat intake.

Fats in Food

The foods with the highest nutrient density for fat are salad oils, butter, margarine, and mayonnaise (see p. 198). All contain close to 100% of energy as fat. Many fat-reduced margarines have been introduced, with water replacing some of the fat. Typical margarines are 80% fat by weight (11 grams per tablespoon). Some fat-reduced margarines are as low as 30% fat by weight (4 grams per tablespoon). The extra water added to these margarines can cause texture and volume changes when used in

Nutrition Insight

Hidden Fat

Some fat in food is obvious: butter on bread, mayonnaise in potato salad, and marbling in raw meat. Fat is harder to detect in other foods that also contribute much fat to our diets. Fat is hidden in whole milk, pastries, cookies, cake, cheese, hot dogs, crackers, french fries, and ice cream. When we try to cut down on fat intake, hidden fats need to be exposed and controlled, along with the more obvious sources.

Finding Hidden Fat

A place to begin searching for hidden fat is on the labels of foods you buy in the grocery store. Some signals that can alert you to the presence of fat are chocolate; animal fats, such as bacon, beef, ham, lamb, pork, chicken, and turkey fats; lard; vegetable oils; nuts; dairy fats, such as butter and cream; egg and egg-yolk solids; and hydrogenated shortening or vegetable oil. Conveniently the label lists ingredients by order of weight in the product. If fat is one of the first ingredients listed, you are probably looking at a high-fat product. Use food labels to learn more about the fat content of the foods you eat (see Figure 6-8). Table 2-7 listed the definitions for various fat descriptors on food labels, such as "low fat," "fat free," and "reduced fat."

Recall that "low fat" signifies in most cases that a product contains no more than 3 grams of fat per serving.

Products claimed to be fat-free must have less than $\frac{1}{2}$ gram of fat per serving. A claim of "reduced fat" means the product has at least 25% less fat than is usually found in that food.

When there is no food label to inspect, moderating portion size is a good way to keep fat intake down. Table 6-3 lists many ways you can avoid eating too much total fat and saturated fat. Whether or not to choose a fat-rich food should depend on how you intend to use it: as a staple item, as an occasional treat, or as a garnish for other foods.

Quick-service foods are notable for their content of hidden fat. (see Appendix A). Quick-service outlets often have nutritional information on their products, but you usually have to ask for it. This literature and your own common sense can help you reduce fat intake from these sources. When you can't find a food label, remember that moderating portion size is a good way to keep fat intake down in foods you suspect are rich in fat.

What to Do

Overall, both visible and hidden sources of fat should be examined when developing a plan to eat less fat. Consider the practical suggestions provided in Table 6-3 for cutting down on visible and hidden fats.

Figure 6-8
Reading labels helps locate hidden fat. Who would think that wieners (hot dogs) can contain 85% of food energy as fat? Looking at the hog dog itself doesn't reveal that almost all of its food energy comes from fat, but the label shows otherwise.

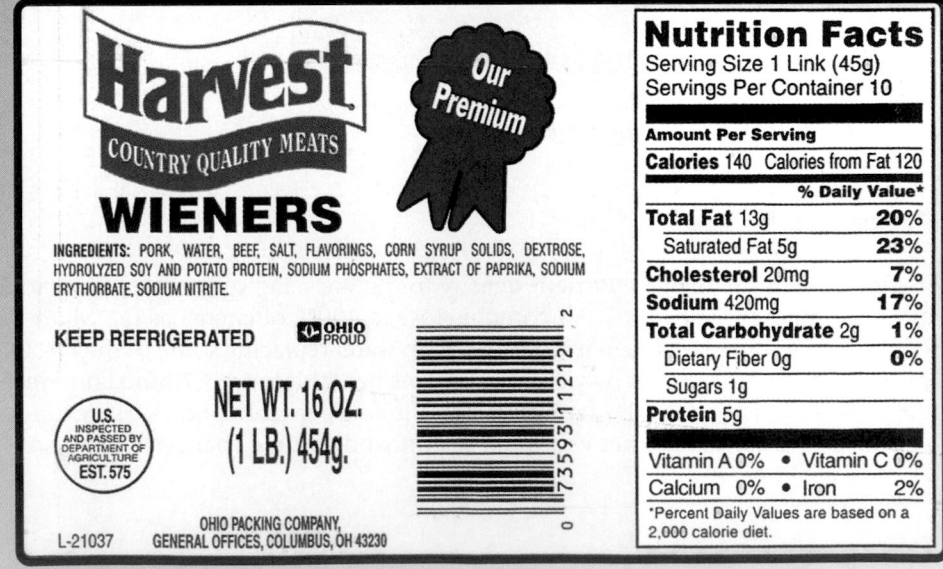

TABLE 6-3

Tips for Avoiding Too Much Fat and Saturated Fat

1. Steam, boil, or bake vegetables. For a change, stir-fry in a small amount of vegetable oil. Consider buying an insert for a pot so you can easily steam your vegetables.

2. Season vegetables with herbs and spices rather than with sauces, butter, or margarine.

3. Try lemon juice on salad or use limited amounts of oil-based salad dressing.

4. To reduce saturated fat, use tub margarine instead of butter or stick margarine in baked products. When possible, use vegetable oil instead of either of these solid fats or hydrogenated shortenings.

5. Limit baked goods made with large amounts of fat, especially saturated fats: croissants, doughnuts, muffins, biscuits, and butter rolls.

6. Try whole-grain flours to enhance flavors when baking goods with less fat. Use applesauce and other fruit purees in place of fat.

7. Replace whole milk with skim or low-fat milk in puddings, soups, and baked products and for use as a beverage.

8. Substitute plain low-fat yogurt, blender-whipped low-fat cottage cheese, or buttermilk in recipes that call for sour cream or mayonnaise.

9. Choose lean cuts of meat. Limit bacon, ribs, and meatloaf.

10. Trim fat from meat before and after cooking.

11. Roast, bake, or broil meat, poultry, and fish so that fat drains away as the food cooks.

12. Remove skin from poultry before cooking. This eliminates the temptation to eat it along with the meat.

13. Use a nonstick pan for cooking so that added fat will be unnecessary; use a vegetable spray for frying.

14. Chill meat or poultry broth until the fat solidifies. Spoon off the fat before using the broth.

15. Eat a vegetarian main dish at least once a week. Include fish (cooked without much added fat) in the diet two times or more a week.

16. Choose fat-reduced ice cream, low-fat frozen yogurt, sorbet, and popsicles as substitutes for regular ice cream.

17. Try angelfood cake, fig bars, and gingersnaps as substitutes for commercial baked goods high in saturated fat.

18. Limit high-fat cheese intake.

19. Read labels on commercially prepared foods to find out what type of fat or how much saturated fat they contain.

20. Use jam, jelly, or marmalade on bread and toast instead of butter or margarine.

21. Buy whole-grain breads and rolls. They have more flavor and do not need butter or margarine to taste good. The dietary fiber present is an added bonus.

22. Think about the balance of fats in the menu. If a meal contains whole milk, cheese, ice cream, a higher-fat meat, or poultry with skin, use margarine and unsaturated vegetable oils for your spreads and dressings. Small amounts of butter, sour cream, or cream cheese can be included if other menu items are low in saturated fat.

recipes. Cookbooks can provide guidance for appropriate use for these products by suggesting alterations in recipes to compensate. You may be surprised to note that some margarines are even advertised as being fat-free. Close inspection of the label shows that these products are made up of monoglycerides and diglycerides. These are not considered to be fats for labeling purposes, as they are not triglycerides, but of course they are still fats and energy dense (Figure 6-9).

Walnuts, bologna, avocados, and bacon have about 80% of energy as fat. Peanut butter and cheddar cheese have about 75%. Marbled steak and hamburgers (ground chuck) have about 60%, and chocolate bars, ice cream, doughnuts, and whole milk have about 50% of energy as fat. Eggs, pumpkin pie, and cupcakes have 35%, as do lean cuts of meat, such as top round (and ground round) and sirloin. Bread contains about 15%. Cornflakes, sugar, and nonfat milk have essentially no fat. Careful label reading is necessary to determine the true fat content of a food—these are only rough guidelines.

Animal fats, which contain about 40% to 60% of total fat as saturated fatty acids, are the chief contributor of saturated fatty acids to the American diet. Saturated fatty acids with 12, 14, and 16 carbons (lauric acid, myristic acid, and palmitic acid, respectively) are the primary contributors to elevated LDL in humans. Of these, the 14-carbon myristic acid is mainly responsible for elevating LDL. Dairy fats are rich sources of myristic acid. The 16-carbon palmitic acid does the same primarily

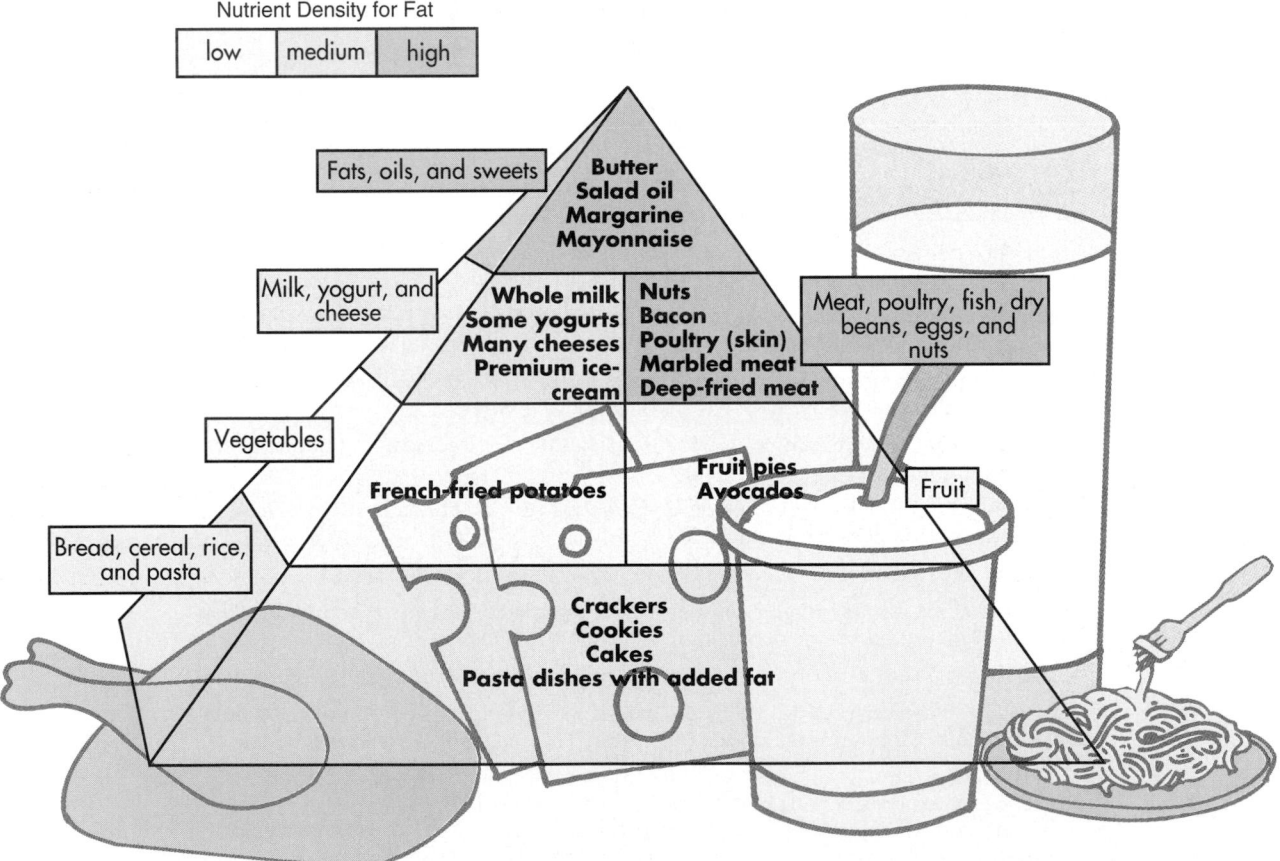

Figure 6-9 *Sources of fats in foods from the Food Guide Pyramid. The background color of each group indicates the average nutrient density for fat in that food group. The fruit group and vegetable group are generally low in fat. In the other groups both high-fat and low-fat choices are available. Careful label reading can lead you along the low-fat path. In general, any type of frying adds significant amounts of fat to a product, as with french-fried potatoes and fried chicken.*

when there is much cholesterol in the diet (>200 to 300 milligrams per day) and blood cholesterol is elevated.[7] In contrast, stearic acid, the saturated fatty acid with 18 carbons, does not raise LDL; it constitutes about 20% of the saturated fat in meats. The saturated fatty acids with 12, 14, or 16 carbons generally constitute about 25% to 50% of the total fat in animal foods. In general, dairy fats and meat are rich in those fatty acids that raise LDL. In some plant oils, these saturated fatty acids also make up a notable percentage of the total fat: for example, cottonseed oil (27%) and coconut oil (89%).

Plant oils contain mostly unsaturated fatty acids, ranging from 73% to 94% of total fat. Canola oil, olive oil, and peanut oil contain moderate to high amounts of total fat as monounsaturated fatty acids (49% to 77%). Some animal fats are also good sources of monounsaturated fatty acids (30% to 47%) (see Figure 6-2). Corn, cottonseed, sunflower, soybean, and safflower oils contain mostly polyunsaturated fatty acids (54% to 77%) in terms of total fat. These plant oils supply the majority of the linoleic acid and alpha-linolenic acid in the U.S. food supply. Note that plant oils vary in their content of polyunsaturated fatty acids. Oils that are similar in appearance still may vary significantly in fatty acid composition

Cholesterol is found only in the animal foods we eat (see Table 6-4). An egg yolk contains about 210 milligrams of cholesterol. This is our main dietary source of cholesterol, along with meats and whole milk. Some plants contain related sterols, but none we typically eat contains cholesterol. Manufacturers who advertise peanut butter, vegetable shortening, margarines, and vegetable oils as containing "no cholesterol" are taking advantage of uninformed consumers. Peanut butter and margarine never contain cholesterol—its not part of their nature!

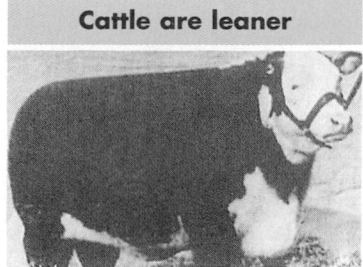

Cattle are leaner

1950s steer

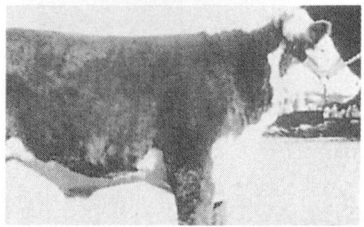

1990s steer

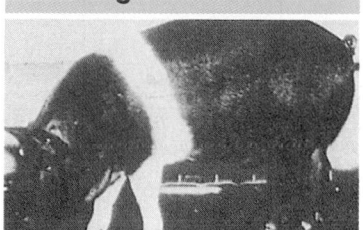

Hogs are leaner

1940s hog

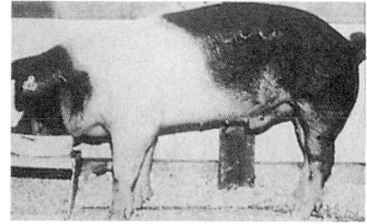

1990s hog

During the past several decades, beef and hog producers have altered breeding and feeding practices to increase muscle mass and decrease body fat.

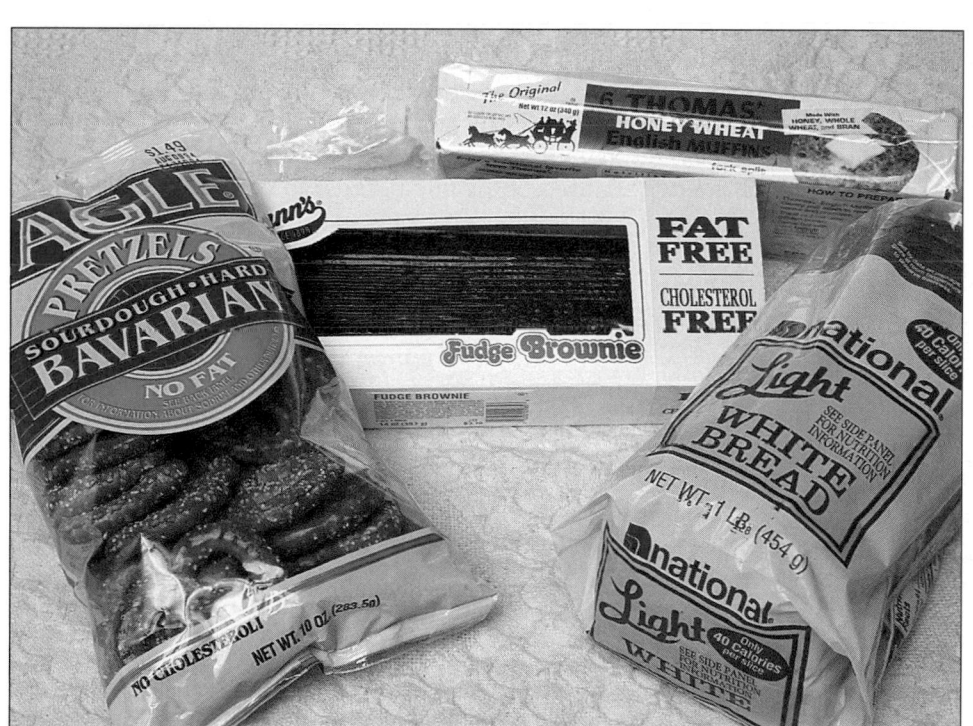

Many manufacturers and food producers are trying to devise products that are lower in fat, particularly saturated fat. Still, read the labels rather than the advertising claims to find out the fat content of products like these.

TABLE 6-4

Cholesterol Content of Common Measurements of Selected Foods (in Ascending Order)

Food	Amount	Cholesterol in milligrams	Food	Amount	Cholesterol in milligrams
Skim milk	1 cup	4	Oysters, salmon	3 oz	40
Mayonnaise	1 tbsp	10	Clams, halibut, tuna	3 oz	55
Butter	1 pat	11	Chicken, turkey (white meat)	3 oz	70
Lard	1 tbsp	12	Beef,* pork*	3 oz	75
Cottage cheese	½ cup	15	Lamb, crab	3 oz	85
Low-fat milk (2%)	1 cup	22	Shrimp, lobster	3 oz	90–110
Half and half	¼ cup	23	Heart, beef	3 oz	165
Hot dog*	1	29	Egg (egg yolk)*	1 each	210
Ice cream, ≈10% fat	½ cup	30	Liver, beef	3 oz	410
Cheese, cheddar	1 oz	30	Kidney	3 oz	540
Whole milk	1 cup	34	Brains	3 oz	2640

*Leading contributors of cholesterol to the U.S. diet.

Using Reduced Fat Foods Wisely

In recent years, manufacturers have introduced reduced fat versions of numerous food products (Figure 6-10). The fat content of these alternatives ranges from 0% in fat-free Fig Newtons to about 75% of the original fat content in other products.. However, the total energy content of most fat-reduced products is not substantially lower than that of their conventional versions (Table 6-5). Generally, when fat is removed from a product, something must be added, commonly carbohydrate, in its place. Generally it is very difficult to reduce both the fat and carbohydrate content of a product at the same time. For this reason, many fat-reduced products (for example, cakes, cookies, and yogurt) are still very energy dense. Don't be fooled into thinking you can eat substantially more of such foods just because some or all of the fat has been removed.[1] "Reduced fat" is not a license to overeat.[2]

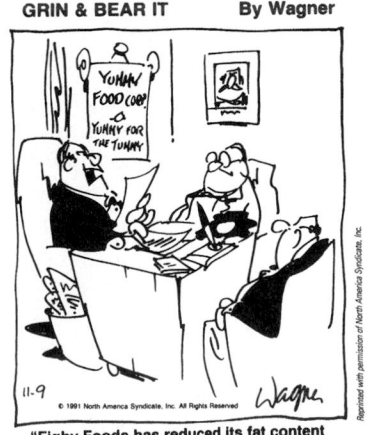

GRIN & BEAR IT By Wagner

"Figby Foods has reduced its fat content by another gram! This is war, gentlemen!"

Figure 6-10
Grin & Bear It.

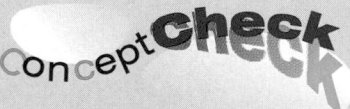

There is no RDA for fat. We need about 4% of total energy intake from plant oils to obtain the needed essential fatty acids. Eating fish about twice a week is also advised to supply omega-3 fatty acids. Many health-related agencies recommend a diet containing no more than 30% of energy intake as fat, with no more than 10% of energy intake as saturated fat. The current American diet contains about 34% of energy content as fat, with about 12% of energy content as saturated fat. Fat-dense foods—those with more than 60% of total energy as fat—include plant oils, butter, margarine, mayonnaise, walnuts, bacon, avocados, peanut butter, cheddar cheese, steak, and hamburger. Of the foods we typically eat, cholesterol is found naturally only in those of animal origin, with eggs being a primary source. Fat free doesn't mean calorie free; moderation in the use of fat-reduced products is still important.

TABLE 6-5

Energy and Fat Content of Original and Fat-Reduced Forms of Some Food Products

Food product	Amounts/serving	Energy (kcal)	Fat (grams)
Nabisco Chips Ahoy! Cookies			
Original	1 each/11 grams	53	3
Reduced fat	1 each/11 grams	50	2
Nabisco Fig Newtons			
Original	1 each/16 grams	55	1
Fat free	1 each/15 grams	50	0
Hostess Cupcakes			
Original	1 each/46 grams	170	5
Low-fat Cupcake Lights	1 each/40 grams	120	2
Hostess Twinkies			
Original	1 each/41 grams	140	4
Low-fat Twinkie Lights	1 each/40 grams	120	2
Nabisco Ritz Crackers			
Original	5 each/16 grams	80	4
Reduced fat	5 each/16 grams	70	3
Nabisco Triscuit Wafers			
Original	5 each/23 grams	100	4
Reduced fat	5 each/22 grams	85	2
Sunshine Cheez-It Snack Crackers			
Original	10 each/11 grams	60	3
Reduced fat	10 each/10 grams	50	2
Kraft Miracle Whip Salad Dressing			
Original	1 tbsp/14 grams	70	7
Light	1 tbsp/15 grams	40	3
Nestle Crunch Vanilla Ice Cream Bars			
Original	1 bar/60 grams	200	14
Reduced fat	1 bar/50 grams	130	7
Breyer's Natural Vanilla Ice Cream			
Original	½ cup/70 grams	150	8
Premium Light	½ cup/68 grams	130	5
Pringles Original Potato Chips			
Original	10 each/20 grams	114	8
Right Crisps Original (reduced fat)	10 each/18 grams	88	4
Betty Crocker Creamy Deluxe Chocolate Frosting			
Original	2 tbsp/36 grams	140	6
Low fat	2 tbsp/36 grams	120	1
Kraft Ranch Dressing			
Original	2 tbsp/29 grams	170	18
Deliciously Right (reduced fat)	2 tbsp/30 grams	110	11
Oscar Meyer Bologna			
Original	1 slice/28 grams	90	8
Light	1 slice/28 grams	50	4
Land O'Lakes Sweet Cream Salted Butter			
Original	1 tbsp/14 grams	100	11
Light	1 tbsp/14 grams	50	6
Cool Whip Topping			
Original	2 tbsp/8 grams	25	2
Lite	2 tbsp/8 grams	20	1
Kraft Singles American Cheese			
Original	1 slice/21 grams	70	5
⅓ less fat	1 slice/21 grams	50	3

Fat Replacement Strategies

Currently five different types of fat replacements are available in the United States. Addition of these substances during manufacture yields products that to varying degrees satisfy consumers' desire for fat-reduced products that are still tasty.

Water, Starch Derivatives, and Gums

The first and simplest fat replacement is water. Addition of water yields a product, such as diet margarine, with less fat per serving than the normal product. Starch derivatives that bind water form a second type of fat replacement. Derivatives commonly used by food manufacturers include cellulose, Maltrin, Stellar, and Oatrim. These substances are used in a variety of foods, including luncheon meats, salad dressings, frozen desserts, table spreads, dips, baked goods, and candies. Gums extracted from plants can also be used to replace fat. They thicken a product and replace some of the body that fat provided. Diet salad dressings have gums added for this reason.

Protein-Derived Fat Replacements

A new type of fat replacement on the market consists of proteins that have been treated to produce microscopic, mistlike protein globules. Both egg and milk proteins can be used. When these substances replace fat in a food product, they feel like fat in the mouth, although the product does not contain any fatty acids. Simplesse is a currently used fat replacement of this type. Since it contains protein, Simplesse yields some energy—but only about 1.3 kcal per gram, much less than the 9 kcal per gram supplied by regular fats. Simplesse has this low energy value primarily for two reasons: proteins contain only 4 kcal per gram, and the product has a high water content.

Simplesse is used primarily in frozen desserts. It reduces the energy content of these products by about one half and fat content to a negligible amount. However, these products tend to develop a grainy texture upon refreezing. This is one reason for their limited acceptance to date. Simplesse can also replace fat in mayonnaise, salad dressing, yogurt, sour cream, cheese, and other dairy products. Because high temperatures alter the structure of Simplesse so much that it no longer resembles fat, it cannot be used for cooking or frying. Note also that people who are allergic to milk or egg proteins should not consume Simplesse.

Engineered Fats

The final form of fat replacement is the engineered fat. This type of product is synthesized in the laboratory from various food constituents. The experimental product olestra (Olean) is a good example. It is made by chemically linking fatty acids to sucrose (table sugar). The resulting product cannot be digested by either human digestive enzymes or bacteria that live in the intestine. Therefore olestra yields no energy to the body.

A highly versatile ingredient, Olestra can replace much of the fat in salad dressings and cakes and can also be used for frying in food manufacturing. Olestra was approved by FDA in 1996 for use in fried snack foods.

Some problems are associated with the use of olestra. It binds the fat-soluble vitamins A, D, E, and K, thus reducing absorption. To compensate, the manufacturer will add these vitamins to olestra. Olestra also may cause abdominal cramping and loose stools in some people, because even though it is not absorbed in the small intestine, it still may influence intestinal function. The problem is mostly seen with intakes of 20 grams at a meal. In

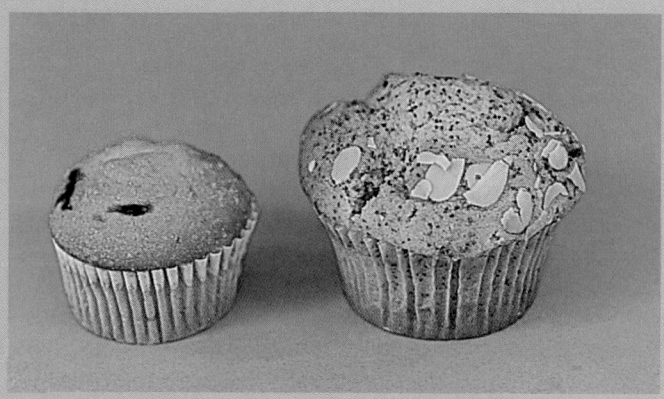

Serving sizes are getting bigger and bigger. A muffin like the one on the right, which once would have looked huge, has now practically become the norm. The smaller muffin provides 180 kcal and 8 grams of fat. Contrast this with the big muffin, which provides 460 kcal and 26 grams of fat.

comparison, a 1-ounce bag of chips will have about 10 grams of olestra.

The following statement will be required on all products made with olestra: "This product contains olestra. Olestra may cause abdominal cramping and loose stools. Olestra inhibits the absorption of some vitamins and other nutrients. Vitamins A, D, E, and K have been added."[20] As a condition of approval, the manufacturer will also conduct studies to monitor olestra consumption and its long-term effects. FDA will review its approval decision by July 1998.

One final problem linked to olestra is its ability to bind carotenoids, the yellow, orange, or red pigments found in many fruits and vegetables. Recall from Chapter 2 the discussion of phytochemicals and their proposed contribution to overall health; one class of phytochemicals is carotenoids. Population studies have linked fruits and vegetables containing carotenoids to reduced risk of heart disease, some forms of cancer, and certain eye disorders. There is no planned attempt to add carotenoids to olestra. This effect of olestra will be most important when it is consumed in large amounts with meals rich in carotenoids. Typical projected intakes of 10 to 20 grams don't have much of an effect. Nevertheless, this ability to bind carotenoids has caused some experts to recommend that we not consume olestra. At the very least, moderate

intake is recommended until we know more about its long-term effects.

Food manufacturers are working on still other types of engineered fats that either wholly or partially escape absorption by the body. One example is Caprenin. This triglyceride product contains two medium-chain fatty acids and a long-chain (22-carbon) saturated fatty acid, called behenic acid. Because of its length and saturation, behenic acid is solid even at body temperature and therefore is difficult to absorb from the small intestine. The fat yields only about 5 kcal per gram to the body, mostly because of the limited absorption of the behenic acid. Caprenin is currently used in reduced-calorie confections. Another example is Salatrim, which yields only about 5 kcal per gram. It is generally composed of stearic acid, which the body absorbs poorly, and short-chain fatty acids. This product is currently used in reduced-fat chocolate chips. A final product is Appetize, which blends animal fats stripped of cholesterol with plant oils. This produces a stable frying fat low in trans fatty acid content. Tests show this fat does not increase LDL.[7]

Fat Replacement in Perspective

So far, fat replacements have had little impact on the American diet, partly because the currently approved forms either are not very versatile or have not been used extensively by manufacturers. In addition, fat replacements are of little use in many foods that contribute the most fat to our diets—hamburgers, hot dogs, whole milk, and beefsteaks and roasts, to name some key players. We consumers must decide to limit our intake of these fat sources; the replacements currently can't help us much.

The main benefit of fat replacements will be in helping people cut some fat from their diets, most important, saturated fat and cholesterol. The reduction in energy intake will probably be less impressive because studies show that people tend to make up the lost energy by increasing their intake of other foods or by eating more of fat-reduced foods than the corresponding conventional foods. However, we won't know the true impact of fat replacements on American diets until they are more widely used. For now they are of limited significance.

Summary

➤ Lipids are a group of compounds that don't readily dissolve in water. Fatty acids can be grouped according to the type of bonds between the carbons: saturated fatty acids contain no double bonds, monounsaturated fatty acids contain one double bond, and polyunsaturated fatty acids contain two or more double bonds.

➤ Fats composed of saturated fatty acids tend to be solid at room temperature. Those with polyunsaturated fatty acids are usually liquid at room temperature.

➤ If the double bonds in a fatty acid begin at the third carbon from the -CH₃ end of the chain, the fatty acid is an omega-3 fatty acid. In omega-6 fatty acids the double bonds begin at the sixth carbon. Both omega-3 and omega-6 fatty acids are essential parts of a diet because our bodies need them but don't produce them.

➤ Body cells use omega-3 fatty acids to synthesize compounds that tend to reduce blood clotting and inflammatory responses. Because many types of fish contain ample amounts of the omega-3 fatty acids, eating fish about twice a week is a recommended dietary practice.

➤ Triglycerides are the major form of fat in our bodies. Besides supplying essential fatty acids to the body, triglycerides supply energy, allow efficient energy storage, insulate and protect the body, transport fat-soluble vitamins, and promote satiety, or a feeling of fullness.

➤ Phospholipids are derived from triglycerides. They form important parts of cell membranes. Some act as efficient emulsifiers, allowing fats to disperse in water.

➤ Cholesterol is in the class of lipids called sterols. It forms part of vital compounds, such as hormones and bile. Cells in the body can make all the cholesterol we need; there is no dietary requirement.

➤ Fat digestion takes place primarily in the small intestine. An enzyme released from the pancreas digests the triglycerides into smaller breakdown products, namely monoglycerides (glycerol backbones with single fatty acids attached) and fatty acids. The breakdown products then are absorbed by the small intestine. These products are mostly resynthesized into triglycerides and combined with cholesterol, protein, and other substances to yield a chylomicron. Chylomicrons enter the lymphatic system, in turn passing into the bloodstream.

➤ Fats are carried in the bloodstream by various lipoproteins: chylomicrons, very low-density lipoproteins (VLDL), low-density lipoproteins (LDL), and high-density lipoproteins (HDL). The greater the amount of triglycerides in the lipoproteins, the less their density. Both elevated LDL and low HDL speed the development of heart disease.

➤ Fats add flavor and texture to foods. Hydrogenation is the process of adding hydrogens to fatty acids to turn many double bonds into single bonds. This process also forms some trans fatty acids. Manufacturers hydrogenate (increase saturation of) fats to solidify vegetable oils for making shortenings and margarine. This practice also reduces the breakdown of polyunsaturated fatty acids, which lessens rancidity.

➤ There is no RDA for fat. We need to eat at least the equivalent of about 1 tablespoon of plant oils daily in foods to get the needed omega-6 essential fatty acids. Fish is a good source of omega-3 fatty acids.

➤ The typical American diet contains about 34% of total energy as fat. Many health agencies and scientific groups suggest reducing fat intake to no more than 30% of energy intake and cholesterol intake to between 200 and 300 milligrams. Some health experts advocate an even greater reduction to 20% of energy intake, but such a diet is generally difficult to plan and follow without some initial professional guidance.

➤ Fat-reduced products aid in the goal of reducing fat intake, but they must be eaten in moderate amounts to maintain control of total energy intake.

Study Questions

1 Describe the chemical structures of saturated and polyunsaturated fatty acids and their different effects in both food and the human body.

2 Relate the need for omega-3 fatty acids in the diet to the recommendation to consume fish about two times per week.

3 Describe the structures, origins, and roles of the four major blood lipoproteins.

4 What are the recommendations of health care professionals regarding fat intake? What does this mean in terms of actual food choices?

5 What are two important functions of fat in food? How are these different from the general functions of lipids in the human body?

6 What are the significance of and possible uses for the new reduced-fat foods?

7 Does the total cholesterol concentration in the bloodstream tell the whole story with respect to heart disease risk?

Read the Nutrition Issue before answering the following questions:

8 List five risk factors for the development of premature heart disease.

9 What actually brings on a myocardial infarction? What dietary practices are thought to help precipitate this event?

References

1 ASCN/AIN Task Force on Trans Fatty Acids: Position paper on trans fatty acids, *American Journal of Clinical Nutrition* 66:663, 1996.

2 Allred JB: Too much of a good thing? *Journal of the American Dietetic Association* 95:417, 1995.

3 Anderson JW and others: Meta-analysis of the effects of soy protein intake on serum lipids, *The New England Journal of Medicine* 333:276, 1995.

4 Drewnowski A: Impact of taste preferences on dietary choices and food consumption patterns, *Food & Nutrition News* 67 (May/June):15 1995.

5 Fuhrman B and others: Consumption of red wine with meals reduces the susceptibility of human plasma and low-density lipoprotein to triple peroxidation, *American Journal of Clinical Nutrition* 61:549, 1995.

6 Havel RJ, Rapaport E: Management of primary hyperlipidemia, *New England Journal of Medicine* 332:1491, 1995.

7 Hayes KC: Designing a cholesterol-removed fat blend for frying and baking, *Food Technology,* April 1996, p 92.

8 Hennekens CH and others: Antioxidant vitamin–cardiovascular disease hypothesis is promising, but unproven: the need for randomized trials, *American Journal of Clinical Nutrition* 62(suppl):1377S, 1995.

9 Herbert V: Iron worsens high-cholesterol–related coronary artery disease, *American Journal of Clinical Nutrition* 60:299, 1994.

10 Howard BV and others: Effects of sex and ethnicity on responses to a low-fat diet: a study of African Americans and whites, *American Journal of Clinical Nutrition* 62:488S, 1995.

11 Iribarren C and others: Serum cholesterol level and mortality due to suicide and trauma in the Honolulu Heart Program, *Archives of Internal Medicine* 155:695, 1995.

12 Jenkins DJA and others: Effect of nibbling versus gorging on cardiovascular risk factors: serum uric acid and blood lipids, *Metabolism* 44:549, 1995.

13 Katan M: Fish and heart disease, *New England Journal of Medicine* 332:1024, 1995.

14 Klatsky AL: Cardiovascular effects of alcohol, *Scientific American Science & Medicine* March/April 1995, p 28.

15 Kris-Etherton P and others: Cardiovascular disease and women's health, *Topics in Clinical Nutrition* 11:8, 1995.

16 Kushi LH and others: Health implications of Mediterranean diets in light of contemporary knowledge, *American Journal of Clinical Nutrition* 61(suppl):1407S, 1995 (Part I); 61(suppl):1416S, 1995 (Part II).

17 Milani RV, Lavie CJ: Pharmacologic prevention of coronary artery disease, *Postgraduate Medicine* 99:109, 1996.

18 Murray RK and others: Harper's Biochemistry, ed 23, Norwalk, CT, 1996, Appleton & Lange.

19 O'Keefe JH and others: Lifestyle change for coronary artery disease, *Postgraduate Medicine* 99:89, 1996.

20 Olestra approved with special labeling, *FDA Consumer,* April 1996, p 11.

21 Renaud S and others: Cretan Mediterranean diet for prevention of coronary heart disease, *American Journal of Clinical Nutrition* 61(suppl):1360S, 1995.

22　Retzlaff BM and others: Changes in plasma triacylglycerol concentrations among free-living hyper-lipidemic men adopting different carbohydrate intakes over 2 years: the Dietary Alternatives Study, *American Journal of Clinical Nutrition* 62:988, 1995.

23　Rich-Edwards JW and others: The primary prevention of coronary heart disease in women, *New England Journal of Medicine* 332:1758, 1995.

24　Ross R: Cell biology of atherosclerosis, *Annual Review of Physiology* 57:791, 1995.

25　Rim EB and others: Vegetable, fruit, and cereal fiber intake and risk of coronary heart disease among men, *Journal of the American Medical Association* 275:447, 1996.

26　Thompson SG and others: Hemostatic factors and the risk of myocardial infarction or sudden death in patients with angina pectoris, *New England Journal of Medicine* 332:635, 1995.

27　Verschuren WMM and others: Serum total cholesterol and long-term coronary heart disease mortality in different cultures, *Journal of the American Medical Association* 274:131, 1995.

28　Walsh JME, Grady D: Treatment of hyperlipidemia in women, *Journal of the American Medical Association* 274:1152, 1995.

29　Wei M and others: The impact of changes in coffee consumption on serum cholesterol, *Journal of Clinical Epidemiology* 48:1189, 1995.

30　WHO and FAO Joint Consultation: Fats and oils in human nutrition, *Nutrition Reviews* 53:202, 1995.

31　Willet WC and others: Coffee consumption and coronary heart disease in women, *Journal of the American Medical Association* 275:458, 1996.

32　Willet WC, Ascherio A: Trans fatty acids: are the effects only marginal? *American Journal of Public Health* 84:722, 1994.

33　Williams RR: Diet, genes, early heart attacks, and high blood pressure. In Kotsonis FN and Mackey MA, eds: *Nutrition in the 90's,* New York, 1994, Marcel Dekker.

What Is Your Fat and Cholesterol Intake?

How do your food practices compare with general guidelines suggested for fat, saturated fat, and cholesterol intake? Refer to the nutritional assessment you completed at the end of Chapter 2, and compare it with the guidelines listed below, issued by the American Heart Association and the National Cholesterol Education Program:

- Limit or reduce total fat intake to 30% or less of total energy intake.
- Reduce saturated fat intake to 7% to 10% of energy intake or less.
- Limit cholesterol to 200 to 300 milligrams per day.

To compare your nutritional assessment with these guidelines, first fill in the values for your intakes of the following:

TOTAL ENERGY: _____   TOTAL FAT: _____   SATURATED FAT: _____   CHOLESTEROL: _____

Now complete the following steps:

1. Multiply your total grams of fat by 9 (kcal per gram of fat). Then divide the result by your total energy intake. Next multiply this number by 100. This will give you the percentage of energy you consumed from fat.

    % OF ENERGY FROM FAT _____   IS IT 30% OR LESS OF TOTAL ENERGY?   YES _____   NO _____

2. Multiply your grams of saturated fat by 9 (kcal per gram of fat). Divide the result by your total energy intake. Now multiply this number by 100. This will give you the percentage of energy you consumed from saturated fat.

    % OF ENERGY FROM SATURATED FAT _____

    IS IT 10% OF ENERGY OR LESS?   YES _____   NO _____

3. Look at your milligrams of cholesterol.

    IS YOUR INTAKE LESS THAN 300 milligrams?   YES _____   NO _____

4. Look back at the foods you ate and notice the foods that contributed the most fat, saturated fat, and cholesterol. If you didn't meet one or more of the guidelines and had elevated LDL, how could you change what you ate that day to improve your diet?

5. Now take the next step. Do you know your HDL and LDL values? If not, have them checked soon. All adults should know whether these values are in the abnormal ranges.

6. Finally, fill in the following assessment of your risk for developing premature heart disease. Decide today how you could modify your diet and lifestyle, if necessary, to reduce your risk.

Do you have . . .	YES	NO		YES	NO
a history of smoking?	____	____	diabetes?	____	____
high blood pressure?	____	____	a history of physical inactivity?	____	____
high LDL?	____	____	a family history of premature heart disease?	____	____
low HDL?	____	____	a history of obesity?	____	____
			a diet that lacks sufficient B vitamins, such as B-6, folate, and B-12?	____	____

Other factors also could be considered, as discussed in the Nutrition Issue, but this provides a good start for assessing your risk.

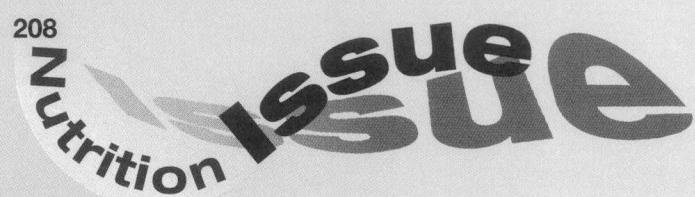

Heart Disease

A heart attack can strike with the sudden force of a sledgehammer, with pain radiating up the neck or down the arm. It can also sneak up at night, masquerading as indigestion, with slight pain or pressure in the chest. Typical warning signs are:

- Intense, prolonged chest pain or pressure, sometimes radiating to other parts of the upper body
- Shortness of breath
- Sweating
- Nausea
- Dizziness
- Weakness

Heart disease—more precisely termed **cardiovascular disease**—is the major killer of Americans. Each year about 500,000 people die of heart disease in the United States, about 60% more than die of cancer. The figure rises to almost 1 million if strokes and other circulatory diseases are included in the more global term cardiovascular disease. The overall male-to-female ratio for heart disease is about 2:1. Women generally lag about 10 years behind men in developing the disease. Still, heart disease eventually kills more women than any other disease— twice as many as cancer.[15]

For each person in America who dies of heart disease, 10 more (over 6 million people) have symptoms of heart disease. In addition, about three times the number who die, 1.5 million, suffer heart attacks each year, accounting for about $47 billion in health-care costs.

Worldwide, the highest number of new cases per year of heart attacks in men—915 per 100,000—is found in Finland. For women, Scotland posts the high—256 per 100,000. The lowest rate for men of 76 per 100,000 is found in China; for women the lowest rate of 30 per 100,000 is found in Spain. In the United States yearly heart-attack incidence per 100,000 is about 500 for men and 140 for women.

DEVELOPMENT OF HEART DISEASE

The symptoms of heart disease develop over many years and often do not become obvious until old age. Nonetheless, autopsies of young adults under 20 years of age have shown that many of them have atherosclerotic plaque in their arteries. This finding indicates that plaque buildup can begin in childhood and continue throughout life, although it usually goes undetected for quite some time.

Preventing premature heart disease—that which appears before age 70 to 80—deserves everyone's consideration. Although we all die, one key to a better life is to prevent premature death and live in good health until essentially the entire body wears out, the heart included. Heart attacks at ages 40 through 60 are closely linked to the risk factors discussed later. Most people at risk can greatly improve their chance to avoid premature heart disease by making some long-term lifestyle changes.[6] (See Chapter 16 for further discussion of the premature appearance of disease in adulthood and how to prevent it.)

Heart disease and strokes are associated with inadequate blood circulation in the heart and brain. Blood supplies the heart muscle and brain—and other body organs—with oxygen and nutrients. When blood flow via the coronary arteries surrounding the heart is interrupted, the heart muscle can be damaged. A heart attack, or **myocardial infarction,** may result (see Figure 6-11). This may cause the heart to beat irregularly or to stop altogether. If blood flow to parts of the brain is interrupted long enough, part of the brain dies, causing a cerebrovascular accident, or stroke. When a stroke causes loss of muscle control, death may occur.

More than 95% of all heart attacks are caused by blood clots that stop blood flow to the heart or brain. Clots form more readily where atherosclerotic plaque has built up in the arteries that serve the heart (coronary arteries) or brain (carotid arteries). Actually, the most dangerous lesions aren't the large, advanced ones, but smaller, unstable lesions covered by a small fibrous cap. In essence, heart attacks are caused not by total blockage of the coronary arteries by plaque, but by disruption of a partial blockage, leading to clot formation.[24] Because aspirin in small doses reduces blood clotting, it is often used under a physician's guidance to treat people at risk for heart attack, especially if one has already occurred.

As mentioned earlier in this chapter, plaque is probably first deposited to repair injuries in a vessel lining.[24] The *athero* in "atherosclerosis" comes from the Greek and means "gruel or paste." Hypertension, diabetes, LDL, and smoking are some of many agents that probably lead to vessel injury, which in turn starts the repair process. Current research also implicates certain bacteria and viruses in vessel injury. This process of damage repair is part of the intiation phase of atherosclerosis. The rate of further plaque deposition in the next phase, called the progression phase, partly depends on the amount of LDL in the

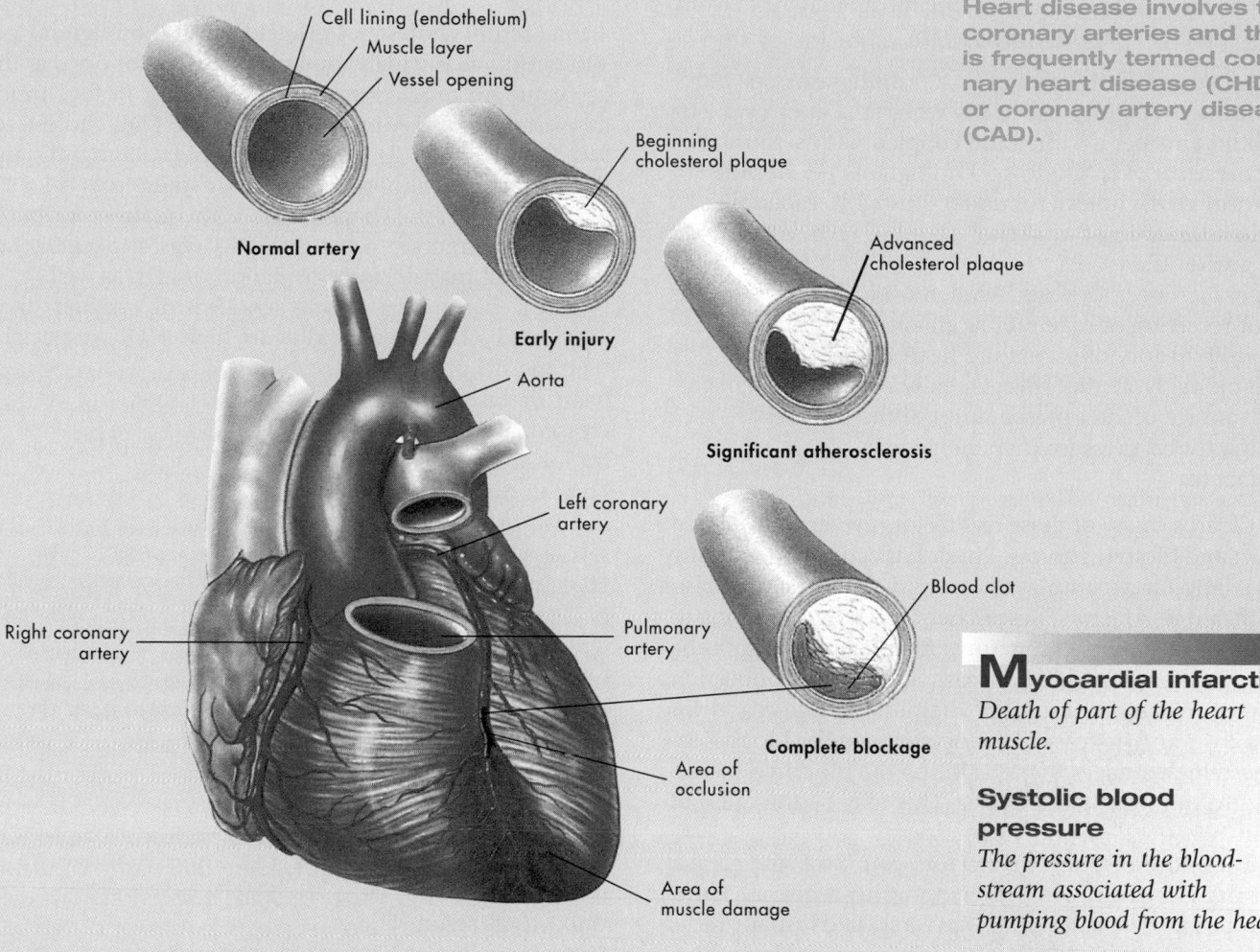

Figure 6-11 *The road to a heart attack. Injury to an artery wall begins the process. This is followed by a progressive buildup of plaque in the artery walls. The heart attack represents the terminal phase of the process. Blockage of the left coronary artery by a blood clot is evident. The heart muscle that is served by the portion of the coronary artery beyond the point of blockage lacks oxygen and nutrients; it is damaged and may die. This can lead to a significant drop in heart function and often total heart failure. Current research suggests that the smaller, early plaques cause most heart attacks as they break up and in turn stimulate blood clotting.*

Myocardial infarction
Death of part of the heart muscle.

Systolic blood pressure
The pressure in the bloodstream associated with pumping blood from the heart.

Diastolic blood pressure
The pressure in the bloodstream when the heart is between beats.

blood. The plaque thickens as layers of cholesterol (part of LDL), protein, smooth muscle, and calcium are deposited. Arteries harden and narrow as plaque builds up, making them less elastic. They are thus unable to expand to accommodate alterations in blood pressure.

Affected arteries become further damaged as blood pumps through them and pressure increases. Finally, in the terminal phase, a clot or spasm in a plaque-clogged artery leads to a myocardial infarction.

Factors that typically bring on a heart attack in a person at risk include dehydration, acute emotional stress, strenuous physical activity (shoveling snow, for example), waking during the night (linked to an abrupt increase in stress), and consuming high-fat meals.

RISK FACTORS FOR HEART DISEASE

Many of us are free of the risk factors that contribute to rapid development of atherosclerosis and premature heart disease. If so, the advice of health experts is to simply consume a balanced diet, perform regular physical activity, and reevaluate risk factors every 5 years.

People who face the highest risk for premature heart disease have one or another rare genetic defect that substantially blocks clearance of chylomicrons and triglycerides from the blood, reduces LDL uptake by the liver, limits synthesis of HDL, or enhances blood clotting.[26,33] Other medical conditions, such as certain forms of liver and kidney disease, low concentrations of thyroid hormone, and use of certain medications to treat hypertension, can increase LDL and thus increase the risk for heart disease.[6]

Continued.

portion of meat can contain 260 milligrams of cholesterol, slightly more than the amount of one egg. If meats have a reputation for being high in cholesterol, it is mainly because of an overly generous portion size.

Increasing monounsaturated and polyunsaturated fats

Until recently, polyunsaturated fatty acids, but not monounsaturated fatty acids, were recommended as a substitute for saturated fatty acids in the diet to lower LDL. However, recent studies show that both monounsaturated and polyunsaturated fatty acids have this effect. In fact, monounsaturated fatty acids may be more beneficial, since LDLs containing these fatty acids are less likely to be oxidized. Recall that oxidized LDL probably contributes more to plaque formation in the arteries than does LDL itself.[24]

However, aside from moving to Crete or some other Mediterranean country where monounsaturated fat-rich olive oil is a major part of the diet, it would be difficult for a typical American to take advantage of this research on monounsaturated fats. Foods and meals rich in monounsaturated fats are not widely available in the United States, nor are they a big part of our cuisine. If you do much of your own cooking, using canola oil, canola oil blended with other vegetable oils, and olive oil on a regular basis will increase your intake of monounsaturated fats. A further emphasis on monounsaturated fat would probably require the counsel of a registered dietitian to design a specific meal pattern.

One approach could be the recently published "Mediterranean Pyramid." This is a plan based on food choices like those traditionally found in the simple

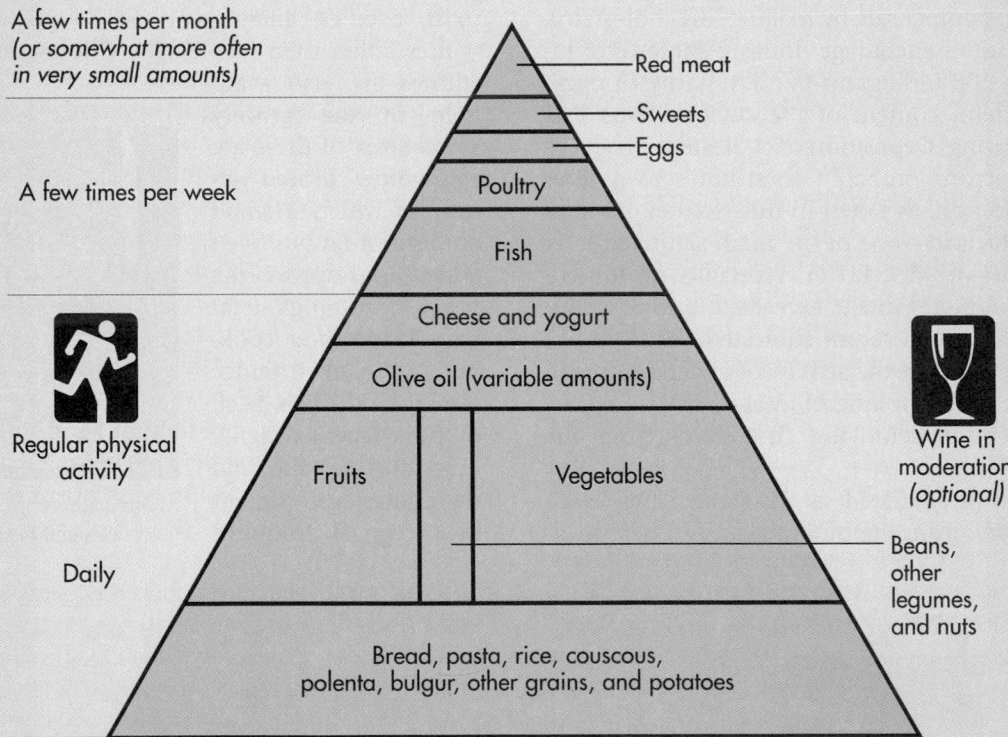

Figure 6-12 *The traditional healthy Mediterranean Diet Pyramid. This plan is based on long-standing eating habits in southern Italy, Crete, and Greece. The base of the diet is bread and grains, fruits and vegetables, and beans and potatoes. Red meat is consumed sparingly—moderate amounts of fish and poultry are preferred. Wine may be included with meals. Most of the fat in this plan comes from olive oil. Cheese and yogurt supply some fat and some calcium. A recommendation for regular physical activity is also made.*

Consider the following suggestions if you want to begin following a more Mediterranean diet:

- Plan meals ahead of time to have better control over food intake.
- Switch to olive oil as a main source of fat. For a less expensive option, canola oil has about the same fatty acid profile, but it does not qualify as the typical Mediterranean fat.
- Reduce intake of butter and margarine.
- Add bread in abundance to each meal.
- Begin or end most meals with a salad.
- Add more vegetables and different vegetables to meals.
- Cut down on the amount of meat consumed.
- Substitute red wine in moderation at meals for other alcoholic beverages.
- Include desserts only occasionally.

cuisines of Greece and southern Italy. In 1994, components of this diet were arranged into a pyramid analogous to the USDA Food Guide Pyramid by respresentatives from the Harvard School of Public Health, the World Health Organization's Regional Office for Europe, and the nonprofit Oldways Preservations & Exchange Trust (Figure 6-12).

The Mediterranean pyramid allows 25% to 35% of total fat in the diet, compared with the typical recommendation of not more than 30%. However, it recommends consuming the type of fat consumed in the Mediterranean region: olive oil. The plan recommends that very small portions of red meat be eaten only a few times a month, and also suggests regular physical activity and modest alcohol intake (wine, preferably red) with meals. Eggs and sweets are to be used sparingly as well.[16, 21]

The Mediterranean pyramid does fall short in some areas. Like the Food Guide Pyramid, it recommends a generous base of grains, fruits, vegetables, and legumes. In contrast, it does not limit fat to the same extent. Olive oil is not rich in saturated fats, but like all fats it is a concentrated source of energy, and obesity is a major public health problem in the United States. The whole-milk cheese and yogurt included in the Mediterranean pyramid contain high amounts of saturated fat, which contribute to heart disease. Recommending reduced-fat varieties of dairy products would improve the plan. Calcium intake is likely to be low in this plan, because low-fat and nonfat milk are omitted. Architects of the plan suggest that calcium supplements be used to meet this shortfall.

Many Americans at risk for premature heart disease consume diets of high-fat convenience foods that offer little variety. The first steps to a better diet should be made away from that pattern and toward the bottom half of either pyramid, where most of the benefits are found.[27] Exactly what the top half looks like is of relatively lesser importance, so long as fat intake is moderate. The inclusion of wine with meals is an interesting twist of the Mediterranean pyramid. The phytochemicals in wine, especially red wine, in some studies are linked to reduced oxidation of LDL in some studies.[5]

Increasing dietary fiber

Another dietary means of reducing LDL is increasing intake of soluble fibers, as discussed in Chapter 5. Although large amounts of fiber must be eaten to have a significant effect on LDL, any amount helps—and has other health benefits as well.[25] Diets with an overall fiber content of 25 to 50 grams per day, especially those that emphasize soluble fiber, are most effective in lowering LDL. Most people would have to change their diets extensively to achieve high intakes of soluble fiber. Instead, the focus could simply be on high-fiber foods—fruits, vegetables, dry beans, and whole grains. Moreover, dietary fiber intake above 35 grams per day may cause binding of dietary minerals, a potentially deleterious side effect. You should consult a physician if considering a very high-fiber diet.

Diets high in soluble fiber probably work by binding cholesterol and bile in the small intestine and carrying them into the large intestine for elimination. Removing bile from the body forces the liver to pull more cholesterol out of the bloodstream to make new bile. This action resembles that of some medications that lower LDL. Other mechanisms have also been suggested to account for the LDL-lowering effect of soluble fiber. For example, fermentation of soluble fiber by bacteria in the large intestine produces short-chain fatty acids that may directly reduce cholesterol synthesis by the liver.

Despite the hoopla by some manufacturers about the ability of oat bran to lower LDL, it clearly is no "magic bullet." You would have to eat about a cup a day to reap a substantial LDL-lowering effect; an oat bran muffin alone won't do much.

RAISING HDL: A MORE DIFFICULT TASK

Scientists believe that raising HDL may be just as important as lowering LDL in reducing the risk of premature heart disease. Physical activity is one way to raise HDL. Exercising for at least 45 minutes four times a week can raise HDL by about 5 mg/dl. Sedentary people in particular should focus on increasing physical activity, because this has other heart-healthy benefits as well. Losing excess weight (especially around the waist) and avoiding smoking also help to maintain or raise HDL.

In addition, eating regularly (three balanced meals daily), matching the amount of energy eaten with that expended, and eating less total fat often raise HDL because these practices lower serum triglycerides. Low serum triglycerides often are associated with higher HDL. The reason for this is not clear. Nevertheless as noted earlier, the goal is to keep fasting serum triglycerides below 150 to 200 mg/dl. Certain medications

Continued.

also act to lower serum triglycerides, thereby indirectly increasing HDL.

Consumption of alcohol is also associated with higher HDL levels and reduced blood clotting—two factors that reduce the risk of heart attack. However, excessive consumption of alcohol has many negative effects. The Dietary Guidelines indicate that most people can consume 1 to 2 drinks daily (no more) without negative health consequences. But for people at risk of alcoholism, any alcohol may be too much (see discussion in Chapter 16).

It is unfortunate that raising HDL is difficult. Lowering LDL is much easier. And sometimes as LDL falls, so does HDL. This often occurs with very low-fat diets. However, if LDL ends up at about 100 mg/dl, the low HDL is not of much concern. Researchers note that people in rural Asia who eat low-fat diets generally have low LDL and HDL, but they also show low risk for premature heart disease.

LDL-LOWERING MEDICATIONS

Medications are a last resort for treating people at high risk for heart disease; most are expensive and all have troublesome side effects.[17] However, sometimes diet changes do not reduce LDL enough, especially in people with strong genetic tendencies toward heart disease. Current medications to lower LDL work in one of two ways. One group inhibits the liver from synthesizing some lipoproteins. The other group of medications bind bile in the small intestine and lead to its elimination, forcing the liver to synthesize new bile. The liver removes LDL from the blood to do this. All these medications work better when a proper diet is followed; they do not substitute for recommended diet changes. Estrogen replacement for women after menopause also deserves consideration, in part because this lowers LDL and raises HDL.[23]

A controversy currently rages about the use of medications and significant diet changes to combat heart disease. The vast majority of researchers in the heart disease arena agree that diet changes and medications (if needed) to lower elevated LDL, ideally to around 100 mg/dl, are especially important for people who already show evidence of heart disease.[6, 23] The current debate concerns how aggressive treatment should be for people who have high LDL but exhibit no symptoms of heart disease and have no other risk factors. Still, mortality from all causes, including that resulting from heart disease, is reduced when treatment to lower elevated LDL in people at high risk for heart disease is followed for a few years or more. Furthermore, new research shows that plaque even regresses in arteries when high LDL is aggressively treated. It is suspected that these aggressive therapies to lower LDL stabilize the development of atherosclerotic plaque, thereby lowering the risk of rupture and in turn reducing the chance of myocardial infarction caused by clot formation.

Some research has suggested that low serum cholesterol itself poses certain risks. These studies indicate that people with total cholesterol less than 160 mg/dl have an increased risk of dying of a certain type of stroke and certain types of cancer. But closer inspection reveals that low serum cholesterol itself isn't the likely culprit.[11] In most cases these people have some underlying medical condition, such as a stomach or liver disorder, that lowers blood cholesterol and increases the risk of death.

In summary, individuals with elevated LDL, in consultation with their physicians, are best suited to determine their desire and ability to make lifestyle changes, supplemented by medications (if necessary) to lower heart disease risk. Some physicians also recommend caution about initiating aggressive LDL-lowering treatment in persons over 65 to 70 years of age because of concern about the safety and cost effectiveness of such inteventions in older people (see Chapter 16).

GENERAL STRATEGY FOR REDUCING HEART DISEASE RISK

Table 6-6 outlines the most effective general strategy for lowering LDL and thus reducing the risk of heart attack. The bottom line is actually quite simple: Remove as much saturated fat from the diet as possible while moderating total fat and cholesterol intake.[22] To do this, you should select foods that are lower in total fat and especially in saturated fat. That means eating fewer high-fat foods of animal origin, such as marbled meat, eggs, and whole-milk dairy products, while eating more plant foods, such as fruits, vegetables, and whole grains.

As mentioned in this chapter, a diet with 30% total energy from fat is an appropriate goal for children age 2 or older. But parents shouldn't go overboard limiting fat intake, because children need to consume about 30% of total energy as fat to grow properly. Experts do not recommend fat-restricted diets in children under the age of 2 (see Chapter 15).

TABLE 6-6

General Diet-Related Strategy for Reducing the Risk of Premature Heart Disease and Heart Attack, Especially for People at Risk.[1, 3, 12, 14, 20, 27, 29, 30, 31, 32]

Action	Rationale
Follow the Food Guide Pyramid, consuming less total fat, especially saturated fat, and less cholesterol. Some researchers advocate a switch to a primary vegetarian diet to help meet this goal (see Chapter 7).	In particular, the bottom half of the pyramid supplies vitamins associated with reduced risk of heart disease. The key focus is on reducing intake of animal fat and hydrogenated fat (especially deep fat-fried foods) as choices from the top half are made.
Meet calcium needs (RDA).	One study has shown that this approach can lower LDL, probably by binding saturated fatty acids in the GI tract and so reducing their absorption.
Eat plenty of fruits, vegetables, and whole grains. Include some soy on a regular basis.	The dietary fiber, antioxidants, and other phytochemical substances present in these foods can contribute to lower risk of heart disease.
Eat regularly spaced meals, not one or two large ones.	The frequency of meals helps determine fasting serum triglycerides. Studies show that increasing meal frequency (from three to nine meals per day or so) can even help reduce LDL.
Lose weight if needed, ideally to attain a healthy body weight (see Chapter 10).	This especially helps reduce blood triglycerides (if elevated), lowers high blood pressure, and can increase HDL, especially if the fat is lost from the abdominal region.
Eat fish about twice a week.	This provides omega-3 fatty acids to reduce blood clotting and thus lessens the risk of heart attack. Regular use of aspirin for people at high risk of a heart attack (under a physician's scrutiny) is promoted for the same reason.
Consume moderate amounts of alcohol with meals if you can control this practice.	Consumption of red wine in particular has been noted to reduce heart disease risk in some studies, but it is speculated that small doses of any form of alcohol may do the same. A reduction in blood clotting is thought to be one mechanism.
Moderate coffee intake.	Heavy coffee use, especially unfiltered (espresso type), increases LDL. Moderate use of filtered coffee appears to be fine for most people.
Use iron supplements with caution.	Although this point is still being debated, some experts recommend that iron-containing supplements not be consumed unless medically needed because this may increase LDL oxidation. This message is especially important for adult men.

Proteins

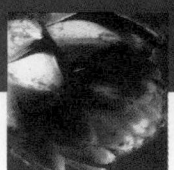

EATING ENOUGH PROTEIN IS vital for maintaining health. Proteins form important structures in the body, make up a key part of the blood, help regulate many body functions, and can fuel body cells.[20]

Americans also eat a lot of protein—generally more than is needed to maintain health. For many of us, protein translates into meat, poultry, fish, and eggs. Turkey, hamburger, cheese, and T-bone steak are some favorite animal protein foods in America. In contrast, our Stone Age ancestors obtained a greater percentage of their protein from vegetables. They primarily picked and gathered their dietary protein, rather than hunted it. Not until *Homo erectus*, our immediate ancestors, emerged about 1.5 million years ago did meat displace other foods in a primarily vegetarian diet. Diets that are mostly vegetarian still predominate in much of Asia and areas of Africa.[21]

Few of us wish to exchange our comfortable modern lifestyles with those of our Stone Age ancestors, and yet we could benefit from eating more plant sources of proteins.[6] It is possible—and desirable—to incorporate the most nutritious practices of both eras and enjoy the benefits of animal and plant protein. Let's see why this is worth your attention.

CHAPTER 7

What Are Your Protein Preferences?

Below is a list of various foods that are good sources of protein. Rank your preferences among them from 1 to 11. A ranking of 1 means you like that particular food the best; a ranking of 11 means you like it the least. The letter before the food represents its origin: (A), Animal source; (P), Plant source.

(A) Eggs _____

(P) Beans (kidney, pinto, navy, or red beans; chick peas) _____

(A) Fish (salmon, halibut, swordfish, tuna) _____

(A) Beef _____

(P) Grains (products made from wheat, corn, oats) _____

(A) Poultry (chicken, turkey) _____

(A) Cheese _____

(P) Nuts and seeds (almonds, sunflower seeds) _____

(A) Milk and milk products (yogurt) _____

(A) Pork _____

(A) Processed meats (pepperoni, bologna, sausage) _____

As previously mentioned, today many rural societies consume more plant than animal sources of protein. This helps diets stay low in saturated fat and cholesterol. In this respect, plant proteins can add a healthful aspect to many typical American diet patterns because their low saturated fat and cholesterol and often high dietary fiber contents help prevent some chronic diseases. Where did the plant sources of protein rank in terms of your preference—high or low? Do you give excellent sources of plant proteins enough attention?

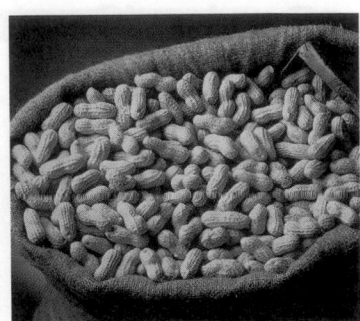

Peanuts are rich in protein but also energy dense. Thus moderation in intake is important.

Both nonessential and essential amino acids are present in foods that contain protein. If you don't eat enough essential amino acids, your body first struggles to conserve what essential amino acids it can. However, eventually your body progressively slows production of new proteins until at some point you will break protein down faster than you can make it. When that happens, as noted, health deteriorates.[14]

Therefore the two main functions of proteins in our diets are (1) to provide the nine essential amino acids needed by our bodies and (2) to provide either the nonessential amino acids our bodies use or nitrogen from an amino acid, which in turn can be used to make the nonessential amino acids. Enough protein must be consumed to serve these two functions. In a practical sense, a key consideration with respect to protein intake is quantity—getting enough protein via the diet to provide enough essential amino acids and enough of the necessary form of nitrogen for use in the production of any missing nonessential amino acid.[4]

Putting Essential and Nonessential Amino Acids into Perspective

Eating a balanced diet can supply us with both the essential and nonessential amino acids (or building blocks needed) to maintain good health. Let's now take a more detailed look at this concept of essential amino acids, especially in relationship to nonessential amino acids.

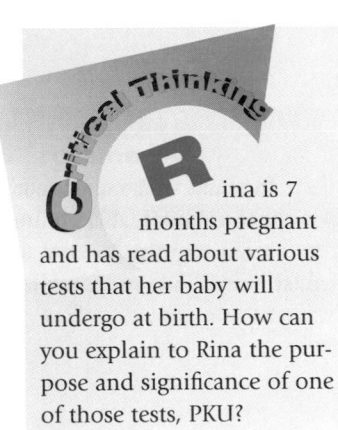

R ina is 7 months pregnant and has read about various tests that her baby will undergo at birth. How can you explain to Rina the purpose and significance of one of those tests, PKU?

Physiological aspects. The disease phenyketonuria (PKU) illustrates the importance of one essential amino acid. This disease was mentioned in Chapter 5. Recall that the person with PKU has a limited ability to metabolize the essential amino acid phenylalanine. Normally the body converts much of this essential amino acid consumed in the diet into the nonessential amino acid tyrosine, because the body's need for phenylalanine is easily exceeded by our typical diets. However, enzymes in the liver of a person with PKU vary in their ability to perform this conversion. Liver enzyme activity may be grossly or mildly insufficient in processing phenylalanine to tyrosine. When the enzymes cannot synthesize enough tyrosine, both amino acids must be derived from foods. The key point here is that both amino acids now end up to be *essential* in terms of dietary needs. Both must be supplied by the diet. In the treatment of PKU, consumption of phenylalanine should also be controlled because it can rise to toxic amounts in the body.

Dietary considerations. Animal and plant proteins can differ greatly in proportions of essential and nonessential amino acids. Animal proteins contain ample amounts of all nine essential amino acids. (Gelatin—made from the animal protein collagen—is an exception because it loses one essential amino acid during processing and is also low in other essential amino acids.) Plant proteins don't match our needs for essential amino acids as precisely as animal proteins. Many plant proteins, especially those found in grains, are low in one or more of the nine essential amino acids.[25]

As you might expect, human tissue composition resembles animal tissue more than it does plant tissue. The similarities enable us to use proteins from single animal sources more efficiently to support human growth and maintenance than we do those from single plant sources. Again, this is because animal proteins closely match the human pattern of essential amino acid composition. For this reason, animal proteins, except gelatin, are considered **high-quality** (also called *complete*) **proteins**—they contain all the amino acids we need in sufficient amounts. Individual plant sources of proteins are considered **lower-quality** (also called *incomplete*) **proteins** because their amino acid patterns can be quite different from ours. A single plant protein, such as corn alone, cannot easily support body growth and

High-quality (complete) proteins *Dietary proteins that contain ample amounts of all nine essential amino acids.*

Lower-quality (incomplete) proteins *Dietary proteins that are low in or lack one or more essential amino acids.*

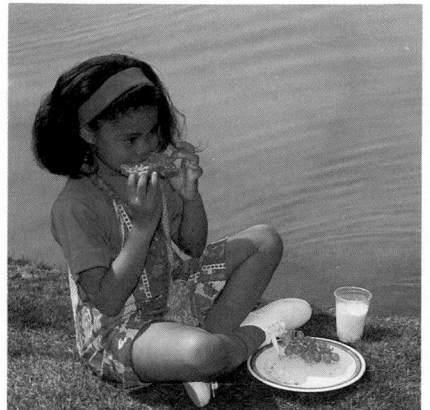

The various plant proteins present in a peanut butter sandwich combine to yield high-quality (complete) protein in the meal.

maintenance. To consume a sufficient amount of amino acids, very large quantities of plant proteins would need to be eaten because each protein lacks adequate amounts of one or more essential amino acids.[14]

If you ate only one food that contained lower-quality protein—that is, one not containing an appropriate balance of all nine essential amino acids—you would need to eat much more than you would eating animal protein sources to obtain enough of the essential amino acids needed for protein synthesis. Moreover, once any of the nine essential amino acids in the plant protein was used up, further protein synthesis would be impossible. The remaining amino acids would be used instead for energy or converted to fat and stored as such. Because the depletion of just one of the essential amino acids prevents protein synthesis, the process illustrates the *all or none principle:* either all essential amino acids acids are available or none can be used. The essential amino acid in smallest supply in a food or diet becomes the limiting factor (called the *limiting amino acid*) because it limits the amount of protein the body can synthesize.

For example, assume the letters of the alphabet represent the 20 or so different amino acids we eat. If A represents an essential amino acid, we would need four of these to spell the hypothetical protein ALABAMA. If the body had an L, B, and M, but only 3 As, the "synthesis" of ALABAMA would not be possible. "A" would then be seen as the limiting amino acid because it is the limiting factor with respect to the body's ability to synthesize ALABAMA.

Most of us eat large enough amounts and such an assortment of protein-rich foods that we easily get a sufficient amount of all nine essential amino acids. That is, Americans eat a diet in which overall protein quality is high. This yields a high-quality (complete) protein diet. Even worldwide, most adults who eat sufficient protein get enough essential amino acids to yield a high-quality protein diet, even if the various protein sources in the diet are of lower quality. This is because the various lower-quality protein sources eaten can make up for deficiencies in essential amino acids that each individual protein presents.[25]

When two or more proteins combine to compensate for deficiencies in essential amino acid content in each individual protein, the proteins are called *complementary proteins*[9] (Table 7-2). Mixed diets generally provide high-quality protein because a complementary protein pattern results. Therefore healthy adults should have little concern about balancing foods to yield the proteins needed to obtain enough of all nine essential amino acids. Even on plant-based diets, complementing proteins need not be consumed at the same meal by adults. Meeting amino acid needs over the course of a day is a reasonable goal for adults because muscles are able temporarily to store essential amino acids.[25]

Limiting amino acid
The essential amino acid in lowest concentration in a food relative to body needs.

Complementary proteins
Two food protein sources that make up for each other's inadequate supply of specific essential amino acids; together they yield a sufficient amount of all nine and so provide high-quality (complete) protein for the diet.

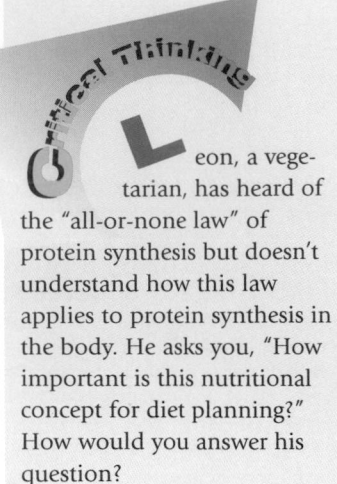

Leon, a vegetarian, has heard of the "all-or-none law" of protein synthesis but doesn't understand how this law applies to protein synthesis in the body. He asks you, "How important is this nutritional concept for diet planning?" How would you answer his question?

TABLE 7-2

Limiting Amino Acids in Plant Foods

Food	Limiting amino acids	Good plant source of the limiting amino acids*	Traditional uses where the proteins complement each other
Beans (legumes)	Methionine	Grains, nuts, and seeds	Red beans and rice
Grains	Lysine, threonine	Legumes	Rice and red beans, lentils, curry, and rice
Nuts and seeds	Lysine	Legumes	Soybeans and ground sesame seeds (miso); peanuts, rice, and black-eyed and green peas; and sunflower seeds
Vegetables	Methionine	Grains, nuts, and seeds	Green beans and almonds
Corn	Tryptophan, lysine	Legumes	Corn tortillas and pinto beans

As you might suspect from the information in this table, the amino acids most likely to be low in a diet are lysine, methionine, threonine, and tryptophan. If a diet is low in an amino acid, nutrition experts recommend finding a good food source to supply it. Forget about amino acid supplements—they can lead to problems, as discussed later in this chapter.
*Animal products in the diet serve the same purpose, such as when fish is consumed with rice.

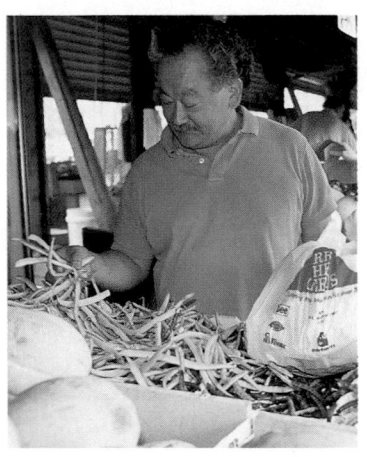

Amino acids in vegetables are best used when a combination of sources is consumed.

Infants and preschool children, on the other hand, need much of their protein supplied by essential amino acids. Consequently, diets for young children must be carefully planned to make sure enough proteins are present to yield high-quality protein intake. Including some animal products in the diet, such as human milk, infant formula, or cow's milk, helps ensure this. Otherwise, complementary amino acids from plant proteins should be consumed in each individual meal or within two subsequent meals.[25] A major health risk for children occurs in famine situations in which only one type of grain is available, increasing the probability that one or more of the nine essential amino acids may be lacking in the total diet. This is discussed further in a later section in the chapter.

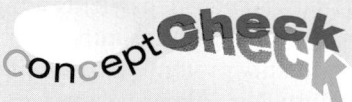

Concept Check

The human body uses 20 or so different forms of amino acids from foods. Because a healthy body can synthesize 11 or so of the different amino acids, it is not necessary to get all amino acids from foods—only the building blocks for protein synthesis of these amino acids are needed. Nine of the various amino acids used by the body must be consumed and are therefore termed *essential (indispensable) amino acids.* Foods that contain all 9 essential amino acids in about the proportions we need are considered high-quality (complete) protein foods. Those low in one or more essential amino acids are lower-quality (incomplete) protein foods. When different lower-quality protein foods are eaten together, the total intake of amino acids generally makes up for the individual foods' shortcomings to yield a high-quality protein meal.

Proteins—Amino Acids Joined Together

Amino acids are joined by chemical links—technically called *peptide bonds*—to form proteins. Although these links are difficult to break, acids, enzymes, and other agents are able to do so, as occurs, for example, during digestion.

Protein Organization

By linking various combinations of the 20 or so types of amino acids, the body synthesizes thousands of different proteins. This process is comparable to using the alphabet to create a dictionary full of words. Amino acids are joined together in specific sequences to form distinct proteins, just as various sequences of letters form specific words. The DNA in a cell directs this ordering during protein synthesis, as noted in Chapter 4. The sequential order of the amino acids determines a protein's shape. The key point is that only correctly positioned amino acids can interact and fold properly to form the intended shape for the protein. The resulting unique three-dimensional form dictates the function of each particular protein. If it lacks the appropriate configuration, a protein cannot function[20] (Figure 7-1).

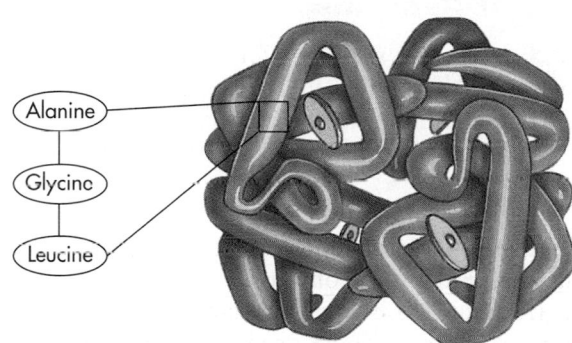

Figure 7-1 *Protein organization. Proteins often form a coiled shape, as shown by this drawing of the blood protein hemoglobin. This shape is dictated by the order of the amino acids in the protein chain. To get an idea of its size, note that each teaspoon (5 milliliters) of blood contains about 10^{18} hemoglobin molecules. Note that one billion is 10^9.*

Sickle cell disease (also called *sickle cell anemia*) illustrates what happens when amino acids are out of order on a protein. African-Americans are especially prone to this genetic disease. It originates in defective production of the protein chains of hemoglobin, a compound found in red blood cells. In two of its four protein chains, a slight error in the amino acid order occurs. This small error produces a profound change in hemoglobin structure: it can no longer form the shape needed to carry oxygen efficiently inside the red blood cell. Instead of forming normal circular disks, the red blood cells collapse into crescent shapes (Figure 7-2). Health deteriorates, and eventually episodes of severe bone and joint pain, abdominal pain, headache, convulsions, and paralysis may occur.[17]

These life-threatening symptoms are caused by a minute but critical error in the hemoglobin amino acid order. Why does this error happen? It results from a defect in a person's genetic blueprint, DNA, which is inherited through one's parents. A defect in the DNA can dictate that a wrong amino acid will be built into the sequence of body proteins. Many diseases stem from incorrect DNA information passed on in the body. Cancer, which is discussed in Chapter 8, is an example.

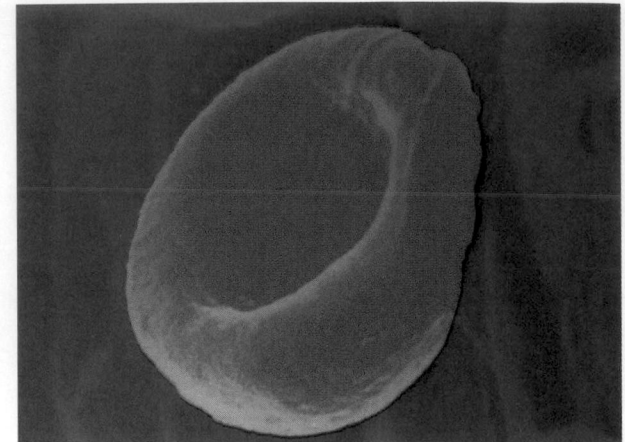
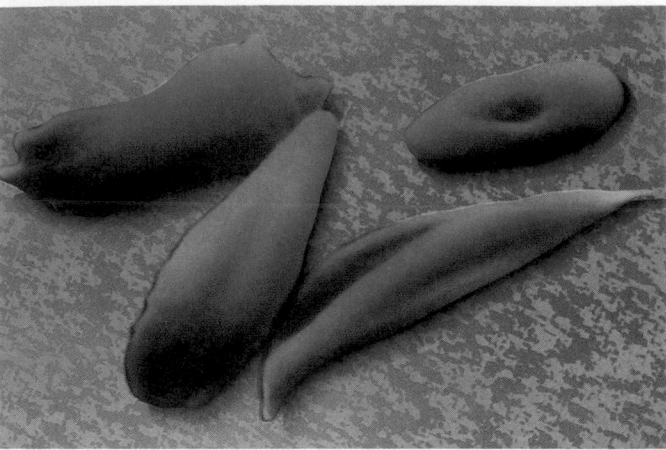

Figure 7-2 *Sickle-cell disease from the perspective of the red blood cell.* **A,** *Normal red blood cell.* **B,** *Blood from a person with sickle-cell disease. Note the abnormal crescent (sicklelike) shape of the red blood cell near the center.*

Denaturation of Proteins

Denature

Alteration of a protein's three-dimensional structure, usually because of treatment by heat, enzymes, acid or alkaline solutions, or agitation.

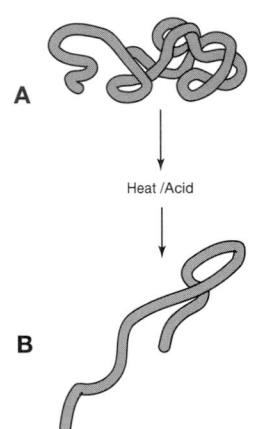

A, Protein showing typical coiled state. B, Protein is now partly uncoiled. This uncoiling can reduce protein function.

Treatment with acid or alkaline substances, heat, or agitation can severely alter a protein's folded structure, leaving it unfolded and in a **denatured** state. The protein now can no longer perform its function. For example, once the bacteria in yogurt have synthesized enough acid and enzymes to precipitate some of the milk protein, the product solidifies irreversibly.

Unraveling a protein's shape often destroys its normal functioning. That characteristic is useful for some body processes, such as digestion. The secretion of stomach acid denatures some bacteria, plant hormones, many active enzymes, and other forms of proteins in foods. The heat produced during cooking likewise denatures these proteins. Both processes make foods safer to eat. Digestion is also enhanced because the unraveling increases exposure of the food to digestive enzymes. Denaturing proteins in some foods can also reduce their tendencies to cause allergic reactions.

Recall that we need proteins in the diet to supply essential amino acids—not the active proteins themselves. We dismantle the proteins we get from foods and use the amino acids to assemble proteins we need.[20]

Protein Digestion and Absorption— Supplying Amino Acids to Body Cells

As discussed in Chapter 4, digestion of protein begins in the stomach (Figure 7-3). Certain cells of the stomach secrete pepsin, a major enzyme used for this digestion. Pepsin attacks all proteins and breaks them down into shorter amino acid units, called *peptones*. Pepsin does not completely separate the protein into amino acids because it can break only a few of the chemical bonds found in protein molecules. Thus it has limited activity. The release of pepsin is controlled by the hormone gastrin. Just thinking about or chewing food stimulates gastrin release. Gastrin also stimulates other cells in the stomach to produce acid. This acid, in turn, activates pepsin and enhances protein digestion. The partially digested proteins now move with the rest of the nutrients in the foods from the stomach into the small intestine.

Once in the small intestine the peptones (and any fats accompanying the incoming peptones produced from a meal) trigger the release of another hormone. This hormone causes the pancreas to release enzyme-rich juice into the small intes-

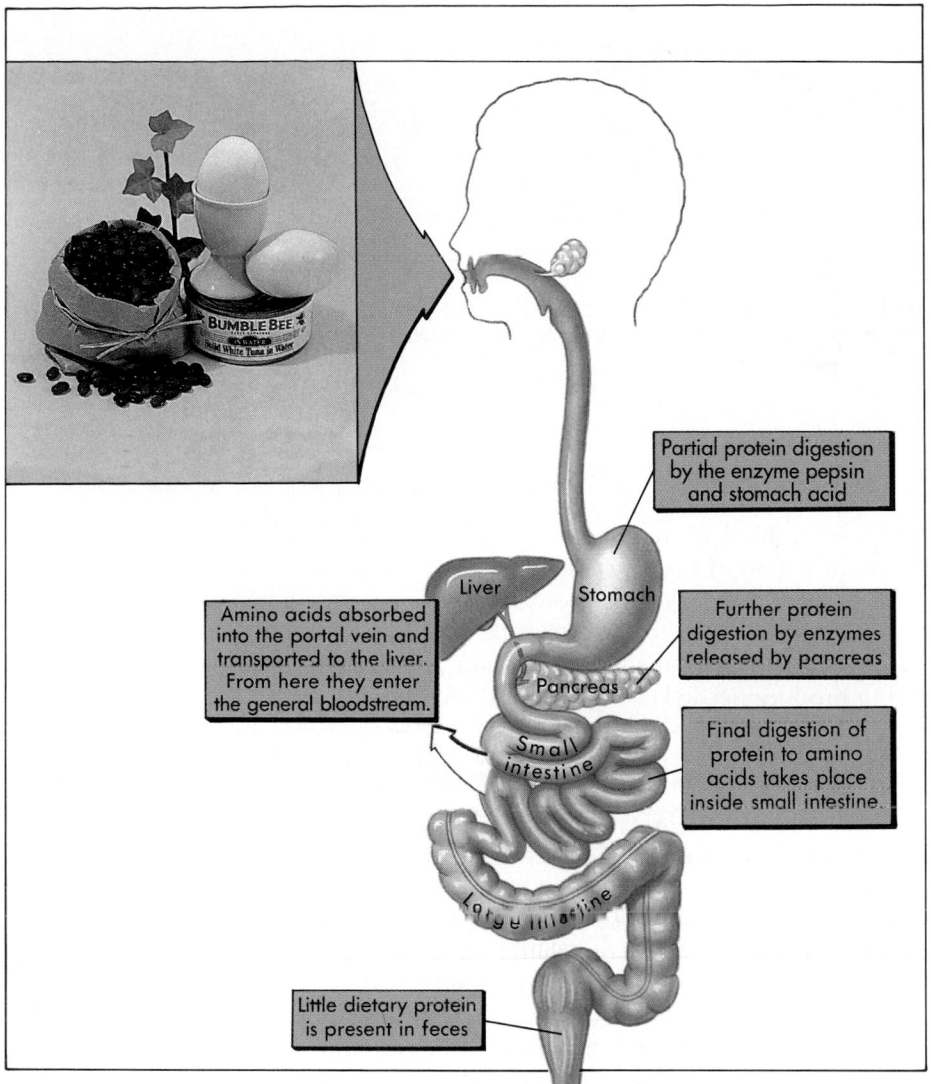

Partial protein digestion by the enzyme pepsin and stomach acid

Liver

Stomach

Amino acids absorbed into the portal vein and transported to the liver. From here they enter the general bloodstream.

Further protein digestion by enzymes released by pancreas

Pancreas

Small intestine

Final digestion of protein to amino acids takes place inside small intestine.

Large intestine

Little dietary protein is present in feces

Figure 7-3
Protein digestion and absorption. Protein digestion begins in the stomach and ends in the absorptive cells of the small intestine, where it is finally broken down into single amino acids. Stomach acid and enzymes from the stomach and pancreas also contribute to protein digestion.

tine. These and other digestive enzymes from the small intestine divide the peptones into shorter products. The eventual digestion of these divided peptones into amino acids occurs inside the absorptive cells of the small intestine. The amino acids travel to the liver via the portal vein, where they are either combined into protein, converted into glucose or fat, used for energy needs, or released into the bloodstream.

ANOTHER Bite

Amino acid supplements are not necessary because we can easily meet our protein needs through diet. This holds true for all of us, including athletes (see Chapter 11). No significant amounts of free amino acids are present in our food. Nor is there any dietary need for or unique dietary value from eating free amino acids. As emphasized earlier, the body is designed to handle whole proteins as a dietary source of amino acids. When individual amino acid supplements are taken, they can overwhelm the absorptive mechanism, triggering amino acid imbalances in the body. These imbalances occur because groups of chemically similar amino acids compete for absorption into the bloodstream. An excess of one can hamper other amino acids from being absorbed. Overall, every amino acid taken in excess can be harmful. In some cases, excess amounts do not vary much above a normal daily intake. Stick to whole foods as your source for amino acids.[2]

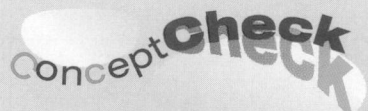

Amino acids are linked together in specific sequences to form distinct proteins. The amino acid order within a protein determines its ultimate shape. Destroying the shape of a protein denatures it. Acid and alkaline conditions present during the body's digestive processes, heat, and other factors can denature proteins, causing them to lose their biological activity. This protein digestion begins in the stomach, producing breakdown products called *peptones.* In the small intestine, peptones separate eventually into amino acids and enter the portal vein en route to the liver.

Functions of Proteins

As you have learned, proteins function in many crucial ways in human metabolism and the formation of body structures. We rely on foods to supply the amino acids needed to form these proteins. Note, however, that only when we also eat enough carbohydrate and fat can food proteins be used most efficiently. If we don't consume enough energy to meet energy needs, some amino acids from proteins are broken down to produce needed energy, rather than used to make needed body proteins.

Producing Vital Body Constituents

Every cell contains protein. Muscles, connective tissue, blood-clotting factors, blood-transport proteins, lipoproteins, enzymes, immune bodies, some hormones, visual pigments, and the support structure inside bones are mainly made of protein. Measurements of the amounts of certain body proteins, particularly some of those in the blood, are used as indicators of health or disease. Excess protein in the diet doesn't enhance the synthesis of body components, but eating too little can impede it.[2]

Most vital body proteins are in a constant state of breakdown, rebuilding, and repair, especially in the bone marrow and the intestine. The GI tract lining is constantly **sloughed** off. The digestive tract treats sloughed cells just like food particles and absorbs the amino acids released during their digestion. In fact, most protein breakdown products—amino acids—released throughout the body can be recycled and are added to the pool of amino acids available for future protein synthesis (Figure 7-4).

However, some protein breakdown products, such as the nitrogen that ends up as **urea,** are lost rather than recycled. If a person habitually doesn't eat enough protein to replace this loss, the protein rebuilding and repairing process slows. Thus for body growth and maintenance, amino acids must be supplied constantly from food. Otherwise, skeletal muscles, heart, liver, blood proteins, and other organs decrease in size or amount. Only the brain resists breakdown. To ensure good health, a person must eat enough protein.

Maintaining Fluid Balance

Blood proteins—albumins and globulins—help maintain body fluid balance. Blood pressure in the arteries forces blood through blood vessels into capillary beds. The blood fluid then enters from the capillary beds into the spaces between nearby cells to provide nutrients to those cells (Figure 7-5). Proteins in the bloodstream are too large to move out of the capillary beds into the tissues. The presence of these proteins in the capillary beds attracts the fluid back to them, partially counteracting the force

Slough
To shed or cast off.

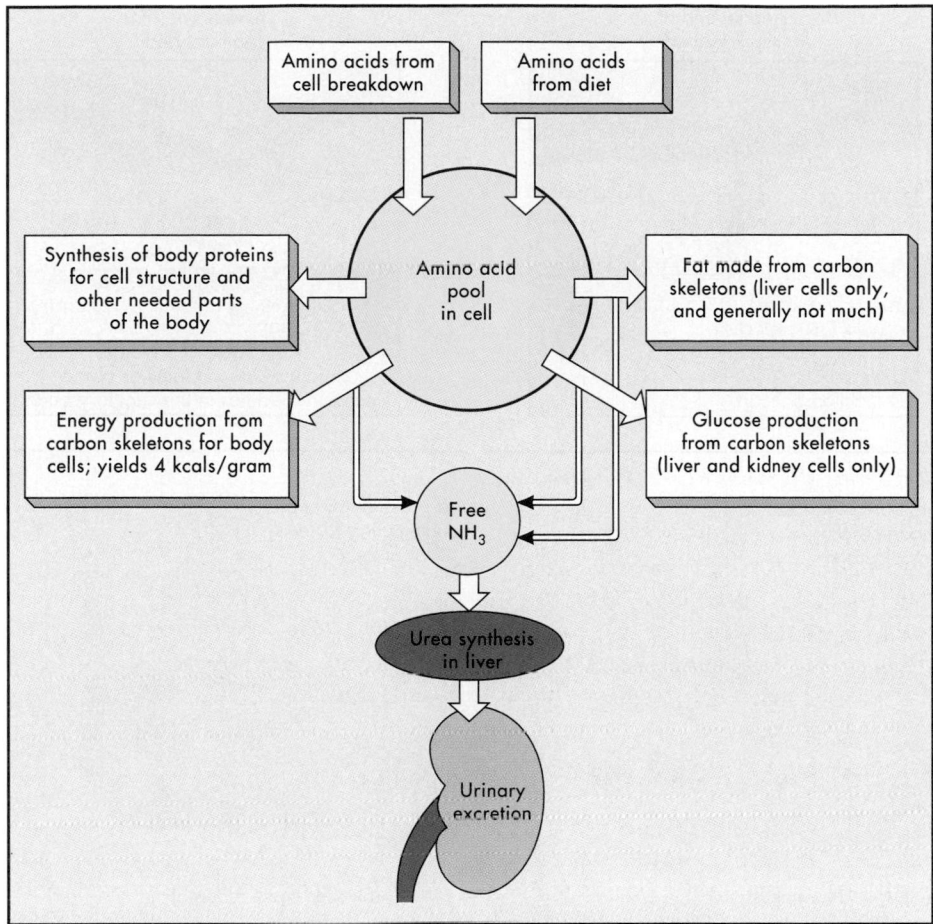

Figure 7-4 *Amino acid metabolism. The amino acid pool in a cell can be used to yield body proteins, as well as a variety of other possible products—from fat and glucose to urea. The urea is a waste product made from the nitrogen-containing ammonia (NH_3) released during amino acid breakdown.*[22]

of blood pressure. This is especially true of the areas of the capillary beds right next to their venous connections. (See Figure 4-2 for a close-up view of a capillary bed.)

Unless enough protein is eaten, the concentration of proteins eventually decreases in the bloodstream. Excessive fluid then builds up in the tissues because the counteracting force produced by the smaller amount of blood proteins is too weak to pull much of the fluid back from the tissues into the bloodstream. As fluids pool in the tissues, the tissues swell. Clinical **edema** results.[14] Because edema sometimes leads to serious medical problems, the cause must be identified. An important step in diagnosing the cause is to measure the concentration of blood proteins.

Contributing to Acid-Base Balance

Proteins help regulate the degree of acidity—the acid-base balance—in the blood. Special proteins located in cell membranes act to pump chemical ions in and out of cells. The pumping action, among other factors, works to keep the blood slightly alkaline. **Buffers**—compounds that maintain acid-base conditions within a narrow range—are another means to regulate acid-base balance in the blood. Some blood proteins are especially good buffers for the body.[20]

Edema
The buildup of excess fluid in the spaces surrounding body cells.

Buffer
Compounds that cause a solution to resist changes in acid-base balance.

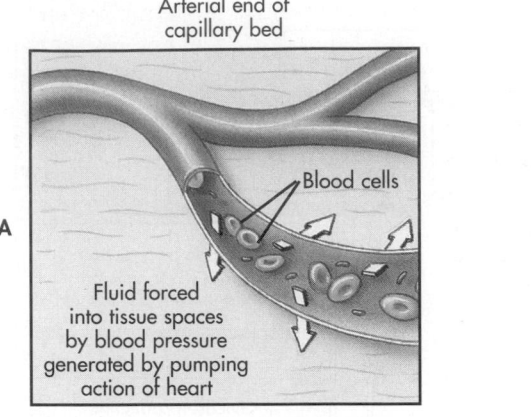
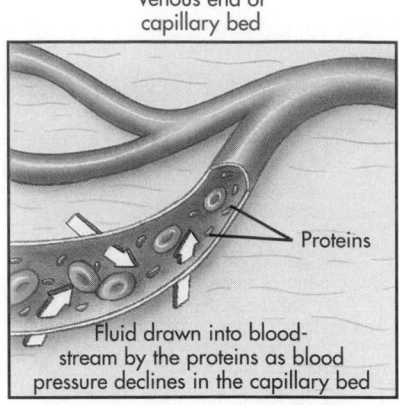

Arterial end of capillary bed

Venous end of capillary bed

Blood cells

Proteins

A

Fluid forced into tissue spaces by blood pressure generated by pumping action of heart

Fluid drawn into bloodstream by the proteins as blood pressure declines in the capillary bed

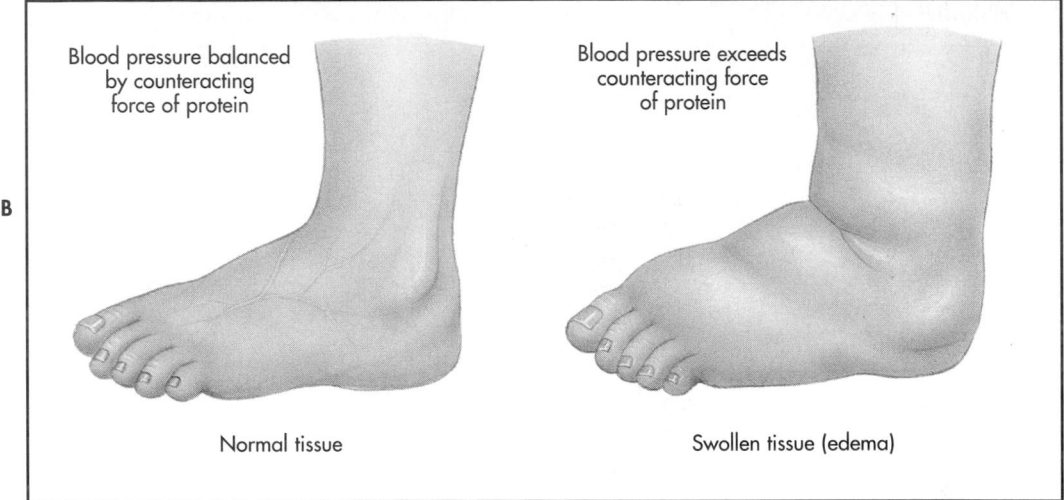

Blood pressure balanced by counteracting force of protein

Blood pressure exceeds counteracting force of protein

B

Normal tissue

Swollen tissue (edema)

Figure 7-5 *Blood proteins in relation to protein balance.* **A,** *Blood proteins are important for maintaining the body's fluid balance.* **B,** *Without sufficient protein in the bloodstream, edema develops.*

Forming Hormones and Enzymes

Protein is required for the synthesis of many hormones—our internal body messengers. Some hormones, such as the thyroid hormones, are made from only one or a few amino acids. Insulin, on the other hand, is composed of 48 amino acids. These and other hormones classified as proteins perform important regulatory functions in the body, such as controlling the metabolic rate and amount of glucose taken up from the bloodstream.

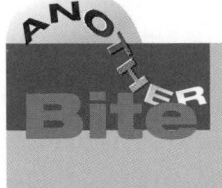

Some hormone medicines from the protein class, such as the insulin used to treat some cases of diabetes, must be injected. If taken orally, insulin would be destroyed: the stomach and small intestine would digest the hormone, dismantling it into amino acids.

Almost all enzymes are proteins. Recall that enzymes are compounds that speed chemical reactions (see Chapter 4). Occasionally a cell lacks the correct genetic information to make needed enzymes. For example, an infant who has the disease **galactosemia** can't make an enzyme needed to metabolize the single sugar galactose. If the infant is not put on a galactose-free diet soon after birth—which in practical terms means no cow's milk, human milk, liver, and certain other foods—its growth and mental development will be depressed. A special infant formula must be used. The galactose-free diet is then continued, ideally throughout life. This example demonstrates the crucial roles that enzymes, and thus proteins, play in cell function.[20]

Contributing to the Immune Function

Proteins make up key parts of the cells used by the immune system. Protein **antibodies** are produced by one type of immune cell. In an important immune response these antibodies bind to foreign proteins in the body. Without enough protein from the diet the immune system will eventually not produce enough of the cells and other tools needed to function properly and resist disease. However, eating more protein than is necessary doesn't boost immune function.

Forming Glucose

In Chapter 5 you learned that the body must maintain a fairly constant concentration of glucose in the bloodstream to supply energy for red blood cells and nervous tissue. At rest the brain uses about 35% of the body's energy requirements, and it gets most of that energy from glucose. If you don't eat enough carbohydrate to supply the glucose, your liver (and kidneys to a lesser extent) will be forced to make glucose from amino acids (see Figure 7-4). Many types of amino acids can be used for this purpose.

Making some glucose from amino acids is normal. For example, when you skip breakfast and haven't eaten since 7 PM the preceding evening, glucose must be manufactured. Taken to an extreme, however, such as occurs in starvation, the conversion of amino acids into glucose wastes much muscle tissue and consequently reduces health.[14]

Providing Energy

Proteins supply about 2% to 5% of the energy the body uses (see Chapter 11 for information about the use of amino acids for energy during exercise). Most cells use primarily carbohydrates and fats for energy. Proteins and carbohydrates contain the same amount of usable energy, 4 kcal per gram. However, proteins are a very costly source of energy, considering the amount of metabolism and processing the liver and kidneys must perform to use this energy source. The monetary cost of protein-rich foods is also a consideration.

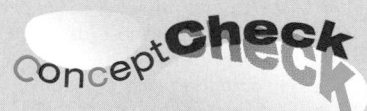

Vital body constituents—such as muscle, connective tissue, blood transport proteins, enzymes, hormones, buffers, and immune factors—are mainly proteins. Proteins can also provide fuel for the body and be used for glucose production.

Galactosemia
A disease characterized by the buildup of the sugar galactose in the bloodstream; the buildup occurs because the liver is unable to metabolize galactose. If present at birth and left untreated, this condition results in severe mental and growth retardation.

Antibodies
Blood proteins that inactivate foreign proteins found in the body. This helps to prevent and control infections.

Neurotransmitters, made by nerve endings, are often derivatives of amino acids. This is true for dopamine (synthesized from tyrosine), epinephrine (synthesized from tyrosine), and serotonin (synthesized from tryptophan). The way in which diet influences the synthesis of some of these neurotransmitters is currently under study. For example, high-carbohydrate meals can induce sleepiness as a result of increased serotonin synthesis in the brain.[5]

The Recommended Dietary Allowance for Protein

How much protein (actually, amino acids) do we need to eat each day? People who aren't growing need to eat only enough protein to match whatever they lose daily in urine, feces, skin, hair, nails, and so on. In short, people need to balance protein intake with output. This maintains a state of protein equilibrium (Figure 7-6).

When a body is growing or recovering from an illness, it needs a positive protein balance to supply raw materials required to build new tissues. To achieve this, a person must eat more protein daily than he or she loses. This positive balance also requires an appropriate hormonal state. The hormones insulin, growth hormone, and testosterone all stimulate positive protein balance. Merely eating more protein does not guarantee a positive balance; building extra body tissues requires the right hormonal condition as well. Resistance exercise (weight training) also works to enhance muscle mass.

Frequently during semistarvation or illness the body loses much more protein than is replaced. The body then falls into a negative protein balance—not enough nitrogen is being obtained from protein foods to maintain normal protein status.

For healthy people the amount of dietary protein needed to maintain nitrogen equilibrium (wherein intake equals output) can be determined by increasing protein intake until it just equals losses. Energy needs must be met so that amino acids are not diverted for energy use. Any protein intake above equilibrium also maintains a balance between intake and output. To estimate the requirement, we need to determine the least amount of protein intake necessary to balance intake with output.[2]

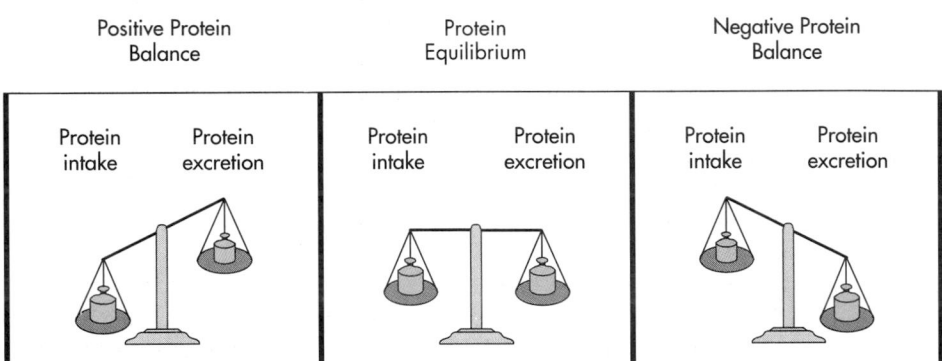

Situations in which protein balance is positive:

Growth
Pregnancy
Recovery stage after illness
Athletic training*
Increased secretion of hormones, such as insulin, growth hormone, and testosterone

Situations in which protein balance is negative:

Inadequate intake of protein (fasting, intestinal tract diseases)
Inadequate energy intake
Conditions such as fevers, burns, and infections
Bed rest (for several days)
Deficiency of essential amino acids
Increased protein loss (as in some kidney disease)
Increased secretion of certain hormones, such as thyroid hormone and cortisol

*Only when additional lean body mass is being gained. Nevertheless, the athlete is probably already eating enough protein to support this extra protein synthesis: protein supplements are not needed.

Figure 7-6 *Protein balance in practical terms.*

Edward Smith, a British physician, studied energy and protein metabolism and in 1862 concluded that a physically active man would need 80 grams of protein daily. During the next 40 years, other estimates of protein needs, based on records of protein amounts consumed by healthy working men, ranged up to 150 grams per day. A controversy developed in the early 1900s after Russell Chittenden, an American chemist, concluded from studies on himself, his colleagues, and students at Yale that only 35 to 45 grams of protein daily was required for healthy adults.

Today the best estimate for the amount of protein required for nearly all adults is 0.8 gram of protein per kilogram (kg) of healthy body weight. This amount at least doubles during infancy. (Specific values for infants and children are discussed in Chapter 15 and the concept of healthy weight in Chapter 10). Healthy weight is used as a baseline because excess fat storage doesn't contribute much to protein needs. This recommended amount works out to about 56 grams of protein daily for a typical 70-kilogram (154-pound) man and about 44 grams of protein daily for a typical 55-kilogram (120-pound) woman.

$$\frac{154 \text{ pounds}}{2.2 \text{ pounds/kg}} = 70 \text{ kg}$$

$$70 \text{ kg} \times \frac{0.8 \text{ gram protein}}{\text{kg healthy body weight}} = 56 \text{ grams protein}$$

$$\frac{120 \text{ pounds}}{2.2 \text{ pounds/kg}} = 55 \text{ kg}$$

$$55 \text{ kg} \times \frac{0.8 \text{ gram protein}}{\text{kg healthy body weight}} = 44 \text{ grams protein}$$

To estimate a recommendation for you, just substitute your body weight in kilograms in the formula listed above. Approximate protein needs based on the 1989 RDA publication are listed in the inside cover of this textbook. Using either method, it is easy to eat the amount of protein suggested each day to meet body needs (Table 7-3). American men typically consume about 105 grams of protein daily, whereas women typically consume 65 grams daily.[15]

Recall that an RDA is an allowance, not a requirement. Some people need less than that amount of protein. Most of us, however, get much more because we like many high-protein foods and can afford to buy them. Excess protein eaten cannot be stored as such, so it is turned into glucose or fat and then either stored or burned for energy needs (see Figure 7-4). Pregnancy raises protein needs by about 10 to 15 grams per day averaged over the 9 months and totaling 60 grams in all for the diet. However, mental stress, physical labor, and routine weekend sports activities do not require an increase in the protein RDA.

To support training needs of endurance athletes, substantial gains in muscle tissue in highly trained athletes, or a large muscle mass formerly acquired, increasing the allowance up to 1.5 times the RDA might be considered. Nevertheless, there is no demonstrated advantage in exceeding 1.5 grams of protein per kilogram of healthy body weight per day. Many Americans, especially men, eat that much protein already.[15] Protein intakes above usual adult intakes are rarely needed for athletes. In addition, as mentioned earlier, athletes do not ordinarily require either protein or individual amino acid supplements. All of us, athletes included, can meet our protein needs using basic foods.

Instead of protein, it is most important for athletes to emphasize carbohydrate and fluid in the diet (see Chapter 11).

Surveys show that only older women as a group fail to eat enough protein to meet the RDA, and the discrepancy is very slight.[15] Older adults may also have slightly higher protein needs than those set by the RDA. Some researchers advocate up to 1.2 grams of protein per kilogram of healthy body weight. If older people eat inadequate amounts of protein, which may happen because their energy intake is so low, they can suffer loss in muscle mass.

TABLE 7-3

The Protein Content of a 140 Kcal Diet and a 2400 Kcal Diet*

1200 kcal diet	Protein (grams)	2400 kcal diet	Protein (grams)
BREAKFAST			
Nonfat milk, 1 cup	8	2% milk, 1 cup	8
Cheerios, ¾ cup	3	Cheerios, ¾ cup	3
Orange	—	Eggs, soft-boiled, 2	12
		Orange	—
LUNCH			
Whole-wheat bread, 2 slices	7	Whole-wheat bread, 2 slices	7
Chicken breast, 2 oz	18	Chicken breast, 2 oz	18
Mayonnaise, 1 tsp	—	Provolone cheese, 2 oz	13
Tomato slices, 2	—	Tomato slices, 2	—
Carrot sticks, 1 cup	1	Mayonnaise, 1 tsp	—
Fig	0.5	Oatmeal-raisin cookies, 2	2
Diet soda	—	Figs, 2	1
		Diet soda	—
DINNER			
Mixed green salad, ½ cup	—	Mixed green salad, ½ cup	—
Italian dressing, 2 tsp	—	Italian dressing, 2 tsp	—
Beef tenderloin, 2 oz	18	Beef tenderloin, 4 oz	36
Spinach pasta, 1 cup, with garlic butter, 1 tsp	7	Spinach pasta, 1 cup, with garlic butter, 1 tsp	7
Zucchini, ½ cup, sautéed in oil, 1 tsp	0.5	Zucchini, ½ cup, sautéed in oil, 1 tsp	0.5
Nonfat milk, 1 cup	8	Carrot sticks, ½ cup	1
Bagel, toasted, ½	4		
Jam, 2 tsp	—	**SNACK**	
		2% milk, 1 cup	8
		Bagel, toasted	7
		Jam, 2 tsp	—
		Fruited yogurt, 1 cup	10
TOTAL	75		134

*This table illustrates how little energy need be consumed while still meeting the RDA for protein. It also shows how much protein we eat when we consume typical energy intakes.

Does Eating a Mainly High-Protein Diet Harm You?

People frequently ask whether the high protein intake of adults in America is harmful. (Getting too much protein can be very harmful to infants. This is discussed in detail in Chapter 15.) The extra vitamin B-6, iron, and zinc that accompany protein foods are often beneficial, but the extra fat—especially saturated fat—found in many high-protein animal foods is not. Research in the 1970s suggested that a diet high in animal protein increased calcium loss in the urine. This finding concerned researchers, who thought that protein caused calcium to leach out of the bones. Animal proteins were singled out because they are rich in sulfur-containing amino acids, and the acidic nature of these amino acids tends to draw calcium out of the body in order to neutralize the acid. Populations in areas of the world where animal protein intake is high also show the highest rates of **osteoporosis,** but this is associated with other factors as well, such as inadequate calcium intake and physical activity, excessive alcohol intake, and smoking.

The RDA for calcium is set high to compensate for the calcium loss induced by the high protein intake of Americans. Also, follow-up studies showed that if extra phosphorus is consumed with animal proteins, urinary calcium does not increase so much. Animal foods are excellent sources of both protein and phosphorus. In addition, women are at highest risk of osteoporosis, and their protein intakes are generally only moderately above RDA guidelines. Thus typical American protein intakes of women probably don't significantly contribute to the risk of osteoporosis, as long as the RDA for calcium is met, but amounts greatly in excess of the RDA may do so.[10]

Excessive intake of red meat is linked to colon cancer in population studies.[8] This link could be attributable to the protein or fat in the food products or to substances that form during cooking of red meat at high temperatures. Excessive fat intake associated with diets rich in red meat, or low dietary fiber intake, may also be contributing factors. More research on this topic is needed before red meat can be singled out as a causative factor in colon cancer.

Some researchers have also expressed the concern that a high protein intake may unduly burden the kidneys to excrete the resulting excess nitrogen (mostly as urea) into the urine. Low-protein diets marginally slow the decline in kidney function in humans if begun early in the course of developing kidney disease, and laboratory animal studies show that protein intakes that just meet nutritional needs preserve kidney function over time better than high-protein diets.[16] Preserving kidney function is especially important for people with diabetes and for people who show signs of kidney disease, such as excess urea in the blood, or who have only one functioning kidney. High-protein diets are discouraged in these cases.[12] For people without diabetes or kidney disease the risk of suffering kidney failure is very low, and thus the risk of a high-protein diet contributing to kidney disease in later life is also low.

Generally speaking, the caution against high protein intake issued by the National Academy of Sciences in their 1989 *Diet and Health Report* deserves consideration. The panel recommended that not more than twice the RDA for protein be consumed on a regular basis. Reducing intake to approximately RDA amounts may benefit some of us, as pointed out above, but the research is still too incomplete to permit a firm conclusion.

Infants' diets must not contain excess protein because their kidneys have difficulty excreting the excess urea and minerals remaining after protein metabolism. Thus regular cow's milk must not be used by itself for feeding young infants—it is too high in protein and other nutrients (see Chapter 15 for details).

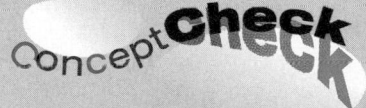

The Recommended Dietary Allowance (RDA) for adults is 0.8 gram of protein per kilogram of healthy body weight. This adds up to 56 grams of protein daily for a 70-kilogram (156-pound) person. The average American man consumes about 105 grams of protein daily, and a woman consumes about 65 grams. So, typically, we eat more than enough protein to meet our needs. Current research has not firmly established that this excess poses a major health risk for most of us, aside from the fat present in most high-protein diets, but it is also not necessary.

Protein in Foods

The most nutrient-dense source of protein is water-packed tuna, which has over 80% of energy as protein. Of the typical foods we eat, those with more than 20% of energy as protein are animal foods. They are also the major sources of protein in the American diet; over 65% of our protein comes from animal sources (Figure 7-7). In the United States, meat, poultry, and fish consumption amounts to about 145 pounds (weight without bones) per person per year. Worldwide, 35% of protein comes from animal sources. In Africa and East Asia, about 20% of the protein eaten comes from animals.[25]

Legumes: They Deserve a Close Look

Legumes are a plant family with pods that contain a single row of seeds: garden and black-eyed peas; green, black, red, great northern, lima, kidney, pinto, and garbanzo beans; lentils; and soybeans. Dried varieties of the mature seeds—what we know as beans—make an impressive contribution to the protein, vitamin, mineral, and dietary fiber content of a meal (Figure 7-7). Regularly consuming these vegetable proteins, as noted in Chapter 2, can add substantial amounts of nutrients to a diet. Moreover, as discussed in Chapters 5 and 6, the soluble fiber in them can help lower blood cholesterol and moderate the swings in blood glucose that occur after eating.

Many people dismiss beans. This unfortunate oversight may be rooted in the Depression of the 1930s, when people could afford little else. Beans, however, are a versatile food: They can anchor or blend into soups, salads, casseroles, sandwich spreads, and cracker dips; they can be added in small quantities wherever extra body, texture, and nutritional value are desired. Because legumes tend to soak up flavors during the cooking process, it is possible to incorporate delicate flavors from combinations of herbs, spices, and broths. Incorporating legumes into your weekly menu can add variety and new flavors.

When you initially add legumes to your diet, they may cause intestinal gas. Split peas, limas, and lentils are

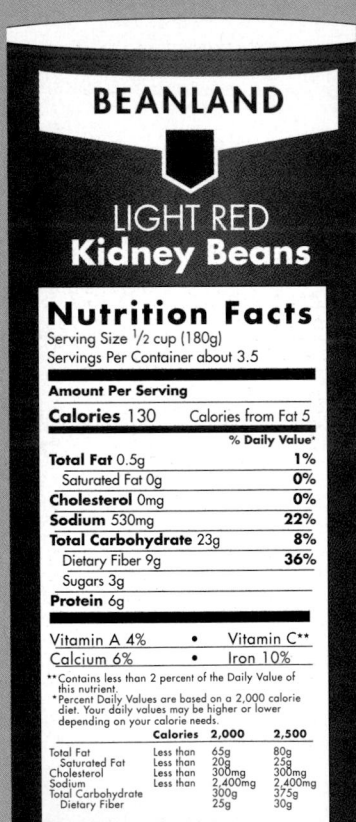

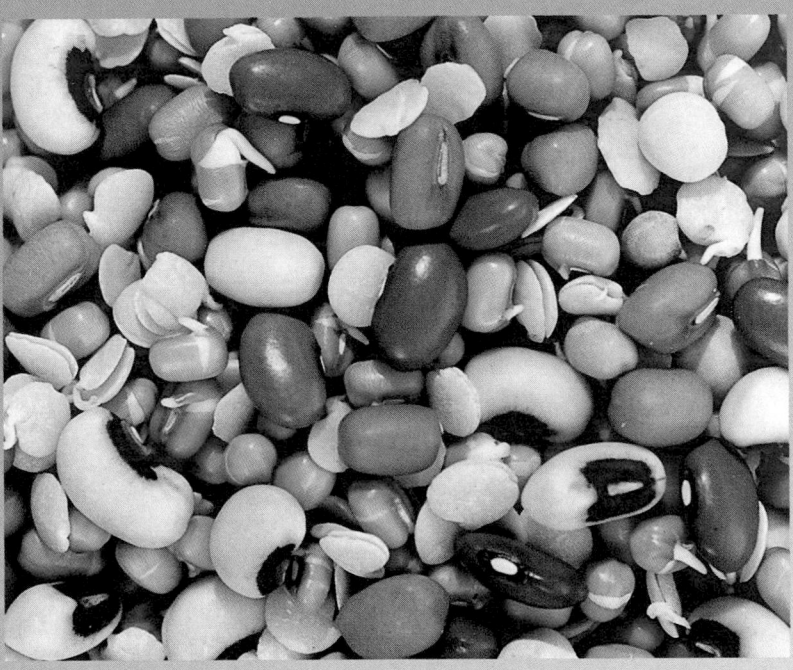

Legumes—another protein source that can meet a body's need. An added bonus is that many other nutrients are also present in legumes.

Figure 7-7
Legumes are rich sources of protein. One half cup meets about 10% of protein needs, and at a "cost" of only about 5% of energy needs.

less likely to cause this problem than the others, so start with them. Eat small servings at first, and give your GI tract a few weeks to adjust.

You can also reduce your risk of getting intestinal gas by cooking dry beans in boiling water for 3 minutes to soften them. Then turn off the heat and let the covered beans soak for a few hours. Much of the indigestible sugars that cause the gas (recall that this happens when certain sugars in beans are broken down by the bacteria in the large intestine) will leach into the water. The water should be poured off and the beans further cooked in fresh water as desired. This practice will lead to some vitamin loss but will not affect protein or dietary fiber content. For canned beans, draining and rinsing with water is an excellent way to lower the content of undigestible sugars.

Many people have no trouble with beans and other legumes, but it's best to be cautious. An enzyme preparation called *Beano* is also available to ease gas symptoms. Taken right before a meal in tablet or liquid form and according to directions, it helps digest the beans' undigestible carbohydrates in the small intestine and thereby lessens the intestinal gas production in the large intes-

tine. Because Beano is made from mold, people sensitive to molds may have allergic reactions and should avoid this product or use it with care. For more information and/or free samples, contact the manufacturer at 1-800-257-8650.

Like all foods, though, legumes do not offer every nutrient and cannot serve as a complete diet by themselves. They contain no vitamin A, vitamin C, or vitamin B-12. The protein in beans is somewhat deficient in methionine, one of the essential amino acids. Serving beans with a food high in methionine, such as meat, eggs, or cheese in typical diets or rice, corn, or other grains in vegetarian diets compensates for this deficiency (see Table 7-2). Many traditional ethnic dishes combine legumes with grains and vegetables to yield a high-quality protein balance: lentil curry on rice, pinto beans and corn tortillas, tofu (soybean curd) and rice, and corn and lima beans (succotash). Try these combinations or create your own.

As you prepare foods or order them in a restaurant, look for beans—salad bars usually provide a few choices. Black bean and other bean soups, baked beans, chili, red beans and rice, and soy burgers are other possibilities.

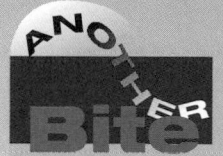

Research over the last few years suggests that soy beans have many unique properties and deserve to be singled out among the legumes as an important part of a diet. The protein in soy can lower blood cholesterol, even beyond the degree that would be expected from its low fat and high dietary fiber content. To reap the benefits requires consuming about 25 grams or more of soy protein per day. This, unfortunately, is no easy feat—10 grams is provided by $^1/_2$ cup tofu, 1 to 2 cups soy milk, or 1 ounce soy flour (read the label, in any case, to be sure).

A compound in soy called genistein—*one of the many phytochemicals discussed in Chapter 2—can reduce cancer risk, most notably breast cancer. Genistein can block cancer development and prevent tumors from creating blood vessels, thus preventing the cells from growing by depriving them of the means to obtain nourishment. The effective dose of soy products is just one serving per day (1 cup soy milk, $^1/_2$ cup tofu, or soybeans). Researchers are investigating still other benefits. Including some soy milk, tofu, or soybeans in your diet is worth considering. In the near future, Food manufacturers will probably make it easier to incorporate soy protein in our diets, as they have with the recent introduction of soy nut butter to be used in place of peanut butter.*

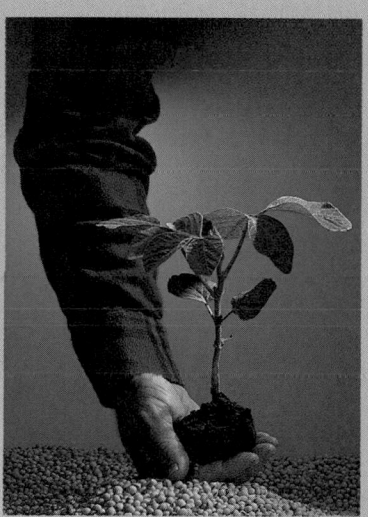

Soybeans make a healthful contribution to a diet.

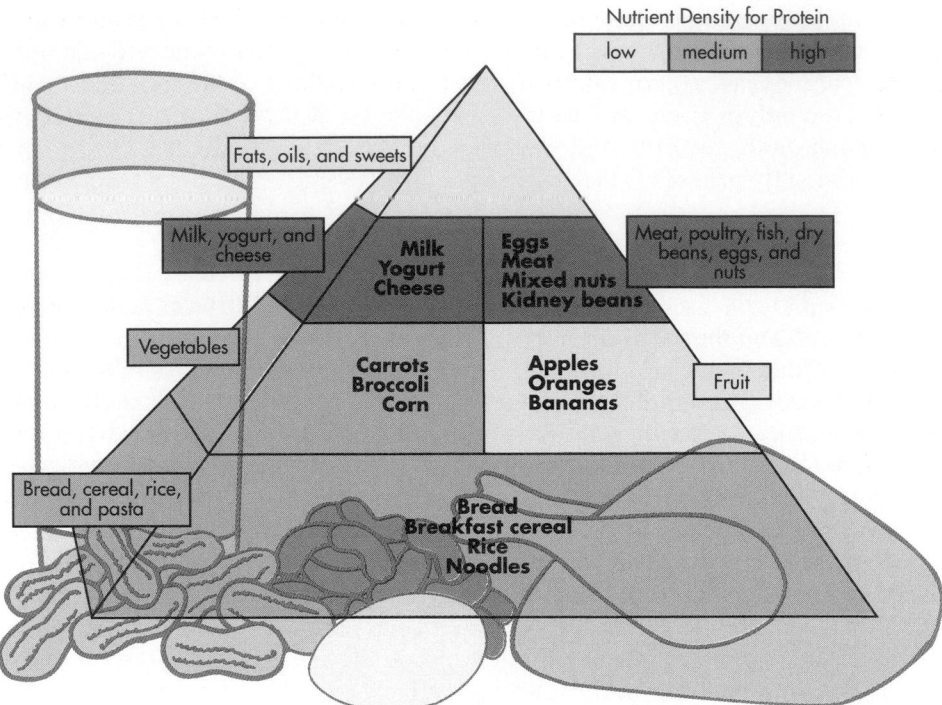

Figure 7-8 *Sources of protein in foods from the Food Guide Pyramid. The fruit group, vegetable group, and fats, oils, and sweet category contain few foods rich in protein, whereas the other groups contain foods with moderate to high amounts. The background color of each group indicates the average nutrient density for protein in that group.*

The Importance of Plant Proteins

Vegetable sources of proteins deserve more attention from Americans. Many plant foods—in proportion to the amount of energy they supply—provide not only much protein but also ample magnesium and dietary fiber, along with other benefits[6] (Figure 7-8). The protein is used somewhat less efficiently by the body than are animal proteins (10% to 20% less), but this drop is not significant enough to influence diet planning when a variety of foods is used. The vegetable proteins we eat also contain no cholesterol and little saturated fat, unless these are added during processing. Regular use of plant foods high in protein makes a valuable addition to the Food Guide Pyramid because these supply a variety of other nutrients. Presently, concentrated sources of plant proteins are not very popular in America, except for maybe peanut butter, baked beans, and refried beans. Should you give them a closer look?

Protein-Energy Malnutrition

Protein-energy malnutrition (PEM)

A condition resulting from regularly consuming insufficient amounts of energy and protein. The deficiency eventually results in body wasting and an increased susceptibility to infections.

Rarely an isolated condition, protein deficiency worldwide usually accompanies a deficiency of dietary energy and other nutrients resulting from insufficient food intake. In developing areas of the world, people often have diets low in energy and protein. This state of undernutrition stunts their growth in childhood and makes them more susceptible to disease throughout life.[14] (Note that undernutrition is a main focus of Chapter 18.) People who eat too little protein and energy food can go on to develop **protein-energy malnutrition (PEM)**, also referred to as *protein-calorie malnutrition (PCM)*. In its milder form, it is difficult to tell if a person with PEM is eating too little energy or protein, or both. But if the nutrient deficiency—

especially for energy—is quite severe, a deficiency disease called *marasmus* can result. On the other hand, when a poor nutrient intake—protein included—is added to other problems from concurrent diseases and infections, a disease called *kwashiorkor* can develop. These two diseases form the tip of the iceberg with respect to all states of undernutrition, and symptoms of these two diseases even can be present in the same person (Figure 7-9).

Kwashiorkor

Kwashiorkor is a word from Ghana that means "the disease that the first child gets when the new child comes." From birth an infant is usually breastfed. By the time the child reaches 1 to 1.5 years, the mother is probably pregnant or has already given birth again, and breastfeeding is no longer possible for the first child. This child's diet abruptly changes from nutritious human milk to native starchy roots and gruels. These foods have low protein densities compared with total energy. The foods are also often so bulky and full of plant fibers that it is difficult for the child to eat enough of them to meet energy needs. The child may also have infections and parasites, which acutely raise energy and protein needs. For these reasons, energy needs of these children are met marginally, at best, and their protein needs are not met, especially when needs are greatly increased by infections and marginal energy

Marasmus
A disease that results from consuming a grossly insufficient amount of protein and energy; one of the diseases classed as protein-energy malnutrition. Victims will have little or no fat stores, little muscle mass, and poor strength. Death from infections is common.

Kwashiorkor
A disease occurring primarily in young children who have an existing disease and consume a marginal amount of energy and considerably insufficient protein despite high needs. The child generally suffers from infections and exhibits edema, poor growth, weakness, and an increased susceptibility to further illness.

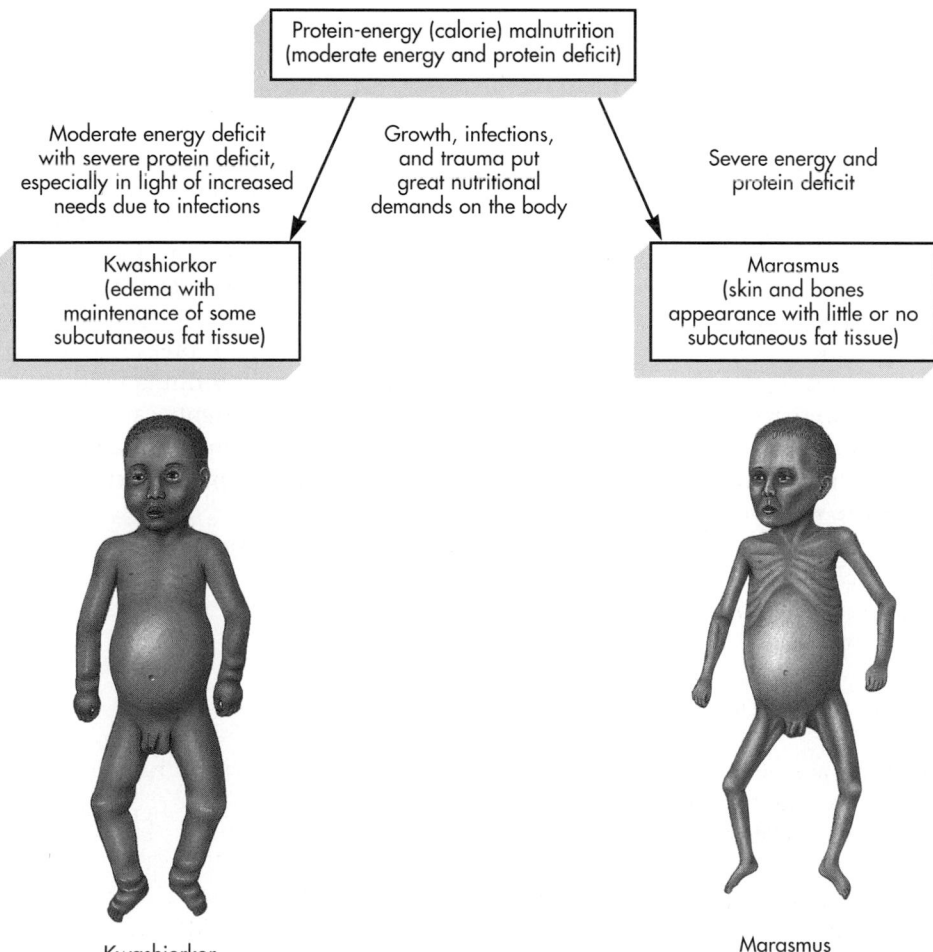

Figure 7-9 *A schema for classifying undernutrition. The presence of subcutaneous fat (directly underneath the skin) is a diagnostic key for distinguishing kwashiorkor from marasmus.*

intakes.[14] Usually many vitamin and mineral requirements are also far from being fulfilled. Famine victims face similar problems.

The major symptoms of kwashiorkor are apathy, listlessness, failure to grow and gain weight, and withdrawal from the environment. These symptoms complicate other diseases present and can make conditions such as measles, a disease that normally makes a healthy child ill for only a week or so, severely debilitating and even fatal. Further signs and symptoms of the disease are changes in hair color, potassium deficiency, flaky skin, fatty infiltration in the liver, reduced muscle mass, and massive edema in the abdomen and legs. The presence of edema in a child who has some subcutaneous fat still present is the hallmark of kwashiorkor (see Figure 7-9). In addition, these children hardly move. If you pick them up, they don't cry. When you hold them, you feel the plumpness of edema, not muscle and fat tissue.

Many symptoms of kwashiorkor can be explained based on what we know about proteins. Proteins play important roles in fluid balance, lipoprotein transport, immune function, and production of tissues such as skin and hair. We should not expect children with an insufficient protein intake to grow and mature normally. And they don't!

If children with kwashiorkor are helped in time—if infections are treated and a diet ample in protein, energy, and other essential nutrients is provided—the disease process reverses. They begin to grow again and may even show no signs of their previous condition, except perhaps shortness of stature. Unfortunately, by the time many of these children reach a hospital or care center, they already have severe infections. In spite of the best care, they still die. Or, if they survive, they return home only to repeat the cycle.

Marasmus

Marasmus typically occurs as an infant slowly starves to death. It is caused by diets containing greatly insufficient amounts of protein, energy, and other nutrients. The condition is also commonly referred to as *protein-energy malnutrition*, especially when experienced by older children and adults. The word *marasmus* means "to waste away." Victims have the "skin and bones" appearance you see on posters from relief agencies (see Figure 7-9). Little or no subcutaneous fat is present.[14]

Marasmus commonly develops in infants who either are not breastfed or have stopped breastfeeding in the early months. Often the weaning formula used is improperly prepared because of unsafe water and because the parents cannot afford sufficient infant formula for the child's needs. The latter problem may lead the parents to dilute the formula to provide more feedings, not realizing that this provides only more water for the infant.

Marasmus in infants commonly occurs in the large cities of poverty-stricken countries. In the cities, bottle-feeding is often necessary because the infant must be cared for by others when the mother is working or away from home. When people are poor and sanitation is lacking, bottle-feeding often leads to marasmus. An infant with marasmus requires large amounts of energy and protein—like a preterm infant—and unless the child receives them, full recovery from the disease may never occur. Most brain growth takes place between conception and the child's first birthday. In fact, the brain is growing at its highest rate at birth. If the diet does not support brain growth during the first months of life, the brain may not grow to its full adult size. This reduced or retarded brain growth may lead to diminished intellectual function.

Both kwashiorkor and marasmus wreak havoc on infants and children; mortality rates in developing countries are often 10 to 20 times higher than in the United States.[14] This high mortality rate in part encourages the high birth rate in developing countries; if a mother wants four children to survive, she had better have ten. The overload of babies makes infant mortality much more likely. Politics and war worsen the problem. Better food availability and sanitation would improve the health of many children worldwide. Chapter 18 examines the issue of undernutrition worldwide in more detail.

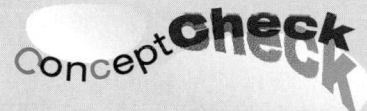

Most undernutrition worldwide consists of mild deficits in energy, protein, and often other nutrients. If a person needs more nutrients because of disease and infection but does not consume enough energy and protein, a condition known as *kwashiorkor* can develop. The person suffers from edema and weakness. Children around age 2 are especially susceptible to kwashiorkor, particularly if they already have other diseases. Famine situations in which only starchy root products are available to eat contribute to this problem. Marasmus is a condition wherein people—infants especially—essentially starve to death. Symptoms include muscle wasting, absence of fat stores, and weakness. Both an adequate diet and treatment of concurrent diseases must be promoted in developing countries to maintain nutritional health.

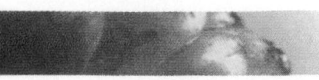

Summary

➤ The building blocks of proteins, amino acids contain a very usable form of nitrogen for us. Of the 20 or so types of amino acids found in food, 9 must be consumed as food and the rest can be synthesized by the body.

➤ High-quality, also called *complete*, protein foods contain ample amounts of all nine essential amino acids. Animal foods typically supply all of them in approximately the right amounts. Lower-quality, also called *incomplete*, protein foods lack sufficient amounts of one or more essential amino acids. This is typical of plant foods, especially cereal grains. Plant foods eaten together often complement each other's amino acid deficits, thereby providing high-quality protein in the diet.

➤ Individual amino acids are linked together to form proteins. The sequential order of amino acids determines the protein's ultimate shape and function. If the three-dimensional shape of the protein eventually formed is unfolded—denatured—by treatment with heat, acid or alkaline solutions, or other processes, the protein loses its biological activity.

➤ Protein digestion begins in the stomach, producing breakdown products called *peptones*. In the small intestine, peptones eventually separate into amino acids. These travel via the portal vein to the liver. Because supplementing the diet with large amounts of individual amino acids can lead to buildup of harmful amounts, they should not be used unless prescribed by a physician.

➤ Important body components—such as muscles, connective tissue, transport proteins, visual pigments, enzymes, some hormones, and immune bodies—are made of proteins. Proteins also provide carbons that can be used to synthesize glucose when necessary.

➤ The protein RDA for adults is 0.8 gram per kilogram of healthy body weight. For a typical 70-kilogram (156-pound) person, this corresponds to 56 grams of protein daily. The American diet generally supplies plenty of protein: men consume about 105 grams of protein daily, and women consume closer to 65 grams. The combined protein intake is also of sufficient quality to support body functions.

➤ Animal products are the most nutrient-dense sources of protein. For example, water-packed tuna contains over 80% of its energy content as protein. The high quality of these proteins means we can easily convert them into body proteins. Plant foods generally contain less than 20% of their energy content as protein; however, legumes are an excellent source of high-quality protein if eaten with grain proteins or animal products.

➤ Undernutrition occasionally leads to kwashiorkor and marasmus. Kwashiorkor results primarily from an inadequate energy and protein intake in comparison to body needs, which often increase with concurrent disease and infection. Kwashiorkor often occurs when a child is taken off human milk and fed mostly starchy gruels. Marasmus results primarily from extreme starvation—a negligible intake of both protein and energy. Marasmus commonly occurs during famine, especially in infants.

Study Questions

1 Discuss the relative importance of essential and nonessential amino acids in the diet. Why is it important for essential amino acids lost from the body to be replaced in the diet?

2 What are four of the functions of proteins? How does the structure of a protein relate to its functions?

3 What factors can denature proteins?

4 What foods provide especially high-quality protein?

5 What are the possible long-term effects of an inadequate intake of dietary protein on children between the ages of 6 months and 4 years?

6 What would be the health benefit of preventing protein-energy malnutrition in children worldwide?

7 What characteristics of vegetable proteins could improve the American diet?

References

1 Craig WJ: Iron status of vegetarians, *American Journal of Clinical Nutrition* 59:1233S, 1994.

2 Crim MC, Munro HN: Protein and amino acids. In Shils ME and others, editors: *Modern nutrition in health and disease,* Philadelphia, 1994, Lea & Febiger.

3 Donovan UM, Gibson RS: Iron and zinc status of young women aged 14 to 19 years consuming vegetarian and omnivorous diets, *Journal of the American College of Nutrition* 14:463, 1995.

4 Dwyer JT: Vegetarianism for women. In Krummel DA, Kris-Etherton PM, editors: *Nutriton in women's health,* Gaithersburg, Md., 1996, Aspen.

5 Fernstrom JD: Dietary amino acids and brain function, *Journal of the American Dietetic Association* 94:71, 1994.

6 Geil PB, Anderson JW: Nutrition and health implications of dry beans: a review, *Journal of the American College of Nutrition* 13:549, 1994.

7 Gibson RS: Content and bioavailability of trace elements in vegetarian diets, *American Journal of Clinical Nutrition,* 59:1223S, 1994.

8 Giovannuci E and others: Intake of fat, meat, and fiber in relation to colon cancer in men, *Cancer Research* 54:2390, 1994.

9 Haddad EH: Development of a vegetarian food guide, *American Journal of Clinical Nutrition* 59:1248S, 1994.

10 Heaney RP: Protein intake and calcium economy, *Journal of the American Diabetes Association* 93:1259, 1993.

11 Herbert V: Staging vitamin B-12 (cobalamin) status in vegetarians, *American Journal of Clinical Nutrition* 59:1213S, 1994.

12 Klahr S and others: The effects of dietary protein restriction and blood-pressure control on the progression of chronic renal disease, *New England Journal of Medicine* 330:877, 1994.

13 Lamberg-Allardt C and others: Low serum 25-hydroxyvitamin D concentrations and secondary hyperparathyroidism in middle-aged white strict vegetarians, *American Journal of Clinical Nutrition* 58:684, 1993.

14 Latham MC: Protein-energy malutrition. In Brown ML, editor: *Present knowledge in nutrition,* Washington, DC, 1990, International Life Sciences Institute-Nutrition Foundation.

15 McDowell MA and others: Energy and macronutrient intakes of persons ages 2 months and over in the United States, *Advance Data,* number 225, October 24, 1994, Centers for Disease Control, USDHHS.

16 Mitch WE: Low-protein diets in the treatment of chronic renal failure, *Journal of the American College of Nutrition* 14:311, 1995.

17 Samuels-Reid JH: Common problems in sickle cell disease, *American Family Physician* 49:1477, 1994.

18 Sanders TA: Vegetarian diets and children, *Pediatric Clinics of North America* 42:955, 1995.

19 Shaw NS and others: A vegetarian diet rich in soybean products compromises iron status in young students, *Journal of Nutrition* 125:212, 1995.

20 Stryer L: *Biochemistry,* ed 4, New York, 1995, WH Freeman.

21 Walker AR: Vegetable and fruit consumption: some past, present and future practices, *Journal of the Royal Society of Health* 115:211, 1995.

22 Waterlow JC: Whole-body protein turnover in humans—past, present, and future, *Annual Review of Nutrition* 15:57, 1995.

23 Weaver CM, Plawecki KL: Dietary calcium: adequacy of a vegetarian diet, *American Journal of Clinical Nutrition* 59:1238S, 1994.

24 Whorton JC: Historical development of vegetarianism, *American Journal of Clinical Nutrition* 59:1103S, 1994.

25 Young VR, Pellett PL: Plant proteins in relation to human protein and amino acid nutrition, *American Journal of Clinical Nutrition* 59:1203S, 1994.

R A T E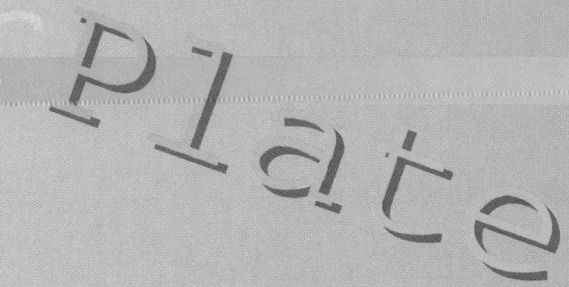

Are You Eating Enough Protein?

I. How much protein do you eat in a typical day? Look at the nutrition assessment you completed at the end of Chapter 2. Review it closely. Find the figure indicating the amount of protein you consumed on that day, and write it in the space below:

TOTAL PROTEIN _____

Compare your protein intake with your RDA for protein. Find your healthy weight for height in pounds using Figure 10-6 in Chapter 10. Choose a midrange value. Divide this number by 2.2 to reveal your healthy weight in kilograms. Next, multiply by 0.8 gram per kilogram of this weight or your current body weight if the numbers are close. This will indicate the RDA for protein for your age and gender. Write it in the space below:

RDA FOR PROTEIN _____

How does your consumption compare with your RDA?

_____
_____
_____

If you consumed either more or less than the RDA, what foods could you add, subtract, or eat more or less of? (Look at the foods you ate.)

_____
_____
_____
_____

Was most of your protein from animal or plant sources?

_____
_____

If your protein intake was primarily from plants, did this come from a wide variety to encourage protein complementarity for the day?

_____
_____
_____

II. Plan a day of meatless meals, using a wide variety of plant-based foods. Can this diet meet your protein needs? A quick calculation using Appendix A or the software for this book will verify the correctness of your assumption.

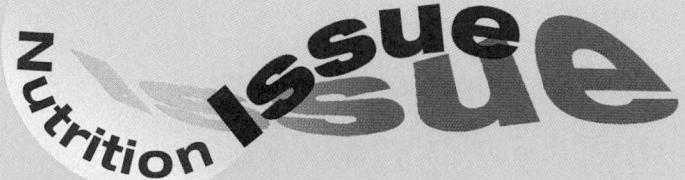

Vegetarianism

Vegetarianism has evolved over the centuries from a necessity into an option (Figure 7-10). Historically, vegetarianism was linked with specific philosophies and religions or with science.[24] In the sixth century BC, Pythagoras advocated a meatless diet for its physical health, ecological, religious, and philosophical benefits.

Today there are about 12 million vegetarians in the United States, about double the number in 1985. Vegetarianism is popular among college students. Fifteen percent of college students in one survey said they select vegetarian options at lunch or dinner on any given day. In response, dining services offer vegetarian options at every meal, the most common being pastas with meatless sauce and pizza. A recent survey by the National Restaurant Association found that 20% of customers want a vegetarian option when they eat out. As nutrition science has grown, new information has enabled the design of adequate vegetarian diets. It is important for vegetarians to take advantage of this information because a diet of only plants can lead to various nutrient deficiencies and to substantial growth retardation in infants and children.[1, 4, 7, 18] People who choose a vegetarian diet can meet their nutritional needs by following a few basic rules and knowledgeably planning their diets.

Recent studies show that death rates from some chronic diseases are lower for vegetarians than for nonvegetarians. Healthful lifestyles (not smoking, abstinence from alcohol and drugs, and increased physical activity) and social class bias probably partially account for these findings.[4] As noted in the last chapter, one study showed that a totally vegetarian diet coupled with physical activity, meditation, and smoking cessation led to regression of atherosclerosis.

WHY DO PEOPLE PRACTICE VEGETARIANISM?

People choose vegetarianism for a variety of reasons. Some believe that killing animals for food is unethical. Hindus and Trappist monks eat vegetarian meals as a practice of their religion. In the United States, many Seventh Day Adventists base their practice of vegetarianism on biblical texts and believe it is a more healthful way to live. Some people might pursue vegetarianism because meat is expensive.

People might choose vegetarianism after realizing that animals are not efficient protein factories. Animals actually use much of the protein they eat just to maintain themselves rather than to synthesize new muscle tissue. Animals that humans eat sometimes eat grasses that humans cannot digest. Many, however, also eat grains humans can eat.

People might also practice vegetarianism because it encourages a high intake of carbohydrates, vitamins A, E, and C, carotenoids, magnesium, and dietary fiber, while limiting saturated fat and cholesterol intake. This produces a diet closely resembling that suggested in the Dietary Guidelines for Americans covered in Chapter 2. Studies confirm that many vegetarians actually do eat nutritious, low-fat diets.[4]

FOOD PLANNING FOR VEGETARIANS

There are a variety of vegetarian styles. **Vegans** eat only plant foods. **Fruitarians** eat fruits, nuts, honey, and vegetable oils. This plan is not recommended because it can lead to nutrient deficiencies in people of all ages. **Lacto-vegetarians** modify vegetarianism a bit—they include dairy products

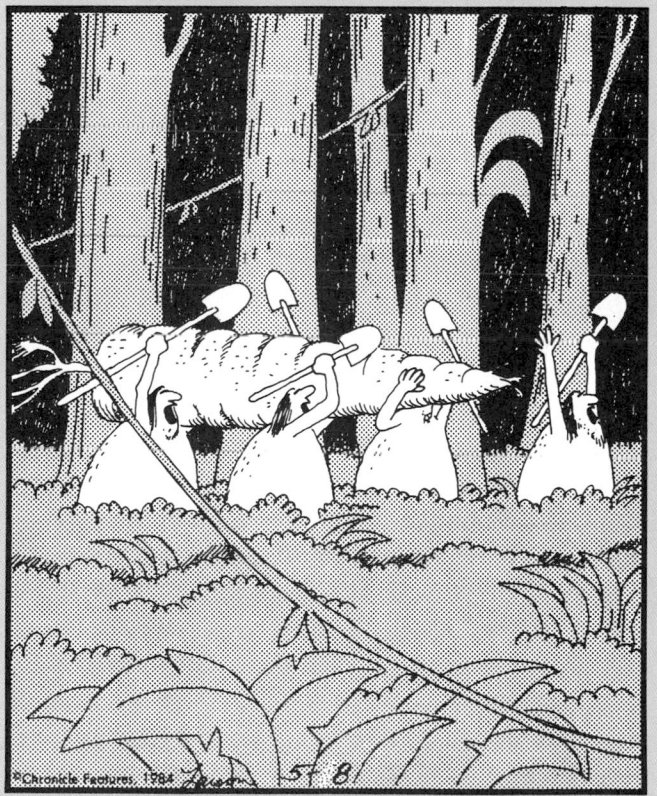

THE FAR SIDE   By GARY LARSON

Early vegetarians returning from the kill.

Figure 7-10 *The Far Side.*

TABLE 7-4

Food-Group Plan for Lacto-Vegetarians and Vegans*⁹

Group†	Lacto-vegetarian‡	Vegan§‖	Key nutrients supplied
	SERVINGS		
Grains¶	6-11	11	Protein, thiamin, niacin, folate, vitamin E, zinc, magnesium, iron, and dietary fiber
Legumes	1-2	2	Protein, vitamin B-6, zinc, magnesium, and dietary fiber
Nuts, seeds	1-2	2	Protein, vitamin E, and magnesium
Vegetables	3-5 (include one dark green or leafy variety daily)	5 (include one dark green or leafy variety daily)	Vitamin A, vitamin C, and folate
Fruits	2-4	4	Vitamin A, vitamin C, and folate
Milk	2-3	—	Protein, riboflavin, vitamin D, vitamin B-12, and calcium

*Base serving size on those listed for the Food Guide Pyramid (see Chapter 2). This plan yields about 1600 to 1800 kcal. Increase the number of servings, or add other foods to meet higher energy needs.
‡Contains about 75 g of protein in 1650 kcal.
§A calcium-fortified food, such as orange juice or soy milk, is needed unless a calcium supplement is used. In addition, use of a vitamin B-12 supplement or foods supplemented with vitamin B-12 is a must. Overall, fortified soy milk makes a valuable contribution to a vegan diet.
‖Contains about 79 g of protein in 1800 kcal.
¶One serving of vitamin- and mineral-enriched cereal is recommended.

and plant foods. **Lacto-ovo-vegetarians** modify the diet even further and eat dairy products and eggs, as well as plant foods. Including these animal products makes food planning easier because they are rich in some nutrients missing or present in low amounts in plants. Overall, the wider the variety of foods eaten, the easier it is to meet nutritional needs. Thus the practice of eating no animal sources of food significantly separates the vegans and fruitarians from all other semivegetarian styles.

Most people who call themselves vegetarians consume at least some dairy products, if not all dairy products and eggs. A food-group plan has been developed for lacto-vegetarians (Table 7-4). This plan includes servings of nuts, grains, legumes, and seeds to help meet protein needs. There is also a vegetable group, a fruit group, and a milk group.

This plan differs a little from the Food Guide Pyramid for **omnivores**. The key to this plan is seeking foods other than meat that supply the nutrients contained in meat. It's not nutritionally sound simply to stop eating meat without making sure the body's needs are still met. Good-quality plant sources of nutrients, such as nuts, grains, legumes, and seeds, should be eaten to supply nutrients that normally come from meat in the diet. By following such a food plan, a lacto-vegetarian should be able to have an adequate diet.⁹

THE VEGAN

A vegan diet requires some creative planning (Table 7-5). A real effort must be made to use grains and legumes to yield high-quality protein and other key nutrients in meals, especially when used with infants and children.¹⁸ Then, if energy needs are satisfied, protein needs should also be met. Including a wide variety of protein sources should provide all amino acids needed for a high-quality protein diet. The essential amino acids deficient from one food protein are supplied by those of another protein in the same meal or in the next.

Table 7-2 lists traditional dishes in which vegetable proteins combine to provide high-quality (complete) protein in the meal.

Purchasing some vegetarian cookbooks will simplify the task of menu planning. They provide numerous

Omnivore
A person who consumes both plant and animal food sources.

TABLE 7-5

Nutrients Likely to be Marginal in the Vegan Diet

Nutrient	Plant sources
Vitamin D	Fortified margarine, fortified breakfast cereal
Riboflavin	Whole and enriched grains, leafy vegetables, mushrooms, beans, nuts, seeds
Vitamin B-12	Fortified breakfast cereal, fortified yeast, fortified soy milk
Iron	Whole grains, prune juice, dried fruits, beans, nuts, seeds, leafy vegetables
Calcium	Fortified soy milk, tofu, almonds, dry beans, leafy vegetables, some fortified breakfast cereals, flour, certain brands of orange juice, and certain snacks
Zinc	Whole grains, wheat germ, beans, nuts, seeds

Be aware that nuts and seeds are very energy dense; watching portion size is important.

ideas for imaginative and nutritious ways to use plant foods.

The vegan diet must also include good sources of riboflavin, vitamins D and B-12, calcium, iron, and zinc.[1, 4, 7, 11, 13, 23] A fortified breakfast cereal provides a good start in meeting those needs. Riboflavin can be obtained from green leafy vegetables, whole grains, yeast, and legumes, part of most vegan diets. A major source of riboflavin in the typical American diet is milk, which is omitted from the vegan diet. Vitamin D can be obtained through regular sun exposure and fortified margarine. Otherwise, a supplement containing vitamin D should be considered[13] (see Chapter 8).

The vegan should find a reliable source of vitamin B-12, such as fortified soybean milk and special yeast grown on media rich in vitamin B-12. Vitamin B-12 occurs naturally only in animal foods; plants can contain soil or microbial contamination that provides at most a trace amount of vitamin B-12. Because the body can store enough vitamin B-12 for about 4 years, a deficiency can take a long time to develop after animal foods are removed from the diet. If a deficiency develops, nerves can be damaged irreversibly and brain function can decrease. Evidence of a vitamin B-12 deficiency has been noted in vegetarian mothers and their infants. The milk produced by the vegetarian mothers was low in vitamin B-12. The earliest sign of a vitamin B-12 deficiency is mental dysfunction. Therefore vegans need to be careful to prevent a vitamin B-12 deficiency[11] (see Chapter 8).

To obtain calcium, the vegan can drink fortified soybean milk or fortified orange juice and consume calcium-rich tofu (check the label) or other calcium-fortified foods, such as certain breakfast cereals and snacks.[23] Green leafy vegetables and nuts also contain calcium, but the calcium is either not well absorbed or not very plentiful. Calcium supplements are another option (see Chapter 9).

For iron the vegan can consume whole grains, dried fruits and nuts, and legumes. The iron in these foods is not absorbed as well as that found in animal foods, but a good source of vitamin C taken with these foods modestly enhances iron absorption. Thus a recommended strategy is to consume vitamin C with every meal that contains adequate iron-rich plant foods. Cooking in iron pots and skillets can also add iron to the diet (see Chapter 9).

The vegan can find zinc in whole grains, nuts, and legumes, but phytic acid and other substances in these foods limit zinc absorption. Grains are most nutritious when leavened, as in bread, because this process reduces the influence of phytic acid.

Of all these nutrients, calcium and iron are the most difficult to consume in sufficient quantities. Special diet planning is required.[1, 19, 23]

Veganism during childhood can pose problems. The sheer bulk of a plant-based diet may make it difficult for a child to eat foods that supply enough energy to permit dietary protein to be used for synthesis of body proteins rather than for energy needs. Vegan children need concentrated sources of energy to avoid this problem.[18] Examples include fortified soybean milk, nuts, dried fruits, avocados, cookies made with vegetable oils or tub margarine, and fruit juices.

Soy milk, soy yogurt, and soy cheese are excellent choices for vegan children (and vegan adults). When fortified with calcium and vitamin B-12, these substitutes can provide many of the key nutrients found in milk.

Finding excellent iron and zinc sources is important in planning vegan diets, especially for infants and children. Pregnancy also deserves special attention. Overall, both infancy and childhood are life stages in which vegetarianism is appropriate, but it must be implemented with knowledge and professional guidance.[4]

Vitamins

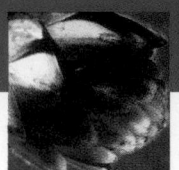

8

WHEN IT COMES TO VITAMINS,
we often hear, "If a little is good, then more must be better." Some people believe that consuming vitamins far in excess of their needs provides them with extra energy, protection from disease, and prolonged youth. Over 50% of adults in the United States take vitamin and mineral supplements on at least an occasional basis. This helps fuel what has become a $4 billion industry.[2]

In stark contrast, our total vitamin needs to prevent deficiency symptoms are really quite small. In general, humans require a total of about 1 ounce (28 grams) of vitamins for every 150 pounds (70 kilograms) of food consumed. Vitamins are found in plants and animals. Plants synthesize all the vitamins they need. Animals vary in their ability to synthesize vitamins. For example, guinea pigs and humans are two of the very few organisms that are unable to synthesize their own supply of vitamin C.[26]

Chapter 3 discussed vitamin supplement use. This chapter first briefly reviews some general properties of the vitamins discussed in Chapter 3. The bulk of this chapter then focuses on the functions and sources of, and the need for, these vitamins and finishes with a look at their role in cancer prevention.

CHAPTER 8

What Do You Believe About Vitamin Supplements?

Below is a brief article about vitamins, typical of one you might find in a popular health and fitness or women's magazine. As you read it, decide whether you think the claims are true or false. A blank is provided next to each claim to record your answers. Write "T" if you think the statement is true or "F" if you think it is false.

Vitamins: Our Health Promoting Allies
by Dr. Wilbert Gruntaloud

Do you take vitamins? If not, you probably aren't doing all you can to promote your health. There are some hidden truths about vitamins that the medical community rarely discloses. Do you suffer from frequent colds and flu? Many people spend their hard-earned dollars for cold medicines and lose a number of workdays because of these ailments. We now know that certain vitamin supplements prevent colds and flu. _____

Do you eat a relatively poor diet because of all the responsibilities you must handle? Vitamin supplements will make up for a poor diet. _____ Do you feel tired and fatigued frequently? You may be one of those people who requires very high intakes of vitamins to be healthy. _____ In addition, vitamin supplements will give you extra energy, especially during times of increased stress. _____ Most of us can't get all the vitamins we need from the food we eat. Plants, potentially rich sources of vitamins, are vitamin deficient today because the soil is so depleted of the nutrients needed for healthy plant growth. _____ Worried about the negative health effects of chemical pollutants in our air and water? Vitamin supplements can protect you. _____

See all the benefits vitamin supplements can bring you? Our Vitablast pack can provide you with all the vitamins you need. These vitamins are from natural sources and are therefore safer and much better than synthetic ones. _____ We at Vitablast Distributors can provide you with a regular supply of vitamins and other supplements for a nominal fee.

Can you afford not to take vitamin supplements? Decide for yourself. Vitamin supplements are harmless, so taking extra amounts will just give extra benefits and security. _____ So what do you have to lose?

Check the answers you gave above against Table 8-1. Then read on to find out more about vitamins.

Key Chapter Concepts

- Vitamins are compounds we generally need daily in small amounts from foods. They yield no energy directly, but many contribute to energy-yielding chemical reactions in the body and promote growth and development.
- Vitamins A, D, E, and K are fat soluble, whereas the B vitamins and vitamin C are water soluble.
- Vitamin A consists of a family of compounds that includes several forms of preformed vitamin A and some carotenoids. Vitamin A, which aids vision, immune function, and cell development, is found in liver and fish oils; carotenoids are especially plentiful in dark green and orange vegetables. Excess vitamin A can be very toxic, especially during pregnancy.
- Vitamin D is both a hormone and a vitamin. Human skin synthesizes it using sunshine and a cholesterol-like substance. If we don't spend enough time in the sun, such foods as fish oils and fortified milk supply the vitamin. The active hormone form of vitamin D helps regulate blood calcium. Excess vitamin D can be very toxic, especially during childhood.
- Vitamin E functions primarily as an antioxidant and is found in plant oils. Claims are made about the curative powers of vitamin E, but to date few have been scientifically validated.
- Vitamin K helps blood clot. Some of the vitamin K absorbed each day comes from bacterial synthesis in the intestine, but most comes primarily from green and leafy vegetables.
- Thiamin, riboflavin, and niacin play key roles in energy-yielding reactions. They help metabolize carbohydrates, fats, and proteins. Enriched grain products are common sources.

- Pantothenic acid, which participates in many aspects of cell metabolism, is widely distributed among foods. Biotin, which participates in glucose and fat metabolism, can be synthesized by bacteria in the intestine. The rest comes from such foods as eggs and cheese.
- Vitamin B-6 performs a vital role in protein metabolism, as well as in other functions. Regular consumption of animal protein foods, cauliflower, and broccoli provides needed vitamin B-6. Taking high doses causes destruction of the nervous system.
- Folate contributes to DNA synthesis. Symptoms of a deficiency are a form of anemia and generally poor cell division in various parts of the body. Excellent food sources are leafy vegetables, organ meats, and orange juice.
- Vitamin B-12 is needed to metabolize the vitamin folate and maintain the insulation surrounding nerves. A deficiency results in a form of anemia (because of its relationship to folate) and nerve degeneration. Vitamin B-12 is highly concentrated in animal foods, our only reliable source. Vegans need a supplemental source.
- Vitamin C is used mainly to synthesize collagen, a major protein for building connective tissue. Vitamin C also modestly enhances iron absorption. Fresh fruits and vegetables, especially citrus fruits, are good sources.
- Cancer is a result of a multistep process in which cells grow excessively. Certain nutrients and other substances—generally present in the bottom half of the Food Guide Pyramid—can impede cancer development. Avoiding obesity and alcoholism and not smoking are also important preventive measures.

Vitamins

Carbon-containing compounds that are needed in very small amounts in the diet to help promote and regulate chemical reactions and processes in the body. Absence from the diet must result in a disease that timely replacement of the vitamin will cure.

Fat-soluble vitamins

Vitamins that dissolve in such substances as ether and benzene but not readily in water. These vitamins are A, D, E, and K.

Vitamins: Vital Dietary Components

By definition, **vitamins** are essential organic (carbon-containing) substances needed in small amounts in the diet for normal function, growth, and maintenance of the body. Although vitamins themselves yield no energy to the body, they often participate in energy-yielding reactions (Table 8-1). Vitamins A, D, E, and K are **fat soluble,** whereas the B vitamins and vitamin C are **water soluble.** In addition, the B vitamins and vitamin K function as parts of **coenzymes** (that is, compounds that help enzymes function)[36] (Figure 8-1).

Vitamins are generally indispensable in human diets because they can't be synthesized in the human body, or because their synthesis can be curtailed by environmental factors. Notable exceptions to a strict dietary need are vitamin D, which may be synthesized by the skin in the presence of sunlight;[20] niacin, which may be synthesized from an amino acid; and vitamin K and biotin, which can be synthesized by bacteria in the intestinal tract.[5]

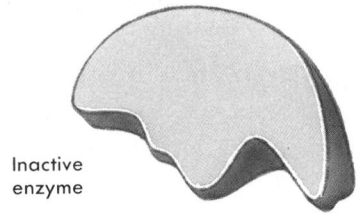

TABLE 8-1

Myths and Facts About Vitamin Supplementation

Most of us view scientific knowledge with awe, and we are quite justified, considering the scientific achievements of our age. Misconceptions about vitamins and their proper functions are understandable. Chapter 3 addressed some misconceptions about vitamins. Let's spend some more time and clear up other misconceptions.

Myth	Fact
Vitamins give you "pep" and "energy."	Vitamins yield no energy. They, of themselves, provide no extra pep or vitality beyond normal expectations, nor do they provide unusual levels of well-being.
Daily timing of vitamin intake is crucial.	There is no medical or scientific basis for this contention.
Some people need very high intakes of vitamins to be healthy.	A multitude of studies have shown that it is rare for anyone to need amounts much higher than the RDA to maintain health.
Vitamin supplements are necessary because today the soil is so depleted.	Crops can't grow in depleted soil. If a nutrient is low, the yield will be low, but the vitamin content will be normal.
Vitamins must be taken in precisely formulated amounts and ratios to each other to have the best effects.	Intake should be adequate, but not excessive, for each. No precise ratios are required.
Organic or natural vitamins are nutritionally superior to synthetic vitamins.	Synthetic vitamins, manufactured in the laboratory, are identical to the natural vitamins found in foods. The body cannot tell the difference and gets the same benefits from either source. Statements to the effect that "nature cannot be imitated" and "natural vitamins have the essence of life" are without meaning.
Vitamin C prevents the common cold.	Too bad, but extensive clinical research fails to support this.
The more vitamins, the better.	The opposite is true. In fact, excess amounts of any of several different vitamins can be harmful.
You cannot get enough vitamins from the conventional foods you eat.	Most people who eat a reasonably varied diet that includes animal products should normally not need supplemental vitamins to maintain health. Studies to date have yet to establish a verifiable benefit from supplement use.
Vitamin supplements are needed to protect against harmful chemicals and pollution.	Vitamin supplements do not have special abilities beyond the vitamins that a healthful diet supplies to ward off harmful agents.

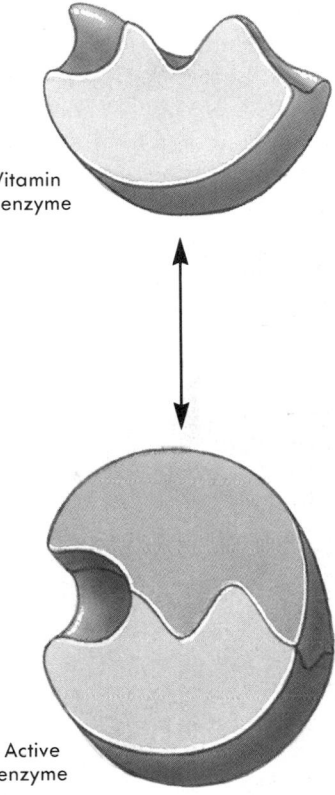

Figure 8-1
Coenzymes, such as those formed from B vitamins, aid in the function of certain enzymes. Without the coenzyme, the enzyme cannot function, and deficiency symptoms associated with the missing vitamin eventually appear.

For a substance to be classified as a vitamin, not only must the body be unable to synthesize it, but its absence from the diet for a defined period of time also must produce deficiency symptoms that, if caught in time, are quickly cured when the substance is resupplied. A substance does not qualify as a vitamin, however, merely because the body can't make it. Evidence must suggest that health declines when the substance is not consumed.

Water-soluble vitamins
Vitamins that dissolve in water. These vitamins are the B vitamins and vitamin C.

As scientists began to identify various vitamins, related deficiencies such as scurvy, beriberi, pellagra, and rickets were dramatically cured. For the most part, as the vitamins were discovered, they were named alphabetically: A, B, C, D, E, and so on. Later many substances originally classified as vitamins were found not to be essential for humans and were dropped from the list. This explains the many gaps in the alphabetical listing. Other vitamins, thought at first to have only one chemical form, turned out to take many forms, so the alphabetical name had to be broken down by numbers (B-6, B-12, and so on).

In addition to their use in correcting deficiency diseases, a few vitamins have also proved useful in treating a limited number of nondeficiency diseases. These medical applications require administration of **megadoses** well above the RDAs for the vitamins. For example, megadoses of niacin are employed as part of blood cholesterol–lowering treatment for appropriately selected individuals. Other examples of medical use include forms of vitamin D in the treatment of psoriasis. Nevertheless, as noted in Chapter 3, any claimed benefits from use of vitamin supplements, especially intakes in excess of 150% of the RDA (or Daily Value listed on a supplement label) should be viewed critically because many unproven claims have been and are continually made.[18]

Have Scientists Found All the Vitamins?

You may wonder whether still more vitamins are lurking in foods that have not been discovered. After all, the first chemical formula of a vitamin (thiamin) was not determined until 1937, and the last structure was characterized in 1948 (vitamin B-12). Though some optimistic researchers hope to discover one or more additional vitamins, most scientists are confident that all vitamins needed by humans have been discovered. Evidence supports this assumption. For example, people have lived well for years on intravenous diets that consist of protein, carbohydrate, fat, all the known vitamins, and the essential minerals. With appropriate medical monitoring, these people not only continue to live but also build new body tissues, have babies, heal wounds, and fight existing diseases. They do not develop deficiency diseases or fail to thrive. Experiences with intravenous diets have also taught us that some lesser known vitamins, such as biotin, are still very important to health.

> Evidence suggests that health declines when choline, a substance the body makes, is not included in a diet. Thus one day choline may be added to the list of known vitamins. This is discussed later in more detail in the section "Vitamin-Like Compounds."

Storage of Vitamins in the Body

Except for vitamin K, the fat-soluble vitamins are not readily excreted from the body. In contrast, the water-soluble vitamins are generally lost from the body quite rapidly, partly because the water in cells dissolves these vitamins and flushes them out of the body via the kidneys. An exception is water-soluble vitamin B-12, which is stored much more readily than both the other water-soluble vitamins.[19]

Because of the limited storage of many vitamins, they should be consumed in the diet daily, although an occasional lapse in the intake of even water-soluble vitamins generally causes no harm. An average person, for example, must consume no thiamin for 10 days or no vitamin C for 20 to 40 days before developing the first symptoms of deficiency of these vitamins. Evidence of a vitamin deficiency occurs only when that vitamin is lacking in the diet and body stores are essentially exhausted.

Vitamin Toxicity

Because fat-soluble vitamins are not readily excreted, some can easily accumulate in the body and cause toxic effects. Although a toxic effect from an excessive intake of any vitamin is theoretically possible, toxicities of the fat-soluble vitamins A and D

[handwritten margin note: Pill form; toxic: Vit E, B6 & C, niacin]

are the most frequently observed.[31] Vitamin E and the water-soluble vitamins niacin, vitamin B-6, and vitamin C can also cause toxic effects but only when consumed in very large amounts.[12] These four vitamins are unlikely to cause toxic effects unless taken in supplement (pill) form. In comparison, vitamins A and D generally are toxic with long-term intake at just five or more times their RDA.

Because regular use of a "one-a-day" type of multivitamin and mineral supplement usually yields less than two times the adult RDAs of the components, this practice is unlikely to cause toxic effects. Consuming many vitamin pills, however, especially highly potent sources of vitamin A and vitamin D, can cause problems. The Nutrition Issue in Chapter 3 should help you determine whether to take a vitamin and mineral supplement and, if so, how to do it safely. Recall that most nutrition scientists agree that a well-chosen diet including some animal products can supply the vitamin needs of almost all people.[18,23] In addition, any supplementation should be approved by your physician because some vitamins and minerals counteract the effect of certain medications. Only with professional advice, which includes evaluation of your current diet, can you best evaluate whether supplementation is in your best interest.[2]

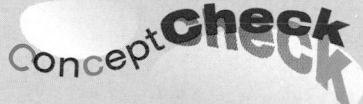

Vitamins are carbon-containing compounds needed in small amounts by the body. Their absence from the diet results in a disease that timely replacement of the vitamin cures. Vitamins do not directly yield energy, but many are needed for energy-yielding reactions in the body. Vitamins A, D, E, and K are fat soluble, whereas the B vitamins and vitamin C are water soluble. In general, the fat-soluble vitamins are not readily excreted from the body and have the potential to build up rapidly to toxic amounts. Water-soluble vitamins are much more readily excreted. Some people take vitamin supplements, believing that they provide health benefits, but most nutrition scientists agree that a well-chosen diet including some animal products can supply the vitamin needs of almost all people.

THE FAT-SOLUBLE VITAMINS— A, D, E, AND K

First, let's look at what we know about the fat-soluble vitamins—vitamins A, D, E, and K (Table 8-2).

Absorption of Fat-Soluble Vitamins

Vitamins A, D, E, and K are absorbed along with dietary fat. These vitamins travel with dietary fats through the bloodstream to reach body cells. Special carriers in the bloodstream help distribute some of these vitamins. Fat-soluble vitamins are stored mostly in the liver and fatty tissues.[12,28]

[handwritten margin note: stored liver & fatty tissues.]

When fat absorption is efficient, about 40% to 90% of the fat-soluble vitamins are absorbed. Anything that interferes with normal digestion and absorption of fats also interferes with fat-soluble vitamin absorption. People who use mineral oil as a laxative at mealtimes risk fat-soluble vitamin deficiencies because the intestine does not absorb mineral oil. Fat-soluble vitamins are simply eliminated with the mineral oil in the feces.

TABLE 8-2

Summary of the Fat-Soluble Vitamins, Their Functions, Deficiency Conditions, and Food Sources

Vitamin	Major functions	Deficiency symptoms	People most at risk	Dietary sources	RDA	Toxicity symptoms
Vitamin A (retinoids) and provitamin A (carotenoids)	Promote vision: light and color Promote growth Prevent drying of skin and eyes Promote resistance to bacterial infection	Night blindness Xerophthalmia Poor growth Dry skin (keratinization)	People in poverty, especially preschool children (still very rare in the United States)	Vitamin A Liver Fortified milk Provitamin A Sweet potatoes Spinach Greens Carrots Cantaloupe Apricots Broccoli	Females: 800 RE* (4000 IU †) Males: 1000 RE* (5000 IU †)	Fetal malformations, hair loss, skin changes, pain in bones
D (chole- and ergocalciferol)	Facilitate absorption of calcium and phosphorus Maintain optimal calcification of bone	Rickets Osteomalacia	Breastfed infants, elderly shut-ins	Vitamin D-fortified milk Fish oils Sardines Salmon	5-10 micrograms (200-400 IU)	Growth retardation, kidney damage, calcium deposits in soft tissue
E (tocopherols, tocotrienols)	Act as an antioxidant: prevent breakdown of vitamin A and unsaturated fatty acids	Hemolysis of red blood cells Nerve destruction	People with poor fat absorption (still very rare)	Vegetable oils Some greens Some fruits	Females: 8 milligrams Alpha-tocopherol equivalents Males: 10 milligrams Alpha-tocopherol equivalents	Muscle weakness, headaches, fatigue, nausea, inhibition of vitamin K metabolism
K (phyllo- and menaquinone)	Help form prothrombin and other factors for blood clotting	Hemorrhage	People taking antibiotics for months at a time (still quite rare)	Green vegetables Liver	60-80 micrograms	Anemia and jaundice

*Retinol equivalents
†International units.

Retinoids

Chemical forms of preformed vitamin A; one source is animal foods.

Carotenoids

Pigment substances in plants that can often form vitamin A. Beta-carotene is the most active form in terms of vitamin A activity.

Vitamin A

The amount of vitamin A you consume is very important. Either too much or too little vitamin A can cause severe problems (Figure 8-2). Vitamin A is found in foods in a variety of forms. Retinol is one example. As a family, the various forms are called *preformed vitamin A* or **retinoids.** Vitamin A activity in the diet also occurs in the form of common plant pigments—**carotenoids**—such as the yellow-orange, beta-carotene pigment in carrots. Carotenoids are also called provitamin A because parts can often be turned into vitamin A. Over 600 carotenoids are found in nature; about 50 of them serve as provitamin A. The most potent form of provitamin A is beta-carotene. The preformed vitamin A and the provitamin A carotenoids both make up what is generically referred to as *vitamin A.*[28]

Functions of Vitamin A

Vitamin A performs many important functions in the body. Although researchers have studied vitamin A since its discovery in 1913, its exact roles in the cell are still baffling. Its importance to vision is perhaps its best-known role and the only role clearly understood. Researchers are investigating other ways that vitamin A functions in the body. Body changes that occur when vitamin A is lacking provide clues to its function.

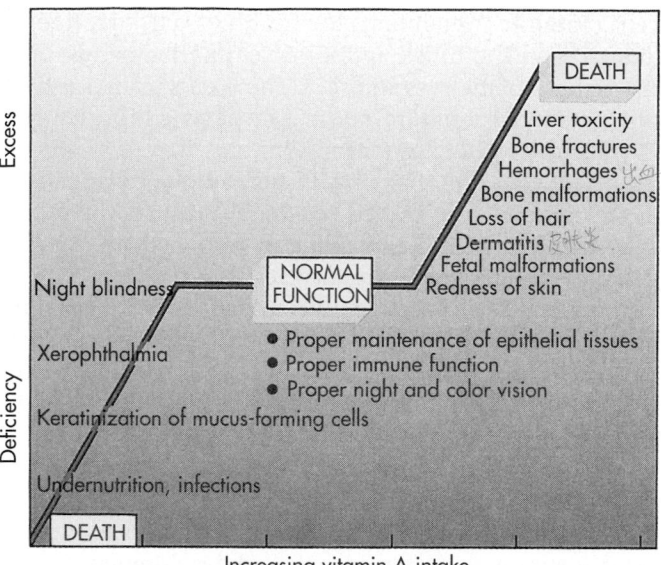

Figure 8-2 *Consuming the right amount of vitamin A is critical to overall health. RDA amounts promote health of a variety of body tissues. A very low (deficient) or a very high (toxic) vitamin A intake can produce damaging symptoms and even lead to death. The severity of effects and the intake range vary among individuals.*

Vision. The link between vitamin A and night vision has been known since ancient Egyptian times, when juice extracted from liver was used as a cure for night blindness. Vitamin A performs important functions in light-dark and color vision. It is a key part of the **visual cycle.**[16] For a person to see in dim light, one form of vitamin A is required to start the chemical process that signals the brain that light is striking the eye. This allows the eye to adjust from bright to dim light (such as after seeing the headlights of an oncoming car). Without sufficient dietary vitamin A, eventually the eye cannot quickly readjust to dim light. The condition is known as **night blindness.** An injection of vitamin A into the bloodstream can cure night blindness in a matter of minutes!

If night blindness is not corrected and vitamin A deficiency progresses, the cells that line the cornea of the eye (the clear window of the eye) also lose their ability to produce mucus. The eye then becomes dry. Eventually, when dirt particles scratch the dry surface of the eye, bacteria infect it. The infection soon spreads to the entire surface of the eye and leads to blindness. This disease process is called *xerophthalmia,* which means *dry eye.*

Vitamin A deficiency is second only to accidents as a worldwide cause of blindness. Americans are at little risk because of generally good diets. However, people—especially children—in less-developed nations are very susceptible to vitamin A deficiency. Poor dietary intakes and low stores of vitamin A fail to meet the children's high needs during rapid childhood growth. About 250,000 children in Asia become blind each year because of vitamin A deficiency.

Today, widespread deficiencies of vitamin A consitute one of the most important public health problems in developing countries. As covered in more detail in Chapter 18, worldwide attempts to reduce this problem have included giving large doses of vitamin A twice yearly and supplementing sugar, margarine, and monosodium glutamate with vitamin A. These food vehicles are used because they are commonly consumed by the populations of less-developed nations. In some countries this effort has proved effective.

A recent study also suggests that deterioration of the retina more likely takes place when a person's diet is low in certain carotenoids (e.g., lutein and zeaxanthin) over an extended period of time. Spinach and other leafy greens are good sources of these carotenoids.[34]

Visual cycle

A chemical process in the eye that participates in vision. Forms of vitamin A participate in the process.

Night blindness

A vitamin deficiency condition in which the retina (in the eye) cannot adjust to low amounts of light.

Xerophthalmia

Literally "dry eye." This is a cause of blindness that results from a vitamin A deficiency. The specific cause is linked to a lack of mucus production by the eye, which then leaves it at a greater risk of damage from surface dirt and bacteria.

In the United States the leading cause of blindness in adults is diabetes; in children, it is accidents.

Epithelial cells
The surface cells that line the outside of the body and all external passages within it.

Health and cells. Vitamin A maintains the health of cells that line internal and external "skin" surfaces in the lungs, intestines, stomach, vagina, urinary tract, and bladder, as well as those of the eyes and skin. These cells (called *epithelial cells*) serve as important barriers to bacterial infection. As just noted for the eye, some epithelial cells secrete mucus, a needed lubricant. Without vitamin A, mucus-forming cells deteriorate and no longer synthesize mucus. Instead, the cells make a protein, typically found in the hair and nails, called *keratin*. This causes the cells to harden and crack, disabling them as barriers to invading microorganisms. First affected by this loss of mucus-synthesizing capacity are the eyes.

Vitamin A deficiency also causes insufficient mucus production in the intestines and lung cells and poor health of cells in general. All of this increases the risk of body infections. Vitamin A deficiency also reduces the activity of certain immune cells. Together, these effects leave the vitamin A–deficient person at great risk for infections.

Growth, development, and reproduction. Vitamin A is necessary for cell growth and development. Vitamin A causes DNA in a cell's nucleus to increase its synthesis of cell proteins that stimulate proper growth and development.[11] One consequence of vitamin A deficiency in laboratory animals is that they cannot reproduce. Resorbing old bone, which must occur before new bone can be deposited, requires bone cells that also use vitamin A. In addition, producing some components of bone requires vitamin A.

Cancer prevention. Most forms of cancer arise from cells that are influenced by vitamin A. Coupled with its ability to aid immune system activity, vitamin A could be a valuable tool in the fight against cancer. This is especially true for skin, lung, bladder, and breast cancers. Scientists have been encouraged by research using laboratory animals.[11]

Cancer research with humans using various forms of vitamin A is under way in research centers throughout the world. The results to date indicate that use of vitamin A supplements can lower the risk of breast cancer among women with very low intakes of dietary vitamin A.[22] However, most studies on prostate cancer indicate no protective effect from dietary vitamin A. The data from colon cancer studies are the same: vitamin A has little protective effect against this form of cancer. Because of the potential for toxicity, use of megadose vitamin A supplements to reduce cancer risk is currently not advised.

Carotenoids by themselves also may help prevent cancer. The many double bonds present in some carotenoids make them effective traps for the energy in certain **free radical** compounds that can probably initiate the cancer process (see the discussion on vitamin E for details). Epidemiological evidence shows that regular consumption of foods rich in carotenoids decreases the risk of lung and oral cancer.[14] However, recall from Chapter 3 that recent studies from here and in Finland failed to show a reduction in lung cancer or heart disease in male smokers and nonsmokers who were given supplements of beta-carotene for 5 or more years. In fact, beta-carotene use increased the lung cancer cases compared with the control groups. No comparable studies have been done with women.

One possible explanation for the absence of a benefit from the beta-carotene supplement may be that it was started too late in the course of the disease or that the supplement interfered with the metabolism of other **antioxidants**. In addition, something else in carotenoid-rich foods—other carotenoids, dietary fiber, various cancer-blocking chemicals (for example, the phytochemical sulphoraphane, isolated from broccoli), or something not yet discovered—may confer the benefit of carotenoids seen in the epidemiological studies.

Much more investigation is needed in this area before specific recommendations regarding carotenoids and cancer prevention—other than eating fruits and

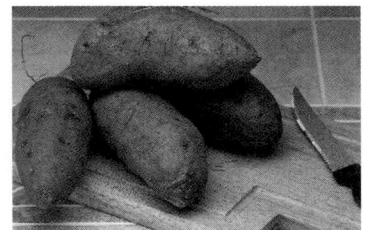

Sweet potatoes are rich in provitamin A carotenoids.

vegetables regularly—can be made.[23] For now the best advice to prevent lung cancer is still to eat a combination of at least 5 fruits and vegetables a day and not smoke.

Vitamin A for acne. The acne medication tretinoin (Retin-A) is made of one form of vitamin A. It has been used as a topical treament (applied to the skin) for acne for more than 10 years. It appears to work by altering cell activity in the skin. Another derivative of vitamin A, 13-cis retinoic acid (Accutane), is an oral drug used to treat serious acne. Note that taking high doses of vitamin A itself would not be safe. Even Accutane, a less toxic form, can induce toxicity symptoms. A person using either Retin-A or Accutane must also limit sun exposure because these drugs cause skin to sunburn easily. Furthermore, Accutane carries such a high risk for fetal malformations when used by pregnant women that women who could become pregnant should not use Accutane (see later section).

Vitamin A in Foods and the RDA

Vitamin A in foods exists in either the animal form (preformed vitamin A) or plant form (provitamin A).[28] Preformed vitamin A is found in liver, fish oils, vitamin A–fortified milk, and eggs. Butter and margarine are also sources because they are fortified with vitamin A. Provitamin A is found mainly in dark green and orange vegetables and some fruits. Carrots, spinach, squash, broccoli, papayas, and apricots are examples of sources. Consuming a varied diet rich in green vegetables and carrots ensures sufficient sources for meeting vitamin A needs (Figure 8-3). About half of the vitamin A in the American diet comes from animal sources, the other half from plants.

Recently, derivatives of vitamin A (Retin-A) have been put into creams (Renova) that reduce some effects of aging on the skin. Note that if the skin is already deeply wrinkled, these creams are ineffective. Limiting sun exposure (especially between 10 AM and 3 PM) and using sunblocks (sun protection factor [SPF] 15 or higher) are much better preventive measures. Also keep in mind that no tan is safe when it comes to protecting skin from damage.

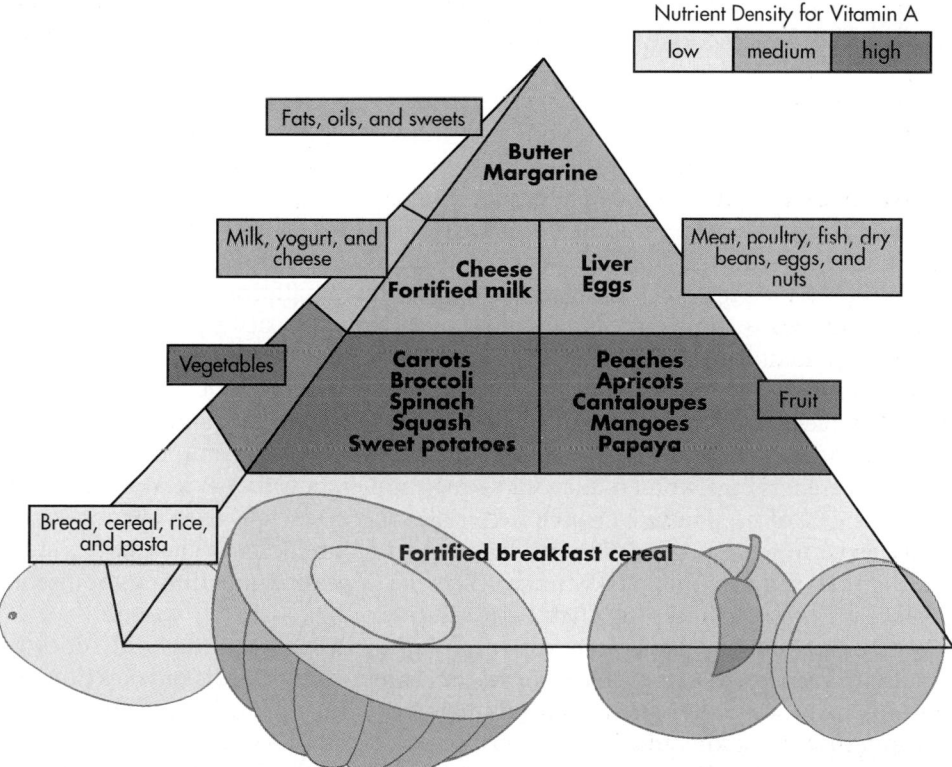

Figure 8-3 *Food sources of vitamin A from the Food Guide Pyramid. The fruit and vegetable groups supply abundant carotenoids if they have an intense yellow-orange or green color. Some of these carotenoids yield vitamin A. Liver is the richest source of preformed vitamin A, because that is the major site of vitamin A storage in animals. Milk is often fortified with vitamin A. The background color of each food group indicates the average number density for vitamin A in that group.*

Retinol equivalents (RE). For vitamin A the current unit of measurement is the retinol equivalent (RE). In this system, all potential forms of vitamin A are scaled based on their activity. Most nutrient amounts in foods, including vitamin A, were formerly expressed in less precise **international units (IU)**. Some supplement labels still show the older IU values for nutrients, but these are being replaced as manufacturers switch to the new Nutrition Facts label. Based on a mixture of preformed and provitamin A, 1 RE of vitamin A is equivalent to 5 IU of vitamin A.

RDA for vitamin A. The RDA for vitamin A is 1000 RE for men and 800 RE for women. (Throughout this and the next chapter, refer to the inside cover for nutrient recommendations for other ages and to Appendix F for Canadian recommendations.) The average intake for adult men and women in the United States is slightly above these values.[1]

In America, poor vitamin A status has been noted among preschool children who do not eat enough vegetables. The urban poor, older people, and people who are alcoholics or who have liver disease (which limits vitamin A storage) can also show poor vitamin A status. Finally, children with severe fat malabsorption, as in cases of cystic fibrosis, may also show a vitamin A deficiency.

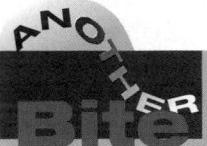

Parents often encourage their children to eat vegetables. Besides contributing to good food habits, this practice helps children consume enough vitamin A. Parents—important role models for children—can positively influence their children's eating interests by eating their own vegetables.

Toxicity of vitamin A. An intake of just 5 times the RDA for vitamin A can cause problems if taken for a prolonged time, especially during pregnancy and in the elderly years. A high preformed vitamin A intake is especially dangerous during the early months of pregnancy because it may cause **fetal** malformations.[31] Birth defects and spontaneous abortions can be caused by vitamin A toxicity, possibly beginning with even as little as 3 times the RDA. In nonpregnant adults, skin, hair, internal organs, and the central nervous system are most affected. These adverse effects in adults generally disappear after the doses stop. Permanent damage to the liver, bones, and eyes and recurrent joint and muscle pain, however, can occur.

Researchers urge women to avoid taking supplements that exceed 1.5 times the RDA (150% of it), and to consume rich food sources, such as liver, in moderation. This also applies to women who may become pregnant. Because vitamin A is stored in the body for long periods, women who take large amounts during the months before pregnancy could place their babies at risk.

The ingestion of large amounts of vitamin A–yielding carotenoids does not cause toxic effects. If someone consumes large amounts of carrots or takes pills containing beta-carotene (more than 30 milligrams daily), or if infants eat a great deal of squash, high carotenoid concentration in the blood can occur. This can turn the skin yellow-orange. The palms of the hand and soles of the feet in particular become colored. This condition does not appear to cause harm and disappears when the excess carotenoids decrease. Dietary carotenoids do not produce toxic effects because (1) their rate of conversion into vitamin A is relatively slow and regulated, and (2) the efficiency of carotenoid absorption from the small intestine decreases markedly as oral intake increases.[28]

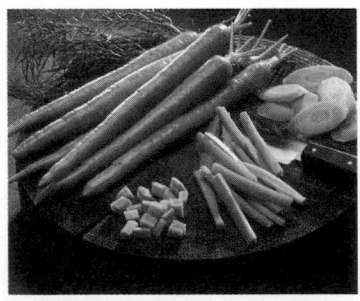

Foods rich in carotenoids pose little threat of vitamin A toxicity.

Vitamin D

Vitamin D is not just a vitamin. It is also considered a hormone because cells in the skin can convert a cholesterol-like substance to vitamin D, using sunlight. These skin cells are different from those cells that respond mostly to vitamin D, namely bone cells and kidney cells (Figure 8-4).

Recall from Chapter 1 that a hormone is a substance made in the body that travels from the point of synthesis through the bloodstream to act at a different site.

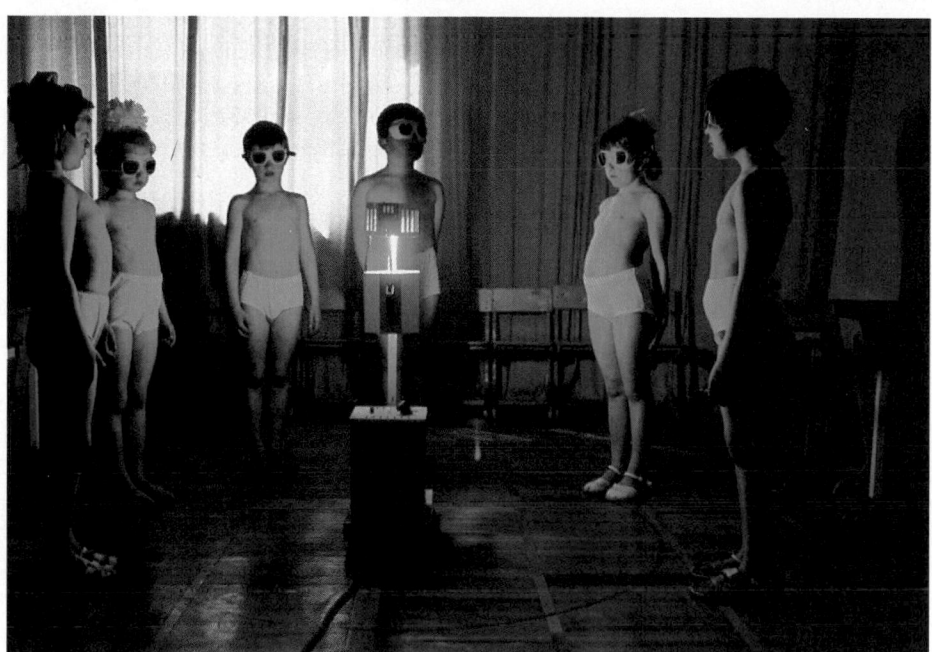

Figure 8-4 *Who's got the tanning oil? Southern Russia endures a long winter. These girls are exposed to a quartz lamp to provide the vitamin D synthesis they would normally experience from playing outdoors.*

The amount of sun exposure people need to produce vitamin D depends on their skin color and their age: young, light-skinned people meet vitamin D needs through casual sun exposure, about 10 minutes per day on the face and hands. Dark-skinned people and older people need more sun exposure than light-skinned and younger people. For example, people with very dark skin, such as those of African descent, need about 10 times more sun exposure. Older people living in northern latitudes during the winter risk not making enough vitamin D because the prevailing sunlight under these conditions is less effective in promoting its synthesis.[20] Anyone who does not receive enough sunshine to synthesize an adequate amount of vitamin D must have a dietary source of the vitamin.

As just noted, the starting product for vitamin D synthesis in the body is a cholesterol-like substance. Ultraviolet light shining on the skin is needed to convert this into vitamin D. Vitamin D toxicity does not result from tanning in the sun too long because the body regulates the amount made in the skin. The same cannot be said for dietary vitamin D sources. Its uptake into the body is not blocked when eaten in high doses. To become the active hormone, vitamin D must be metabolized by the liver and then the kidneys.

Vitamin D
↓ *action by the liver*

25-hydroxy vitamin D
↓ *action by kidney*

1,25 dihydroxy vitamin D (active hormone form, also called calcitriol)

Function of Vitamin D

The main function of the vitamin D hormone (called *calcitriol*)—produced by this two-step process—is to help regulate calcium and bone metabolism. In concert with other hormones, especially **parathyroid hormone (PTH),** vitamin D closely regulates

Calcitriol
The active hormone form of vitamin D (1,25-dihydroxy-vitamin D).

Rickets

A disease characterized by softening of the bones because of poor calcium content. This deficiency disease arises from insufficient vitamin D activity in the body.

Osteomalacia

Adult form of rickets. The weakening of the bones that is seen in this disease is caused by poor calcium content. A reduction in the amount of the vitamin D hormone activity in the body is the cause.

Be careful not to confuse osteomalacia with osteoporosis, another type of bone disorder discussed in Chapter 9.

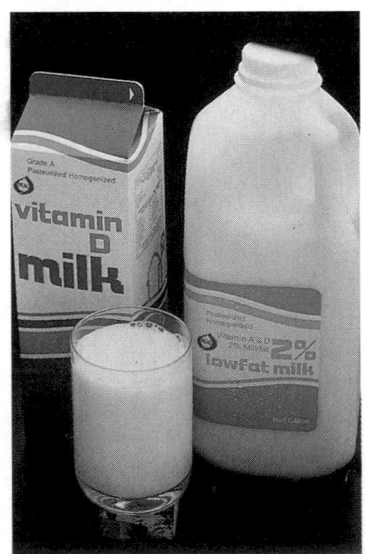

Milk is fortified with vitamin D.

blood calcium to supply appropriate amounts of it to all cells. This task entails a variety of processes: the vitamin D hormone helps regulate absorption of calcium and phosphorus from the intestine, it reduces kidney excretion of calcium, and it helps regulate the deposition of calcium in the bones.[20]

Even tissues in the brain, pancreas, and pituitary gland appear to be influenced by the vitamin D hormone. More interestingly, vitamin D is capable of influencing development in some cancer cells, such as skin, bone, and breast cancer cells.[4] Indeed, adequate vitamin D status has been linked to a reduced risk for developing breast, colon, and prostate cancer. Recent studies have also shown that the vitamin D hormone controls the growth of the parathyroid gland, aids in the function of the immune system, and contributes to insulin secretion and skin cell development. The latter reason is why a form of vitamin D is used in a topical preparation to help treat the skin disorder psoriasis.[4]

Rickets and osteomalacia. The net result of vitamin D hormone action is increased calcium and phosphorus deposition in bones. Without adequate calcium and phosphorus, bones weaken and bow under pressure. A child with these symptoms has the disease **rickets.** Symptoms also include enlarged head, joints, and rib cage and a deformed pelvis.

For the prevention of rickets, infant diets, especially those of breastfed infants after their first 9 months of life, should contain a food source or supplement of vitamin D (the latter under a physician's guidance) if sufficient exposure to sunlight is not possible. Keep in mind that supplements should be used very carefully to avoid vitamin D toxicity. Vitamin D fortification of milk has greatly reduced the risk of rickets in children. Today, rickets is most commonly associated with fat malabsorption, such as occurs in children with cystic fibrosis. It is important to maximize the amount of vitamin D these children make using sunlight.

An adult disease comparable to rickets is **osteomalacia,** which means *soft bones.* It results when calcium is withdrawn from the bones to make up for inefficient absorption in the intestine or poor conservation by the kidneys. Both of these calcium-related problems can be caused by vitamin D deficiency. Bones then lose their minerals and become porous and weak and break easily. This leads to fractures in the hip and other bones.

Osteomalacia in adults occurs most commonly in people with kidney, stomach, gallbladder, or intestinal disease (especially when most of the intestine has been removed) and in people with cirrhosis of the liver. These diseases affect both vitamin D metabolism and calcium absorption. Adults with limited sun exposure may also develop the disease. In fact, current studies show that osteomalacia is present among some older people. Combinations of sun exposure (about 20 minutes per day), vitamin D intake, or both should be used to prevent this problem.[32]

Vitamin D in Foods and the RDA

When exposure to sunshine does not create sufficient vitamin D, fatty fish (and fish oils) and fortified milk serve as the most nutrient-dense sources. Although milk is not a naturally rich source of vitamin D, it is fortified in the United States by adding 10 micrograms (400 IU) of vitamin D to each quart. Eggs, butter, and liver contain vitamin D but require too great a serving size to be considered significant sources. So few other foods contain vitamin D that food tables do not list sources.

The RDA of vitamin D for adults varies from 5 to 10 micrograms (200 to 400 IU) per day. Recall that young, light-skinned people are able to make this amount of vitamin D from casual sun exposure. Infants, children, and adolescents have higher RDAs because of their growing bones. As noted, anyone who both stays inside most of the day and ingests little or no vitamin D is at risk for developing vitamin D deficiency. This includes older people and infants who are fed only human milk. These groups of people need either a more predictable amount of sun exposure or a regular food source of vitamin D or both. For older people, a supplement of 10 to 20 micrograms (400 to 800 IU) should suffice.[20]

Toxicity of vitamin D. As little as five times the RDA of vitamin D taken regularly can create an overdose, especially in children. Consuming more than 25 micrograms (1000 IU) of vitamin D per day requires close monitoring by a physician. Toxicity particularly results in overabsorption of calcium and eventual calcium deposits in the kidneys and other organs. The person also suffers the typical symptoms of high blood calcium: weakness, loss of appetite, diarrhea, vomiting, mental confusion, and increased urine output. Calcium deposits in organs cause metabolic disturbances and cell death.

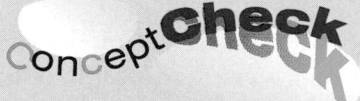

Vitamin A is found in foods as preformed vitamin A and as provitamin A carotenoids. The most fully understood function of vitamin A is its importance in vision. Blindness caused by vitamin A deficiency is a major problem in many parts of the world. Vitamin A is also needed to maintain the health of many types of cells, support the immune system, and promote proper growth and development. Vitamin A may be important in preventing cancer. However, because taking supplements of preformed vitamin A can be toxic, especially in pregnancy, the best recommendation is to focus primarily on eating plenty of provitamin A–rich foods, such as fruits and vegetables.

Vitamin D is a true vitamin only for people who fail to produce enough from sunlight, such as some older people. Using a cholesterol-like substance, people synthesize vitamin D by the action of sunlight on their skin. The vitamin D is later metabolized by the liver and kidneys to form the active hormone calcitriol. This hormone increases calcium absorption in the intestine and works with another hormone to maintain proper calcium metabolism in bones and other organs in the body. Significant food sources of vitamin D are fish oils and fortified milk. Dietary vitamin D can be quite toxic.

Vitamin E

Vitamin E has been called the "vitamin in search of a deficiency disease." However, growing evidence suggests that an inadequate intake increases the risk for heart disease and cancer.[8]

Functioning as a fat-soluble antioxidant, vitamin E resides mostly in cell membranes. As discussed in Chapter 6, an antioxidant can form a barrier between a target molecule—an unsaturated fatty acid in a cell membrane, for example—and a compound seeking its electrons (Figure 8-5). The antioxidant donates electrons or hydrogens or both to the electron-seeking compound (called an *oxidizing compound*) to neutralize it. This protects other molecules or parts of a cell from having electrons nabbed.[15] Note that vitamin C is a water-soluble antioxidant.

If vitamin E is not available to do its job, an electron-seeking compound can pull electrons from cell membranes, DNA, and other electron-dense cell components.[13] This either alters the cell's DNA, which may increase the risk for cancer, or injures cell membranes, possibly causing the cell to die.

One group of electron-seeking compounds found in cells is the free radicals. These were mentioned in Chapter 6 in relation to heart disease. Recall that free radicals are highly reactive compounds containing an unpaired electron. Carbon and

Sunblock agents with an SPF of 8 or above reduce vitamin D synthesis in the skin. Use of these agents is recommended during prolonged sun exposure to reduce the risk of skin cancer. Such use is unlikely to result in low vitamin D status in children, because they undoubtedly spend some time each day in the sun without sunblock protection (for example, during school recess or traveling to and from school). In addition, children often drink vitamin D–fortified milk. In contrast, elderly people should be sure to spend about 20 minutes each day in the sun without sunblock protection or seek a dietary source of vitamin D.[20]

oxygen often form free-radical species. Free radicals seek electrons by attacking other compounds. Often a free radical is generated by cleavage of a chemical bond, with each breakdown product taking an electron from the original pair. This action yields two compounds, each having one unpaired electron.

Free-radical production is a normal result of cell metabolism and immune-system function. For example, white blood cells generate free radicals as part of their action to stop infection. Some exposure to free radicals, then, is part of life. Overall, the body just needs to carefully regulate this exposure to avoid their undesirable effects.[18]

One reason that free radicals are destructive to cells is that they can set off a chain reaction in which thousands of free radicals are generated within minutes of starting from a single one. Vitamin E is one of the body's primary means of interrupting free-radical chain reactions (see Figure 8-5). Once vitamin E acts, some of it is excreted and some of it is recycled by the addition of an electron from other antioxidants (for example, vitamin C).[15]

Many other antioxidant systems exist in cells as well. Cells do not rely exclusively on vitamin E for protection from free radicals. Systems also exist in cells to repair molecules (such as DNA) that have been damaged by free radicals.[36]

This discussion raises the question of the relative role of vitamin E in oxidant protection in the body. Experts do not know whether taking vitamin E supplements confers any additional protection against heart disease and cancer than that achieved by improving diet (especially fruit and vegetable intake), performing regular physical activity, not smoking, and maintaining a healthy body weight. This advice has the widest scientific support in the battle against these diseases.[23,37] Furthermore, the proven benefits of these lifestyle changes are far greater than the postulated benefits of supplemental antioxidants, including vitamin E. Thus even if antioxidant supplements are determined to be effective in preventing heart disease and cancer, they should be used (even in people at high risk) only as an adjunct—not as an alternative—to a healthful lifestyle.

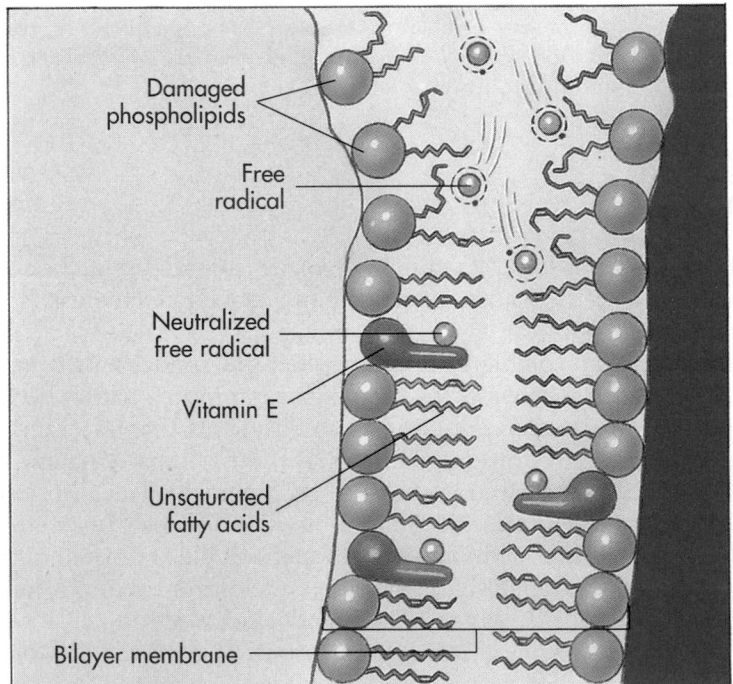

Figure 8-5 *Fat-soluble vitamin E can insert itself into cell membranes, where it helps stop free-radical chain reactions. If not interrupted, these reactions cause extensive oxidative damage to cells and ultimately cell death.*

Vitamin E can help improve vitamin A absorption if the dietary intake of vitamin A is low. In addition, vitamin E is used to metabolize iron in the cell and help maintain nervous tissue, immune, and insulin function.[13]

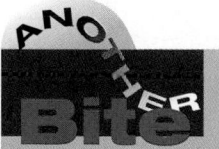

The mineral selenium can spare some of the body's need for vitamin E. Selenium enables an enzyme in cells to decrease the formation of certain oxidizing compounds. Thus an adequate dietary intake of selenium (from cereals, meats, and seafood) reduces the need for vitamin E, whereas low selenium intake in the diet increases it.

A deficiency of vitamin E causes cell membrane breakdown, especially in red blood cells of premature infants. Unsaturated fatty acids in the red blood cell membrane are very sensitive to attack by oxidizing compounds. Because vitamin E neutralizes these agents, it protects the red blood cell membrane from damage. Red blood cell breakage, called *hemolysis,* commonly occurs in premature infants because they did not receive sufficient vitamin E from their mothers. The rapid growth of premature infants, coupled with the high oxygen concentration found in infant incubators, greatly increases the stress on red blood cells. This raises the risk of cell damage. Special formulas and supplements designed for premature infants can help compensate for lack of vitamin E.[13]

Vitamin E has been promoted as an antiaging vitamin. As cells age, they accumulate lipid-oxidation products. The accumulation of *lipofuscin (ceroid pigments)* in cells and increased opacity of the eye lens are examples of aging caused by oxidative damage to tissues. Although these oxidative changes might indicate a nutrient deficiency, no clear evidence suggests that supplementation with vitamin E and other antioxidants slows the aging process; however, an inadequate intake likely promotes this oxidative damage.

Vitamin E in Foods and the RDA

The most nutrient-dense food sources of vitamin E are plant oils; some fruits and vegetables, such as asparagus and green leafy vegetables; and margarine. The vitamin E in plant oils is used to protect the unsaturated fats present in plant oils. Animal fats and fish oils, on the other hand, have practically no vitamin E (Figure 8-6). The actual vitamin E content of a food depends on how it was harvested, processed, stored, and cooked because vitamin E is very susceptible to destruction by oxygen, metals, light, and especially repeated use of oils in deep-fat frying.

The RDA of vitamin E for adults is 8 to 10 milligrams per day of **alpha-tocopherol,** the most active form of what is called vitamin E. This is about the amount we eat each day.[1] To convert from the older IU system, 10 milligrams equals about 10 IU, based on the usual form of vitamin E found in supplements.

The likelihood of finding signs of a vitamin E deficiency in the United States among healthy nonsmokers is very low. However, the beneficial effects of vitamin E and other antioxidants in counteracting free radical damage in biological systems is most apparent when viewed on a long-term basis because free radical–related damage to cells occurs over time. Thus current research can't rule out that some benefit—heart disease and cancer reduction included—may occur from intakes of vitamin E in excess of the RDA. Studies continue, using megadoses from 100 to 800 milligrams (IU) per day. However, current evidence is insufficient to convince many scientists or FDA that this practice is entirely safe or effective.[2, 18]

To postpone the effects of aging, the following practices are recommended: consume a diet based on the Food Guide Pyramid; see your physician regularly (for early diagnosis of health problems); avoid smoking; limit your alcohol intake; maintain a healthy body weight; and stay physically active. These factors have a much greater influence on the rate of aging than does vitamin E.

Hemolysis
Destruction of red blood cells. The red blood cell membrane breaks down, allowing cell contents to leak into the fluid portion of the blood.

Lipofuscin (ceroid pigments)
Lipid breakdown products in cells. These compounds have fluorescence, and in that way can be detected in aged cells, such as those in the eye, the heart, and the brain.

Tocopherols
The chemical name for some forms of vitamin E. The alpha form is the most potent.

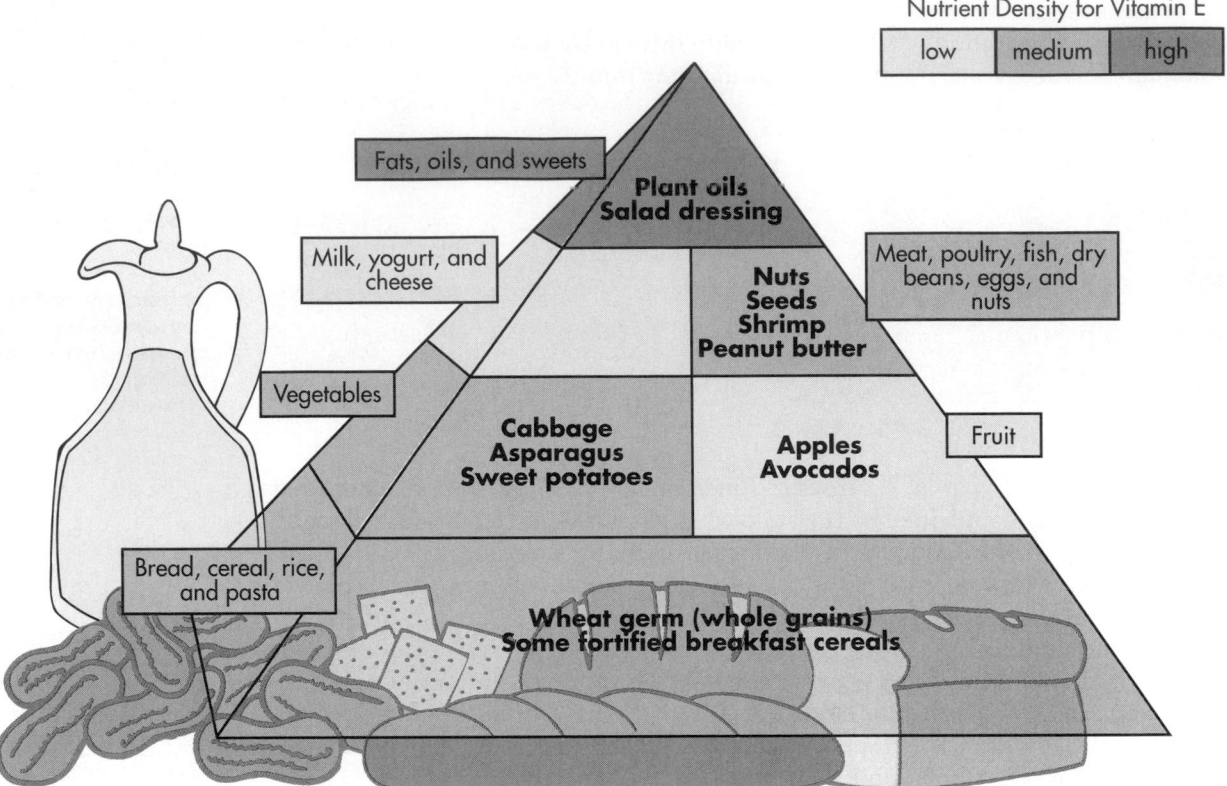

Figure 8-6 *Food sources of vitamin E from the Food Guide Pyramid. Vitamin E is concentrated in plant oils, nuts, seeds, and some vegetables. The background color of each food group indicates the average nutrient density for vitamin E in that group.*

The Daily Value for vitamin E printed on food labels and supplement bottles (30 IU) is at least 3 times the current RDA. This is because the Daily Values are still based on the 1968 RDAs, which listed a higher RDA for vitamin E (see Chapter 2 for further details). Therefore, 100% of the Daily Value on a label corresponds to 3 or more times the current RDA for vitamin E.

Excessive amounts of vitamin E can antagonize vitamin K's role in the clotting mechanism. The risk of insufficient blood clotting is especially high if vitamin E is taken in conjunction with anticoagulant medications (this will be discussed in the next section). Otherwise, daily intakes of vitamin E of 800 milligrams (IU) are probably safe for people who are not taking anticoagulant medicines.[12] Vitamin E megadose studies should settle this question of the potential toxicity of vitamin E from long-term use.

Vitamin K

A family of compounds known collectively as vitamin K is found in plants, fish oils, and meats. One form is synthesized by bacteria in the human intestine. These bacteria supply us with some of the vitamin K we absorb every day. Most, however, comes from diet.[5]

Vitamin K is vital for blood clotting. The *K* stands for *koagulation,* as it is spelled in Denmark. This spelling is used because a Danish researcher first noted the relationship between vitamin K and blood clotting. Vitamin K contributes to the synthesis of several blood-clotting factors, including **prothrombin.**[29]

A newborn's intestinal tract lacks sufficient vitamin K–producing bacteria to allow for blood to clot effectively if the infant is injured. Therefore vitamin K injections are routinely given shortly after birth to bridge the gap until enough bacteria are present to synthesize the vitamin K needed by the infant. In adults, deficiencies of vitamin K have occurred when a person takes antibiotics for a long period and in the presence of severe long-standing fat malabsorption. Long-term antibiotic use most likely leads to this problem because it destroys many of the intestinal bacteria that normally account for some of the vitamin K absorbed.

Inactive blood-clotting factors
↓ Action of
vitamin K
Active blood-clotting factors

Vitamin K in Foods and the RDA

The most nutrient-dense food sources of vitamin K are liver, green leafy vegetables (for example, kale, turnip greens, cabbage, and spinach), broccoli, peas, and green beans. One reason to consume a diet rich in green vegetables is to obtain sufficient vitamin K. Most vitamin K consumed in a day disappears from the body by the next day. Nevertheless, vitamin K is abundant in a balanced diet, and a deficiency is uncommon. Vitamin K is quite resistant to cooking losses.

The RDA of vitamin K for adults is 60 to 80 milligrams per day. Most Americans consume at least this much.[5] As just noted, excessive amounts of vitamin E are known to antagonize the actions of vitamin K. Vitamin E can lead to a decrease in vitamin K–dependent clotting factors and increased bleeding tendency.

Oral vitamin K poses no risk of toxicity. The main problem with megadose use is reduced effectiveness in oral anticoagulants used by some people, especially those with blood-clotting disorders or who have undergone recent heart surgery.[29]

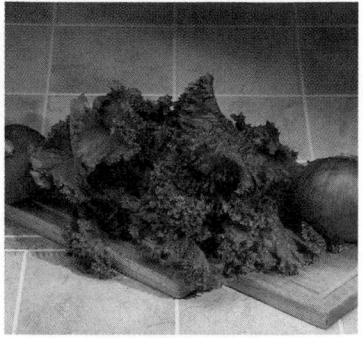

Green vegetables are rich sources of vitamin K.

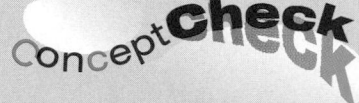

Vitamin E functions primarily as an antioxidant. It can donate electrons to electron-seeking free radical (oxidizing) compounds. By neutralizing these compounds, vitamin E helps prevent cell destruction, especially the destruction of red blood cell membranes. The richest sources of vitamin E are plant oils, but it occurs in a wide variety of foods.

Vitamin K plays a key role in efficient blood clotting; it contributes to the synthesis of certain blood-clotting proteins, such as prothrombin. Some of the vitamin K we absorb every day is synthesized by intestinal bacteria; most comes from our diets. The amount in the diet alone generally meets our daily needs. Thus, except for newborns, a deficiency of vitamin K is unlikely when one consumes some vegetables on a regular basis, even though it is readily excreted from the body.

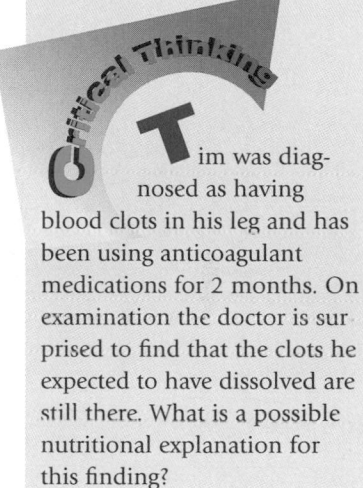

Critical Thinking

Tim was diagnosed as having blood clots in his leg and has been using anticoagulant medications for 2 months. On examination the doctor is surprised to find that the clots he expected to have dissolved are still there. What is a possible nutritional explanation for this finding?

THE WATER-SOLUBLE VITAMINS—THE B VITAMINS AND VITAMIN C

Water-soluble vitamins are more readily excreted than fat-soluble vitamins. Any excess generally ends up in the urine or stool, so consuming the water-soluble vitamins regularly is important. Because they dissolve in water, large amounts of these vitamins can be lost during food processing and preparation. A summary of much of what we know about water-soluble vitamins is presented in Table 8-3.

The B Vitamins

The B vitamins are thiamin, riboflavin, niacin, pantothenic acid, biotin, vitamin B-6, folate, and vitamin B-12. Because they often occur in the same foods, a lack of one B vitamin may mean other B vitamins are also low. The B vitamins are all changed into coenzymes, small molecules that can interact with enzymes to enable enzymes to function. In essence, the coenzymes contribute to enzyme activity[36] (see Figure 8-1).

The B vitamins play many key roles in metabolism. The metabolic pathways used by carbohydrates, fats, and amino acids together require input from B vitamins in their coenzyme forms. This makes many B vitamins interdependent because they participate in the same processes (Figure 8-7).

Vitamin status can be tested by measuring enzyme activities in red blood cells that require vitamins to function. Such biochemical tests for enzyme activity can be used to determine thiamin, riboflavin, and vitamin B-6 status.

TABLE 8-3

A Summary of the Water-Soluble Vitamins, Their Functions, Deficiency Conditions, and Food Sources

Name	Major functions	Deficiency symptoms	People most at risk	Dietary sources	RDA or ESADDI	Toxicity
Thiamin	Coenzyme involved in carbohydrate metabolism; nerve function	Beriberi: nervous tingling, poor coordination, edema, heart changes, weakness	People with alcoholism or in poverty	Sunflower seeds, pork, whole and enriched grains, dried beans, peas, brewer's yeast	1.1-1.5 milligrams	None possible from food
Riboflavin	Coenzyme involved in energy metabolism	Inflammation of mouth and tongue, cracks at corners of the mouth, eye disorders	Possibly people on certain medications if no dairy products consumed	Milk, mushrooms, spinach, liver, enriched grains	1.2-1.7 milligrams	None reported
Niacin	Coenzyme involved in energy metabolism, fat synthesis, fat breakdown	Pellagra: diarrhea, dermatitis, dementia	Severe poverty where corn is the dominant food; alcoholism	Mushrooms, bran, tuna, salmon, chicken, beef, liver, peanuts, enriched grains	15-19 milligrams	Flushing of skin at >100 milligrams
Pantothenic acid	Coenzyme involved in energy metabolism, fat synthesis, fat breakdown	Tingling in hands, fatigue, headache, nausea	People with alcoholism	Mushrooms, liver, broccoli, eggs; most foods have some	4-7 milligrams	None
Biotin	Coenzyme involved in glucose production, fat synthesis	Dermatitis, tongue soreness, anemia, depression	People with alcoholism	Cheese, egg yolks, cauliflower, peanut butter, liver	30-100 micrograms	Unknown
Vitamin B-6,* pyridoxine, and other forms	Coenzyme involved in protein metabolism, neurotransmitter synthesis, hemoglobin synthesis, many other functions	Headache, anemia, convulsions, nausea, vomiting, flaky skin, sore tongue	Adolescent and adult women; people on certain medications; alcoholism	Animal protein foods, spinach, broccoli, bananas, salmon, sunflower seeds	1.8-2 milligrams	Nerve destruction at doses >500 milligrams
Folate* (folic acid)	Coenzyme involved in DNA synthesis, other functions	Megaloblastic anemia, inflammation of tongue, diarrhea, poor growth, mental disorders	People with alcoholism, pregnancy, people on certain medications	Green leafy vegetables, orange juice, organ meats, sprouts, sunflower seeds	180-200 micrograms	None; nonprescription vitamin dosage is controlled by FDA
Vitamin B-12* (cobalamins)	Coenzyme involved in folate metabolism, nerve function, other functions	Macrocytic anemia, poor nerve function	Elderly people because of poor absorption; vegans	Animal foods, especially organ meats, oysters, clams (not natural in plants)	2 micrograms	None
Vitamin C (ascorbic acid)	Collagen synthesis, hormone synthesis, neurotransmitter synthesis	Scurvy: poor wound healing, pinpoint hemorrhages, bleeding gums	People with alcoholism, elderly men living alone	Citrus fruits, strawberries, broccoli, greens	60 milligrams	Doses >1-2 grams cause diarrhea and can alter some diagnostic tests

*These vitamins also participate in homocysteine metabolism, which in turn limits its ability to promote heart disease.

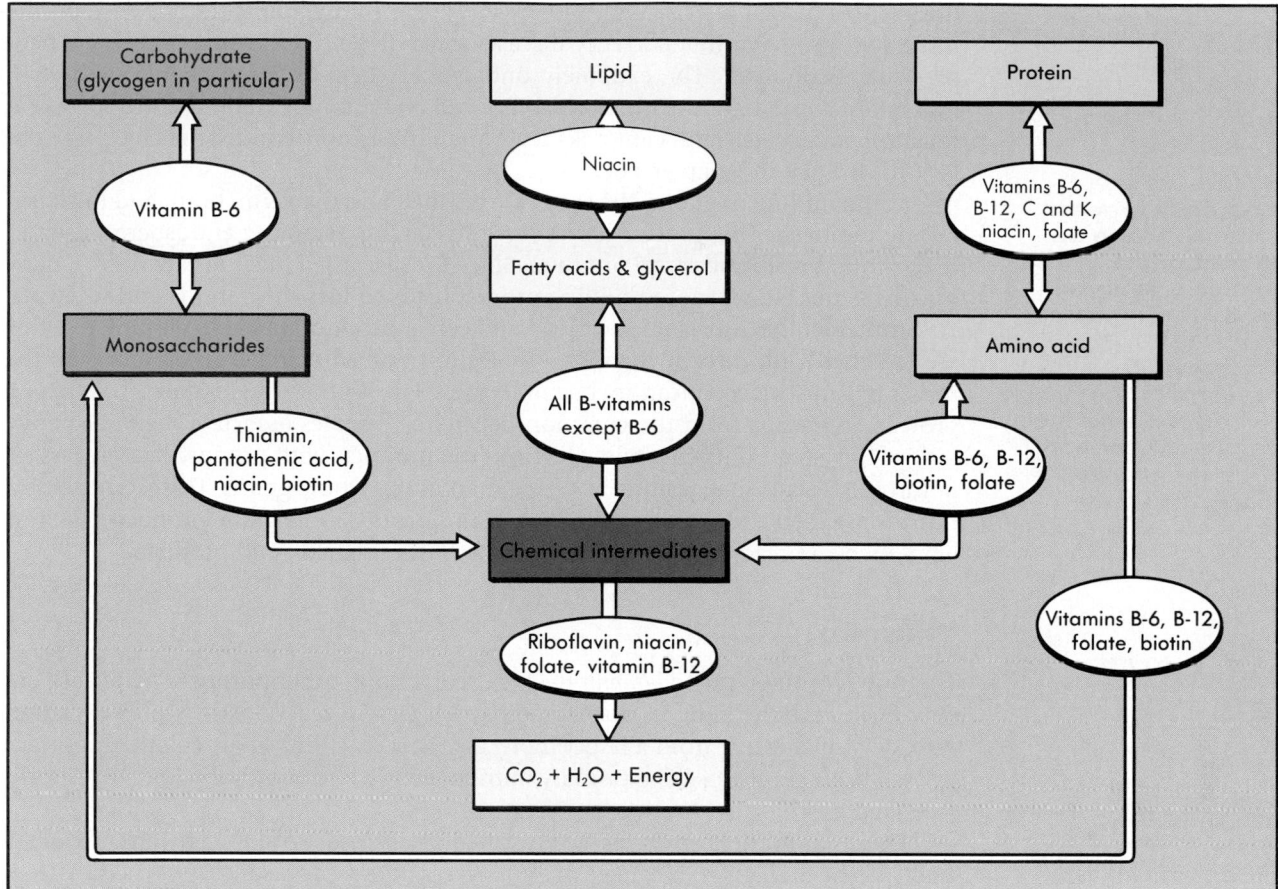

Figure 8-7 *Examples of metabolic pathways for which vitamins are essential. The metabolism of energy-yielding nutrients requires vitamin input.*

After being ingested, the B vitamins are first broken down from their coenzyme forms into free vitamins in the stomach and small intestine. The vitamins are then absorbed, primarily in the small intestine. Typically, about 50% to 90% of the B vitamins in the diet are absorbed. Once inside cells the coenzyme forms are resynthesized. Because we make them when needed, we don't need to consume the coenzyme forms themselves.

B Vitamin Status of Americans

The nutritional status of most Americans with regard to the B vitamins is generally good. Typical diets in the United States contain plentiful and varied natural sources of these vitamins.[1] In addition, many common foods are fortified with one or more of the water-soluble vitamins. In some developing countries, however, deficiencies of the water-soluble vitamins are more common, and the resulting deficiency diseases pose significant public-health problems. (A detailed discussion of nutritional deficiencies worldwide is presented in Chapter 18.)

Despite the generally good B vitamin status of Americans, marginal deficiencies of the water-soluble vitamins may occur in some Americans and others in the western world, especially older people. The long-term effects of such marginal deficiencies are as yet unknown, but increased risk of heart disease, cancer, and cataracts of the eye is suspected.[12, 35] However, in the short run, such a marginal deficiency in most people likely leads only to fatigue or other bothersome and

FDA has recently ordered that the vitamin folate be added as part of the enrichment of grain products. This will be in place by January 1, 1998. The intent is to provide adequate folate in the diets of women during the weeks before conception so as to reduce the risk of birth defects in their offspring (see section on folate).

Beriberi

The thiamin deficiency disorder characterized by muscle weakness, loss of appetite, nerve degeneration, and sometimes edema.

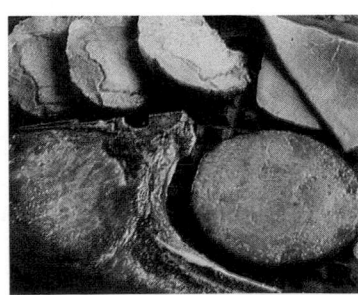

Pork is a good source of thiamin.

unspecific physical effects. With rare exceptions, healthy adults do not develop the more serious B vitamin deficiency diseases from diet alone. The exceptions are people with alcoholism. The extremely unbalanced diets of some people with alcoholism, in combination with alcohol-induced alteration of vitamin absorption and metabolism, create significant risks for some serious nutrient deficiencies[33] (see the Nutrition Issue in Chapter 16).

In the milling of grains, the seeds are crushed and the germ, bran, and husk layers are removed. This process leaves just the starch-containing endosperm, used to make flour, bread, and cereal products. Since the discarded fractions are rich in many nutrients, the time-honored milling process leads to loss of vitamins and minerals. To counteract this nutrient loss, bread and cereal products made from milled grains are enriched with three B vitamins—thiamin, riboflavin, and niacin—and with the mineral iron. This fortification, begun in the 1940s in the United States, has helped protect Americans from the common deficiency diseases associated with a dietary lack of the added nutrients but still leaves the products with proportionately less vitamin B-6, folate, magnesium, and zinc than in the whole grains. This is one reason nutrition experts advocate regular consumption of whole-grain products, such as whole-wheat bread, rather than consuming only enriched grain products.

Thiamin

Thiamin (formerly called *vitamin B-1*) is used, among other purposes, to release energy from carbohydrate. Its coenzyme participates in reactions in which a carbon dioxide (CO_2) is lost from a larger molecule. This reaction is particularly important in metabolizing glucose, the primary nutrient yielded from carbohydrate digestion[36] (see Figure 8-7).

The thiamin deficiency disease is called *beriberi*, a word that means "I can't, I can't" in the Sri Lankan language of Sinhalese. The symptoms include weakness, loss of appetite, irritability, nervous tingling throughout the body, poor arm and leg coordination, and deep muscle pain in the calves. A person with beriberi often develops an enlarged heart and sometimes severe edema (wet beriberi).

Beriberi is seen where rice is a staple and the polished (white) form is consumed rather than the brown (whole grain) form. In most parts of the world, brown rice has had its bran and germ layer removed to make white rice, a poor source of thiamin, unless later enriched.

Beriberi results when glucose, the primary fuel for brain and nerve cells, is poorly metabolized. Because the thiamin coenzyme participates in glucose metabolism, body functions associated with brain and nerve action quickly show signs of a thiamin deficiency. Symptoms of depression and weakness can be seen after only 10 days on a thiamin-free diet. This shows how limited the body's stores of thiamin are and how important it is to consume thiamin-rich foods daily. Thiamin probably also contributes in other ways to nerve function.

Thiamin in foods and the RDA. Foods that contain a very high nutrient density of thiamin include pork products and sunflower seeds. Whole grains (wheat germ), enriched grains, green beans, organ meats, peanuts, dried beans, and other seeds are also good sources.

Major contributors of thiamin to the American diet are white bread and rolls, crackers, pork, hot dogs, luncheon meat, cold cereals, orange juice, and dairy products. White bread, bakery products, and cereals are usually enriched with thiamin. They serve as important sources because many people eat them so often (Figure 8-8).

The adult RDA for thiamin is about 1.5 milligrams per day for men and 1.1 milligrams per day for women. Average daily intakes for men and women exceed the RDA values by 25%.[1] Some groups, such as poor people and older people, may

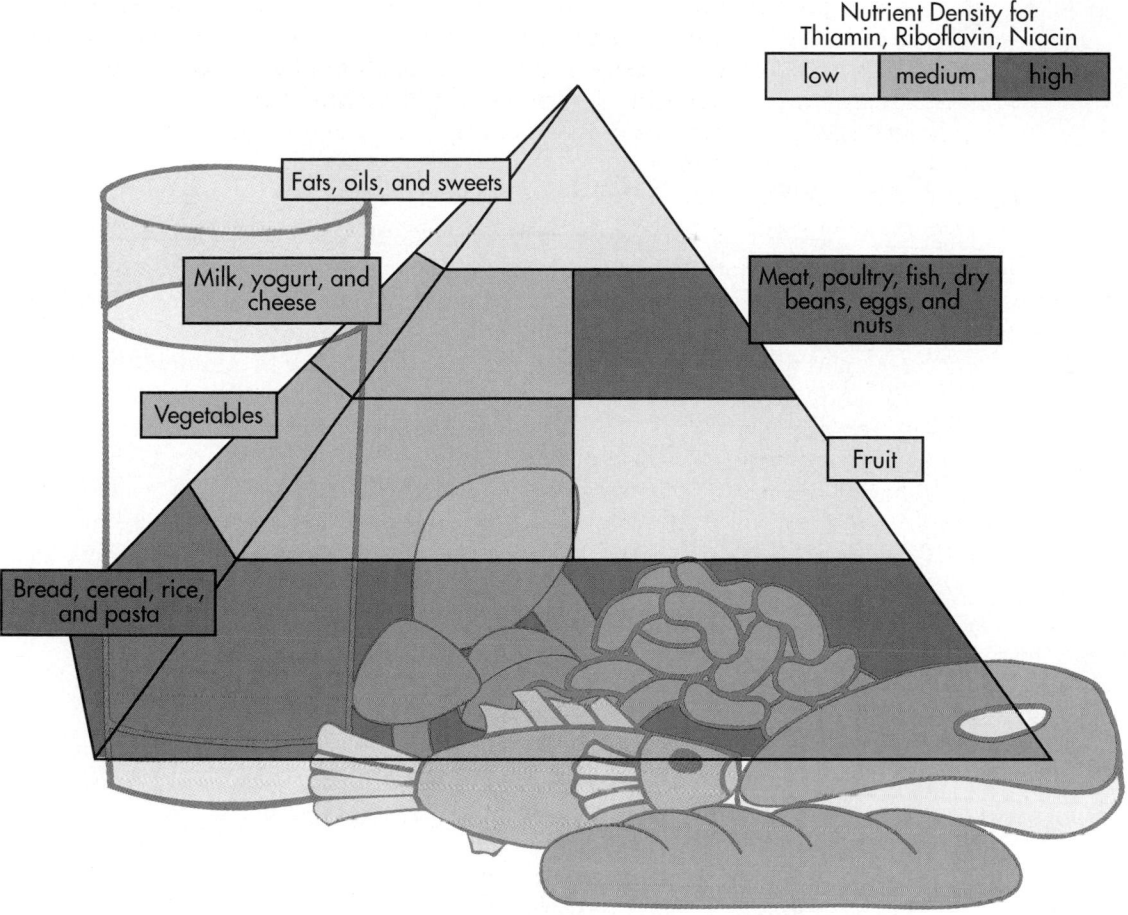

Figure 8-8 *Food sources of thiamin, riboflavin, and niacin from the Food Guide Pyramid. The meat, poultry, fish, dry beans, eggs, and nuts group and the bread, cereal, rice, and pasta group are especially rich sources of these nutrients. The background color of each food group indicates the average nutrient density for the nutrients in that group.*

barely meet their needs for thiamin. A diet dominated by highly processed and un-enriched foods, sugar, fat, and alcohol also creates a potential for thiamin deficiency. Oral thiamin supplements are essentially nontoxic.

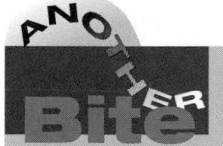

People with alcoholism are at great risk for thiamin deficiency because alcohol profoundly diminishes the ability to absorb and use thiamin. Furthermore, they often eat poorly. An alcohol-related thiamin deficiency can lead to a cluster of symptoms, including mental confusion, memory loss, and poor nervous system control of arms and legs.

Riboflavin

The name *riboflavin* comes from its yellow color (*flavus* means yellow in Latin). Riboflavin was formerly referred to as *vitamin B-2*.

The coenzymes of riboflavin participate in many energy-yielding metabolic pathways. When cells form cellular energy using oxygen-requiring pathways, such as

Preserving Vitamins in Food

Substantial amounts of vitamins in foods can be lost from the time a fruit or vegetable is picked until it is eaten. The water-soluble vitamins—particularly thiamin, vitamin C, and folate—can be destroyed with improper storage and excessive cooking. Heat, light, exposure to the air, cooking in water, and alkalinity are all factors that can destroy vitamins. The sooner the food is eaten, the less chance of nutrient loss.

In general, if the food is not to be eaten within a few days, freezing is the best method to retain nutrients. In fact, frozen vegetables and fruits are often as nutrient rich as supermarket-fresh ones. Frozen foods are often processed immediately after harvesting. As part of the freezing process, vegetables are quickly blanched in boiling water. This destroys the enzymes that would otherwise degrade the vitamins.

Below are some tips to aid in preserving the vitamins in food:

- Keep fruits and vegetables cool. Enzymes in foods begin to degrade vitamins once the fruit or vegetable is picked. Chilling reduces this process, so refrigerating these foods until they are consumed is important.
- Refrigerate foods in moisture-proof containers. Nutrients keep best at temperatures near freezing, at high humidity, and away from exposure to air.
- Avoid trimming and cutting fruits and vegetables into small pieces as much as possible: the more surface exposed, the faster oxygen breaks down vitamins. Keep in mind the outer leaves of lettuce and other greens have higher values of vitamins and minerals than the inner, tender leaves or stems. In addition, the skins of potatoes and apples and the outer layer of carrots are higher in vitamins and minerals than the center part.
- To retain the high amounts of nutrients in vegetables, microwave cooking, steaming, or using a pan or wok with very small amounts of water and a tight-fitting lid is best. The less contact with water and the shorter the cooking time, the more nutrients retained. Whenever possible, cook fruits or vegetables in their skins.
- Minimize reheating food, which reduces the vitamin content.
- Don't add baking soda to vegetables to enhance the green color. The alkalinity destroys much vitamin C, thiamin, and other vitamins.
- Store canned goods in a cool place. To get maximal nutritive value from the canned goods, serve any liquid packed with the food whenever possible. Canned foods vary in the amount of nutrients lost, largely because of differences in storage time and temperatures in the canning process.
- Keep milk cold, covered, and away from strong light. Riboflavin may be lost in direct light. Pasteurizing raw milk does not destroy the main nutrients that milk products provide (protein, riboflavin, and calcium, among others).

when fats are broken down and burned for energy, the coenzymes of riboflavin are used (see Figure 8-7). Some vitamin and mineral metabolism also requires riboflavin. In addition, because of its link to activity of certain enzymes, riboflavin is believed to have an antioxidant role in the body.[30]

The symptoms associated with riboflavin deficiency include inflammation of the mouth and tongue, **dermatitis,** cracking of tissue around the corners of the mouth (called *cheilosis*), various eye disorders, sensitivity to the sun, and confusion. The first symptoms of a deficiency are inflammation of the mouth and tongue. All symptoms associated with deficiency develop after approximately 2 months on a riboflavin-poor diet (containing one fourth or less of the RDA).

Clinicians have great difficulty identifying true riboflavin deficiency because it shares symptoms with deficiencies of other B vitamins, such as thiamin, vitamin B-6, and folate. In addition, riboflavin deficiencies probably do not exist by themselves. Instead, a riboflavin deficiency would occur with deficiencies of niacin, thiamin, and vitamin B-6 because these nutrients often occur in the same foods.

Riboflavin in foods and the RDA. Most riboflavin in the U.S. diet comes from one of the primary nutrient-dense sources: milk and milk products. The remainder of the U.S. riboflavin intake comes from enriched white bread, rolls, and crackers, as well as meat and eggs (see Figure 8-8). For some people a high meat consumption partially offsets a low intake of dairy products in terms of their meeting riboflavin needs.

The adult RDA of riboflavin is 1.4 to 1.7 milligrams per day for men and 1.2 to 1.3 milligrams per day for women. On average, daily intakes of riboflavin are slightly above the RDA.[1] Athletes at the outset of a training program may need extra riboflavin (about 1.5 times the RDA), partly because of their increased use of fatty acids as fuel and of all the energy-yielding pathways. As mentioned earlier, the riboflavin coenzymes are crucial to the operation of these pathways. The higher energy intakes typical of athletes should easily meet any additional riboflavin needs. People with alcoholism are the ones who primarily risk riboflavin deficiency because they generally eat nutrient-poor diets. No specific symptoms indicate that riboflavin taken in megadoses is toxic.

Niacin

Niacin is actually composed of a pair of related compounds. Both can function as niacin in the body. Niacin was formerly referred to as *vitamin B-3.*

The coenzyme forms of niacin function in many cellular metabolic pathways. In general, when cell energy is being formed, a niacin coenzyme is used. Synthetic pathways in the cell—those that make new compounds—also often use a niacin coenzyme. This is especially true for fat synthesis[36] (see Figure 8-7).

Because almost every cellular metabolic pathway uses a niacin coenzyme, a deficiency causes widespread changes in the body. The entire group of symptoms is known as *pellagra,* which means rough or painful skin. The symptoms of the disease are known as the three Ds—**dementia,** diarrhea, and dermatitis (especially on areas of skin exposed to the sun). Later, death often results. Early symptoms include poor appetite, weight loss, and weakness.

Pellagra became epidemic in southern Europe in the early 1700s when corn, a poor source, became a staple food. It became a major problem in the southeastern United States in the late 1800s and persisted until the late 1930s when standards of living and diets improved. In fact, pellagra is the only dietary deficiency disease ever to reach epidemic proportions in the United States. The pellagra epidemic in the United States in the early 1900s gave impetus to a federally sponsored program in 1941 to enrich grains. Pellagra is extremely uncommon today.

Dermatitis
Inflammation of the skin.

Dementia
A general loss or decrease in mental function.

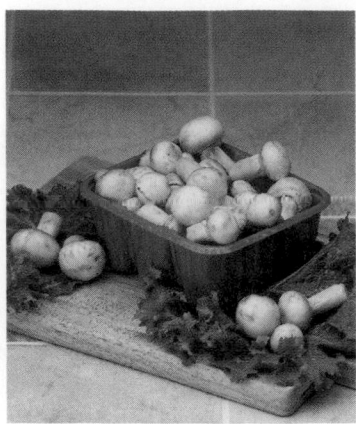

Mushrooms are a nutrient-dense source of niacin.

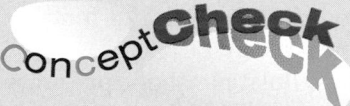

Niacin in corn is bound by a protein that hampers its absorption. Soaking corn in an alkaline solution, such as lime water (water with calcium hydroxide), releases bound niacin and renders it more usable. Hispanic people traditionally soak corn in lime water before making tortillas. This treatment is one reason Hispanic populations never suffered much pellagra.

Niacin in foods and the RDA. The most nutrient-dense sources of niacin are mushrooms, wheat bran, tuna and other fish, chicken, asparagus, and peanuts. Most niacin in the American diet comes from enriched white bread, rolls, crackers, and breakfast cereals (to which niacin is added as part of the enrichment process), beef, chicken, and turkey (see Figure 8-8). Niacin is very heat stable, so little is lost in cooking.

Besides the preformed niacin found in protein foods, every 60 milligrams of the amino acid tryptophan remaining after protein synthesis is metabolized into about 1 milligram of niacin.

The adult RDA of niacin is 15 to 19 milligrams per day for men and 13 to 15 milligrams per day for women. The RDA is expressed as niacin equivalents to account for niacin received intact from the diet, as well as that made from tryptophan. Intakes of niacin by adults average about 40% greater than the RDA, without considering the contribution from tryptophan.[1] Note that tables of food values also ignore this contribution. Thus a niacin deficiency is unlikely to develop in people who consume a wide variety of foods. People with alcoholism and those with rare disorders of tryptophan metabolism are generally the only groups to show a niacin deficiency.

Niacin becomes toxic at intakes of 100 milligrams or more of the nicotinic acid form. Effects include headache, itching, and increased blood flow to the skin, causing a general blood vessel dilation or flushing in various parts of the body. This excessive intake is sometimes used, under a physician's guidance, to lower blood cholesterol.

Concept Check

The B vitamins thiamin, niacin, and riboflavin are all important in the metabolism of carbohydrates, proteins, and fats. Energy metabolism in particular requires adequate amounts of coenzymes of these three vitamins. Enriched grains are adequate sources of all three vitamins. Otherwise, pork is an excellent source of thiamin, milk is an excellent source of riboflavin, and protein foods in general—such as chicken—are excellent sources of niacin. Deficiencies of all three vitamins can occur with alcoholism; a thiamin deficiency is the most likely.

Pantothenic Acid

Like the other B vitamins, pantothenic acid helps release energy from carbohydrates, fats, and protein. By forming its coenzyme, called coenzyme A, pantothenic acid allows many important energy-yielding metabolic reactions to occur. Coenzyme A makes other molecules much more reactive. For example, coenzyme A must activate fatty acids before they can break down to yield energy. It is also used in the beginning steps of fatty acid synthesis.[36]

Pantothenic acid is so widespread in foods that a nutritional deficiency among healthy people who eat varied diets is unlikely. A full-blown deficiency is so rare that it has possibly been observed only during World War II. Prisoners in the Philippines and Japan displayed a "burning foot" syndrome described as numbness and tingling in the toes and burning and shooting pains in the feet, in addition to other mental and nervous system problems. To study possible consequences of a pantothenic acid deficiency, researchers induce it in subjects by having them consume an antagonist to the vitamin. When antagonists are given, people suffer from such general symptoms as tingling hands, fatigue, headache, sleep disturbances, nausea, and abdominal distress.

Pantothenic acid in foods and the ESADDI. Pantothenic acid is present in all foods. *Pantothen* actually means "from every side" in Greek. Nutrient-dense sources of pantothenic acid are mushrooms, peanuts, and eggs. Other good sources are meat, milk, and many vegetables.

The **estimated safe and adequate daily dietary intake (ESADDI)** of pantothenic acid is 4 to 7 milligrams per day for adults. Not enough is known about this nutrient to set an RDA (see Chapter 2). The average intake for people in the United States is about 6 milligrams of pantothenic acid per day. A deficiency of pantothenic acid might occur in alcoholism along with a very nutrient-deficient diet. However, the symptoms would probably be hidden among deficiencies of thiamin, riboflavin, vitamin B-6, and folate, so the pantothenic acid deficiency might be unrecognizable. No toxicity level is known for pantothenic acid.

Biotin

Biotin exists in two active forms in foods. In the ultimate coenzyme form, biotin acts in fat and carbohydrate metabolism. Specifically, biotin assists the addition of carbon dioxide to other compounds. By doing so, it promotes the synthesis of glucose, fatty acids, and DNA, while helping to break down certain amino acids.[36]

Symptoms of biotin deficiency include a scaly inflammation of the skin, changes in the tongue and lips, decreased appetite, nausea, vomiting, a form of **anemia,** depression, muscle pain and weakness, and poor growth.

Biotin in foods and the ESADDI. Cauliflower, egg yolks, peanuts, and cheese are the most nutrient-dense sources of biotin. Intestinal bacteria synthesize and supply some biotin, making a biotin deficiency unlikely. However, scientists are not sure how much of the bacteria-synthesized biotin in our intestines is actually absorbed. If the intestinal bacteria are not sufficient, as in people who are missing a large part of the small intestine or who take antibiotics for many months, special attention should be paid to eating good food sources of biotin.

A protein called *avidin* in raw egg whites binds biotin and inhibits its absorption. Feeding many raw egg whites to animals leads to a deficiency disease. An occasional raw egg in eggnog is unlikely to cause this disease because it would take a regular daily consumption of 12 or more raw eggs to produce a biotin deficiency. Biotin deficiency resulting from consuming raw eggs has been reported, however, in people with alcoholism who eat as few as three raw eggs a day. These people probably also had extremely deficient diets. The main concern about eating raw eggs for healthy people is the risk of food-borne illness caused by *Salmonella* bacteria, which may contaminate eggs (see Chapter 17).

The ESADDI for biotin is 30 to 100 milligrams per day for adults. Our food supply is thought to provide 100 to 300 milligrams per person per day. Biotin is relatively nontoxic. Large doses have been given over an extended period without harmful side effects to children who exhibit defects in biotin utilization from foods.

Estimated safe and adequate daily dietary intake (ESADDI)
Nutrient intake recommendations made by the Food and Nutrition Board where a range for intake of some nutrients is given, because not enough information is available to set an RDA (see Chapter 2).

Anemia
Generally refers to a decreased oxygen-carrying capacity of the blood. This can be caused by many disorders.

Avidin
A protein found in raw egg whites that can bind biotin and inhibit absorption; cooking destroys avidin.

Vitamin B-6

Vitamin B-6 is actually a family of three compounds. All can be changed to the active vitamin B-6 coenzyme. The general vitamin name is *pyridoxine*.

The coenzymes of vitamin B-6 are needed for the activity of numerous enzymes involved in carbohydrate, protein, and fat metabolism. Because vitamin B-6 is needed in so many areas of metabolism, a deficiency results in widespread symptoms, such as depression, vomiting, skin disorders, irritation of the nerves, and impaired immune response.

The most important function of vitamin B-6 concerns protein because metabolizing any amino acid requires the vitamin B-6 coenzyme. By helping to split the nitrogen group ($-NH_2$) from an amino acid, the coenzyme participates in reactions that allow a cell to synthesize nonessential (dispensable) amino acids.[36]

Another important role of vitamin B-6 is to reduce an important cause of heart disease. As noted in Chapter 6, scientists estimate that about 10% of heart disease in the United States results from excess homocysteine in the blood. Vitamin B-6 is needed to recycle this compound back to a common food constituent, the amino acid methionine. If not recycled, homocysteine is thought to damage the cells that line the blood vessels and in turn trigger the process of atherosclerosis.[27] Consuming adequate amounts of the vitamin folate and vitamin B-12 is also important because these participate with vitamin B-6 in the recycling process. Older people who underconsume these vitamins have been shown to run higher risks of heart disease and strokes.[35]

The synthesis of many **neurotransmitters** requires the vitamin B-6 coenzyme. Neutrotransmitters allow nerve cells to communicate with each other and with other body cells. Recall that deficiency of vitamin B-6 results in depression, headaches, confusion, and seizures. These results are predictable, given the importance of vitamin B-6 in the metabolism of key nervous system regulators. In the 1950s, infants fed oversterilized commercial formulas developed vitamin B-6 deficiency symptoms, particularly convulsions. Heat destroyed vitamin B-6 in the formulas, possibly contributing to the infants' decreased ability to synthesize a vital neurotransmitter. Today, manufacturers are more careful to maintain adequate vitamin B-6 content in formulas.

The link between vitamin B-6 and neurotransmitters suggested to some researchers that vitamin B-6 might be helpful in the treatment of **premenstrual syndrome (PMS).** This disorder appears in some women a few days before the menstrual period begins and is characterized by depression, irritability, anxiety, headache, bloating, and mood swings. Researchers thought that increasing vitamin B-6 intake might increase the synthesis of serotonin and thereby decrease the depression and confusion associated with premenstrual syndrome. However, vitamin B-6 has not proved to be a reliable treatment for PMS. In addition, use of megadoses can cause serious side effects (see the next section).

Currently, a nutrition-related approach to treating PMS, the cause of which is not well understood, is initially to recommend a nutrient-rich diet, especially with regard to carbohydrate, calcium, and magnesium; a decrease in alcohol, caffeine, and nicotine usage to decrease nervousness; a decrease in salt intake to decrease bloating; an increase in physical activity to stimulate relaxation; and adequate sleep. If such therapy is not helpful, women with premenstrual syndrome should consult a physician, who may suggest trying various forms of antidepressant or antipanic medications. Women should definitely avoid the widely available PMS "cures" sold primarily in drug stores and through mail-order catalogues.

Similarly the benefits of using vitamin B-6 to treat **carpal tunnel syndrome** have been promoted. This nerve disorder of the wrist has been effectively treated in some studies with a daily dosage of 100 to 200 milligrams of vitamin B-6 for 3 months. Pain diminished with vitamin treatment. However, other clinical trials demonstrate no therapeutic effect of vitamin B-6. Because of potential toxicity, any therapy must be supervised by a physician.

The vitamin B-6 coenzyme is important for the synthesis of hemoglobin, the oxygen-carrying part of the red blood cell. Vitamin B-6 is also necessary for the synthesis of white blood cells, which perform a major role in the immune system.[36]

Neurotransmitter
A compound made by a nerve cell that allows for communication between it and other cells.

Premenstrual syndrome (PMS)
A disorder occurring in some women a few days before a menstrual period begins. It is characterized by depression, anxiety, headache, bloating, and mood swings. Severe cases are currently termed premenstrual dysphoric disorder (PDD).

Carpal tunnel syndrome
A disease in which nerves that travel to the wrist are pinched as they pass through a narrow opening in a bone in the wrist.

Vitamin B-6 in foods and the RDA. The most nutrient-dense sources of vitamin B-6 are such fruits and vegetables as bananas, cantaloupe, broccoli, and spinach. Animal foods remain the best sources, however, because the vitamin B-6 they contain is often more absorbable than that in plant foods. Rich animal sources include meat, fish, and poultry (vitamin B-6 is stored in muscles) (Figure 8-9). Vitamin B-6 is not added to foods as part of an enrichment process for grains. Food tables listing vitamin B-6 are often incomplete because measuring this vitamin in foods is difficult.

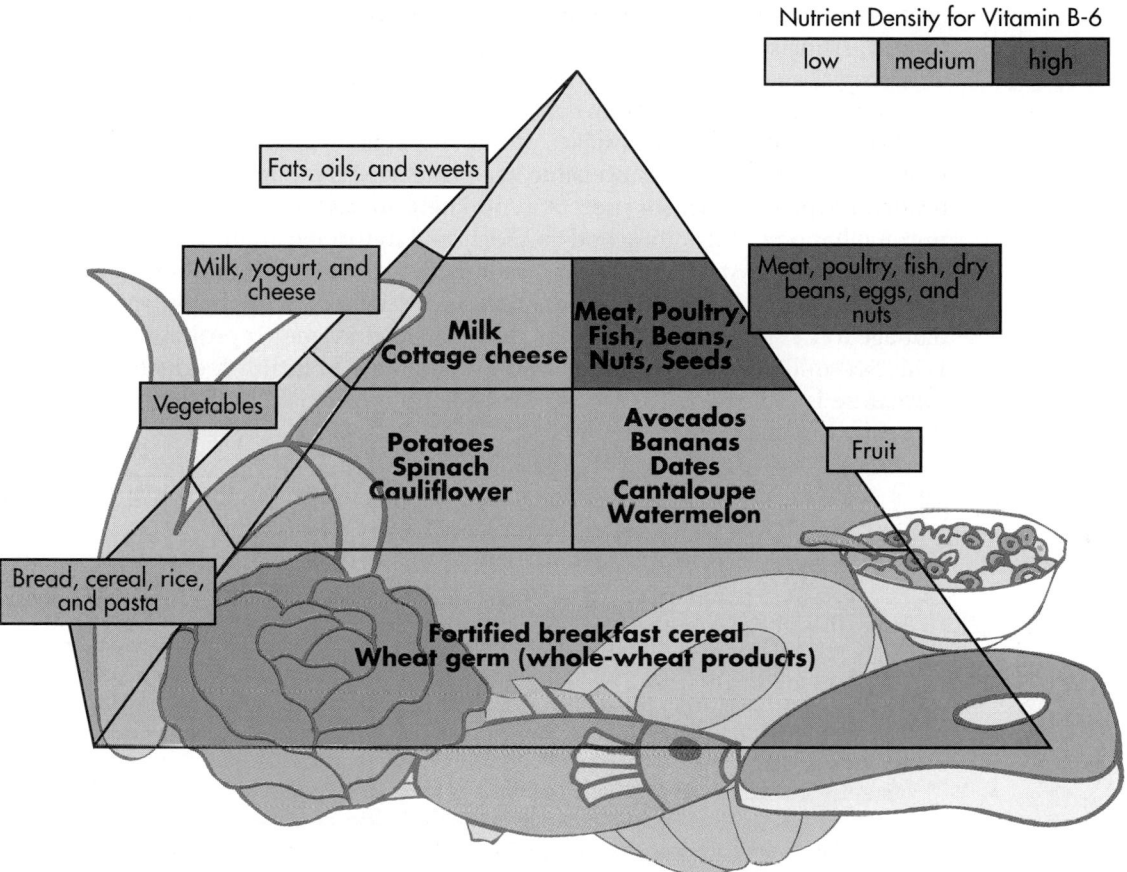

Figure 8-9 *Food sources of vitamin B-6 from the Food Guide Pyramid. The meat, poultry, fish, dry beans, eggs, and nuts group is an especially rich source of this nutrient. The background color of each food group indicates the average nutrient density for vitamin B-6 in that group.*

The adult RDA of vitamin B-6 is 2 milligrams per day for men and 1.6 milligrams per day for women. The RDA is set high in response to high protein intakes (which leads to more protein metabolism) of people in the United States. The 2.0 milligram value for men corresponds to a protein intake of 126 grams—approximately twice the RDA of protein for adult men. Average daily consumption of vitamin B-6 for men and women is about equal to the RDA.

Athletes may need slightly more vitamin B-6 because of their increased use of glycogen as a fuel (glycogen metabolism requires vitamin B-6), their increased use of amino acids for fuel, and their high protein intakes. Still, the protein foods in their diets should supply any extra vitamin B-6 needed.

Numerous studies have shown that some adolescent, adult, and older women have vitamin B-6 intakes below the RDA. However, because the vitamin B-6 values of many foods are not known, intake is probably greater. Routine multivitamin supplement use, which many women follow, probably also makes up for the deficit in many cases. In addition, the basis for the vitamin B-6 RDA assumes a daily intake of 100 grams of protein. Women, on average, consume only about 65 grams of protein daily and thus generally have lower needs for vitamin B-6 than the RDA suggests.

Reliably separating adequate vitamin B-6 status from an abnormal or deficient state is not yet possible. Still, scientists are concerned that the vitamin B-6 status of many women and older people in general warrants more attention.

People with alcoholism are susceptible to a vitamin B-6 deficiency because acetaldehyde, a metabolite formed in ethanol metabolism, can displace the coenzyme form from enzymes, increasing its tendency to be destroyed. In addition, alcohol decreases the absorption of vitamin B-6 and decreases the synthesis of its coenzyme form. **Cirrhosis** and hepatitis (both of which may accompany alcoholism) also disable liver tissue from actively metabolizing vitamin B-6, which in turn decreases synthesis of its coenzyme form.

With regard to toxicity, intakes of 2 to 6 grams of vitamin B-6 per day for 2 or more months can lead to irreversible nerve damage, as can long-term intakes of 500 milligrams per day. Use, or more appropriately, misuse, of such high doses of vitamin B-6 has occurred among body builders and in women attempting to treat themselves for PMS. Symptoms include walking difficulties and hand and foot numbness. Some nerve damage in individual sensory neurons is probably reversible, but damage to the ganglia (where many nerve fibers converge) is probably permanent. With 500 milligram tablets of vitamin B-6 available in health food stores, taking a toxic dose is quite easy. To be safe, consume no more than 200 milligrams per day if considering megadose use.

Cirrhosis

A loss of functioning liver cells, which are replaced by nonfunctioning connective tissue. Any substance that poisons liver cells can lead to cirrhosis. The most common cause is a longstanding, excessive alcohol intake.

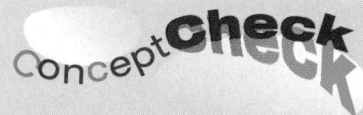

Pantothenic acid and biotin both participate in the metabolism of carbohydrate and fat. A deficiency of either vitamin is unlikely; pantothenic acid is found widely in foods, and our need for biotin is probably partially met by intestinal synthesis from bacteria. Vitamin B-6 is important for protein metabolism, neurotransmitter synthesis, and other key metabolic functions. Headache, a form of anemia, nausea, and vomiting can result from a vitamin B-6 deficiency. Increased risk of heart disease is also likely. Animal protein foods, broccoli, spinach, and bananas are some food sources.

Megaloblast

A large, immature red blood cell that results from the particular cell's inability to divide when it normally should.

Macrocyte

A greatly enlarged mature red blood cell; it has a short life span.

Erythrocytes

Mature red blood cells. These have no nucleus and a life span of about 120 days; they contain hemoglobin, which transports oxygen and carbon dioxide.

Folate

In the past, folate was referred to as *folic acid* and *folacin*. Today the term *folate* is preferred because it encompasses the variety of food forms of the vitamin.

A key role of the folate coenzymes is helping to form DNA. The active coenzymes help in this synthesis by supplying or accepting single carbon compounds. The coenzymes also help metabolize various amino acids and their derivatives.[19]

One major result of a folate deficiency is that in the early phases of red blood cell synthesis the immature cells cannot divide because they cannot form new DNA. The cells grow progressively larger because they can still synthesize enough protein and other cell parts to make new cells. When the time comes for the cells to divide, however, the amount of DNA is insufficient to form two nuclei. The cells then remain in a large immature form, known as a **megaloblast.** Megaloblasts can convert to abnormally large red blood cells, called *macrocytes.*[10]

Because the bone marrow of a folate-deficient person produces mostly immature megaloblast cells, few mature red blood cells (called *erythrocytes*) arrive in the bloodstream. When fewer mature red blood cells are present, the blood's capacity to carry oxygen decreases, causing a form of anemia. In short, a folate deficiency causes megaloblastic anemia.

The changes in red blood cell formation occur after 7 to 16 weeks on a folate-free diet, depending on the person's folate stores. White blood cell formation is also affected but to a lesser degree. In addition, cell division throughout the entire body is disrupted. Clinicians focus primarily on red blood cells because they are easy to examine and have a relatively short life span. The need to continually replenish red blood cells leads to a great demand for folate, making anemia the first major symptom of folate deficiency. Other symptoms of folate deficiency are inflammation of the tongue, diarrhea, poor growth, mental confusion, and problems in nerve function.[19]

Some forms of cancer therapy provide a vivid example of the effects of a folate deficiency on DNA metabolism. A cancer drug, methotrexate, closely resembles a form of folate but cannot act in its place. Because of this resemblance, when methotrexate is taken in high doses, it hampers folate metabolism. In essence, methotrexate crowds out folate in the metabolic pathways. The result is less formation of the active folate coenzymes. DNA synthesis, and consequently cell division, then decreases. Because cancer cells are among the most rapidly dividing cells in the body, they are among those first affected. However, other rapidly dividing cells, such as intestinal cells and skin cells, are also affected. Not surprisingly, typical side effects of methotrexate therapy are diarrhea, vomiting, and hair loss. These are also typical symptoms of folate deficiency.

A maternal deficiency of folate and a genetic predisposition have been linked to development of a variety of birth defects, such as **neural tube defects**[7] (Figure 8-10). This includes spina bifida (spinal cord or spinal fluid bulge through the back) and anencephaly (absence of a brain). About 2500 infants are affected annually in the

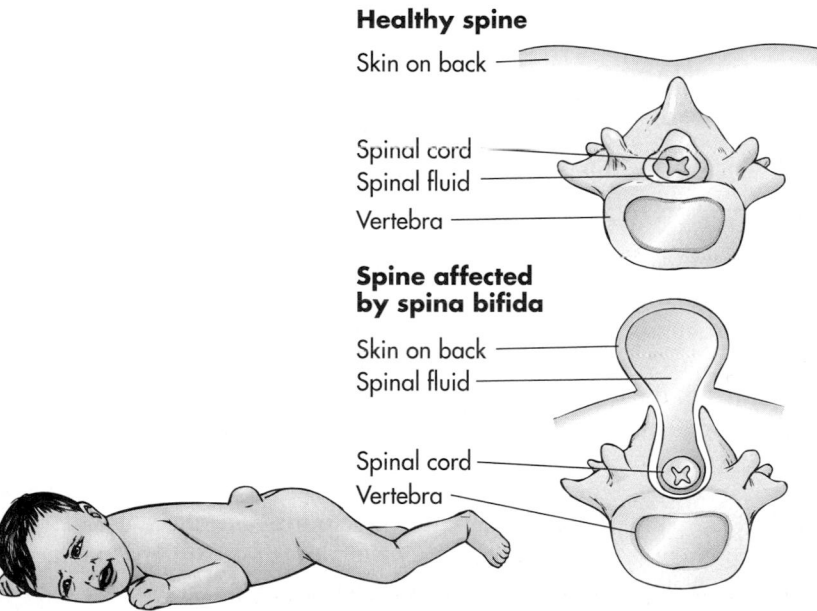

Figure 8-10 *Neural tube defects result from a developmental failure affecting the spinal cord or brain in the embryo. Very early in fetal development a ridge of neural-like tissue forms along the back of the embryo. As the fetus develops, this material develops into both the spinal cord and body nerves at the lower end, and into the brain at the upper end. At the same time, the bones that make up the back gradually surround the spinal cord on all sides. If any part of this sequence goes awry, many defects can appear. The worst is total lack of a brain (anencephaly). Much more common is spina bifida, in which the back bones do not form a complete ring to protect the spinal cord. Deficient folate status in the mother during the beginning of pregnancy increases the risk of neural tube defects.*

United States. Victims of spina bifida exhibit paralysis, incontinence, **hydrocephalus,** and learning disabilities. Children born with anencephaly die shortly after birth. The neural tube closes by the 28th day of gestation, a time when a woman would generally not know that she is pregnant. Hence the recommendation that ample folate be consumed at least 6 weeks before conception.

FDA recently ordered fortification of grain products with folate to help prevent neural tube defects. This law goes into effect January 1, 1998. Foods required to be fortified are enriched bread, rolls, and buns; enriched flour; enriched corn grits and corn meals; enriched farina and rice; and all enriched macaroni and noodle products. In addition, breakfast cereals can add folic acid up to 400 micrograms per serving.

Scientists suggest that about half of all neural tube defects could be prevented by ample folate intake.[7] Currently about half of all pregnancies in the United States are unplanned. Thus all women of child bearing age should make sure their diets are adequate in folate. The U.S. Public Health Service recommends that all women capable of becoming pregnant consume 400 micrograms of folate daily. Current intakes average about half this amount.[1]

Women with a family history of neural tube defects should consume even more folate: 4 milligrams for at least 6 weeks before pregnancy and the first three months of pregnancy. The use of vitamin supplements would be the only way to achieve that goal but should be attempted only under the direction of a physician.

Finally, folate is thought to aid in reducing colon cancer risk. Studies show that the risk of colon cancer is lower among people who both consume a liberal amount of fruits and vegetables and minimize animal fat intake. Studies are under way to determine whether regular folate consumption reduces colon cancer in adults.

Folate in foods and the RDA. Green, leafy vegetables (*folate* is derived from the Latin word *folium*, which means *foliage*), organ meats, sprouts, other vegetables, and orange juice are the most nutrient-dense sources of folate (Figure 8-11). The vitamin C in orange juice also reduces folate destruction. Ready-to-eat breakfast cereals are also a rich source of folate for many adults.

Food processing and preparation destroy 50% to 90% of the folate in food. Folate is very susceptable to destruction by heat. This underscores the importance of regularly eating fresh fruits and raw or lightly cooked vegetables. As mentioned before, vegetables retain their nutrients best when cooked quickly in minimal water—steaming, stir-frying, or microwaving.

The RDA of folate for adults is 180 to 200 micrograms per day. Average daily folate intake in the United States is approximately 20% above the RDA values.[1]

Folate deficiencies sometimes appear in pregnant women. They need extra folate to meet an increased rate of cell division and thus of DNA synthesis in their own bodies and that of the developing fetus. Today, prenatal care often includes vitamin and mineral supplements enriched with folate to compensate for the extra needs associated with pregnancy.

Young women in general often register low serum folate values. They should seek out and eat regularly foods that are good sources of folate. Use of a balanced vitamin supplement is another option (see the Nutrition Issue in Chapter 3).

Older people are also at risk for folate deficiency. Some studies have linked low folate status with severe vascular disease and heart disease (the homocysteine link discussed earlier), probably because of inadequate folate intake and absorption.[27,35] Perhaps these people failed to consume sufficient amounts of fruits and vegetables because of poverty or physical problems, such as a lack of teeth.

FDA limits the amount of folate in a vitamin supplement to 400 micrograms. This measure is taken to prevent excess folate from masking a vitamin B-12 deficiency. The metabolisms of folate and vitamin B-12 are linked, as noted earlier. Regular consumption of large amounts of folate can prevent the appearance of the

Folate deficiencies also often occur with alcoholism. Symptoms of a folate-related anemia can alert a physician to the possibility of alcoholism.[10]

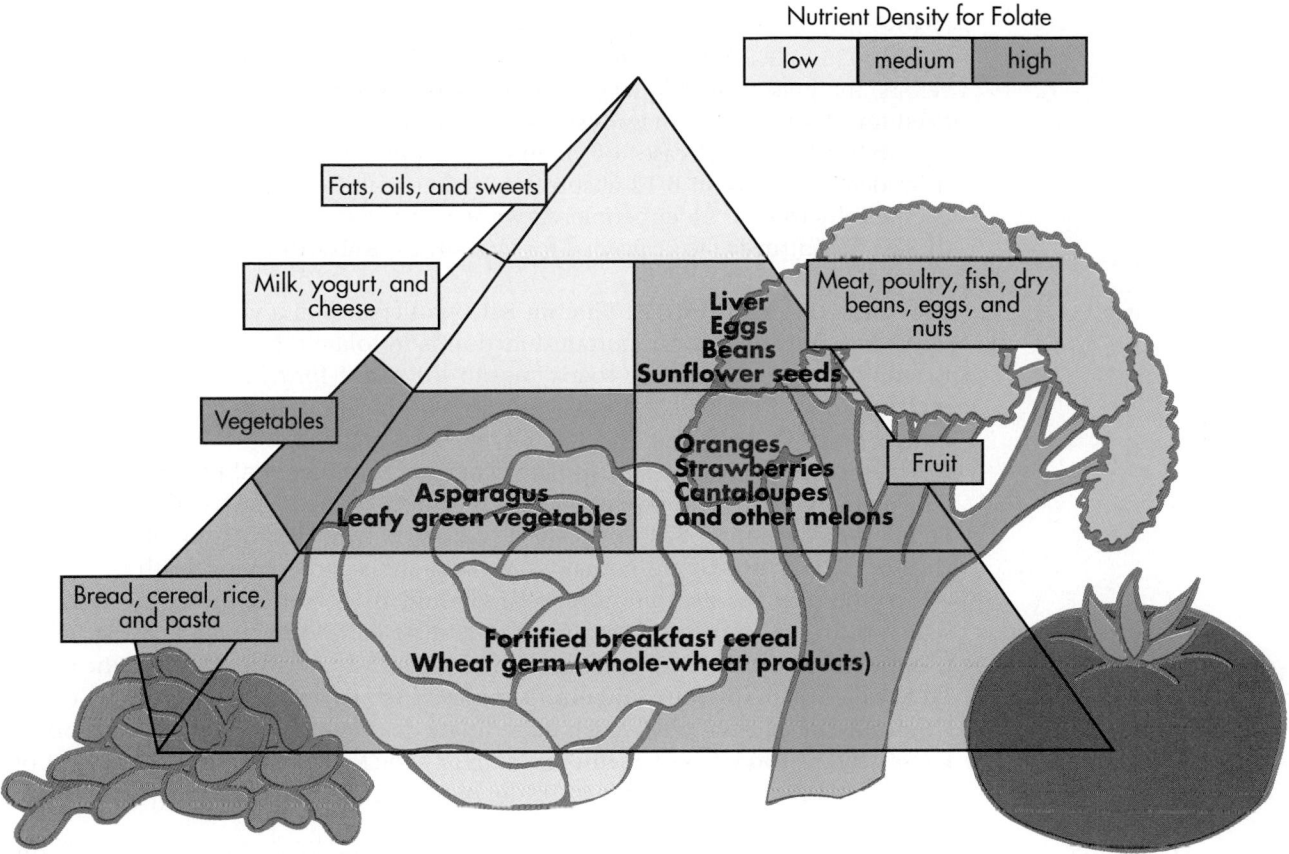

Figure 8-11 *Food sources of folate from the Food Guide Pyramid. The vegetable group is an espe-cially rich source of this nutrient. The background color of each food group indicates the average nutrient density for folate in that group.*

primary early warning sign of vitamin B-12 deficiency—alteration in red blood cell formation. A lack of vitamin B-12, however, has other effects that may ultimately lead to paralysis and death. Thus early detection and treatment of a vitamin B-12 deficiency is critical. Note that the recent FDA order to enrich grain products with folate has set a prescribed limit with the intent of not raising folate intakes above 1 milligram per day. This keeps folate intake below the amount needed to mask a vitamin B-12 deficiency.

Vitamin B-12

Vitamin B-12 represents a family of compounds that contain the mineral cobalt. All vitamin B-12 compounds are synthesized by bacteria, fungi, and other lower organisms.[19]

The body's complex means of absorbing vitamin B-12 is unique to this vitamin. Vitamin B-12 in food enters the stomach and is released from other materials by digestion, especially by stomach acid. The free vitamin B-12 binds with a substance produced by salivary glands in the mouth and then later with **intrinsic factor** pro-duced in the stomach. The resulting intrinsic factor–vitamin B-12 complex travels to the last portion of the small intestine, called the *ileum.* Ileum cells absorb vitamin B-12. According to this system, approximately 30% to 70% of dietary vitamin B-12

Intrinsic factor
A proteinlike compound produced by the stomach that enhances vitamin B-12 absorption.

Ileum
Essentially, the area consisting of the last half of the small intestine.

In the 1920s, researchers noted that they could cure a vitamin B-12 deficiency with massive amounts of liver or with concentrated water extracts of liver. In this case, the researchers cured a vitamin B-12 absorption defect by providing enough of the vitamin via simple diffusion across the intestinal tract.

Pernicious anemia
The anemia that results from a lack of vitamin B-12 absorption; it is pernicious because of associated nerve degeneration that can result in eventual paralysis.

is absorbed, depending on the body's need for it. Any failure in this system results in only 1% to 2% absorption of dietary vitamin B-12. If a defect in absorption develops, the person usually takes monthly injections of vitamin B-12 to bypass the need for absorption, or megadoses of a supplemental form.

About 95% of all cases of vitamin B-12 deficiencies in healthy people result from defective vitamin B-12 absorption, rather than from inadequate intakes. This is especially true for older people. As we age, our stomachs lose their ability to synthesize the intrinsic factor needed for vitamin B-12 absorption.[19]

Functions of vitamin B-12. Vitamin B-12 participates in a variety of cellular reactions. Probably its most important function is in folate metabolism. Vitamin B-12 is required to convert folate coenzymes to the active forms needed for important metabolic reactions, such as DNA synthesis. Without vitamin B-12, reactions that require certain active forms of folate do not take place in the cell. Thus a vitamin B-12 deficiency contributes to a folate deficiency. Another vital function of vitamin B-12 is maintaining the myelin sheaths that insulate nerve fibers from each other. People with vitamin B-12 deficiencies show patchy destruction of the myelin sheaths. This destruction eventually causes paralysis and perhaps death.[19]

In the past the inability to absorb vitamin B-12 eventually led to death. Researchers in mid-nineteenth century England noted a form of anemia that caused death within 2 to 5 years of the initial illness, mainly because it destroyed the nerves. They called it **pernicious anemia** (*pernicious* literally means "leading to death"). Clinically the anemia looks much like a folate deficiency anemia. You can probably guess why the two types of anemia are similar—the folate–vitamin B-12 connection. Because many macrocytes appear in the bloodstream, the vitamin B-12 anemia is called a **macrocytic anemia.**[10]

Besides the anemia, symptoms of pernicious anemia include weakness, sore tongue, back pain, apathy, and tingling in the extremities. Symptoms of nerve destruction generally develop after about 3 years from the onset of the disease. Unfortunately, significant nerve destruction often occurs before the anemia, which a physician can easily recognize, is seen, and this destruction is irreversible. When a vitamin B-12 deficiency is caused strictly by a lack of the vitamin in the diet, evidence of significant nerve damage takes even longer to show up because whenever absorption is possible, tiny amounts suffice.[19]

Infants who are breastfed by vegetarian or vegan mothers are at risk for vitamin B-12 deficiency accompanied by anemia and long-term nervous system problems, such as diminished brain growth, degeneration of the spinal cord, and poor intellectual development. The problems may have their origins during pregnancy, when the mother is deficient in vitamin B-12. Vegan diets supply little vitamin B-12 unless they include vitamin B-12–enriched food or supplements.[19]

Vitamin B-12 in foods and the RDA. Important sources of vitamin B-12 include meat, poultry, seafood, and eggs. The most nutrient-dense sources of vitamin B-12 are organ meats (especially liver, kidneys, and heart), seafood, beef, eggs, hot dogs (they contain many organ meat scraps), and ham. A final source of vitamin B-12 is milk and milk products.

The RDA of vitamin B-12 for adults is 2 milligrams. On average, men consume 3 times the RDA and women consume two times the RDA.[1] This high intake provides the average meat-eating person with 2 to 3 years' storage of vitamin B-12 in the liver.

It takes approximately 20 years of consuming a diet essentially free of vitamin B-12 for a person to exhibit nerve destruction caused by a diet deficiency. Vegans, who eat no animal products, should find a reliable source of vitamin B-12. As noted earlier, older persons are at significant risk for developing pernicious anemia; regular physical examinations should test for this possibility.[10] Vitamin B-12 supplements are essentially nontoxic.

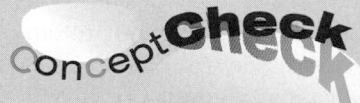

Folate is needed for cell division because it influences DNA synthesis. A folate deficiency results in megaloblastic anemia, as well as inflammation of the tongue, diarrhea, and poor growth—all signs of poor cell division. Folate is found in fresh vegetables and organ meats. Emphasizing fresh and lightly cooked vegetables is important because much folate is lost during cooking. Folate needs during pregnancy are especially high; deficiency may lead to neural tube defects in the fetus.

Vitamin B-12 is necessary for the formation of some of the active coenzymes of folate. Without dietary vitamin B-12, folate deficiency symptoms, such as macrocytic anemia, develop. In addition, vitamin B-12 is necessary for maintaining the nervous system. Paralysis can develop from a vitamin B-12 deficiency. The absorption of vitamin B-12 requires a number of specific factors. If absorption is inhibited, the resulting deficiency can lead to pernicious anemia and its associated nerve destruction. Concentrated amounts of vitamin B-12 are found only in animal foods; meat eaters generally have a 2- to 3-year supply stored in the liver. Vitamin B-12 absorption may decline as we age. Monthly injections can make up for this. Both folate and vitamin B-12 participate with vitamin B-6 in homocysteine metabolism; an adequate intake of all three vitamins minimizes the possibility of development of heart and blood vessel disease related to excess blood homocysteine.

Vitamin C

Scurvy, the vitamin C deficiency disease, was long ago a constant threat to the health of sailors. Its symptoms include weakness, opening of previously healed wounds, slower wound healing times, bone pain, fractures, bleeding gums, diarrhea, and pinpoint hemorrhages around hair follicles on the back of the arms and legs. On long sea voyages, captains often lost half or more of their crews to scurvy. Epidemics of scurvy occurred in Europe from 1556 to 1857, and soldiers in the U.S. Civil War died of it. In 1740 the Englishman Dr. James Lind first showed that citrus fruits—two oranges and one lemon a day—could cure scurvy. Fifty years after Lind's discovery, rations for British sailors included limes to prevent scurvy. That's how the British earned the nickname "limey"—and one reason for their preeminence at sea during the nineteenth century.

Vitamin C (ascorbic acid) is a puzzling vitamin. It is found in all living tissues, and most animals synthesize their own from the simple sugar glucose. Only guinea pigs, monkeys, some birds, a few fish, and humans need vitamin C in their diets. What is strange is that animals who synthesize vitamin C often make quite a lot of it. For instance, a pig produces 8 grams per day (though we do not benefit from it when we eat pork because it is lost in processing). This amount is over 130 times our human RDA of 60 milligrams, and even 60 milligrams appears to be quite a generous intake for humans. As little as 10 milligrams daily can prevent scurvy.[26]

Why some animals make so much vitamin C whereas other animals, including humans, appear to need so little has fueled much controversy. Is the amount of vitamin C that prevents scurvy the same amount that promotes optimal health? This question hasn't been fully answered.

Vitamin C is absorbed in the small intestine. About 80% to 90% of vitamin C is absorbed when a person eats between 30 and 120 milligrams of it per day. If someone ingests 6 grams (6000 milligrams) per day, absorption efficiency drops to about 20%. A common side effect of high vitamin C intake is diarrhea. The unabsorbed vitamin C stays in the small intestine and attracts water, finally causing diarrhea.[26]

Scurvy
The deficiency disease that results after a few weeks of consuming a diet that lacks vitamin C.

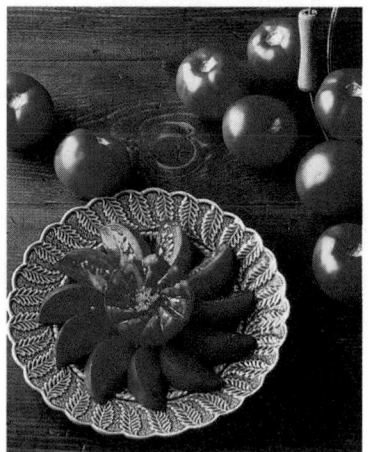

Tomatoes and tomato juice are major contributors of vitamin C to American diets.

Functions of Vitamin C

The best understood function of vitamin C is its role in synthesizing the protein collagen. This protein is highly concentrated in connective tissue, bone, teeth, tendons, and blood vessels. It is very important for wound healing. Vitamin C increases the cross-connections between amino acids in collagen, greatly strengthening the tissues it helps form.

A vitamin C deficiency can cause widespread changes in tissue metabolism. Most symptoms of scurvy are linked to a decrease in collagen synthesis. About 20 to 40 days with no vitamin C intake are required for the first symptoms of scurvy to appear.

Vitamin C is one of the cell's water-soluble antioxidants. Recall that vitamin E is a fat-soluble antioxidant for the cell membrane. The antioxidant capabilities of vitamin C can reduce the formation of cancer-causing nitrosamines in the stomach and also keep the folate coenzymes intact, preventing their destruction. Vitamin C and vitamin E work together as free-radical scavengers.[8] Vitamin C also aids in reactivating oxidized vitamin E so that it can be reused. Finally, epidemiological studies suggest that vitamin C is effective in helping prevent certain cancers (such as esophageal, oral, and stomach cancers), heart disease, and cataracts in the eye, probably because of its antioxidant capabilities.[8,14] Some researchers, however, are skeptical about the true degree of these effects.[18]

Vitamin C enhances iron absorption by keeping iron in its most absorbable form. The iron in the small intestine's alkaline environment is much more usable than other forms of iron. Thus iron absorption is modestly enhanced. Increasing intake of vitamin C–rich foods is beneficial for those people with poor iron stores. However, one symptom of vitamin C toxicity—with doses of 1 to 2 grams per day—can be overabsorption of iron, with the potential for iron toxicity.[18]

Vitamin C is vital for the function of the immune system, especially for the activity of certain cells in the immune system. Thus disease states can increase the need for vitamin C, although we don't know what amount above the RDA is needed (if any). Partly on the basis of this observation, Dr. Linus Pauling gained great notoriety by claiming that vitamin C could combat the common cold. He claimed that 1000 milligrams (1 gram) or more of vitamin C daily could reduce the number of colds for most people by nearly half. As a result of the popularity of his books and the respectability of his scientific credentials, millions of Americans supplement their diets with vitamin C.

But does vitamin C reliably and effectively work against colds and other infections? Most medical and nutrition scientists strongly disagree with Pauling's views of vitamin C. Numerous well-designed, double-blind studies have not shown megadoses of vitamin C to reliably prevent colds, though it seems to reduce duration of symptoms by a day or so.

Most vitamin C consumed in large doses ends up in the feces or the urine. Only a small fraction of such large doses can be used. The body is saturated at intakes of about 200 milligrams per day. This means that if more than 200 milligrams of vitamin C is ingested, it is quickly excreted. In addition, no credible evidence suggests that a dose even as high as 10 grams a day will cure colon cancer.

Vitamin C in Foods and the RDA

The most nutrient-dense sources of vitamin C are green peppers, cauliflower, broccoli, cabbage, strawberries, papayas, and romaine lettuce. Citrus fruits, potatoes, and other green vegetables are also good sources of vitamin C (Figure 8-12). The five to nine servings of fruits and vegetables from the Food Guide Pyramid can easily provide enough vitamin C. The major contributors of vitamin C to the diets of people in the United States are orange juice, grapefruit and grapefruit juice, tomatoes and tomato juice, fortified fruit drinks, oranges, tangerines, and potatoes.

Vitamin C is also necessary for the synthesis of a number of hormones, neurotransmitters, and other vital compounds, such as bile acids and DNA.[26]

Critical Thinking

Carlos just returned from a local mall and is excited because he saw an advertisement claiming that vitamin C will cure just about everything, from colds to heart disease. How would you explain to him vitamin C's main functions in the human body?

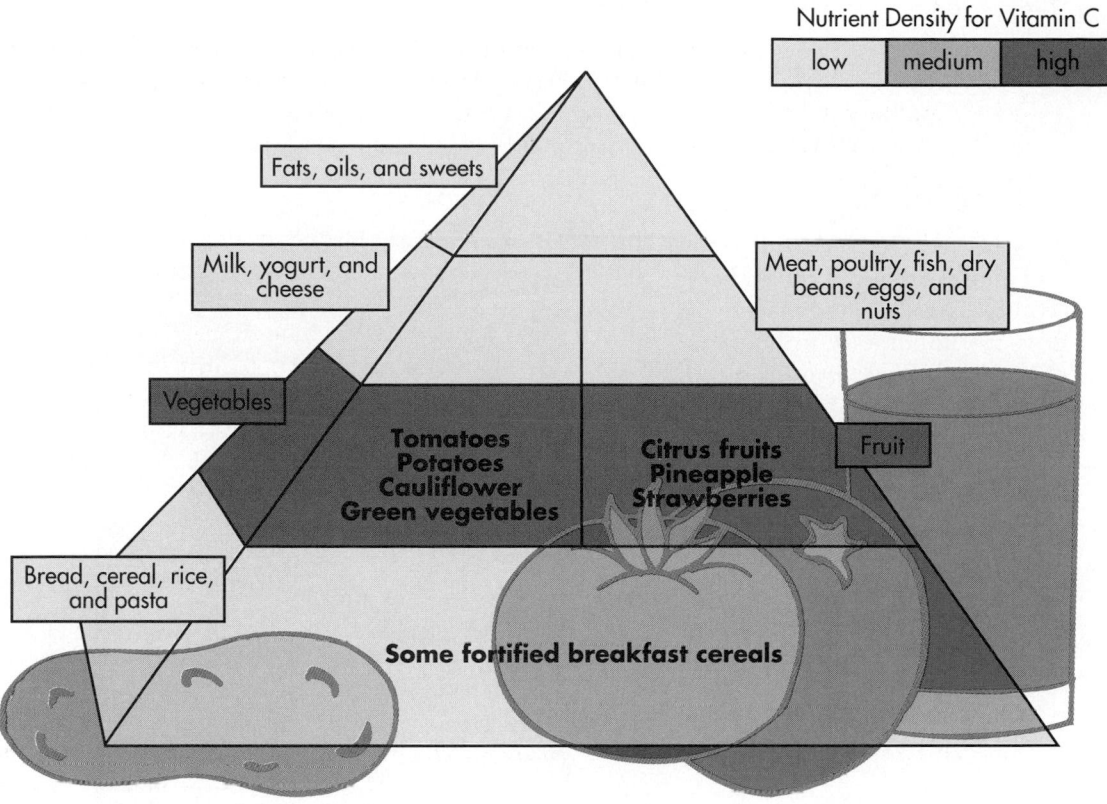

Nutrient Density for Vitamin C

| low | medium | high |

Fats, oils, and sweets

Milk, yogurt, and cheese

Meat, poultry, fish, dry beans, eggs, and nuts

Vegetables

Tomatoes Potatoes Cauliflower Green vegetables

Citrus fruits Pineapple Strawberries

Fruit

Bread, cereal, rice, and pasta

Some fortified breakfast cereals

Figure 8-12 *Food sources of vitamin C from the Food Guide Pyramid. The fruit group and the vegetable group are especially rich sources of this nutrient. The background color of each food group indicates the average nutrient density for vitamin C in that group.*

Vitamin C is easily lost in processing and cooking. Juices are good foods to fortify with vitamin C because their acidity reduces vitamin C destruction. Vitamin C is very unstable in contact with heat, iron, copper, or oxygen.

The adult RDA of vitamin C is 60 milligrams per day. The 1989 RDA publication recommends that cigarette smokers consume 100 milligrams per day because of the great stress on their lungs from oxygen and toxic by-products of cigarette smoke. Our food supply yields about twice the adult RDA (120 milligrams) of vitamin C per day. Approximately 80 milligrams is derived naturally from foods; the remainder comes from vitamin C added to foods. Nearly all nonsmoking Americans likely meet their daily needs for vitamin C because men consume an average of 120 milligrams per day and women consume 100 milligrams per day.[1] Respected nutrition experts who advocate increased use of vitamin C often recommend intakes of about 200 milligrams per day.[26] Still, this amount is easily obtained by sufficient fruit and vegetable intake, and data supporting the benefits of this dosage are sketchy.

Today vitamin C deficiency appears mostly in alcoholic people who eat nutrient-poor diets and in older men who live alone and also eat poorly.[33] Men are more susceptible to vitamin C deficiency than are women because, as a group, they tend to smoke more and are less apt to consume vitamin supplements. Generally, a diet with limited fruit and vegetable consumption puts a person at risk of deficiency. Worldwide, scurvy is associated with poverty. It is especially common in infants who are fed boiled milk (all forms of milk are poor sources of vitamin C) and not provided with a good food source of vitamin C or a supplement.

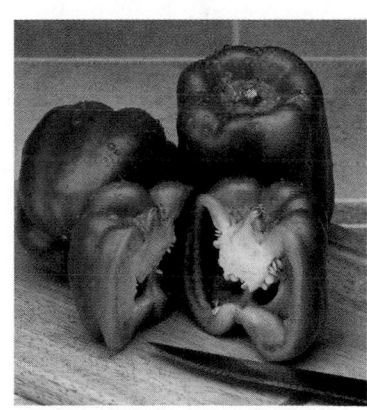

Green peppers are one vegetable source of vitamin C.

Nutrition **Insight**

Bogus Vitamins

ealth food enthusiasts promote a variety of compounds as vitamins even though these substances have no importance in human nutrition. Because some of these so-called vitamins may cause increased growth in lower organisms, some vitamin marketers try to promote them as important for humans.

The list of these pseudovitamins changes frequently. The following are some of the more persistent pseudos:

- Paraaminobenzoic acid (PABA): Although this compound is part of the vitamin folate, humans can't use it to make folate. Entrepreneurs represent PABA as "a member of the B complex family," omitting the words "for bacteria" when they sell it as a food supplement. If consumed along with sulfa antibiotics, it can defeat the effect of the antibiotic (Figure 8-13).
- Laetrile: This cyanide-containing compound, wrongly labeled vitamin B-17, is promoted as a cure for cancer. FDA does not recognize it as a legitimate cancer therapy. Chronic cyanide intoxication from laetrile in the diet has produced cases of slowly progressing nerve damage, resulting in blindness, deafness, and muscle weakness.
- Bioflavonoids: These compounds, wrongly labeled vitamin P, include rutin and hesperidin. They were originally thought to be more effective than vitamin C alone for treating fragile blood vessels in scurvy. Today, no nutritional requirement for bioflavonoids is recognized, although they may enhance vitamin C absorption, and epidemiological evidence links consumption of foods rich in these substances with decreased risk from some cancers (the phytochemical link discussed in Chapter 2).
- Pangamic acid: This bogus compound, wrongly labeled vitamin B-15, has no link to nutrition and deserves no attention from anyone, including athletes. Its roots are in quackery, pure and simple.

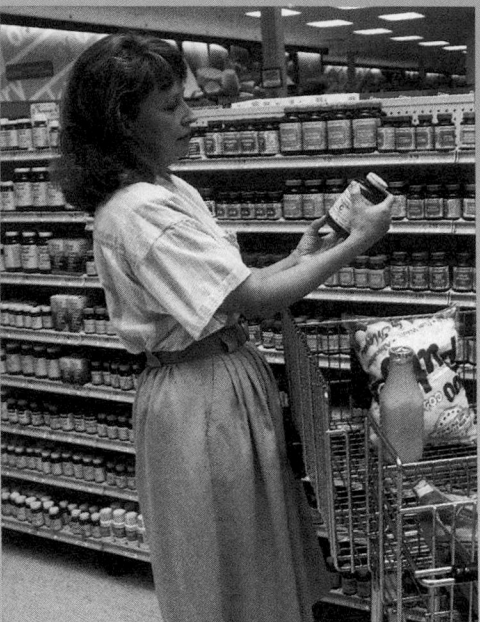

Figure 8-13 *Don't be misled by the inclusion of nonvitamins in supplements. This is a common practice, but it serves no nutritional need.*

Other compounds will surely come and go in the next few years. Again, because people have been maintained for years on intravenous feedings that contain all the known essential nutrients without developing deficiency symptoms, the discovery of any new vitamin is unlikely. You can be sure that if a new compound has the potential to be a vitamin, the Food and Nutrition Board of the National Academy of Sciences will closely examine it. If it then appears with the rest of the nutrients that have an RDA or ESADDI, you can be confident that the compound can be called a vitamin and merits your attention.

Vitamin C is probably not toxic when consumed in amounts less than about 1 to 2 grams per day. Regularly consuming more than that may cause stomach inflammation, diarrhea, and iron toxicity (again, caused by overabsorption of iron). This last point is important to note, however, because some people suffer from **hemochromatosis,** a disease characterized by overstorage of iron (see Chapter 9). These people may be harmed if an increased vitamin C intake increases their iron absorption. This is just one of many examples in which recommending a vitamin intake well above the RDA can have conflicting results. Some people may benefit, whereas others may be injured.[18]

If people want to experiment with large doses of vitamin C, they should alert their physician, primarily because high doses of vitamin C can change reactions to medical tests for diabetes or blood in the feces. Physicians may misdiagnose conditions when large doses of vitamin C are consumed without their knowledge.[2]

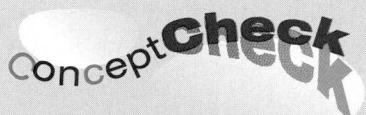

Vitamin C is important in the synthesis of collagen, a major connective tissue protein. A vitamin C deficiency, known as scurvy, causes many changes in the skin and gums, such as small hemorrhages. This is mainly because of poor collagen synthesis. Vitamin C also modestly improves iron absorption, is involved in synthesizing certain hormones and neurotransmitters, and acts as a general body antioxidant. Citrus fruits, green peppers, cauliflower, broccoli, and strawberries are good sources of vitamin C. As with folate, eating fresh or lightly cooked foods is important because vitamin C loses a lot of its potency in cooking. High doses of vitamin C can lead to diarrhea and foil various medical tests. These high doses do not prevent the common cold or cure cancer. However, consuming the RDA of vitamin C is part of the general approach to good health.

Now that we have discussed the vitamins, review the Food Guide Pyramid in Chapter 2 and note how each group makes an important vitamin contribution (Figure 8-14).

VITAMIN-LIKE COMPOUNDS

A variety of vitamin-like compounds are found in the body. These include the following:

- Choline
- Carnitine
- Inositol
- Taurine
- Lipoic acid

All these vitamin-like compounds are necessary to maintain proper metabolism in the body. They can be synthesized by cells using common building blocks, such as amino acids and glucose. In disease states, synthesis of vitamin-like compounds may not meet needs, so dietary intake can be crucial. For example, liver dysfunction similar to that seen in choline-deficient test animals has developed in humans fed choline-deficient diets.[40] We make all these substances each day, and our diets are also a source. Because of this, the needs for choline, carnitine, and taurine in certain conditions, such as for premature infants, are being investigated. Although promoted and sold by health food stores, these vitamin-like compounds need not be included in the diet of the average healthy adult.

Hemochromatosis
A disorder of iron metabolism characterized by increased iron absorption and deposition in the liver tissue. This eventually poisons the liver cells.

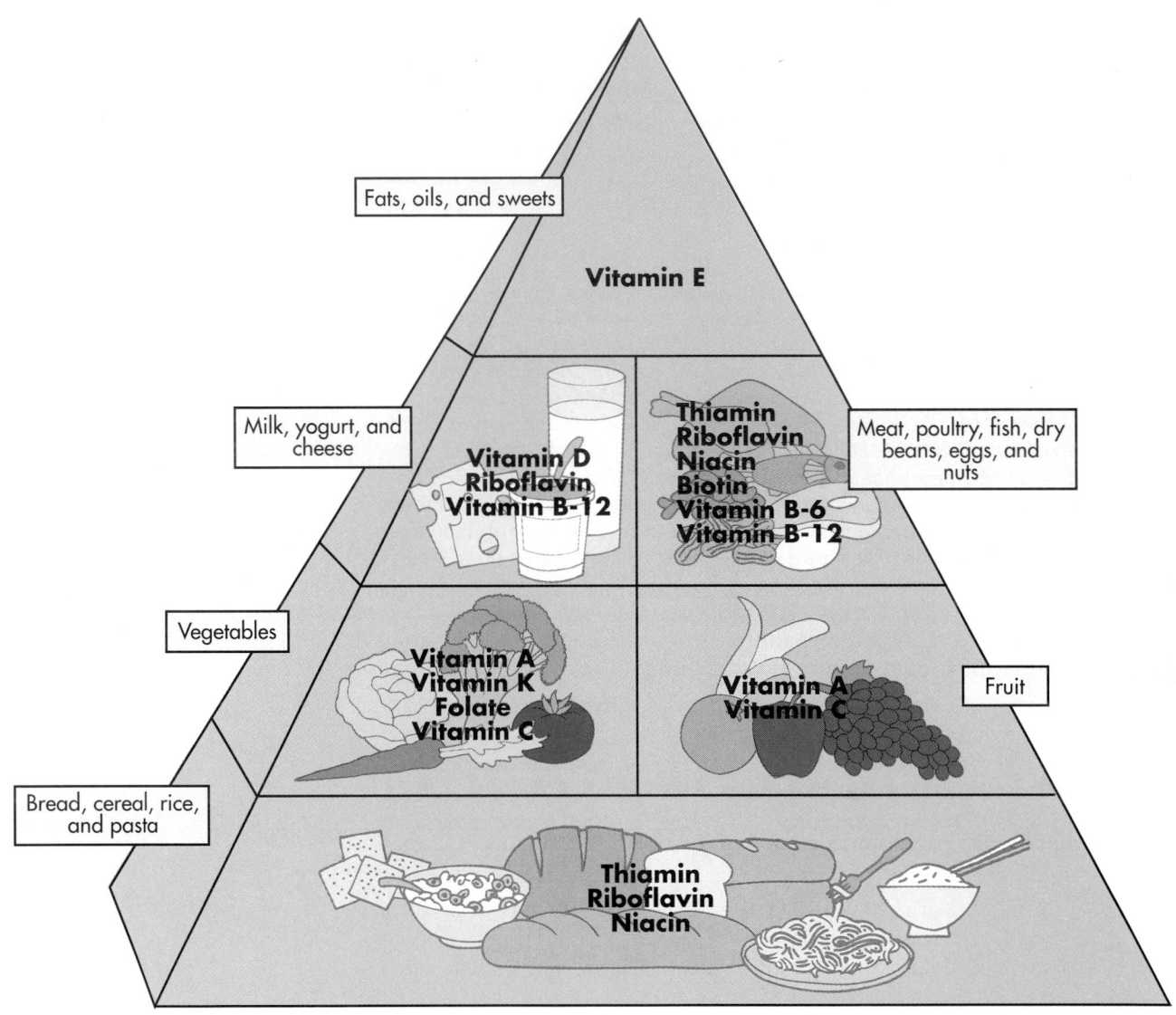

Figure 8-14 *Certain groups of the Food Guide Pyramid are especially rich sources of various vitamins. This is true for the vitamins listed. Each vitamin may be also found in other groups but in lower amounts. Pantothenic acid is also present in moderate amounts in many groups.*

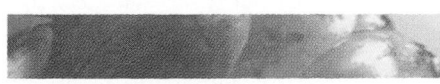

Summary

➤ Vitamins are compounds we generally need daily in small amounts from foods. They yield no energy directly, but many contribute to energy-yielding chemical reactions in the body and promote growth and development. Many vitamins act as coenzymes, which help enzymes function. Vitamins A, D, E, and K are fat soluble, whereas the B vitamins and vitamin C are water soluble.

➤ Vitamin A consists of a family of compounds that includes several forms of preformed vitamin A. Some carotenoids function as antioxidants and can also yield vitamin A. Vitamin A contributes to vision, immune function, and cell development. Vitamin A is found in liver and fish oils; carotenoids are especially plentiful in dark green and orange vegetables. Vitamin A can be quite toxic, even when taken at just 5 times the RDA. High vitamin A intakes are especially dangerous during pregnancy because they can lead to fetal malformations.

➤ Vitamin D is both a hormone and a vitamin. Human skin synthesizes it using sunshine and a cholesterol-like substance. If we don't spend enough time in the sun, such foods as fish oils and fortified milk can supply the vitamin. The active hormone form of vitamin D helps regulate blood calcium in part by influencing calcium absorption from the intestine. Children who don't get enough vitamin D may develop rickets, and adults with inadequate amounts in the body develop osteomalacia. Vitamin D is a very toxic substance. An intake just 5 times the RDA can cause problems, especially in childhood.

➤ Vitamin E functions primarily as an antioxidant and is found in plant oils. By donating electrons to electron-seeking free-radical (oxidizing) compounds, it neutralizes them. This effect shields cell membranes and red blood cells from breakdown. Claims are made about the curative powers of vitamin E, but few have been scientifically validated. Studies are in progress.

➤ Vitamin K helps blood clot. Some vitamin K absorbed each day comes from bacterial synthesis in the intestine, but most comes from foods, primarily green, leafy vegetables. Vitamin K is poorly stored in the body, but our dietary intake alone is usually sufficient. People who can't absorb fat well or who are on antibiotics for long periods may need extra vitamin K.

➤ Thiamin, riboflavin, and niacin play key roles as coenzymes in energy-yielding reactions. They help metabolize carbohydrates, fats, and proteins. Alcoholism and a poor diet can create deficiencies of these three nutrients. Enriched grain products are common sources of all three of these vitamins.

➤ Pantothenic acid, which participates in many aspects of cell metabolism, is widely distributed among foods. Biotin, which participates in glucose production, fat synthesis, and DNA synthesis, can be synthesized by bacteria in the intestine. We probably synthesize about half our requirement for biotin. The rest comes from foods such as eggs and cheese.

➤ Vitamin B-6 performs a vital role in protein metabolism, especially in synthesizing nonessential amino acids. It also helps synthesize neurotransmitters and performs other metabolic roles, such as metabolism of homocysteine. Headaches, a form of anemia, nausea, and vomiting result from a B-6 deficiency. Increased risk of heart disease is also possible, especially when coupled with inadequate folate or vitamin B-12 intake or both. Generally, women are more likely to have poor vitamin B-6 stores than are men. Regular consumption of animal protein foods, cauliflower, and broccoli provides needed vitamin B-6. Taking high doses causes malfunction of the nervous system.

➤ Folate plays an important role in DNA synthesis. Symptoms of a deficiency are generally poor cell division in various areas of the body, megaloblastic anemia, tongue inflammation, diarrhea, and poor growth. Pregnancy puts high demands for folate on the body. A deficiency is most likely to occur in people with alcoholism. Excellent food sources are leafy vegetables, organ meats, and orange juice. Great amounts of folate can be lost in prolonged cooking.

➤ Vitamin B-12 is needed to metabolize folate and maintain the insulation surrounding nerves. A deficiency results in anemia (because of its relationship to folate) and nerve degeneration. Older people often absorb vitamin B-12 inefficiently. If so, they can benefit from monthly injections of the vitamin. Generally a deficiency is unlikely because vitamin B-12 is highly concentrated in animal foods, which constitute a major part of the American diet. Vitamin B-12 does not occur naturally in plant foods. Vegans need a supplemental source.

➤ Vitamin C is mainly used to synthesize collagen, a major protein for building connective tissue. A vitamin C deficiency results in scurvy, which is evidenced by poor wound healing, pinpoint hemorrhages in the skin, and bleeding gums. Vitamin C also modestly enhances iron absorption and is needed for synthesizing some hormones and neurotransmitters. Fresh fruits and vegetables, especially citrus fruits, are generally good sources. Because a great amount of vitamin C is lost in cooking, a good diet should emphasize fresh or lightly cooked vegetables. Deficiencies can occur in people with alcoholism and those whose diets lack sufficient fruits and vegetables. Smoking makes matters worse for people already at risk.

Study Questions

1 Why is the risk of toxicity greater with fat-soluble vitamins than with water-soluble vitamins?

2 How would you determine which fruits and vegetables displayed in the produce section of your supermarket are likely to provide plenty of carotenoids?

3 Older people living in nursing homes are most likely to have a deficiency of which vitamin? Why?

4 What is the primary function of the vitamin D hormone? Discuss the specific mechanism involved in this function.

5 Describe how vitamin E functions as an antioxidant. Use the term *free radical.*

6 Why is it critical for a surgeon to know the vitamin K status of a patient before operating?

7 The need for certain vitamins increases as energy expenditure increases. Name two such vitamins and explain why this is the case.

8 Take one of the B vitamins that might be deficient in the American diet and explain why the lack might occur.

9 Which vitamins are lost from cereal grains as a result of the "refining" process? Which vitamins must be replaced by law in the subsequent enrichment process?

10 Although folate itself is not known to have any toxic effects, FDA limits the amount that may be included in supplements. Why?

11 Is it necessary for Americans to consume a great excess of vitamin C to avoid the possibility of a deficiency? Does the intake of vitamin C well above the RDA have any negative consequences?

References

1   Alaimo K and others: Dietary intake of vitamins, minerals, and fiber of persons age 2 months and over in the United States: Third National Health and Nutrition Examination Survey, Phase 1, 1988-91, *Advance Data* 258:1, 1994.

2   ADA Reports: position of The American Dietetic Association: vitamin and mineral supplementation, *Journal of The American Dietetic Association* 96:73, 1996.

3   Belury MA: Conjugated dienoic linoleate: a polyunsaturated fatty acid with unique chemoprotective properties, *Nutrition Review* 53:83, 1995.

4   Bikle DD: A bright future for the sunshine hormone, *Scientific American Science & Medicine,* p 58, March/April 1995.

5 Booth SL and others: Food sources and dietary intakes of vitamin K-1 (phylloquinone) in the American diet: data from the RDA Total Diet Study, *Journal of The American Dietetic Association* 96:149, 1996.

6 Bostick RM and others: Calcium and colorectal epithelial cell proliferation in sporadic adenoma patients: a randomized, double-blinded, placebo-controlled clinical trial, *Journal of the National Cancer Institute* 887:1307, 1995.

7 Bowers C: Folate and neural tube defects, *Nutrition Reviews* 53:S33, 1995.

8 Byers T, Guerrero N: Epidemiologic evidence for vitamin C and vitamin E in cancer prevention, *American Journal of Clinical Nutrition* 62(suppl):1385S, 1995.

9 Cave WT: Dietary ω3 polyunsaturated fats and breast cancer, *Nutrition* 12:S39, 1996.

10 Davenport J: Macrocytic anemia, *American Family Physician* 53:155, 1996.

11 De Luca LM and others: Retinoids in differentiation and neoplasia, *Scientific American Science & Medicine*, p 28, July/August 1995.

12 Diplock AT: Safety of antioxidant vitamins and β-carotene, *American Journal of Clinical Nutrition* 62(suppl):1510S, 1995.

13 Farrell PM, Roberts RJ: Vitamin E. In Shils ME and others, editors: *Modern nutrition in health and disease*, ed 8, Philadelphia, 1994, Lea & Febiger.

14 Flagg EW and others: Epidemiologic studies of antioxidants and cancer in humans, *Journal of the American College of Nutrition* 14:419, 1995.

15 Frei B: Reactive oxygen species and antioxidant vitamins: mechanisms of action, *American Journal of Medicine* 97(suppl 3A):5S, 1994.

16 Ganong WF: *Review of medical physiology*, ed 16, Norwalk, Conn, 1995, Appleton & Lange.

17 Greider CW, Blackburn EH: Telomeres, telomerase and cancer, *Scientific American*, p 92, February 1996.

18 Herbert V: The antioxidant supplement myth, *American Journal of Clinical Nutrition* 60:157, 1994.

19 Herbert V: Folic acid and vitamin B-12. In Shils ME and others, editors: *Modern nutrition in health and disease*, ed 8, Philadelphia, 1994, Lea & Febiger.

20 Holick MF: Vitamin D and bone health, *Journal of Nutrition* 126:1159S, 1996.

21 Hunter DJ and others: Cohort studies of fat intake and the risk of breast cancer: a pooled analysis, *The New England Journal of Medicine* 334:356, 1996.

22 Hunter DJ and others: A prospective study of the intake of vitamins C, E, and A and the risk of breast cancer, *The New England Journal of Medicine* 329:234, 1993.

23 Jacob RA, Burri BJ: Oxidative damage and defense, *American Journal of Clinical Nutrition* 63:985S, 1996.

24 Langston AA and others: BRCAI mutations in a population-based sample of young women with breast cancer, *The New England Journal of Medicine* 334:137, 1996.

25 Levine AJ: The genetic origin of neoplasia, *Journal of the American Medical Association* 273:592, 1995.

26 Levine M and others: Determination of optimal vitamin C requirements in humans, *American Journal of Clinical Nutrition* 62(suppl):1347S, 1995.

27 Morrison HI and others: Serum folate and risk of fatal coronary heart disease, *Journal of the American Medical Association* 275:1893, 1996.

28 Olsen JA: Needs and sources of carotenoids and vitamin A, *Nutrition Reviews* 52:S67, 1994.

29 Olsen RE: Vitamin K. In Shils ME and others, editors: *Modern nutrition in health and disease*, ed 8, Philadelphia, 1994, Lea & Febiger.

30 Rivlin RS, Dutta P: Vitamin B2 (riboflavin), *Nutrition Today* 30:62, 1995.

31 Rothman KJ and others: Teratogenicity of high vitamin A intake, *The New England Journal of Medicine* 333:1369, 1995.

32 Ryan C and others: Vitamin D in the elderly, *Nutrition Today* 30:228, 1995.

33 Scully RE and others: Case 39-1995, *The New England Journal of Medicine* 333:1695, 1995.

34 Seddon JM and others: Dietary carotenoids, vitamins A, C, and E, and advanced age–related macular degeneration, *Journal of the American Medical Association* 272:1413, 1994.

35 Selhub J and others: Association between plasma homocysteine concentrations and extracranial carotid-artery stenosis, *The New England Journal of Medicine* 332:286, 1995.

36 Stryer L: *Biochemistry*, ed 4, New York, 1995, WH Freeman.

37 Voelker R: Ames agrees with mom's advice: eat your fruits and vegetables, *Journal of the American Medical Association* 273:1077, 1995.

38 Weindruch R: Caloric restriction and aging, *Scientific American*, p 46, January 1996.

39 Winawer SJ and others: Risk of colorectal cancer in the families of patients with adenomatous polyps, *The New England Journal of Medicine* 334:82, 1996.

40 Zeisel SH, Blusztajn JK: Choline and human nutrition, *Annual Review of Nutrition* 14:269, 1994.

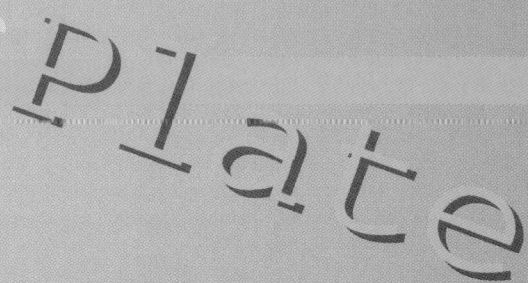

RATE

Measuring Your Vitamin Intake Against the RDA

This activity requires you to reexamine the nutritional assessment you completed in Chapter 2. You recorded the types, quantities, and amounts of nutrients in the foods and drinks you consumed for one day. Then you assessed your intake by recording the total amounts of nutrient you consumed. You were then asked to compare your intake of nutrients with certain standards. Many of the standards you used were the 1989 RDA found on the inside cover of this book. Using your completed assessment, record your intakes of vitamins A, E, C, B-6, B-12, thiamin, riboflavin, niacin, and folate in the table below. Next, record the RDA for each nutrient from your assessment. Then, record the percentage of the RDA you had for each vitamin. Last, place a +, −, or = in the space provided, reflecting an intake higher, lower, or equal to the RDA.

Vitamin	Intake	RDA	% of RDA	+/−/=
A				
E				
C				
THIAMIN				
RIBOFLAVIN				
NIACIN				
B-6				
FOLATE				
B-12				

ANALYSIS

1. Which of your vitamin intakes equaled or exceeded your RDA? Are any excesses in a possibly toxic range?

   _____

2. Which of your vitamin intakes were below the RDA?

   _____

3. What foods could you eat to improve your dietary intake of vitamins? (Review sources of certain vitamins in the text.)

   _____

   _____

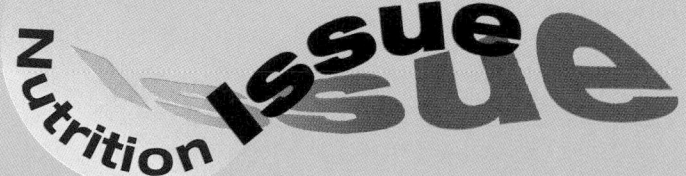

Nutrition and Cancer

Cancer is currently the second leading cause of death for American adults. It is projected to be the number-one cause of early death in the next century, in part because as people live longer the risk of developing cancer increases. Cancer comprises many diseases; these differ in the types of cells affected and, in some cases, in the factors contributing to cancer development (Figure 8-15). For example, the factors leading to skin cancer differ from those leading to breast cancer. Similarly the treatments for the different types of cancer may differ.

Cancer essentially represents abnormal and uncontrollable division of cells; if untreated or not treatable, it leads to death. Most cancers take the form of **tumors,** although not all tumors are cancers. A tumor is simply spontaneous new tissue growth that serves no functional purpose. It can be **benign,** like a wart, or **malignant,** like most lung cancers. The term *malignant tumor* is synonymous with cancer. Malignant tumors can also spread, or *metastasize,* to distant sites via the blood and lymphatic circulation, thereby producing tumors in almost any part of the body[16] (Figure 8-16).

Recent evidence indicates that many cancers can keep growing because they contain an enzyme called telomerase. Typically as cells divide, the DNA shortens. When it becomes too short, the cell can no longer divide. Telomerase prevents the shortening by replacing DNA lost at each cell division. Thus cancer cells can keep growing. Scientists speculate that drugs that inhibit telomerase may be future tools for treating cancer.[17]

Tumor
Mass of cells; may be cancerous (malignant) or noncancerous (benign).

Benign
Noncancerous; tumors that do not spread.

Malignant
Essentially to do anything malicious. In reference to a tumor, the property of spreading locally and to distant sites.

Metastasis
Spread of cancerous cells from their site of origin to other areas of the body.

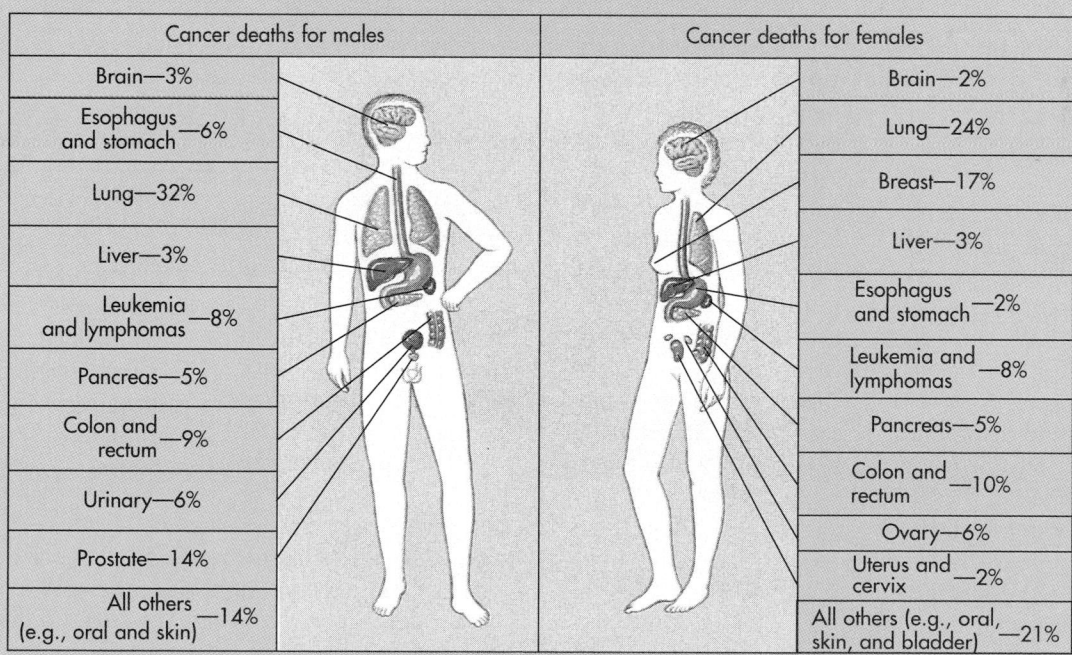

Cancer deaths for males		Cancer deaths for females
Brain—3%		Brain—2%
Esophagus and stomach—6%		Lung—24%
Lung—32%		Breast—17%
Liver—3%		Liver—3%
Leukemia and lymphomas—8%		Esophagus and stomach—2%
Pancreas—5%		Leukemia and lymphomas—8%
Colon and rectum—9%		Pancreas—5%
Urinary—6%		Colon and rectum—10%
Prostate—14%		Ovary—6%
All others (e.g., oral and skin)—14%		Uterus and cervix—2%
		All others (e.g., oral, skin, and bladder)—21%

Figure 8-15 *Cancer is actually many diseases. Numerous types of cells and organs are its target. Note that about one third of all cancers arise from smoking.*

Continued.

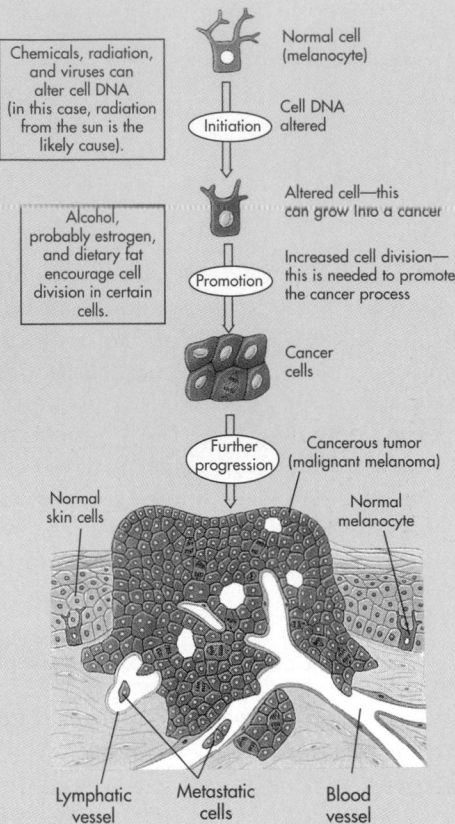

Chemicals, radiation, and viruses can alter cell DNA (in this case, radiation from the sun is the likely cause).

Normal cell (melanocyte)

Initiation — Cell DNA altered

Altered cell—this can grow into a cancer

Alcohol, probably estrogen, and dietary fat encourage cell division in certain cells.

Promotion — Increased cell division—this is needed to promote the cancer process

Cancer cells

Further progression — Cancerous tumor (malignant melanoma)

Normal skin cells   Normal melanocyte

Lymphatic vessel   Metastatic cells   Blood vessel

Figure 8-16 *Progression from a normal skin cell to skin cancer through the initiation, promotion, and progression stages. The ball of cells is a developing tumor. As the mass of cells grows, it can invade surrounding tissues, eventually penetrating into both lymph and blood vessels. These vessels carry spreading (metastatic) cancer cells throughout the body, where they can form new cancer sites.*

Both genetics and lifestyle are potent forces that influence the risk of cancer developing. Certain cancers tend to occur in some families more than in others. About 30 cancer-susceptibility **genes** have been isolated.[25] People within high-risk families are said to be genetically predisposed, or at risk, for developing specific types of cancer. A genetic predisposition is especially important in development of colon cancer and some types of breast cancer.[24,39] People in these families should be more vigilant in trying to prevent the cancer and should stay under close surveillance for its occurrence. For example, a history of breast cancer should encourage a woman to maintain a healthy weight, limit alcohol intake, and have regular mammograms.

Lifestyle is also a critical factor in most forms of cancer, as evidenced by the variation in cancer rates from country

Genes

The genetic material on chromosomes that make up DNA. Genes provide the blueprints for the production of cell proteins.

to country. The Japanese, for example, have higher rates of stomach cancer than Americans, whereas Americans tend to have higher rates of colon cancer than the Japanese. When Japanese people immigrate to the United States, their risk of stomach cancer decreases but their risk of colon cancer increases. In addition, women who have borne many children experience a reduced risk for endometrial cancer. Finally, people living in poverty show higher cancer death rates than middle- and upper-income groups, probably because of inadequate health care and deficient diets.

Although we have little control over our genetic risks for cancer, we do have a great deal of choice in deciding which lifestyle risks to take, especially with regard to smoking, alcohol abuse, and nutrient intake (food choice). That one third of all cancers in the United States are due directly to tobacco use is well established. About half of the cancers of the mouth, pharynx, and larynx are associated with heavy use of alcohol. A combination of alcohol use and smoking increases cancer risks even higher. Moreover, that certain dietary factors either promote or inhibit cancer has become increasingly apparent. With diet, as with tobacco and alcohol use, imprudent choices today likely cause medical problems tomorrow.[37]

CANCER-CAUSING MECHANISMS

To understand how cancer can be prevented, first examine how cancer develops in the body. Cancer initiation begins with multiple steps, starting with exposure of a cell to a **carcinogen.** Subsequent steps are cancer promotion and finally cancer progression (see Figure 8-16).

Carcinogens

Compounds that have potential to cause cancer.

Cancer initiation

The initiation stage begins with alterations—called **mutations**—in DNA, the genetic material in a cell. As a result, the cell no longer responds to normal controls on cell division. Initiation can develop spontaneously or be induced by carcinogens. The affected cell now can dictate its own rate of division and is not inhibited from doing so at the expense of surrounding cells. Alteration of DNA can occur within a few minutes to days. Among the carcinogens that can initiate cancer development are radiant energy, chemical agents, and biological agents.

Mutation

A permanent change in a cell's DNA; includes changes in sequence, alteration of gene position, gene loss or duplication, and insertion of foreign gene sequences.

Radiation can alter DNA by cross-linking the double strands or breaking the strands into fragments. Damaging free radicals can also form as a result of radiation and can consequently alter DNA. As a practical example, various skin cancers often begin with overexposure to the sun. The altered skin cells may then begin to multiply out of control.

Cancer can be induced by various chemicals, especially multi-ring chemicals, such as aflatoxin and benzo-(a)pyrene. Aflatoxin, which is produced by molds present in peanuts and cereal grains, is a potent carcinogen for rats. For this reason, FDA regulates the amount of aflatoxin that can be present in peanut products (see Chapter 17). Rejecting moldy foods is one way to avoid possible carcinogens. Benzo(a)pyrene is formed as meat fat drips onto hot coals when foods are charcoal-broiled. If smoke containing the carcinogen penetrates the meat and the meat is consumed, benzo(a)pyrene is absorbed into the body. To limit this, trim fat from meat before cooking, cut barbecuing time by partially cooking meat in a microwave oven before finishing it off on the grill, and don't nibble on really black bits.

Biological agents such as viruses can also initiate cancer development. Viruses insert their genetic material into target cells within the body. Alteration of the target-cell DNA by the viral information can transform a normal target cell into a cancer cell.

Potentially thwarting this process of cancer development are other human genes, called *tumor suppressors*. These may step in to prevent the abnormal growth. An important tumor-suppressor gene, p53, provides a check on inappropriate cellular division. However, if mutations also cause the tumor suppressor to fail, this block against cancer development also fails. Mutations of this and other tumor-suppressor genes are often linked to cancer.[25] Generally speaking, one or more mutations of various genes may be required for a tumor to develop.

To review, three basic agents can alter DNA: radiation, chemicals, and biological agents such as viruses. However, alteration of DNA does not necessarily mean cancer will develop. As you'll see, along with suppressor genes, some other substances also inhibit cancer development. In addition, special enzymes travel up and down the DNA to repair breaks and correct defects.[36] About 99% of the time the repair enzymes find alterations caused by chemicals or radiation and correct them before the altered cell divides to begin its unrestrained growth. A key function of the p53 tumor-suppressor gene is to allow time for that to take place before the next cell division.[25]

Alcohol in large amounts is toxic to cells. The resulting cell death creates a need for new cell division. In this way, alcohol can increase cell division and therefore the risk for cancer, especially in the mouth and esophagus.

Cancer promotion

The initiation stage of carcinogenesis, during which DNA is altered, is relatively short (minutes to days). In contrast, the promotion stage may last for months or years

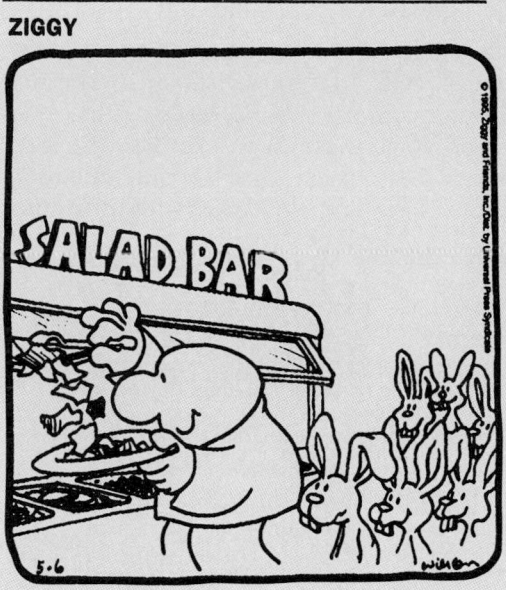

ZIGGY

Figure 8-17 *Ziggy.*

before the final stage, progression, appears. During the promotion stage the DNA alterations are "locked" into the genetic material of cells. Once a cell multiplies and incorporates its newly altered DNA into its genetic instructions, the repair enzymes can no longer detect the changes in DNA. Anything that increases the rate of cell division decreases the chance that the repair enzymes will find the altered part of the DNA in time to do their work. Compounds that increase cell division—called *cancer promoters*—are thought to promote cancer either by decreasing the time available for repair enzymes to act or encouraging cells with altered DNA to develop and grow.

These altered cells may develop and grow for 10 to 30 years before they become cancerous. We know this because increased lung cancer rates lagged about 30 years behind the increase in cigarette smoking that started in World War II. Common promoters are estrogen, alcohol, and probably high intakes of fat and total energy (kcals). Bacterial infections in the stomach are also suspected agents.

Experimental studies with animals have revealed that some substances, called *antipromoters*, can inhibit carcinogenesis during the promotion stage. Compounds present in cruciferous vegetables, onions, garlic, and citrus fruits—as well as vitamin A, vitamin D, and calcium—are thought to have antipromoter activity (see the discussion on phytochemicals in the Nutrition Insight in Chapter 2). Cancer experts agree that a diet rich in fruits and vegetables is a key cancer-preventive measure[37] (Figure 8-17). Supplementation with individual nutrients, such as vitamin C, does not receive as much support, partly because this practice doesn't contribute phytochemicals, as food choices supplying these nutrients do.[2]

Continued.

Cancer progression

The final stage in carcinogenesis begins with the appearance of cells that can grow autonomously (that is, without normal controls on growth). During the progression stage these cancer cells proliferate, invade the surrounding tissue, and spread (metastasize) to other sites. Early in this stage the immune system may find the altered cells and destroy them. Another possibility is that the cancer cells are so defective that their own DNA limits their ability to grow, and they die. If nothing impedes growth of cancer cells, one or more tumors eventually develop that are large enough to affect body functions, and symptoms of cancer appear.

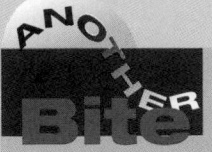

Remember that if a cancer is left untreated, it can spread quickly throughout the body. When this happens, it is much more likely to lead to death. Thus early detection is critical. Aids in early detection include the following warning signs:

- *Unexplained weight loss*
- *A change in bowel or bladder habits*
- *A sore that does not heal*
- *Unusual bleeding or discharge*
- *A thickening or lump in the breast or elsewhere*
- *Indigestion or difficulty in swallowing*
- *An obvious change in a wart or mole*
- *A nagging cough or hoarseness*

Other ways exist to detect cancer early. Colonoscopy examinations for middle-age and older adults, PSA (prostate-specific antigen) tests for men, and Papanicolaou tests (Pap smears) and regular breast examinations for women are recommended by the American Cancer Society.

DIET AND CANCER

Cancer quackery aside, a nutritious diet, as well as other lifestyle characteristics, can reduce the risk of cancer initiation and promotion. For example, both obesity and physical inactivity are linked to an increased risk for many types of cancer. Some food constituents may contribute to cancer development, whereas others have a protective effect (Table 8-4).

Contribution of fat and energy intakes to cancer risk

Obesity, especially excess fat storage in the abdominal region, is related to all major forms of cancer except lung cancer, including cancer of the breast, colon, endometrium, and prostate. The link probably occurs between adipose tissue and the synthesis of estrogen from other hormones in the blood. High concentrations of circulating estrogen in the blood are thought to promote cancer. A long-standing excess energy intake may also promote cancer. When animals are fed diets high in fat or total energy, they tend to experience more cancers, especially in the colon and breast. The effect is most apparent when a carcinogen is used to deliberately initiate the cancer process, and the animals are then fed a high-fat or energy-rich diet.[38] Fat and total energy intakes are not considered initiators of cancer but rather promoters.

The National Cancer Institute (NCI) believes the link between dietary fat and cancer is sufficient to encourage Americans to reduce fat intake. The NCI recommends initially decreasing dietary fat to 30% of total energy intake and eventually to 20% or less of total energy if the person is at high risk and can follow such a dietary pattern. Some scientists, however, believe that the NCI has overreacted to the fat and cancer issue. Although epidemiological evidence does link fat and certain forms of cancer, the evidence is not strong.

A stronger link actually exists between cancer and total energy in the diet. If rats or mice are treated with a carcinogen to promote either breast or colon cancer and then one group consumes a typical energy intake while a second group consumes a reduced energy intake, the group with the low energy intake will exhibit about a 40% reduction in tumor development. The amount of fat in the diet is not important, as long as energy intake is about 70% of the usual intake of the animals. Energy restriction is currently the most effective technique for preventing cancer in laboratory animals.[38]

A large scale study called the Women's Health Initiative is testing the hypothesis that a diet with 20% or less energy from fat reduces cancer occurrence in the breast and other sites in adult women (ages 59-70 years). The study is due for completion in 2005. Currently the research community is divided on whether this will be an effective therapy for reducing breast cancer.[21]

TABLE 8-4

Some Food Constituents Suspected of Having a Role in Cancer[4, 6, 8, 9, 14, 22, 37]

Constituent	Dietary sources	Action
POSSIBLY PROTECTIVE*		
Vitamin A	Liver, fortified milk, fruits, vegetables	Encourages normal cell development
Vitamin E	Whole grains, vegetable oil, green leafy vegetables	Antioxidant
Vitamin C	Fruits, vegetables	Antioxidant; can block conversion of nitrites and nitrates to potent carcinogens
Folate	Fruits, vegetables, whole grains	Encourages normal cell development
Selenium	Meats, whole grains	Part of antioxidant system
Carotenoids	Fruits, vegetables	Tend to be antioxidants; some possibly influencing cell metabolism
Indoles, phenols, and other plant substances	Vegetables, especially cabbage, cauliflower, brussels sprouts, garlic, onions, tea (especially green tea)	May reduce carcinogen activation
Dietary fiber	Whole grains, fruits, vegetables, beans	May bind carcinogens in the feces, decrease stool transit time, thus lowering risk of colon and rectal cancer
Calcium	Dairy products, green vegetables	Slows cell division in the colon, binds bile acids and free fatty acids
Omega-3 fatty acids	Cold-water fish, such as salmon and tuna	May inhibit tumor growth
Soy products		Phytic acid present possibly binding carcinogens in the intestinal tract; the genistein component possibly reducing growth and metastasis of malignant cells
Conjugated linoleic acid	Dairy products, meats, fish	May inhibit tumor development and act as an antioxidant
POSSIBLY CARCINOGENIC		
Fats	Meats, high-fat milk and milk products, vegetable oils	Linked to increased synthesis of estrogen and other sex hormones, which in excess may themselves increase the risk for cancer
Alcohol	Beer, wine, liquor	Contributes to cancers of the throat, liver, and bladder and very likely the breast; increased cell turnover and liver metabolism of carcinogens are the main mechanism
Nitrites, nitrates	Cured meats, especially ham, bacon, and sausages	Under very high temperatures will bind to amino acid derivatives to form nitrosamines, potent carcinogens
Multi-ring compounds: Aflatoxin	Formed when mold is present on peanuts and other grains	May alter DNA structure and inhibit its ability to properly respond to physiologic controls; aflatoxin linked to liver cancer
Benzo(a)pyrene	Charcoal-broiled foods, especially meats	Benzo(a)pyrene linked to stomach and other intestinal cancers

*Many of the actions listed for these possibly protective agents are speculative and have been verified only by animal studies.

Continued.

The mechanism behind this effect of total energy intake is probably hormonal changes that inhibit tumor growth. Slowing cell division, which allows more time for any needed DNA repair, is another possible mechanism. Moreover, reduced cell metabolism from caloric restriction may reduce free radical damage to DNA.[38]

Can we apply this evidence from animal studies to ourselves? We don't want to suffer from cancer, but very few of us want to eat only 70% of our usual energy intake. Despite the evidence of a strong link between some types of cancer and obesity, many Americans are still overweight and have not slimmed down to a healthier body weight. Furthermore, reducing dietary energy to 70% of usual intake is very difficult. So while the data obtained from animal studies are interesting, scientists do not see any practical way to make recommendations on the basis of these studies. Moreover, once cancer is present, energy restriction is no longer helpful.

Cancer-inhibiting food constituents

Many single nutrients may have cancer-inhibiting properties. These anticarcinogens include antioxidants, certain phytochemicals, and dietary fiber[8,14] (see Table 8-4). The antioxidant activity of vitamin C and vitamin E helps prevent formation of **nitrosamines** in the GI tract, thus preventing formation of a potent carcinogen. Vitamin E also helps protect unsaturated fatty acids from damage by free radicals. Generally, carotenoids, vitamin E, vitamin C, and selenium function as or contribute to antioxidant systems in the body. These antioxidant systems help prevent the alteration of DNA by electron-seeking compounds.

Nitrosamine

A carcinogen formed from nitrates and breakdown products of amino acids; can lead to stomach cancer.

In addition, phytochemicals from fruits and vegetables in some cases block cancer development. Numerous studies suggest that fruit and vegetable intake reduces the risk of cancers of the mouth, pharynx, larynx, esophagus, stomach, colon, rectum, bladder, and cervix.[8,37] These foods are normally rich in carotenoids and vitamin C, plus dietary fiber and vitamin E. Inadequate vitamin D intake (coupled with little sun exposure) is suspected of fostering breast, colon, and prostate cancer. In sum, a diet that follows the Food Guide Pyramid, so that fruits, vegetables, whole

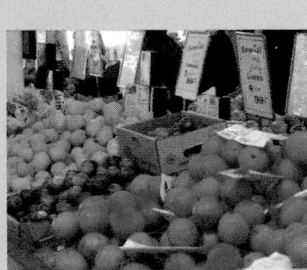

A diet rich in fruits and vegetables may reduce the risk of some forms of cancer.

grains, low-fat and nonfat dairy products, and some plant oils are eaten daily, is a rich source of anticarcinogens (Table 8-5).

Chapter 5 introduced the possible role of fiber in preventing colon cancer. Insoluble fiber decreases transit time so that the stool is in contact with the colon wall for a shorter period of time, thus reducing contact with carcinogens. Soluble fibers may bind bile acids and thus block some recycling of these by the body. Bile acids are thought to contribute to cancer risk by irritating the colon cells, thereby increasing cell division. In addition, dietary fiber (specifically the insoluble fiber content) may increase the binding and excretion of the sex hormones testosterone and estrogen from within the intestines. This is important because of the links between excessive amounts of sex hormones and certain types of cancer, specifically prostate and colon cancer. The evidence regarding the importance of fiber in preventing colon cancer is still inconclusive. For now the recom-

A current nationwide study designed to reduce the risk of colon cancer is under way in the United States. It employs a diet having five to eight daily servings of fruits and vegetables in which fat is 20% of the energy intake. This diet also aims for about 30 grams of dietary fiber daily.

TABLE 8-5

One Example of a Diet Intended to Limit Risk for Cancer. This is Low in Fat and Rich in Foods with Anticancer Properties.

BREAKFAST

1 cup nonfat milk
1 cup Crispy
   Wheat N' Raisins
1 orange
1 slice whole wheat
   toast with 2 tea-
   spoons fruit jam
Hot tea

LUNCH

Sandwich:
   2 slices whole wheat
   bread
   ¾ oz Monterey Jack
   cheese
   ½ cup alfalfa sprouts
   red onion slices
   mustard
1 cup lowfat yogurt
   (with fruit)
3 fig bar cookies
1 cup apple juice

SNACK

½ cup nonfat milk
3 graham crackers

DINNER

Salad:
   1½ cups romaine lettuce
   ½ tomato
   3 sliced mushrooms
   2 tablespoons oil and
   vinegar dressing
3 ounces broiled salmon
¾ cup brown rice
¾ cup green beans
Hot tea

SNACK

1 banana
¼ cup roasted soy beans

NUTRIENT BREAKDOWN

2200 kcal; 22% kcal as fat

mendation to consume 20 to 35 grams a day is reasonable advice. Liberal use of whole grains, fruits, and vegetables should be sufficient to meet guidelines.

Calcium is also linked to a decreased risk for developing colon cancer. As with fiber the evidence is inconclusive. Some studies show that calcium decreases the growth of cells in the colon; therefore it probably decreases the risk of a genetically altered cell developing into a cancer. Calcium may also bind free fatty acids and bile acids in the colon, so they are less apt to interact with cells located there and induce cancer.[6] More research is needed before calcium can be promoted as a cancer-preventing agent.

If you have a question about cancer, call the National Cancer Institute hotline at 1-800-4-CANCER.

Many other important reasons exist, of course, for consuming the RDA of calcium (see Chapter 9).

THE BOTTOM LINE

Table 8-6 lists a variety of dietary changes that can reduce your risk for cancer. View this as a total diet and lifestyle approach. Start by making sure that your diet is moderate in energy and fat content and that you consume many fruits, vegetables, whole grains, beans, and low-fat or nonfat dairy products. In other words, follow the Food Guide Pyramid. In addition, remain physically active; avoid smoking, excessive sun exposure and obesity; and consume cured meat and alcohol only moderately if at all. Until more definitive information about diet and cancer is available, that is all the diet and related lifestyle advice scientists can offer.[37]

TABLE 8-6

General Dietary Recommendations to Reduce the Risk of Cancer*

1. Avoid obesity.
2. Reduce fat intake to 30% of total energy intake as a start. Then consider a reduction closer to 20% of total energy intake if at high risk, such as a family history of cancer.
3. Eat more higher-fiber foods, such as fruits, vegetables, and whole-grain cereals.
4. Include foods rich in vitamins A, E, and C, as well as carotenoids, in the daily diet.
5. If alcohol is consumed, do not drink excessively.
6. Use moderation when consuming salt-cured, smoked, and nitrite-cured foods.

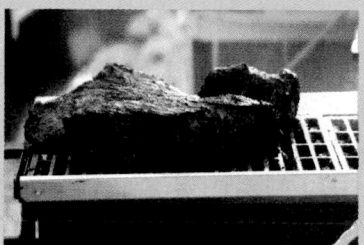

Moderation in consumption of charbroiled meat is advocated as part of a plan to reduce cancer risk.

*The National Cancer Institute (U.S.) endorses all the above but warns not to exceed 35 grams of dietary fiber intake.
The American Cancer Society endorses all the above but sets no percentage for fat intake and adds a recommendation to include cruciferous vegetables in the diet (cabbage, broccoli, and brussels sprouts). These may decrease carcinogen activation.
The Canadian Dietetic Association generally endorses all of the above, but the specific language differs.

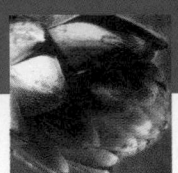

Water and Minerals

WATER—THE MOST VERSATILE

medium for all kinds of chemical reactions—constitutes the major portion of our bodies. Without water, our life processes would cease in a matter of days. We lose about 2 quarts (2 liters) of water daily, and this should be replenished daily because the body does not store water well. We know the resulting constant demand for water as *thirst*.

Many minerals, like water, are vital to health. They are key players in body growth and metabolism, muscle movement, and water balance, among other wide-ranging processes. Researchers are still defining what minerals the body requires and the quantities needed for good health. We are not sure that all the minerals found in our bodies—for example, vanadium and tin—are necessary to sustain human life.[26] Some minerals, such as lead, may be found in humans only as a contaminant. The mere presence of a mineral in our bodies is not proof that we need it.

Based on the amount we need each day, minerals are categorized as major (requiring >100 milligrams per day) or trace (requiring ≤100 milligrams per day). These categories do not reflect the importance of those minerals to the body; deficiencies of some trace minerals can cause severe health problems.[1,3,13] In this chapter, you will see why the study of water and minerals is critical for understanding human nutrition.

ASSESS yourself

yourself

Working For Denser Bones

In this chapter you will learn important information about the disease osteoporosis, characterized by thinning and brittle bones.

Osteoporosis affects more than 25 million people in the United States. One third of all women experience fractures because of this disease, amounting to 1.2 million bone fractures per year. In addition, 12% to 20% of all elderly people who suffer hip fractures die from complications. Given the rise in the number of elderly people in the United States, osteoporosis-related illness and death are anticipated to increase dramatically in coming years.

This is a disease you can do something about. Some risk factors can't be changed, but others can. To what degree are you doing the things that can help prevent this debilitating disease? Answer "yes" or "no" to the following questions by placing an "X" in the appropriate blank:

	YES	NO
1. Do you average at least 10-20 minutes of sun exposure per day to at least your hands and face to get vitamin D, or do you drink vitamin D–fortified milk regularly?	_____	_____
2. Do you engage in weight-bearing physical activity (jogging, brisk walking, etc.) for at least 30 minutes on most or all days of the week?	_____	_____
3. If you are a woman, do you experience regular menstruation?	_____	_____
4. Do you avoid smoking cigarettes?	_____	_____
5. Do you avoid regular consumption of large amounts (greater than 1-2 drinks per day) of alcohol?	_____	_____
6. Do you consume milk and other dairy products regularly, or substitute other sources to meet at least the RDA for calcium?	_____	_____
7. Do you moderate intake of phosphorus, sodium, protein, and caffeine?	_____	_____

The more *yes* answers you have, the more you are actively preserving your bone density for the future. Also, remember that this is not just a consideration for women, because if men plan to live well into their 80s and 90s they are at risk for osteoporosis. In fact, about 14% of all spine fractures and 25% of all hip fractures linked to osteoporosis occur in men.

Key Chapter Concepts

- Water constitutes 50% to 70% of the human body. It serves as a medium for chemical reactions, temperature regulation, and lubrication. For adults, daily water needs are estimated at 1 milliliter per kcal expended. Sources include all beverages.
- Many minerals are vital for sustaining life. For humans, animal products are the most bioavailable sources for most minerals. Supplements of minerals exceeding 150% of recommended amounts should be taken only under a physician's supervision, because toxicity and nutrient interactions are a likely possibility.
- Sodium is the major positive ion (Na⁺) found outside cells. The typical American's diet provides abundant sodium; about 10% to 15% of adults are at risk for developing high blood pressure if they consume too much sodium.
- Potassium is the major positive ion found inside cells. Milk, fruits, and vegetables are good sources.
- Chloride, which is part of table salt (NaCl), is the major negative ion found outside cells.
- Calcium forms a vital part of bone structure and is also very important for blood clotting, muscle contraction, nerve transmission, and cell metabolism. Dairy products are important calcium sources. Women are particularly at risk for inadequate calcium intake.
- Phosphorus aids enzyme function and forms part of key metabolic compounds, cell membranes, and bone. Good food sources are dairy products, bakery products, and meats.
- Magnesium is important for nerve and heart function and as an activator for many enzymes. Whole grains (such as bran), vegetables, nuts,

seeds, milk, and meats are good food sources.
- Iron helps to synthesize hemoglobin and myoglobin. Women are at great risk for developing iron deficiency. When severe, this condition decreases the amount of oxygen in the blood and results in iron-deficiency anemia. Iron absorption depends primarily on the form of iron present in food and the body's need for it. Iron toxicity usually results from a genetic disorder called *hemochromatosis.*
- Zinc aids the action of more than 300 enzymes that are important for growth, development, immune function, wound healing, and taste. The most nutrient-dense sources of zinc are oysters, shrimp, crab, and beef. Good plant sources are whole grains, peanuts, and beans.
- Selenium decreases the action of free radical (oxidizing) compounds. Meats, eggs, fish, and shellfish are good animal sources of selenium. Good plant sources include grains and seeds.
- Iodine forms part of the thyroid hormones. A lack of dietary iodine results in the development of an enlarged thyroid gland or goiter. Iodized salt is a good food source.
- Copper is important for iron and protein metabolism, among other functions. Copper is found mainly in liver, seafood, legumes, and whole grains.
- Fluoride that is incorporated into dietary intake during development makes teeth resistant to dental caries. Most of us receive the bulk of our fluoride from fluoridated water and toothpaste.
- Chromium aids action of the hormone insulin. Egg yolks, meats, and whole grains are good sources of chromium. Human needs for other trace minerals are so low that deficiencies are uncommon.

WATER

To appreciate how minerals operate in the body, we must understand the nature and general chemical properties of water, as well as specific nutrient-related functions.

Water is the perfect medium for body processes because it enables chemical reactions to occur. Water even participates directly in many of these reactions. It forms the greatest component of the human body, making up 50% to 70% of the body's weight (about 10 gallons or 40 liters). Lean muscle tissue contains about 73% water. Adipose tissue is about 20% water. Thus, as fat content increases (and the percentage of lean tissue decreases) in the body, total body water content drifts toward 50%.[14]

Depending on how much fat has been stored, an adult can survive for about 8 weeks without eating food but only a few days without drinking water. This occurs not because water is more important than carbohydrate, fat, protein, vitamins, or minerals, but rather because we can neither store nor conserve water as well as we can the other components of our diet.

Water in the Body—Intracellular and Extracellular Fluid

Water flows in and out of body cells through cell membranes. Water inside cells forms part of the intracellular fluid—the fluid within the cells. When water is outside cells or in the bloodstream, it is part of the extracellular fluid—that outside cells (Figure 9-1). Because cell membranes are permeable to water, water shifts freely in and out of cells. For example, if blood volume decreases, water can move from the areas inside and around cells to the bloodstream to increase blood volume. On the other hand, if blood volume increases, water can shift out of the bloodstream into cells and the surrounding areas.

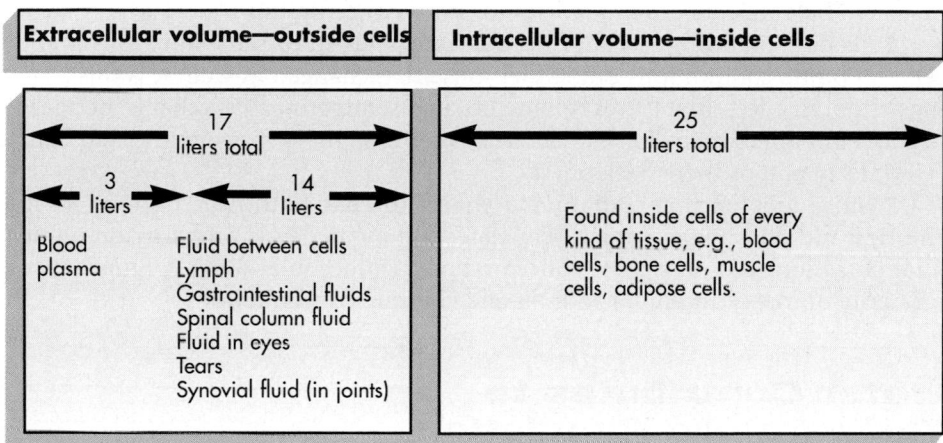

Figure 9-1 *The fluid compartments in the body.*

The body controls the amount of water in the intracellular and extracellular compartments mainly by controlling ion concentrations. Ions have electrical charges. Water is attracted to ions, such as sodium, potassium, chloride, phosphate, magnesium, and calcium. By controlling the movements of ions in and out of the cellular compartments, the body maintains the appropriate amount of water in each compartment. Where ions go, water follows.[14]

Osmosis

Osmosis is the process that regulates and equalizes the proportion of water in cells and in the bloodstream. Osmosis operates when fluids containing different ion concentrations are separated by a semipermeable membrane. In the body, for example, a semipermeable cell membrane separates cells from the fluid-filled spaces (compartments) surrounding cells. The semipermeable membrane allows water to passively diffuse into cells but controls the flow of ions. This passage in the body actually uses certain channels through which water can move. If adjoining fluid compartments contain dissimilar concentrations of particles (have different total ion concentrations), water flows through the cell membrane channels to equalize the particle concentrations in each compartment.

Osmosis
Passive diffusion of a solution (water) through a semipermeable membrane from a less concentrated compartment to a more concentrated compartment.

Examples that demonstrate osmosis are sugar pulling fluid from strawberries and a salty salad dressing wilting lettuce.

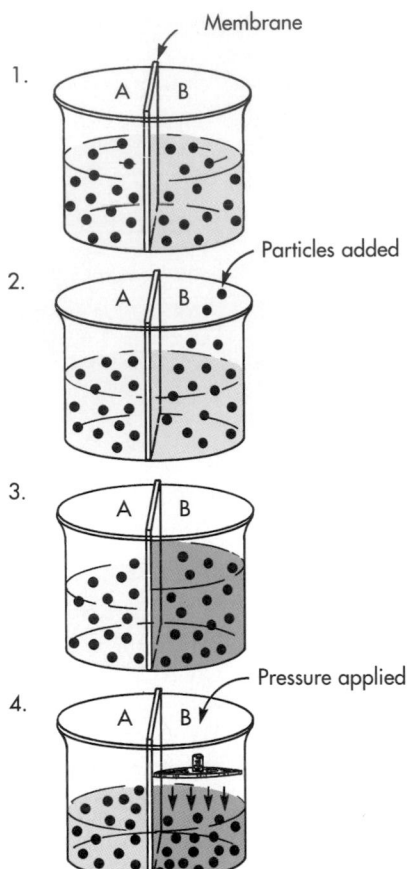

Figure 9-2

A graphic representation of osmosis and osmotic pressure. 1. An equal number of particles on each side allows equal amounts of water. 2. Now additional particles are added to side B, but the particles cannot flow across the membrane, 3. Water can flow across the membrane, so it flows to side B, where there are more particles. The volume of water becomes greater on side B, causing the particle concentrations on sides A and B to again become equal. 4. If physical pressure (such as a pump) compressed the fluid on side B to restore its original volume, that pressure would equal the osmotic pressure exerted by the added particles.

Figure 9-2 illustrates osmosis. Adding particles to the right compartment increases its particle concentration and, in turn, decreases its relative water concentration. This happens in the bloodstream when you eat sodium. Because most particles cannot easily pass through the membrane depicted in Figure 9-2, water shifts from the compartment with a low particle concentration (the more diluted compartment) to the more highly concentrated one. To counteract a high sodium concentration in the bloodstream, one body response is to shift fluid from cells into the bloodstream.[14]

Water and Ions in the Body—A Balancing Act

Adding water—instead of particles—to a compartment dilutes its particle concentration, and so the compartment tends to donate water to more concentrated compartments near-by. This happens when you drink water. Some water absorbed by the body moves from the bloodstream into body cells, which in turn equalizes the particle concentration in the cells with that in the various nearby body compartments. Therefore, because of the action of osmosis, water is forced to move across membranes to balance changes in particle—or ion—concentrations.

Cells have pumping mechanisms that constantly draw potassium ions into the cell and pump sodium ions out. Other ions are exchanged as well. It is this pumping action, in effect, that leaves cell membranes semipermeable—that is, permeable to water but not to many ions. Ions, such as sodium, may cross into the cell, but the cell quickly pumps them back out.

Positive ions, such as sodium and potassium, pair with negative ions, such as chloride and phosphate. Intracellular water volume depends primarily on intracellular potassium and phosphate concentrations. Extracellular water volume depends primarily on the extracellular sodium and chloride concentrations.[14]

Water Contributes to Temperature Regulation

Water changes temperature slowly because it has a great ability to hold heat. It takes much more energy to heat water than it does to heat fat. Compare the time it takes to melt ice cubes with the time it takes to melt frozen butter in a microwave oven. Foods with high water content heat up and cool down slowly. Because water requires so much energy to change states—for example, from a liquid to a gas—it forms an ideal medium for removing heat from the body.

The body secretes fluids in the form of perspiration, which evaporates through skin pores. To evaporate water, heat energy is required. So, as perspiration evaporates, heat energy is taken from the skin, cooling it in the process. Each quart (liter) of perspiration evaporated represents approximately 600 kcal of energy lost from the skin and surrounding tissues.[16] For this reason, fever increases one's need for energy.

However, to cool efficiently, perspiration must be allowed to evaporate. If it simply rolls off the skin or soaks into clothing, perspiration doesn't cool us much. Evaporation of perspiration occurs readily when humidity is low. This is why humans often tolerate hot, dry climates far better than they do hot, humid climates.

Water Helps Remove Waste Products

Water is an important vehicle for ridding the body of waste products. Most unusable substances in the body can dissolve in water and exit the body through the urine.

A major body waste product is **urea.** This by-product of protein metabolism contains nitrogen. The more protein we eat in excess of needs, the more nitrogen we excrete—in the form of urea—in the urine. Likewise, the more sodium we consume, the more sodium we excrete in the urine. Overall, the amount of urine a person needs to produce is determined primarily by excess protein and sodium chloride (salt) intake. By limiting excess protein and sodium intakes, it is possible to limit urine output—a useful practice, for example, in space flights. This type of diet is also used to treat some kidney diseases where the ability to produce urine output is hampered.

A typical urine volume is about 1 to 2 liters (1 to 2 quarts) per day, depending mostly on the amount of fluid, protein, and sodium intake. Somewhat more urine output than that is fine, but less—especially less than 600 milliliters ($2^{1}/_{2}$ cups)—forces the kidneys to form a very concentrated urine. The heavy ion concentration increases the risk of kidney stone formation in susceptible people, generally men. Kidney stones are simply minerals and other substances that have precipitated out of the urine and accumulated in kidney tissues.

How Much Water Do We Need?

Adults need roughly 1 milliliter of water per kcal expended. We consume about 1 liter (1 quart) of water a day in various liquids, such as fruit juice, coffee, tea, soft drinks, and water itself (Figure 9-3). Foods supply another liter of fluid; many fruits, vegetables, and beverages are more than 80% water. Water as a by-product

Urea
A by-product of protein metabolism that contains nitrogen.

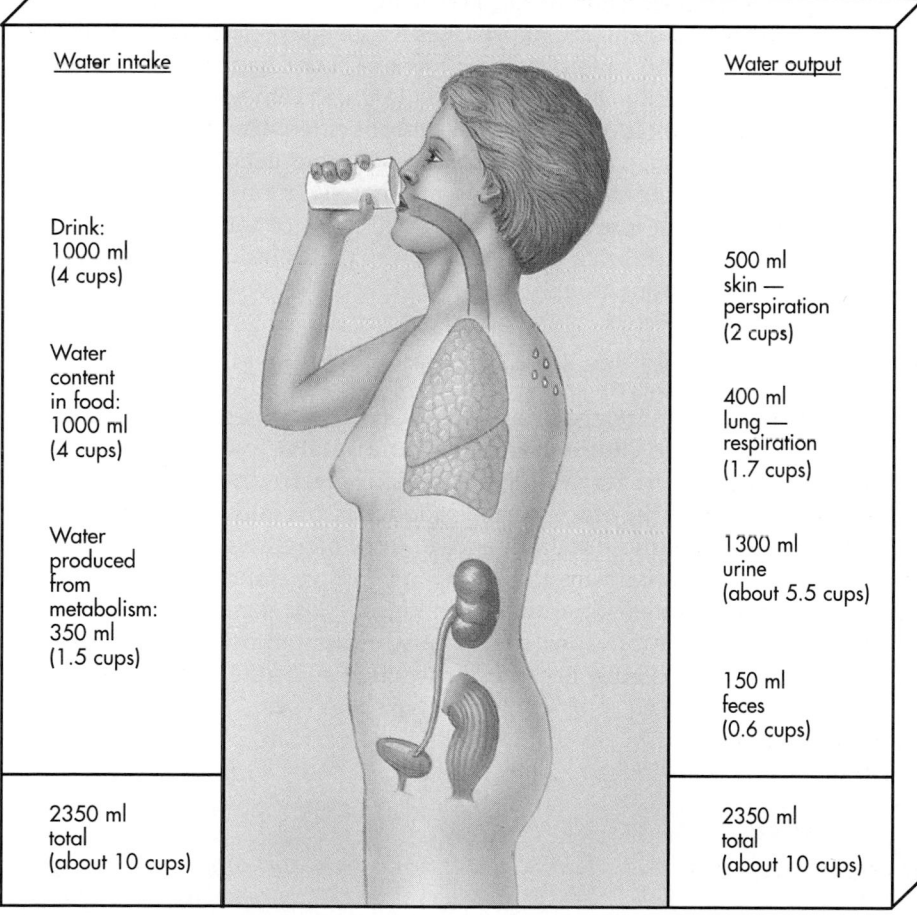

Figure 9-3 *Water balance—intake versus output. We maintain body fluids at an optimum amount by adjusting water intake and output. Most water comes from the liquids we consume. Some comes from the moisture in more solid foods, and the remainder is manufactured during metabolism. Water output includes that lost via lungs, kidneys, skin, and bowels. (Note that ml is the abbreviation for milliliter.)*

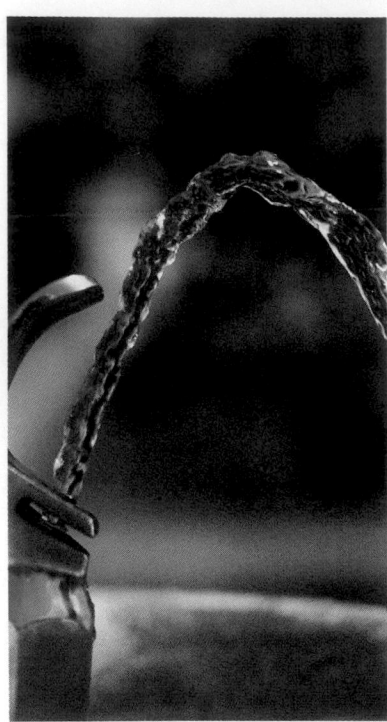

We need water in our diets every day.

of metabolism provides approximately 350 milliliters (1¹/₂ cups) of additional water. This yields a total of about 2.4 liters (10 cups) of water for a 2400 kcal diet, or about 1 milliliter per kcal expended.

Of the 2.4 liters of water needed, about 1.4 liters is used to produce urine. The rest, about 1 liter, compensates for typical water losses through the lungs (400 milliliters), feces (150 milliliters), and skin (500 milliliters) (see Figure 9-3). We are not normally aware of these **insensible** water losses. Note also that when we consider the large amount of water used to lubricate the gastrointestinal (GI) tract, the loss of only 150 milliliters of water a day through the feces is remarkable. About 8000 milliliters of water enters the GI tract daily via secretions from the mouth, stomach, intestine, pancreas, and other organs. The diet supplies an additional 2000 milliliters or more. The kidneys also greatly conserve water. They reabsorb about 97% of the water filtered from waste products.[14]

Thirst

If you don't drink enough water and total body water falls by 1% to 2%, your body often lets you know by signaling thirst. Your brain is communicating the need to drink. This thirst mechanism is not always reliable, however, especially during illness, in later years, and during vigorous exercise, such as in athletic events.[16] Athletes should weigh themselves before and after training sessions to determine their rate of water loss and thus their water needs. Replacing at least 75% of this weight loss is advised, especially as weight loss approaches 3% or more. Two cups (¹/₂ liter) of water weigh about a pound (about half a kilogram) (see Chapter 11 for details on fluid use in athletics). Ailing children—especially those with fever, vomiting, diarrhea, and increased perspiration—and older persons often need to be reminded to drink plenty of fluids. As Chapter 15 discusses in further detail, infants easily become dehydrated. Long airplane flights are another situation that demands extra fluid intake: a traveler can lose about 6 cups (1.5 liters) of water during a 3-hour flight. The dehumidified air in an airplane is so dry that it induces excessive insensible perspiration and evaporation.

What If the Thirst Message Is Ignored?

Once the body registers a shortage of available water, it increases fluid conservation. The pituitary gland releases **antidiuretic hormone (ADH)** to force the kidneys to conserve water. The kidneys respond by reducing urine flow. At the same time, as fluid volume decreases in the bloodstream, blood pressure falls. This eventually signals the kidneys to retain more sodium and, in turn, more water.

However, despite mechanisms that work to conserve water, fluid is constantly lost via the insensible routes—feces, skin, and lungs. Those losses must be replaced. In addition, there is a limit to how concentrated urine can become. Eventually, if fluid is not consumed, the body becomes dehydrated and suffers ill effects.[16]

Antidiuretic hormone (ADH)
A hormone that is secreted by the pituitary gland and that acts on the kidneys to cause a decrease in water excretion.

Insensible
In this case, not perceived by the person, such as water lost with each breath.

ANOTHER Bite

Too much water—whatever amount the kidneys are unable to excrete—can also lead to ill health. However, an excessive amount would have to approach many quarts (liters) each day. Most people have little risk of drinking too much water, but problems do accompany some disease states and mental disorders. When excessive water overwhelms the kidneys' capacity to excrete, blurred vision is one resulting symptom.

Again, by the time a person loses 1% to 2% of body weight in fluids, he or she will be thirsty. At a 4% loss of body weight, muscles lose significant strength and endurance. By the time body weight is reduced by 10% to 12%, heat tolerance is decreased and weakness results. At a 20% reduction, coma and death may soon follow (Figure 9-4).

Alcohol inhibits the action of antidiuretic hormone (ADH). One reason people feel so bad the day after heavy drinking is that they are very dehydrated. Even though they may have consumed a lot of liquid in their drinks, they have excreted even more liquid because alcohol has inhibited ADH.

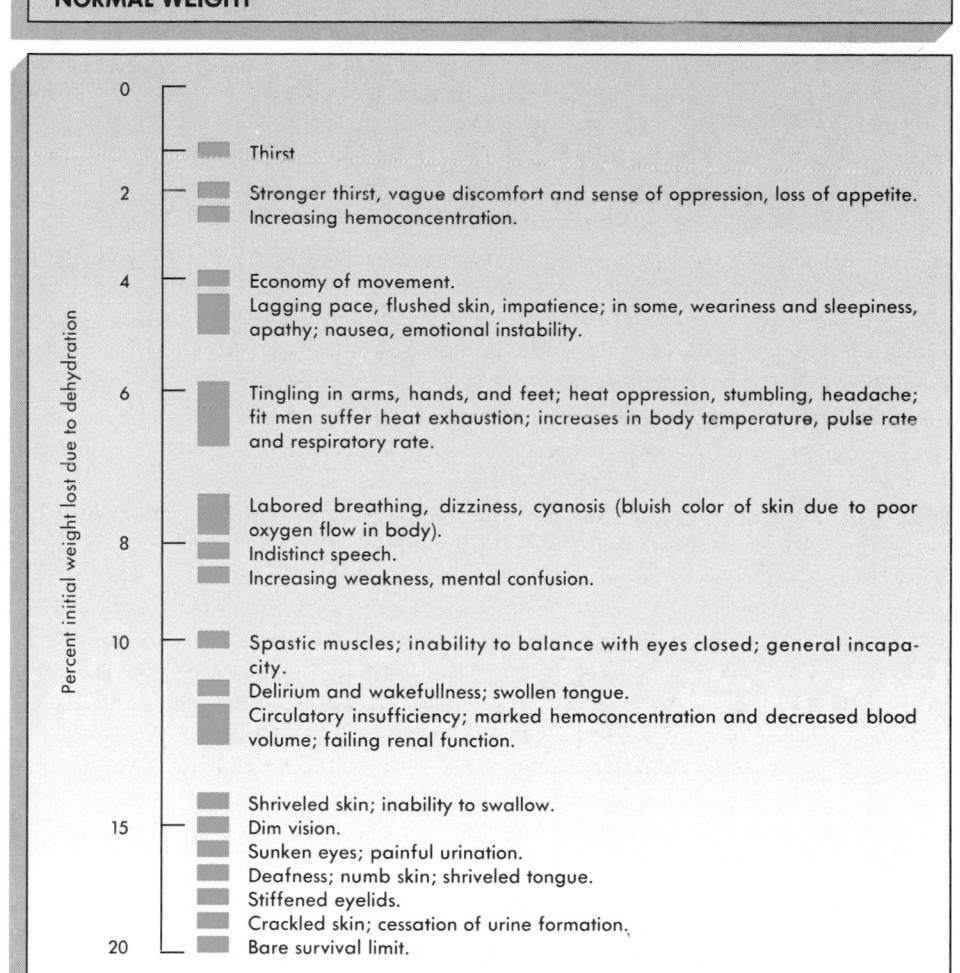

NORMAL WEIGHT

Percent initial weight lost due to dehydration

0

— Thirst

2 — Stronger thirst, vague discomfort and sense of oppression, loss of appetite.
Increasing hemoconcentration.

4 — Economy of movement.
Lagging pace, flushed skin, impatience; in some, weariness and sleepiness, apathy; nausea, emotional instability.

6 — Tingling in arms, hands, and feet; heat oppression, stumbling, headache; fit men suffer heat exhaustion; increases in body temperature, pulse rate and respiratory rate.

Labored breathing, dizziness, cyanosis (bluish color of skin due to poor oxygen flow in body).
8 — Indistinct speech.
Increasing weakness, mental confusion.

10 — Spastic muscles; inability to balance with eyes closed; general incapacity.
Delirium and wakefullness; swollen tongue.
Circulatory insufficiency; marked hemoconcentration and decreased blood volume; failing renal function.

Shriveled skin; inability to swallow.
Dim vision.
15 — Sunken eyes; painful urination.
Deafness; numb skin; shriveled tongue.
Stiffened eyelids.
Crackled skin; cessation of urine formation.
20 — Bare survival limit.

DEATH

Figure 9-4 *The effects of dehydration range from thirst to death, depending on the extent of body weight loss.*

Critical Thinking

Stacy has been working in the yard with her brother Tom. They have been busy mowing the lawn and pulling weeds since noon. Tom tells Stacy that he is feeling weak and has a headache. Stacy is concerned that her brother might be somewhat dehydrated. How can his symptoms be explained? How could Tom's risk of dehydration have been decreased?

Bottled Water

These days, it is common to see 5-gallon bottles of water being delivered to homes. Grocery store shelves are now stocked with all kinds of bottled waters—more than 700 brands in the United States—ranging from simple plastic jugs containing "pure spring water" to fancier, imported varieties of mineral water in glass bottles. In Europe, bottled water is an institution, as popular as soft drinks are in the United States.

Currently, it is quite fashionable to order a bottle of Evian at a restaurant or bar. Not only are people looking for alternatives to alcoholic beverages and soft drinks, but they are also attracted to the perceived health value or taste of bottled water. This popularity has turned the bottled water industry into a business that rakes in more than $3 billion a year.

Bottled waters vary, depending on the source, use, mineral content, and carbonation. All bottled waters must list the source of the water on the label. This can include wells, spas, springs, geysers, and quite often, the public water supply. Some bottled water companies add minerals—such as calcium, magnesium, and potassium— to give the water a better taste. But the term *mineral water* is misleading, because all water (except distilled and specially purified water) contains minerals. In fact, FDA notes that a number of bottled water products on the market have misleading labels. In response, FDA recently set definitions for such claims as "artesian water," "distilled water," "purified water," "spring water," "mineral water," and others. In essence, the source must be the same one that is listed on the label. Thus "spring water" must come from an underground spring. The presence of carbon dioxide gas in the water source results in carbonation. Bottled waters from this type of source are said to be naturally sparkling. Other carbonated waters have had carbon dioxide added during bottling.

Many people choose bottled water over tap water because they doubt the safety of public drinking water. Some concern over municipal water supplies is warranted. For example, in 1993 about 400,000 people became ill in Milwaukee, Wis., from contamination of the public water supply caused by the parasite *Cryptosporidium*. This parasite is usually found in lakes and rivers; the typical chlorination procedures used to treat public water supplies do not kill *Cryptosporidium*. This parasite poses little risk to healthy people—other than a case of diarrhea—but this is not true for people who have AIDS or other diseases that compromise function of the immune system (such as some forms of cancer therapy or organ transplant therapy). Recently, these high-risk people have, in fact, been advised to boil for at least 1 minute any tap water they use for cooking or drinking to ensure the parasite gets destroyed. Alternatively, you can purchase a water filter that screens out *Cryptosporidium* (the National Sanitation Foundation at (800) 673-8010 can provide a list of manufacturers) or use bottled water that is certified to be free of the parasite (contact the supplier if in doubt). Generally distilled water or that which has undergone reverse osmosis is parasite free.

Under the Safe Water Drinking Act, all public drinking water supplies are monitored for contaminants, such as bacteria, various chemicals, and toxic metals (such as lead and mercury). The local municipal water department can provide results of these tests. According to the Environmental Protection Agency (EPA), the U.S. water supply ranks among the safest in the world. Nevertheless, this water does sometimes fail to meet the agency's standards for contaminants, such as lead and nitrates. Generally the public will be warned about the latter, as it is dangerous to use nitrate-rich water for mixing baby formulas (see Chapter 15). Some studies indicate that in a year about one in five Americans consumes water that is not up to standards, especially in rural areas. These people could consider using a home water filter or bottled water. The local water department can help a person evaluate whether health risks are worth the cost of home water filters or bottled water.

Keep in mind that, by most standards, bottled water ranges from moderately expensive to expensive. In many cases, you are paying for water that is not much different from the water you get from your tap. If you are concerned about the safety of your tap water, you can ask the municipal water department for the most current recent test results mentioned above, or you can have the water tested yourself. A local testing laboratory or state health department can be of service, as well as the EPA at (800) 426-4791. This testing can point out whether there are indeed health risks associated with your water supply. Compared with the cost of bottled water, the testing fee will be insignificant. As noted in Chapter 17, letting cold water run for a minute or so before taking a drink or before using it in meal preparation is a good way to limit possible lead exposure, especially if the water has been off for more than an hour. In addition, do not use hot tap water for food preparation.

It is necessary to closely monitor the purity of our drinking water. However, Congress is currently debating whether such standards should be relaxed. Expressing your opinion on this matter to your congressional representative is one way to become involved in this issue.

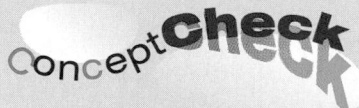

Minerals
The basic chemical elements, such as calcium and iron, needed by the body. These contribute to body structure and regulation of body processes.

Bioavailability
The degree to which the amount of an ingested nutrient is absorbed and is available to the body.

ConceptCheck

Because the body can neither readily store nor entirely conserve water, we can survive only a few days without it. Water dissolves substances, serves as a medium for chemical reactions and as a lubricant, and aids in temperature regulation. Water accounts for 50% to 70% of body weight and distributes itself all over the body: among lean and other tissues (in both intracellular and extracellular fluids) and in urine and other body fluids. Adults need about 1 milliliter of water or other fluids for each kcal expended. Thirst is the body's first sign of dehydration. If this thirst mechanism is faulty, as it may be during illness or vigorous exercise, hormonal mechanisms also help conserve water by reducing urine output. Excess fluid intake can be hazardous to a person's health.

MINERALS

The metabolic roles of **minerals** and the amounts of them in the body vary considerably (Figure 9-5). Some minerals, such as copper and selenium, work as cofactors, which by definition enable enzymes to function. Minerals also contribute to important body compounds. For example, iodine is a component of the hormone thyroxine that comes from the thyroid gland. Iron is a component of hemoglobin in red blood cells. Sodium, potassium, and calcium aid in the transfer of nerve impulses throughout the body. Calcium is also a key participant in muscle contraction. Body growth and development (such as the bony skeleton) also depend on certain minerals, such as calcium and phosphorus. Water balance requires sodium, potassium, calcium, and phosphorus. At all levels—cellular, tissue, organ, and whole body—minerals clearly play important roles in maintaining body functions.

Mineral Bioavailability

Foods contain and supply us with many minerals, but our bodies vary in their capabilities to absorb and use available minerals. Although minerals may be present in foods, they are not **bioavailable** unless a body can absorb them. The ability to absorb minerals from a diet depends on many factors. The number listed in a food composition table for the amount of a mineral in a food is just a starting point for estimating the actual contribution the food will make to our mineral needs. Spinach is a good example. It contains plenty of calcium, but only about 5% of it can be absorbed because of the vegetable's high concentration of *oxalic acid*, a calcium-binder. Usually, about 20% to 40% of dietary calcium is absorbed by adults, with the higher percentage coming from dairy products.[23]

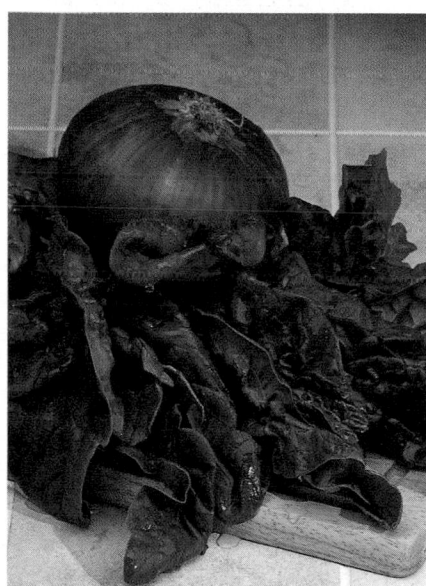

Spinach contains plenty of calcium, but only about 5% of it can be absorbed because of the vegetable's high concentration of oxalic acid. Usually, about 30% of calcium is absorbed from foods.

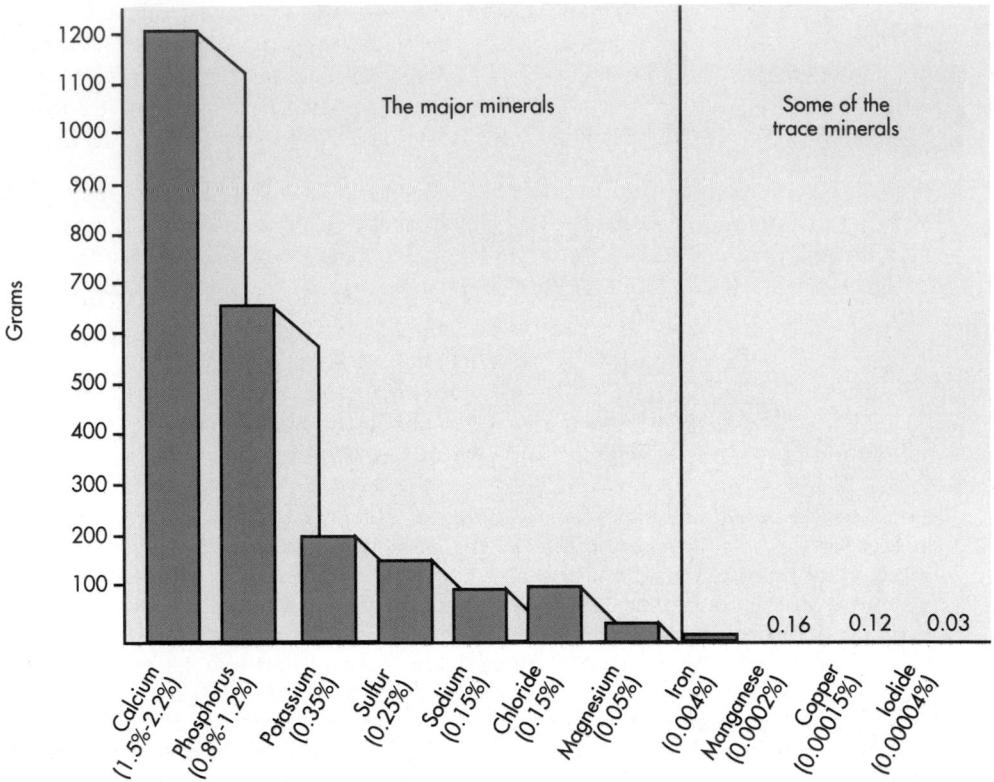

Figure 9-5 *Approximate amounts of various minerals present in the average human body. The percent values in parentheses indicate the amounts as percentages of body weight. Other trace minerals of nutritional importance not listed include chromium, fluoride, molybdenum, selenium, and zinc.*

Minerals in the average American's diet come from both plant and animal sources. Overall, minerals from animal products are absorbed better, because binders and dietary fiber (as will soon be discussed) are not present to hinder absorption. The mineral content of plants depends on mineral concentration in the soil. Animals, however, may consume foods from multiple soil conditions and may eat a variety of plant products, because the animals are often shipped across country during their growth, so soil conditions have less of an influence.

Generally the more refined a plant food—as in the case of white flour—the lower its content of minerals. The enrichment process for grains adds only the mineral iron. The selenium, zinc, copper, and other minerals lost when grains are refined are not replaced.

Fiber-Mineral Interactions

Oxalic acid (or oxalate)

An organic acid that is found in spinach, rhubarb, and other leafy green vegetables and that can depress the absorption of certain minerals.

Mineral bioavailability can be greatly affected by nonmineral substances in the diet. Components of fiber, especially phytic acid (phytate) in grain fiber, can limit absorption of some minerals by binding to them. Oxalic acid, mentioned before, is another substance in plants that binds minerals and makes them less available to the body. High-fiber diets can decrease the absorption of iron, zinc, magnesium, and probably other minerals. An intake above the recommendation of 20 to 35 grams of dietary fiber per day then can cause problems with mineral status of the body, as noted in Chapter 5.

If grains are leavened with yeast, as they are in bread, enzymes produced by the yeast can break some of the bonds between phytic acid and minerals. This increases mineral absorption. The zinc deficiencies found among some Middle Eastern populations are attributed partly to their consumption of unleavened breads, resulting in low bioavailability of dietary zinc.[1] This is discussed in detail in a later section.

Mineral-Mineral Interactions

Many minerals are of similar sizes and chemical charges, such as magnesium, calcium, iron, and copper. Having similar sizes and the same chemical charge causes these minerals to compete with each other for absorption, and so they affect each other's bioavailability. Because of this, people should avoid taking individual mineral supplements, unless a medical condition specifically warrants it. This is because an excess of one mineral influences the absorption and metabolism of other minerals. For example, the presence of a large amount of zinc in the diet decreases copper absorption. High doses of calcium supplements can interfere with iron absorption when both are consumed in the same meal.[20]

Mineral Toxicities

Excess mineral intake can lead to toxic results, especially with the trace minerals, such as iron and copper.[13,34] This potential for toxicity is yet another reason to carefully consider the use of mineral supplements. Every year, people poison themselves using mineral supplements, even though their intent is to maximize health. Many trace minerals are quite toxic at doses not much above the RDA or the estimated safe and adequately daily dietary intake (ESADDI). Mineral supplements exceeding 150% (1.5 times) of nutrient recommendations should be taken only under a physician's supervision, because toxicity and nutrient interactions are possible. This concept will be discussed further as each individual mineral is reviewed.

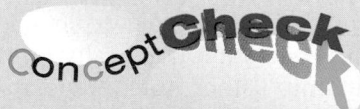

Minerals are vital to the functioning of many body processes. Their bioavailability depends on many factors, including a mineral's interaction with dietary fiber and other minerals. Animal products often yield better mineral absorption than do plants. Still, both animal and plant sources help us meet our mineral needs. Taking an individual mineral supplement can greatly diminish the absorption and metabolism of other minerals. In addition, some minerals are potentially toxic. These are two good reasons to consider carefully any use of mineral supplements.

MAJOR MINERALS

Up to now some general characteristics of minerals and how some of them interact with water in the body have been covered. Now let us review the individual properties of the **major minerals** in the context of the American diet. Recall that these are the minerals we need in excess of 100 milligrams each day (Figure 9-5).

Major mineral
A mineral vital to health and required in the diet in amounts greater than 100 milligrams per day.

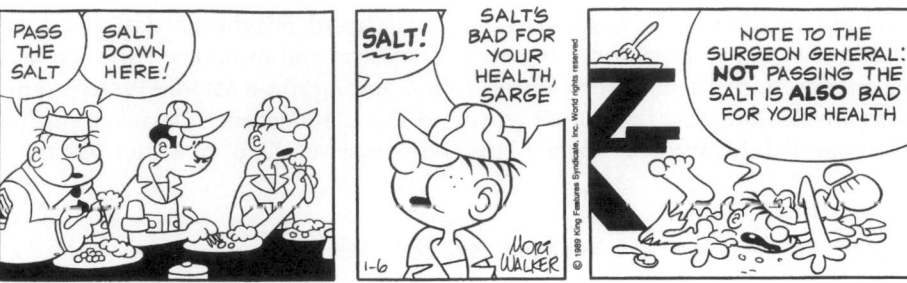

Figure 9-6 *Beetle Bailey.*

Sodium (Na)

We both crave and hear concerns about sodium and its primary dietary source, table salt. Some of this concern is warranted, and some is not (Figure 9-6).

Functions of Sodium

The human body absorbs almost all sodium that gets eaten. This sodium then becomes the major positive ion in extracellular fluid and a key factor for retaining body water. Fluid balance throughout the body depends partly on varied sodium and other **electrolyte** concentrations among the water-containing compartments in the body. Sodium ions also function in nerve impulse conduction and absorption of some nutrients (for example, glucose).

A low-sodium diet—coupled with excessive perspiration, persistent vomiting, or diarrhea—has the ability to deplete the body of sodium. This state can lead to muscle cramps, nausea, vomiting, dizziness, and later to shock and coma. The likelihood of this happening, however, is low because early kidney responses to low sodium status eventually trigger the body to conserve sodium. In addition, people generally eat a lot of sodium.

Only when weight loss from perspiration exceeds 3% of total body weight (or about 5 to 6 pounds) should sodium losses raise concern. Even then, merely salting foods is sufficient to restore body sodium for most people. Endurance athletes, however, may need to consume sports drinks during competition to avoid depletion of sodium (see Chapter 11). Note also that although perspiration tastes salty on the skin, sodium is not highly concentrated in perspiration. Rather, water evaporating from the skin leaves concentrated sodium behind. Perspiration contains about two-thirds the sodium concentration found in blood.

Sodium in Foods and Minimum Sodium Requirements

About one third to one half the sodium we consume is added during cooking or at the table. Most of the rest is added during food manufacturing. Many health authorities are calling for manufacturers to use less sodium so that our total sodium intakes fall. To some extent this is taking place (for example, low sodium soups and crackers). Almost all foods naturally contain a little sodium; the higher amount found in milk (about 120 milligrams per cup) is one exception. The more home cooking a person does, the more sodium control that person has. Major contributors of sodium in the adult diet are white bread and rolls, hot dogs and lunch meats, cheese, soups, and spaghetti with tomato sauce, partly because these foods are eaten so often. Other foods that generally are especially high in sodium include tomato-based products, salted snack foods, french fries and potato chips, and sauces and gravies (Figure 9-7).

For your information, the chemical symbols for the minerals we discuss are given next to each mineral heading.

Electrolytes
Substances that break down into ions in water and, in turn, are able to conduct an electrical current. These include sodium, chloride, and potassium.

The importance of salt to human health has been recognized since antiquity. Salt was a commodity in the classical world. Indeed, the Latin word *salary* reflects the way a soldier's wages were paid.

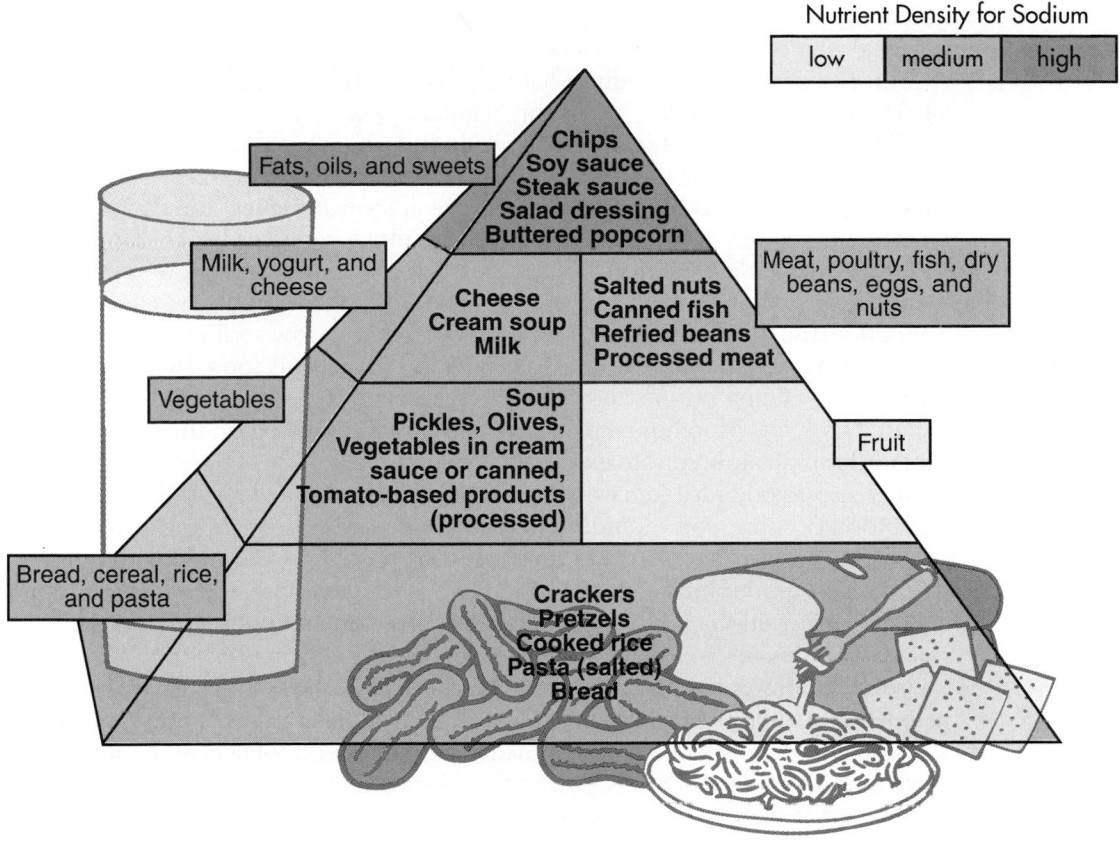

Nutrient Density for Sodium

| low | medium | high |

Figure 9-7 *Food sources of sodium from the Food Guide Pyramid. All groups except fruit contain foods that are rich sources of this nutrient, most of which is added in food processing. The background color of each food group indicates the average nutrient density for sodium in that group. The salt shaker can add considerably more sodium, depending on use.*

If we ate only unprocessed foods and added no salt, we would consume about 500 milligrams of sodium per day. This is also the recommended minimum sodium requirement for adults as set by the current RDA publication (see the inside cover for references to mineral needs for other age-groups). Even this is a generous amount, considering that we really need only about 100 milligrams a day.

If we compare 500 milligrams of sodium from unprocessed food with the 3000 to 6000 milligrams or more typically eaten by adults, it is clear that food processing and cooking contribute most of our dietary sodium.[2] As discussed in Chapter 2, nutrition labels list a food's sodium content. When dietary sodium must be severely restricted, these labels become very helpful. Under FDA food-labeling rules, the Daily Value for sodium is 2400 milligrams. FDA established this value because it is consistent with government reports that encourage reduced sodium intakes.

In cases where sodium intake must be very limited, even contributions from tap water (especially from softened water), as well as medicines that contain sodium, must be considered.

Most humans can adapt to various dietary salt intakes, though very high intakes can be toxic. For most people who eat a typical diet, today's sodium intake is simply tomorrow's urine output. However, approximately 10% to 15% of adults are sodium sensitive. For these people, high sodium intakes contribute to high blood pressure, and lower sodium diets (about 2 to 3 grams daily) often help correct the problem[24] (see the Nutrition Insight on page 312). Scientific groups typically suggest

Table salt is 40% sodium and 60% chloride. The range of sodium intakes seen in adults of 3 to 6 grams per day translates to 7.5 to 15 grams of salt. A teaspoon of salt contains about 2 grams of sodium (2000 milligrams).

As noted later in this chapter, a sodium intake greater than about 2 grams per day increases urinary calcium loss as it is excreted, providing another reason to control sodium intake.

that all adults reduce intake to 2.4 to 3 grams, mostly to limit the risk of later developing high blood pressure.

You can evaluate your sodium habits by completing the questionnaire in Table 9-1. The more checks in the "often" or "regularly" columns, the higher your dietary sodium intake. However, not all the habits in the table contribute the same amount of sodium. For example, many natural cheeses are relatively moderate in sodium, whereas processed cheeses and cottage cheese are much higher. You can choose to reduce your sodium intake by cutting back on those items for which you checked "often" or "regularly." You needn't suddenly eliminate foods from your diet. Rather, to moderate sodium intake, choose lower-sodium foods from each food group more often and balance high-sodium food choices with low-sodium ones. It is also important to pay attention to the sodium values listed on food labels, and taste foods before adding salt. In addition, when eating out, avoiding foods commonly prepared with lots of sodium and asking to have sauces served on the side and then using only small amounts are two good ideas.

It is also a good idea to have your blood pressure checked regularly. If you have high blood pressure, you should try to reduce your sodium intake and to determine what effect this can have. If you don't have this problem, you might still consider slowly reducing your intake to build good habits for the future. If your daily sodium intake is already in the range of less than 3 grams, you are meeting that objective.

Adapting to a lower sodium intake. If you choose to eat less sodium, you can eventually adapt to a low-sodium diet. At first, foods will taste quite bland, but eventually you will perceive more flavor as the tongue's salt receptors become more sensitive to the salt content of foods. By slowly reducing dietary sodium and substituting garlic, oregano, lemon juice, and other herbs and spices, you can eventually become accustomed to a diet that contains only 3 grams of sodium daily but does not result in much of a flavor trade-off. Many new cookbooks offer excellent recipes for flavorful low-sodium foods. Except when baking breads with yeast, omitting salt from food preparation can still yield excellent-tasting products.

Commercially prepared condiments, sauces, and seasonings are often high in sodium. Examples include onion, celery, garlic, seasoned, and sea salts; baking powder; salad dressings; pickles; soy, steak, barbecue, chili, and Worcestershire sauces; meat tenderizer; baking soda; salt pork; brine; catsup; mustard; bouillon; monosodium glutamate (MSG); and relish.

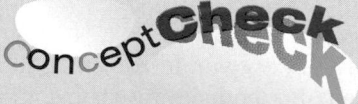

Concept**check**

Sodium is the major positive ion of extracellular fluid. It is important for maintaining fluid balance and conducting nerve impulses. Sodium depletion is unlikely, since the typical American's diet has abundant sources of sodium and most of it gets absorbed. The more foods we prepare at home, the more control we have over our sodium intake. The minimum sodium requirement for adults is 500 milligrams per day. The average adult consumes 3000 to 6000 milligrams or more daily. About 10% to 15% of the population is sensitive to sodium. In these people, high blood pressure can develop as a result of high-sodium diets. Many scientific groups suggest that for all adults sodium intake should be limited to about 3 grams (3000 milligrams) per day, but there is not universal support for this recommendation.

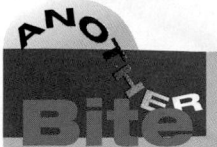

Some experts argue that there is no justification for recommending that the general population should restrict its salt intake to avert future high blood pressure. These experts suggest caution when issuing nationwide recommendations to reduce dietary sodium intake, preferring instead to provide advice on an individual basis, especially to people with high blood pressure who are also salt sensitive.[8] In addition, the Nutrition Insight on page 312 addresses several other factors that should be evaluated when determining the cause of high blood pressure. These other factors include inadequate intakes of potassium, calcium, and magnesium as well as inactivity, obesity, and excessive alcohol consumption.

TABLE 9-1

Questionnaire for Evaluating Your Sodium Habits with Respect to Typically Rich Sources

HOW OFTEN DO YOU:	Rarely	Occasionally	Often	Regularly (daily)
1. Eat cured or processed meats, such as ham, bacon, sausage, frankfurters, and other luncheon meats?	☐	☐	☐	☐
2. Choose canned or frozen vegetables with sauce?	☐	☐	☐	☐
3. Use commercially prepared meals, main dishes, or canned or dehydrated soups?	☐	☐	☐	☐
4. Eat cheese, especially processed cheese?	☐	☐	☐	☐
5. Eat salted nuts, popcorn, pretzels, corn chips, or potato chips?	☐	☐	☐	☐
6. Add salt to cooking water for vegetables, rice, or pasta?	☐	☐	☐	☐
7. Add salt, seasoning mixes, salad dressings, or condiments—such as soy sauce, steak sauce, catsup, and mustard—to foods during preparation or at the table?	☐	☐	☐	☐
8. Salt your food before tasting it?	☐	☐	☐	☐
9. Ignore labels for sodium content when buying foods?	☐	☐	☐	☐
10. When dining out, choose foods at restaurants with sauces, or foods that are obviously salty?	☐	☐	☐	☐

The more checks you have in the last two columns, the higher your dietary sodium intake.

Adapted from *USDA Home and Garden Bulletin* No. 232-6, April 1986.

Nutrition Insight

Minerals and High Blood Pressure

About 50 million Americans suffer from some degree of high blood pressure (more technically called hypertension) that warrants therapy. In 1994 more than 500,000 Americans suffered a **stroke,** which is typically associated with long-standing high blood pressure.

Blood pressure is expressed by two different numbers. The higher number represents **systolic blood pressure,** which is the pressure in the arteries when the heart actively pumps blood. The second value is for **diastolic blood pressure,** which is the artery pressure when the heart is relaxed. Normal systolic blood pressure varies from 100 to 140 millimeters of mercury. Normal diastolic blood pressure varies from 60 to 90 millimeters of mercury.[14] A high diastolic pressure shows a strong relationship to various diseases, as does a high systolic pressure.

High blood pressure is defined as sustained systolic pressure exceeding 140 millimeters of mercury or diastolic blood pressure exceeding 90 millimeters of mercury. Stages are defined as mild, moderate, severe, and very severe:

Mild	Diastolic 90 to 99 millimeters of mercury
	Systolic 140 to 159 millimeters of mercury
Moderate	Diastolic 100 to 109 millimeters of mercury
	Systolic 160 to 179 millimeters of mercury
Severe	Diastolic 110 to 119 millimeters of mercury
	Systolic 180 to 209 millimeters of mercury
Very severe	Diastolic ≥120 millimeters of mercury
	Systolic ≥210 millimeters of mercury

Most high blood pressure (about 90% of cases) has no clear-cut cause. It is described as primary, or essential, in nature (for example, essential hypertension). Kidney disease often causes the other 10% of cases, known as secondary hypertension. African-Americans are more likely than whites to develop high blood pressure and to do so earlier in life. As a result, they also suffer more from high blood pressure–related diseases.

Unless blood pressure is measured periodically, development of high blood pressure is easily overlooked. Thus it's described as a "silent" disorder. A physician usually does not treat high blood pressure with medication until the diastolic blood pressure measures at least 95 millimeters of mercury (or the systolic blood pressure reaches 160) on three or more occasions. Still, a diastolic value more than 90 millimeters of mercury is actually too high and deserves dietary and lifestyle interventions as a start.

Why Control High Blood Pressure?

High blood pressure needs to be controlled mainly to prevent heart disease, kidney disease, strokes and related declines in brain function, poor blood circulation in the legs, and sudden death. All these diseases are much more likely to be found in people with high blood pressure than in people with normal blood pressure. Smoking and elevated blood lipoproteins make these diseases even more likely. People with high blood pressure need to be diagnosed and treated as soon as possible, as the condition generally progresses to a more serious stage over time.

Causes of High Blood Pressure

Blood pressure usually increases as a person ages. Some increase is caused by atherosclerosis. As plaque builds up in the arteries, the arteries become less flexible and cannot expand. When vessels remain rigid, blood pressure remains high. Eventually the plaque begins to choke off blood supply to the kidneys, decreasing their ability to control blood volume, and in turn, blood pressure.

Obesity is often associated with high blood pressure, especially in women. High blood insulin associated with insulin-resistant adipose cells is one reason for this. Insulin increases sodium retention in the body and speeds atherosclerosis.[30] Inactivity also is associated with high blood pressure. If an obese person can lose weight and engage in regular physical activity, blood pressure often returns to normal. A weight loss of as little as 10 to 15 pounds often can help.[28]

The enzyme renin (secreted by the kidneys) and some hormonelike compounds affect blood pressure.[14] Medications are available to reduce their effect.

Sodium and Blood Pressure

Sodium intake tends to increase blood pressure, particularly in those who are susceptible to developing it. However, only some Americans with high blood pressure are very susceptible to sodium-linked high blood pressure. Ideally dietary advice concerning sodium should be determined on an individual basis, once the response to treatment is verified.[8,24] Physicians usually resort to a combination of antihypertensive medications such as **diuretics** and moderate sodium restriction as an initial form of therapy. This reduces blood volume, and therefore is often effective in controlling blood pressure.

Other Minerals and Blood Pressure

Minerals such as calcium, potassium, and magnesium also deserve attention when it comes to high blood pressure.[31] People often register slightly lower blood pressures—especially the systolic component—when they consume at least the RDA of calcium per day, as compared with one third to one half that amount.[7] It is reasonable for a person with high blood pressure to experiment, in consultation with a physician, with increasing calcium intake to see if that produces the desired effect.

Potassium supplementation in the range of 4 grams—about 1 to 2 grams above our typical intakes—also has been shown to moderately decrease blood pressure in people currently consuming far below this amount. Some studies indicate that magnesium also is capable of lowering blood pressure at intakes of about twice the RDA, but overall the results of these studies are inconsistent.

Alcohol and High Blood Pressure

Excess alcohol intake is responsible for about 10% of cases of high blood pressure, especially in middle-aged males and in African-Americans in general.[28] A prudent intake is two or fewer drinks per day for people with high blood pressure.

Preventing High Blood Pressure

Many of these and other risk factors for high blood pressure and stroke are controllable, and appropriate lifestyle changes can reduce a person's risk (Table 9-2). A reduction in stress adds to the list of preventive measures. And even if antihypertensive medications are still needed, a proper diet and lifestyle approach can often reduce the dosage, and in turn, the expense and side effects of medications.[30]

TABLE 9-2

A Nutritional Plan to Minimize Hypertension and Stroke Risk

1. Follow the Food Guide Pyramid.
2. Make sure to meet the RDA for calcium, potassium, and magnesium.
3. Attain and maintain a healthy body weight.
4. Incorporate regular physical activity (at least 5 times per week).
5. Consume alcoholic beverages in moderation, if at all (two drinks per day maximum).
6. Consume moderate amounts of sodium and see if this helps.
7. Don't smoke.
8. Maintain blood lipoproteins in the normal range (see Chapter 6).

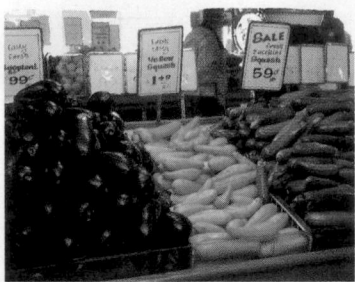

Many vegetables are good sources of potassium.

Potassium (K)

Potassium performs many of the same functions as sodium, such as fluid balance and nerve impulse transmission. However, it operates inside, rather than outside, cells. Intracellular fluids—those inside cells—contain 95% of the potassium in the body. Also, unlike sodium, potassium is associated with lower rather than higher blood pressure values. We absorb about 90% of the potassium we eat.

Low blood potassium is a life-threatening problem. Symptoms often include a loss of appetite, muscle cramps, confusion, and constipation. Eventually, the heart beats irregularly, decreasing its capacity to pump blood.

Potassium in Foods and Minimum Potassium Requirements

Generally, fruits and vegetables are nutrient-dense sources of potassium. Milk, whole grains, dried beans, and meats are also good sources. Major contributors of potassium to the adult diet include coffee, tea, milk, potatoes, orange juice, and various animal products (Figure 9-8).

The adult minimum potassium requirement for health set by the current RDA is 2000 milligrams (2 grams) per day. Typically an adult gets enough potassium by eating a wide variety of foods. Americans average 2 to 3 grams per day.[2] If kidneys function normally, typical intakes of dietary potassium are not toxic; otherwise, high amounts in the body can lead to heart failure.

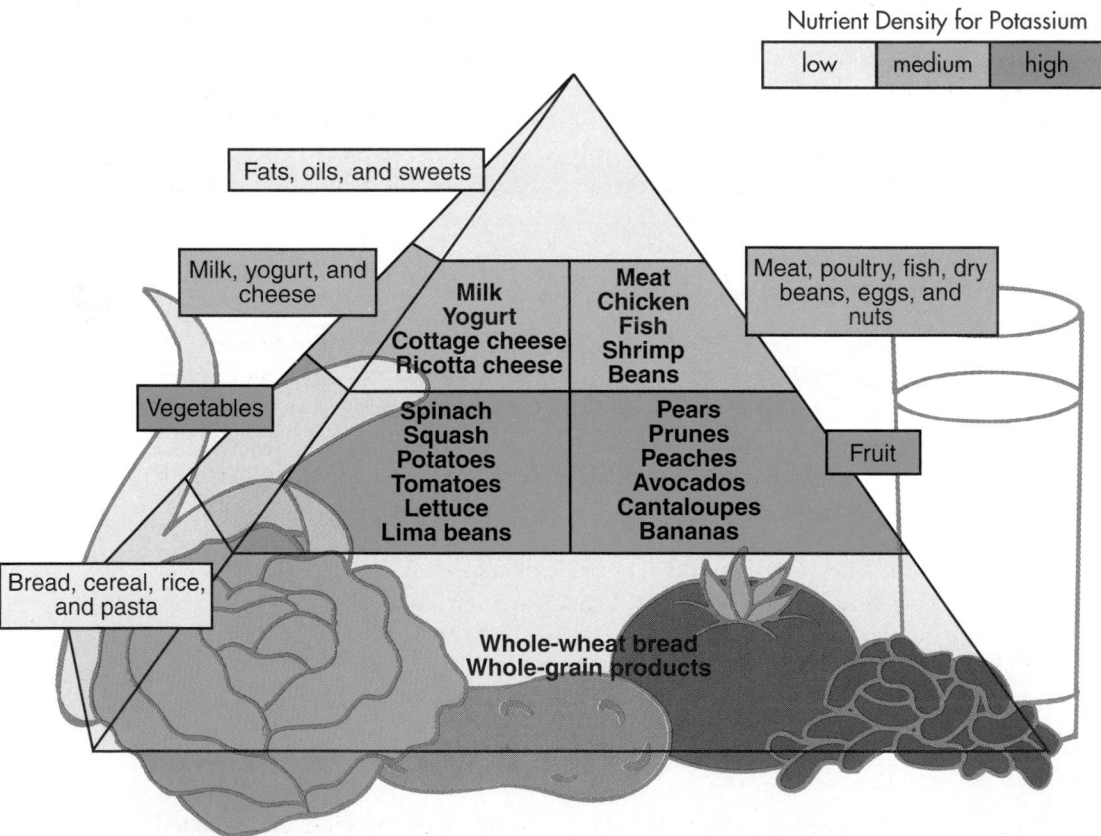

Figure 9-8 *Food sources of potassium from the Food Guide Pyramid. The fruit group and the vegetable group are the best dietary sources of this nutrient, but is is widely distributed in foods. The background color of each food group indicates the average nutrient density for potassium in that group.*

Our diets are more likely to be low in potassium than sodium because we generally do not add potassium to foods. Some diuretics used to treat high blood pressure deplete the body's potassium. People who take potassium-wasting diuretics need to monitor their potassium intakes carefully. For these people, high-potassium foods—such as fruits, fruit juices, and vegetables—are good additions to the diet, and if recommended by a physician, so are potassium chloride supplements.

A continual deficient food intake, as may be the case in alcoholism, can also result in potassium deficiency. People with anorexia nervosa and bulimia, whose diets are poor and whose bodies can be depleted of nutrients because of vomiting, are also at risk for potassium deficiency (see Chapter 13). People on very low-calorie diets are also at risk and so are athletes who exercise heavily. As covered in Chapters 10 and 11, all of these people should compensate for potentially low body potassium by consuming potassium-rich foods.

Chloride (Cl)

Chlorine is a very poisonous gas. Public water utilities often rely on it to kill bacteria in water supplies. Consequently, many water-borne diseases are rare in America. Chlorinated water is generally harmless to humans in dilute concentrations, although some researchers suspect it may be linked to a slight risk for rectal and bladder cancer. The federal government limits the amount of certain chlorination by-products that can be present in drinking water; a still greater reduction is possible but would be expensive for utilities to institute. Currently it is unclear whether the slight decrease in cancer risk is worth the effort and expense.[9]

If you find the taste of chlorinated water unpleasant or are concerned about the slight cancer risk, you can remove the chlorine from tap water by boiling it or by letting a large container filled with water stand uncovered overnight. In both cases the chlorine will evaporate, taking its characteristic flavor with it. Alternatively, you can install a filter on the household spigot from which you obtain your water. It should be designed to remove trihalomethanes, common chlorine by-products. It is possible to obtain a list of water filter manufacturers by calling the telephone number listed earlier in the chapter.

In our bodies, chloride—an ion form of chlorine—forms an important negative ion for the extracellular fluid. These ions are a component of the hydrochloric acid produced in the stomach and are also used during immune responses as white blood cells attack foreign cells. In addition, nerve function relies on the presence of chloride.[14] As is the case with sodium, most of the body's chloride is excreted by the kidneys; some is lost in perspiration. It is also implicated in the blood pressure–raising ability of sodium chloride.

A chloride deficiency is unlikely, because our dietary sodium chloride (salt) intake is so high. Frequent and lengthy bouts of vomiting—if coupled with a nutrient-poor diet—can contribute to a deficiency, because stomach secretions contain much chloride. During the late 1970s, insufficient chloride added to a brand of infant formula caused severe convulsions and other health problems in the infants who consumed it. This incident showed what can happen when the need for a nutrient normally abundant in our diet is not given adequate attention.

Chloride in Foods and Minimum Chloride Requirements

A few fruits and some vegetables are naturally good sources of chloride. Chlorinated water is also a source. However, we consume most chloride as salt added to foods. If we know a food's salt content, we can predict closely its chloride content; recall salt is 60% chloride. Naturally occurring sodium or chloride won't significantly affect the prediction.

Diuretic
A substance that increases the flow of urine.

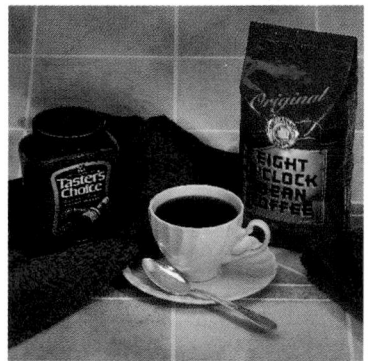

Coffee is a major contributor of potassium to the American diet.

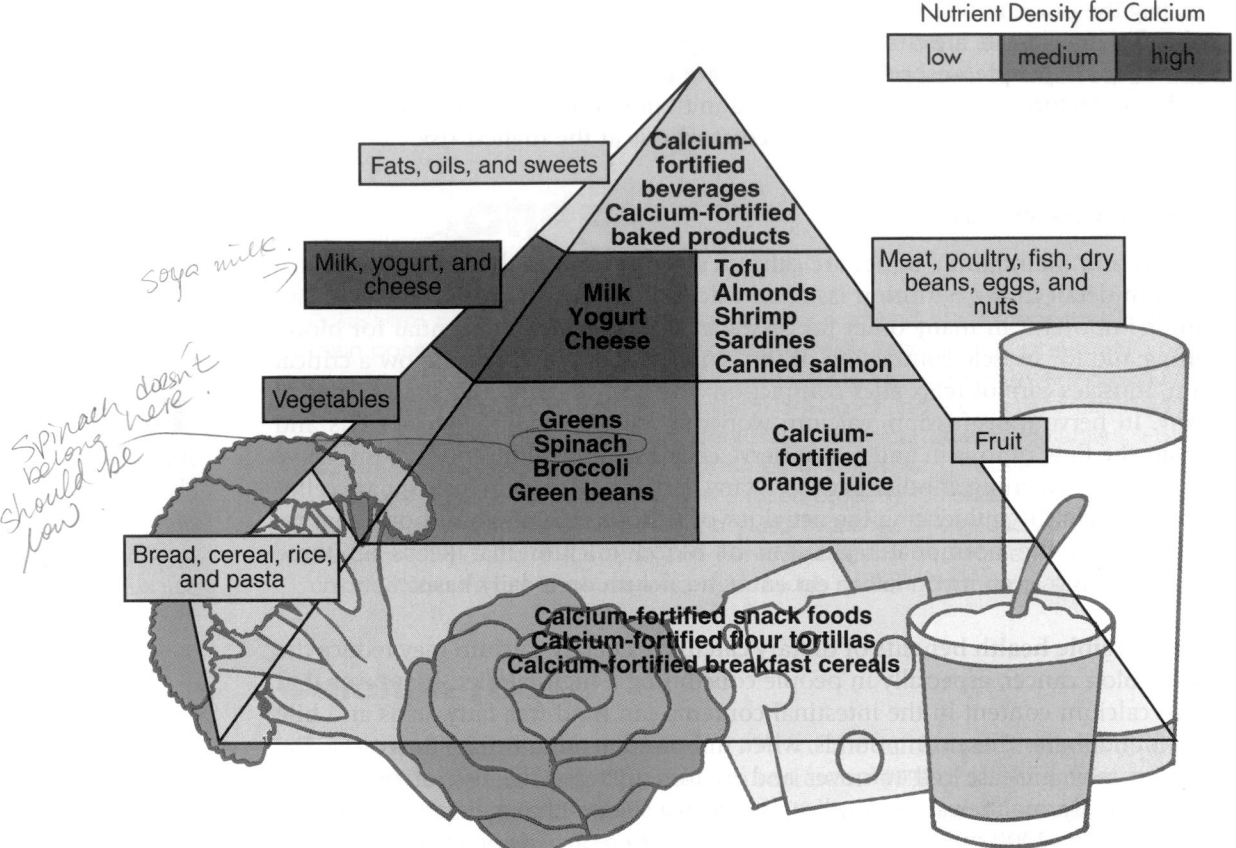

Nutrient Density for Calcium

| low | medium | high |

soya milk. →

Spinach doesn't belong here! should be low.

Figure 9-9 *Food sources of calcium from the Food Guide Pyramid. The milk, yogurt, and cheese group includes the best dietary sources of this nutrient. The background color of each food group indicates the average nutrient density for calcium in that group. Additional calcium-fortified foods appear in stores each year and thus will add to the food sources currently listed for various groups.*

as well as calcium-fortified cottage cheese, breakfast cereals, breakfast bars, and snacks, also follow as close competitors. Another good source of calcium is soybean curd (tofu) if it is made with calcium carbonate (check the label). Note that it is the bones in canned fish, such as salmon and sardines, that supply the calcium.

One reason the Food Guide Pyramid contains a milk, yogurt, and cheese group is to supply calcium to the diet. In addition, this group provides protein, vitamin A, vitamin D, riboflavin, potassium, magnesium, and zinc. People who do not like milk can use products made with milk, such as chocolate milk, yogurt, cheese, and ice cream. All forms of milk, yogurt, and cheese allow about the same degree of calcium absorption. Moderation in use of either cheese or ice cream as a calcium source is advised, because they are usually high in total and saturated fat. However, some low-fat cheeses and frozen desserts are good calcium sources and have a low fat content.

Information about calcium is mandatory on food labels. The Daily Value for calcium used for food labels is 1000 milligrams.

The RDA for calcium for adults is 800 milligrams per day. The current RDA extends the 1200 milligram standard used for the teenage years to age 25, in order to contribute to building and maintaining a higher **bone mass.**

A recent National Institutes of Health (NIH) Consensus Development Panel on Optimal Calcium Intake recommended even higher intakes of calcium than those specified by the RDAs[27] (Table 9-3).

In the United States, average calcium intakes range from only approximately 600 to 800 milligrams per day for women and 800 to 1000 milligrams per day for

Bone mass

Total mineral substance (such as calcium or phosphorus) in a cross section of bone, generally expressed as grams per centimeter of length.

TABLE 9-3

Recent Recommendations for Optimal Daily Calcium Intakes to Reduce Risk for Osteoporosis

Age (years) or condition	Calcium intake (milligrams per day)
Children	
1-5	800
6-10	800-1200
11-24	1200-1500
Adults	
Women 25-50	1000
Women >50 (postmenopausal)	
Taking estrogen	1000
Not taking estrogen	1500
Women >65	1500
Men 25-65	1000
Men >65	1500

Adapted from NIH Consensus Development Panel on Optimal Calcium Intake: Optimal calcium intake, *Journal of the American Medical Association* 272:1909, 1994.

men.[2] About 25% of women consume only about 300 milligrams per day. Thus dietary intakes of calcium by many women, especially young women, are well below the RDA, whereas intakes by most men are roughly equivalent to the RDA. The greater food consumption by men, to support their higher energy outputs, accounts for part of the difference. An easy way for women to increase calcium intake is to increase their physical activity and in turn their food consumption.

To estimate your calcium intake, use the rule of 300s. Give yourself 300 milligrams to account for calcium in the small amounts provided by a moderate energy intake from foods scattered throughout the diet. Add to that another 300 milligrams for every cup of milk or yogurt or 1.5 ounces of cheese. If you eat a lot of tofu, almonds, or sardines, or drink calcium-fortified beverages, use Table 9-4 or food consumption tables to get a more accurate account of your calcium intake.[37]

It is especially important for vegetarians to focus on eating good plant sources of calcium as well as on the total amount of calcium ingested.

Calcium supplements can be used by people who don't like milk or who can't incorporate enough milk products, foods made with milk, or calcium-fortified foods into their diet.[25] Calcium carbonate, the form commonly found in calcium-based antacid tablets, is the most common supplement used. People with ample output of gastric acid should take this supplement between meals in doses of about 500 milligrams. This practice enhances absorption and limits its negative impact on iron absorption.[27] People with low acid production should take the calcium carbonate supplement with meals, so that what little acid is produced during digestion can aid absorption. It is best, however, not to include the supplement with the meal richest in iron for that day. People with low acid production also can use a supplement containing calcium citrate, which is acidic itself, between meals. The lower percentage of calcium in calcium citrate, however, requires using a greater number or size of pills, or consuming it in a tablet form that is designed to first be dissolved in water. Note that decreased output of gastric acid is common among elderly people.

Overall, taking 1000 milligrams of calcium daily in divided doses in the form of calcium carbonate or calcium citrate is probably safe, but people using a supplement should notify their physician of the practice.

Critical Thinking

Manuela is a vegan. She stopped eating meat and dairy products when she was 12 years old and is now in her mid-twenties. She wants to start a family but is concerned about whether she can obtain enough calcium from her diet to ensure her baby's health. She is also concerned that she may be at risk for osteoporosis. How can she consume enough calcium to meet her own and her baby's needs?

TABLE 9-4

A Tool for Estimating Current Calcium Intake

For all of the following foods, write the number of servings eaten in a day. Total the number of servings in each category and then multiply the totals by the milligrams of calcium for each category. Finally, add the total milligrams to estimate calcium intake for that day.

Food	Serving size	No. serv.	Calcium (mg)	Total calcium (mg)
Plain low-fat yogurt	1 cup	_____		
Nonfat dry milk powder	½ cup	_____		
Total servings		_____	× 400	= _____ milligrams
Canned sardines (with bones)	3 oz	_____		
Fruit flavored yogurt	1 cup	_____		
Skim or low-fat milk, buttermilk	1 cup	_____		
Whole milk, chocolate milk	1 cup	_____		
Parmesan cheese (grated)	¼ cup	_____		
Swiss cheese	1 oz	_____		
Total servings		_____	× 300	= _____ milligrams
Cheese (all other hard cheese)	1 oz	_____		
Pancakes	3	_____		
Total servings		_____	× 200	= _____ milligrams
Canned pink salmon (with bones)	3 oz	_____		
Spinach, cooked	½ cup	_____		
Tofu (processed with calcium)	4 oz	_____		
Total servings		_____	× 150	= _____ milligrams
Collards or turnip greens, cooked	½ cup	_____		
Ice cream or ice milk	½ cup	_____		
Almonds	1 oz	_____		
Total servings		_____	× 75	= _____ milligrams
Chard, cooked	½ cup	_____		
Cottage cheese	½ cup	_____		
Corn tortilla	1 med	_____		
Orange	1 med	_____		
Total servings		_____	× 50	= _____ milligrams
Kidney, lima, or navy beans, cooked	½ cup	_____		
Broccoli	½ cup	_____		
Carrot, raw	1 med	_____		
Dates or raisins	¼ cup	_____		
Egg	1 large	_____		
Whole wheat bread	1 slice	_____		
Peanut butter	2 tbsp	_____		
Total servings		_____	× 25	= _____ milligrams
Calcium-fortified orange juice	6 oz	_____		
Calcium-fortified snack bars	1 each	_____		
Calcium-fortified breakfast bars	½ bar	_____		
Total servings		_____	× 200	= _____ milligrams
Calcium supplements	1 each	_____	× 500	= _____ milligrams
Total calcium intake				= _____ milligrams

Other calcium sources to consider include many breakfast cereals (100 to 250 milligrams per cup) and some vitamins/ mineral supplements (up to 500 milligrams per tablet)

From Wardlaw GM, Weese N: Putting calcium into perspective for your clients, *Topics in Clinical Nutrition* 11:23, 1995.

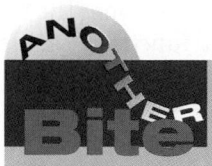

Some calcium supplements are poorly digested, because they do not readily dissolve. To test for this, put a supplement in 6 ounces of cider vinegar. Stir every 5 minutes. It should dissolve within 30 minutes.

Some calcium supplements pose a risk for lead toxicity. Chapter 17 points out that lead produces an array of deleterious effects on the body, especially in children. Currently FDA has no standards for lead in food supplements. However, FDA does plan to regulate the lead content of supplements, including calcium, in the future. Until then, it is important to avoid bonemeal, the worst offender when it comes to lead. Tablet or liquid calcium supplements with the USP (United States Pharmacopeia) seal of approval are less likely than others to contain high concentrations of lead or other contaminants.

The major risk from taking excess calcium supplements is development of one form of kidney stones, as well as constipation, intestinal gas, and interference with absorption of other minerals. However, sticking to a daily limit of 2000 milligrams from diet plus any supplement use poses little risk for developing these problems.[27]

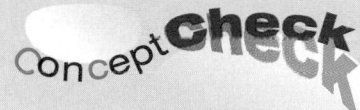

About 99% of calcium in the body is found in the bones. Aside from its critical role in bone, calcium also functions in blood clotting, muscle contraction, nerve-impulse transmission, and cell metabolism. Calcium requires a slightly acid pH and the vitamin D hormone for efficient absorption. Factors that reduce calcium absorption include large amounts of dietary fiber (especially wheat bran), decreased estrogen in the bloodstream, and a great excess of phosphorus in the diet. Blood calcium is regulated primarily by hormones and does not closely reflect daily intake.

Dairy products are rich food sources of calcium. Certain calcium-fortified foods, such as beverages, are rich sources as well. Supplemental forms, such as calcium carbonate, are well-absorbed by most people. However, overzealous supplementation can also result in the development of one form of kidney stones and other health problems.

Phosphorus (P)

Although no disease is currently associated with a poor phosphorus intake, a deficiency may contribute to bone loss in elderly women. The body absorbs phosphorus quite efficiently, about 70% of dietary intake. This high absorption, plus the wide availability of phosphorus in foods, makes this mineral less important than is calcium in diet planning. The active vitamin D hormone enhances phosphorus absorption, as it does for calcium. Kidney excretion primarily regulates blood phosphorus. This regulating mechanism differs from that of calcium, where changes in the rates of absorption are a more significant factor.

Phosphorus is a component of enzymes, other key metabolic compounds (many of which are involved in energy metabolism), DNA (genetic material), cell membranes, and bone. About 85% of the body's phosphorus is inside bone. The remaining phosphorus circulates freely in the bloodstream and functions inside cells.[14]

Phosphorus in Foods and the RDA

Milk, cheese, bakery products, and meat provide most of the phosphorus in the adult diet. Cereals, bran, eggs, nuts, and fish are also good sources. About 20% to 30% of dietary phosphorus comes from food additives, especially in baked goods, cheeses, processed meats, and many soft drinks (about 75 milligrams per 12-ounce—$^1/_3$-liter—serving of soft drinks). Next time you have a soft drink, look for a listing of phosphoric acid on the label.

The same amounts of phosphorus and calcium intake are recommended by the current RDA—800 milligrams per day for adults older than 24. Adults eat about 900 to 1700 milligrams of phosphorus per day.[2] Thus deficiencies of phosphorus are unlikely in healthy adults, especially because it is so efficiently absorbed.

Marginal phosphorus status can be found in premature infants, vegans, people with alcoholism, elderly people on nutrient-poor diets, people with long-term bouts of diarrhea, and people who use aluminum-containing antacids daily (these bind phosphorus in the small intestine).

Phosphorus does not appear to be toxic for healthy adults, but high amounts can lead to problems in people with certain kidney diseases. A chronic imbalance in the calcium to phosphorous ratio in the diet, resulting from a high phosphorus intake coupled with a low calcium intake, also can contribute to bone loss.[4] This situation most likely arises when the RDA for calcium is not met, as can occur in adolescents and adults who regularly substitute soft drinks for milk, or otherwise underconsume calcium.

Magnesium (Mg)

Magnesium is important for nerve and heart function and aids many enzyme reactions. It is found mostly in the plant pigment chlorophyll, where it functions in respiration. We normally absorb about 30% to 40% of the magnesium in our diets, but absorption efficiency can increase up to about 80% if intakes are low. The active vitamin D hormone appears to enhance magnesium absorption.

Bone contains 60% of the body's magnesium. The rest circulates in the blood and operates inside cells. Over 200 enzymes use magnesium, and many energy-yielding compounds in cells require magnesium to function properly.[12]

Animals deficient in magnesium become very irritable and, with severe deficiency, eventually suffer convulsions and often die. In humans a magnesium deficiency causes an irregular heartbeat, sometimes accompanied by weakness, muscle pain, disorientation, and seizures. However, a magnesium deficiency develops very slowly, because our bodies store it readily. A link between magnesium deficiency and sudden heart attacks has been observed, and so now an intravenous dose is being investigated as part of the treatment during the early phases of a heart attack.[33]

Magnesium in Foods and the RDA

The best sources for magnesium are plant products, such as whole grains (like wheat bran), broccoli, squash, beans, nuts, and seeds. Animal products, such as milk and meats, and even chocolate supply some magnesium although less than the foods in the previous list (Figure 9-10). Another surprising source of highly concentrated magnesium is hard tap water, which contains a high mineral content.

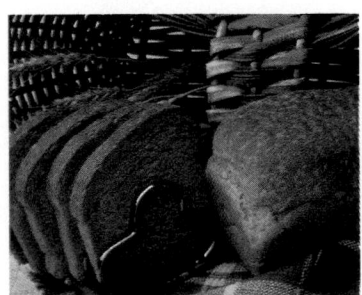

Whole-grain foods, such as bread, are good sources of magnesium.

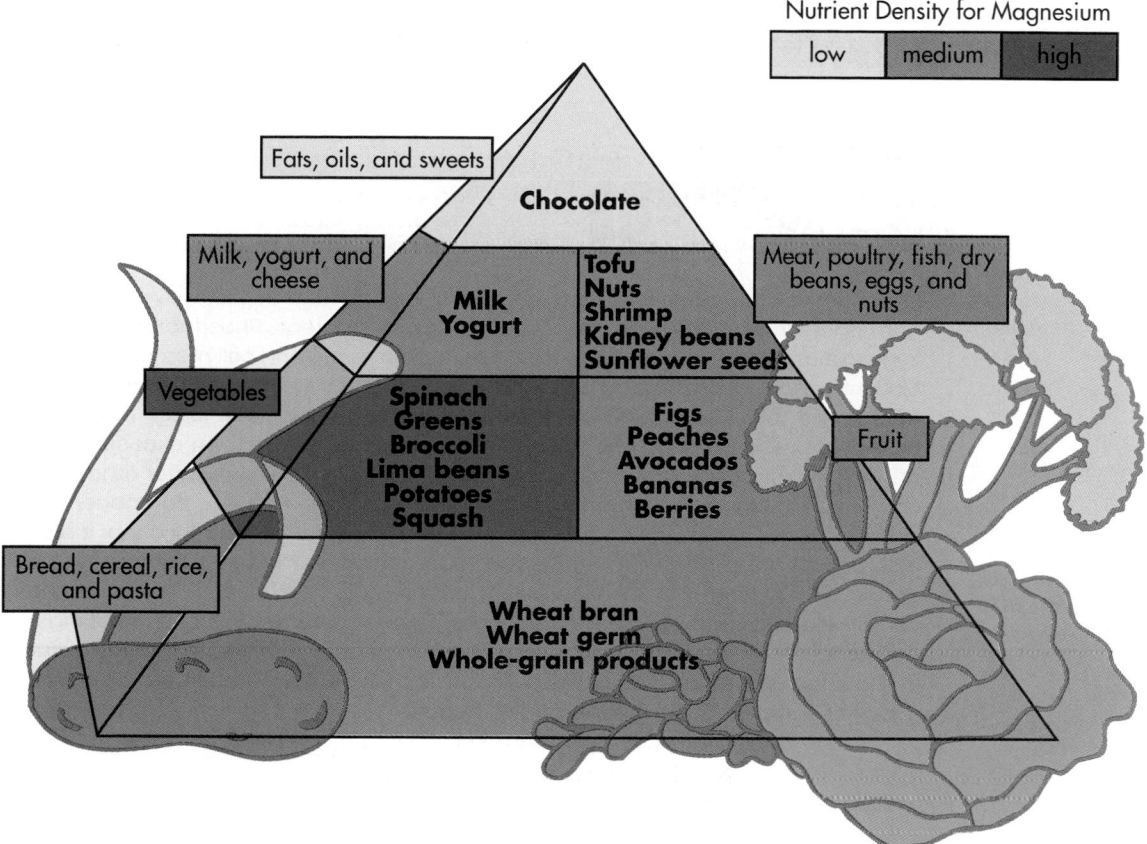

Nutrient Density for Magnesium

| low | medium | high |

Fats, oils, and sweets

Chocolate

Milk, yogurt, and cheese

**Milk
Yogurt**

**Tofu
Nuts
Shrimp
Kidney beans
Sunflower seeds**

Meat, poultry, fish, dry beans, eggs, and nuts

Vegetables

**Spinach
Greens
Broccoli
Lima beans
Potatoes
Squash**

**Figs
Peaches
Avocados
Bananas
Berries**

Fruit

Bread, cereal, rice, and pasta

**Wheat bran
Wheat germ
Whole-grain products**

Figure 9-10 *Food sources of magnesium from the Food Guide Pyramid. The vegetable group and whole-grain choices in the bread, cereal, rice, and pasta group are the best dietary sources of this nutrient. The background color of each food group indicates the average nutrient density for magnesium in that group.*

The adult RDA for magnesium is 350 milligrams per day for men and 280 milligrams per day for women. Adult men consume an average of 350 milligrams daily, whereas women consume closer to 250 milligrams daily.[2] Poor magnesium status is found among users of certain diuretics; some diuretics increase magnesium excretion in the urine. In addition, heavy perspiration for weeks in hot climates and bouts of long-standing diarrhea or vomiting all cause significant magnesium loss.[12] Alcoholism also increases the risk of a deficiency because dietary intake may be poor and because alcohol increases magnesium excretion in the urine. The disorientation and weakness associated with alcoholism closely resemble the behavior of people with low blood magnesium. Magnesium toxicity typically occurs only in people who have kidney failure or who overuse over-the-counter medications that contain magnesium, such as certain antacids and laxatives.

Sulfur (S)

Sulfur is found in many important compounds in the body, such as some amino acids (like methionine) and the vitamins biotin and thiamin. Sulfur helps in the balance of acids and bases in the body and is an important part of the liver's drug-detoxifying pathways. Because proteins supply the sulfur we need, sulfur is naturally a part of a healthful diet. Sulfur compounds are also used to preserve foods (see Chapter 17).

Hemoglobin

The iron-containing part of the red blood cell that carries oxygen to the cells and some carbon dioxide away from the cells. It is also responsible for the red color of blood.

Myoglobin

Iron-containing compound that binds oxygen in muscle tissue.

Heme iron

Iron provided from animal tissues in the form of hemoglobin and myoglobin. Approximately 40% of the iron in meat is heme iron; it is readily absorbed.

Nonheme iron

Iron provided from plant sources and animal tissues other than in the forms of hemoglobin and myoblogin. Nonheme iron is less efficiently absorbed than heme iron.

Absorption and Distribution of Iron

The body uses several mechanisms to regulate iron absorption. Controlling absorption is important, because our bodies cannot easily eliminate excess iron once it is absorbed. Iron absorption from foods varies from about 5% to 10% in healthy people, and 10% to 20% in people with iron deficiency. Overall, iron absorption depends on its form in the food, the body's need for it, and a variety of other factors.[13]

The form of iron in foods especially influences how much is absorbed. About 40% of the total iron in animal flesh is in the form of **hemoglobin** (the same form as in red blood cells) and **myoglobin** (pigment found in muscle cells). This **heme iron** is absorbed more than twice as efficiently as the simple elemental iron, called **nonheme iron.** Nonheme iron is also present in animal flesh, as well as in eggs, milk, vegetables, grains, and other plant foods.

About 10% to 15% of iron in the typical adult diet is heme iron, and usually about 20% is absorbed. Nonheme iron makes up the rest, and usually 2% to 20% is absorbed. Therefore animal flesh, especially red meat, is the best source of iron in the adult diet, because of both its iron content and the amount in the heme form. Consuming heme iron and nonheme iron together increases nonheme iron absorption. A protein factor in meats may also aid nonheme absorption. Overall, eating meat with vegetables and grain products enhances the absorption of all nonheme iron present.

Vitamin C can modestly increase nonheme iron absorption.[17] So when taking an iron supplement, consider drinking a glass of orange juice with it. Consuming more foods rich in vitamin C is particularly desirable if dietary iron is inadequate or if blood iron is low. Iron use in the body is also aided by copper, as explained in a later section.

Several dietary factors interfere with our ability to absorb iron. Phytic acid and other factors in grain fibers and oxalic acid in vegetables can all bind iron and reduce its absorption. Polyphenols (tannins) found in tea also reduce iron absorption. It is a good idea to moderate intake of tannins and keep dietary-fiber intake within 35 grams a day to reduce this effect of dietary fiber. Zinc also interferes with iron by competing with it for absorption. Finally, high-dose calcium supplements can also bind with iron—an important consideration when taking more than 500 milligrams in supplement per occasion.[27]

Overall, the most important factor influencing iron absorption is the body's need for it. In a deficiency state, iron absorption can increase. When iron stores are inadequate, the main blood protein that carries iron, transferrin, readily binds more iron, shifting it from intestinal cells into the bloodstream. If iron stores are adequate and the transferrin protein in the blood is fully saturated with iron, little will be absorbed from the intestinal cells. It stays bound as a ferritin protein in the intestinal cells.

By this mechanism, in normal circumstances, iron is absorbed only as needed. If not needed, when intestinal cells are shed at the end of their 2- to 5-day life cycle, the iron returns to the lumen of the intestinal tract. This whole process is referred to as a mucosal block against excess iron absorption.[6] High doses of iron can still be toxic, but absorption is carefully regulated under typical dietary conditions in most people.

Most iron in the body is contained in the hemoglobin molecules of the red blood cells. Some iron is stored in the bone marrow, and a small portion goes to other body cells, such as the liver, for storage. As iron is needed, it can be mobilized from body stores. If dietary intake is inadequate, these iron stores become depleted. Only then do signs of an iron deficiency appear.

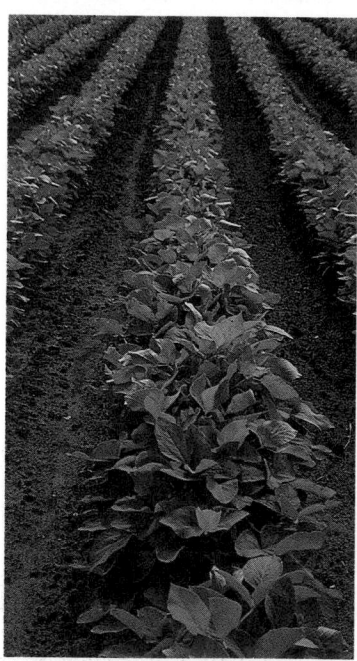

The trace mineral content of plant foods reflects the trace mineral concentration in the soil in which they were grown.

Functions of Iron

Iron forms part of the hemoglobin in red blood cells and myoglobin in muscle cells. Hemoglobin molecules in red blood cells transport oxygen (O_2) from the lungs to cells and assist in the return of some carbon dioxide (CO_2) from cells to the lungs for excretion. In addition, iron is used as part of many enzymes, some proteins, and compounds that cells use in energy production. Iron is also needed for immune function and contributes to drug detoxification pathways in the liver.[13]

Iron-deficiency anemia. If neither the diet nor body stores can supply the iron needed for hemoglobin synthesis, the number of red blood cells decreases in the bloodstream. The blood hemoglobin concentration also falls. When both the percentage of red blood cells (called the *hematocrit*) and the hemoglobin concentration fall, a physician would suspect iron deficiency.[14] In severe deficiency, hemoglobin and hematocrit fall so low that the amount of oxygen carried in the bloodstream is decreased. Such a person has anemia, defined as a decreased oxygen-carrying capacity of the blood. While there are many types of anemia, iron-deficiency anemia is the major type worldwide. About 30% of the world's population is anemic, and about half of those cases are caused by an iron deficiency. Probably about 7% to 12% of Americans in high risk categories indicated below have iron-deficiency anemia.[39]

Iron-deficiency anemia appears most often in infancy, the preschool years, and at puberty for both males and females.[36] Growth, with accompanying expansion of blood volume and muscle mass, increases iron needs, making it difficult to consume enough iron. Women are also very vulnerable during childbearing years when menstruation occurs. In addition, anemia is often found in pregnant women, as discussed in Chapter 14. Iron-deficiency anemia in adult men is usually caused by blood loss from ulcers, colon cancer, or hemorrhoids. Finally, athletes can incur anemia, as discussed in Chapter 11.

Clinical symptoms of iron-deficiency anemia primarily include pale skin, fatigue, poor temperature regulation, loss of appetite, and apathy. Insufficient iron for the synthesis of red blood cells and key cell compounds may cause the fatigue. Researchers suspect that poor iron stores may also decrease learning ability, attention span, work performance, and immune status even before a person is actually anemic[13,36] (see Chapter 18).

More Americans have an iron deficiency than iron-deficiency anemia. Their blood hemoglobin values are still normal, but they have no stores to draw from in times of pregnancy or illness, and basic functioning may not be up to par. That could mean anything from too little energy to perform everyday tasks in an efficient manner to difficulties staying alert in school or on the job.[39]

To speed the cure of iron-deficiency anemia, a person needs to take iron supplements. A physician should also find the cause—an inadequate diet or a bleeding ulcer, for example—so that the anemia does not recur. Changes in diet may prevent iron-deficiency anemia, but supplemental iron is the only reliable cure.

Iron in Foods and the RDA

The most nutrient-dense iron sources are spinach, oysters, liver, clams, peas, and legumes. However, total iron content and nutrient density of foods are not the only considerations when choosing dietary iron sources. Serving size and bioavailability are probably more important.[6] For example, although spinach is rich in iron, the body absorbs very little of it. Animal sources contain some heme iron, the most bioavailable form. These then are our best iron sources. Iron present in iron supplements is also absorbed well. The major iron sources in the adult diet are animal and grain products (Figure 9-11). Most of the iron in bakery products has been added to refined flour in the enrichment process.

The use of iron-fortified formulas and cereals in the Special Supplemental Food Program for Women, Infant, and Children (WIC) in the United States is probably a major contributor to decreasing rates of iron-deficiency anemia in preschool children (see Chapter 15). Another possible iron source is cooking utensils. When

Hematocrit
The percentage of blood that is made up of red blood cells.

A red blood cell has a life span of approximately 120 days. A rapid cell turnover such as this puts great nutrient demands on the body, and iron is one of those nutrients in great demand.

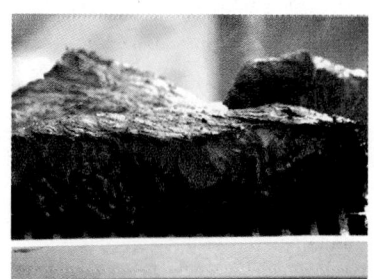

Red meat is a major source of iron in the American diet.

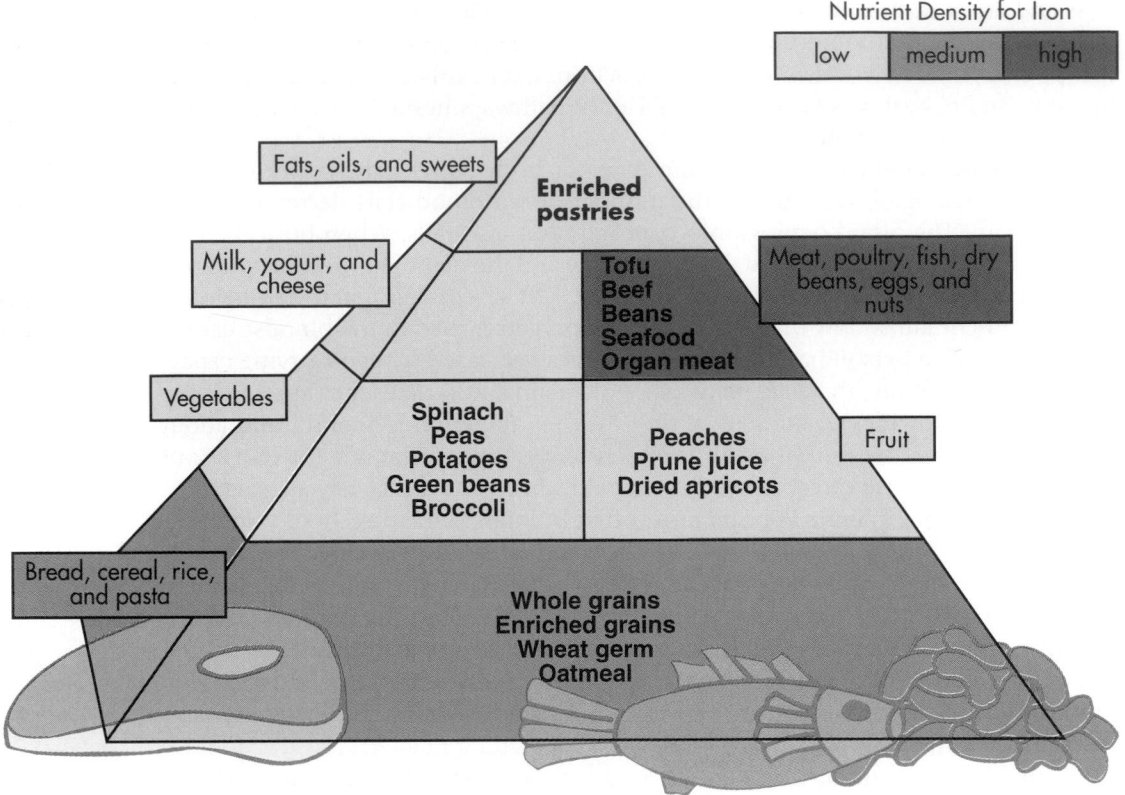

Figure 9-11 *Food sources of iron from the Food Guide Pyramid. The meat, poultry, fish, dry beans, eggs, and nuts group and the bread, cereal, rice, and pasta group are the best dietary sources of this nutrient. The heme iron in the meat, poultry, fish, dry beans, eggs, and nuts group is especially well absorbed. The iron content of a food containing mostly nonheme iron is only an approximate measure of the amount delivered to body cells, as body need greatly influences the absorption of nonheme iron. The background color of each food group indicates the average nutrient density for iron in that group.*

acidic foods, such as tomato sauce, are cooked for prolonged times in iron pots and cast iron frying pans, some iron from the cookware is taken up by the food. Breakfast cereals are generally rich iron sources, too (Figure 9-12).

Milk is a very poor source of iron. A common cause of iron-deficiency anemia in children is an overreliance on milk, coupled with an insufficient meat intake. Total vegetarians (vegans) are particularly susceptible to iron-deficiency anemia, because of their lack of dietary heme iron.

The daily adult RDA for iron is 10 milligrams for men and 15 milligrams for women. The RDA value assumes that about 10% of dietary iron is absorbed. If iron absorption exceeds that, less dietary iron is needed.

The higher RDA for women is primarily because of menstrual blood loss. Women who menstruate more heavily and longer than average may need even more dietary iron, and those who have lighter and shorter flows may need less iron. The variation in menstrual blood loss, and hence, loss of iron, makes it difficult to set an RDA for iron for women.

By recording dietary intakes from a variety of women, researchers find that most women do not consume 15 milligrams of iron daily. The average daily value is closer to 12 milligrams, while in men it is about 17 milligrams per day.[2] Of course, not all women need 15 milligrams of iron daily, because the RDA is set high enough to allow for variations in menstrual flow and absorption rates. Whether male or female, if you are not consuming the RDA for iron, you should be concerned, but not

Hemochromatosis
A disorder of iron metabolism characterized by increased absorption and deposition of iron in liver and heart tissue.

alarmed. Try to consume a diet that meets the RDA for iron; and make sure your physician checks your iron status during regular physical examinations. It is difficult to tell whether a lower iron intake is actually harmful. Although we have very sensitive measures of iron stores in the body, we lack the knowledge to reliably predict the resulting effects on health status when people register low values.

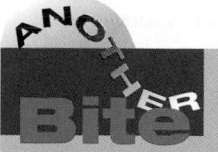

The adult human body contains about 21 cups (5 liters) of blood. Blood donations are generally 2 cups (500 milliliters). Thus a blood donor gives about a tenth of his or her total supply. Healthy people generally can donate blood two to four times a year without harmful consequences. As a precaution, blood banks first screen potential donors' blood for the presence of anemia.

Toxicity of Iron

Although not as common as iron deficiency, iron overload can be serious because it can easily lead to toxic symptoms. Even a large single dose of iron of 60 milligrams can be life-threatening to a 1-year-old. Children are frequently victims of iron poisoning because iron pills and nutrient supplements containing iron are tempting targets on kitchen tables and in cabinets. FDA has proposed a rule that would require label warnings on iron supplements with 30 milligrams of iron or more per tablet, stating that iron may be lethal to children who ingest the product.

Smaller doses of iron (but still greater than what is needed) over a long period can also cause problems. A form of iron toxicity, for example, has been observed in an African tribe that brews beer in iron pots.[22] Some people of Mediterranean descent have a type of anemia caused by increased destruction of red blood cells; low-dose iron therapy used to treat this disease can lead to toxicity symptoms. Repeated blood transfusions can also lead to iron toxicity.

In addition, iron toxicity accompanies the genetic disease called hereditary *hemochromatosis.* The disease is associated with a substantial increase in iron absorption. For people with this disease, iron in the body eventually builds up to dangerous amounts, especially in the blood and liver. Some iron is deposited in the muscles, pancreas, and heart. If not treated, the excess iron deposits contribute to severe organ damage, especially in the liver and heart.

Hereditary hemochromatosis requires that a person carry two defective copies of a particular gene to develop the disease. People with one defective gene and one normal gene, called carriers, may also absorb excess dietary iron but not to the same extent as those with two defective genes. About 5% to 10% of Americans of Northern European extraction are carriers of hemochromatosis. An estimated 0.25% to 0.4% of this population carries two defective genes and therefore has the potential for developing the disease.[22]

Carriers of hemochromatosis may be prime candidates for heart disease, especially men. As noted in Chapter 6, excess iron in the blood may accelerate atherosclerosis in people with elevated LDL by contributing to oxidation of lipids in the LDL particles. This in turn allows LDL to be taken up more readily by scavenger cells in the blood vessels. However, the importance of iron in stimulating atherosclerosis is still hotly debated.[29] Because of its relatively efficient absorption, dietary heme iron, such as that found in red meats, poses the greatest risk in this regard.[22] To put

Figure 9-12 *Breakfast cereals are often enriched in many trace minerals, including iron.*

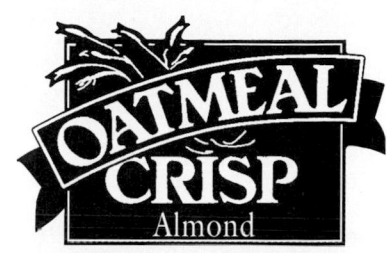

Nutrition Facts

Serving Size 1 cup (55g)
Servings Per Container About 8

Amount Per Serving	Oatmeal Crisp with Almonds	with ½ cup skim milk
Calories	230	270
Calories from Fat	50	50

	% Daily Value**	
Total Fat 6g*	9%	9%
Saturated Fat 0.5g	3%	4%
Cholesterol 0mg	0%	1%
Sodium 320mg	13%	16%
Potassium 150mg	4%	10%
Total Carbohydrate 39g	13%	15%
Dietary Fiber 3g	12%	12%
Sugars 11g		
Other Carbohydrate 25g		
Protein 6g		

Vitamin A	25%	30%
Vitamin C	25%	25%
Calcium	10%	25%
Iron	90%	90%
Vitamin D	10%	25%
Thiamin	25%	30%
Riboflavin	25%	35%
Niacin	25%	25%
Vitamin B$_6$	25%	25%
Folic Acid	25%	25%
Phosphorus	15%	25%
Magnesium	10%	15%
Zinc	25%	30%
Copper	8%	8%

*Amount in Cereal. A serving of cereal plus skim milk provides 6g fat (1g saturated), less than 5mg cholesterol, 380mg sodium, 360mg potassium, 45g carbohydrate (17g sugars), and 10g protein.

**Percent Daily Values are based on a 2,000 calorie diet. Your daily values may be higher or lower depending on your calorie needs:

	Calories:	2,000	2,500
Total Fat	Less than	65g	80g
Sat Fat	Less than	20g	25g
Cholesterol	Less than	300mg	300mg
Sodium	Less than	2,400mg	2,400mg
Total Carbohydrate		300g	375g
Dietary Fiber		25g	30g

INGREDIENTS: ROLLED OATS, RICE, ALMOND PIECES WITH FRESHNESS PRESERVED BY BHT, BROWN SUGAR, SUGAR, HONEY, SALT, CORN SYRUP, SUNFLOWER OIL, ARTIFICIAL AND NATURAL FLAVORS, CALCIUM CARBONATE.

VITAMINS AND MINERALS: IRON AND ZINC (MINERAL NUTRIENTS), VITAMIN C (SODIUM ASCORBATE), A B VITAMIN (NIACINAMIDE), VITAMIN B$_6$ (PYRIDOXINE HYDROCHLORIDE), VITAMIN A (PALMITATE), VITAMIN B$_2$ (RIBOFLAVIN), VITAMIN B$_1$ (THIAMIN MONONITRATE), A B VITAMIN (FOLIC ACID), VITAMIN D.

General Mills, Inc.
GENERAL OFFICES
MINNEAPOLIS, MINNESOTA 55440
Made in U.S.A.

© 1994 General Mills, Inc.

this relatively new research area into perspective, a reasonable approach is for you to ask to be screened for iron overload at your next visit to a physician. If you show evidence of this it would be wise to undergo therapy, especially if you have high LDL as well.

Ideally, consent of a physician should precede any use of iron supplements. When iron supplements are advised, there should be adequate follow-up so that supplementation does not exceed what is necessary. Probably the only factor keeping many people with hemochromatosis and carriers of one gene from experiencing serious effects of the disease is that they consume only a moderate amount of iron.

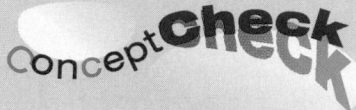

Iron is absorbed depending mostly on its form and the body's need for it. Absorption is affected by a "mucosal block," but excess iron intake can override the system, leading to toxicity. Iron absorption increases somewhat in the presence of vitamin C and meat protein and decreases in the presence of large amounts of calcium and some components of grain fiber, such as phytic acid. Iron is most important in synthesizing hemoglobin and myoglobin, in supporting immune function, and in energy metabolism. An iron deficiency can cause decreased red blood cell synthesis, which can lead to anemia. It is particularly important for women of childbearing age to consume adequate iron, primarily to replace that lost in menstrual blood. Good sources include red meat, pork, liver, enriched grains and cereals, and oysters. Iron toxicity usually results from a genetic disorder called hemochromatosis. This disease causes overabsorption and accumulation of iron, which can result in severe liver and heart damage. Because of the risk of toxicity, any use of iron supplements, especially by men, should be supervised by a physician.

Zinc (Zn)

Although zinc has been recognized as an essential nutrient in farm animals since the early 1900s, zinc deficiency was first recognized in humans in the early 1960s in Egypt and Iran. Zinc deficiencies were determined to cause growth retardation and poor sexual development in some groups of people, even though the zinc content of their diets was fairly high. However, the customary diet contained unleavened bread almost exclusively and little animal protein. Unleavened bread is very high in phytic acid and other factors that decrease zinc bioavailability. Parasite infestation and the practice of eating clay and other parts of soil also probably contributed to the severe zinc deficiency.

In America, zinc deficiencies were first observed in the early 1970s in hospitalized patients who were fed only intravenously. Zinc was not added to solutions at that time, but the protein source in the solutions was based on milk protein or a blood protein, which are both naturally rich in zinc. When the solutions were changed in the early 1970s to include mostly individual amino acids as the protein source, deficiency symptoms quickly developed because amino acid formulas are low in zinc.

Symptoms of adult zinc deficiency include an acnelike rash, diarrhea, lack of appetite, reduced sense of taste and smell, and hair loss. In children and adolescents with zinc deficiency, growth, sexual development, and learning ability may also be hampered.[1] When children show poor growth, they should be checked for inadequate zinc status.

Like iron, zinc absorption is influenced by the foods a person ingests. About 10% to 35% of dietary zinc is absorbed; the higher figure is more likely when ani-

A rare disease, acrodermatitis enteropathica, results from an inherited inability to absorb zinc. Symptoms in infants include rash, hair loss, depressed immune response, decreased sense of taste, lack of appetite, and poor growth. This disease can be treated with supplements of zinc in amounts of about twice the RDA.

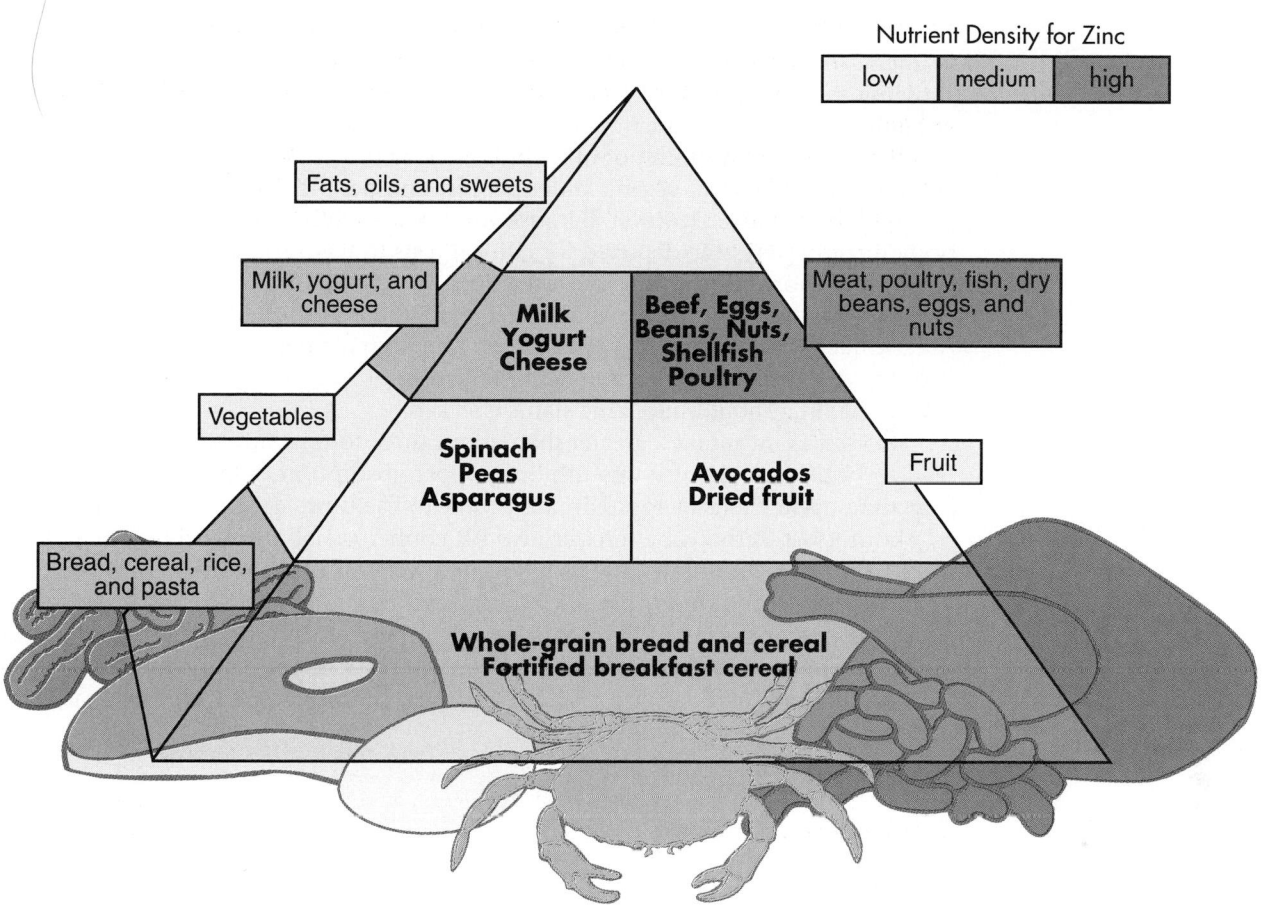

Nutrient Density for Zinc

| low | medium | high |

Fats, oils, and sweets

Milk, yogurt, and cheese

Milk Yogurt Cheese

Beef, Eggs, Beans, Nuts, Shellfish Poultry

Meat, poultry, fish, dry beans, eggs, and nuts

Vegetables

Spinach Peas Asparagus

Avocados Dried fruit

Fruit

Bread, cereal, rice, and pasta

Whole-grain bread and cereal Fortified breakfast cereal

Figure 9-13

Food sources of zinc from the Food Guide Pyramid. The meat, poultry, fish, dry beans, eggs, and nuts group includes the best dietary sources of this nutrient. Some zinc is supplied by whole grains and fortified breakfast cereals from the bread, cereal, rice, and pasta group. The background color of each food group indicates the average nutrient density for zinc in that group.

mal protein sources are used and when the body needs more zinc. Most people worldwide rely on cereal grains (low in zinc) for their source of protein, energy, and zinc. This makes consuming adequate zinc a problem.

Functions of Zinc

More than 300 enzymes require zinc for optimal activity. Adequate zinc intake is necessary to support many bodily functions, including the following:

- DNA and protein metabolism, wound healing, and growth
- Proper immune function (taking more than the RDA does not provide extra benefit to immune function)
- Proper development of sexual organs and bone
- Storage and release of the hormone insulin
- Alcohol metabolism
- Taste sensation

Zinc in Foods and the RDA

In general, protein-rich diets are also rich in zinc. Animal foods supply almost half our zinc intake. The most nutrient-dense sources of zinc are oysters, shrimp, crab, lean beef, lamb, turkey, beans, and mushrooms. As with iron, nutrient density is not the only issue; bioavailability is probably more important. Animal foods are again our best sources because zinc from animal sources is not bound by phytic acid. However, good plant sources of zinc—such as whole grains, peanuts, and beans—should not be discounted. They can deliver substantial amounts of zinc to body cells (Figure 9-13).

The daily adult RDA for zinc is 15 milligrams for men and 12 milligrams for women. The average American takes in 9 to 15 milligrams of zinc a day, with men showing the higher values.[2] This raises concern that many women do not consume enough zinc. Still, there are no indications of moderate or severe zinc deficiencies in an otherwise healthy adult population. It is likely that many Americans—especially women, poor children, vegans, older people, and people with alcoholism—have a marginal zinc status. However, because we lack a sensitive marker for zinc status, a body must be very zinc-depleted for clinical tests to register a deficiency.

Furthermore, absorption and excretion can maintain an adequate zinc status even when intakes are somewhat lower than those furnished by typical diets of Americans. However, the long-term effects of marginal zinc intakes are not known.[1] People who show deterioration in taste sensation, recurring infections, or poor wound healing should have zinc status checked.

Excessive zinc intakes, greater than about three to four times the RDA, can also lead to problems, because this inhibits copper absorption.[1] One study has shown that zinc supplements at approximately three to five times the RDA can reduce HDL by about 15%, perhaps by interfering with copper metabolism. That is disturbing for two reasons. First, low HDL is associated with an increased risk of developing heart disase. Second, many people who take zinc supplements do in fact consume an excessive amount. The RDA publication recommends not exceeding the RDA for zinc with supplements unless under close medical supervision. Zinc intakes over 50 to 100 milligrams per day also result in diarrhea, cramps, nausea, vomiting, and depressed immune system function.

Selenium (Se)

Selenium exists in many forms that are readily absorbed. Selenium's best understood role is aiding the activity of an enzyme that participates in reducing the damage that electron-seeking free radical (oxidizing) compounds can do to cell membranes.[19]

In Chapter 8 you saw that vitamin E helps prevent attacks on cell membranes by electron-seeking compounds. Thus vitamin E and selenium work together toward the same goal. Chapter 8 also discussed how free radical compounds can cause cancer. Although selenium could prove to have a role in cancer prevention, it is premature to recommend selenium supplementation for this purpose. Animal studies in this area are conflicting, and current studies with humans are under way to help clarify what role, if any, selenium plays in cancer prevention. The effect of selenium on other metabolic functions, such as with thyroid hormone metabolism, is still under investigation.[19]

Selenium deficiency symptoms in farm animals and humans include muscle pain and wasting and a form of heart disease. Farm animals in areas with low selenium soil concentration, such as New Zealand, and humans in some areas of China develop characteristic muscle and heart disorders associated with inadequate selenium intake. Other factors probably also contribute.

Selenium in Foods and the RDA

Fish, meats (especially organ meats), eggs, and shellfish are good animal sources of selenium. Grains and seeds grown in soils containing selenium are good plant sources. Major selenium contributors to the adult diet are animal and grain products. Because we eat a varied diet of foods supplied from many geographic areas, it is unlikely that low soil selenium in a few locations will mean inadequate selenium in our diets.

The RDA for selenium is 55 to 70 micrograms per day for adults. In general, adults meet the RDA, consuming on average 110 micrograms of selenium each day.[19]

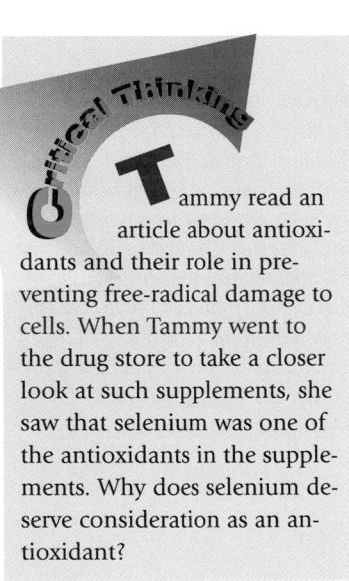

Critical Thinking

Tammy read an article about antioxidants and their role in preventing free-radical damage to cells. When Tammy went to the drug store to take a closer look at such supplements, she saw that selenium was one of the antioxidants in the supplements. Why does selenium deserve consideration as an antioxidant?

Selenium at daily intakes as low as 900 micrograms per day (15 times the RDA) can cause toxicity symptoms if taken for many months. These symptoms include garlicky breath odor, changes in fingernails, hair loss, nausea and vomiting, and general weakness. Rashes and cirrhosis of the liver may also develop. Selenium clearly illustrates the saying: "It's the dose that makes the poison."

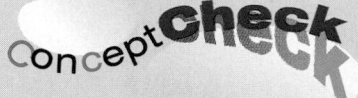

Zinc functions as a cofactor for many enzymes and is important for growth, immune function, and sense of taste. Beef, seafood, and whole grains are good food sources. As in the case of iron, the intestinal cells regulate zinc absorption according to the body's needs for the mineral. If taken in excess amounts, copper competes with zinc for absorption. Selenium activates an enzyme that helps change electron-seeking free radical (oxidizing) compounds into less toxic compounds so these do not attack and break down cell membranes. By helping to dismantle the free radical compounds, selenium works toward the same goal as vitamin E. A selenium deficiency results in muscle and heart disorders. Animal products and grains are good selenium sources; however, the selenium content in plants depends on the selenium concentration in the soil. The misuse of both selenium and zinc supplements can lead to toxic results.

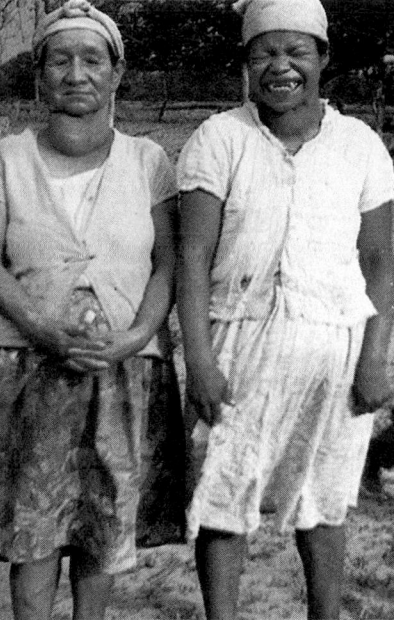

Figure 9-14
Goiter and cretinism in Bolivia. The mother on the left is goitrous, but otherwise normal. The daughter is goitrous, mentally retarded, deaf, and mute.

Iodine (I)

Iodine in foods is actually found in an ion form, called iodide. During World War I, a link was discovered between a deficiency of iodide and the production of a **goiter,** an enlarged thyroid gland (Figure 9-14). Men drafted from the Pacific Northwest and the Great Lakes Region of the United States had a much higher rate of **goiter** than did men from other areas of the country. The soils in these areas have very low iodide contents. In the 1920s, researchers in Ohio found that low doses of iodide given to children over a 4-year period could prevent goiter. That finding led to the addition of iodide to salt beginning in the 1920s.

Today, many nations require iodide fortification of salt. In the United States, salt can be purchased either iodized or plain. Check for this on the label of a package of salt next time you are in a grocery store. Some areas of Europe, such as northern Italy, have very low soil levels of iodide, but have yet to adopt the practice of fortifying salt with iodide. People in these areas, especially women, still suffer from goiter, as do people in areas of Central America, South America, and Africa. The World Health Organization estimates that millions of people in the world have varying degrees of iodide deficiency. Eradication of iodide deficiency is a goal of many health-related organizations worldwide.[3]

Goiter
An enlargement of the thyroid gland; this is often caused by insufficient iodide in the diet.

Function of Iodide

The thyroid gland actively accumulates and traps iodide from the bloodstream to support its hormone synthesis. Thyroid hormones, such as thyroxine, are synthesized using iodide. These hormones help regulate metabolic rate and promote growth and development throughout the body, including the brain.

If a person's iodide intake is insufficient, the thyroid gland enlarges as it attempts to take up more iodide from the bloodstream. This eventually leads to goiter.

Goitrogens

Substances in food that interfere with the absorption and use of iodide. They therefore may cause goiter if consumed in large amounts.

Cretinism

Stunting of body growth and poor mental development that result from inadequate maternal intake of iodide during pregnancy.

Although iodide can prevent goiter formation, it does not shrink a goiter once it has formed. Goiters have been described in people—usually women—as far back as 3000 BC.

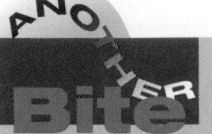

*Goiters are sometimes found in people who consume large amounts of raw turnips and rutabagas. These vegetables contain compounds called **goitrogens,** which inhibit the function of the thyroid gland and, in turn, thyroid hormone synthesis. However, goitrogens are generally not an important cause of goiter because the cooking process destroys them, and turnips and rutabagas are not typically staples in human diets.*

If a woman has an iodide-deficient diet during the early months of her pregnancy, the fetus suffers iodide deficiency because the mother's body uses up the available iodide. The infant then may be born with short stature and develop mental retardation.[5] This stunted growth that results is part of what is known as *cretinism.* Cretinism appeared in America before iodide fortification of table salt began. Today, cretinism still appears in Europe, Africa, Latin America, and Asia.

Food Sources of Iodide and the RDA

Saltwater fish, seafood, iodized salt, dairy products, and grain products contain various forms of iodide. Sea salt found in health food stores, however, is not a good source because the iodide is lost during processing.

The RDA for iodide for adults is 150 micrograms. A half teaspoon of iodide-fortified salt (about 2 grams) supplies that amount. Most adults consume much more iodide than the RDA—an estimated 170 to 250 micrograms daily, not including that from use of iodized salt at the table. This extra amount adds up because dairies and quick-service restaurants use it as a sterilizing agent, bakeries use it as a dough conditioner, food producers use it as part of food colorants, and it is added to salt.

Reports in scientific literature raise concern about a high iodide intake. Amounts of up to 1 to 2 milligrams per day appear to be safe. However, when very high amounts of iodide are consumed, thyroid gland function is hampered. This can occur in people who eat a lot of seaweed, because some seaweeds contain so much iodide; total iodide intake can then add up to 60 to 130 times the RDA. Because it is potentially toxic, manufacturers are currently working to reduce unnecessary iodide use in dairies, restaurants, and bakeries.

Copper (Cu)

Copper is a critical element in the metabolism of iron; it operates in processes that form hemoglobin and transport iron. A copper-containing enzyme aids in the release of iron from storage. Copper also is needed by enzymes that create cross-connections in collagen and elastin, connective tissue proteins.[34] In laboratory animals with copper deficiencies, blood vessels rupture because collagen is unavailable to form the important connective tissue network that strengthens blood vessels.

Copper is also needed by other enzymes, such as those that defend the body against free radical (oxidizing) compounds and those that act in the brain and central nervous sytem. In addition, copper performs in immune system function, blood clotting, and blood lipoprotein metabolism. Symptoms of copper deficiency include a form of anemia, low white blood cell count, bone loss, poor growth, and some forms of heart disease.

Copper in Foods and Needs

Copper is found primarily in liver, seafood, cocoa, legumes, nuts, seeds, and whole-grain breads and cereals.

The ESADDI for copper is 1.5 to 3 milligrams daily for adults. The average adult intake is about 1 to 1.5 milligrams per day.[2] Women generally consume the smaller amount. Even so, the copper status of adults appears to be good, though we lack sensitive measures for copper status. It is wise, however, to regularly eat good sources of copper.

The groups most likely to develop copper deficiencies are premature infants, infants recovering from semistarvation on a milk-dominated diet (which is a poor source of copper), and people recovering from intestinal surgery (during which time copper absorption decreases). Recall that a copper deficiency can also result from overzealous supplementation of zinc, because zinc and copper compete with each other for absorption.

Copper can cause toxicity, including vomiting, at single doses of greater than 10 to 30 milligrams. When copper is used to treat a deficiency, it must be given in divided doses to limit this effect. An inherited condition called Wilson's disease results in accumulation of copper in the liver, brain, kidneys, and corneas. If recognized early, treatment that binds copper in the bloodstream and increases its excretion in the urine can prevent damage to these tissues and reduce the mental degeneration commonly seen in active cases.

An inherited condition known as Menkes' kinky hair syndrome is characterized by slow growth, brain degeneration, kinky white hair, and low blood copper levels. This condition results from a defect of copper absorption and incorporation into proteins. Supplemental copper is given in an attempt to partially reverse this condition.

Fluoride (F)

Dentists in the early 1900s noticed a lower rate of dental caries (cavities) in the southwestern United States. These areas contained high amounts of fluoride in the water. The amounts were sometimes so high that small spots on the teeth, called *mottling*, appeared. Even though mottled teeth were quite discolored, they contained very few dental caries. After experiments showed that fluoride in the water did indeed decrease the rate of dental caries, controlled fluoridation of water in parts of the United States began in 1945.

Those of us who grew up drinking fluoridated water generally have 40% to 60% fewer dental caries than people who did not drink fluoridated water as children. Dentists can provide fluoride treatments, and schools can provide fluoride tablets, but it is much less expensive and more reliable to simply add fluoride to a community's drinking water. State and private water sources do not always contain enough fluoride, however. When in doubt, contact your local water plant or have the water in your home analyzed for fluoride content. If it is less than 1 part fluoride per million parts of water (1 ppm), talk to your dentist about the best means for your children to obtain the fluoride they need.[10]

Functions of Fluoride

Dietary fluoride consumed during childhood, when bones and teeth are developing, aids the synthesis of tooth crystals that strongly resist acid. Therefore teeth become very resistant to dental caries. Fluoride also inhibits metabolism and growth of the bacterium that causes dental caries, and fluoride present in saliva directly inhibits tooth demineralization and enhances tooth remineralization.[18]

Fluoride applied to the surface of the teeth by dentists or from toothpaste adds additional protection against dental caries. Thus people of all ages benefit from the topical effects of fluoride, whether or not they consumed fluoridated water or fluoride supplements as children. Dietary fluoride also improves growth rate in rats, but scientists are not sure if fluoride is actually necessary for growth in humans.

High doses of fluoride (≥20 milligrams per day) are being used experimentally in adults to treat severe **osteoporosis**, especially that seen in the spine. Such high fluoride dosages can cause significant side effects, such as stomach upset and bone pain. Ongoing research is attempting to establish a dose, form, and duration of treatment that aid bone mass accretion and contribute to reduced fracture risk.

Fluoride in Foods and Needs

Tea, seafood, seaweed, and some natural water supplies are the only good food sources of fluoride. Most fluoride consumed in America comes from water fortification, toothpaste, and fluoride treatments performed by dentists. No credible evidence shows that water fluoridation is harmful at levels currently used in the United States.

The ESADDI for fluoride for adults is 1.5 to 4 milligrams. This amount provides resistance to dental caries without causing mottling of the teeth or other toxicity symptoms. Adults generally meet this amount of intake.

A fluoride intake greater than 6 milligrams per day can mottle teeth during their developmental stage, as mentioned above. Children who consume large amounts of fluoridated toothpaste as part of daily tooth care are at greatest risk. Not swallowing toothpaste and limiting the amount used to "pea" size are the best ways to prevent this problem. In addition, children under 6 years should have toothbrushing supervised by an adult.[10] High fluoride intake in adults does not cause mottling. When fluoride intakes reach 20 milligrams per day during tooth development, the tooth structure is weakened and can crumble.

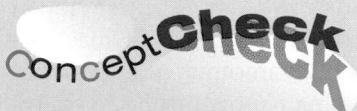

Iodide is vital for the synthesis of thyroid hormones. A prolonged insufficient intake causes the thyroid gland to enlarge, resulting in a goiter. The use of iodized salt in America has virtually eliminated this condition. Copper functions mainly in iron metabolism and in the cross-bonding of collagen. A deficiency can result in an iron-deficiency type of anemia. Good food sources of copper are seafoods, legumes, nuts, dried fruits, and whole grains. Fluoride aids in tooth and bone development. When incorporated into the diet during development, fluoride makes teeth resistant to acid and bacterial growth, in turn reducing development of dental caries. Fluoride also aids in remineralization of teeth once decay begins. Most of us receive adequate amounts of fluoride from that added to drinking water and toothpaste. A high fluoride intake during tooth development can lead to spotted, or mottled, teeth.

Chromium (Cr)

The importance of chromium in human diets has been recognized only in the past 20 years. There is much we do not understand about this mineral, but chromium deficiency may be related to diabetes in some individuals.

The most-studied function of chromium is the maintenance of glucose uptake into cells. Our current understanding is that chromium enters the cell and likely increases the number of insulin receptors or enhances the transport of glucose across the cell membrane.[26]

In both animals and humans, a chromium deficiency is characterized by impaired blood glucose control and elevated blood cholesterol and triglycerides. The mechanism by which chromium influences cholesterol metabolism is not known but may involve enzymes that control cholesterol synthesis. Chromium deficiency appears in people maintained on intravenous solutions not supplemented with chromium and in children with malnutrition. Because sensitive measures of chromium status are not available, marginal chromium deficiencies may go undetected.[26]

Food Sources of Chromium and Needs

Specific data regarding the chromium content of various foods are scant, and most food composition tables do not include values for this trace mineral. Egg yolks, whole grains (bran), organ meats, other meats, mushrooms, nuts, and beer are good sources. Yeast is also a source. The amount of chromium in foods is closely tied to the local soil content of chromium. To provide yourself with a good chromium intake, regularly choose whole grains in preference to refined grains.

The estimated safe and adequate daily dietary intake of chromium is 50 to 200 micrograms per day. Average adult intakes in the United States are estimated at about 30 micrograms per day, but could be somewhat higher. Marginal to low chromium intakes in the elderly may contribute to their increased risk for developing diabetes. Chromium intakes of less than 20 micrograms per day may be detrimental to a significant portion of the population that has marginally elevated blood glucose.[26]

Some research also shows that an intake at the high end of the ESADDI, or slightly above 200 micrograms per day, may raise HDL. More studies are needed on this effect. Chromium toxicity has been reported in people exposed to industrial waste and in painters who use art supplies with a very high chromium content. Liver damage and lung cancer can result. Because of the risk of toxicity, any supplement use should not exceed 200 micrograms per day.

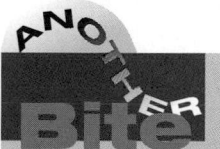

The current promotion of chromium picolinate as an agent to increase lean body mass or act as a weight-loss inducer provides a typical example of misleading use of research results by the health-food industry. The scant positive findings have come from the laboratory of the originator of chromium picolinate. Several well-designed controlled studies, however, have failed to duplicate these findings or have found only a select few individuals (possibly with initially low chromium status) whose body composition responded significantly to chromium supplementation.[21] As noted in Chapter 10, any claims for chromium picolinate are speculative at best.

Manganese (Mn)

The mineral manganese is easily confused with magnesium. Not only are their names similar, but they also often substitute for each other in metabolic processes. Manganese is needed by some enzymes, such as those used in carbohydrate metabolism. Manganese is also important in bone formation.

No human deficiency symptom is associated with a low manganese intake. Animals on manganese-deficient diets suffer alterations in brain function, bone formation, and reproduction. If human diets were low in manganese, these symptoms would probably appear as well. As it happens, our need for manganese is very low, and our diets tend to be adequate in manganese.

Good food sources of manganese are nuts, rice, oats and other whole grains, beans, and leafy vegetables. The estimated safe and adequate daily dietary intake of manganese is 2 to 5 milligrams. Average intakes fall within this range. Manganese is toxic at high doses, so be cautious with supplement use that exceeds body needs.

Molybdenum (Mo)

Molybdenum interacts with iron and copper, especially to inhibit copper absorption. Several human enzymes use molybdenum. No molybedenum deficiency has been noted in people who consume normal diets, though deficiency symptoms have appeared in people maintained on intravenous feedings. These symptoms include increased heart and respiration rates, night blindness, mental confusion, edema, and weakness.

Good food sources of molybdenum include milk and milk products, beans, whole grains, and nuts. The ESADDI for molybdenum is 75 to 250 micrograms, about the same as typical intakes. In addition, the ESADDI may be quite generous compared to our needs.[35] When consumed in high doses, molybdenum causes toxicity in laboratory animals, with weight loss and decreased growth.

Other Trace Minerals

Although a variety of other trace minerals is found in humans, many of them have not yet been shown to be required. The list of minerals in this category includes boron, nickel, vanadium, arsenic, lithium, silicon, tin, and cadmium. Widespread deficiency symptoms in humans have never been noted, probably because typical diets provide adequate amounts and they are needed by very few enzymes and metabolic systems. Their potential for toxicity should make one question any supplementation not supervised by a physician. These trace minerals may achieve more importance as more research is reported.

See Table 9-6 to review what has been discussed about the trace minerals.

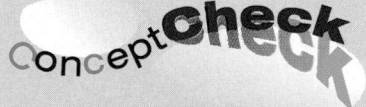

Chromium acts to increase the action of the hormone insulin. The amount of chromium found in food depends on soil content. Meats, whole grains, and egg yolks are some good sources. Manganese is a component of bone and used by many enzymes, including those involved in glucose production. Because our need for manganese is low, deficiencies are rare. Nuts, rice, oats, and beans are good food sources. Molybdenum is another trace mineral required by a few enzymes. Good sources include milk, beans, whole grains, and nuts. Deficiencies appear only with intravenous diets. The needs for some other trace minerals—such as boron, nickel, arsenic, and vanadium—have not been fully established in humans. If required, these minerals are needed in such small amounts that our current diets are probably adequate sources of them.

TABLE 9-6

A Summary of Key Trace Minerals

Mineral	Major functions	Deficiency symptoms	People most at risk	RDA or ESADDI	Nutrient-dense dietary sources	Results of toxicity
Iron	Used for hemoglobin and other key compounds used in respiration; used for immune function	Low blood iron; small, pale red blood cells; low blood hemoglobin values	Infants, preschool children, adolescents, women in childbearing years	Men: 10 milligrams Women: 15 milligrams	Meats, spinach, seafood, broccoli, peas, bran, enriched breads	Toxicity seen when children consume ≥60 milligrams in iron pills; also in people with hemochromatosis
Zinc	Required for more than 300 enzymes, including enzymes involved in growth, immunity, alcohol metabolism, sexual development, and reproduction	Skin rash, diarrhea, decreased appetite and sense of taste, hair loss, poor growth and development, poor wound healing	Vegetarians, elderly people	Men: 15 milligrams Women: 12 milligrams	Seafoods, meats, greens, whole grains	Reduces copper absorption; can cause diarrhea, cramps, and depressed immune function
Selenium	Aids antioxidant system	Muscle pain, muscle weakness, heart disease	Unknown	55-70 micrograms	Meats, eggs, fish, seafoods, whole grains	Nausea, vomiting, hair loss, weakness, liver disease
Iodide	Aids thyroid hormone	Goiter; poor growth in infancy when mother is iodide deficient during pregnancy	None in America, because salt is usually fortified	150 micrograms	Iodized salt, white bread saltwater fish, dairy products	Inhibition of function of the thyroid gland
Copper	Aids in iron metabolism; works with many enzymes, such as those involved in protein metabolism and hormone synthesis	Anemia, low white blood cell count, poor growth	Infants recovering from semi-starvation, people who use overzealous supplementation of zinc	1.5-3 milligrams	Liver, cocoa, beans, nuts, whole grains, dried fruits	Vomiting; nervous system disorders
Fluoride	Increases resistance of tooth enamel to dental caries	Increased risk of dental caries	Areas where water is not fluoridated and dental treatments do not make up for a lack of fluoride	1.5-4 milligrams	Fluoridated water, toothpaste, dental treatments, tea, seaweed	Stomach upset; mottling (staining) of teeth during development; bone pain
Chromium	Enhances blood glucose control	High blood glucose after eating	People on intravenous nutrition, and perhaps elderly people with non-insulin-dependent diabetes	50-200 micrograms	Egg yolks, whole grains, pork, nuts, mushrooms, beer	Caused by industrial contamination, not dietary excess
Manganese	Aids action of some enzymes, such as those involved in carbohydrate metabolism	None in humans	Unknown	2-5 milligrams	Nuts, oats, beans, tea	Unknown in humans
Molybdenum	Aids action of some enzymes	None in humans	Unknown	75-250 micrograms	Beans, grains, nuts	Unknown in humans

Summary

➤ Water constitutes 50% to 70% of the human body. Its unique chemical properties enable it to dissolve substances as well as serve as a medium for chemical reactions, temperature regulation, and lubrication. Water also helps regulate the acid-base balance in the body. For adults, daily water needs are estimated at 1 milliliter per kcal expended.

➤ Many minerals are vital for sustaining life. For humans, animal products are the most bioavailable sources of most minerals. Supplements of minerals exceeding 150% of recommended amounts should be taken only under a physician's supervision, because toxicity and nutrient interactions are a likely possibility.

➤ Sodium, the major positive ion found outside cells, is vital in fluid balance and nerve impulse transmission. The American diet provides abundant sodium through processed foods and table salt. About 10% to 15% of the adult population is sodium-sensitive and is at risk for developing high blood pressure from consuming excessive sodium.

➤ Potassium, the major positive ion found inside cells, has a similar function to sodium. Milk, fruits, and vegetables are good sources. Chloride is the major negative ion found outside cells. It is important in digestion as part of gastric hydrochloric acid and in immune and nerve functions. Table salt supplies most of the chloride in our diets.

➤ Calcium forms a vital part of bone structure and is also very important in blood clotting, muscle contraction, nerve transmission, and cell metabolism. Calcium absorption is enhanced by stomach acid and the active vitamin D hormone. Dairy products are important calcium sources. Women are particularly at risk for not meeting calcium needs.

➤ Phosphorus aids enzyme function and forms part of key metabolic compounds, cell membranes, and bone. It is efficiently absorbed, and deficiencies are rare, although there is concern about possibly poor intake by some elderly women. Good food sources are dairy products, bakery products, and meats. Sulfur is incorporated into certain vitamins and amino acids. Magnesium is a mineral found mostly in plants. It is important for nerve and heart function and as an activator for many enzymes. Whole grains (bran portion), vegetables, nuts, seeds, milk, and meats are good food sources.

➤ Iron absorption depends mainly on the form of iron present and the body's need for it. Heme iron from animal sources is better absorbed than the nonheme iron obtained primarily from plant sources. Consuming vitamin C simultaneously with iron modestly increases nonheme absorption. Iron operates mainly in synthesizing hemoglobin and myoglobin and in the action of the immune system. Women are at great risk for developing iron deficiency, which decreases blood hemoglobin and red blood cell number. When this condition is severe enough to decrease the amount of oxygen carried in the blood, iron-deficiency anemia develops. Iron toxicity usually results from a genetic disorder called hemochromatosis. This disease causes overabsorption and accumulation of iron, which can result in severe liver and heart damage.

➤ Zinc aids in the action of more than 300 enzymes that are important for growth, development, immune function, wound healing, and taste. A zinc deficiency results in poor growth, loss of appetite, reduced sense of taste and smell, hair loss, and a persistent rash. Zinc is best absorbed from animal sources. The most nutrient-dense sources of zinc are oysters, shrimp, crab, and beef. Good plant sources are whole grains, peanuts, and beans.

➤ An important role of selenium is decreasing the action of free radical (oxidizing) compounds. In this way, selenium acts along with vitamin E. Muscle pain, muscle wasting, and a form of heart disease may result from a selenium deficiency. Meats eggs, fish, and shellfish are good animal sources of selenium. Good plant sources include grains and seeds.

➤ Iodide forms part of the thyroid hormones. A lack of dietary iodide results in the development of an enlarged thyroid gland or goiter. Iodized salt is a major food source.

➤ Copper is important for iron metabolism, collagen cross-linking, and other functions. A copper deficiency can result in an iron-deficiency–type anemia. Copper is found mainly in liver, seafood, cocoa, legumes, and whole grains.

➤ Fluoride incorporated into dietary intake during development makes teeth resistant to dental caries. Most Americans receive the bulk of their fluoride from fluoridated water and toothpaste.

➤ Chromium aids action of the hormone insulin. Egg yolks, meats, and whole grains are good sources of chromium. Manganese and molybdenum are used by various enzymes. Clear deficiencies in otherwise healthy people are rarely seen for any of these three nutrients. Human needs for other trace minerals are so low that deficiencies are uncommon.

Study Questions

1 Approximately how much water do you need each day to stay healthy? Identify at least two situations that increase the need for water. Then list three sources of water in the average person's diet.

2 Why are most minerals generally present in higher concentrations in animal foods than in plant foods?

3 Identify four factors that influence the bioavailability of minerals from food.

4 What is the relationship between sodium and water balance, and how is that relationship monitored as well as maintained in the body?

5 Within what physiological system do potassium, chloride, and calcium interact? What are the individual roles of these minerals in this system?

6 In terms of total amounts in the body, calcium and phosphorus are the first and second most abundant minerals, respectively. Name two ways in which phosphorus and calcium are alike and two ways in which they differ.

7 Describe how a "mucosal block" lessens the risk of developing an iron toxicity state.

8 Describe the symptoms of iron-deficiency anemia and explain possible reasons why they occur.

9 Which trace minerals are lost from cereal grains when they are refined? Are any of these nutrients replaced by enrichment?

10 Describe the chief function of fluoride, copper, and chromium in the body.

References

1 Aggett P, Comerford JG: Zinc and human health, *Nutrition Reviews* 53:S16, 1995.

2 Alaimo K and others: Dietary intake of vitamins, minerals, and fiber of persons ages 2 months and over in the United States, Third National Health and Nutrition Examination Survey, Phase 1, 1988-91, *Advance Data* 258(Nov 14):1, 1994.

3 Ali O: Iodine deficiency disorders: a public health challenge in developing countries, *Nutrition* 11:517, 1995.

4 Anderson JJB: Calcium, phosphorus, and human bone development, *Journal of Nutrition* 126:1153S, 1996.

5 Bleichrodt N and others: The benefits of adequate iodine intake, *Nutrition Reviews* 54(4): S72, 1996.

6 Bothwell TH: Overview and mechanisms of iron regulation, *Nutrition Reviews* 53:237, 1995.

7 Bucher HC and others: Effects of dietary calcium supplementation on blood pressure, *Journal of the American Medical Association* 275:1016, 1996.

8 Callaway W: Reexamining cholesterol and sodium recommendations, *Nutrition Today,* 29(Sept/Oct):32, 1994.

9 Cantor KP: Water chlorination, mutagenicity, and cancer epidemiology, *American Journal of Public Health* 84:1211, 1994.

10 Clark MM and others: Preventive dentistry and the family physician, *American Family Physician* 53:619, 1996.

11 Cummings SR and others: Risk factors for hip fracture in white women, *New England Journal of Medicine* 332:767, 1995.

12 Dreosti IE: Magnesium status and health, *Nutrition Reviews* 53:S23 (Sept), 1995.

13 Fairbanks VF: Iron in medicine and nutrition. In Shils ME and others, editors: *Modern nutrition in health and disease*, Philadelphia, 1994, Lea & Febiger.

14 Ganong WF: *Review of medical physiology*, ed 17, Norwalk, Conn, 1995, Appleton & Lange.

15 Gilman MW and others: Protective effect of fruits and vegetables on development of stroke in men, *Journal of the American Medical Association* 273:1113, 1995.

16 Greenleaf JE: Problem: thirst, drinking behavior, and involuntary dehydration, *Medicine and Science in Sports and Exercise* 24:645, 1993.

17 Hunt JR and others: Effect of ascorbic acid on apparent iron absorption by women with low iron stores, *American Journal of Clinical Nutrition* 59:1381, 1994.

18 Konig KG, Navia JM: Nutritional role of sugars in oral health, *American Journal of Clinical Nutrition* 62 (suppl):275S, 1995.

19 Levander OA, Burk RF: Selenium. In Shils ME and others, editors: *Modern nutrition in health and disease*, Philadelphia, 1994, Lea & Febiger.

20 Levenson DI, Bockman RS: A review of calcium preparations, *Nutrition Reviews* 52:221, 1994.

21 Lukaski HC and others: Chromium supplementation and resistance training: effects on body composition, strength, and trace element status of men, *American Journal of Clinical Nutrition* 63:954, 1996.

22 Lynch SR: Iron overload: prevalence and impact on health, *Nutrition Reviews* 53:255, 1995.

23 McBean LD: Osteoporosis: boning up on the latest facts, *Dairy Council Digest* 67(1):1, 1996.

24 Midgeley JP and others: Effect of reduced dietary sodium on blood pressure, *Journal of the American Medical Association* 275:1590, 1996.

25 Mortensen L, Charles P: Bioavailability of calcium supplements and the effect of vitamin D: comparisons between milk, calcium carbonate, and calcium carbonate plus vitamin D, *American Journal of Clinical Nutrition* 63:354, 1996.

26 Nielsen FH: Chromium and ultratrace minerals. In Shils ME and others, editors: *Modern nutrition in health and disease*, Philadelphia, 1994, Lea & Febiger.

27 NIH Consensus Development Panel on Optimal Calcium Intake: Optimal calcium intake, *Journal of the American Medical Association* 272:1909, 1994.

28 Preuss HG and others: Association of macronutrients and energy intake with hypertension, *Journal of the American College of Nutrition* 15:21, 1996.

29 Proulx MR, Weaver CM: Ironing out heart disease, *Nutrition Today* 30(Jan/Feb):16, 1995. (See also Sempos CT and others: Iron and heart disease: the epidemiologic data, *Nutrition Reviews* 54:73, 1996.)

30 Reaven GM and others: Hypertension and associated metabolic abnormalities—the role of insulin resistance and the sympathoadrenal system, *New England Journal of Medicine* 334:374, 1996.

31 Reusser ME, McCarron DA: Micronutrient effects on blood pressure regulation, *Nutrition Reviews* 52:367, 1994.

32 Riggs BL, Melton LJ: The prevention and treatment of osteoporosis, *New England Journal of Medicine* 327:620, 1992.

33 Seelig MS: ISIS 4: Clinical controversy regarding magnesium infusion, thrombolytic therapy, and acute myocardial infarction, *Nutrition Reviews* 53:261, 1995.

34 Turnlund JR: Copper. In Shils ME and others, editors: *Modern nutrition in health and disease*, Philadelphia, 1994, Lea & Febiger.

35 Turnlund JR and others: Molybdenum absorption, excretion, and retention studied with stable isotopes in young men during depletion and repletion, *American Journal of Clinical Nutrition* 61:1102, 1995.

36 US Public Health Service: Anemia in children, *American Family Physician* 51:1121, 1995.

37 Wardlaw GM, Weese N: Putting calcium into perspective for your clients, *Topics in Clinical Nutrition* 11:23, 1995.

38 Writing Group for the PEPI Trial: Effects of estrogen or estrogen/progestin regimens on heart disease risk factors in postmenopausal women, *Journal of the American Medical Association* 273:199, 1995.

39 Yip R: Iron deficiency: contemporary scientific issues and international programmatic approaches, *Journal of Nutrition* 124:1479S, 1994.

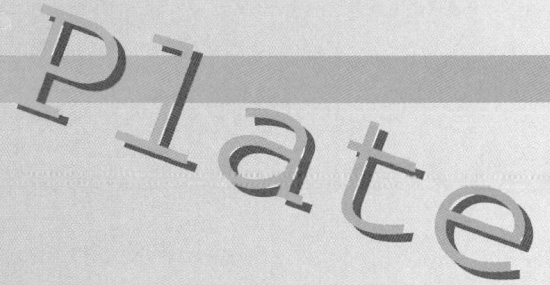

RATE Your Plate

How Does Your Mineral Intake Measure Up?

To complete this activity, you must reexamine your nutritional assessment from Chapter 2. Compare your intake of selective minerals with the RDA (or other standards given). Use your completed nutritional assessment to complete the table below. For each mineral, record your intake, the RDA, the percentage of the RDA you consumed, and a +, −, or = to indicate an intake higher, lower, or equal to the RDA. Note that for sodium and potassium, minimum requirements for health are designated and already recorded in the table (these can also be found on the inside front cover of the book). RDAs have not been established for these two minerals.

Mineral	Intake	RDA/other	% of RDA/other	+/−/=
Calcium				
Phosphorus				
Sodium		500 mg		
Potassium		2000 mg		
Iron				
Zinc				

ANALYSIS

1. Which of your mineral intakes equaled or exceeded the RDA (or other standard given)? Do the nutrients for which you exceeded the RDA pose a likely risk for toxicity, based on the total amount consumed?

   _____

2. Which of your intakes were below the RDA (or other standard given)?

   _____

3. What foods and cooking practices could be emphasized or deemphasized to modify your weaknesses? Indicate for each food the specific amount of the missing nutrient(s) supplied.

   _____

   _____

   _____

   _____

   _____

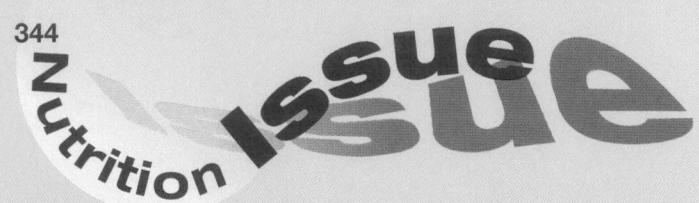

Calcium and Osteoporosis

Widespread advertising has made it almost impossible for women to ignore **osteoporosis.** The crippling effect this disease has on older persons is now recognized as a major medical problem. The disease affects more than 25 million people in the United States, most of them women. Osteoporosis leads to approximately 1.5 million bone fractures per year, usually in the hip, spine, or wrist. About one third of all women experience osteoporosis-related fractures in their lifetimes.[23]

Scientific estimates of the physical activity and dietary patterns of humans living at the end of the Stone Age suggest that their calcium intake was twice that of contemporary humans and physical exertion was also greater than at present. Bony remains from that period also suggest that Stone Age humans developed a greater bone mass in young adulthood and experienced less age-related bone loss than do humans in the twentieth century. Does this tell you something?

The slender, inactive woman who smokes is most susceptible to osteoporosis, but any person who lives long enough can suffer from the disease, including men. About 25% of women older than 50 develop osteoporosis. Among people older than 80, osteoporosis becomes the rule—not the exception. The spine fractures commonly found in women with osteoporosis cause considerable pain and deformity and decrease physical ability (Figure 9-15); hip fractures are seen in both men and women with osteoporosis. Not only is this disease debilitating, it also can be fatal. Between 12% and 20% of all older persons who suffer hip fractures eventually die from fracture-related complications.

A QUICK LOOK AT BONE STRUCTURE AND STRENGTH

To better understand the role calcium plays in bone health and osteoporosis, it is important to understand how bone is constructed. Visual observation of the cross-sections of a bone reveals two primary bone structural types: **cortical bone** and **trabecular bone.** These interact within each bone to form quite an engineering marvel of strength (Figure 9-16).

The entire outer surface of all bones is composed of cortical (compact) bone, which is very dense. The shafts of long bones, such as those of the arm, are almost entirely cortical bone. Trabecular (spongy) bone is found in the ends of the long bones, inside the spinal vertebrae, and inside the flat bones of the pelvis. Trabecular bone forms an internal scaffolding network for a bone. It supports the outer cortical shell of the bone, especially in heavily stressed areas, such as joints.[14]

Bone strength depends on a person's **bone mineral density.** The more densely packed the bone crystals are, the stronger the bone structure. Another important element of bone strength is the trabecular bone support network inside a bone. It is especially critical for the horizontal trabeculae to extend continuously—without breaks—between the areas of vertical trabeculae. Any break in either the horizontal or more vertical trabecular beams weakens the support system of a bone and increases the risk for bone fracture. And once these beams are broken, there is no way to rebuild them. This is why it is so important to limit bone loss as people age.

BONE MASS IS RELATED TO AGE AND GENDER

The question of how and why osteoporosis takes place is largely a matter of one's bone mass. Rapid and continual bone growth and calcification occur throughout the adolescent years, utlimately resulting in what is called *peak bone mass.* In the adolescent growth spurt, bone mass is increasing at the rate of about 8.5% per year. Small increases in bone mass then continue between 20 and 30 years of age.[23]

The ultimate amount of bone built by a person is clearly dependent on gender, race, familial patterns seen in the mother and father, and probably other genetically determined factors. In addition, men have higher bone mass value than women, and blacks have heavier skeletons than whites. As a direct consequence, men and blacks have a lower risk of fractures than other populations. Slender, small-framed whites and Asian women show the lowest bone mass values. Peak bone mass is also related to dietary intake of calcium and other nutrients, such as vitamin K, magnesium, zinc, and copper.[1,12,23,34]

Bone mass varies among young adults; some have much denser bone than others, perhaps because they built more bone when they were young. Some people also may more easily adapt to lower-calcium diets. People who have developed more bone by early adulthood can sustain greater age-related bone loss with less fracture risk compared with those who have less bone.

For women, bone loss begins about age 30 and proceeds slowly and continuously to menopause (approximately age 50). It often speeds up at menopause and continues at a high rate for the next 10 years. By age 65 to

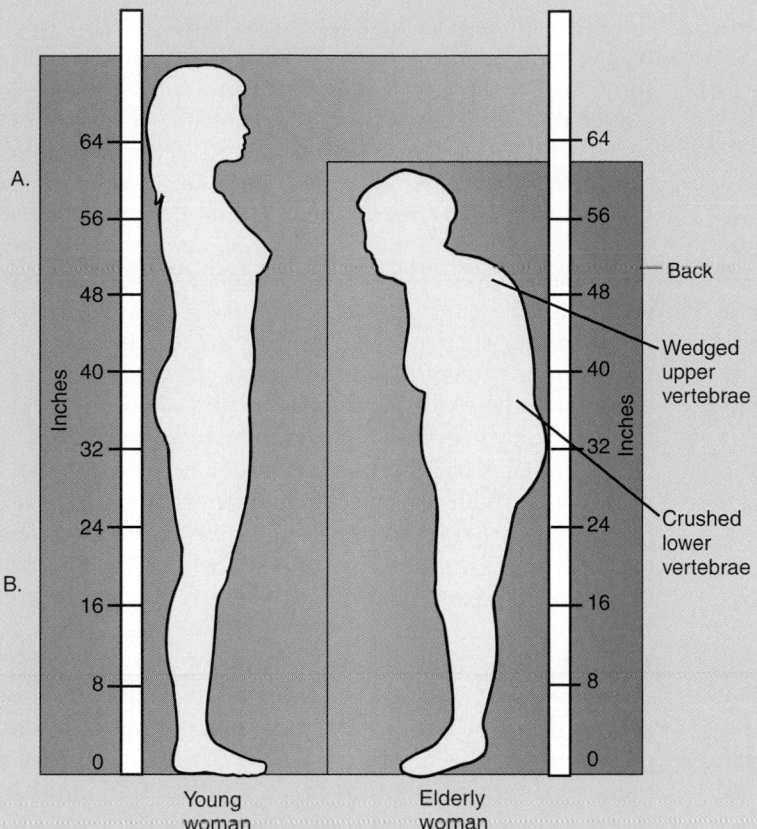

Researchers in Australia have uncovered what they think is one reason hip fractures are more common in Western countries than in the developing world. Because children in Western countries have higher average nutrient intakes than those in developing countries, they grow faster and to a greater extent. As a result, the part of the thigh bone that fits into the pelvis becomes quite long. The greater the length of this part, called the hip axial length, the more fragile this region of the hip is, and in turn the higher the risk for hip fracture, especially as bone mass decreases with advanced age. This suggests that people in Western countries especially must pursue strategies to avert hip fracture, notably in later years.

Figure 9-15 *A loss of height and a distorted body shape are commonly seen in osteoporosis. Monitoring adult height changes is one way to detect early osteoporosis.*

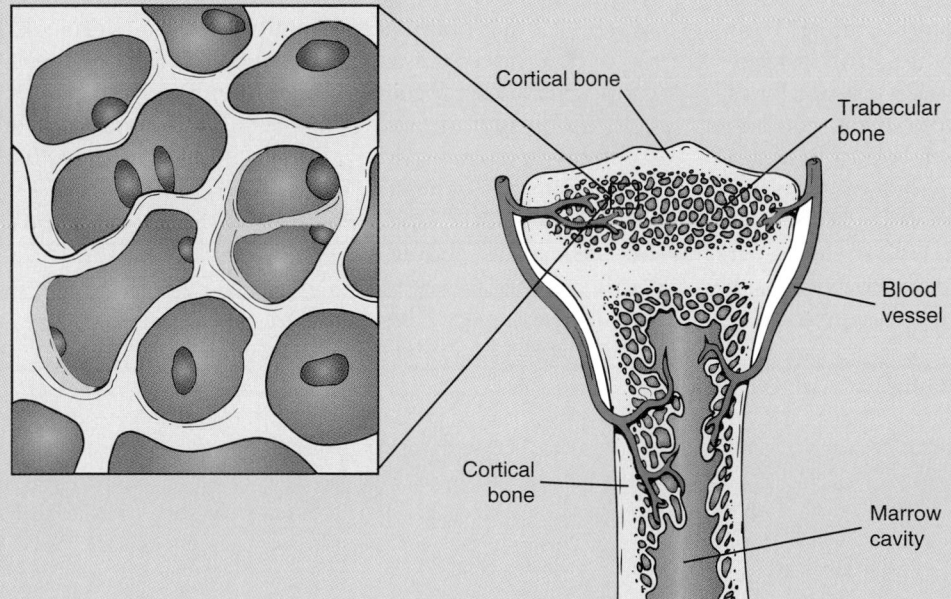

Figure 9-16 *Cortical and trabecular bone. Cortical bone forms the shafts of bones and the outer mineral covering. Trabecular bone supports the outer shell of cortical bone in various bones of the body, as in the bone pictured.*

Osteoporosis

Decreased bone mass where no outward cause can be found. Related to effects of aging, poor diet, and hormonal effects of menopause in women.

Bone mineral density

Total mineral content of bone at a specific bone site divided by the width of the bone at that site, generally expressed as grams per cubic centimeter.

Continued.

70, the rate of bone loss falls to about the same rate as before menopause. In men, bone loss is slow and steady from around age 30. Overall, this bone loss in both males and females progresses without noticeable symptoms.[23]

OSTEOPOROSIS

Failure to maintain enough bone mass in the body eventually results in **osteopenia** (from the Greek words *osteo* meaning "bone" and *penia* meaning "poverty"). Osteopenia can be caused by the vitamin D deficiency disease osteomalacia, the use of certain medications (such as cortisol, antiseizure drugs, and thyroid hormones), and cancer. If these or similar causes are not present, the diagnosis is osteoporosis. Osteoporosis can be roughly classified as type I (postmenopausal), which appears in women in the years right after menopause, and type II (senile), which is found in both men and women of advanced age.[32]

Recall from Chapter 8 that in osteomalacia the bone is abnormal because it contains too little calcium. In contrast, bone composition in osteoporosis is essentially normal. The bone may contain some extra sodium, but basically there is just less bone throughout the body. Because these bones have less substance, osteoporosis can lead to fractures in old age, distorted body shape, and loss of teeth (Figure 9-15).

ESTROGEN REPLACEMENT PLUS CALCIUM IS THE BEST APPROACH FOR REDUCING POSTMENOPAUSAL BONE LOSS

Hormone replacement therapy with estrogen (and often with added progestins) is widely recommended for women at menopause to prevent osteoporosis, especially if (1) they have no contraindications to use and (2) they fall in the lower third of bone mass values for their age.[32] Women with intermediate values who do not opt for estrogen treatment should have their bone mass values remeasured at their physician's discretion, typically in 2 or so years. However, women postponing therapy should realize that alteration of the internal trabecular support system of the bone as a result of bone loss is currently a permanent phenomenon. No therapy can reverse this problem. Estrogen is also used to reduce the symptoms of menopause.[32]

Estrogen replacement at menopause greatly slows further bone loss in women. Thus it is reasonable to assume that estrogen replacement therapy will significantly reduce the risk of osteoporosis and related fractures, especially in the spines of women who begin treatment right after menopause and continue it for 20 years or so. Estrogen also helps reduce bone loss in older women.

Estrogen aids bone maintenance in a number of ways. Some studies show that estrogen is associated with greater synthesis of the active vitamin D hormone. Estrogen also may increase the sensitivity of the intestine to this hormone, in turn improving the action of this hormone and therefore increasing calcium absorption. Finally, the binding of estrogen to these receptors on bone cells stimulates or inhibits synthesis of local factors that, respectively, influence bone maintenance.[32]

Estrogen therapy is relatively safe for most women but still must be closely supervised by a physician. Resumption of menstruation with some forms of therapy is common, but it subsides after a few years or so. A slight increased risk for certain forms of cancer, notably in the breast and endometrium (the latter if the woman has not had a **hysterectomy),** and gallbladder problems has been observed in women on estrogen therapy. Thus close monitoring is needed. Adding progestins to the regimen greatly reduces the risk of endometrial cancer.[32]

An additional benefit of estrogen replacement therapy is a significant reduction in the risk of heart disease. Heart disease risk climbs sharply after menopause. Estrogen blunts this change in part by lowering LDL and raising HDL,[38] as noted in Chapter 6. A direct benefit of estrogen on cells lining the blood vessels is also suspected, as well as other possible explanations for the effect.

When the decreased risks for osteoporosis and heart disease are added together, estrogen replacement therapy ends up greatly improving the overall health risk profile for many women, especially those with many risk factors for osteoporosis or heart disease. A woman and her physician should work together to see if that is true for her. The Women's Health Initia-

Estrogen replacement therapy is also associated with decreased risk of developing Alzheimer's disease.

tive trial, currently under way, is designed to help pinpoint the actual net benefit from estrogen replacement experienced by a wide variety of women, and should in turn contribute to this decision making. Results are due by 2006.

Some women cannot take estrogen because they have estrogen-sensitive breasts or uterine tumors. Other therapies, such as taking certain **bisphosphonate compounds,** are available and quite effective. However, these treatments are still relatively new, more expensive, and more cumbersome than estrogen therapy.

The question that often arises is whether an increased calcium intake can substitute for the use of estrogen or other medications in reducing bone loss in postmenopausal women. Overall, studies have found that taking as much as 2000 milligrams of extra calcium daily (equal to about 7 cups of milk) after menopause does not prevent bone loss in the spine, hip, or wrist as successfully as estrogen replacement does. Although such high intakes of dietary calcium do reduce bone loss in some areas, they are no more effective than calcium intakes closer to the RDA in reducing the often significant loss of spinal bone that occurs in the 5 to 10 years immediately after menopause.

Earlier it was noted that spinal fractures cause considerable pain and deformity and decrease physical ability. Because no reliable cure exists for osteoporosis, it is very important to prevent these fractures. Thus for most women at high risk for osteoporosis it is not a question of estrogen versus calcium. Rather, estrogen plus calcium probably constitutes the most effective treatment currently available. Also, as women who are not on estrogen therapy 10 years beyond menopause, consumption of 1500 milligrams of calcium and maintenance of adequate vitamin D nutriture lead to less bone loss throughout the body than if this intervention is not undertaken. This therapy in turn can lead to a significant reduction in the risk of hip fracture.[23]

WILL A NUTRITIOUS DIET IN YOUTH HELP PREVENT OSTEOPOROSIS LATER?

Meeting at least the RDA for calcium from childhood through adolescence builds a stronger bone structure than does a lower calcium intake. The extent and importance of this difference in bone strength are currently under study. Some researchers think that the RDA for women ages 11 through 24 is too low. Note that a recent NIH Consensus Conference on Optimal Calcium Intake recommended up to an additional 300 milligrams (to a total of 1500 milligrams per day) through age 24, suspecting that such higher calcium intakes will result in greater bone mass compared with just following the RDA.[27] Researchers are likely to have the answer to this question in about 1997, once current studies are completed.

ARE ALL WOMEN AT RISK FOR OSTEOPOROSIS?

Only about one-third of all women experience osteoporosis-related fractures in their lifetimes. Some women just do not live long enough to suffer from osteoporosis. They may experience some bone loss, but their bones still remain reasonably strong throughout their lives. This is especially true of women who die before the age 75.

In addition, some women have much denser bone than others. They probably built more bone when they were young, so they are able to endure greater bone loss without experiencing more fractures. Actually, the reason for such variations in bone mass and fracture risk in women of any age still needs more research. However, researchers have identified numerous factors—including physical activity, body weight, and calcium intake throughout life—associated with higher bone mass values in some studies (Table 9-7). Even more factors are associated with low bone mass in women: slim figure; a family history of osteoporosis; irregular menstruation; premature menopause; use of certain medications; excess dietary protein, caffeine, and sodium, which increase calcium loss in the urine; and prolonged bed rest.[23,37] We clearly can't focus only on calcium when discussing this disease—many factors are involved.

PROPER PLANNING HELPS PREVENT FRACTURES IN LATER LIFE

As women mature, different strategies for preventing osteoporosis are needed, based on the risk factors present. Young women should see a physician upon any sign of irregular menstruation and should pursue an active lifestyle that includes sun exposure (to promote synthesis

Continued.

of vitamin D) and weight-bearing physical activity (to build/maintain muscle mass). Greater muscle mass linked to physical activity is associated with greater bone mass, as this keeps tension on bone.

In young women, regular menstruation is a main contributor to bone maintenance, as evidenced by low bone mass in some nonmenstruating female athletes and other women with irregular menstruation, such as those with anorexia nervosa. Physical activity cannot prevent the bone loss associated with irregular menstruation. It is also important to at least meet the RDA for calcium, and possibly consume more, as recommended by the recent NIH Consensus Conference on Optimal Calcium Intakes.

Smoking and excessive alcohol intake work against bone strength. Smoking lowers estrogen in the blood in women, increasing bone loss. Alcohol is toxic to all cells, including bone cells, and alcoholism is probably a major undiagnosed and unrecognized cause of osteoporosis today. Moderation in phosphorus, caffeine, sodium, and protein intake is also advised. These are especially problematic when insufficient calcium is consumed.[4,23]

At menopause, women should discuss estrogen replacement therapy with a physician. They also need to accurately track their height. A decrease of more than 1 inch from premenopausal values is a sign that significant bone loss is taking place.

Older men and women need to stay physically active (if possible)—including some weight-bearing and resistance activities—and they should meet their RDA for calcium at the very least; a higher goal of 1500 milligrams per day is advocated by many researchers. As mentioned previously, this physical activity and calcium intake are most likely to limit bone loss in some areas of the body, such as the hip. Older people also need to minimize the risk for falls, especially by limiting their use of medications and alcohol, which might disturb coordination, and should take corrective measures if visual function is impaired.[11] Getting regular sun exposure and consuming food sources of vitamin D also are very important. Supplements containing about 10 to 20 micrograms (400 to 800 IU) are also appropriate (see Chapter 8).

TABLE 9-7

Some Factors Associated with Bone Accretion/Maintenance Versus Bone Loss

Accretion/maintenance	Loss	
Normal menses	Lack of menses	Cigarette smoking
Estrogen replacement	(generally from post-	Slender figure
African ethnic origin	menopausal status)	Bed rest (months)
Thiazide diuretics	Early menopause	Excessive wheat bran in-
Physical activity	Glucocorticoid use	take
Dietary calcium	Hyperparathyroidism	Anorexia nervosa
Vitamin D nutriture	Hyperthyroidism	Excessive sodium intake
Body weight	Thyroid hormone replace-	Excessive caffeine intake
Overall adequate diet	ment	Excessive phosphorus
Parents with large bone	Factors made by white	consumption if calcium
mass	blood cells	RDA is not met
	Alcoholism	Excessive protein intake

For a recent review of many of the factors influencing bone health, see Heaney RP: Bone mass, nutrition, and other lifestyle factors, *Nutrition Reviews* 54(4):S3, 1996.

Osteopenia
Decreased bone mass caused by cancer, hyperthyroidism, or other reasons.

Hysterectomy
Surgical removal of the uterus.

Bisphosphonates
Compounds primarily composed of carbon and phosphorous that bind to bone mineral and in turn reduce bone breakdown.

The National Osteoporosis Foundation will answer your questions about the disease ([800] 464-6700).

ENERGY

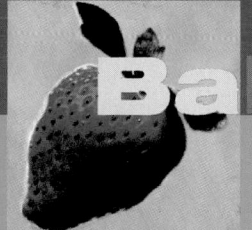

Balance and Imbalance

PART 3

Weight Control

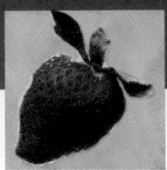

IMAGINE A MAGIC PILL OR potion melting away unwanted pounds. No sweat or starvation, just a sleek body in a few quick swallows. Many proponents of magical drinks and diet programs erroneously claim they eliminate excess fat forever. Consumers presently pour $33 billion into the diet industry, a business predicted to increase by $20 billion within 5 years.[22] The diet industry digests dollars, and consumers lose not only pounds. They often lose cash—and sometimes good health—needlessly.

Of people you see on the street, one fourth of the men and nearly half the women are struggling to control their weight. Still, despite all their efforts, the ranks of the obese in America are still growing. Currently, about 33% of adult Americans are obese. The highest proportion of obesity, 42% of men and 52% of women, occurs in those age 50 to 59.[21] This disorder increases the likelihood of many health problems, such as heart disease, cancer, high blood pressure, bone and joint disorders, and the major form of diabetes.[7]

Most diets fizzle before bodies become slim. Monotonous, ineffective, and confusing, fad diets even endanger some populations, such as children, teenagers, pregnant women, and people with various health disorders. Yet the secret to weight loss is actually very straightforward: (1) eat less, especially fat, (2) increase physical activity, and (3) change problematic eating behaviors. This chapter discusses these recommendations to help you understand obesity's effects, causes, and potential treatments.

A S S E S S

Is the TTFV Lipoloss Weight Loss Plan for You?

Read the following discussion of the TTFV Lipoloss Weight Loss Plan. See whether it is one you would want to follow.

Do you want to turn your body into a high-powered fat burner? Try the TTFV Lipoloss Weight Loss Plan, scientifically proven to be the quickest and most permanent fat loss miracle in America. The nutritional part of the TTFV Plan consists of eating 800 kcal of delicious tuna, turkey, fruits, and vegetables. Combine the fruits with the turkey and the vegetables with the tuna to achieve the greatest lipoloss effect (remember, *lipo* means fat).

We encourage at least 30 minutes of physical activity—brisk walking, jogging, swimming, or biking—at least five times per week. And we haven't forgotten those diet-wrecking urges and cravings. Fight them with our high-fiber Urge-Smasher Wafers. These wafers fill you up, fighting the gnaw of hunger.

If you have any health problems, see your physician for approval and clearance for regular exercise. Overall, with the TTFV LipoLoss Plan you can lose 3 to 5 pounds each week and enjoy a variety of tasty food.

Now rate this diet based on the following questions; a perfect score of 100 points indicates a good weight loss plan. Start at 100 points.

1. Will the diet meet all nutritional needs with a wide variety of foods? IF NOT, SUBTRACT 10 POINTS.
2. Does the program stress slow and steady weight loss of about 1 to 2 pounds per week rather than rapid loss? IF NOT, SUBTRACT 10 POINTS.
3. Is the diet tailored to individual habits and tastes, diminishing feelings of deprivation? IF NOT, SUBTRACT 10 POINTS.
4. Does the plan avoid rigid rituals, such as eating fruits only in the morning or not eating meat after milk products? IF NOT, SUBTRACT 10 POINTS.
5. Does the diet minimize hunger and fatigue by containing at least 1000 kcal per day? IF NOT, SUBTRACT 10 POINTS.
6. Does the diet include readily obtainable foods, with no special products to buy to speed weight loss? IF NOT, SUBTRACT 10 POINTS.
7. Is the diet socially acceptable, allowing the dieter to attend parties, eat at restaurants, and participate in normal daily activity? IF NOT, SUBTRACT 10 POINTS.
8. Does the plan promote changes in eating habits and lifestyle so that weight maintenance will be possible? IF NOT, SUBTRACT 10 POINTS.
9. Does the plan emphasize regular physical activity? IF NOT, SUBTRACT 10 POINTS.
10. Does the plan encourage the dieter to see a physician before starting if the person has existing health problems, wants quick weight loss, is over 35 years of age, or plans to perform vigorous physical activity? IF NOT, SUBTRACT 10 POINTS.

Now, having assessed the TTFV Lipoloss Weight Loss Plan, how many points would you give it? SCORE _____
Would you choose this weight loss plan if you were attempting to lose fat and keep it off? YES _____   NO _____
To assess the legitimacy of any weight loss plan, ask yourself questions like those above. With so many competing diet plans available, you can save yourself money, disappointment, effort, and time by asking the right questions.

Key Chapter Concepts

- Energy balance is energy intake minus energy output. Positive energy balance occurs when energy intake is greater than energy output. The result is weight gain.
- Total energy use by the body is accounted for by basal metabolism, the thermic effect of food, physical activity, and adaptive thermogenesis. The first two factors account for about 70% to 80% of energy use in a primarily sedentary person.
- Energy use by the body can be measured directly from heat output or indirectly from oxygen uptake. Energy needs can be estimated using formulas based on various combinations of body weight with degree of physical activity and age.
- A variety of related forces promote feeding. In America the major determinants of food intake are most likely availability, habits, and various social factors, rather than hunger per se.
- A person of healthy weight shows good health and performs daily activities without weight-related problems. A body mass index (weight [in kilograms] divided by height² [in meters]) of 19 to 25 is one measure of healthy weight, although weight in excess of this value may not necessarily indicate ill health.
- Obesity can be defined as total body fat percentage over 25% in men and 30% to 35% in women. A body mass index over 27 to 30 also represents obesity.
- Fat distribution partially determines health risks from obesity. Upper body fat storage distribution suggests higher risks of high blood pressure, heart disease, and diabetes associated with obesity than does lower body fat distribution.
- Genetic factors influence the tendency to develop obesity. How a person is raised (or nurtured) is also an influence. Obesity can be viewed as nurture allowing nature to be expressed.
- When considering a treatment for obesity, remember these important points: (1) the emphasis should be on preventing obesity, because curing the disorder is very difficult; (2) the body resists weight loss; and (3) rapid weight loss and quick regain can be harmful to physical and emotional health.
- A sound weight-loss diet recommends regular physical activity and meets the dieter's nutritional needs by emphasizing low-fat and nonfat food choices from the Food Guide Pyramid.
- Modifying problem behaviors is a vital part of a weight-loss program because the dieter may have many habits that encourage overeating and discourage weight loss and subsequent weight maintenance.

ENERGY BALANCE

Energy balance
State in which energy intake, in the form of food and/or alcohol, matches the energy expended, primarily through basal metabolism and physical activity.

Positive energy balance
State in which energy intake is greater than energy expended, generally resulting in weight gain.

Negative energy balance
State in which energy intake is less than energy expended, resulting in weight loss.

Does your weight yo-yo up and down while you aim for your ideal? If the scales keep you emotionally off balance, consider another scale—that of **energy balance.** This balance depends on energy input and energy output. These in turn influence energy stores, primarily in adipose tissue (Figure 10-1). Energy balance can be thought of as an equation: energy consumed minus energy expended. You are in positive energy balance when energy consumed is greater than energy expended. The result of positive energy balance is storage of the excess energy, mostly in the form of triglycerides in adipose (fat) tissue.[18]

Positive energy balance is necessary during pregnancy because the surplus of energy supports the developing fetus. Infants and children also need to be in positive energy balance to grow. In adults, however, positive energy balance causes creeping weight gain.

Negative energy balance results from an energy deficit. Energy consumed is less than energy expended. Weight loss occurs when a person is in a state of negative energy balance. In adulthood, however, the weight that is lost consists of a combination of lean and adipose tissue. In positive energy balance, fat stores are primarily affected.

As noted in the overview, maintenance of energy balance—energy intake matches energy output—substantially contributes to health and well-being in adults by minimizing the risk for developing many common health problems.[7] Maintenance of

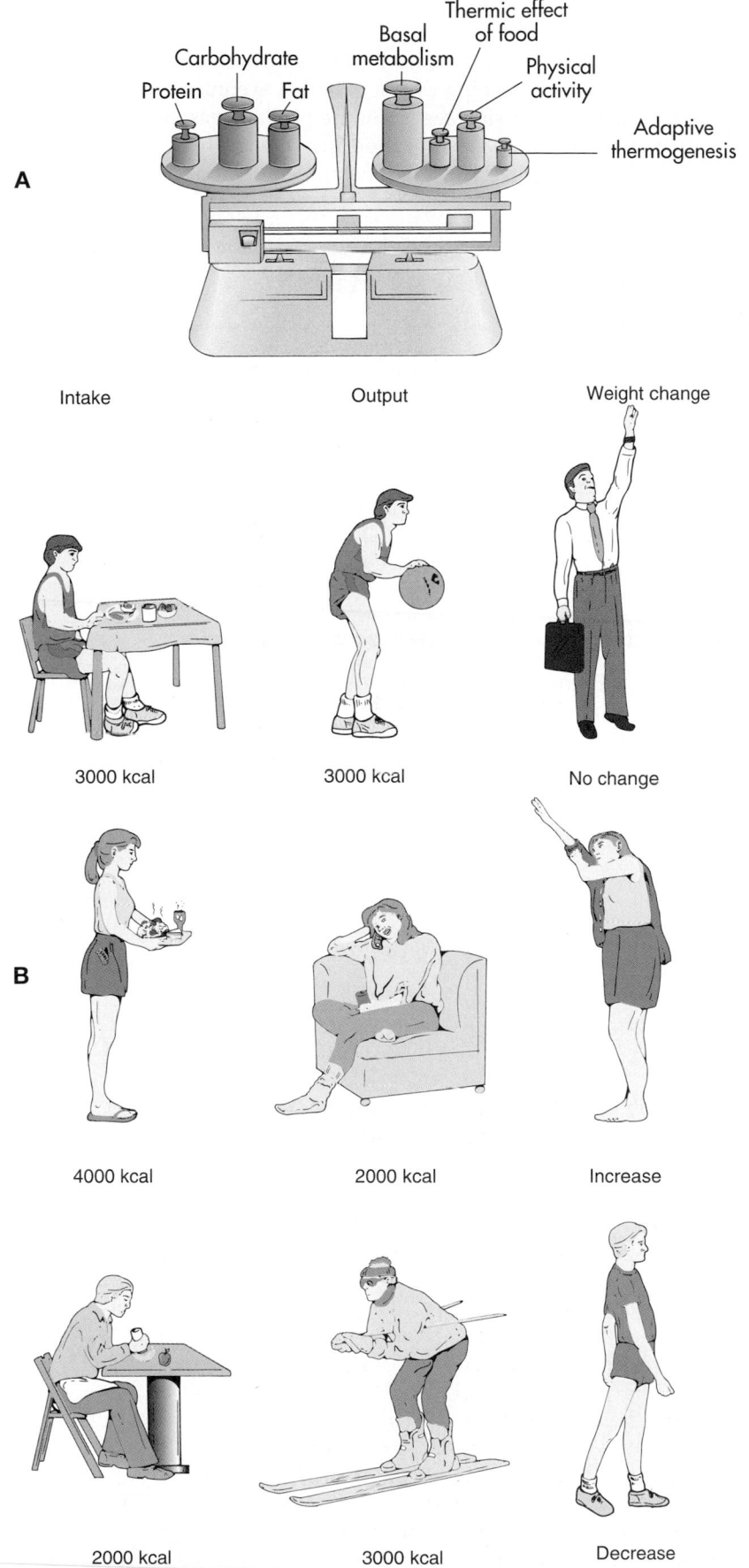

A

Protein
Carbohydrate
Fat
Basal metabolism
Thermic effect of food
Physical activity
Adaptive thermogenesis

Intake
Output
Weight change

3000 kcal
3000 kcal
No change

B

4000 kcal
2000 kcal
Increase

2000 kcal
3000 kcal
Decrease

Figure 10-1 *A model for energy balance. The model of a laboratory scale in* **(A)** *incorporates the major variables that influence energy balance. Note that alcohol is an additional source of energy for some of us. The different states of energy balance are shown in* **(B).**

energy balance is an important goal for everyone who is interested in a long, healthy life. Adulthood can be a time of creeping weight gain that eventually turns into obesity if not checked. However, increasing age is not the primary reason for this weight gain; it is caused primarily by the pattern of food intake and physical activity. Let's look in detail at the factors that affect the relationship between positive and negative energy balance.

Energy Intake: The First Half of Energy Balance

Energy needs are met by food intake, represented by the number of kcal eaten each day. Determining the appropriate amount and type of food to match energy needs is a challenge for many of us. Our ability to consume food and use it efficiently is an evolutionary survival mechanism. However, given modern American food supplies, many of us are now too successful in attaining food energy. Early people hunted food. Today, it is more likely that food hunts us, given its wide availability in vending machines, drive-up windows, social gatherings, and covenient quick-service restaurants.

Determining the Energy Content of Foods

How much food energy is contained in a meal? A bomb calorimeter is used to determine the amount of energy in a food (Figure 10-2). The process involves burning a portion of food inside a chamber of the calorimeter that is surrounded by water. As the food burns, it gives off heat, which raises the temperature of the water surrounding the chamber. The increase in water temperature measured after the food

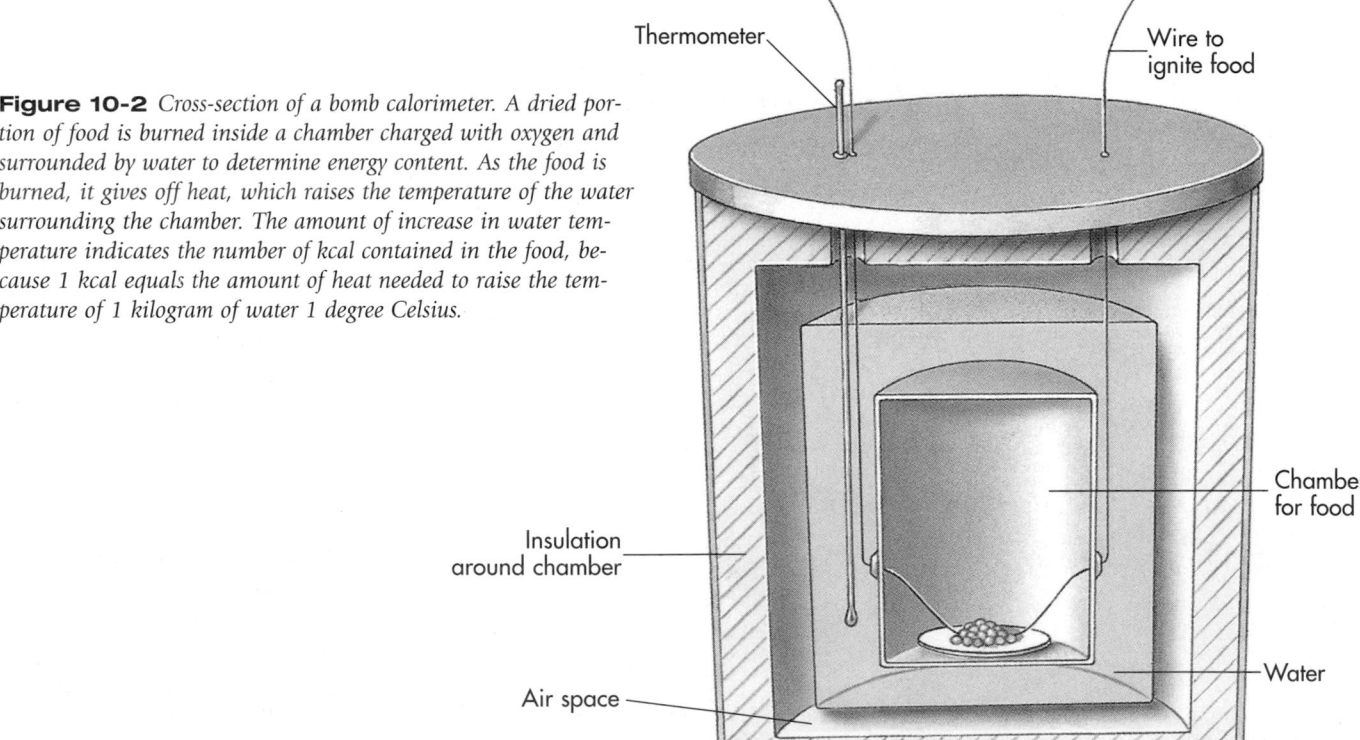

Figure 10-2 *Cross-section of a bomb calorimeter. A dried portion of food is burned inside a chamber charged with oxygen and surrounded by water to determine energy content. As the food is burned, it gives off heat, which raises the temperature of the water surrounding the chamber. The amount of increase in water temperature indicates the number of kcal contained in the food, because 1 kcal equals the amount of heat needed to raise the temperature of 1 kilogram of water 1 degree Celsius.*

Thermometer

Wire to ignite food

Chamber for food

Insulation around chamber

Water

Air space

has burned indicates the amount of energy in the food. One kilocalorie (kcal) is the amount of energy required to increase the temperature of 1 kilogram (about 2.2 pounds) of water 1° Celsius. Any food can be burned in the calorimeter to determine energy content, although some foods must be dried first.

The bomb calorimeter provides values for the amount of energy that can be derived from carbohydrate, fat, protein, and alcohol. Recall that carbohydrates yield 4 kcal per gram, proteins yield 4 kcal per gram, fats yield 9 kcal per gram, and alcohol yields 7 kcal per gram. These energy figures have been adjusted for (1) digestibility and (2) substances in food, such as fibrous plant parts, that burn in the bomb calorimeter but are unusable by the human body for energy needs. The figures are then rounded to whole numbers.

As pointed out in Chapter 1, once you know the gram quantities of the energy-yielding substances in a food, you can estimate the total energy content in that food using the energy values. For example, if a banana milk shake contains 45 grams of carbohydrate, 7 grams of protein, and 10 grams of fat, it contains 298 kcal ([45 × 4] + [7 × 4] + [10 × 9] = 298). If a banana-flavored rum drink has 10 grams of carbohydrate, 1 gram of protein, 1 gram of fat, and 15 grams of alcohol, it contains 158 kcal ([10 × 4] + [1 × 4] + [1 × 9] + [15 × 7] = 158).

Energy Use: the Other Side of Energy Balance

So far, some factors that encourage energy intake have been discussed. Now let's look at the other side of the relationship—energy output.

The body uses energy for three general purposes: basal metabolism, physical activity, and the thermic effect of food. Shivering, the body's reflex to cold, demonstrates another minor form of energy turned into heat production, often called *adaptive thermogenesis* (see Figure 10-1).

Basal Metabolism

Basal metabolism represents the minimal energy expended to keep a resting, awake body alive. This requires about 60% to 70% of total energy use by the body. The processes involved include maintaining a heartbeat, respiration, temperature, and other functions. It does not include energy used for physical activity or digesting foods. Basal metabolism accounts for about 1 kcal per kilogram of body weight per hour, or about 1600 kcal per day.

The amount of energy used for basal metabolism depends primarily on **lean body mass.** The participating tissues—such as muscle, liver, brain, and kidney—show high metabolic activity at rest and have high energy needs. Other influences that determine basal metabolism include the following:

- The amount of body surface (the greater the area, the greater the heat loss)
- Gender (males average higher energy use, because of greater lean body mass)
- Body temperature (fever increases metabolic rate)
- Thyroid hormone (higher amounts increase metabolic rate)
- Aspects of nervous system activity
- Age (metabolic rate falls as we age through adulthood)
- Nutritional state (eating less slows metabolic rate in the short term)
- Pregnancy (increases metabolic rate)
- Caffeine and tobacco use (increases metabolic rate)

A low energy intake decreases the basal metabolic rate (BMR) by about 10% to 20%, or about 150 to 300 kcal per day.[32] This lowered BMR makes losing weight difficult. In addition, the effects of aging make weight maintenance hard. BMR declines

While a person is resting, the percentage of total energy use by various organs is about as follows:

Liver	29%
Muscle	18%
Brain	19%
Heart	10%
Kidney	7%
Other	17%

Basal metabolism
The minimal energy the body requires to support itself when resting and awake. It amounts to roughly 1 kcal per minute, or about 1400 kcal per day.

Lean body mass
Body weight minus fat storage weight equals lean body mass. This includes organs such as the brain, muscles, and liver, as well as blood and other body fluids.

about 2% each decade past age 30 as activity metabolizing cells slowly and steadily decrease. However, because physical activity helps maintain lean body mass, remaining active as one ages helps maintain a high basal metabolism and, in turn, aids in weight control.[7]

Energy for Physical Activity

Basal metabolism uses roughly the same proportion of energy in most people (usually varies ±25% to 30% between individuals). Physical activity then increases energy expenditure above and beyond basal energy needs by as much as 25% to 40%. In choosing to be inactive or active, we determine much of our total energy expenditure for a day. Unlike basal metabolism, energy expenditure from physical activity varies widely among people.

Climbing stairs rather than riding the elevator, walking rather than driving to the store, and standing in a bus rather than sitting increase physical activity and, hence, energy use. People who fidget and can't sit still use more energy (an extra 100 to 800 kcal daily in one study) than do those who readily relax.

The alarming rate of obesity in America is caused in part by our inactivity.[9] We eat little more than people did at the turn of this century, but we are less active. Jobs demand less physical activity, and leisure time is usually spent slouched before a television or computer. What are the alternatives to obesity and inactivity? One answer is *movement!*

Thermic Effect of Food

In addition to basal metabolism and physical activity, the body uses energy to digest, absorb, and further process food nutrients. Energy used for these tasks contributes the **thermic effect of food.** The energy cost of this thermic effect is analogous to a sales tax. It is like being taxed about 5% to 10% for the total energy you eat. The charge covers the cost of processing that energy. To supply the body with 100 kcal for basal metabolism and physical activity, you must eat between 105 and 110 kcal. The processes of digestion, absorption, and metabolism use the extra 5 to 10 kcal to modify the energy-yielding nutrients for use. Given a daily energy intake of 3000 kcal, the thermic effect of food would use 180 to 300 kcal. However, the total amount can vary somewhat among individuals.

Adaptive Thermogenesis

The body expends some energy to produce heat in response to a cold environment and as a result of overfeeding. This process is known as *adaptive thermogenesis.* Some studies of overfeeding show that heat is produced without work being done. This subject has produced much controversy and interest. In some cases, people who were overfed did not gain the amount of weight that might be expected.[18] Though adaptive thermogenesis probably does not play a major role in weight regulation, it appears to represent a small portion of energy use; about 7% of the total.

In many animals, including humans to an undetermined extent, adaptive thermogenesis is linked to the presence of **brown adipose tissue.** Most fat is stored in white adipose tissue. Brown adipose tissue, so named because of its appearance, is less than 1% of body weight in humans. This tissue represents a specialized form of fat storage found primarily in the shoulder area. For hibernating animals, it is a main source of heat during their long winter sleep. Brown adipose tissue fails to use energy in the same manner as other body tissues do. Most brown adipose cell energy is lost in the form of heat; little is used to perform useful work beyond simply warming the body. Therefore these cells can produce a lot of heat and, in turn, "waste" a lot of potentially useful energy. If you touch an infant's back, you can feel

---

Smoking cessation increases the risk of adult weight gain and obesity. Smoking cessation is still advised, but a plan to limit weight gain should also be implemented (see later section).

Thermic effect of food
The increase in metabolism occurring during the digestion, absorption, and metabolism of energy-yielding nutrients. This represents 5% to 10% of energy consumed.

Adaptive thermogenesis
Adaptive energy expended in heat production, such as when subjected to a cold environment or to overfeeding.

Brown adipose tissue
A specialized form of adipose tissue that produces large amounts of heat by metabolizing energy-yielding nutrients inefficiently. The energy is mostly released as heat.

the heat produced by brown adipose tissue. The extent to which brown adipose tissue is both present and operative in adults has not been clearly determined.

Decreased activity of brown adipose tissue during overfeeding and cold adaptation is associated with obesity in rats. Some evidence suggests that impaired adaptive thermogenesis resulting from abnormalities in the functioning of brown adipose tissue may also contribute to human obesity.[3]

Overall, a sedentary person uses about 70% to 80% of energy for a combination of basal metabolism and the thermic effect of food. The remainder is used for physical activity and adaptive thermogenesis.

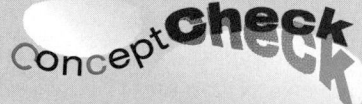

Energy balance compares energy intake with energy output. Energy content of food is expressed in kcal and determined using a bomb calorimeter. This analysis yields the 4-9-4-7 rule for carbohydrate, fat, protein, and alcohol.

The body uses this energy for four main purposes.

• Basal metabolism represents the minimal amount of energy needed to maintain a body in a resting state. The rate of a person's basal metabolism depends greatly on the amount of lean body mass, the amount of body surface, and thyroid hormone.

• Physical activity expenditure represents energy use for total body cell metabolism above what is needed during rest (that is, basal metabolism).

• The thermic effect of food represents the energy needed to digest, absorb, and process absorbed nutrients. This corresponds to about 5% to 10% of energy used for basal metabolism and physical activity.

• Adaptive thermogenesis is heat production in response to cold or overfeeding. This phenomenon may be linked to the presence of brown adipose tissue.

In a sedentary person, about 70% to 80% of energy is used for basal metabolism and the thermic effect of food; the remainder is used for physical activity and adaptive thermogenesis.

Determining Energy Use by the Body

The amount of energy a body uses can be measured by both direct and indirect calorimetry or simply estimated based on weight, degree of physical activity, and age.

Direct and Indirect Calorimetry

To understand the method used in **direct calorimetry,** imagine a science fiction film in which a creature is submerged in ice water. The creature gradually raises the water temperature to a tropic warmth simply by releasing body heat. Direct calorimetry uses this concept to measure the body heat released by a person. The subject is put into an insulated chamber, often the size of a small bedroom, and body heat released raises the temperature of a layer of water surrounding the chamber. A kcal, as you recall, is related to the amount of heat available to raise the temperature of the water. By measuring the water temperature in the direct calorimeter before and after the body releases heat, scientists can determine the energy expended. This method resembles the bomb calorimeter method for measuring the energy content in food.

Direct calorimetry
A method of determining a body's energy use by measuring heat that emanates from the body, usually using an insulated chamber.

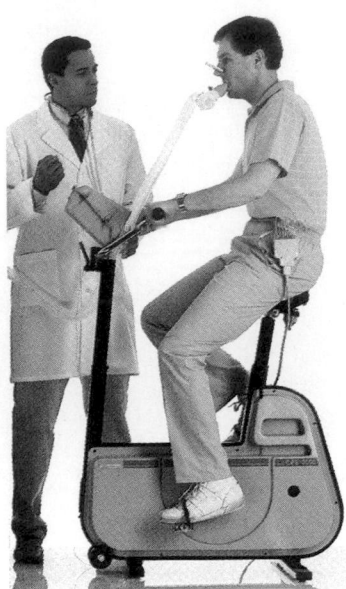

Figure 10-3
Indirect calorimetry. The method of measuring oxygen use can determine energy output during daily activities.

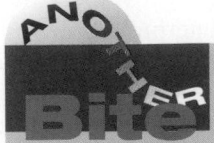

Today, scientific journals often express energy intake and output in kjoules, rather than kcal. A kjoule is a measure of work, not heat. It is the amount of work involved in moving 1 kilogram for 1 meter with the force of 1 newton. Heat and work are just two forms of energy. Energy expressions in the form of either heat or work can be exchanged for each other; 4.18 kjoules equals 1 kcal.

Direct calorimetry works because almost all the energy used by the body eventually leaves as heat. However, few studies use direct calorimetry, mostly because of its expense and complexity.

For **indirect calorimetry,** instead of measuring heat output, the most commonly used method; a technician measures the amount of oxygen a person uses (Figure 10-3). A predictable relationship exists between the body's use of energy and oxygen. For example, when metabolizing a mixed diet of carbohydrate, fat, and protein—a typical blend of nutrients we use—the human body needs 1 liter of oxygen to burn about 4.85 kcal.

Instruments used to measure oxygen consumption for indirect calorimetry have great versatility. They can be mounted on carts and rolled up to a hospital bed or carried in backpacks while a person plays tennis or jogs. Tables showing energy demands of exercises rely on information gained from indirect calorimetry studies.

Estimating Energy Needs

A rough estimate for energy needs uses a person's weight and degree of physical activity. Total energy needs for a sedentary person are set at 9 to 10 kcal per pound (20 kcal per kilogram). The value is then decreased by 100 kcal for every 10 years of age over age 30. People performing light activity, such as routine walking, start with 12 to 13 kcal per pound (30 kcal per kilogram); those regularly performing heavy activity, as required in some sports play, start at 20 kcal per pound (45 kcal per kilogram). These values are then adjusted for age, as mentioned previously. For example, a 150-pound, 40-year-old woman performing light activity needs to eat about 1850 kcal ([13 × 150] − 100) to meet total energy needs.

Rough guidelines for energy needs found in the Food Guide Pyramid publication are as follows:

• Sedentary women and some older adults	1600 kcal
• Children, teenage girls, active women, most men	2200 kcal
• Teenage boys, active men, very active women	2800 kcal
• Young children, pregnant and breast-feeding women	Check with a registered dietitian

These values then need to be fine-tuned based on personal characteristics and experiences, such as amount of physical activity performed.

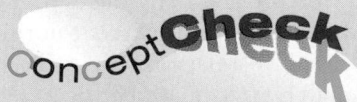

Energy use by the body can be measured by direct calorimetry as heat given off and by indirect calorimetry as oxygen used. Total energy needs can be estimated based on a person's weight, age, and amount of physical activity practiced. In addition, the RDA and Food Guide Pyramid publications both provide rough guidelines for energy intake.

Recall from Chapter 2 that the RDA publication also lists recommendations for energy intake for lightly to moderately active persons (see the inside cover of this textbook).
Men ages 19 to 50: 2900 kcal
Women ages 19 to 50: 2200 kcal

Why Am I Hungry?

Two drives influence our desire to eat and thus take in food energy, **hunger** and **appetite.** These differ dramatically (Figure 10-4). Hunger, our physiological drive to eat, is controlled by internal body mechanisms. Appetite, our psychological drive to eat, is affected by external food choice mechanisms, such as seeing a tempting dessert. Fulfilling either or both drives by eating sufficient food normally brings a state of **satiety,** temporarily halting our desire to continue eating.[19]

Hunger
The primarily physiological drive to find and eat food, mostly regulated by internal cues to eating.

Appetite
The external (psychological) influences that encourage us to find and eat food, often in the absence of obvious hunger.

Satiety
State in which there is no longer a desire to eat.

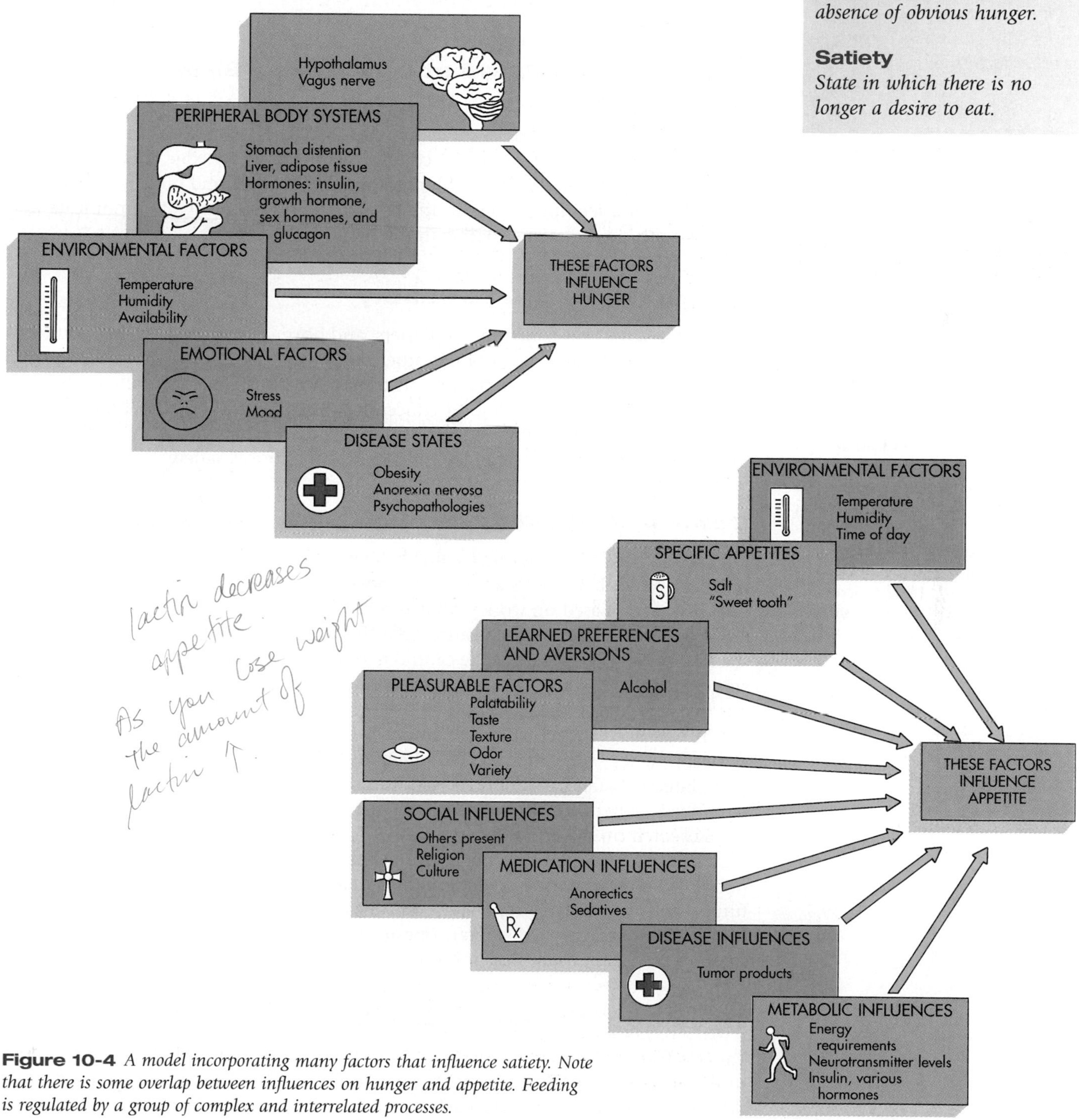

lactin decreases appetite. As you lose weight the amount of lactin ↑

Figure 10-4 *A model incorporating many factors that influence satiety. Note that there is some overlap between influences on hunger and appetite. Feeding is regulated by a group of complex and interrelated processes.*

Hypothalamus

A grouping of cells at the base of the brain. These cells participate in many body functions, such as in the regulation of hunger.

Stomach distention

Expansion of the walls of the stomach (intestines as well) from the pressure caused by the presence of gases, food, drink, or other factors.

Satiety cascade

early	taste of food
	↓
	knowing a meal was just eaten
	↓
	influence of stomach distention and receptors in the intestinal tract
	↓
late	influence of nutrient metabolism in liver and resulting communication with the brain

The Hypothalamus: a Satiety Regulator

The **hypothalamus,** a portion of the brain, helps regulate satiety. When stimulated, cells in the feeding centers of the hypothalamus signal us to eat. Then as we eat, hunger decreases. Eventually, we stop eating as cells in the satiety centers of the hypothalamus are stimulated. The amount of blood glucose probably stimulates both groups of centers. When glucose drops, we eat. Other cues to eat come from amino acids and fatty acids in the bloodstream and from various hormones and other substances. Such internal signals both inhibit and encourage food intake.[19]

Chemicals, surgery, and some cancers can destroy the feeding and satiety centers in the hypothalamus. Without satiety-center activity, laboratory animals (and humans) eat their way to obesity. Without feeding-center activity, animals eat little and eventually lose weight.

Satiety Is Regulated at Other Body Sites

Satiety is controlled by a network of mechanisms spread throughout the body that regulate the desire to either eat or avoid food. Satiety is maintained first by the sensory stimulation that food elicits, coupled with the knowledge that a meal was eaten. Second, the effects of nutrient digestion, absorption, and metabolism are felt. The satiety and feeding centers in the hypothalamus especially communicate and interact with other decision points in the brain, small intestine, and liver.[30]

Hormones Regulate Satiety

Endorphins, the body's natural painkillers, and hormones, such as high amounts of cortisol, can prod us to eat. On the other hand, other hormones, hormone-related compounds, and still other chemical factors in the body can contribute to the feeling of satiety. With eating, blood concentrations of some digestive hormones increase. This increase, combined with **stomach distention,** helps shut off hunger. Certain parts of the nervous system also contribute to this satiety.[19]

Control of Feeding Through Body Composition

One recent observation is that feeding behavior also changes in response to body fat content. When body fat is surgically removed from animals, their food consumption increases. Based on work with genetic forms of obesity in animals, researchers have identified a group of substances that circulates in the blood and communicates the degree of body fatness to the central nervous system. The gene for one such substance in mice and humans has been isolated. The product produced by the gene has been named *leptin.*

Theoretically, when adipose tissue stores are increasing, leptin (or related substances) causes satiety. Conversely, when adipose tissue stores are decreasing, leptin (or related substances) is not released into the bloodstream and the desire to eat is enhanced.

Research on this topic is in progress. To date, it appears that some obese people may not readily respond to the leptin signal and so may eat more food than those people who do respond.[8] Treatment for obesity with leptin is still 5 to 7 years in the future, and then only if it is found to be a safe and effective treatment. Researchers hope that some cases of human obesity will respond as certain species of mice have—with a significant loss of body fat.

Does Appetite Regulate What We Eat?

Various feeding and satiety messages from body cells do not singlehandedly determine what we eat. Almost everyone has encountered a mouthwatering dessert and devoured it, even on a full stomach. Appetite can be affected by a great variety of external forces, such as environmental and psychological factors and social customs (Figure 10-5).

We often eat because food confronts us. It smells good, tastes good, and looks good. We might eat because it is the right time of day, we are celebrating, or we are trying to overcome the blues. Appetite may not be a biological process, but it does influence food intake. After a meal, memories of pleasant tastes and feelings reinforce appetite. If stress or depression sends you to the refrigerator, you are mostly seeking comfort, not energy.

Internal and external signals—driving hunger and appetite—generally operate simultaneously and combine into a momentary decision whether to reject or eat a food item.[19] Often we don't think about why or what we eat, but a simple reconsideration of what motivates your food choices may show you whether you respond to hunger or to external factors linked to appetite, such as what you feel like eating. American prosperity and ample food supply set the stage for a population that eats primarily from appetite and habit, not hunger. If you rarely feel real hunger, you probably reach for food mostly as a reflex.

THE MIDDLETONS

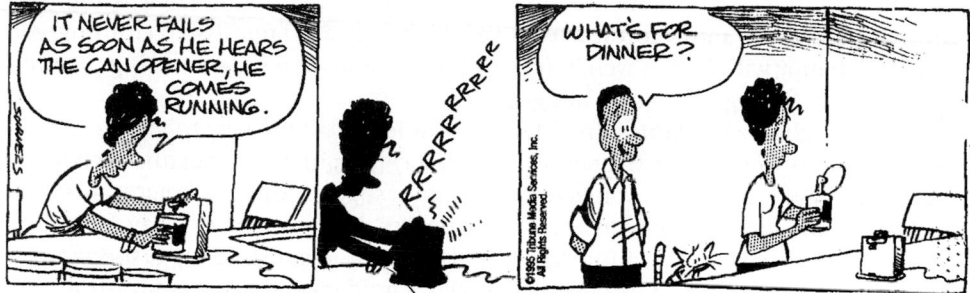

Figure 10-5 *The Middletons.*

Social customs, peers, and authority figures can influence the desire to eat. Concern about appearance when on a date can influence the food choices made. A woman concerned about looking "petite" in company may choose a smaller portion of food than when alone. We are also likely to eat more at a meal when with a large group of people than when with a few people or alone.

Putting Hunger and Appetite into Perspective

The next time you pick up a candy bar or ask for second helpings, remember the physiological and psychological influences on eating behavior. Body cells (brain, stomach, intestine, liver, and other organs), hormones (like cortisol), and social customs all influence food intake. Where food is ample, appetite—not hunger—mostly triggers eating. Keep track of what triggers your eating for a few days. Is it primarily hunger or appetite? Note as well that this system is not perfect; body weight can fluctuate.

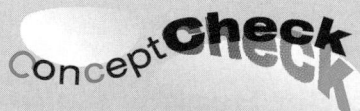

Hunger, the physiological drive to find and eat food, is regulated by internal mechanisms, such as the brain, adipose tissue, liver, and hormones. Appetite, the psychological drive to find and eat food, is affected mostly by external factors, such as social custom, time of day, and food palatability. Internal and external factors influence decisions about food intake. Appeasing both hunger and appetite typically leaves us in a state of satiety. Americans probably respond more to external, appetite-related forces than to hunger-related ones in choosing when and what to eat.

Estimating a Healthy Weight

Over the long run, energy balance influences body weight. Numerous methods are used to set what body weight should be, often called *healthy body weight*.[10] Several tables exist, based on weight and one or more factors, including height, age, and body frame size. These tables arise from studies of large population groups. When applied to a population, they provide good estimates of weight associated with good health and longevity. These tables, however, do not necessarily refer directly to an individual's weight and health status.[1]

Ideally, family history of obesity-related disease and current health parameters should be considered when establishing a healthy weight for an individual, in addition to weight-for-height. Evidence of the following obesity-related conditions is important:

- High blood pressure
- Elevated LDL
- Family history of obesity, heart disease, or cancer
- Pattern of fat distribution in the body
- Elevated blood glucose

On a more practical note, other questions can be pertinent: What is the least you weighed as an adult, for at least a year? What is the largest size clothing you would be happy with? What weight have you been able to maintain during previous diets without feeling constantly hungry?

Thus height/weight tables don't tell the whole story. One way to view a height/weight table is to consider the values a "statistical" estimate of healthy weight.[1] If you weigh somewhat more or less than the tables suggest for your height, this does not necessarily imply adverse health consequences. However, extra body fat can set the stage for future disease, although even that is not guaranteed for a specific person. Overall, the individual, under a physician's guidance, should establish a "personal" healthy weight (or need for weight reduction) based on weight history, fat distribution patterns, family history of obesity-related disease, and current health status. Current height/weight standards are only a rough guide.[12]

Striving for body weights and shapes presented in the media is not the way to establish healthy weight. For example, consider a woman who is 5 feet 2 inches tall and has weighed 250 pounds for 25 years. Theoretically she should weigh about 125 pounds according to height and weight tables, but this is not necessarily a realistic weight goal for her. Attempting massive weight loss almost invariably results in rapid weight regain. The most important factor in determining healthy weight for this person is the amount of weight loss that results in a final body weight that is not an impediment to health, employment, or life's normal activities.

Furthermore, a healthy lifestyle may make a more important contribution to a person's health status than the number on the scale.[5] This topic is discussed at greater length later in the chapter with regard to appropriateness of weight loss. In sum, height/weight tables provide a guide for healthy weight, but some fine-tuning is often necessary.[12]

Using Body Mass Index (BMI) to Set Healthy Weight

Body mass index (BMI) is currently the preferred weight-for-height standard used to define healthy weight. This is calculated as:

$$\frac{\text{body weight (in kilograms)}}{\text{height}^2 \text{ (in meters)}}$$

Table 10-1 lists BMI for various heights and weights. Health risks from excess weight begin when the body mass index exceeds 25. A healthy weight for height

Body mass index (BMI)
Weight (in kilograms) divided by height (in meters) squared; a value greater than 25 indicates a higher risk for obesity-related health disorders.

TABLE 10-1

Body Weights in Pounds According to Height and Body Mass Index (BMI)

| | BMI (kg/m²) | | | | | | | | | | | | | |
| Height (inches) | 19 | 20 | 21 | 22 | 23 | 24 | 25 | 26 | 27 | 28 | 29 | 30 | 35 | 40 |
						Body weight (pounds)								
58	91	96	100	105	110	115	119	124	129	134	138	143	167	191
59	94	99	104	109	114	119	124	128	133	138	143	148	173	198
60	97	102	107	112	118	123	128	133	138	143	148	153	179	204
61	100	106	111	116	122	127	132	137	143	148	153	158	185	211
62	104	109	115	120	126	131	136	142	147	153	158	164	191	218
63	107	113	118	124	130	135	141	146	152	158	163	169	197	225
64	110	116	122	128	134	140	145	151	157	163	169	174	204	232
65	114	120	126	132	138	144	150	156	162	168	174	180	210	240
66	118	124	130	136	142	148	155	161	167	173	179	186	216	247
67	121	127	134	140	146	153	159	166	172	178	185	191	223	255
68	125	131	138	144	151	158	164	171	177	184	190	197	230	262
69	128	135	142	149	155	162	169	176	182	189	196	203	236	270
70	132	139	146	153	160	167	174	181	188	195	202	207	243	278
71	136	143	150	157	165	172	179	186	193	200	208	215	230	286
72	140	147	154	162	169	177	184	191	199	206	213	221	258	294
73	144	151	159	166	174	182	180	197	204	212	219	227	265	302
74	148	155	163	171	179	186	194	202	210	218	225	233	272	311
75	152	160	168	176	184	192	200	208	216	224	232	240	279	319
76	156	164	172	180	189	197	205	213	221	230	238	246	287	328

From Bray GA, Gray DS: *Western Journal of Medicine* 148:429, 1988.
Each entry gives the body weight in pounds for a person of a given height and BMI. Pounds have been rounded off. To use the table, find the appropriate height in the far left column. Move across the row to a given weight. The number at the top of the column is the BMI for the height and weight.

is a BMI 19 to 25. What is your BMI? How much would your weight need to change to yield a BMI of 27? 30? These are general cut-off values for the presence of obesity[10] (see later section).

The concept of body mass index is convenient to use because the values apply to both men and women. However, any body weight-for-height standard is actually a crude measure because we are concerned about overfat, not simply overweight, individuals when setting guidelines for healthy weight. The husky athlete is a notable exception; he or she may be overweight but not overfat. Still, overfat and overweight conditions almost always appear together. The focus is on body weight-for-height standards in clinical settings mainly because these are easier to measure than total body fat.

Using the Metropolitan Life Insurance Table to Estimate Healthy Weight

The Metropolitan Life Insurance Table (see inside cover) provides another common standard for estimating healthy weight. The tables lists for any height the weight that is associated with a maximum lifespan. The table does not tell the healthiest weight for a living person; it simply lists the weight associated with longevity.

There are many criticisms of this method. One is that the table's data are derived only from purchasers of life insurance, so the results underrepresent poor people

BMI is not a standard for everyone. BMI should not be applied to children, adolescents who are still growing, adults over 65, pregnant and lactating women, and highly muscular individuals.

and many minorities. Smokers are included in the table, and they often have both lower body weights and earlier ages of death because of their increased risk for lung cancer and heart disease. This distortion may mean that the table overestimates the best weight for maximum longevity. Another problem, body weight, is determined only at the time the insurance policy is purchased; no follow-up weights are recorded.

The weight and height values in the Metropolitan Life Insurance Table assume the subject is wearing clothes and shoes. The table also refers only to people under 60 years old. An overweight elderly person may have already avoided the typical causes of death, such as stroke, heart disease, and cancer, to which obesity contributes. The fact that they have survived into their 70s and 80s suggests that they are somewhat resistant to the effects of obesity (see Chapter 16 for a further discussion).

The Metropolitan Life Insurance Table adjusts for small, medium, and large frames. Methods for estimating frame size use measurements of wrist width or elbow breadth (see Appendix I). Overall, obviously small and thin people have a small frame, obviously big and bulky people who have large bones have a large frame, and everyone else has a medium frame.

Weighing slightly more or less than the range listed in the table is not necessarily cause for alarm. In addition, the weight ranges listed do not guarantee health. They simply attempt to maximize the chances of a long life.

Additional Methods of Setting Healthy Weight

Another height/weight table currently in use is from the USDA/DHHS Dietary Guidelines (Figure 10-6). This method considers age but not gender or frame size. The range-suggested weight for height is very large because both males and females and various frame sizes are included.

Still another method of estimating healthy body weight is the pounds per inch of height method. For women, allow 100 pounds for the first 5 feet, then add 5 pounds for every inch thereafter. To estimate a man's healthy body weight, allow 106 pounds for the first 5 feet and then add 6 pounds for each inch thereafter. Based on this system, a 6-foot-tall man should weigh about 178 pounds ($106 + [12 \times 6]$).

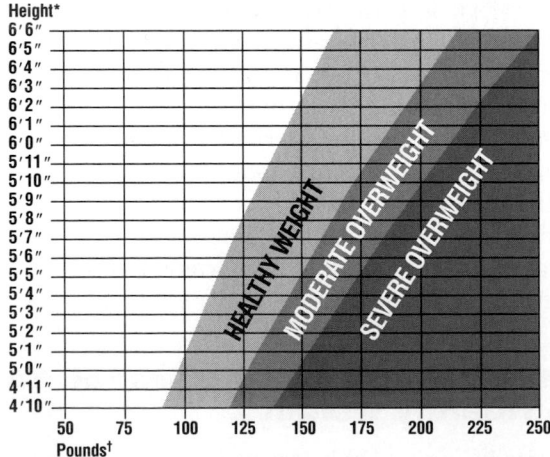

* Without shoes.

† Without clothes. The higher weights apply to people with more muscle and bone, such as many men.

Figure 10-6 *Height/weight table included as part of the latest Dietary Guidelines publication. The upper ends of the "healthy weight" ranges correspond to a body mass index of about 25.*

Putting Healthy Weight into Perspective

One current school of thought is to let nature takes its course with regard to body weight.[5] According to this proposal, by trying to lose weight in order to fall within a specific height-weight range, people often regain their original weight plus more. In contrast, listening to the body for hunger cues, eating a healthy diet, and remaining physically active eventually maintain an appropriate height-weight value.

Overall, the clearest idea regarding a healthy weight is that it is personal. Weight has to be considered in terms of health, not simply fashion. A BMI of 19 to 25 is a reasonable goal but is not a rigid value for a person's healthy weight.[1]

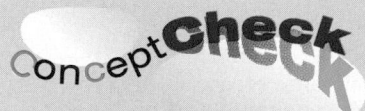

Healthy body weight is generally determined in a clinical setting using a body mass index or some other weight-for-height standard. The presence of existing weight-related disease should be considered in determining healthy body weight. Total health and a healthy lifestyle, not simply fashion, should be the major considerations when determining healthy weight.

Energy Imbalance

If energy intake exceeds expenditure over time, **obesity** is likely to result. Often, health problems soon follow (Table 10-2). In this context, medical experts recommend that an individual's cut-off for obesity should not be based primarily on body weight but rather on the total amount of fat in the body, the location of body fat, and the presence or absence of weight-related medical problems.

Obesity
A condition characterized by excess body fat. In clinical settings it is often defined in one of two ways: (1) a body mass index above 27 to 30; or (2) weighing 20% above healthy weight, based on height-weight tables.

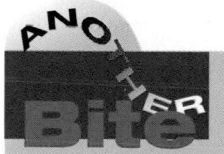

Former Surgeon General C. Everett Koop is currently spearheading a campaign, called "Shape Up America," to convince overweight people to lose weight and increase physical activity. According to Dr. Koop, obesity is the number-two killer in the United States. What many Americans don't understand, he explains, is how serious the problem of excess pounds is: Although many Americans are aware that smoking is responsible for more than 400,000 deaths per year, they are not aware that obesity is responsible for nearly as many—300,000— deaths annually in the United States. Before long, obesity will surpass cigarette smoking as a leading cause of death.

Typical health problems associated with obesity include the following[7]:

- Increased risk in surgery
- Non–insulin-dependent (adult-onset) diabetes
- High blood pressure
- Heart disease
- Arthritis
- Gallstones
- Pregnancy risks
- Premature death
- Various forms of cancer, such as colon, rectal, and prostate cancer in men and breast (especially after menopause), uterine, and ovarian cancer in women
- Sleep disorders

TABLE 10-2

Health Problems Associated with Excess Body Fat

Health problem	Partially attributable to:
Surgical risk	Increased anesthesia needs and greater risk of wound infections
Pulmonary disease and sleep disorders	Excess weight over lungs and pharynx
Adult-onset diabetes (non–insulin-dependent diabetes mellitus)	Enlarged fat cells, which poorly bind insulin and also poorly respond to the message insulin sends to the cell
Hypertension and stroke	Increased miles of blood vessels found in the adipose tissue; increase blood volume; increased resistance to blood flow
Heart disease	Increases in blood cholesterol (LDL) and triglyceride values, low HDL values, decreased physical activity
Bone and joint disorders	Excess pressure put on knee, ankle, and hip joints
Gallstones	Increased cholesterol content of bile
Skin disorders	Trapping of moisture and microbes in tissue folds
Various cancers	Estrogen production by adipose cells; animal studies suggest excess energy intake encourages tumor development
Shorter stature (in some forms of obesity)	Earlier onset of puberty
Pregnancy risks	More difficult delivery, increased number of birth defects, and increased needs for anesthesia
Reduced physical agility and increased risk of accidents and falls	Excess weight impairs movement
Premature death	A variety of risk factors for disease, listed above

The greater the degree of obesity, the more likely and the more serious these health problems generally become. They are much more likely to appear in people who show an upper body fat distribution pattern and/or greater than twice healthy body weight (see later chapter discussions).

Furthermore, discrimination against obese people is very common. Overweight women have lower household incomes (averaging $6700 less) and are 10% more likely to be poor than women who are not obese. Other examples of discrimination include decreased chance of marriage, fewer choices in clothing, and rude remarks.

Obesity Signifies an Overfat State

Health risks associated with obesity actually apply only to people who are overfat. Body fat can range from 2% to 70% of body weight. In this regard, men with over 25% body fat and women with over 30% to 35% body fat are considered obese. Desirable amounts are 12% to 20% body fat for men and 20% to 30% fat for women.[1] Women need more body fat because some "sex-specific" fat is associated with reproductive functions. This fat is normal and factored into calculations (Figure 10-7).

Various methods are used to estimate body fat content. Underwater weighing (most accurate) works because fat tissue is less dense than lean tissue; because fat floats, the more fat tissue present, the less a person weighs when submerged. This procedure requires a trained technician and submersion.

Though there are some limits to its accuracy, skinfold thickness is the method most widely used to estimate total body fat. Clinicians use special calipers to measure the fat layer directly under the skin at multiple sites (Figure 10-8).

Other methods to estimate body fat include using instruments to measure air displacement by the body (plethysmography) or total-body electrical conductance when placed in an electromagnetic field (TOBEC).

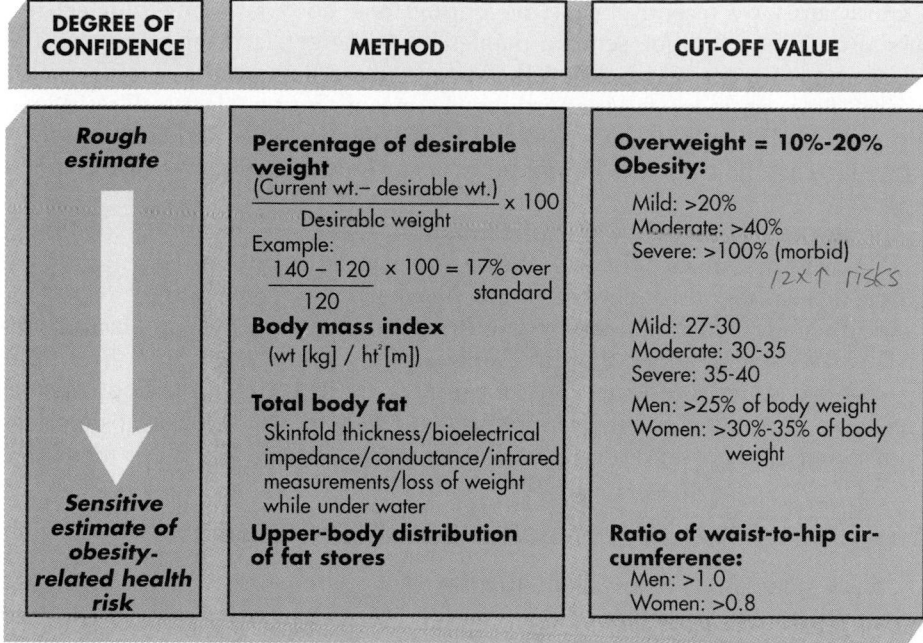

DEGREE OF CONFIDENCE	METHOD	CUT-OFF VALUE

Rough estimate

⬇

Sensitive estimate of obesity-related health risk

Percentage of desirable weight

$$\frac{(\text{Current wt.} - \text{desirable wt.})}{\text{Desirable weight}} \times 100$$

Example:

$$\frac{140 - 120}{120} \times 100 = 17\% \text{ over standard}$$

Body mass index
(wt [kg] / ht²[m])

Total body fat
Skinfold thickness/bioelectrical impedance/conductance/infrared measurements/loss of weight while under water

Upper-body distribution of fat stores

Overweight = 10%-20%
Obesity:

Mild: >20%
Moderate: >40%
Severe: >100% (morbid)

12× ↑ risks

Mild: 27-30
Moderate: 30-35
Severe: 35-40
Men: >25% of body weight
Women: >30%-35% of body weight

Ratio of waist-to-hip circumference:
Men: >1.0
Women: >0.8

Figure 10-7 *Methods used to establish obesity in a person. A person is generally considered obese if any one of these measures is met. If the person has upper body distribution of fat stores, the risk of complications is greater than when the fat distribution is held lower in the body.*

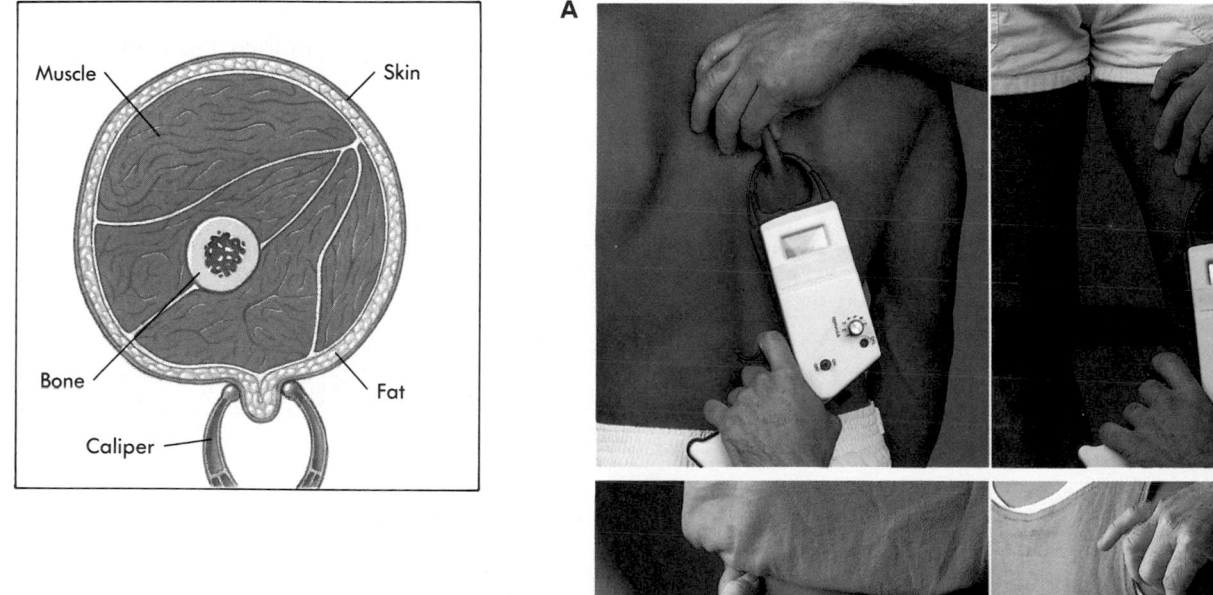

Figure 10-8 *Skinfold measurements. Use of proper technique, calibrated equipment, and standards in multiple skinfold measurements can accurately predict body fat content in about 10 minutes. Commonly measured skinfolds for this method are (A) subscapular, (B) thigh, (C) suprailiac, and (D) triceps.*

Bioelectrical
impedance
A method to estimate total body fat that uses a low-energy electrical current. The more fat storage a person has, the more impedance (resistance) to electrical flow will be exhibited.

Clinicians have recently begun measuring total body fat using **bioelectrical impedance.** This technique sends a painless, low-energy electrical current to and from the body via wires and electrode patches. Researchers surmise that fat resists electrical flow, so more fat proportionately means greater electrical resistance. Within a few minutes, bioelectrical impedance analyzers convert body electrical resistance into a good estimate of total body fat, as long as body hydration status is normal.[17]

Another new method for estimating total body fat exposes the biceps to infrared light, assessing the interactions with the fat and protein in arm muscle. After only 2 seconds, this flashlight-size device can give an estimate.

A further advance in determining body fat is use of x-ray photon absorptiometry. This x-ray system allows the clinician to separate body weight into three components—fat, fat-free soft tissue, and bone mineral.[28] The usual whole-body scan requires 15 to 20 minutes and delivers a minimal radiation dose. Obesity, osteoporosis, and other aspects of nutritional health can be investigated using this method.

Using Body Mass Index to Establish Obesity

Body mass index (BMI) offers an alternative way to define obesity. This measure is highly predictive of the degree of body fatness. When BMI begins to exceed 25 to 27, obesity-related health risks often begin for men and women and the person is said to be overweight.[10] At a BMI of about 27 the risk for diabetes and high blood pressure is three times greater than normal, and the risk for high blood cholesterol is two times normal. A BMI above 30 poses even greater health risks and is typically defined as obesity. A value this high suggests that a treatment program should be considered, especially if obesity-related health problems are present. About 10% of Americans exceed this value. A BMI above 40 represents a severe health risk. Note again that these BMIs for health risks are the same for both men and women.

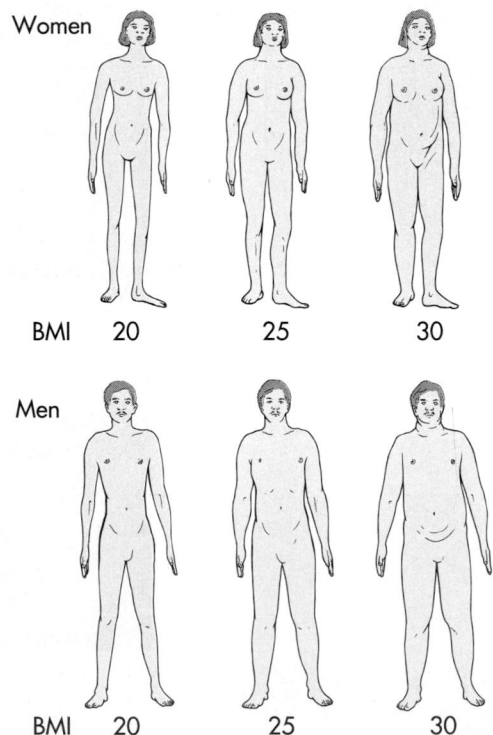

For your reference, estimates of body shapes at different BMI values.

Using Body Fat Distribution to Establish Obesity

Where we store fat, as well as how much, can predict health risks. Some people store fat in upper body areas. Others hold fat low. Excess fat in either place generally spells trouble, but each storage space also has its unique risks.[36] Fat deposited in the lower body often resists being shed. However, **upper-body obesity** is related to more heart disease, high blood pressure, and diabetes. Whereas other fat cells empty fat directly into general circulation, the fat contents of abdominal fat cells go straight to the liver, by way of the portal vein, before being circulated to the muscles. This process likely interferes with the liver's ability to clear insulin and also alters lipoprotein metabolism by the liver. Both changes spell trouble for the body.

High blood testosterone (a primarily male hormone) levels apparently encourage upper-body obesity, as does alcohol intake. This characteristic male pattern of fat storage appears in the "apple-on-a-stick" shape (large abdomen [pot belly] and small buttocks and thighs). A ratio of waist circumference (at the level of the umbilicus) to hip circumference more than 1.0 in men and 0.8 in women indicates upper body fat storage[26] (Figure 10-9).

Estrogen and progesterone (primarily female hormones) encourage lower body fat storage and **lower-body obesity**—the typical female pattern. The familiar small abdomen and much larger buttocks and thighs give a pearlike appearance. After menopause, blood estrogen falls, encouraging upper body fat distribution.

Overall, researchers suggest that women with lower body fat distribution must be about 20 pounds more obese than men with a "pot belly" shape before they show the same health risks from an overfat state. Only a small percentage of women have upper body obesity.

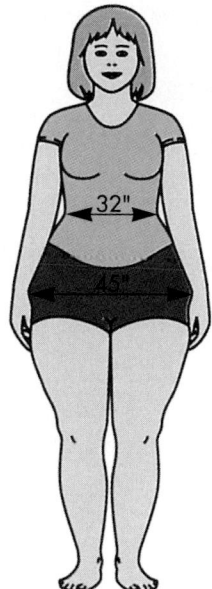

Lower-body obesity

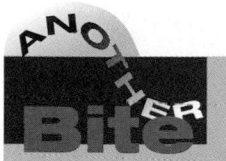

In the future we may have obesity standards that apply more strictly to upper-body fat distribution and more leniently to lower-body fat distribution. For now it is best to consider one's BMI and pattern of fat distribution when assessing possible health risks from obesity.

Using Body Weight to Establish Obesity

Body weight is actually a crude measure of obesity, because it can miss the critical factor—being overfat. Given that, overweight can be defined as weighing at least 10% more than healthy body weight. Obesity weighs in at 20% more than healthy weight.[10] Moreover, this measure of obesity comes in degrees. Whereas mild obesity carries little risk, severe (morbid) obesity raises overall health risk twelvefold.

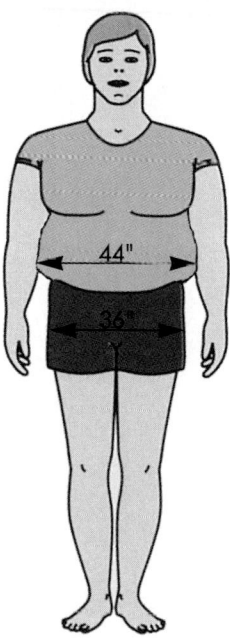

Upper-body obesity

Figure 10-9
Body fat distribution, showing upper body and lower body obesity. The upper body form brings higher risks for ill health associated with obesity. The woman has an approximate waist-to-hip ratio of 32 inches by 45 inches, or 0.7. The man has an approximate waist-to-hip ratio of 44 inches by 36 inches, or 1.2. Thus the man has upper body obesity, but the women does not, based on a cutoff of 0.8 for women and 1.0 for men.

Degrees of obesity

% Over healthy body weight	% of cases	Form of obesity
20%–40%	90	MILD
41%–99%	9.8	MODERATE
100%+	0.2	SEVERE (MORBID)

To determine healthy body weight for this calculation, many clinicians and research scientists use the current (1983) Metropolitan Life Insurance Table. In the United States, about 90% of obese people are mildly obese. This condition carries little health risk. About 0.2% of cases are severe.

Using Age of Onset as a Measure of Obesity

Obesity can be classified as juvenile-onset or adult-onset. When obesity develops in infancy or childhood, numerous adipose cells develop, each with the ability to grow larger. (This is discussed further in Chapter 15, particularly in reference to weight control in childhood.) In adult obesity, fewer adipose cells are usually present, but these contain an excess amount of fat. Still, as obesity progress in adulthood, adipose cells can increase in number again.

Juvenile-onset obesity presents a special concern because the greater number of adipose cells may increase the body's resistance to cutting down fat stores. Adipose cells have a long life span and apparently need to store some fat. If more adipose cells automatically require more fat storage, reducing total body fat becomes a tough task. Though the reasons are still puzzling, long-term obesity appears to make losing weight more difficult.[7]

Obesity in Perspective

Obesity is a very personal disorder. It may be measured in many ways, but statistics aside, each person has unique characteristics and problems. Treatment needs to account for current energy expenditure, weight range in adulthood, fasting blood glucose, family history of obesity, number of years the person has been obese, and the extent of erroneous nutrition practices. Each person faces possible complications requiring individual treatment plans.[7]

On a positive note, however, only about a 10% weight loss is often needed for people to experience improvement in health and self esteem. Researchers are calling this a "healthier" weight. Although you might not achieve a BMI of 25, you might still be healthier after a small weight loss.[26]

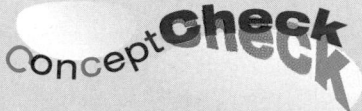

Genetic background plays a role in obesity, influencing body shape, sites of fat deposition, and rate of basal metabolism. The role of nurture is evident in families, who tend to have similar eating habits, activity patterns, and degrees of fatness. Men tend to develop obesity after age 30, and women tend to have both childhood and adult roots for obesity; this suggests an especially important influence of nurture in men. Because both factors have an impact, it makes sense to assume that nurture serves as a catalyst for expressing or denying a genetic tendency toward obesity.

Why Some People Are Obese— Nature Versus Nurture

Both genetic traits and psychological factors can increase the risk for obesity. These diverse influences spark controversies concerning which factor yields the greater influence.

How Does Nature Contribute to Obesity?

Identical twins raised apart tend to show similar weight gain patterns, whether lean or obese. It appears that nurture—what we learn about eating habits and nutrition, which varies with twins who are raised apart—has less to do with obesity than genes. In fact, research using twins suggests genetic background accounts for about 50% of weight differences between people. Twins even tend to accumulate

Identical twins
Two offspring that develop from a single ovum and sperm and consequently have the same genetic makeup.

fat in the same body sites. Our genes help determine rates of metabolism and differences in brain chemistry. Both affect weight.[3]

We also inherit specific body types, such as pencil-thin or muscular. The specific body types—known as endomorphs, mesomorphs, and ectomorphs—greatly determine human size and shape. Endomorphs, with their stocky builds, have short, stubby bones, short trunks, round heads, wide chest and hips, and very short fingers. Ectomorphs, like Abraham Lincoln, are tall and slender with long, thin bones and narrow chests, hips, heads, and fingers. Mesomorphs exhibit a medium, muscular build.

Some rare medical disorders can lead to obesity. This includes Prader-Willi Syndrome, in which the drive to eat is so powerful and unrelenting that food may need to be locked up between meal times. Low thyroid hormone output can also lead to obesity, but this is rarely the cause of typical cases.

Ectomorph   Mesomorph   Endomorph

Ectomorphs appear to have an inherently easier time maintaining healthy body weight. Basal metabolism increases as body surface increases. Tall people have more body surface (based on body weight comparisons) than short, stocky people. Therefore taller people use more energy than do shorter ones, even when resting.

You've heard of fat cats, but have you heard of fat rats? Some rats and mice have a genetic predisposition to obesity. They inherit a **thrifty metabolism,** one that uses energy frugally. This enables them to store fat more readily than the typical animal. Some people probably inherit a thrifty metabolism as well. Farmers once bred cows and hogs based on their ability to acquire fat. Today, because we know that eating too much animal fat can increase the risk for heart disease, farmers breed leaner animals.

A thrifty human metabolism requires less energy to get through the day. In earlier times, when food supplies were scarce, a thrifty metabolism helped protect against starvation. With today's general abundance of food, operating in this low gear requires a high-energy output and wise food choices to prevent obesity.[34]

We cannot measure small differences in energy efficiency among humans. In the long run, however, even a 1% or 2% difference in metabolic rate may be a decisive factor between massive weight gain and healthy weight maintenance. Resting metabolic rates among family members tend to be more similar than a comparison with those of the general population. Families with lower resting metabolic rates have higher rates for obesity. Even after adjusting for the amount of body fat, research shows that resting metabolic rate varies as much as 30% between leaner and more obese families. Some Native American tribes also show a high rate of obesity, linked in part to lower metabolic rates and reduced fat use for body fuel.[23]

If you think your metabolism promotes weight gain, you may have inherited a thrifty metabolism to some extent. A child with no obese parent has only a 10% chance of becoming obese. A child with one obese parent has a 40% risk, and one with two obese parents an 80% risk. It can be argued that these probabilities are

Thrifty metabolism
A metabolism that characteristically conserves more energy than normal so that it increases the risk of weight gain and obesity.

Fraternal twins

Offspring that develop from two separate ova and sperm and therefore have separate genetic identities, although they develop simultaneously in the mother.

related, in part, to the eating behaviors a child learns. **Fraternal twins** vary less in weight than do two unrelated people. This pattern supports the theory that environment, or nurture, affects obesity. Still the close association of body weights between identical twins strongly supports the genetic explanations. This varied evidence shows how complicated it is to separate nature from nurture when searching for the causes of obesity.

Does Nurture Have a Role?

Genetic factors determine some differences in energy metabolism and explain certain weight gain variations among people. However, environmental factors, such as high-fat diets and inactivity, can literally shape us as well. Consider that our gene pool hasn't changed much in the last 50 years, but the ranks of obese people have grown.

Family members often have similar eating habits and choose similar foods. Even husbands and wives—who have no genetic link—may behave similarly toward food and eventually assume similar degrees of leanness or chunkiness. Therefore the family that bonds at the quick-service restaurant counter can influence each other's eating habits and, ultimately, fatness.

Is poverty associated with obesity? Ironically, the answer is often yes. Americans of lower socioeconomic status, especially females, are more likely to be obese than those in upper socioeconomic groups. Are cultural expectations or socioeconomic stress the cause of this?

Adult obesity in women is often rooted in childhood obesity. In addition, periods of stress and boredom and excess weight gain in pregnancy contribute to female obesity. Relative inactivity further adds to the problem. These patterns suggest both social and genetic links. Male obesity, however, is not strongly linked to childhood obesity and instead tends to appear after age 30 (Figure 10-10). In part, a working life encourages a sedentary life for men. This powerful and prevalent pattern suggests a primary role of nurture in obesity, with less genetic influence.[3]

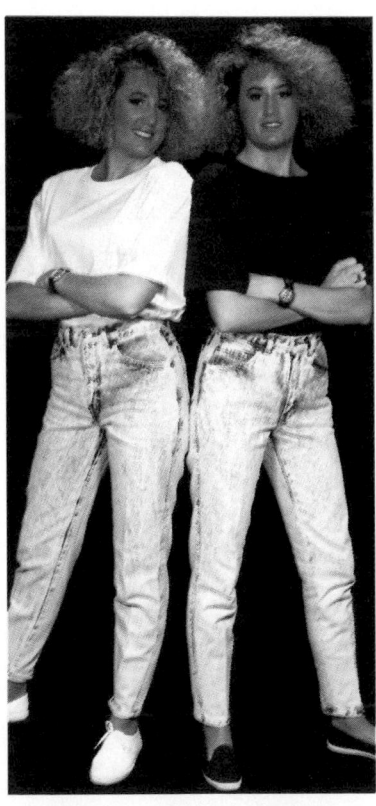

Figure 10-10

Nature or nurture: what causes these twins to have similar body weights?

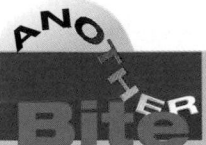

Early research suggested that infant feeding practices, such as introducing solid foods and bottle feeding before age 6 months, encourage infant weight gain and higher risk of obesity later in life. However, many recent studies reexamining this issue show very little relationship between how an infant was fed or how much weight was gained in the first year of life and the presence or absence of obesity in later childhood. The exception could be the infant who gains weight very rapidly in the first 6 weeks of life. Most overweight or obese infants become normal-weight schoolchildren. However, if a child has become obese by 5 years of age, immediate attention is necessary. Obesity in childhood is strongly related to obesity in adulthood.

Nature and Nurture Together

Evidence suggests that both nature and nurture influence the tendency toward obesity (Table 10-3). Consider the possibility that obesity is nurture allowing nature to express itself, like an accident waiting to happen. Some people begin with a slower metabolism. Put these people in an inactive environment, feed them high-calorie foods, and praise them for eating. Like any of us, they can be nurtured into gaining

TABLE 10-3

What Encourages Excess Body Fat Stores and Obesity?

Factor	How fat storage is affected
Age	Excess body fat is more common in adults and middle-aged individuals.
Menopause	Increase in abdominal fat deposition is favored.
Gender	Females have more fat.
Insulin resistance	This often develops as obesity develops.
Positive energy balance	This is especially important if over a relatively long period.
Composition of diet	High fat intake, excess alcohol intake, and preference for sugary, fat-rich foods are likely to contribute to obesity.
Physical activity level	Low or decreasing amount of physical activity affects energy balance and body fat stores.
Resting metabolic rate	A low value with respect to lean body mass is linked to weight gain.
Sympathetic nervous system	Low activity may favor weight gain.
Thermic effect of food	This is low for some obesity cases.
Use of fat for energy	There is limited fat release into the bloodstream.
Total fat mass	Leptin, produced by adipose tissue, affects food intake. Greater fat mass leads to greater loptin production.
Ratio of fat to lean tissue	A high ratio of fat mass to lean body mass is correlated with weight gain.
Fat uptake by adipose tissue	This is high in some obese individuals and remains high (perhaps even increases) with weight loss.
Blood cortisol value	Elevated values promote weight and fat gain.
Variety of social and behavioral factors	Obesity is associated with socioeconomic status, familial conditions, network of friends, busy life-styles that discourage balanced meals, binge-eating, easy availability of inexpensive, high-fat food (such as in quick-service restaurants), pattern of leisure activities, television time, smoking cessation, alcohol intake, and number of meals eaten away from home. These meals are often high in fat and energy content.
Undetermined genetic characteristics	These affect energy balance, particularly via the energy expenditure components, the deposition of the energy surplus as fat or as lean tissue, and the relative proportion of fat and carbohydrate use by the body.
Race	In some races, higher body weight may be more socially acceptable.
Certain medications	Food intake increases.
Childbearing	Women may not lose all weight gained in pregnancy, leading to creeping weight gain.
National region	Regional differences, such as high-fat diets and sedentary lifestyles in the Midwest, cause different rates of obesity in different places.

Modified from Bouchard C: Current understanding of the etiology of obesity: genetic and nongenetic factors, *American Journal of Clinical Nutrition* 53:1561S, 1991.

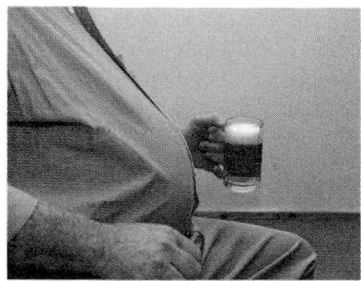

Alcohol intake encourages fat deposition, especially in the abdominal region.

Nutrition Insight

Do You Have a Set Point for Body Weight?

William Bennett and Joel Gurin popularized the "**set-point** theory of weight maintenance" in 1982 in their book *The Dieter's Dilemma*. This theory espouses the notion that weight is closely regulated by the body. It proposes that humans have a genetically predetermined body weight or body fat content that the body attempts to defend. Some research suggests that the hypothalamus monitors the amount of body fat in humans and tries to keep that amount constant over time.[8] This regulation of body fat content is referred to as a "set point." You have already seen in this chapter that the protein called *leptin* may form one communication link between adipose cells and the brain that allows for some weight regulation.

Analogies to the tight regulation of blood pressure and body temperature are used to support this concept. You could view the set point as a coiled spring: the further you stray from your usual weight, the harder the force acts to pull you back to that weight.

In the major studies of humans cited to support the set-point theory, volunteers who lost weight through starvation later ate in a way to regain their original weight or a little more. In addition, studies in the 1960s using prisoners with no history of obesity found it was hard for the men to gain weight, and after gaining weight, they quickly returned to their previous weight when returning to their previous habits. Also, after an illness is resolved, a person generally gains lost weight.

Sound physiological evidence also suggests that body weight tends to be regulated. If energy intake is reduced, the blood concentration of thyroid hormone falls, and the metabolic rate slows.[24] In addition, lower body weight decreases the energy cost of each future weight-bearing activity, and the total energy used by lean tissues falls because some of these tissues are also lost. Furthermore, the enzyme used by adipose and muscle cells to take up fat from the bloodstream often increases its activity. Through these changes the body resists further weight loss.

If a person overeats, in the short run the metabolic rate tends to increase because total body mass increases. This causes some resistance to further weight gain. People often recognize the body's resistance to weight loss when dieting but do not think much about the resistance to weight gain after eating a big holiday meal. However, in the long run resistance to weight gain is much less than resistance to weight loss. When a person gains weight and stays at that weight for a while, the body tends to defend the new weight.[24]

Let's explore set-point regulation of weight in concrete terms. The amount we eat varies from day to day. Daily energy intake varies from about 20% (about 400 kcal) below to 20% above a person's 28-day average energy intake. In comparison, even as little as a 2% (40 kcal) overconsumption of energy per day, if continued for 20 years, could result in an over 100-pound gain in fat stores. This significant effect from such a small variation demonstrates how easy it is to become obese. However, the average weight gain between the ages of 18 and 54 is only 15 to 20 pounds. It appears that some powerful forces encourage a balance of overeating with undereating. Thus, over time, daily energy imbalances cancel each other, with high energy intake days balancing low energy intake days. Considering that over a 35-year period an adult eats about 35 tons of food (yielding 30 million kcal), the ability to regulate weight, though imperfect, is still quite impressive.

Arguments against the set-point theory cite the fact that during pregnancy women slowly increase body weight and fat. Also, an average person's weight does not remain constant throughout adulthood; it usually increases slowly, at least until old age. This means that a person must be able to shift his or her set point. It is also argued that if an individual is placed in a different social, emotional, or physical environment, weight can become markedly higher or lower and is maintained. These arguments suggest that humans, rather than having a set point determined by genetics or number of adipose cells, actually settle into a particular stable weight based on an interaction between nature and nurture influences.

Other researchers argue that the concept of a set point can actually undermine therapy for those who are obese. The idea that the body strongly resists changes in weight can be discouraging and depressing. Obese individuals may fall victim to a self-fulfilling prophecy. A person may believe that maintenance will be so difficult or impossible that he or she may give up at the slightest lapse or weight gain.

In the final analysis, we must bear much of the responsibility for weight maintenance ourselves. The odds are against the likelihood that, even with a set point helping us, we can avoid creeping weight gain in adulthood without great attention to this tendency. Ideally this includes following a diet both moderate in fat and ample in complex carbohydrates and dietary fiber and a lifestyle rich in opportunities for physical activity.[7]

weight, which allows their natural tendency for obesity to blossom. The eventual location of fat storage is strongly influenced by genetics.[14] Weight gain in adulthood often alternates with periods of weight maintenance. This suggests that for some of us a natural tendency to gain weight persists, and changes in our nurturing environment, such as frequent high fat choices as part of regular visits to quick-service restaurants, can cause spurts of weight gain.

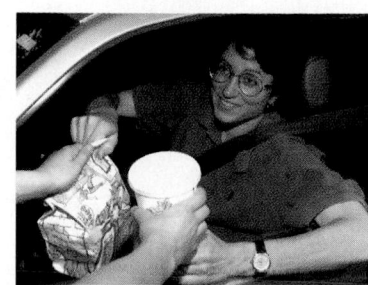

The easy availability of quick-service food has made weight control even harder for many people.

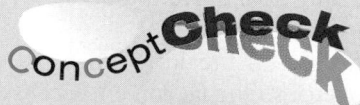

TIPS TO FIGHT THE "FRESHMAN FIFTEEN"

The freshman fifteen is the weight students frequently gain during their first year of college. Freedom from parents, all-you-can-eat meal plans, and nighttime snacking are the chief culprits. The key to avoiding this trap is to choose foods wisely, paying particular attention to fat-rich and sugar-rich foods, such as desserts and soft drinks. Saving enough time for regular physical activity is also important. "Late-night" snackers should turn to plain popcorn and pretzels. Regular meals may also help you avoid snacking.

If your parents are obese, you're likely to be at risk for obesity all your life. To avoid it will require eternal vigilance. Eat the right foods at the right times for the right reasons. Remember that genes do not control your destiny. With increased physical activity and decreased food consumption (especially fats), even those with a genetic tendency toward obesity can maintain a healthy body weight.[33]

Concept Check

Obesity refers to a state of excessive body fat storage. The risk of health problems related to obesity increases under the following conditions:
- A man's percent of body fat exceeds 25%; a woman's exceeds 30% to 35%.
- Body mass index (BMI) is over 25 to 27 (calculated as weight in kilograms divided by height squared in meters).
- Scale weight is 20% above healthy body weight as predicted by the 1983 Metropolitan Life Insurance Table.

However, if a healthy lifestyle is being followed and no current health problems exist, these guidelines need to be reevaluated.

Body fat storage can be estimated clinically using skinfold thickness or bioelectrical impedance. Fat storage distribution further specifies an obese state as either upper body or lower body. Obesity leads to an increased risk for heart disease, some types of cancer, high blood pressure, adult-onset diabetes, bone and joint disorders, and some digestive disorders. The risks for some of these diseases are greater with upper-body fat storage.

TREATMENT OF OBESITY

Obesity should be considered similar to any chronic disease. Treatment requires long-term lifestyle changes, rather than simply taking medicine for 2 weeks, as for a sore throat, or following some quick fix promoted by a fad diet book. Chronic diseases such as high blood pressure and diabetes require lifelong dietary management and ample physical activity, in addition to medical care. Let's explore why obesity must be regarded and treated in the same way.

Some Basic Premises

As you begin to consider current treatment options for obesity, you should first focus on five important general principles concerning weight loss for adults. (Chapter 15 provides weight-loss strategies for children.)

Much of the Current Mania Surrounding Dieting Is Misdirected

People on diets often fall within a BMI of 25. Instead of worrying about weight loss, these individuals should be focusing on a healthy lifestyle that allows for weight maintenance. Incorporating necessary lifestyle changes and learning to live with your particular body characteristics—such as an endomorphic shape—should be your overriding goal.

Actually, this dieting mania can be viewed as mostly a social problem, stemming from unrealistic weight expectations (especially for women) and lack of appreciation for the natural variety in body shape and weight. Not every woman can be a size 10, nor can every man look like a Greek god, but all of us can strive for good health and, if physically possible, an active lifestyle.[12]

The Body Defends Itself Against Weight Loss

As noted in the Nutrition Insight earlier in this chapter, thyroid hormone concentrations and, consequently, basal metabolism drop during weight loss. This fall in metabolic rate is also a consequence of weight loss, caused by a loss of metabolizing tissue. Declines in basal metabolism average 8% to 22% in some studies.[24] This drop makes it difficult to lose weight.

In addition, the activity of the enzyme responsible for breaking down triglyceride from lipoproteins into free fatty acids and glycerol so the fat can enter cells increases. Now the body more efficiently takes up fat from the bloodstream for storage. Often, fat use for energy needs also remains depressed in people who have recently lost weight.[14] This is a good reason to stay on a low-fat diet and remain physically active for weight maintenance. Insulin action on adipose cells also improves with weight loss, which reduces fat release by these cells.

Weight Cycling Is a Common Phenomenon

Only about 5% of people who follow commercial diet programs actually lose weight and then remain close to that weight. Typically, one third of the weight lost during dieting is regained within 1 year of the end of dietary restriction, and almost all weight lost is regained within 3 to 5 years. Some programs have slightly higher success rates than 5%, as do some people who simply lose weight on their own without enrolling in any supervised plan.[6] Overall, however, the statistics are grim. Dieting often results in eventual weight regain. Essentially only the surgical approaches to obesity treatment (discussed later) show much success in maintaining the weight loss.[13] Moreover, the weight gained after dieting includes not only the weight that was lost but often additional weight as well, causing the dieter to be worse off than before. Furthermore, the weight gained may consist primarily of adipose tissue, whereas the weight that was lost consisted of a mix of adipose and lean tissue. Therefore the long-term effect is not only an increase in total weight but also an increase in percentage of body fat.

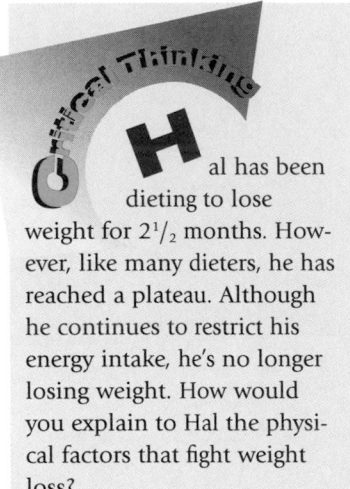

Critical Thinking

Hal has been dieting to lose weight for 2½ months. However, like many dieters, he has reached a plateau. Although he continues to restrict his energy intake, he's no longer losing weight. How would you explain to Hal the physical factors that fight weight loss?

This gain-and-lose predicament is referred to as *weight cycling* or *yo-yo dieting*. Additional negative health consequences are associated with weight cycling, such as an increased risk for upper body fat deposition and profound discouragement and erosion of self-esteem.[35] Nevertheless, experts still encourage obese people to attempt weight loss, with a strong focus on maintaining that lower weight.[7] Still, dieters need to be aware of the trap of today's crash diet, which too often leads to the next month's weight gain. A weight-loss program should be considered successful only when the subjects involved in the process remain at or close to their lower weights.

Overall, current treatments for obesity are deceptively simple but usually unsuccessful in the long term. We are groping in the dark in our search for an effective obesity treatment.[16] Keep in mind that (1) no single approach to weight loss is suitable for everyone; (2) the more knowledge a person has about weight loss interventions, the better; and (3) we are still a long way from knowing which individuals benefit most from specific approaches.

Weight Gain in Adulthood Is All Too Common

From ages 25 to 44, danger of weight gain exists, especially for women. Particular prudence should be practiced in these decades, although childhood and adolescent years also deserve attention. Adults should generally set a goal of not gaining more than about 10 to 16 pounds more than their weight was upon reaching age 21.[26] People who gain weight rapidly should closely monitor food intake and activity patterns to discover the causes and then moderate the increases or reverse the trend in appropriate ways. Later in this chapter, you'll learn how to do this.

Changes in Body Composition Deserve a Primary Focus in Weight Loss

Weight should be lost mostly from adipose stores, not from muscle and other lean tissues. Rapid weight loss at the start of a diet program often represents fluid lost as a result of decreased salt intake and loss of glycogen from the liver and muscles. Much muscle tissue may be lost as well, and this is mostly (about 73%) water. People are fooled when they weigh themselves after starting a fad diet. They lose weight, but very little of it represents fat loss. Any loss of lean tissue means a decrease in basal metabolism and thus a decrease in overall energy expenditure.

All this shows the importance of preventing obesity, because curing the disorder is very difficult. Only the very motivated should try to lose weight, and ideally this attempt should be preceded by a period of weight maintenance in order to begin the process of balancing energy intake with a degree of energy output that can be maintained.[26] Nutrition experts strongly endorse this point and state, as noted at the outset, that many people would be healthier if they simply focused on improving food habits, minimizing symptoms of any weight-related chronic disease present (such as high blood pressure) and increasing physical activity rather than remaining focused on a particular body weight and shape.[31] This conclusion is partly made by nutrition experts because obtaining and maintaining a substantially lower body weight are so difficult.

Weight loss and subsequent maintenance of a lower weight are possible. Many of us know people who have done so, but this takes great motivation. Nutrition science can provide the tools for weight maintenance and loss. The missing ingredients are the motivation and the supportive environment needed to put these tools to use for a lifetime.[11] Obviously, knowledge alone is not enough, because some nutrition and other health professionals are themselves obese. This brings us back to an earlier concept that is worth repeating—prevention of obesity is the most reliable therapy. Overall, an ounce of prevention is worth a pound of cure.

It was once thought that weight cycling—weight loss followed by regain—contributed to a decrease in basal metabolism. However, many current studies have not been able to demonstrate this effect.

Wishful Shrinking—Why Quick Weight Loss Can't Be Mostly Fat

We know that rapid weight loss cannot consist mostly of fat loss because of the high energy deficit needed to lose a large amount of adipose tissue. The body fat present in adipose tissue contains about 3500 kcal per pound. Fat storage, which includes body fat tissue plus supporting lean tissues, contains approximately 2700 kcal per pound.[29] To lose 1 pound of fat stores per week, energy intake must be decreased by approximately 400 kcal per day (2700/7 = 386) to account for the loss of both body fat and associated lean support tissues. Diets that promise 10 to 15 pounds of weight loss per week can't ensure that the weight loss is from fat stores alone. Producing an energy deficit sufficient to lose that amount of fat storage simply isn't practical. Lean tissue, rather than fat, accounts for the major part of the weight lost.

What to Look for in a Sound Weight-Loss Diet

A dieter can try to devise a plan of action by seeking advice from professionals or consulting current books. Either way, a sound weight-loss program should include three components: control of energy intake, especially fat intake; increased energy expenditure through physical activity; and acknowledgment that life-long change in habits is required, not simply a short-term weight-loss period.[7, 13, 31] Focusing on just eating less energy represents a difficult path to success, as will be shown. Adding regular physical activity and an appropriate psychological component contributes to success and later maintenance of the weight loss.

Specifically, any weight-loss plan should include the following characteristics:

1. The plan should meet nutritional needs, except for energy. To do that, it should follow the Food Guide Pyramid, emphasizing low-fat choices. Overall, this controlled eating should remain a satisfying and pleasurable experience.
2. Slow and steady weight loss, rather than rapid weight loss, should be stressed. A loss of 1 or so pounds of fat storage per week is desirable. Once about 10% of excess weight is lost, maintenance of that loss for about 6 months is desirable before more weight loss is attempted.[10] That may seem like a disappointing prescription, but a more radical approach to weight loss is likely to produce a yo-yo episode. Recall that the person could view this as a "healthier" weight, because it will probably lead to health improvement. Then careful evaluation should be made to determine whether further weight loss is needed, based on current health state.
3. The plan should allow adaptations to individual habits and tastes. The same plan does not work for everyone.
4. The plan should minimize hunger and fatigue. To do this, it should contain at least 1200 to 1500 kcal per day. Otherwise, consuming sufficient vitamins and minerals, especially enough iron for young women, is difficult. In reality, however, 1000 kcal per day is generally regarded as the minimum energy intake because many dieters perform so little physical activity and therefore need very restricted energy allowances. If the eating plan calls for an energy intake below 1200 to 1500 kcal per day, it should recommend use of either fortified foods (breakfast cereals, for example) or a balanced vitamin and mineral supplement (see Chapter 3 for advice on supplements).
5. The plan should contain common foods. There is no magical food that can speed weight loss. If a diet suggests that there is, whether ginseng, tofu, or garlic, advice should be sought elsewhere. Furthermore, if special foods were required, maintaining this practice indefinitely would be difficult.

6. The plan should fit into any social situation. The healthier lifestyle should allow attendance at parties, eating at restaurants, and participation in normal daily activities.

7. The plan should help change problem eating habits. It should promote reshaping food habits and lifestyle to make weight loss, and then weight maintenance, possible and so thwart weight regain. Eating at least three meals per day and avoiding binge eating are two important considerations. Maintenance should be a key concern of any plan—the plan must have a lifetime focus. For example, a 150-pound person should reduce energy intake, increase physical activity, and start eating like a 130-pound person to become a 130-pound person. Moreover, once the weight is lost, the person can't go back to the habits of his or her 150-pound self. The program should also focus on changing obesity-promoting beliefs and rallying healthy social support.

8. The plan should improve overall health. It should emphasize proper rest, stress reduction, and other healthy changes in lifestyle. All too often people know how to diet, but they don't know how to live. They find it easier to count calories and follow a plan than to deal with underlying issues that encourage eating, such as stress.

9. The plan should insist that the person see a physician before starting if any of the following are true:
   - He or she has existing health problems
   - He or she plans to lose weight as quickly as possible
   - He or she is over 35 years of age and plans to perform substantially increased physical activity

When you read brochures or research reports about specific diet plans, ask not only whether the people lost weight but also whether they maintained much of that weight loss. If this did not happen, then the entire dieting program was in vain.

Controlling Energy Intake—The First Key to Weight Loss

A goal of losing 1 to 2 pounds of stored fat per week often requires limiting energy intake to 1000 to 1600 kcal per day for women and 1600 to 2000 kcal for men, with less than 30% of energy intake coming from fat. Recall that adults currently consume about 34% of energy as fat. The range for each gender is due to the varying amounts of physical activity that may be performed. It could also be higher for very active people.

Another approach to setting energy needs is to allow 10 kcal per pound of desirable weight for sedentary people and 13 kcal per pound for active people. Then subtract 400 kcal for each pound per week of fat tissue loss desired. For example, an active 160-pound woman who should weigh 140 pounds and wants to lose 1 pound per week could start with 1820 kcal (13×140) and then subtract 400 kcal, which allows about 1400 kcal for her diet.

Traditionally dieters have counted calories. Many experts recommend counting mostly fat grams, assuming that control of energy intake follows. This makes sense, because a life-long restriction of energy intake is almost impossible, whereas a low-fat diet is easy to follow indefinitely if it allows consumption of enough food—especially fruits, vegetables, and whole grains—to satisfy hunger. The new food labels simplify the task of counting fat grams.[22] Note that not all food choices need to be low fat. Total fat intake for the day is the focus.

As discussed in Chapter 6, many of the fat-reduced products flooding the market substitute sugar for fat in order to maintain flavor and consequently end up not much lower in energy content. This makes it easy to gain weight, even on a low-fat diet, without careful portion control of fat-reduced foods. A better low-fat diet focuses primarily on foods that are naturally low in fat—such as fruits, vegetables, plain breads and cereals, lean cuts of meats, and low-fat/nonfat dairy products—rather than foods that have been "tweaked" a bit to reduce fat content enough to satisfy food labeling regulations. This low-fat approach helps train the palate to enjoy a leaner diet and generally increases vitamin and mineral content of the diet, while reducing saturated fat and total fat intake.

Some experts think that certain fat-reduced foods, such as nonfat sour cream, serve merely to remind dieters what they are missing, driving them back to the high-fat food choice. In addition, some studies have shown that people eat more when told a food is fat-reduced, even if it is not. This suggests it may be better to avoid high-fat foods and their fat-reduced counterparts, instead replacing them with a food choice naturally low in fat, such as nonfat yogurt for sour cream or a plain warm bagel for a doughnut.

In any case, dieters should consume at least 1000 kcal daily; fewer than that causes so much hunger that they will probably not be able to stick to the plan. A better idea is to first increase physical activity, allowing at least 1000 kcal (ideally, closer to 1500 kcal) to be eaten each day.

Two ways for a dieter to monitor energy intake are reading labels and learning the exchange system. Label reading is important, because many foods are more energy-dense than people suppose (Figure 10-11). See the menu patterns listed in Appendix D for some possible exchange system approaches.

Another method is to write down food intake throughout the day and then calculate energy intake from the food table in Appendix A in the evening, adjusting future food choices as needed. Because people often underestimate portion size when recording food intake, measuring cups can help. A kitchen scale may be as important as the bathroom scale in helping to control body weight. Overall, if your eating plan allows only 3 ounces of skinless chicken breast, you should realize that this amount is not much bigger than a pack of playing cards or the palm of your hand. A kitchen scale will make this abundantly clear.

One of the biggest obstacles to staying on a reduced-fat diet is lack of taste. One way to overcome this is to savor foods:
- Choose foods with eye appeal. They will stimulate saliva.
- Serve foods hot or warm to increase their aroma.
- Take time to smell the food.
- Enjoy the flavor by holding the food in your mouth before swallowing.
- Chew foods thoroughly to release their flavor.
- Eat several foods at each meal, and alternate foods as you eat to reduce taste bud fatigue.

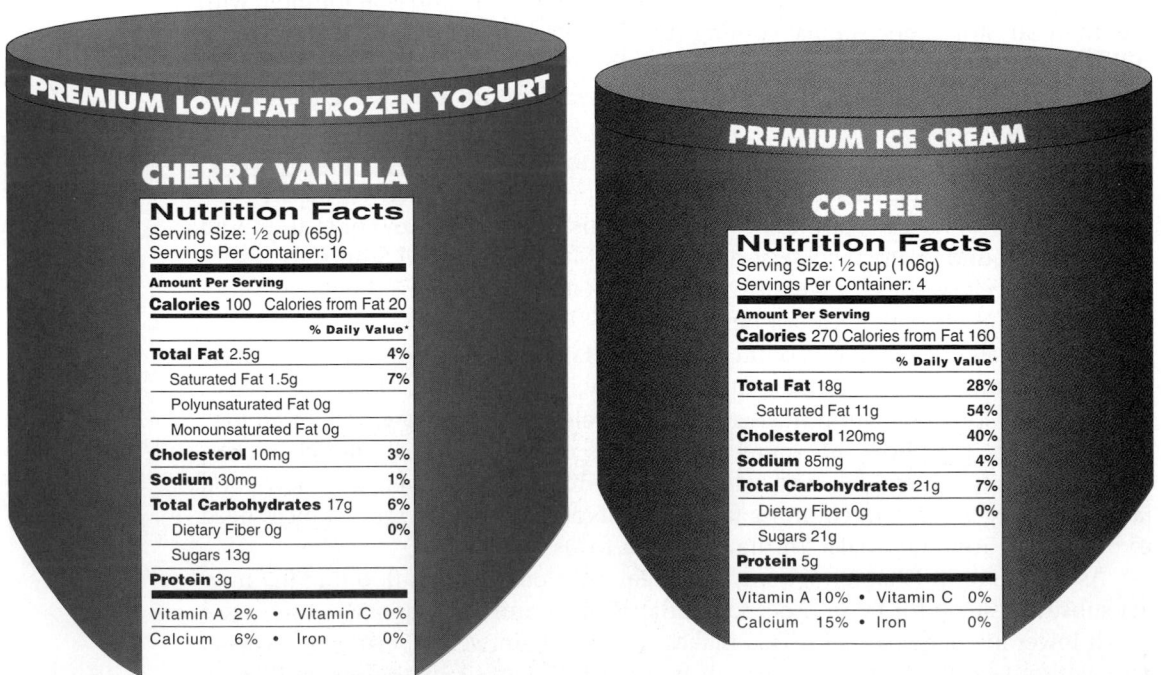

Figure 10-11 *Reading labels helps you choose foods with less fat and energy. Which frozen dessert is the better choice for a person on a weight-loss diet? The % Daily Values are based on a 2000 kcal diet.*

Minimizing fat intake is a very important goal when trying to lose body fat.[15] Diets containing as little as 20% of energy from fat are well tolerated, especially when they are high in complex carbohydrates and dietary fiber. Complex carbohydrates and dietary fiber in a diet help ensure adequate satiety when less total energy intake comes from fat. One study showed that when energy intake from fat was reduced from 40% to 30% and then to 20%, subjects ate slightly more food on the lower-fat diet. However, the end result was that the lower-fat diet provided far less energy, allowing more weight loss even though more food was consumed.[25]

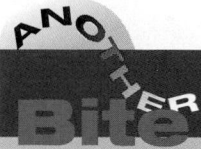

HERE ARE SOME PRACTICES THAT CAN STIMULATE METABOLISM WHILE ONE IS DIETING:[18]

- *Perform physical activity regularly throughout the day. Find opportunities for increasing activity, such as quick walks, stair climbing, or calisthenics (sit-ups, push-ups, etc.)*
- *Fidget when sitting and standing.*
- *Eat breakfast, so food intake is spread throughout the day. Each time food is consumed, metabolism increases.*
- *Follow a carbohydrate-rich diet; much of this is further processed by the liver, which uses energy.*
- *Avoid "crash" dieting. Slow weight loss is a better idea because it leads to a smaller decline in metabolism during a diet.*

What Should Be Eaten?

The easiest and healthiest way to eat is to begin with the Food Guide Pyramid, spreading out the food choices into a regular meal pattern (3 or more meals). To review, this consists of 6 servings ($1/2$ cup, 1 ounce, or 1 slice) of breads, cereals, rice, and pasta. An emphasis on whole grains, with limited amounts of sugar and fat, is important. The dietary fiber helps us feel full longer. Then add between 2 and 4 servings (one medium or $1/2$ cup) of fruit and 3 and 5 servings of vegetables. To finish, add 2 to 3 servings of nonfat or low-fat milk/dairy products (1 cup) and about 4 ounces of lean meat or alternatives each day. Sweets and fats should be restricted. Remember that potato chips and cheese are rich in fat, and fruit punches are considered a sweet. Table 10-4 shows how to start reducing energy intake.

As you should realize by now, it is best to consider healthy eating a lifestyle change rather than simply a weight-loss plan. You should make reasonable choices, consume adequate portions, and not expect a miracle overnight (Figure 10-12).

SHOE

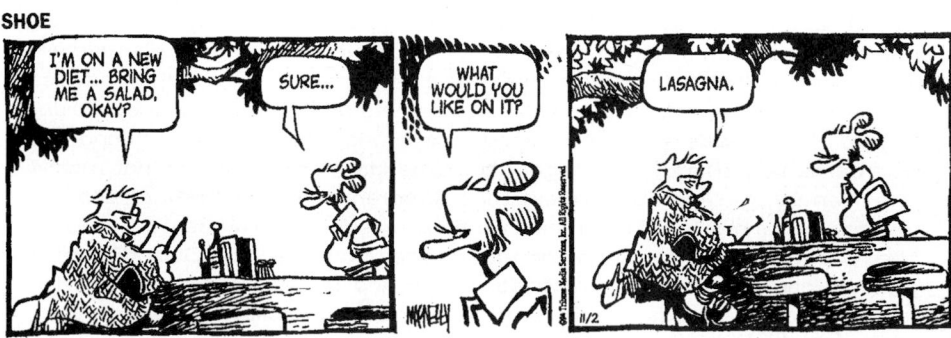

Figure 10-12 *Shoe.*

TABLE 10-4

Reducing Energy Intake Begins with Moderating High-Fat Foods

The chart below can help plan meals that encourage healthful eating. When you select a variety of foods from those listed in the far left column, you'll be eating foods that are low in fat and/or high in dietary fiber.

Types of food	Select most often	Select moderately often	Select least often
Animal protein	Lean cuts of beef/pork Salmon, halibut (broiled) Canned tuna in water Poultry (without skin) Egg Crab	Untrimmed beef and pork Canned tuna in oil Poultry (with skin) Lobster, shrimp Canadian bacon	Fatty beef, lamb, pork Luncheon meats/hot dogs Fried chicken Fried fish Liver, kidneys Bacon

Dairy	Nonfat yogurt
	Nonfat milk (or ½%)
	Nonfat dry milk
	Nonfat frozen yogurt
		Reduced-fat and part-skim
		  cheeses
		Low-fat cottage cheese
		Low-fat milk
		Low-fat yogurt
		95% fat-free frozen yogurt
			Whole-milk cheese (cheddar,
			  Muenster)
			Whole-milk
			Sour cream, ice cream
			Cream, half-and-half

Vegetable protein	Dried beans and peas (kidney,
	  lima, and soy beans; lentils;
	  split peas)
	Tofu (bean curd)
		Raw or dry-roasted nuts and
		  seeds
		Peanut and other nut butters
		  (moderate amounts)
			Oil-processed nuts and seeds

Vegetables	Raw, fresh vegetables
	Fresh or frozen, slightly
	  cooked vegetables
		Canned vegetables
		Canned tomato or vegetable
		  juice
			Vegetables in cream or butter
			  sauces
			Fried vegetables

Fruits	Fresh, raw fruit Dried fruit Frozen and fresh fruit juices	Canned fruit packed in juice Canned fruit juices Frozen fruit	Fruit-flavored beverages Canned fruit packed in syrup Avocados Olives
Grain products	Shredded wheat, oats Whole-grain cereals Whole-grain breads Brown rice Wheat bran, oat bran Bagels Fig bars	Refined cereals Enriched white breads Refined pasta White rice Granola Toast with margarine Plain cookies	Cookies, cakes, pies Sweetened cereals Tortilla chips Oil-processed crackers Cream-filled cookies Croissants, doughnuts Fat-rich salad dressings
Other (limit quantity)	Popcorn (air popped)	Low-fat salad dressing Low-fat mayonnaise Pretzels	Mayonnaise Gravies, cream sauce Potato chips

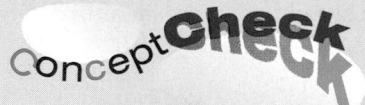

Concept Check

Obesity is a chronic disease that necessitates lifelong treatment. Key points to consider when attempting to treat obesity include the following: (1) The primary focus should be on a healthy lifestyle that can be maintained; (2) the body resists weight loss; (3) typical weight-loss attempts often are followed by weight regain; (4) emphasis should be placed on preventing obesity, since curing this disorder is very difficult; (5) weight should be lost from fat stores, not mostly from lean tissues. Appropriate weight-loss programs have the following characteristics in common: (1) They meet nutritional needs—this can be evaluated by checking for mostly low-fat and non-fat choices from the Food Guide Pyramid; (2) they can adjust to accommodate habits and tastes; (3) they emphasize readily obtainable foods; (4) they promote changing habits that lead to overeating; (5) they encourage regular physical activity; and (6) they help change obesity-promoting beliefs and rally healthy social support.

Regular Physical Activity—A Second Key to Weight Loss and Later Weight Maintenance

Regular physical activity is very important for everyone, especially those who are trying to lose weight or maintain a lower body weight. Fat burning is enhanced. Therefore it greatly complements a reduction in energy intake, but does not substitute for it.[37] Many of us rarely do more than sit, stand, and sleep. Obviously, much more energy is used during physical activity than at rest. In addition, expending only 200 to 300 extra kcal per day above and beyond normal activity level, while controlling energy intake, can lead to about a half pound of fat loss per week, or about 25 pounds of fat loss per year. Furthermore, physical activity often boosts overall self-esteem.[20]

Adding any of the activities in Figure 10-13 to your lifestyle leads to expenditure of an extra 200 kcal; note that sitting is not a recommended "activity." Duration and regular performance, rather than intensity, are the keys to success with this approach to weight loss. You should search for activities that can be continued over time.[31] In this regard, walking vigorously 2 miles per day can be as helpful as aerobic dancing or jogging if it is maintained. Moreover, walking is less likely to lead to injuries. Some strength training can also be added to increase lean body mass and, in turn, fat use (see Chapter 11).

The easiest way to increase physical activity is to make it part of a daily routine. To start, you could consider walking every day and then incorporating some regular stair climbing. A simple trick is to park your car farther from school, work, and the shopping mall so you must walk farther.

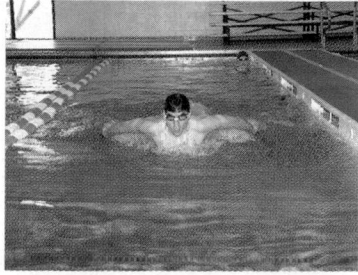

Regular physical activity is one component of a healthy weight-loss plan.

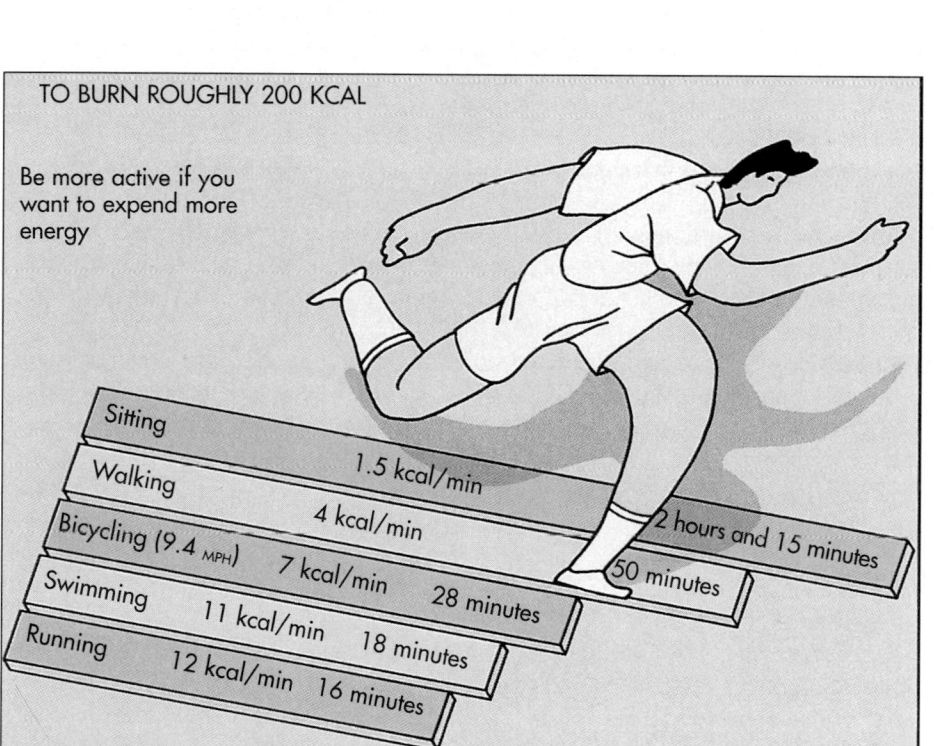

TO BURN ROUGHLY 200 KCAL

Be more active if you want to expend more energy

Sitting	1.5 kcal/min	2 hours and 15 minutes
Walking	4 kcal/min	50 minutes
Bicycling (9.4 MPH)	7 kcal/min	28 minutes
Swimming	11 kcal/min	18 minutes
Running	12 kcal/min	16 minutes

Figure 10-13
Physical activity improves any diet strategy. Weight loss is enhanced because much more energy is used in physical activity than at rest. In addition, physical activity facilitates fat loss while preserving most lean body mass. Each of these activities uses approximately 200 kcal.

Behavior Modification—What Makes Us Tick?

Does dieting test your self-control? Do you know what habits sabotage your good intentions? Controlling energy intake, so important to weight loss, means modifying *problem* behaviors. Only you can decide what behaviors keep you from reaching for the wrong foods at the wrong times for the wrong reasons.

TABLE 10-5

Behavior Modification Principles for Weight Loss

STIMULUS CONTROL
Shopping

1. Shop for food after eating—buy nutritious foods
2. Shop from a list; limit purchases of irresistible "problem" foods.
3. Avoid ready-to-eat foods.
4. Put off shopping until absolutely necessary.

Plans

1. Plan to limit food intake as needed.
2. Substitute periods of physical activity for snacking.
3. Eat meals and snacks at scheduled times; don't skip meals.

Activities

1. Store food out of sight, preferably in the freezer, to discourage impulsive eating.
2. Eat all food in the same place.
3. Keep serving dishes off the table, especially dishes of sauces and gravies.
4. Use smaller dishes and utensils.

Holidays and parties

1. Drink fewer alcoholic beverages.
2. Plan eating behavior before parties.
3. Eat a low-calorie snack before parties.
4. Practice polite ways to decline food.
5. Don't get discouraged by an occasional setback.

EATING BEHAVIOR

1. Put fork down between mouthfuls.
2. Chew thoroughly before taking the next bite.
3. Leave some food on the plate.
4. Pause in the middle of the meal.
5. Do nothing else while eating (for example, reading, watching television).

REWARD

1. Solicit help from family and friends and suggest how they can help you.
2. Help family and friends provide this help in the form of praise and material rewards.
3. Use self-monitoring records as basis for rewards.
4. Plan specific rewards for specific behavior (behavioral contracts).

SELF-MONITORING
Diet diary

1. Note time and place of eating.
2. List type and amount of food eaten.
3. Record who is present and how you feel.
4. Use diet diary to identify problem areas.

COGNITIVE RESTRUCTURING

1. Avoid setting unreasonable goals.
2. Think about progress, not shortcomings.
3. Avoid imperatives like "always" and "never."
4. Counter negative thoughts with positive restatements.

From Frankle RT, Yang M: *Obesity and weight control*, Rockville, Md, 1988, Aspen Publishers.

What events start (or stop) your eating? What factors influence food choices? Psychologists often use terms like *chain-breaking, stimulus control, cognitive restructuring, contingency management,* and *self-monitoring* when discussing behavior modification (Table 10-5). This terminology, as will be covered in detail in Chapter 12, helps place the problem in perspective and organize the intervention strategy into manageable steps.

Chain-breaking separates behaviors that tend to occur together—for example, snacking on chips while watching television. Although these activities do not have to occur together, they often do. Dieters may need to break the chain reaction.

Stimulus control puts us in charge of temptations. Options include pushing tempting food to the back of the refrigerator, removing fat-laden snacks from the kitchen counter, and avoiding the path by the vending machines. Provide a positive stimulus by keeping low-fat snacks ready to satisfy hunger/appetite. Note that alcohol and foods offer quick, easy stress relief. We need to plan healthful alternatives.

Cognitive restructuring changes our frame of mind. For example, after a hard day, respond with a walk or satisfying talk with a friend instead of a binge. Replace eating reactions to stress with healthful, relaxing alternatives.

Decreeing some food off limits sets up an internal struggle to resist the urge to eat that food. This hopeless battle can keep us feeling deprived. We lose the fight. Managing food choices with the principle of moderation is best. If a favorite food becomes troublesome, place it off limits only temporarily, until you can enjoy it in moderation.

Contingency management prepares us for potential pitfalls and high-risk situations. We might rehearse in advance appropriate responses to pressure—like food being passed at a party.

Did you keep a record of what you ate and what catalysts urged you to pick up the fork or put it down as suggested in Chapter 1? If so, you already know one key tool in modifying behavior—self-monitoring. A self-monitoring record can reveal patterns—such as unconscious overeating—that may explain problem eating habits. This record can encourage new habits to counteract unwanted behaviors.

New habits often need to replace defeating ones. For example, limiting eating to a single room in the house might eliminate television snacking. Eating rapidly, holding an ever-ready forkful of food while chewing, outpaces the natural satiety response. The brain requires about 20 minutes to register satiety. Put the fork down! Because appetite, not physical hunger, often makes us eat, we may need to simply stop purchasing irresistible foods.

Overall, it is important to analyze shortcomings that make dieting difficult, and *address specific* problems, such as snacking, compulsive eating, or mealtime overeating. Consult Chapter 12 for a more detailed discussion of how to develop a plan to change behavior.

Chain-breaking
Breaking the link between two or more behaviors that encourage overeating, such as snacking while watching television.

Stimulus control
Altering the environment to minimize the stimuli for eating—for example, removing foods from sight and storing them in kitchen cabinets.

Cognitive restructuring
Changing one's frame of mind regarding eating—for example, instead of using a difficult day as an excuse to overeat, substituting other pleasures for rewards, such as a relaxing walk with a friend.

Contingency management
Forming a plan of action to respond to a situation in which overeating is likely, such as when snacks are within arm's reach at a party.

Self-monitoring
A process of tracking foods eaten and conditions affecting eating; actions are usually recorded in a diary, along with location, time, and state of mind. This is a tool to help people understand more about their eating habits.

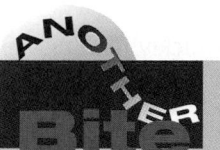

People carry on an internal dialogue—self-talk—to sort out their own truth, beliefs and attitudes, and responses to events around them. Positive self-talk leads us kindly through changes, like choosing to lose weight. We praise ourselves for success. Negative self-talk is different. Praise is replaced with self-deprecating remarks; self-blame; and angry, guilt-producing put-downs. Negative self-talk undermines efforts at self-control—dieting included—and leads to anxiety and depression. Beliefs and self-talk influence how we interpret events of today and expectations of the future, as well as how we feel and react. Positive self-talk and problem-solving efforts and realistic beliefs and goals lead us to a healthful, self-caring lifestyle.

Relapse Prevention is Important

A dieter can tolerate an occasional lapse but needs to plan for lapses, encouraging calm, but taking charge immediately. Change responses like "I ate that cookie; I'm a failure," to "I ate that cookie, but I did well to stop after only one!" An occasional cookie is fine; a pound of cookies in an afternoon deserves reconsideration. When dieters lapse from their diet plan, newly learned food habits should steer them back toward the plan. This should enable dieters to avoid the lapse-relapse-collapse trap. Without a strong behavioral plan, a lapse frequently turns into a relapse. Once a pattern of poor food choices begins, dieters may feel that they have failed and stray further from the plan. As the relapse lengthens, the diet plan collapses, and the dieters fall short of their weight-loss goal. Even with a good behavioral plan, you may fail at a diet. Losing weight is difficult.

Social Support Aids Behavior Change

Healthy social support is helpful in weight control. Helping others understand how they can be supportive can make weight control easier.[11] Family and friends can provide praise and encouragement. A weight-control professional can keep dieters accountable and help them learn from difficult situations. Long-term contact with a professional can be quite helpful for later weight maintenance.[6] Groups of individuals attempting to lose weight or maintain losses can provide empathetic support.

A Recap

When weight-loss experts pool their collective experience, they identify certain factors that characterize success and failure in weight loss and later weight maintenance. As you've learned from this chapter, that success is encouraged by the following measures[7, 11]:

1. Moderation in fat/energy intake. A first step should be use of this intervention to establish weight maintenance behavior before attempting to lose weight.
2. Time and inclination to perform regular physical activity.
3. A sense of control of personal destiny and likelihood of success.
4. Taking charge of the plan with a strong motivation to succeed.
5. Focusing on improved health status to spur success.
6. Positive self-talk.
7. Social support via family/friends, in turn balancing life with friendships, work, hobbies, and other interests.
8. Sustained vigilance in pursuit of goals—realizing it is a lifetime pursuit that must be suited to one's specific needs. It's not a diet but a permanent lifestyle change.
9. Realistic goals that promote gradual change.
10. Keeping track of body weight and body measurements and quickly making changes in a plan if relapse is noticed.

Failure is encouraged by the following factors[4, 11]:

1. Negative feelings.
2. Out-of-control situations, such as family life or lifestyle that constantly challenges the will to succeed; prior or current practices of bingeing, laxative abuse, or induced vomiting. In these cases professional help should be sought.
3. Reverting to old habits, such as eating primarily foods rich in fat and abusing alcohol.

A disturbing fact about dieting for weight loss is that often the weight is quickly regained. Dieters may then end up with a greater percentage of body fat and be less

A good idea is to keep low-fat snack foods close at hand, especially during peak snacking periods. Reaching for fruit by the refrigerator may prevent snacking on fat-laden foods. While having the willpower to resist high-fat foods is desirable, a better alternative is to avoid the temptation.

healthy after their diet-and-regain cycle than when they began. Based on this information, it appears that dieting itself can promote obesity. Thus dieting should not be undertaken lightly. If you are not highly motivated and do not have the needed social support, delay dieting for weight loss until a more appropriate time. There is no reason to add more failure to your life. In the meantime, strive to give up unrealistic weight goals that you may have harbored for a lifetime.

Would-be dieters should choose and follow diet plans that are appropriate for them. They have a smorgasbord of options: lowered energy and fat intakes, behavior modification, increased physical activity, and group or individual counseling. Many tools are effective, but some are more useful than others, depending on the dieter's lifestyle, personality, and motivation.

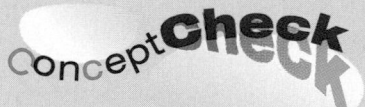

Increasing physical activity as part of daily life should be part of any weight-loss plan. A goal of 200 or more kcal spent in daily activity such as walking and stair climbing is recommended. Behavior modification can improve conditions for losing weight. One behavior area that requires change is habit chains that encourage overeating, such as snacking while watching television. Another tactic is to modify the environment to reduce temptation; for example, put foods into cupboards to keep them out of sight. In addition, rethinking attitudes about eating—for example, substituting pleasures other than food as a reward for coping with a stressful day—can be important for altering undesirable eating behavior. Advance planning to prevent and deal with lapses is vital, as is rallying healthy social support. Finally, careful observation and recording of eating habits can reveal subtle cues that lead to overeating.

Professional Help for Weight Loss

The first professional to see for advice about a weight-loss program is the family physician. Doctors are best equipped to assess overall health and the appropriateness of weight loss. The physician may recommend a registered dietitian for a specific weight-loss plan and answers to diet-related questions. Registered dietitians are uniquely qualified to help design a weight-loss plan because they understand both food composition and the psychological importance of food. Exercise physiologists can provide advice about programs to increase physical activity.

Many communities have a variety of weight-loss organizations. These may include self-help groups, such as Take Off Pounds Sensibly and Weight Watchers.[6] Other programs, such as Jenny Craig and Physicians' Weight Loss Center, are less desirable for the average dieter. Often the employees are not dietitians or other appropriately trained health professionals. These programs also tend to be expensive because of their requirements for intense counseling or mandatory diet foods and supplements. In addition, the Federal Trade Commission has charged these and other commercial diet-program companies with misleading consumers through unsubstantiated weight-loss claims and deceptive testimonials.

Treating Severe Obesity

Severe (morbid) obesity—weighing at least 100 pounds over healthy body weight (or twice one's healthy body weight)—requires professional treatment. Because of the severe health problems related to severe obesity, drastic measures may be necessary. Such treatments are recommended only when traditional diets fail. Drastic

Nutrition Insight

Medications to Aid Weight Loss

Over-the-counter medications that claim to facilitate weight loss are very profitable. Some can be effective, but so far none can substitute for the basic approach outlined in this chapter to promote weight loss. Diet aids include fiber pills, **phenylpropanolamine,** and benzocaine.[22] Phenylpropanolamine is an epinephrine-like drug that can cause a slight decrease in food intake. At a typical dose the degree of appetite suppression varies among people. FDA recommends that phenylpropanolamine be used with caution in people with hyperthyroidism, cardiovascular disorders (including high blood pressure), and diabetes. Adverse reactions may also occur in people taking various other medications or consuming caffeine at the same time. Benzocaine numbs the tongue, so a person tends to eat less.

Fiber pills can increase bulk in the stomach and ideally lead to satiety. Only soluble fiber, the type found in beans, oats, and guar gum, is effective in decreasing food intake. Bran fiber, such as that found in fiber pills, is not effective. However, when people consume enough soluble fiber (23 grams) incorporated into crackers to decrease food intake, they also experience significant intestinal gas.

Physicians sometimes, prescribe amphetamines for weight loss. Amphetamines cause a person to eat less, but they can also be addictive. In addition, amphetamines can increase heart rate and nervousness and lead to insomnia. Work on related medications continues. Thyroid hormone preparations were once popular, but these caused significant loss of lean tissue.

Fenfluramine (Pondimin) and related medications, such as dexfenfluramine (Redux), are prescribed by physicians to promote weight loss. These drugs increase the action of serotonin in the brain, which may lead to less food craving, especially for high-carbohydrate foods. Rapid weight gain after discontinuing the drug is a problem. Addition of behavioral therapy to this approach may improve weight maintenance. Some medication regimens add a form of amphetamine-like medications (phentermine [Fastin]) as well to increase efficacy. These therapies are effective for some people in the short run, but have not yet been proved safe and effective in the long run. Studies are ongoing. Most state medical boards currently limit use to 12 weeks unless the person is participating in a medical study using the product. FDA has approved use of dexfenfluramine for up to 1 year.

Researchers are studying a medication that inhibits fat digestion in the small intestine (Orlistat). This drug reduces absorption of dietary fat. The drawback is that it is only 30% effective, no matter what the dose is, so a reduced-energy diet is also needed for this approach to work. Therefore, this product has the potential to give only a slight boost to someone already following a healthy lifestyle for weight loss. A common side effect of this drug is diarrhea; a low-fat diet reduces this problem.

A medication used for treatment of ulcers, cimetidine, is being tested as a hunger-suppressing agent. Cimetidine reduces acid output by the stomach, as described in Chapter 4. Experts suggest that if there is reduced acid in the stomach, the sensation of hunger will decrease. Further studies are needed before the overall efficacy of this drug is known, but results are promising to date.

Overall, in skilled hands, prescription medications can aid weight loss.[2] However, they do not supplant the need for reducing energy and fat intake, modifying problem behavior, and increasing physical activity, both during and after therapy.

weight-loss procedures are not without side effects, both physical and psychological, making careful physician monitoring a necessity.

Gastroplasty. Stomach stapling, or **gastroplasty,** is the most common surgical procedure for treating severe obesity. The procedure works by reducing the stomach to the size of a shot glass, about 50 milliliters (2 ounces). Overeating of solid foods is consequently less likely, because rapid vomiting would result. The smaller stomach also promotes more rapid satiety. With the enforced food reduction, about 75% of people with severe obesity eventually lose 50% or more of excess body weight. The surgery's success at long-term loss maintenance often leads to dramatic health improvements, such as reduced blood pressure and correction of adult-onset diabetes. Risk of death from the surgery itself is about 1%.[13]

Gastroplasty has disadvantages. The surgery is costly and often not covered by medical insurance. Months of difficult adjustments face the dieter who has chosen this drastic approach to weight loss. Nutrient deficiencies are also possible if an appropriate diet and nutrient supplement plan is not followed. This surgery is not reversed, even after the desired weight loss is attained. Thus, however successful for weight loss, gastroplasty still requires major, life-long lifestyle changes.

Very-low-calorie diets. If more traditional diet changes have failed, treating severe obesity with a **very-low-calorie diet (VLCD)** is possible.[27] Optifast is one such commercial program. Some researchers believe people with body weight greater than 30% above their healthy weight are also appropriate candidates. The diet allows a person to eat 400 to 800 kcal per day, often in liquid form. (These diets were known earlier as protein-sparing modified fasts.) Of this amount, about 30 to 120 grams (120 to 480 kcal) is carbohydrate. The rest is high-quality protein, which supplys about 70 to 100 grams per day (280 to 400 kcal). This low carbohydrate intake often causes ketosis, which may decrease hunger. However, the main reasons for weight loss are the minimal energy allowed and the absence of food choice. About 3 to 5 pounds can be lost per week; men tend to lose at a higher rate than women. When physical activity and weight training augment this diet, a greater loss of adipose tissue occurs. Careful physician monitoring is crucial throughout this very restrictive form of diet therapy.

Weight regain remains a nagging problem with this type of therapy. If behavioral therapy and physical activity supplement a long-term support program, maintenance of the weight loss is more likely but still difficult. Any program under consideration should include a maintenance plan.

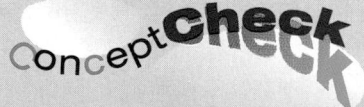

Severely obese people who have failed to lose weight with conservative weight-loss strategies may consider other options. Their doctors may recommend undergoing surgery to reduce the volume of the stomach to approximately 50 milliliters or following a very-low-calorie diet plan containing 400 to 800 kcal per day. Careful physician monitoring is crucial in both cases.

TREATING UNDERWEIGHT

Underweight can be caused by a variety of factors, such as anorexia nervosa, cancer, infectious disease, digestive tract disorders, and excessive physical activity. Genetic background may also lead to a higher resting metabolic rate, a slight body frame, or both. Significant underweight is also associated with increased death rates, especially

Very-low-calorie diet (VLCD)
Also known as a protein-sparing modified fast (PSMF), this diet allows the consumption of 400 to 800 kcal per day, generally in a liquid form. Of this, about 120 to 480 kcal comes from carbohydrate; the rest comes from mostly high-quality protein.

Spot-reducing using diet and physical activity is not possible. Physical activity may firm the tissue by tightening the muscles present, but the fat decreases only as other fat stores in the body generally decrease. "Problem" local fat deposits can be reduced in size, however, using suction lipectomy. Lipectomy means surgical removal of fat. A pencil-thin tube is inserted into an incision in the skin, and the fat tissue, such as that in the buttocks and thigh area, is suctioned. This procedure carries risks such as infection, lasting depressions in the skin, and blood clots that can lead to kidney failure. It can also be quite painful. It is designed to help a person lose about 4 pounds per treatment. It can be used as part of cosmetic surgery by an experienced physician to help reduce localized fat deposits that are very diet resistant, such as those in the outer and inner thighs and stomach. Cost is about $1600 per site.

Underweight

Body weight for height about 15% to 20% below healthy weight, or a body mass index below about 19. These cut-offs are less precise than for obesity because this condition has been less studied.

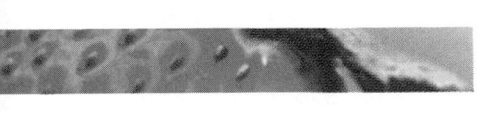

when combined with cigarette smoking. Health problems associated with underweight include the loss of menstrual function, complications with pregnancy and surgery, and slow recovery after illness. We frequently hear about the risks of obesity, but seldom of underweight. In our culture, being underweight is much more socially acceptable than being obese.

Sometimes being underweight requires medical intervention. A physician should be consulted first to rule out hormonal imbalances, depression, cancer, infectious disease, digestive tract disorders, excessive physical activity, and other hidden disease, such as anorexia nervosa and bulimia nervosa.

The causes of underweight are not altogether different from the causes of obesity. Internal and external satiety-signal irregularities, rate of metabolism, hereditary tendencies, and psychological traits can all contribute to underweight.

In growing children the demand for energy to support physical activity and growth can cause underweight. During growth spurts in adolescence, active children may not take the time to consume enough energy to support their energy needs. Moreover, gaining weight can be a formidable task for an underweight person. More than 500 extra kcal per day may be required to gain weight, even at a slow pace, in part because of the expenditure of energy in adaptive thermogenesis. In contrast to the weight loser, the weight gainer may need to increase portion sizes and learn to like new energy-dense foods.

When underweight requires a specific intervention, one approach for treating adults is to gradually increase their consumption of energy-dense foods (foods that provide a great deal of energy in a small volume), especially those high in vegetable fat. Italian cheeses, nuts, and granola can be good energy sources with low saturated fat content. Dried fruit and bananas are energy-dense fruit choices. If eaten at the end of a meal, they don't cause early satiety. Underweight people should replace such foods as diet soft drinks with good energy sources like fruit juices.

Keeping a daily food record for weekly review can help point toward wise high-energy food choices (the right side of Table 10-4 lists some possible choices). In addition, encouraging a regular meal and snack schedule aids in weight gain and maintenance. Sometimes people who are underweight have experienced stress at work or have been too busy to eat. Making regular meals a priority may not only help them attain an appropriate weight, but may also help with digestive disorders, such as constipation, which are sometimes associated with irregular eating times.

Physically active people can reduce activity. If their weight remains low, they may add muscle mass through a resistance (weight-lifting) program, but they must increase their energy intake to support that physical activity. Otherwise, weight gain will be hindered.

If these efforts fail to achieve the desired weight, they should at least prevent health problems associated with being underweight. After achieving that, they may have to accept their very lean frames.

Summary

➤ Energy balance is energy intake minus energy output. Negative energy balance occurs when energy output surpasses energy intake, resulting in weight loss. Positive energy balance occurs when energy intake is greater than energy output. The result is weight gain.

➤ Groups of cells in the hypothalamus and other regions in the brain affect hunger, the primarily internal desire to find and eat food. These cells monitor nutrients and other substances in the blood and read low amounts as a signal to promote feeding.

➤ A variety of external (appetite-related) forces affect satiety. Hunger cues combine with appetite cues, such as easy availability of food, to promote feeding.

➤ In America the major determinants of food intake are probably appetite-driven forces because food is so readily available. The physiological influences affecting food consumption are often suppressed or ignored.

➤ Basal metabolism, the thermic effect of food, physical activity, and adaptive thermogenesis account for total energy use by the body. Basal metabolism, which represents the minimum energy expenditure needed to keep the resting, awake body alive, is primarily affected by lean body mass, surface area, and thyroid hormone concentrations. Physical activity represents energy use above that expended at rest. The thermic effect of food represents the increase in metabolism to facilitate the digesting, absorbing, and processing of nutrients recently consumed. Adaptive thermogenesis is heat production caused by overfeeding or a cold environment. Brown adipose tissue may be the active heat-producing tissue in adaptive thermogenesis. About 70% to 80% of energy use is accounted for by basal metabolism and the thermic effect of food in a primarily sedentary person.

➤ Energy use by the body can be measured directly from heat output or indirectly from oxygen uptake, carbon dioxide output, or both. Energy use by the body can be estimated using formulas based on various combinations of body weight with degree of physical activity and age.

➤ A person of healthy weight shows good health and performs daily activities without weight-related problems. A body mass index (weight [in kilograms] ÷ height^2 [in meters]) of 19 to 25 is one measure of healthy weight, although weight in excess of this value may not lead to ill health. This suggests that healthy weight is best determined in conjunction with a thorough health evaluation by a physician.

➤ Obesity is usually defined as total body fat percentage over 25% in men and 30% to 35% in women. A body mass index over 27 to 30 also represents obesity. Being 20% over healthy body weight is another measure of obesity.

➤ Fat distribution partially determines health risks from obesity. Upper body fat storage distribution (waist-to-hip circumference ratio greater than 1.0 in men or greater than 0.80 in women) suggests higher risks of hypertension, heart disease, and diabetes associated with obesity than does lower body fat distribution.

➤ Genetic factors influence the tendency toward obesity. Basal metabolism and body fat distribution both have genetic links. How a person is raised (or nurtured) also influences the tendency toward obesity, because family members often develop similar eating habits and activity patterns. Obesity can be viewed as nurture allowing nature to be expressed.

➤ Those in search of a treatment for obesity should remember these five points: (1) a focus on healthy lifestyle rather than weight loss per se is more appropriate for many potential and current dieters; (2) the body resists weight loss; (3) the emphasis should be on preventing obesity because curing the disorder is very difficult; (4) weight loss should represent mostly a loss of fat storage and not primarily the loss of muscle and other lean tissues; and (5) rapid weight loss and quick regain can be harmful to physical and emotional health.

➤ A sound weight-loss diet meets the dieter's nutritional needs by emphasizing low-fat and nonfat food choices from the Food Guide Pyramid; it adapts to the dieter's habits, consists of readily obtainable foods, strives to change poor eating habits, stresses regular physical activity, and stipulates the participation of a physician if weight is to be lost rapidly or if the person is over 35 years of age and plans to perform substantially greater physical activity than usual.

➤ A pound of adipose tissue lost or gained—the fat itself plus lean support tissue—represents approximately 2700 kcal. Thus if energy output exceeds energy intake by about 400 kcal per day, a pound of fat storage can be lost per week. Decreasing the intake of high-fat foods is probably the best way to obtain this energy deficit, along with increasing physical activity.

➤ Physical activity as part of a weight-loss program should be focused on duration rather than intensity. Ideally, approximately 200 or more kcal should be expended in vigorous activity each day.

➤ Behavior modification is a vital part of a weight-loss program because the dieter may have many habits that encourage overeating and thus discourage weight maintenance. Specific behavior-modification techniques, such as stimulus control and self-monitoring, can be used to help change problem behavior.

➤ Treatment of severe obesity includes surgery to reduce stomach volume to approximately 50 milliliters or very-low-calorie diets containing 400 to 800 kcal per day. Both these measures should be reserved for people who have failed at more conservative approaches to weight loss. They require close medical supervision.

➤ Underweight can be caused by a variety of factors, such as excessive physical activity and genetic background. Sometimes being underweight requires medical intervention. A physician should be consulted first to rule out ongoing disease. The underweight person may need to increase portion sizes and learn to like new energy-dense foods. In addition, encouraging a regular meal and snack schedule aids in weight gain and maintenance. A physically active person can reduce aerobic activity and substitute some resistance exercise (weight training).

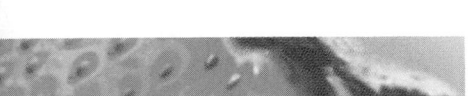

Study Questions

1 After reexamining the internal and external forces associated with hunger, satiety, and food intake, propose two hypotheses for the development of obesity.

2 Knowing the four contributors to human energy expenditure, propose four hypotheses for the development of obesity, based on the classes of energy expenditure.

3 Define a way to achieve a healthy weight that makes the most sense to you.

4 Describe a practical method to define obesity in a clinical setting.

5 What are the two most convincing pieces of evidence that both genetic and environmental factors play significant roles in the development of obesity?

6 What three health problems do obese people typically face? Describe a possible reason that each problem arises.

7 When searching for a sound weight-loss program, what three key characteristics would you look for?

8 Define the term *behavior modification*. Relate it to the terms *stimulus control, self-monitoring, chain breaking, relapse prevention,* and *cognitive restructuring*. Give examples of each.

9 Describe the type of physical activity you would suggest for someone who is obese.

10 Why should the treatment of obesity be viewed as a lifelong commitment rather than just a short episode of weight loss?

11 If a friend or relative told you he or she had found a great new vitamin and mineral supplement that allows the loss of 12 pounds in 2 weeks, how would you respond?

References

1 Abernathy RP, Black DR: Healthy body weights: an alternative perspective, *American Journal of Clinical Nutrition* 63(suppl):448S, 1996.

2 Atkinson RL, Hubbard VS: Report on the NIH workshop on pharmacologic treatment of obesity, *American Journal of Clinical Nutrition* 60:153, 1994.

3 Bourchard C: Long-term programming of body size, *Nutrition Reviews* 54(2)S8, 1996.

4 Bruce B, Wilfley D: Binge eating among the overweight population: a serious and prevalent problem, *Journal of the American Dietetic Association* 96:58, 1996.

5 Cassell JA: Social anthropology and nutrition: a different look at obesity in America, *Journal of the American Dietetic Association* 95:424, 1995.

6   Christakis G, Miller-Kovach K: Maintenance of weight goal among Weight Watchers lifetime members, *Nutrition Today* 31:29, 1996.

7   Committee to Develop Criteria for Evaluating the Outcomes of Approaches to Prevent and Treat Obesity, Food and Nutrition Board, Institute of Medicine, National Academy of Sciences: Summary: weighing the options—criteria for evaluating weight-management programs, *Journal of the American Dietetic Association* 95:96, 1995.

8   Considine RV and others: Serum immunoreactive-leptin concentrations in normal-weight and obese humans, *New England Journal of Medicine* 334:292, 1996.

9   de Groot LC, van Staveren WA: Reduced physical activity and its association with obesity, *Nutrition Reviews* 53:11, 1995.

10   Dwyer J: Policy and healthy weight, *American Journal of Clinical Nutrition* 63(suppl):415S, 1996.

11   Fletcher AM: *Thin for life: 10 keys to success from people who have lost weight and kept it off*, Shelburne, Vt., 1994, Chapters Publishing.

12   Fraser L: Who's the healthiest of them all? *Health*, p 76, May/June.

13   Gastrointestinal surgery for severe obesity: National Institutes of Health Consensus Development Conference Statement, *American Journal of Clinical Nutrition* 55:615S, 1992.

14   Heitmann BL and others: Dietary fat intake and weight gain in women genetically predisposed for obesity, *American Journal of Clinical Nutrition* 61:1213, 1995.

15   Hill JO, Prentice AM: Sugar and body weight regulation, *American Journal of Clinical Nutrition* 62(suppl):264S, 1995.

16   Hirsh J: Herman Award Lecture, 1994: Establishing the biological basis for obesity, *American Journal of Clinical Nutrition* 60:613, 1994.

17   Holt TL: Clinical applicability of bioelectric impedance to measure body composition in health and disease, *Nutrition* 10:221, 1994.

18   Horton TJ and others: Fat and carbohydrate overfeeding in humans: different effects on energy storage, *American Journal of Clinical Nutrition* 62:19, 1995.

19   Kaiyala KJ and others: New model for the regulation of energy balance and adiposity by the central nervous system, *American Journal of Clinical Nutrition* 62(suppl):1123S, 1995.

20   Kempen KPG and others: Energy balance during an 8-wk energy-restricted diet with and without exercise in obese women, *American Journal of Clinical Nutrition* 62:722, 1995.

21   Kuczmarski RJ and others: Increasing prevalence of overweight among U.S. adults, *Journal of the American Medical Association* 272:205, 1994.

22   Larkin M: Losing weight safely, *FDA Consumer*, January/February 1996.

23   Larson DE and others: Energy metabolism in weight stable postobese individuals, *American Journal of Clinical Nutrition* 62:735, 1995.

24   Leibel RL and others: Changes in energy expenditure resulting from altered body weight, *New England Journal of Medicine* 332:621, 1995.

25   Lewitsky DA: Imprecise control of food intake on low-fat diets. In Kotsonis FN, Mackey MA, editors: *Nutrition in the 90's*, New York, 1994, Marcel Dekker.

26   Meisler JG, St Jeor S: Summary and recommendations from the American Health Foundation's Expert Panel on Healthy Weight, *American Journal of Clinical Nutrition* 63(suppl):474S, 1996.

27   National Task Force on the Prevention and Treatment of Obesity: Very low-calorie diets, *Journal of the American Medical Association* 270:967, 1993.

28   Ogle GD and others: Body-composition assessment by dual-energy x-ray absorptiometry in subjects aged 4-26, *American Journal of Clinical Nutrition* 61:746, 1995.

29   Owen OE: Regulation of energy and metabolism. In Kinney JM and others, editors: *Nutrition and metabolism in patient care*, Philadelphia, 1988, WB Saunders.

30   Read N and others: The role of the gut in regulating food intake in man, *Nutrition Reviews* 52:10, 1994.

31   Rippe JM: Overweight and health: communications, challenges, and opportunities, *American Journal of Clinical Nutrition* 63(suppl):470S, 1996.

32   Saltzman E, Roberts SB: The role of energy expenditure in energy regulation: findings from a decade of research, *Nutrition Reviews* 53:209, 1995.

33   Saris WHM: Physical inactivity and metabolic factors as predictors of weight gain, *Nutrition Reviews* 54(4): S110, 1996.

34   Weinsier RL and others: Metabolic predictors of obesity, *Journal of Clinical Investigations* 95:980, 1995.

35   Williamson DF: "Weight cycling" and mortality: how do the epidemiologists explain the role of intentional weight loss? *Journal of the American College of Nutrition* 15:6, 1996.

36   Young TK, Geiskey DE: Is noncentral obesity metabolically benign? *Journal of the American Medical Association* 274:1939, 1995.

37   Zelasko CJ: Exercise for weight loss: what are the facts? *Journal of the American Dietetic Association* 95:1414, 1995.

R A T E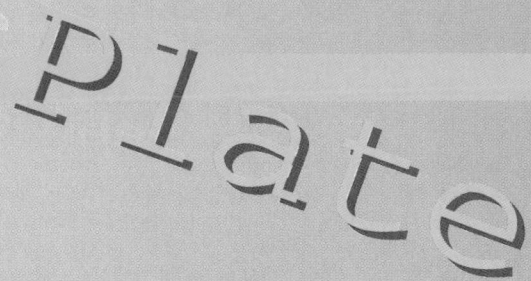

A Close Look at Your Weight Status

Determine the following two indices of your body status: body mass index and waist-to-hip ratio.

BODY MASS INDEX (BMI)

Record your weight in pounds: _____ lb.

Divide your weight in pounds by 2.2 to determine your weight in kilograms (kg): _____ kg.

Record your height in inches: _____ in.

Divide your height in inches by 39.3 to determine your height in meters (m): _____ m.

Calculate your BMI using the following formula:

BMI = Weight (kg)/height(m)^2

BMI = _____ kg/ _____ m^2 = _____

WAIST-TO-HIP RATIO

Use a tape measure to measure the circumference of your waist (at the umbilicus with stomach muscles relaxed) and hips (widest point).

Circumference of waist (umbilicus) = _____ in.

Circumference of hips = _____ in.

Calculate your waist-to-hip ratio using the following formula:

Circumference of waist/circumference of hips

Waist to hip ratio = _____ in/ _____ in = _____

INTERPRETATION

1. When BMI is greater than 25, health risks from obesity begin. It is especially advisable to attempt weight loss if your BMI exceeds 30. Does yours exceed 25?

   Yes _____   No _____

2. When a person is greater than 20% above healthy weight, a waist-to-hip ratio exceeding 1.0 in men and 0.8 in women suggests upper body obesity. This is associated with an increased risk of heart disease, high blood pressure, and diabetes.

   If appropriate, does your ratio exceed the standard for your gender?

   Yes _____   No _____

3. Do you feel you need to pursue a program of weight loss?

   Yes _____   No _____

APPLICATION

From what you've learned in this chapter, what habits could you change in patterns of eating and physical activity to lose weight and help ensure maintenance of any loss?

_____

_____

_____

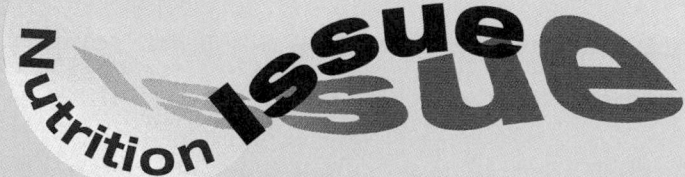

Fad Diets—Why All the Commotion?

Many overweight people try to help themselves using the latest **fad** diet book. But as you will see, most of these diets do not help, and some can actually harm those who follow them (Table 10-6).

You may wonder why fad diet books exist at all. Why doesn't the government put a stop to them? Many contain blatant misinformation. However, FDA concerns itself only when products are suspected of doing serious harm, as in the case of earlier forms of liquid protein diets. FDA is too busy to pursue every new fad diet plan. Ancient advice is still valid: "Let the buyer beware." Responsibility rests with the authors and publishers, who want to sell books and earn money and know there is little risk involved. Making outrageous claims sells more books than writing "eat less fat and walk more."

It is illegal in the United States to falsely represent worthless or dangerous cures and medical devices. Thus U.S. citizens can use their rights under federal law to have FDA pursue a seller of a dangerous fad diet book in an attempt to have it removed from the market.

HOW TO RECOGNIZE A FAD DIET

Earlier in this chapter are listed criteria for evaluating weight-loss programs with regard to their safety and effectiveness. In contrast, fad diets typically share some different common characteristics. We list a few here:

1. They promote quick weight loss. As mentioned before, this loss primarily results from glycogen, sodium, and lean muscle mass depletion. All lead to a loss of body water.
2. They limit food selections and dictate specific rituals, such as eating only fruit for breakfast.
3. They use testimonials from famous people and tie the diet to well-known cities, such as Beverly Hills and New York.
4. They bill themselves as "cure-alls." These diets claim to work for everyone, whatever the type of obesity or whatever the person's specific strengths and weaknesses.
5. They often recommend expensive supplements. Some of these supplements can be harmful because of high doses of vitamin A, vitamin D, or vitamin B-6.
6. No attempts are made to permanently change eating habits. Dieters follow the diet until the desired weight is reached and then revert to old eating habits—they are told to eat rice for a month, lose weight, and then return to old habits.
7. They are generally critical of and skeptical about the scientific community. They suggest that physicians and registered dietitians do not really want people to lose weight. They encourage people to look outside the medical establishment for correct advice.

Probably the cruelest characteristic of fad diets is that they essentially guarantee failure for the dieter. These diets are not designed for permanent weight loss. Habits are not changed, and the food selection is so limited that the person cannot follow the diet in the long run (Figure 10-14). Although dieters assume they have lost fat, they have actually lost mostly muscle and other lean tissue mass. As soon as they begin eating normally again, the lost tissue is replaced. In a matter of weeks, most of the

B.C.

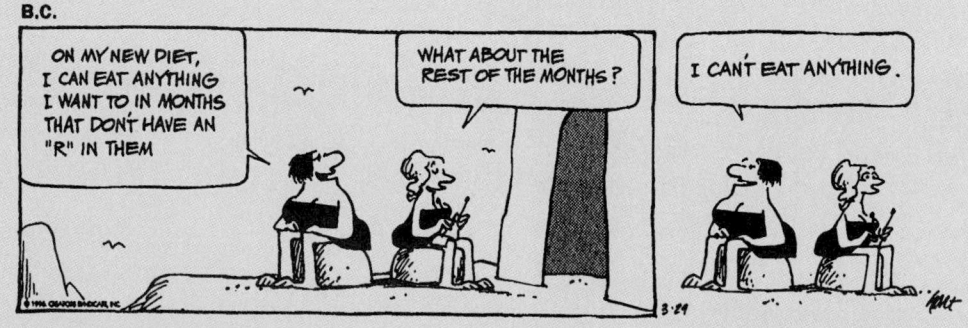

Figure 10-14 *B.C.*

Continued.

TABLE 10-6

Summary of Popular Diet Approaches to Weight Control

Approach and examples*	Characteristics and possible negative health consequences
MODERATE CALORIE RESTRICTION	
The Setpoint Diet	Usually 1000-1800 kcal per day, with moderate fat intake
Slim Chance in a Fat World	Reasonable balance of macronutrients
Weight Watcher's Diet	Encourage exercise
The American Heart Association Diet	May employ behavioral approach
Mary Ellen's Help Yourself Diet Plan	
The Beyond Diet	Acceptable if vitamin and mineral supplement is used and permission of family physician is granted
Staying Thin	
Nutripoints	
The Good Calorie Diet	
The Callaway Diet	
Living Without Dieting	
Fast Food Diet	
50 Ways to Lose Your Blubber	
Take It Off. Keep It off	
MACRONUTRIENT RESTRICTION **Low or restricted carbohydrate**	
Dr. Atkins' Diet Revolution	Less than 100 g of carbohydrate per day
Calories Don't Count	
Wild Weekend Diet	Ketosis; reduced exercise capacity due to poor glycogen stores in the muscles; excessive animal fat intake
Miracle Diet for Fast Weight Loss	
Drinking Man's Diet	
Woman Doctor's Diet for Women	
The Doctor's Quick Weight Loss Diet	
The Complete Scarsdale Medical Diet	
Four Day Wonder Diet	
Endocrine Control Diet	
Air Force Diet	
Enter the Zone	
Protein Power	
The Five-Day Miracle Diet	
Low fat	
The Rice Diet Report	Less than 20% of energy from fat
The Macrobiotic Diet (some versions)	Limited (or elimination of) animal protein sources; also all fats, nuts, seeds
The Pritikin Diet	
The Tokyo Diet	
The Palm Beach Lifelong Diet	Little satiety; flatulence; possibly poor mineral absorption from excess dietary fiber; limited food choices sometimes leads to deprivation
The James Coco Diet	Not necessarily to be avoided, but certain aspects of the plan possibly unacceptable
The 35+ Diet	
7-Week Victory Diet	
Fat to Muscle Diet	
T-Factor Diet	
Fit or Fat	
Two Day Diet	
Complete Hip and Thigh Diet	
The Maximum Metabolism Diet	
The Pasta Diet	
The McDougall Plan	
Ultrafit Diet	
Stop the Insanity	
G-Index Diet	
Eat More, Weigh Less	
Outsmarting the Female Fat Cell	
Foods that Cause You to Lose Weight	
Lean Bodies	

*Diets may be listed in more than one category if multiple characteristics apply.

TABLE 10-6—CONT'D

Summary of Popular Diet Approaches to Weight Control

Approach and examples	Characteristics and possible negative health consequences
NOVELTY DIETS	
Dr. Abravenel's Body Type and Lifetime Nutrition Plan (or his other books)	Promotes certain nutrients, foods, or combinations of foods as having unique, magical, or previously undiscovered qualities
Dr. Berger's Immune Power Diet	Malnutrition; no change in habits leads to relapse; unrealistic food choices lead to possible bingeing
Fit for Life	
The Rotation Diet	
The Hilton Head Metabolism Diet	
The Junk Food Diet	
The Beverly Hills Diet	
Dr. Debetz Champagne Diet	
Sun Sign Diet	
F-Plan Diet	
Fat Attack Plan	
Popcorn Plus Diet	
Jean Simpson's Numbers Diet	
Autohypnosis Diet	
The Ultrafit Diet	
The Princeton Diet	
The Diet Bible	
Bloomingdale's Diet	
The Love Diet	
Eat to Succeed	
The Underburner's Diet	
Eat to Win	
Two Day Diet	
Paris Diet	
Cabbage-Soup Diet	
VERY-LOW-CALORIE DIETS (VLCDS)	
Optifast	
Cambridge Diet	Less than 800 kcal per day
The Last Chance Diet	Also known as protein-sparing modified fasts
Genesis	
Medifast	Must be under close physician scrutiny
New Direction	Organ tissue loss—especially from the heart; low blood potassium leads to heart failure; expense; kidney stones; gout
HMR	
Ultrafast	
Thin So Fast	
FORMULA DIETS	
U.S.A. (United States of America), Inc.	
Optifast	Can help people who find it easier not to eat whole foods while dieting to lose weight
Genesis	
Cambridge Diet	Based on formulated or packaged products
Herbalife	
The Last Chance Diet	Tend to be very low-calorie diet regimens (see above); no change in habits possibly leading to increased chance of relapse; expense; constipation
Slimfast	
PREMEASURED DIETS	
Jenny Craig	Most food supplied in premeasured servings to take much of the decision making out of the process of eating
	Expense; may not allow for easy sound eating later

lost weight is back. The dieter appears to have failed, when actually the diet has failed. This whole scenario can add more blame and guilt, challenging the self-worth of the dieter—and that is very unfortunate. If someone needs help losing weight, professional help is advised. Sound nutrition and regular physical activity are the only interventions that come close to offering hope for weight loss and later weight management, and that is something fad diets rarely offer.

TYPES OF FAD DIETS
Low- or restricted-carbohydrate approaches

This is the most common form of fad diet. The low carbohydrate intake forces the liver to produce needed glucose. The source of carbons for this glucose is mostly protein tissue. Thus a low carbohydrate diet results in protein tissue loss, as well as urinary loss of essential ions, such as potassium. Since protein tissue is mostly water, the dieter loses weight very rapidly. When a normal diet is resumed, the protein tissue is rebuilt and the weight is regained.

There is nothing special about a low-carbohydrate diet in terms of weight loss. If the diet is also low in energy, it is likely to result in weight loss. However, a low-carbohydrate diet by itself does not result in more weight loss than any other type of diet.

Critical Thinking

Jenny's been invited to be a guest speaker at a very important social event at work. Looking at her wardrobe, she realizes that she's gained 10 pounds since she wore her special black dress. Because she has only 1 week to lose the excess weight, she's going to resort to a low-carbohydrate diet. What could the consequences be if Jenny goes on this diet?

Diet plans that use a low-carbohydrate approach are the Dr. Atkins' Diet Revolution, Dr. Stillman's Calories Don't Count Diet, the Scarsdale Diet, the Drinking Man's Diet, Four Day Wonder diet, and the Air Force Diet. When you see a new fad diet advertisement, look first to see how much carbohydrate it contains. If breads, cereals, fruits, and vegetables are extremely limited, you are probably looking at a low- or restricted-carbohydrate diet.

Low-fat approaches

The very-low-fat diet turns out to be a very-high-carbohydrate diet. These diets contain approximately 5% to 10% of energy intake as fat. The most notable is the Pritikin Diet. This approach is not harmful for healthy adults, but it is extremely difficult to follow. People get bored with this type of diet very quickly because they can't eat many of their favorite foods. Dieters primarily eat grains, fruits, and vegetables, which most people cannot do for very long. Eventually the person wants some foods higher in fat or protein. Thus the dieter suffers a lapse, then a relapse, and probably a collapse. These diets are just too different from the typical American diet to follow consistently. A popular diet marketed recently, the T-Factor Diet, focuses on restricting fat but is a more moderate approach than the Pritikin diet.

Novelty diets

A whole variety of diets are built on gimmicks. The Rotation Diet, for example, rotates the amount of energy ingested in an attempt to prevent the usual drop in basal metabolism associated with dieting. A woman is supposed to eat 600 kcal per day for 3 days, then 900 kcal per day for 4 days, and then 1200 kcal per day for 7 days, repeating this cycle over and over again. For men, the levels are 1200, 1500, and 1800 kcal. No scientific data show that this diet works or even how it could work. Thus it must be considered a fad diet.

Other novelty diets emphasize one food or food group and exclude almost all others. A rice diet was designed in the 1940s to lower blood pressure; now it has resurfaced as a weight-loss diet. The first phase consists of eating only rice and fruit until you can't stand them any longer. Another novelty diet is the egg diet, on which you eat all the eggs you want. On the Beverly Hills Diet, you eat mostly fruit.

The rationale behind these diets is that you can eat only eggs, fruit, or rice for just so long before becoming bored and, in theory, reducing your energy intake. However, chances are that you will abandon the diet entirely before losing much weight.

Since the 1960s grapefruits have been touted for their supposed unique ability to cause weight loss. No studies back up this claim. To add appeal to a grapefruit diet, proponents even suggest adding several "diet aids": lecithin to help release fat from the tissues, vitamin B-6 to act as a diuretic, vinegar to provide potassium, and kelp to stimulate the thyroid gland.

The most bizarre of the novelty diets proposes that "food gets stuck in your body." Fit for Life and the Beverly Hills Diet are examples. The supposition is that food gets stuck in the intestine, putrefies, and creates toxins that invade the blood and cause disease. This is utter nonsense. Nevertheless, the same idea has been promoted in health food books since the 1800s. Today, Fit for Life suggests that meat eaten with potatoes is not digested and that fresh fruit should be consumed only before noon. These recommendations are absurd. They are gimmicks that appear controversial but are really designed to sell books.

Finally, some commercial schemes are used to sell diet books. Books describing the allergy approach to dieting, for instance, suggest that diseases, including obesity, are due to food allergies. Supposedly, once your food allergies are found and treated, you will no longer have the disease. However, there is no research that supports the claim that 30% of people have food allergies, as suggested in Dr. Berger's Immune Power Diet Book. In addition, see the Sun Sign Diet if you believe in astrology, the Champagne Diet if you need a drink, or the Body Type and Lifetime Nutrition Diet if you have a "dominant" gland.

QUACKERY IS CHARACTERISTIC OF FAD DIETS

Fad diets fall under the category of quackery, people taking advantage of others. They usually involve a product or service that costs a considerable amount of money. Often those offering the product or service don't realize that they are promoting quackery, because they were victims themselves. For example, they tried the product and by pure coincidence it worked for them, so they wish to sell it to all their friends and relatives.

Recent examples of quackery in the field of weight loss are thigh-reducing creams, chromium picolinate, and "Quickly." The thigh-reducing creams contain aminophylline, an asthma drug, that is thought to increase fat metabolism. The product was in fact developed by obesity researchers famous in the scientific community; there is a legitimate science behind the concept. However, the researchers did not intend their work to be on the market yet. Few people using the product have been carefully studied, and there are still many other unanswered questions that have serious implications, such as "Where does the fat go?" Allergic reactions to the product are also possible.

Numerous other gimmicks for weight loss have come and gone and are likely to resurface. If in the future an important aid for weight loss is discovered, you can feel confident that major journals, such as the *Journal of the American Dietetic Association*, the *Journal of the American Medical Association*, or the *New England Journal of Medicine*, will report it. You don't need to rely on paperback books or newspaper advertisements for information about weight loss.

Chromium picolinate, a nutritional supplement, has been touted as an aid for reducing body fat, increasing lean body mass, suppressing hunger, and increasing metabolic rate. However, chromium picolinate has not been approved for weight loss by FDA, nor has the agency seen any convincing data on the claims being made.

"Quickly" is a product that was marketed for weight loss. After about 5000 containers were sold, they were found to contain significant amounts of the prescription drug furosemide, a powerful diuretic. Furosemide is used for people who have congestive heart failure and liver and kidney disease. The unsupervised use of this product could have serious health implications.

Usually, quackery harms only the bank account. However, it can lead to life-threatening results. The rule of thumb upon seeing a new diet aid on the market is that if it sounds too good to be true, it is.

NUTRITION

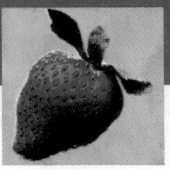

Athletics and Fitness

YOUR MUSCLES AND ORGANS use a lot of energy when you dash across the street or smash a backhand across the net. Have you wondered what your body does to transform food into this energy? Understanding where this energy comes from and how it is used is fascinating even if you don't compete in sports.

Then, once your muscles have energy available to them, what determines the type of fuel they use? *You* do, to an extent, depending on how physically fit you are and how hard you perform. Physical fitness, defined as the ability to do moderate to vigorous activity without undue fatigue, affects your fuel use. Diet also has an effect, especially for athletes who expend 2000 or more kcal per day in physical activity.[22]

In this chapter, you will also discover how physical fitness benefits the entire body; it is an essential ingredient in achieving maximal health.[20] Another basic reason to be physically fit is, of course, that it's fun and it feels good. Some people are active simply because they're enjoying it, whether they're swimming, playing basketball, or engaging in any of innumerable other activities. Let's now look further at nutrition as it relates to fitness.

CHAPTER 11

How Physically Active Are You?

How physically active are you really? Here are five activity levels: (1) sedentary, (2) mostly inactive, (3) moderately active, (4) active, and (5) superactive. Each category is defined below. Your task is to track your activities for the next 3 weeks (even if this class ends before 3 weeks). Assign yourself an activity level each week. Then average the three values and place yourself (X) in the appropriate place on the ladder. Note that you may end up halfway between two classifications.

(5) Superactive—

One hour of vigorous activity at least 5 days per week. Examples are full-court basketball, mountain climbing, treadmill work, soccer, and other similar activities.

(4) Active—

Thirty minutes of sustained activity at least 5 days per week. Examples are swimming, tennis singles, cycling, jogging, cross-country skiing, and walking briskly.

(3) Moderately Active—

Twenty minutes of sustained activity at least 3 days per week or 10 to 15 minutes of sustained activity at least 4 days a week. Examples include tennis doubles, downhill skiing, skating, aerobic dancing, golf, and similar activities.

(2) Mostly Inactive—

Sustained activity fewer than 3 days per week that usually involves mostly walking. Examples include fishing, bowling, and sporadic jogging.

(1) Sedentary—

Most activities are limited to sitting or minimal walking.

What kind of program of regular physical activity would allow you to move up the ladder, if appropriate?

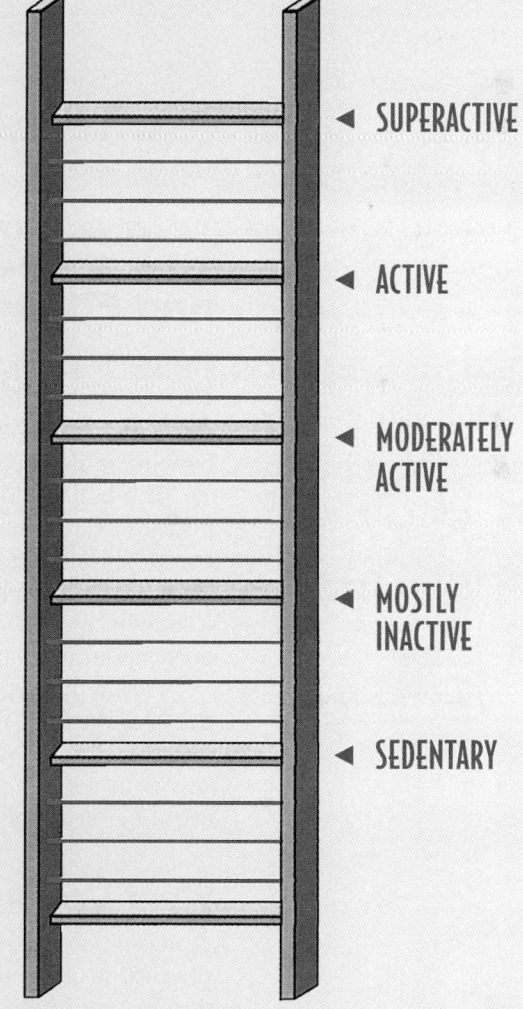

◄ SUPERACTIVE

◄ ACTIVE

◄ MODERATELY ACTIVE

◄ MOSTLY INACTIVE

◄ SEDENTARY

Key Chapter Concepts

- A gradual increase to regular physical activity is recommended for all healthy persons. Any one over age 35 is recommended to consult a physician first.
- A minimum plan for physical activity includes a total of at least 30 minutes per day. A more intense program should begin with warm-up exercises to increase blood flow and warm the muscles and end with cool-down exercises.
- Human metabolic pathways extract chemical energy from foodstuffs and transfer it into ATP, the compound that provides energy for body functions.
- In glycolysis, glucose is broken down into a three-carbon compound, yielding some ATP. The three-carbon compound is metabolized further via the aerobic pathway to form carbon dioxide (CO_2) and water (H_2O) or via the anaerobic pathway to form lactic acid.
- At rest, muscle cells mainly use fat for fuel, forming carbon dioxide (CO_2) and water (H_2O). For intense exercise of short duration, muscles use mostly phosphocreatine (PCr) for energy.

During more sustained intense activity, muscle glycogen breaks down into lactate.
- For endurance exercise, both fat and carbohydrate are used as fuels; carbohydrate is used increasingly as activity intensifies. Little protein is used to fuel muscles.
- Anyone who exercises regularly should consume a diet that is moderate to high in carbohydrates and that follows the Food Guide Pyramid. Weekend athletes are advised to do the same, because the many health benefits experienced add to those from the physical activity.
- Athletes should consume enough fluid to minimize loss of body weight and ultimately restore preexercise weight. Sports drinks aid fluid, electrolyte, and carbohydrate replacement. Their use should be considered when continuous activity lasts beyond 60 to 90 minutes.
- Rather than waiting for a magic bullet to enhance performance, athletes should concentrate their efforts on improving training routines and sport technique and consuming well-balanced diets. Adequate fluid and carbohydrate are the primary diet-related ergogenic (work-producing) aids.

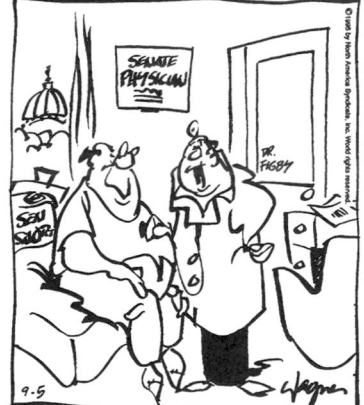

GRIN AND BEAR IT

"You need to get less rest."

Figure 11-1
Grin and Bear It.

The Close Relationship Between Nutrition and Fitness

The ability to engage routinely in vigorous physical activity requires good health. The ability to perform also depends on a nutritious diet that supplies all the needed nutrients. Adequate fluid and carbohydrate intakes are especially important for enhancing athletic performance.[12,16]

The benefits of regular physical activity are many: improvement in several aspects of heart function, fewer injuries, better sleep habits, and improvement in body composition (less body fat, more muscle mass). Physical activity can also reduce stress and positively affect blood pressure and blood glucose regulation. In addition, it aids in weight control and later weight maintenance, by both raising resting energy expenditure and increasing overall energy expenditure.[2]

For the most part, nutrition influences physical activity, and physical activity influences nutrient use and general health.[27] Unfortunately, as noted in Chapter 10, many American adults lead sedentary lives. Did that discussion motivate you to assess your activity patterns and improve them as needed? In other words, will you avoid being simply a spectator throughout your life (Figure 11-1)?

What Can a Physically Active Lifestyle Promise?

Many Americans have become interested in the potential health benefits of regular physical activity. Increasing evidence suggests that physical activity may delay the onset of and help treat many chronic diseases that plague adults. Furthermore, although increasing your physical activity is hardly a cure-all, moderate physical activity can improve your health and your chance of living longer.[20] The best news is that you do not have to work out like a world-class athlete to reap most of the benefits. "No pain–no gain" does not apply—a moderate approach suffices.[17]

Improving overall physical fitness. Physical fitness can be divided into two components: skill-related fitness and health-related fitness. The elements composing skill-related fitness include agility, balance, coordination, speed, power, and reaction time. Skill-related fitness is more important for athletic competition. Health-related fitness—a more important focus for the general population—includes the elements of endurance, body composition, and muscular-skeletal fitness. The last consists of flexibility, muscular strength, and muscular endurance. In general, a program of regular physical activity **(aerobic training)** will produce beneficial **cardiovascular** changes, including increases in heart size and strength. Muscle strength and flexibility should also improve, especially if resistance activities **(anaerobic training)** are added, such as work with dumbbells.[14] In all, these attributes allow a person to do everyday tasks such as climbing stairs and carrying books or groceries with ease; they enhance the enjoyment of recreational sports by making it possible to achieve high degrees of performance; and they provide protection against injury and improve body composition by increasing lean body mass and decreasing fat mass. All of this promotes a more positive self-image.[2]

Reducing heart-disease risk. Regular physical activity can produce changes in the cardiovascular system that decrease the risk of heart attack, such as increasing heart size and pumping capacity and enlarging the arteries that supply the heart with blood. Exercise also has a favorable effect on many risk factors for cardiovascular disease, including high blood pressure, blood lipids, obesity, diabetes, and stress, and it even helps to control smoking.[28]

Prevention and treatment of obesity. Although obesity is most commonly treated with energy restriction (that is, dieting), a combination of dieting and physical activity is preferable to dieting alone. Losing weight solely by dieting usually entails losing lean tissue as well as body fat. Performing regular physical activity in addition to dieting usually spares some of this lean tissue loss, while promoting the loss of fat tissue.[29]

Physical activity stimulates fat mobilization and the preferential use of fat for energy, assists in better control of appetite, increases energy expenditure during and after exercise, and helps the body more precisely balance energy intake and expenditure after a meal. All these factors help maintain optimal body composition.[25] Physical activity can also help prevent or reverse development of other diseases associated with obesity, including diabetes, high blood pressure, and heart disease.

Preventing and controlling diabetes. Physical activity contributes to weight loss in obesity, which in turn enhances the action of the hormone insulin. Blunted insulin action is characteristic of the adult-onset form of diabetes (NIDDM), the predominant type of diabetes in the United States. Enhancing insulin sensitivity in those who have NIDDM and use insulin can also make possible a reduction in insulin dosage. The benefits of insulin action are also short-lived, so regular moderate physical activity is encouraged.[28]

To perform exercise safely, a person with diabetes must work with a physician to make the correct alterations in diet and medications. This precaution is necessary because physical activity can adversely affect some people by inducing low blood glucose.

Reducing osteoporosis risk. Osteoporosis is a disease that leads to a high risk for bone fracture caused by bone loss. Physical activity, particularly moderate weight-bearing exercise, can help prevent osteoporosis. An extremely sedentary lifestyle

Aerobic training
In common usage this refers to activities that work the lungs and heart at a moderate to vigorous pace for a continuous period of time, such as brisk walking, jogging, swimming, or cycling. Duration is a key attribute of these types of activities

Cardiovascular
Pertaining to the heart and blood vessels.

Anaerobic training
In common usage this refers to activities that consist of bursts of energy expenditure followed by a rest period, such as weightlifting or sprinting. Intense, short-term exertion is a key attribute of these types of activities.

Regular physical activity is also linked to a decreased risk of colon cancer and possibly breast cancer.

causes bone loss. Bone loss also occurs under conditions of prolonged bed rest or weightlessness, such as that experienced by astronauts in space. Experts agree that regular moderate physical activity is important for bone health, especially among older persons, who are generally at great risk of osteoporosis. The agility and strength developed from regular physical activity can reduce the likelihood of both falls and injuries caused by falls.[29]

Enhancing psychological health. One of the most important habits that anyone can develop to improve mood state and manage stress is regular physical activity. Good scientific evidence supports regular physical activity as a means of reducing depression, anxiety, and mental stress, while increasing psychological well-being and mental cognition. It may even make us feel good simply because we believe it will.[2]

Designing a Fitness Program

For healthy people, a gradual increase in regular physical activity is recommended. People who are 35 years or older, who have been inactive for many years, or who have an existing health problem should talk to a physician before increasing activity. Health problems that require medical evaluation before beginning an exercise program are obesity, heart disease (or family history of it), high blood pressure, diabetes (or family history), shortness of breath after mild exertion, and arthritis.[14]

Phase I: Getting Started Means Getting Going

During the first phase of a fitness program, you should begin to incorporate short periods of physical activity into your daily routine. This includes brisk walking, stair climbing, house cleaning, gardening, and other activities that cause you to "huff and puff" a bit. The goal is a total of 30 minutes of this moderate type of physical activity each day—in bursts lasting at least 10 minutes—expending an average of 200 total kcal[20] (Table 11-1). Experts suggest starting small, building up to a total of 30 minutes of activity incorporated into each day's tasks, such as gardening, raking leaves, and climbing stairs. If you can't find this much time for activity, go for more intensity in the activities you can fit in to get the same benefits.

Any physical activity that leads to energy use of more than 300 kcal per hour in a typical woman or 350 kcal per hour in a typical man is especially helpful (Table 11-2). These vigorous activities are especially effective for establishing and maintaining fitness. Note that only about 1 in 10 adults practices vigorous activities daily.

The easiest way to increase physical activity is to make it part of your daily routine, similar to other regular activities, such as eating. Many people find that the best time to exercise is when they need an energy pick-me-up or a break from work. Rather than abandon an exercise program entirely when obstacles impede, strive to use any small periods of available time. As you begin to enjoy exercising and reaping its benefits, you'll tend to spend more time at it.

Clearly, many of the activities recommended for Phase I are not very vigorous. By recommending Phase I for those starting an exercise program, fitness experts have not given up on the value of vigorous physical activity. They're just making concessions to human nature.[20]

Phase II: Seeking Greater Fitness Requires Greater Exertion

Once on the path of regular moderate-intensity activity, you can add more intense activities to reap even more health benefits. Suggested activities include brisk walking, jogging, cycling, and swimming. The goal is 30 minutes of such vigorous activity

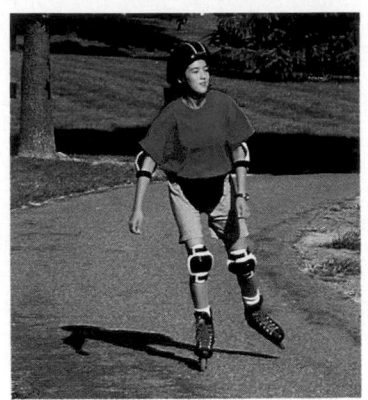

Your goal should be to stay physically active throughout your life.

TABLE 11-1

Your Exercise Prescription

Fitness component	Definition	Activities
Flexibility	The ability to bend without injury; it is dependent on elasticity of muscles, tendons, and ligaments, and condition of joints.	Stretches will enhance flexibility. They should be held for 10 to 20 seconds. Never use bouncy, choppy, or painful stretches that twist or put pressure on joints.
Strength	The ability to work against resistance.	Using 1 to 5 sets (8 to 12 repetitions per set) with weights as heavy as is safely possible will increase strength. The more sets the better, but even one aids in muscle development and later maintenance.
Muscle endurance	The ability of a muscle to sustain effort over a period of time.	Repetitive exercises, such as push-ups, pull-ups, sit-ups.
Cardiovascular endurance	The ability of the cardiovascular system to sustain effort over a period of time; it should involve larger muscle groups and be performed at 65% to 80% of maximum heart rate (220 − your age).	Activities include fast walking, jogging, swimming, bicycling, and stair climbing. These can provide the needed sustained, submaximal work if the exercise is performed at an appropriate pace.

THE PLAN

Warm-up: 5-10 minutes of stretching the whole torso. Start with smaller muscle groups (arms) and work toward larger muscle groups (legs and abdomen).

5-10 minutes more of exercises, such as walking, slow jogging, or any slow version of anticipated activity. Low-intensity movement literally warms up muscles so that muscle filaments slide more easily over one another and will gradually bring heart rate up to target range.

Workout: 20 or more minutes of rhythmic continuous activity 5 or more times a week at a pace that raises heart rate to within target range. Modify pace or workload as necessary so that the heart rate reaches and does not exceed target range. A good rule of thumb is that you should still be able to converse. Popular aerobic conditioning activities include brisk walking, jogging, swimming, cycling, cross-country skiing, and aerobic dance. Activities such as basketball and racquetball provide a good workout, but because the heart rate jumps up high and then drops and then goes up again, they do not condition the heart as rhythmic continuous activities do. Exercises that develop muscular strength and endurance can follow the aerobic session or alternate with it on different days. Resistance exercises, such as weight training or calisthenics, encourage muscle maintenance and are particularly important in weight-reducing diets in order to maintain muscle mass.

Cool-down: Follow a reverse pattern of warm-up: 5-10 minutes of low-intensity activity and 5-10 minutes of stretching. The same exercises performed during warm-up are appropriate. The cool-down is essential to the prevention of injury and soreness.

TABLE 11-2

Approximate Energy Costs of Various Activities for a 150-Pound (68-Kilogram) Person

Activity	Kcal per hour
Aerobics—heavy	544
Aerobics—light	204
Aerobics—medium	340
Backpacking	612
Basketball—vigorous	680
Bicycling (5.5 MPH)	204
Bowling	265
Calisthenics—heavy	544
Calisthenics—light	272
Canoeing (2.5 MPH)	224
Cleaning (female)	253
Cleaning (male)	236
Cooking	190
Cycling (13 MPH)	659
Dressing/showering	106
Driving	117
Eating (sitting)	93
Food shopping	245
Football—touch	476
Golf	244
Horseback trotting	346
Ice skating (10 MPH)	394
Jogging—medium	612
Jogging—slow	476
Lying—at ease	89
Racquetball—social	544
Roller-skating	346
Running or jogging (10 MPH)	897
Skiing (10 MPH)	598
Sleeping	80
Swimming (.25 MPH)	299
Tennis	414
Volleyball	346
Walking (2.5 MPH)	204
Walking (3.75 MPH)	299
Water skiing	476
Weight lifting—heavy	612
Weight lifting—light	272
Window cleaning	240
Writing (sitting)	118

From *Mosby Diet Simple,* Salem, Oregon N-Squared Computing..

at least 5 days per week. Some resistance exercise, (for example, push-ups, sit-ups, and weight training) should also be performed at least 2 to 3 days per week. Pushing a little past fatigue is fine, but when arms or legs start shaking uncontrollably, it's time to ease up. Ignoring pain can almost guarantee an injury.

This basic exercise program should begin with warm-up exercises, primarily designed to increase blood flow and warm the muscles.[14] Warming up reduces the risk of injuries (Figure 11-2). Activities to increase muscular strength, endurance, and flexibility should follow. Cool-down exercises finish the program. Table 11-1 shows how to design a cardiovascular workout program. Fitness target heart rates for adults are about 65% to 80% of predicted maximum heart rate (220 minus current age).

GARFIELD   *BY JIM DAVIS*

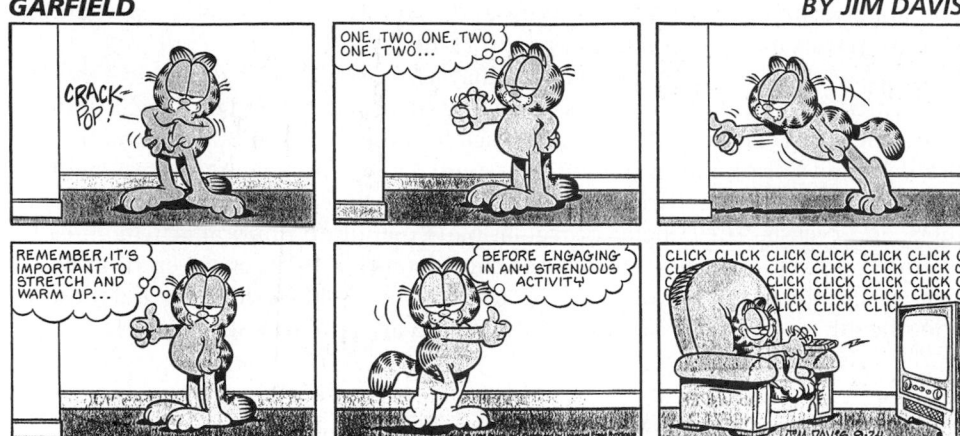

Figure 11-2 *Garfield.*

To determine whether you are in the target exercise zone, learn to count your pulse. Placing a hand over your heart is a simple method. However, because clothing may obscure the beat, putting light pressure on either large artery at the side of your neck is best. You can also feel a full pulse at your wrist or inside the bend of the elbow. Count your pulse immediately after stopping exercise because the rate changes very quickly once exercise slows or stops. Find the beat within a second, and count for 10 seconds . Multiply this number by 6 to obtain the count for a minute. Do not count for the whole minute or even for 15 seconds, because the fall-off rate after exercise is too fast.

Including several types of enjoyable physical activities in a fitness program is important, as is making sure to start gradually and work up to longer times. Doing too much too soon is a quick way to extinguish enthusiasm and determination. A new trend in exercising is cross-training, in which a variety of exercises are incorporated into a fitness program. For example, instead of jogging for 30 minutes, you might swim for 15 minutes and then jog for 15 minutes. Adding variety to a program not only keeps you mentally fresh but also strengthens different muscle groups and reduces risk of injury. Variety also keeps the program interesting. An exercise partner may offer additional motivation.

Brisk walking is a good way to ease into a regular aerobic exercise routine.[2] After a few weeks, you can speed up to a jog or start an aerobic dance program. Vigorous programs for overweight people should be non–weight-bearing activities, such as swimming and bicycling.

In moderate activity a good pace should allow you to talk comfortably without becoming short of breath. This minimizes muscle fatigue. A beginner could switch from brisk walking to jogging and back again every couple of minutes. Gradually the walking time can be decreased and the jogging time extended. Because jogging or running may be stressful to the knees, selecting proper shoes is very important, as is seeking an appropriate running surface, such as a track.

Whatever physical activities you include in your fitness program, they should be enjoyable and done regularly and willingly. This way they can become routine. Consider convenience, cost, and options for bad weather so that when motivation wanes, you are not adding further obstacles. Overall, do what you enjoy, but start

The next chapter lists many guidelines for setting goals and sticking to them. These suggestions are useful in meeting the goal to perform regular physical activity.

out small, committing to keep on track and maintaining reasonable expectations. Positive results may take a month or so to be noticeable.

Realize also that harmful side effects may accompany excessive physical activity. The list of complications includes an increased risk of muscular-skeletal injuries, heat illness, sudden death from heart attack, respiratory infections, gastrointestinal problems, and disturbances in mood, sleeping habits, and appetite, not to mention impaired performance. These complications are most common in runners, swimmers, and cyclists. The benefits of regular participation in physical activity must be balanced against these risks, which rise considerably with excessive exertion or activity. Still, although vigorous exercise involves minimal health risks for those in good health, far greater risks exist for those who are primarily sedentary.[20]

Metabolism Sets the Stage for Physical Activity

Like all cells, muscle cells need energy to perform work. Cells need to capture this energy and then release it to do the work demanded.

A discussion of this process—energy **metabolism**—must start with the definition of *metabolism*. This term refers to all chemical processes that take place in the body. Any sequence of a chemical process from beginning to end (for example, burning glucose for fuel) is called a *pathway.*

Metabolic pathways can produce both **anabolic** and **catabolic** results. Anabolic pathways build compounds. In these pathways the typical building blocks—oxygen (O_2), water (H_2O), and carbon dioxide (CO_2)—are used to form new, larger compounds. These parts can be combined to form a fatty acid or glucose. Energy input is required to fuel the building process.

Conversely, catabolic pathways—which break down compounds into smaller units—often release energy. Glucose and fatty acids, for example, are catabolized when broken down into carbon dioxide and water. Energy is released as a by-product. Anabolic and catabolic pathways take place simultaneously in cells.[26]

Generally speaking, the catabolism needed for energy producton from food-stuffs occurs in two stages. In the first stage, large compounds in food—proteins, starches, and triglycerides—are broken down during digestion into smaller units, such as amino acids, simple sugars, and fatty acids. These units are then delivered to working cells, such as muscle cells, via the bloodstream. In this second stage these compounds are eventually broken down into carbon dioxide and water inside the cell. During this second process, large amounts of energy are released to power the cell.[26]

ATP: Energy a Cell Can Use

The energy that fuels the body originates as solar energy. Plants capture the energy through the process of **photosynthesis.** As discussed in Chapter 5, plants use solar energy to produce carbohydrates, proteins, and fats. In essence, plants trap solar energy and store it as chemical energy in these nutrients. Every amino acid, glucose, and fatty acid molecule contains a specific amount of chemical energy stored within the chemical bonds that hold the substance together. When these bonds are broken, the energy that is released can be used to perform cellular work.

One key function of metabolism is to convert energy stored in foodstuffs to a form human cells can use. Generally, each cell must first break down glucose, fatty acids, or other energy-rich sources to release stored energy and then convert that energy into usable and smaller energy packets.

As you may have guessed from the discussion so far, however, cells can't directly use the energy released from breaking down glucose or fat. Rather, the energy must

---

Metabolism

Chemical reactions occur in the body, enabling cells to release energy from foods, convert one substance into another, and prepare end products for excretion.

Pathway

A metabolic progression of individual steps from starting materials to end products, such as glucose → CO_2 + H_2O

Anabolism

The process of building compounds.

Catabolism

The process of breaking down compounds.

Almost every step in any metabolic pathway depends on input from an enzyme to allow the step to take place.

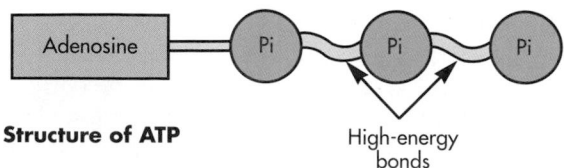

Structure of ATP

High-energy bonds

first be stored in a special form known as **adenosine triphosphate (ATP)**. To store chemical energy, our cells make ATP from its breakdown product **adenosine diphosphate (ADP)** and a phosphate group (abbreviated as Pi). Again, the cells are using the energy obtained from foodstuffs. Conversely, to release energy from ATP, cells partially break down ATP to ADP and Pi. This releases usable energy for cell functions.[26]

ADP + Energy from foodstuffs + Pi → ATP

ATP → Energy to do work + ADP + Pi

Essentially, ATP is the immediate source of energy for body functions. This includes locomotion. The primary goal in the use of any fuel, whether carbohydrate, fat, or protein, is to make ATP. A resting muscle cell has only a small amount of ATP that can be used. If no resupply of ATP were possible, this stored ATP could keep the muscle working maximally for only about 2 to 4 seconds. Fortunately, several types of chemical compounds—**phosphocreatine (PCr)**, carbohydrates, fats, and proteins—can be broken down to release enough energy to make more ATP. Cells must constantly and repeatedly use and then re-form ATP.[26]

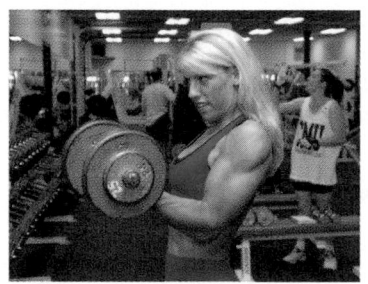

Bursts of muscle activity use a variety of fuel sources (see Table 11-3).

ANOTHER Bite

Think about ATP the next time you race after a bus. When you finally sit down, you are exhausted, you breathe hard, and your heart races. Your muscle cells have used up most of their ATP and other high-energy compounds. While you rest, muscle cells begin to resynthesize the ATP used up during your run. Reforming ATP requires energy. Again, cells can get this energy from foodstuffs. If you sit long enough, you can then race off to class using some of the newly formed ATP.

Phosphocreatine Is the First Line of Defense for Resupplying ATP in Muscles

The instant that breakdown products of ATP begin to accumulate in the contracting muscle, an enzyme is activated to split PCr. This releases energy that can be used to re-form ATP from its breakdown products. If no other source of energy for ATP resupply were available, PCr could probably maintain maximal muscle contractions for about 10 seconds. Because other ATP resupply sources kick in, however, PC ends up the major source of energy for all events lasting up to about 1 minute[14] (Figure 11-3).

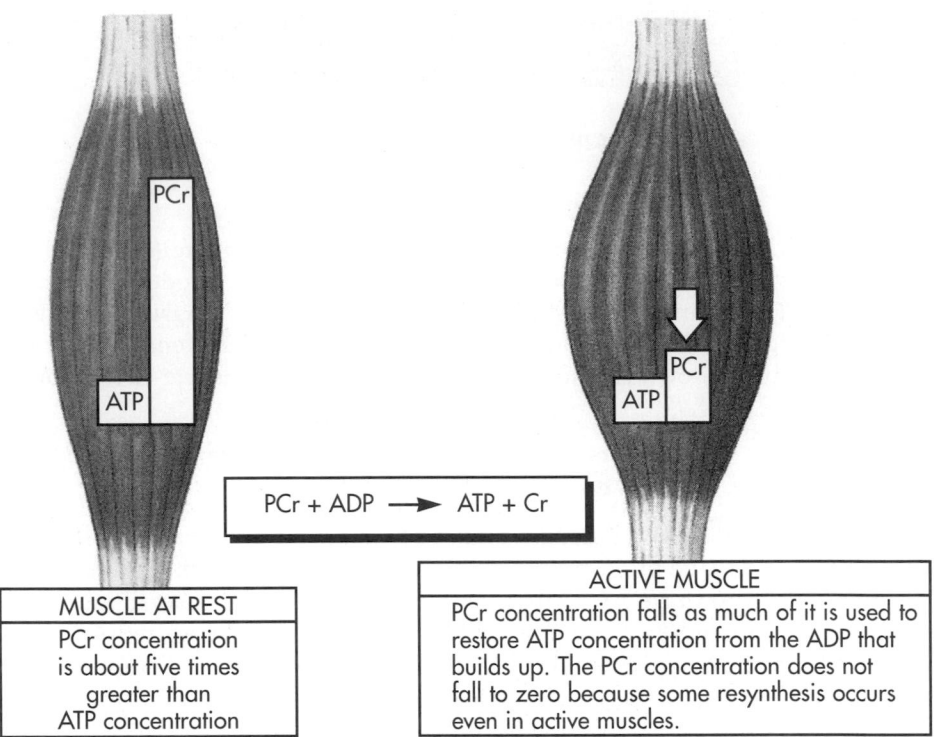

Figure 11-3
Quick energy for muscle use includes a supply of phosphocreatine (PCr). This can rapidly replenish adenosine triphosphate (ATP) stores as activity begins. PCr can be almost totally depleted in maximally contracting human forearm muscles in less than 60 seconds. Replenishing 95% of the PCr then takes 4 minutes of rest. Similarly, about 7 minutes of rest are required to replenish 95% of the PCr depleted with repeated knee extensions against resistance.

PCr + ADP ⟶ ATP + Cr

MUSCLE AT REST
PCr concentration is about five times greater than ATP concentration

ACTIVE MUSCLE
PCr concentration falls as much of it is used to restore ATP concentration from the ADP that builds up. The PCr concentration does not fall to zero because some resynthesis occurs even in active muscles.

The main advantage of PCr is that it can be activated instantly and can replenish ATP at rates fast enough to meet the energy demands of the fastest and most powerful actions, including jumping, lifting, throwing, and sprinting. The disadvantage of PCr is that not enough of it is made and stored in the muscles to sustain a high rate of ATP resupply for more than a few minutes.

Releasing the Energy in Carbohydrate Begins with Glycolysis

Carbohydrates are an important fuel for muscles. The most useful form of carbohydrate fuel is the simple sugar glucose, available to all cells from the bloodstream. The breakdown of liver glycogen (a storage form of glucose) helps maintain blood glucose. Breakdown of glycogen stored in a particular muscle also helps meet the carbohydrate demand of that muscle. In the catabolic pathway that breaks down glucose—called *glycolysis* (*glyco* means sugar, and *lysis* means breakdown)—the six-carbon glucose splits into two three-carbon compounds. The net energy released equals two ATPs, or about 5% of the total number of ATPs that can be made from one glucose.[26]

Although this phase of glucose metabolism does not extract much energy from a single glucose molecule, a muscle cell can break down thousands of glucose molecules per second. Therefore this form of glucose metabolism can resupply ATP at a very high rate for a brief period.

When glucose breaks down, the resulting three-carbon compound follows one of two main routes. When oxygen supply in the muscle is limited (**anaerobic** conditions) and when the exercise is intense (for example, running 400 meters or swimming 100 meters), the three-carbon compound accumulates in the muscle and is converted to **lactic acid.** No further ATP is directly formed. This conversion of glucose to lactic acid is called *anaerobic glycolysis.* Carbohydrate is the only fuel that can be used for this process[26] (Table 11-3).

If plenty of oxygen is available in the muscle (**aerobic** conditions) and the exercise is of moderate to low intensity (for example, jogging or distance swimming), the bulk of the three-carbon compound is shuttled to the **mitochondria** of the cell,

Glycolysis
The pathway that results in the breakdown of glucose into two three-carbon compounds.

Anaerobic
Not requiring oxygen.

Lactic acid
A three-carbon acid formed during anaerobic cell metabolism; a partial breakdown product of glucose; also called lactate.

Aerobic
Requiring oxygen.

Mitochondria
The main sites of energy production in a cell. Structure inside most cells, including muscle cells. Mitochondria also contain the pathway for burning fat for fuel, among other metabolic pathways.

TABLE 11-3

Energy Sources Used by Resting and Working Muscle Cells

Source/system*	When in use	Examples of an exercise
ATP	At all times	All types
Phosphocreatine (PCr)	All exercise initially; extreme exercise thereafter	Shotput, jumping
Carbohydrate (anaerobic)	High-intensity exercise, especially lasting 30 seconds to 2 minutes	200-yard (20-meter) sprint
Carbohydrate (aerobic)	Exercise lasting 2 minutes to 4 to 5 hours; the higher the intensity (for example, running a 6-minute mile), the greater the use	Basketball, swimming, jogging
Fat (aerobic)	Exercise lasting more than a few minutes; greater amounts are used at lower exercise intensities	Long-distance running, long distance cycling; much of the fuel used in a brisk walk is fat
Protein (aerobic)	Low quantity during all exercise; moderate quantity in endurance exercise, especially when carbohydrate fuel is lacking	Long-distance running

*Note that at any given time more than one system is operating.

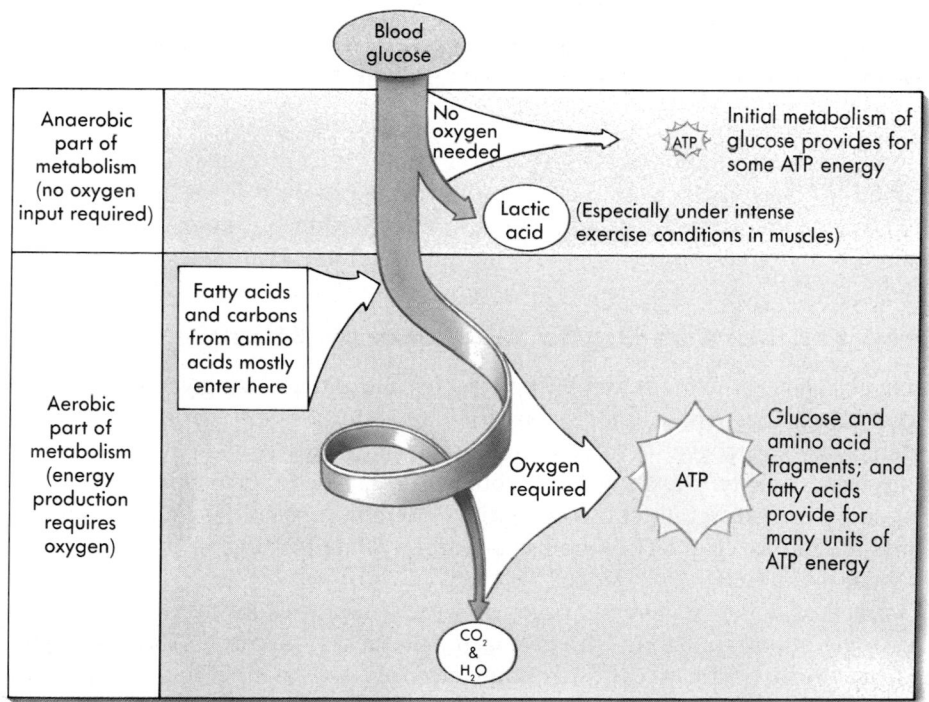

Figure 11-4

Carbohydrate, fat, and protein fuels can all supply energy to form ATP for a muscle cell. Carbohydrate can follow both aerobic and anaerobic pathways, whereas fat and protein are limited for the most part to the aerobic pathway.

where it is further metabolized into carbon dioxide (CO_2) and water (H_2O). This process is known as aerobic glycolysis, because the breakdown of glucose in this manner uses oxygen. This aerobic stage of glycolysis forms approximately 95% of the ATP made from complete glucose metabolism to carbon dioxide and water[26] (Figure 11-4).

Anaerobic Glycolysis Yields Energy Fast

The advantage of anaerobic glycolysis is that it is the fastest way to resupply ATP, other than PCr breakdown. Anaerobic glycolysis provides most of the energy for events ranging from about 30 seconds to 2 minutes. The two major disadvantages of anaerobic glycolysis are that (1) the high rate of ATP production cannot be sustained for long events and (2) the rapid accumulation of lactic acid greatly increases the acidity of the muscle. This acid inhibits the activities of key enzymes in the glycolysis pathway, slowing anaerobic ATP production and causing fatigue.[26]

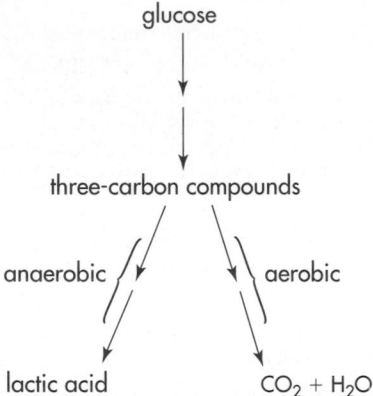

For the most part, lactic acid accumulates in active muscle cells until it is released into the bloodstream. The liver picks up the lactic acid and resynthesizes it into glucose. Glucose can then reenter the bloodstream, where it is available for cell uptake and breakdown. The heart can also use the lactic acid directly for its energy needs, as can less active muscle cells situated near active ones.[14]

Aerobic Glycolysis Yields Energy More Slowly But Does Not Produce Lactic Acid

Aerobic glycolysis supplies ATP more slowly than does anaerobic glycolysis but releases more energy. Furthermore, the slower rate of aerobic energy supply can be sustained for hours. Moreover, the end products are carbon dioxide and water, not lactic acid. Aerobic glycolysis makes a major energy contribution to activities that last anywhere from 2 minutes to 4 or 5 hours[14] (see Table 11-3).

Glycogen Versus Blood Glucose As Muscle Fuel

Muscle glycogen is the main fuel for both anaerobic and aerobic glycolysis in fairly intense muscular activities that last for less than about 2 hours. For these activities the depletion of glycogen fuel in the muscle can cause fatigue and cut in half maximal exercise capacity. Diets high in carbohydrate can be used to build up muscle glycogen stores before athletic competition, thereby forestalling fatigue and improving endurance. The technique used—carbohydrate loading—is discussed in a later section.

As exercise duration increases beyond 20 to 30 minutes, blood glucose becomes increasingly important, along with glycogen, as a fuel for glycolysis. The use of glucose from the bloodstream can spare some glycogen use, saving it in the muscle for sudden bursts of effort that may be required (for example, a sprint to the finish in a marathon race). When carbohydrate fuel (glycogen) in muscles is eventually used up, maintaining the high initial work load is difficult unless normal blood glucose concentrations are maintained by carbohydrate feedings.[10] Athletes call this point of glycogen depletion "hitting the wall," because further exertion is hampered. Thus when exertion meets or exceeds about 90 minutes, athletes (for example, long-distance runners or cyclists) should consider increasing the amount of carbohydrates stored in muscles, as mentioned before.

As people start exercising regularly four or five times a week, they experience a "training effect." Initially these people might be able to exercise for 20 minutes before tiring. Months later exercise can be extended to an hour before they feel tired. During the months of training, muscle cells have produced more mitochondria and can burn more fat. As a result, lactic acid production decreases. Because it contributes to muscle fatigue, the less lactic acid produced, the longer the exercise can continue. Part of the training effect derives also from the increased aerobic efficiency of heart and muscle action.

Many researchers have studied various types of carbohydrate feedings during exercise to maximize glucose supply to muscles. Overall, the techniques have succeeded. Carbohydrate feedings of about 30 to 80 grams per hour during strenuous endurance exercise can aid in maintaining adequate blood glucose, resulting in delay of fatigue by 30 to 60 minutes.[18] This issue is also discussed in a later section.

Fat: The Main Fuel for Prolonged Low-Intensity Activity

When fat stores in body tissues are broken down for energy, one triglyceride molecule first yields three fatty acids and a glycerol. The majority of the stored energy is found in the fatty acids. During physical activity the fatty acids are released from various fat depots into the bloodstream and travel to the muscles, where they are taken into each cell and broken down aerobically to carbon dioxide and water (see Figure 11-4).

The rate at which muscles use fatty acids partly depends on the concentration of fatty acids in the bloodstream. In other words, the more fatty acids that are released from fat stores into the bloodstream, the more fat will be used by the muscles. Recently, some athletes have attempted to raise their blood concentrations of fatty acids by consuming caffeinated beverages. This practice can actually increase fatty-acid release from the fat depots and is therefore helpful to some athletes, but it is illegal under International Olympic rules if the amount of caffeine in the body exceeds the equivalent of 6 to 8 cups of coffee (see the Nutrition Issue in this chapter).

Fat is ultimately not a very useful fuel for intense, brief exercise, but it becomes a progressively more important energy source as duration increases, especially when exercise remains at a low or moderate (aerobic) rate for more than 20 minutes[10] (Figure 11-5). The reason for this is that some of the steps involved in fat breakdown simply cannot occur fast enough to meet the ATP demands of short-duration, high-intensity exercise. If fat were the only available fuel, we would be unable to exercise beyond a fast walk or jog.

The advantage of fat fuel is that it provides tremendous stores of energy in a relatively concentrated form, and we generally have a lot stored. For a given weight of fuel, fat supplies more than twice as much energy as carbohydrate. For very lengthy activities at a moderate pace (for example, hiking), manual labor in a foundry, or even sitting at a desk for 8 hours a day, fat supplies about 70% to 90% of the energy required. Carbohydrate use is much less. As intensity increases, such as in a 3-hour marathon run at a competitive pace, muscles use about a 50:50 ratio of fat to carbohydrate.[14] In comparison, for short events, such as a 100-meter sprint or even a 1500-meter race, the contribution of fat used to resupply ATP is minimal. Keep in mind that the only fast-paced (anaerobic) fuel we eat is carbohydrate; slow and steady (aerobic) activity uses carbohydrate, fat, and protein for energy sources.

Does This Mean We Use Protein to Fuel Activity?

Protein—actually amino acids—can be used for fueling muscles, but in most circumstances protein contributes only about 2% to 5% of the body's general energy needs. This is also true for the typical energy needs of exercising muscles. However, proteins can contribute somewhat more to energy needs in endurance exercise, perhaps as much as 10%, especially as carbohydrate stores in the muscles are exhausted. We easily eat enough to supply this amount of fuel.[16,19] Protein or amino acid supplements are not needed. Contrary to what many athletes believe, protein is used less for fuel in resistance types of exercise, such as weight lifting, than for endurance exercise, such as running. The primary fuels for the actual act of weight lifting are PCr and carbohydrate.[14] Recent research shows that carbohydrate even enhances the anabolic effect of weight-training, probably by increasing insulin and growth hormone release into the bloodstream.[6]

The fatty acids can come from all over the body, not necessarily from depots near the active muscles. This is why spot reducing does not work. Exercise can tone the muscles underlying adipose tissue but does not preferentially use those stores. If this was not the case, we would all have lean cheeks and necks, because muscles in that vicinity are regularly used!

In terms of body fat loss, whether the activity uses primarily carbohydrate or fat as a fuel is not very important. Studies show that people who exercise hard and those who move at a more leisurely pace lose the same amount of adipose stores over time if the number of kcals expended is the same.

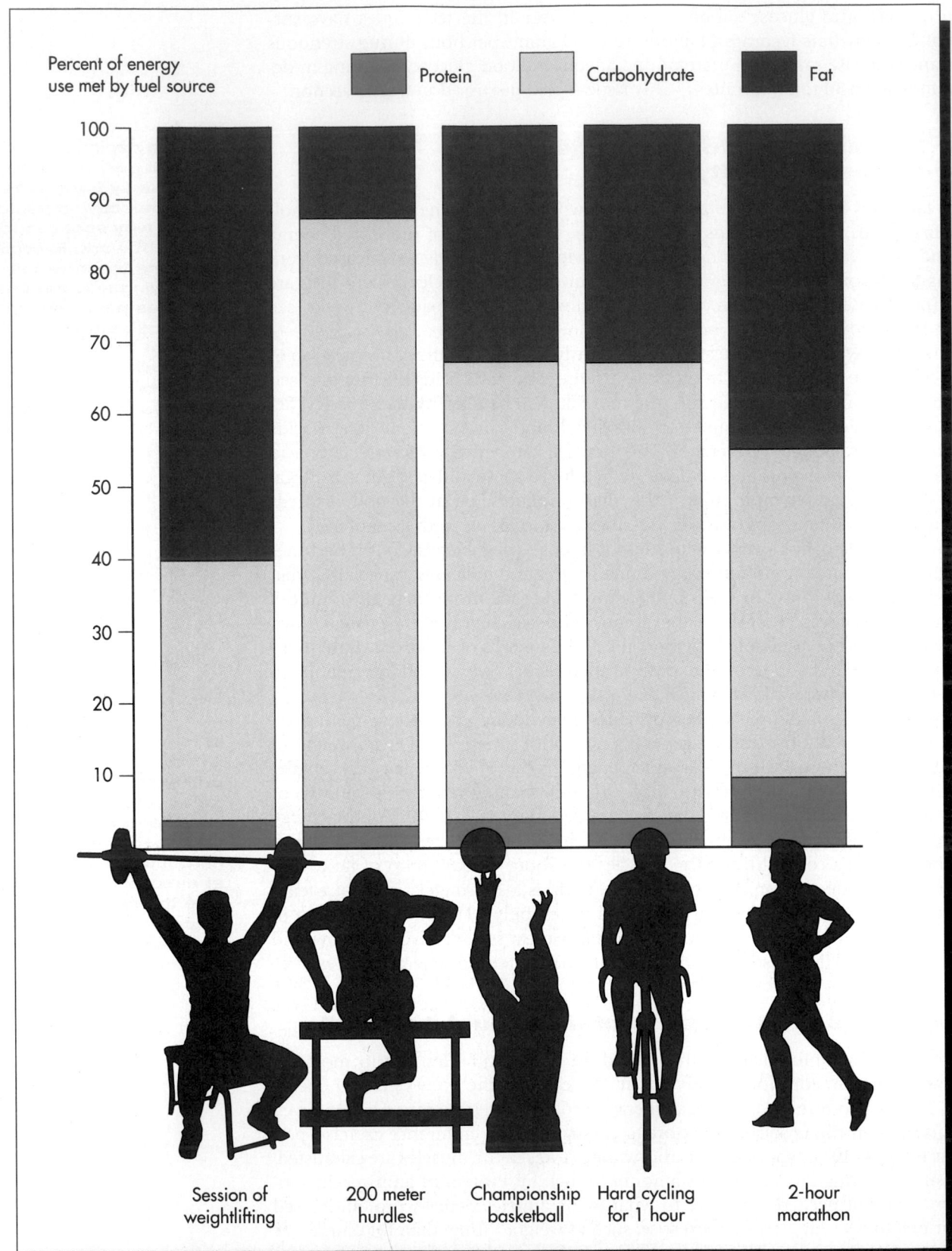

Figure 11-5 *Rough estimates of food fuel use during various forms of physical activity.*

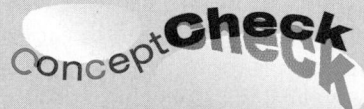

Adenosine triphosphate (ATP) is the main form of energy used by cells. Metabolic pathways use food energy to form ATP. Phosphocreatine (PCr) can rapidly reform ATP from its breakdown product adenosine diphosphate (ADP), but PCr supplies are limited. Carbohydrate metabolism to form ATP begins as glucose becomes available from the bloodstream or glycogen breakdown. In a muscle cell, each glucose molecule is broken down through a series of steps to yield either lactic acid or carbon dioxide (CO_2) plus water (H_2O). The process that occurs when glucose is broken down into carbon dioxide and water is called *aerobic glycolysis* because oxygen is used. The conversion of glucose to lactic acid is called *anaerobic glycolysis*, because no oxygen is used. This latter process allows the cell to quickly re-form ATP and supports the demand for energy during intense exercise. Fat is a key aerobic fuel for muscle cells, especially at low exercise outputs. At rest, muscles burn primarily fat for energy needs. In comparison, little protein is used to fuel muscles. Protein supplies about 2% to 5% of energy needs and, at most, 10% of energy needs during endurance events.

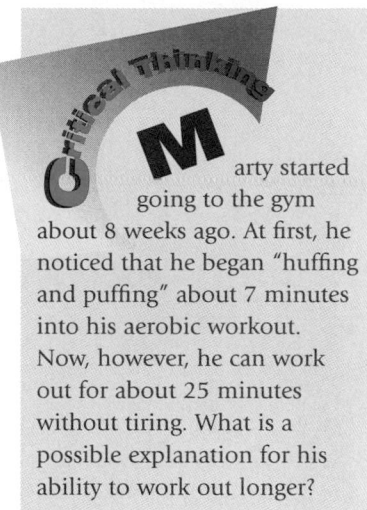

Marty started going to the gym about 8 weeks ago. At first, he noticed that he began "huffing and puffing" about 7 minutes into his aerobic workout. Now, however, he can work out for about 25 minutes without tiring. What is a possible explanation for his ability to work out longer?

Power Food: Dietary Guidelines for Athletes

Athletic training and genetic makeup are two important determinants of athletic performance. A good diet won't substitute for either factor, but as previously mentioned, diet can enhance and maximize an athlete's potential. More important, a poor diet can certainly harm performance.[22]

Determining Needed Food-Energy Intake

Athletes need varying amounts of food energy, depending on each athlete's body size and current body composition and on the type of training or competition being considered. A small person may need only 1700 kcal daily to sustain normal daily activities without losing body weight; a large, muscular man may need 4000 kcal. These rough estimates can be viewed as starting points that each athlete needs to individualize by trial and error.

The energy required for sports training or competition has to be added to the basal energy that is needed just to carry on normal activities. Energy use averages 5 to 8 kcal per minute for moderate activity; again, this is just an estimate. For example, an hour of bowling requires little energy above that which is required to sustain normal daily living. At the other extreme, a 12-hour endurance bicycle race over mountains can require an additional 4000 kcal per day.[8] Therefore some athletes may need as much as 7000 kcal daily just to maintain body weight while training, whereas others may need 1700 kcal or less.

How Can We Know Whether an Athlete Is Consuming Enough Food Energy?

The first step in assessing energy status is to estimate the athlete's body fat percentage by measuring skinfold thicknesses or using bioelectrical impedance or the underwater weighing technique (see Chapter 10). Body fat should be in the desirable range—that is, about 5% to 15% for most male athletes and 10% to 25% for most female athletes.[22] The next step is daily or weekly monitoring of body weight changes. If body weight starts to fall, food energy should be increased; if weight rises because of increases in body fat, the athlete should be encouraged to eat less.

If the body composition test shows that an athlete has too much body fat, the athlete should lower food intake by about 200 to 500 kcal per day, while maintaining a regular exercise program, until reaching the desirable fat percentage. Reducing fat intake is the best nutrient-related approach. On the other hand, if an athlete needs to gain weight, increasing food intake by 500 to 700 kcal per day will eventually lead to the needed weight gain. A mix of carbohydrate, fat, and protein is advised, coupled with enough training to make sure this gain is mostly from lean tissue, not mostly from added fat stores.

Rapid weight loss by dehydration is risky. Wrestlers, boxers, judoists, and oarsmen often try to lose weight so that they can be certified to compete in a lower weight class. This helps them gain a mechanical advantage over an opponent of smaller stature. They usually lose this weight only a few hours before stepping on the scale for weight certification. Athletes can lose up to 22 pounds (10 kilograms) of body water in 1 day by sitting in a sauna, exercising in a plastic sweat suit, or taking diuretic drugs that speed water loss from the kidneys. Losing as little as 3% of body weight by dehydration can adversely affect endurance performance.[1] A pattern of repeated weight loss or gain of more than 5% of body weight by dehydration carries some risk of kidney malfunction and heat illness (see Figure 9-4 in Chapter 9).

The practice of losing weight by dehydration is especially common in sports such as interscholastic and intercollegiate wrestling. Most competitive wrestlers probably face an opponent who has gone through the same misery to gain an "advantage." If athletes wish to compete in a lower body weight class and have enough extra fat stores, they should begin a gradual, sustained reduction in food-energy intake long before the competitive season starts. In so doing, the athlete attains a healthier body composition (less fat) while avoiding the potentially harmful and certainly misery-creating effects of severe dehydration. Athletes who have no extra body fat should not attempt to compete at a lower body weight class. Coaches and trainers must be aware of the decreased performance and serious side effects of severe dehydration.[1]

Meeting Carbohydrate Needs in the Training Diet

Anyone who exercises regularly, including the dieter, needs to consume a diet that includes moderate to high amounts of carbohydrates. The diet should include a variety of foods, in accordance with the Food Guide Pyramid. Numerous servings of starches and fruits will provide enough carbohydrate to maintain adequate liver and muscle glycogen stores, especially for replacing glycogen losses from the previous day.[3]

Carbohydrate intake should be at least 5 grams per kilogram of body weight. People engaged in aerobic training and endurance athletes (duration >60 minutes per day) may need as much as 8 to 10 grams per kilogram.[24] In other words, triathletes and marathon runners should consider eating close to 600 grams of carbohydrates daily, and even more if necessary, to (1) prevent chronic fatigue and (2) load the muscles and liver with glycogen.[10] This is especially important when performing multiple training bouts in a day, such as swim practices, or heavy training on successive days, as in cross-country running. Table 11-4 shows sample menus, based on the Food Guide Pyramid, for diets providing food energy ranging from 1500 to 5000 kcal per day. Figure 11-6 provides a number of carbohydrate-rich options for meals. In addition, the Exchange System shown in Appendix D is a very useful tool for planning all types of diets, including high-carbohydrate diets for athletes.

Note that you do not have to give up any specific food when planning a high-carbohydrate diet. Just turn to more of the best (high-carbohydrate foods) and

Critical Thinking

Joe is a wrestler who qualified for the lightweight division in his annual high school competition. After a few matches, Joe began to feel dizzy and faint. He was disqualified because he was unable to continue the match. Later, the coach found out that Joe had spent 2 hours in the sauna before weighing in, which had made him dehydrated. What are the consequences of dehydration? What can you suggest as an alternative way to lose weight?

TABLE 11-4

Sample Daily Menus Based on the Food Guide Pyramid That Provide Various Total Energy Intakes

1500 KCAL DIET
Breakfast

Skim milk, 1 cup
Cheerios, ½ cup
Bagel, ½
Cherry jam, 2 tsp
Margarine, 1 tsp

Lunch

Chicken breast (roasted), 2 oz
Figs, 1
Skim milk ½ cup
Banana, 1

Snack

Oatmeal-raisin cookie, 1
Low-fat fruit yogurt, 1 cup

Dinner

Spaghetti w/meatballs, 1 cup
Romaine lettuce, 1 cup
Italian dressing, 2 tsp
Green beans, ½ cup
Cranberry juice, 1½ cups

———
18% protein (68 grams)
64% CHO (240 grams)
19% fat (32 grams)

2000 KCAL DIET
Breakfast

Skim milk, 1 cup
Cheerios, 1 cup
Bagel, ½
Cherry jam, 1 tbsp
Margarine, 1 tsp

Lunch

Chicken breast (roasted), 2 oz
Wheat bread, 2 slices
Mayonnaise, 1 tsp
Figs, 2
Cranberry juice, 1½ cups
Banana, 1

Snack

Oatmeal-raisin cookies, 3
Low-fat fruit yogurt, 1 cup

Dinner

Broiled beef sirloin, 3 oz
Romaine lettuce, 1 cup
Italian dressing, 2 tsp
Green beans, 1 cup
Skim milk, ½ cup

———
17% protein (85 grams)
63% CHO (315 grams)
20% fat (44 grams)

3000 KCAL DIET
Breakfast

Skim milk, 1 cup
Cheerios, 2 cups
Bagel, 1
Cherry jam, 2 tsp
Margarine, 1 tsp
Oat bran muffins, 2

Lunch

Chicken breast (roasted), 2 oz
Wheat bread, 2 slices
Provolone cheese, 1 oz
Mayonnaise, 1 tsp
Figs, 3
Cranberry juice, 1½ cups
Low-fat fruit yogurt, 1 cup

Snack

Banana, 1
Oatmeal-raisin cookies, 3

Dinner

Broiled beef sirloin, 3 oz
Romaine lettuce, 1 cup
Garbanzo beans, 1 cup
Italian dressing, 2 tsp
Spinach pasta noodles, 1½ cups
Margarine, 1 tsp
Green beans, 1 cup
Skim milk, ½ cup

———
17% protein (128 grams)
62% CHO (465 grams)
21% fat (70 grams)

4000 KCAL DIET
Breakfast

Orange, 1
Cheerios, 2 cups
Skim milk, 1 cup
Bran muffins, 2

Snack

Chopped dates, ¾ cup

Lunch

Romaine lettuce, 1 cup
Garbanzo beans, 1 cup
Alfalfa sprouts, ½ cup
French dressing, 2 tbsp
Macaroni and cheese, 3 cups
Apple juice, 1 cup

Snack

Wheat bread, 2 slices
Margarine, 1 tsp
Jam, 2 tbsp

Dinner

Skinless turkey breast, 2 oz

Mashed potatoes, 2 cups
Peas and onions, 1 cup
Banana, 1
Skim milk, 1 cup

Snack

Pasta, 1 cup
Margarine, 2 tsp
Parmesan cheese, 2 tbsp
Cranberry juice, 1 cup

———
14% protein (140 grams)
61% CHO (610 grams)
26% fat (116 grams)

5000 KCAL DIET
Breakfast

Cheerios, 2 cups
Bran muffins, 2
Orange, 1
2% milk, 1 cup

Snack

Low-fat yogurt, 1 cup
Chopped dates, 1 cup

Lunch

Apple juice, 1 cup
Chicken enchilada, 1
Romaine lettuce, 1 cup
Garbanzo beans, 1 cup
Alfalfa sprouts, ¾ cup
Grated carrots, ½ cup
Seasoned croutons, 1 oz
French dressing, 2 tbsp
Wheat bread, 2 slices
Margarine, 1 tbsp

Snack

Banana, 1
Bagel, 1
Cream cheese, 1 tbsp

Dinner

2% milk, 1 cup
Beef sirloin, 5 oz
Mashed potatoes, 2 cups
Spinach pasta noodles, 1½ cups
Grated parmesan cheese, 2 tbsp
Green beans, 1 cup
Oatmeal-raisin cookies, 3

Snack

Cranberry juice, 2 cups
Air-popped popcorn, 4 cups
Figs, 3

———
14% protein (175 grams)
63% CHO (813 grams)
24% fat (136 grams)

Figure 11-6

Foods rich in carbohydrate are characteristically included in our typical meals. For the specific amount of carbohydrate in each food choice, one can use either the Exchange System to provide an estimate or Appendix A for a more exact value.

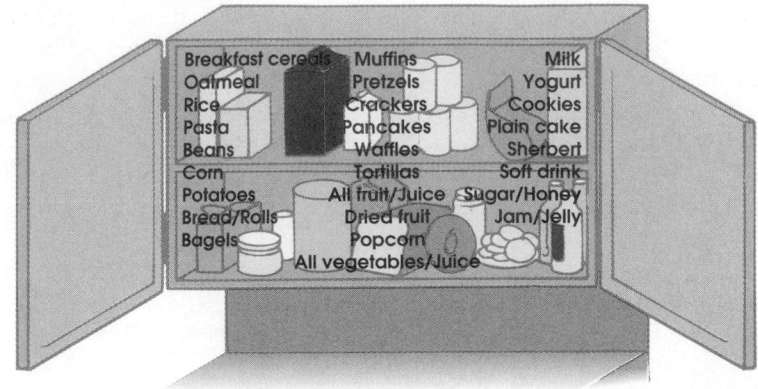

moderate the rest (concentrated fat sources). Sports nutritionists emphasize the difference between a high-carbohydrate meal and a high-carbohydrate–high-fat meal. Before endurance events, such as marathons or triathalons, some athletes seek to increase their carbohydrate reserves by eating potato chips, french fries, banana cream pie, and pastries. Although such foods contain carbohydrate, they also contain a lot of fat. Better high-carbohydrate food choices include pasta, rice, potatoes, bread, and many breakfast cereals (check the label for carbohydrate content). Sports drinks appropriate for carbohydrate loading, such as GatorLode and UltraFuel, can also help. Consuming only a moderate amount of dietary fiber during the final day of training is a good precaution to reduce the risk of bloating and intestinal gas during the next day's event.[1]

As a general rule, athletes should obtain about 60% to 70% of their total energy needs from carbohydrate, rather than the 50% typical of most American diets. Endurance athletes should meet the higher value, especially when exercise duration exceeds 2 hours. With carbohydrate intakes in this range, intake of fat should fall so that fat provides 20% to 30% of total energy needs, rather than the typical 34%. Protein then provides the rest of the total energy—about 12% to 15% of total needs.[1] This approach yields a training diet that is about two-thirds carbohydrate-rich foods and one-third protein-rich foods, with fat mainly from the many other food choices.

A further look at carbohydrate: carbohydrate loading. For athletes who compete in continuous events lasting more than 90 minutes or in shorter events repeated over a 24-hour period, undertaking a **carbohydrate-loading** regimen is often advantageous to maximize muscle glycogen stores. One possible regimen includes a gradual reduction or "tapering" of exercise intensity and duration, coupled with a gradual increase in dietary carbohydrate as a percentage of energy intake. The procedure can begin 6 days before competition, with the athlete completing a hard workout lasting about 60 minutes. Workouts for the next 4 days then last about 40, 40, 20, and 20 minutes respectively, with exercise intensities being progressively reduced each day. On the final day before competition the athlete rests.[1]

The dietary carbohydrate on the first 3 days of this regimen (about 450 grams per day) contributes 45% to 50% of energy intake. The carbohydrate contribution rises to 65% to 75% (about 600 grams per day) for the last 3 days before competition. This carbohydrate-loading technique usually increases muscle glycogen stores by 50% to 85% over typical conditions (that is, when dietary carbohydrate constitutes about 50% of the total energy intake). The greater carbohydrate stores often result in improved athletic endurance. A typical carbohydrate-loading schedule would look like this:

Carbohydrate-loading

A process in which a very high-carbohydrate diet is consumed for about 3 days before an athletic event while tapering exercise duration to try to increase muscle glycogen stores.

Days before competition	6	5	4	3	2	1
Exercise time (minutes)	60	40	40	20	20	REST
Carbohydrate (grams)	450	450	450	600	600	600

A potential disadvantage of carbohydrate loading is that some water is stored in the muscles with the extra glycogen. In some individuals this additional water weight is sufficient to detract from their sport performance, making carbohydrate loading inappropriate. Athletes considering carbohydrate loading should try it during training (and well before an important competition) to experience its effects on performance. They can then determine whether it is worth the effort.

Carbohydrate loading is safe for adolescents, but the activities for which this technique is useful, such as marathon runs, may not be. Adolescents should obtain the approval of their physician's before participating in such a regimen.

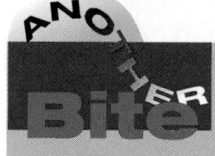

APPROPRIATE ACTIVITIES FOR CARBOHYDRATE LOADING	INAPPROPRIATE ACTIVITIES FOR CARBOHYDRATE LOADING
Marathons	American football games
Long-distance swimming	10-kilometer runs
Cross-country skiing	Walking and hiking
30-kilometer runs	Most swimming events
Triathalons	Single basketball games
Tournament-play basketball	Weight lifting
Soccer	Most track and field events
Cycling time trials	
Long-distance canoe racing	

Protein Needs Are Generally Met by a Balanced Diet That Meets Energy Needs

Typical protein-intake recommendations for athletes range from 1.2 to 1.6 grams of protein per kilogram of body weight, considerably higher than the RDA of 0.8 gram per kilogram[13,16] (Table 11-5). Athletes engaged in endurance sports should aim for the higher value, because protein supplies a greater percentage of the energy used (up to 10%) in these sports than in other athletic endeavors. Overall, the vast majority of athletes can meet protein needs without having to exceed twice the RDA (1.6 grams per kilogram).[19]

For athletes beginning a weight-training program, some experts recommend 2 to 2.5 grams of protein per kilogram of body weight, or approximately three times the RDA for protein.[3] To date, the importance of such an excessive protein intake during the initial phases of weight training has not been supported by sufficient research. Note that energy needs for weight lifting are not the reason for the high protein recommendation, because the fuel used in this activity is primarily carbohydrate. Theoretically the extra protein is required for the synthesis of new tissue brought on by the loading effect of weight training, which is the greatest during the initial phases of weight training. Once the desired muscle mass is achieved, protein intake need not exceed twice the RDA.[13,16]

Any athlete can easily have a protein intake twice the RDA by eating a variety of foods (see Table 11-4). Generally speaking, many athletes routinely consume an unnecessary amount of protein. Again, athletes do not need protein or amino acid supplements, because their diets can easily meet their protein needs.

Consuming excessive amounts of protein is not without its drawbacks. As noted in Chapter 7, it increases calcium loss in the urine.

TABLE 11-5

Grams of Protein That Meet Recommendations for Individuals of Different Weights

BODY WEIGHT		PROTEIN ALLOTMENT (GRAMS)	
Pounds	Kilograms	RDA (0.8 gram per kilogram)	2 × RDA (1.6 grams per kilogram)
110	50	40	80
130	60	48	96
155	70	56	112
175	80	64	128
200	90	72	144
220	100	80	160

Compare these quantities with protein intake from the diets listed in Table 11-4. Note that diets supplying enough total energy for athletes yield plenty of protein, even for those who make no special attempt to consume high-protein foods.[16,19]

However, athletes who feel they must significantly limit their energy intake or who are vegetarians should specifically determine how much protein they eat, making sure to choose foods that provide a daily protein intake of at least 1.2 grams per kilogram of body weight. Skimping on protein is not a good idea.

Vitamin and Mineral Intakes for Athletes: Diet Can Meet Extra Needs

Vitamin and mineral needs are the same or slightly higher for athletes compared with sedentary adults. Athletes' needs for vitamin E and vitamin C may be somewhat greater because of the antioxidant protection these nutrients provide in the face of high oxygen use by muscles.[4] Still, use of megadoses of vitamin E and vitamin C requires more study and is not currently an accepted part of dietary guidance for athletes. Riboflavin, vitamin B-6, potassium, magnesium, iron, zinc, copper, and chromium needs may also increase somewhat; these vitamins and minerals, which play a role in energy metabolism, are lost in sweat[3] (Table 11-6). Current available research suggests that any extra needs can be met by diet. In addition, because athletes usually have high food-energy intakes, they tend to consume plenty of vitamins and minerals.

Athletes who reduce their energy intake to less than 1500 to 1800 kcal to lose weight should pay close attention to their vitamin and mineral intake. Vegetarian athletes should heed the same warning, as well as athletes undergoing intense training. A good approach for such athletes is to focus on nutrient-dense foods, such as low-fat and nonfat milk, broccoli, tomatoes, oranges, strawberries, whole grains, and kidney beans. Meat-eaters should emphasize lean meat, such as lean beef, turkey, fish, and chicken. Vitamin- and mineral-fortified foods, including many breakfast cereals, are also good choices. Supplemental use of vitamins and minerals greatly exceeding 150% of the Daily Values listed on the labels is not advised.

Iron deficiency impairs performance. Athletes, especially female and adolescent athletes, should pay special attention to their iron intake.[23] In all athletes, iron stores can be depleted by both the loss of iron in sweat, urine, and gastrointestinal blood and the increased use of iron required for the elevated production of red blood cells associated with physical fitness. Another less important mechanism of iron loss is foot-strike destruction of red blood cells in the blood passing through the feet; this results from the trauma created at the point of impact when a foot strikes the ground. Young women are at special risk of iron deficiency because of the additional iron loss during menstruation.[9]

At one time in his career, long-distance runner Alberto Salazar experienced problems sleeping and performed poorly because of low iron intake and related iron-deficiency anemia. Both men and women are at risk and should regularly monitor iron status.

TABLE 11-6

Vitamins and Minerals: Functions and Usage with Regard to Exercise

Vitamins and minerals	Exercise-related function	Proposed benefit to performance	Effects of supplementation in excess of RDA/ESADDI
Thiamin	Carbohydrate metabolism	Enhances endurance performance	Likely does not enhance performance
Riboflavin	Energy metabolism	Enhances aerobic performance	Does not enhance performance; needs may increase to 1.5 times the RDA at outset of training program.
Niacin	Energy metabolism	Enhances energy metabolism	Does not enhance performance and may even impair performance by reducing fatty acid release.
Vitamin B-6	Formation of hemoglobin	Enhances exercise performance	Does not enhance performance
Pantothenic acid	Energy metabolism	Enhances aerobic performance	Does not enhance performance
Vitamin B-12	Red blood cell development	Enhances endurance performance	Does not enhance performance
Folate	Cell synthesis; red blood cell formation		Does not enhance performance
Biotin	Fat and glycogen synthesis		No studies available
Vitamin C	Antioxidant capability	Prevents tissue damage; speeds repair	Well-controlled studies show no effect on performance, but some researchers think extra amounts may reduce oxidative damage to muscle from exercise. However, diet can easily supply the 200 milligrams it takes to saturate body tissues.
Vitamin A and carotenoids	Antioxidant capability	Prevents tissue damage; speeds repair	Enhanced performance unlikely, but some researchers think extra amounts of carotenoids may reduce oxidative damage to muscle from exercise.
Vitamin D	Bone mineral metabolism	Bone formation and muscle repair	Does not affect work performance, may affect muscle building (one study), but needs likely do not exceed the RDA. Note that excess intakes can be toxic.
Vitamin E	Antioxidant capability	Prevents tissue damage; speeds repair	Does not enhance performance; may reduce exercise damage caused by breakdown in fat structure in cell membranes; research is ongoing. Needs may approach 2 times the RDA.
Zinc	Carbohydrate, fat, and protein metabolism; tissue repair	Repair of exercise damage	Does not enhance performance if diet meets the RDA.
Copper	Red blood cell synthesis; energy metabolism	Enhances aerobic performance	No studies available to show enhanced performance, but sweating increases copper losses.
Chromium	Carbohydrate metabolism; increases effects of insulin	Enhances muscle gain	Currently conflicting results in literature. May enhance muscle gain during weight training, but a study of football players did not support this hypothesis.[7] Any use should be considered experimental and should not exceed 200 micrograms per day.
Selenium	Antioxidant capability	Protects against exercise damage; delays fatigue	No conclusive studies available; note that it has a high potential for toxicity
Iron	Oxygen transport and delivery	Reduces fatigue; enhances endurance	No effect on performance in nonanemic or non–iron-deficient subjects

Primarily from Brouns F: *Nutritional needs of athletes,* Chichester, England, 1993, John Wiley & Sons.

If iron stores are not replenished, iron-deficiency anemia and markedly impaired endurance performance can eventually result. Although true anemia (noted as a depressed blood hemoglobin concentration) isn't widespread among athletes, having the blood hemoglobin concentration checked annually and monitoring dietary iron intake is wise, especially for adult women athletes. Vegetarian female athletes should be especially careful to watch iron status. If blood iron is consistently low, athletes are advised to use iron supplements. Iron supplements can improve athletic performance if an athlete is truly anemic, but indiscriminate use of iron supplements is not advised because toxic effects are possible[1] (see Chapter 9).

Calcium intake deserves attention, especially in women. Athletes, especially women trying to lose weight by restricting their intake of dairy products, can have marginal or low dietary intakes of calcium.[9] This practice compromises optimal bone health. Of still greater concern are women athletes who have stopped menstruating because their arduous training interferes with the normal secretion of the reproductive hormones. Disturbing reports show that female athletes who do not menstruate regularly have far less dense spinal bones than both nonathletes and female athletes who menstruate regularly.[11] This diminished bone density places them at increased risk for osteoporosis in later life, a subject that is discussed further in the section on the female athlete triad in Chapter 13.

Current studies suggest that a female runner who does not menstruate regularly may also be more likely to develop a **stress fracture.** Female athletes whose menstrual cycles become irregular should consult a physician to ascertain the cause. Decreasing the amount of training or increasing energy intake and body weight (or doing both) often restores regular menstrual cycles. If irregular menstrual cycles persist, severe bone loss and osteoporosis can result. Extra calcium in the diet does not necessarily compensate for the effects of menstrual loss, but inadequate dietary calcium makes matters worse. Calcium intakes up to 1500 milligrams per day have been suggested, but the most effective measure is to have menstruation resume.

Stress fracture

A fracture that occurs from repeated jarring of a bone. Common sites include bones of the foot.

Meals Before Events Should Emphasize Carbohydrate

To top off muscle and liver glycogen stores, prevent hunger during an event, and provide extra fluid (see next section also), a light meal supplying 300 to 1000 kcal should be eaten about 2 to 4 hours before the event.[1] The longer the period before an event, the larger the meal can be, because more time is available for digestion. A preevent meal should consist primarily of carbohydrate (about 70% of energy: 70 to 175 grams or more), have little dietary fiber, and include a moderate amount of fat and protein (Table 11-7). A preeevent meal eaten 1 to 2 hours before an event should be blended or liquefied to promote rapid stomach emptying.[1]

Good food choices for a preevent meal include spaghetti, bagels, muffins, bread, and breakfast cereals with low-fat or nonfat milk. Liquid meal replacement formulas, such as Carnation Instant Breakfast, can also be used. Foods rich in dietary fiber should be eaten the previous day to help clear the bowels before an event, but they should not be eaten the night or morning before the event. Foods to avoid are those that are fatty or fried, such as sausage, bacon, sauces, and gravies. A meal high in carbohydrate is quickly digested, promotes maintenance of blood glucose, and prevents the body from dipping immediately into glycogen stores. If an athlete believes a preevent meal harms performance, eating a high-carbohydrate diet the day and night before can help meet the same goal.

Because it increases release of insulin, which causes blood glucose to fall, specific carbohydrate feeding an hour or so before competition was previously thought to adversely affect performance. However, we know now that this practice causes neither premature fatigue nor decreased endurance for most people, especially if

TABLE 11-7

Convenient PreEvent Meals*

BREAKFAST (MCDONALD'S)	ENERGY CONTENT

Hot cakes with syrup and margarine
Orange juice, 2 servings
English muffin (whole) with 2 tsp margarine
  and 2 tsp jam
	900 kcal
	67% from carbohydrate
	  (150 grams)

Cheerios, $3/4$ cup Low-fat milk, 1 cup Bluberry muffin Orange juice, 1 serving	450 kcal 82% from carbohydrate (92 grams)
LUNCH OR DINNER (WENDY'S)	
Chili, 8 oz portion Baked potato with sour cream and chives Chocolate Frosty, 10 ounces	900 kcal 65% from carbohydrate (150 grams)
Grilled chicken sandwich Cola, 12 ounces	425 kcal 65% from carbohydrate (70 grams)

*Extra water would also be helpful.

they have eaten breakfast and performed adequate warm-up exercises. In fact, recent studies show positive benefits from preevent carbohydrate feeding.[16] However, some athletes are extremely sensitive to an insulin surge. Athletes should therefore experiment with preevent carbohydrate feedings to determine whether their performance is adversely or positively affected.

ANOTHER Bite

It cannot be emphasized enough that any nutrition strategies should be tested during practice and trial runs before being used in a meet or key event. An athlete should never try a new food or beverage on the day of competition. Some food items and beverages may not be well tolerated, and the day of competition is not the time to find this out.

Maximizing Body Fluids and Energy Stores During Exercise

Water (fluid) needs for an average adult are about 1 milliliter per kcal expended, or about 6 to 8 cups of fluid per day. Athletes need this and generally even more water to maintain the body's ability to regulate its internal temperature and keep itself cool. Much energy released during metabolism appears immediately as heat. Unless this heat is quickly dissipated, **heat exhaustion, heat cramps,** and deadly **heatstroke** may ensue.[15] Virtually all body heat is lost through the evaporation of sweat from the skin. Sweat loss during prolonged exercise ranges from 3 to 8 cups per hour. As the humidity rises, especially when it rises above 75 percent, evaporation slows and sweating becomes inefficient.

Increased body temperature associated with dehydration is most evident when the amount of water lost exceeds 3% of body weight. This dehydration then leads

Heat exhaustion
Heat illness that occurs when heat stress causes depletion of blood volume from fluid loss by the body. This increases body temperature and can lead to headache, dizziness, muscle weakness, and visual disturbances, among other effects.

Heat cramps
Heat cramps are a frequent complication of heat exhaustion. They usually occur in people who have experienced large sweat losses from exercising for several hours in a hot climate and have consumed a large volume of unsalted water. The cramps occur in skeletal muscles and consist of contractions for 1 to 3 minutes at a time.

Heatstroke
Heatstroke can occur when internal body temperature reaches 105°F. Sweating generally ceases if left untreated, and blood circulation is greatly reduced. Nervous system damage may ensue, and death is likely. Often the skin of individuals who suffer heatstroke is hot and dry.

Nutrition **Insight**

Sports Drinks: Most Helpful for Endurance Activities

A question that often arises is whether to drink water or a sports-type drink, such as All Sport, Exceed Energy Drink, Gatorade, Power-Ade, and Amino Force, during competition. For sports that require less than 30 minutes of exertion or when total weight loss is less than 5 to 6 pounds, the primary concern is replacing the water lost in sweat, because losses of body carbohydrate stores and **electrolytes** (sodium, chloride, potassium, and other minerals) are not usually too great. Although electrolytes are lost in sweat, the quantities lost in exercise of brief to moderate duration can be easily replaced later by consuming normal foods, such as orange juice, potatoes, and tomato juice.[12] Keep in mind that sweat is about 99% water and only 1% electrolytes and other substances.

The use of sports drinks is most critical for athletes engaged in sports events lasting longer than 60 to 90 minutes.[12] Prolonged exercise results in large sweat losses, and some of the fluid for sweating comes from the bloodstream. If plain water is used to replace the fluid lost from the blood, the concentration of essential electrolytes in the bloodstream may become too diluted. Thus when sports drinks are used to help maintain blood volume, they must contain small amounts of sodium and potassium to avoid electrolyte imbalance. Generally speaking, beverages for the endurance athlete must provide water for hydration, electrolytes to both enhance water and glucose absorption from the intestine and help maintain blood volume, and carbohydrate to provide energy. Beyond 2 to 4 hours of exertion, electrolyte and carbohydrate replacement becomes increasingly important, especially in hot weather. In fact, sports drinks that contain carbohydrate have been found to delay fatigue during endurance sports with exercise intensities of a 3-hour marathon pace.

The following is but one possible protocol for using sports drinks as part of fluid replacement[12]:

- About 20 to 30 minutes before endurance exercise, consume 1 to 2 cups of water. However, some experts recommend consuming instead the same amount of a 10% to 20% solution of carbohydrate (25 to 50 grams of carbohydrate per 8-ounce cup of fluid). Drinks such as GatorLode, UltraFuel, and CarboForce have carbohydrate concentrations in the higher range.
- Once exercise begins, consume 1 cup of a 6% to 8% carbohydrate solution (14 to 19 grams per cup of fluid) every 15 to 20 minutes, totaling about 45 to 60 grams of carbohydrate and up to 4 cups (1 liter) per hour. The carbohydrate concentration of many common sports drinks is 6% to 8%, but check the label to be sure (Figure 11-7).
- After $1\frac{1}{2}$ to 2 hours of exertion, switch back to a drink with a higher carbohydrate concentration (10% to 20%), and continue consuming 1 cup every 15 to 20 minutes.

Comparisons of drinks containing **glucose polymers** (glucoses linked together, more properly known as *maltodextrins*), glucose, and sucrose show that all of these carbohydrates have similar positive effects on exercise performance and physiologial function as long as the carbo-

Glucose polymer
Carbohydrate sources used in some sports drinks that consist of a grouping of a few glucose molecules.

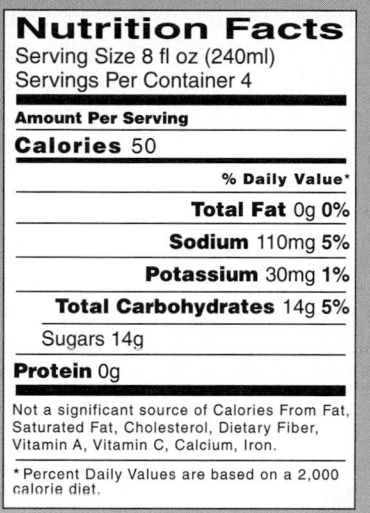

Nutrition Facts

Serving Size 8 fl oz (240ml)
Servings Per Container 4

Amount Per Serving

Calories 50

	% Daily Value*
Total Fat 0g	0%
Sodium 110mg	5%
Potassium 30mg	1%
Total Carbohydrates 14g	5%
Sugars 14g	
Protein 0g	

Not a significant source of Calories From Fat,
Saturated Fat, Cholesterol, Dietary Fiber,
Vitamin A, Vitamin C, Calcium, Iron.

* Percent Daily Values are based on a 2,000
calorie diet.

NO FRUIT JUICE

INGREDIENTS: WATER, SUCROSE SYRUP, GLUCOSE-
FRUCTOSE SYRUP, CITRIC ACID, NATURAL ORANGE
FLAVOR WITH OTHER NATURAL FLAVORS, SALT,
SODIUM CITRATE, MONOPOTASSIUM PHOSPHATE,
YELLOW 6, ESTER GUM, BROMINATED VEGETABLE OIL

Figure 11-7 *Sports drinks for fluid and electrolyte replacement typically contain a form of simple carbohydrate plus sodium and potassium. The various sugars in this product total 14 grams per 1 cup (240 milliliters) serving. In percentage terms based on weight, the sugar content is about 6% ([14 grams of sugar per serving ÷ 240 grams per serving] × 100 = 5.8%). Sports drinks typically contain about 6% to 8% sugar, which provides ample glucose and other monosaccharides to aid in fueling working muscles, and are well tolerated. Drinks with a higher sugar content may cause stomach distress.*

hydrate concentration is in the 6% to 8% range.[11] Drinks in which fructose is the only carbohydrate source are the only exception to this rule. Fructose is absorbed from the intestine more slowly than glucose and often causes bloating and diarrhea.

For the most part, then, the decision to use a sports drink depends primarily on the duration of the activity. As the duration of continuous activity approaches 60 to 90 minutes or longer, the advantages from use of a sports drink over plain water begin to emerge.[12]

to a fall in endurance, strength, and overall performance. Wearing football equipment in hot weather can lead to a loss of 2% of body weight in 30 minutes. Marathon runners have been shown to lose 6% to 10% of body weight during a race.

Common symptoms of heat illness include profuse sweating, headache, dizziness, nausea, vomiting, muscle weakness, visual disturbances, and flushing of the skin. Anyone experiencing such symptoms should be taken to a cool environment immediately and stripped of excess clothing. Immediate administration of ice packs or cold water is the usual treatment until medical help can be summoned.

To decrease the risk of developing heat-related illness, athletes should replace lost fluids, watch for rapid body-weight changes (3% or more of body weight), and avoid exercise under extremely hot, humid conditions.[1] Athletes must avoid becoming dehydrated because dehydration during exercise sets the stage for heat illness. When possible, fluid intake during exercise should be adequate to minimize body-weight loss; this practice is a good idea even in the winter, when sweating can go unnoticed. The recommended goal is a loss of no more than 3% of body weight during exercise.[11]

Athletes should first calculate 3% of their body weight and then by trial and error determine how much extra fluid they need to compensate for the amount lost during exercise. This determination will be most accurate if the athlete is weighed before and after a typical workout. For every 1 pound lost, 2 cups of water should be consumed during exercise or immediately afterward. However, most athletes find that replacing more than about 75% to 80% of this sweat loss during exercise is uncomfortable.

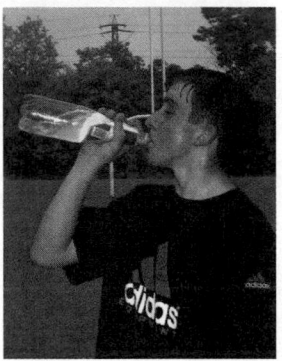

Attention to fluid consumption is one key for the person seeking peak athletic performance—or for anyone who exercises, for that matter.

Thirst is not a reliable indicator of an athlete's need to replace fluid during exercise. An athlete who drinks only when thirsty is likely to take 48 hours to replenish fluid loss. After several days of training, an athlete relying on thirst as an indicator can build up a fluid debt large enough to impair performance.

The following fluid-replacement approach can meet athletes' fluid needs in most cases[12,21]:

• Freely drink beverages (for example, water, diluted fruit juice, and sports drinks) until 2 hours before an event, even when not particularly thirsty. For events lasting less than 60 to 90 minutes, water is sufficient to meet fluid needs.

- About 20 to 30 minutes before an event, consume about $1^1/_2$ to 2 cups of these fluids. This is called *hyperhydration*. The extra fluid in the body will be ready to replace sweat losses as needed.
- During events lasting more than 30 minutes, consume about $^1/_2$ to 1 cup of fluid every 15 to 20 minutes as possible, totaling about 4 cups (1 liter) per hour. Consuming more than this can cause discomfort. On hot days, cold drinks are preferable because they help cool the body. Again, athletes should not wait until they feel thirsty.
- After exercise about 2 cups of fluid should be consumed for every pound lost.

If the weather is hot or humid, even more fluids may be required. Skipping fluids before or during events will almost certainly cause problems!

Carbohydrate Intake During Recovery from Exercise

Carbohydrate-rich foods yielding about 50 to 100 grams of carbohydrate should be consumed within 2 hours after extended (endurance) exercise—the sooner the better, because this is when glycogen synthesis is greatest.[24] This process should then be repeated over the next 2 hours. Athletes who are training intensively can consume a simple sugar candy, sugared soft drink, fruit or fruit juice, or a sports-type carbohydrate supplement immediately after training as they attempt to reload their muscles with glycogen. At quick-service restaurants, athletes can order thicker crust on pizza and extra rolls and muffins.

Fluid and electrolyte (that is, sodium and potassium) intake is also an essential component of an athlete's recovery diet. Fluids and electrolytes help replenish body fluids as quickly as possible, which is especially important if the athlete works out twice a day and the environment is hot and humid. If food and fluid intake are sufficient to restore weight loss, they generally also supply enough electrolytes to meet needs during recovery from endurance activities.

The symptoms of heat-stroke include
- Nausea
- Confusion
- Irritability
- Poor coordination
- Seizures
- Elevated body temperature
- Coma (in severe cases)

Alcohol and caffeine both have a dehydrating effect on the body, so fluids containing them should not be part of any hydration plan for exercise.

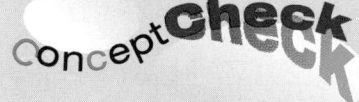

Concept Check

All athletes would do well to plan a diet that follows the Food Guide Pyramid. They should emphasize high-carbohydrate foods, especially in the preevent meal. Protein intake above that available in the usual American diet is generally unnecessary. Nutrient supplements need be taken only to correct actual nutrient deficiencies or to compensate for a low nutrient intake. Fluid should be consumed as liberally as possible before, during, and after an event. Endurance athletes may find that a sports-type drink can be helpful for activity lasting more than 60 to 90 minutes.

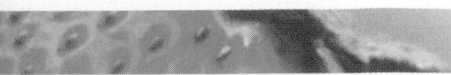

Summary

➤ Regular physical activity is a vital part of a healthy lifestyle, ideally constituting a total of at least 30 minutes per day of aerobic and resistance activities. People over 35 years should first discuss plans with a physician. Physically active people show lower risks of premature heart disease, diabetes, and other common chronic diseases.

➤ All energy available to humans comes from solar energy. Adenosine triphosphate (ATP) is the major form of energy used for cellular metabolism. Plants capture solar energy using photosynthesis. Human metabolic pathways are able to extract that energy from foodstuffs and convert it into ATP energy. Phosphocreatine (PCr) can also provide the energy needed to form ATP in a human cell.

➤ In glycolysis, glucose is broken down into three-carbon compounds, yielding some ATP. The three-carbon compounds can then proceed to an aerobic pathway to form carbon dioxide (CO_2) and water (H_2O) or to an anaerobic pathway to form lactic acid.

➤ At low workloads, muscle cells use mainly fat for fuel. For high-output exercise of short duration, muscles use PCr for energy.

➤ For more sustained high-output activity, muscle glycogen breaks down into lactic acid. For endurance exercise, fat and carbohydrate are used as fuels; carbohydrate is used increasingly as activity intensifies. Little protein is used to fuel muscles.

➤ Anyone who exercises regularly needs to consume a diet that is moderate to high in carbohydrates and consistent with the Food Guide Pyramid. Vitamin and mineral supplements are indicated if a low energy intake makes it difficult to meet nutrient needs or a nutrient deficiency exists.

➤ Carbohydrate loading can increase usual stores of muscle glycogen by 50% to 85%. Participants in endurance events that last more than 2 hours benefit most from carbohydrate loading, which basically involves eating a diet very high in carbohydrate for about 3 days before the event.

➤ Athletes should consume enough fluid both to minimize loss of body weight from fluid loss and to ultimately restore preexercise weight. A sports-type drink can be helpful for endurance athletes participating in activities lasting more than 60 to 90 minutes.

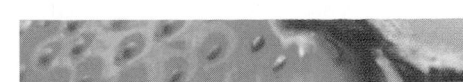

Study Questions

1 How does greater physical fitness contribute to greater overall health? Explain the process.

2 The store of ATP in muscle is rapidly depleted once contraction begins. For physical activity to continue, ATP must be resupplied immediately. Describe how this occurs after initiation of exercise and at various times thereafter.

3 What is the difference between anaerobic and aerobic exercise? Explain why aerobic metabolism is increased by a regular exercise routine.

4 What is glycogen? How does the body obtain it? How is it used during exercise?

5 Are fat stores used as an energy source during exercise? If so, when?

6 What are some typical measures used to assess whether an athlete's energy intake is adequate.

7 List five specific nutrients that athletes need and appropriate food sources from which these nutrients can be obtained.

8 What advice would you give your neighbor, who is planning to run a 50-kilometer (km) race, concerning fluid intake before and during the event?

9 One of your friends, a competitive athlete, asks your opinion about a nutritional supplement sold in a local sporting-goods store. She has read that such supplements, which contain vitamins, minerals, and amino acids, can help improve athletic performance. What would you tell her about the general effectiveness of such products?

References

1 Benardot D: *Sports nutrition,* Chicago, 1993, The American Dietetic Association.

2 Blair SN: Diet and activity: the synergistic merger, *Nutrition Today* 30:108, 1995.

3 Brouns F: *Nutritional needs of athletes,* Chichester, England 1993, John Wiley.

4 Bucci LR: Nutritional ergogenic aids. In Wolinsky I, Hickson JF, editors: *Nutrition in exercise and sport,* ed 2, Boca Raton, Fla, 1994, CRC Press.

5 Burke LM, Read RS: Dietary supplements in sport, *Sports Medicine* 15:43, 1993.

6 Chandler RM and others: Dietary supplements affect the anabolic hormones after weight-training exercise, *Journal of Applied Physiology* 76:839, 1994.

7 Clancy SP and others: Effects of chromium picolinate supplementation on body composition, strength, and urinary chromium loss in football players, *International Journal of Sports Nutrition* 4:142, 1994.

8 Clarkson PM, Haymes EM: Exercise and mineral status of athletes: calcium, magnesium, phosphorus, and iron, *Medicine and Science in Sports and Exercise* 27:831, 1995.

9 Coyle EF: Substrate utilization during exercise in active people, *American Journal of Clinical Nutrition* 61(Suppl):968S, 1995.

10 DiFiori JP: Menstrual dysfunction in athletes, *Postgraduate Medicine* 97:143, 1995.

11 Gisolfi CV: Fluid balance for optimal performance, *Nutrition Reviews* 54:S159, 1996.

12 Hawley JA and others: Carbohydrate, fluid, and electrolyte requirements during prolonged exercise. In Kies CV, Driskell JA, editors: *Sports nutrition,* Boca Raton, Fla, 1995, CRC Press.

13 Hickson JF: Research directions in protein nutrition for athletes. In Wolinsky I, Hickson JF, editors: *Nutrition in exercise and sport,* ed 2, Boca Raton, Fla, 1994, CRC Press.

14 Katch FI, McArdle WD: *Introduction to nutrition, exercise, and health,* ed 4, Philadelphia, 1993, Lea & Febiger.

15 Lee-Chiong TL, Stitt JT: Heatstroke and other heat-related illnesses, *Postgraduate Medicine* 98:26, 1995.

16 Lemon PWR: Is increased dietary protein necessary or beneficial for individuals with a physically active lifestyle? *Nutrition Reviews* 54:S169, 1996.

17 Manson JE, Lee IM: Exercise for women—how much pain for optimal gain, *The New England Journal of Medicine* 334:1325, 1996.

18 Maughan RJ: Nutritional aspects of endurance exercise in humans, *Proceedings of the Nutrition Society* 53:181, 1994.

19 Millward DJ and others: Physical activity, protein metabolism, and protein requirments, *Proceedings of the Nutrition Society* 52:223, 1994.

20 Pate RR and others: Physical activity and public health: a recommendation from the Centers for Disease Control and Prevention and the American College of Sports Medicine, *Journal of the American Medical Association* 273:402, 1995.

21 Pivarnik JM, Palmer RA: Water and electrolyte balance during rest and exercise. In Wolinsky I, Hickson JF, editors: *Nutrition in exercise and sport,* ed 2, Boca Raton, Fla., 1994, CRC Press.

22 Position of the American Dietetic Association and the Canadian Dietetic Association: Nutrition for physical fitness and athetic performance for adults, *Journal of the American Dietetic Association* 93:691, 1993.

23 Rajaram S and others: Effects of long-term moderate exercise on iron status in young women, *Medicine and Science in Sports and Exercise* 27:1105, 1995.

24 Sherman WM: Metabolism of sugars and physical performance, *American Journal of Clinical Nutrition* 62:228S, 1995.

25 Skender ML and others: Comparison of 2-year weight loss trends in behavioral treatments of obesity: diet, exercise, and combination interventions, *Journal of the American Dietetic Association* 96:342, 1996.

26 Stryer L: *Biochemistry,* ed 4, New York, 1995, WH Freeman.

27 Tucker LA and others: Participation in a strength training program leads to improved dietary intake in adult women, *Journal of the American Dietetic Association* 96:388, 1996.

28 Will PM and others: Prescribing exercise for health: a simple framework for primary care, *American Family Physician* 53:579, 1996.

29 Wilmore JH: Increasing physical activity: alterations in body mass and composition, *American Journal of Clinical Nutrition* 63(suppl):456S, 1996.

30 Yesalis CE and others: Anabolic-androgenic steroid use in the United States, *Journal of the American Medical Association* 270:1217, 1993.

RATE 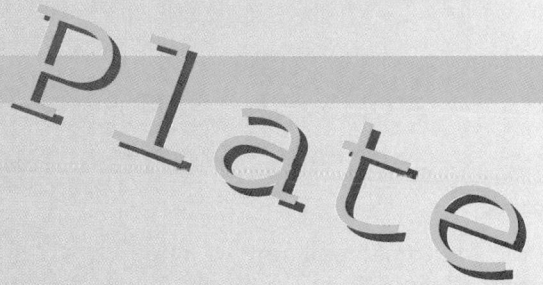 Your Plate

Are You Measuring Up to the Numbers?

In this chapter, several key nutrients were discussed in relation to exercise performance. The following guidelines were mentioned, not only for athletes but for everyone maintaining generally good fitness:

- **Eat a moderate to high amount of carbohydrates (55% or more of total energy intake).**
- **Athletes should eat a minimum of 1.2 grams of protein per kilogram of body weight.**
- **Consume the RDA of vitamins and minerals.**
- **Make sure iron and calcium intake is at RDA amounts (especially for women).**
- **Consume enough fluid to maintain weight during exercise.**

Review the results of the dietary assessment you completed in Chapter 2. Remember that you assessed 1 day's food intake. Now answer the following questions, whether or not you consider yourself an athlete:

1. What percentage of your energy intake came from carbohydrate? Was your carbohydrate intake 55% or more of your total energy intake?
   _____

2. Did you eat at least 0.8 gram of protein per kilogram of body weight? If you are an athlete, did you consume 1.2 grams per kilogram of body weight?
   _____
   _____

3. Did you consume at least the RDA of all vitamins and minerals assessed, especially iron and calcium? Which ones were below the RDA?
   _____
   _____

4. For nutrients below the RDA, list one rich food source (see Chapters 8 and 9).
   _____

5. Did you consume enough fluid—about 6 to 8 cups for a good starting point?
   _____
   _____

6. What can you do to improve your dietary intake to aid general fitness and, if you are an athlete, to promote maximal performance in your chosen event(s)?
   _____
   _____
   _____
   _____

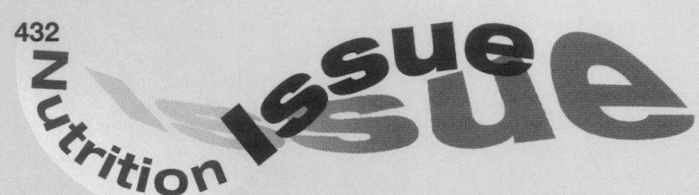

Evaluating Ergogenic Aids to Enhance Athletic Performance

Diet manipulation to improve athletic performance is not a recent innovation. As long as 30 years ago, American football players were encouraged on hot practice days to "toughen up" for competition by liberally consuming salt tablets before and during practice and by not drinking water. Now it is widely recognized that this practice can be fatal. Today's athletes are as likely as their predecessors to experiment; artichoke hearts, bee pollen, dried adrenal glands from cattle, seaweed, freeze-dried liver flakes, gelatin, and ginseng are just some of the worthless substances now used by athletes in hopes of gaining an **ergogenic** (work-producing) edge.

Still, today's athletes can benefit from recent scientific evidence documenting the ergogenic properties of a few dietary substances. These ergogenic aids include sufficient water, lots of carbohydrates, and a balanced and varied diet consistent with the Food Guide Pyramid.[1,5,12,24] Protein and amino acid supplements are not among these aids, because athletes can easily meet protein needs from foods, as Table 11-4 demonstrated. Clearly, changing average athletes into champions is not possible simply by altering their diets. The use of nutrient supplements should be designed to meet a specific dietary weakness, such as an inadequate iron intake.[23] These and other aids, which often have dubious benefits and may pose health risks, must be given close scrutiny before use. The risk-benefit ratio of these ergogenic aids especially needs to be examined.

As summarized in Table 11-8, no scientific evidence supports the effectiveness of many substances touted as performance-enhancing aids. Athletes should avoid these substances until their ergogenic effects are scientifically verified. Even substances whose ergogenic effects have been supported by systematic scientific studies should be used with caution. Finally, rather than waiting for a magic bullet to enhance performance, athletes are advised to concentrate their efforts on improving their training routines and sport technique and consuming well-balanced diets as described in this chapter. Adequate fluid and carbohydrate are the primary diet-related ergogenic aids.

Carnitine
A compound used to shuttle fatty acids into the cell mitochondria. This allows for the fatty acids to be burned for energy.

Sodium bicarbonate
An alkaline substance basically made of sodium and carbon dioxide ($NaHCO_3$).

Anabolic steroids
A general term for hormones that stimulate development in male sex organs and such male characteristics as facial hair (for example, testosterone).

Growth hormone
A pituitary hormone that produces body growth and release of fat from storage, among other effects.

Blood doping
A technique by which an athlete's red bood cell count is increased. Blood is taken from the athlete. The red blood cells are concentrated by removing fluid from that blood sample, which is later reintroduced into the athlete.

TABLE 11-8

Some Substances and Practices That Are Claimed to Have Ergogenic Effects*

Substance/ practice	Rationale	Reality
Carnitine	Shuttles fatty acids into mitochondria of cells	Body cells produce enough; therefore ineffective.
Bicarbonate	Counters lactic acid buildup	Partially effective in some circumstances, such as wrestling, but induces nausea and diarrhea.[17]
Alcohol	Reduce fatigue, provide energy	Actually impairs performance; can lead to hypoglycemia.
MCT oil (medium chain triglyceride)	Excellent fuel for muscles; transfers directly from GI tract into bloodstream	Can provide a source of energy for muscles, but provides no advantage over carbohydrate intake alone
Caffeine	Increased use of fatty acids to fuel muscles, promote psychological effects	Drinking 2 to 3 5-ounce cups of coffee (equivalent to 3 to 6 milligrams of caffeine per kilogram body weight) about 1 hour before events lasting about 5 minutes or longer than 30 minutes useful for some athletes; benefits less apparent in those who have ample stores of glycogen, are highly trained, or habitually consume caffeine; intake of more than about 600 milligrams eliciting a urine concentration illegal under Olympic rules.
Anabolic steroids	Increase muscle mass and strength	Although effective, illegal in the United States; numerous potential side effects, such as premature closure of growth plates in bones (thus possibly limiting the adult height of a teenage athlete), bloody cysts in the liver, increased risk of heart disease, high blood pressure, and reproductive dysfunction. Possible psychological consequences, including increased aggressiveness, drug dependence (addiction), withdrawal symptoms (such as depression), sleep disturbances, mood swings[30]
Growth hormone	Increase muscle mass	At critical ages may increase height; may also cause uncontrolled growth of the heart and other internal organs and even death; potentially dangerous; requires careful monitoring by a physician.
Arginine, ornithine, and glycine	Increase growth hormone output	Increases rather modest, probably of little physiological consequence
Blood doping	Injection of red blood cells harvested earlier from the athlete into the bloodstream to try to enhance aerobic capacity.	May offer aerobic benefit; very serious heatlh consequences possible, including thickening of the blood, which puts extra strain on the heart; an illegal practice under Olympic guidelines.
Phosphate loading	Improves oxygen delivery to muscles	Not effective
Inosine	Increase protein and ATP synthesis	Not effective
Coenzyme Q-10	Increase energy metabolism	Sufficient amount produced by body
Aspartates	Reduce ammonia accumulation in muscles	Mixed results to date.
Creatine	Increase phosphocreatine (PcR)	May improve performance in those who undertake repeated bouts of activity.

From Lamb D: Ergonemic aids In Wardlaw GM, Insel PM, *Perspectives in nutrition*, ed 3, St Louis, 1996, Mosby .
*Besides carbohydrate loading and meeting fluid electrolyte and nutrient/energy needs.

Charting a Course for Change

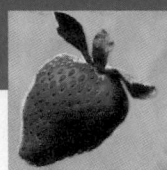

WHEN YOU THINK OF AN IDEAL

diet, what do you see? Imagine the shapes and colors of the foods chosen. Smell the aromas of a nutritious hot meal. Savor the sweetness of vegetables fresh from a garden. These *mind pictures* help us visualize the appeal of healthy foods. The senses of sight, smell, and taste are strategic guides to our nutrition goals.

Imagery, such as mind pictures, is a useful technique in changing eating behaviors. This chapter presents such strategies to help you make choices about your eating habits. You'll learn how to set goals for food choices and weight change. These techniques are powerful tools for changing eating and related behaviors important to you.[3]

Any diet or nutrition book can give you the basics. But how many of those books speak to you as an individual? Do they consider the fact that you're pressed for time and eat most meals on the run? Is the author aware that you eat when you're "stressed out"? Does the diet advice take into consideration your family history, health status, or how work affects your eating habits? An important goal of this chapter is to offer you a way to tailor nutrition and health goals to your needs. You are in control of your diet. Is it time to become more involved?

A S S E S S *Your self*

Wise Shopper Inventory

Most of us follow a routine when shopping for food. Circle the numbers below that best describe what you do before, during, and after each trip to the supermarket. Total them to find your score. Small changes in your shopping habits can make it easier to prepare nutritious meals at home.

	Hardly ever	Sometimes	Most of the time
A. Before shopping I check to see what foods I have on hand.	1	2	3
B. Before shopping I plan meals to include a variety of foods from each major food group.	1	2	3
C. Before shopping I plan food purchases to restrict nutrients I'm trying to limit in my diet, such as fat, sugar, and sodium.	1	2	3
D. Before shopping I consider how much money I have to spend on food.	1	2	3
E. Before shopping I make a shopping list.	1	2	3
F. While shopping I read food labels, watching for ingredients I'm trying to limit.	1	2	3
G. While shopping I use the Nutrition Facts printed on labels to help select food products.	1	2	3
H. While shopping I use product dating information to ensure quality and freshness.	1	2	3
I. While shopping I use unit pricing (when available) to compare prices.	1	2	3
J. After shopping I store foods promptly and properly to maintain their nutritive value and quality.	1	2	3
K. After shopping I place newer foods in the back of refrigerator, freezer, and cabinet shelves, so older foods will be used first.	1	2	3
L. After shopping I use fresh foods promptly to avoid waste.	1	2	3

Score:

12-18 You are not practicing wise shopping skills. What habits should you focus on to improve your score?

19-27 You tend to be a wise shopper but could do better.

28-36 You are a super-wise shopper. Keep up the good work!

Key Chapter Concepts

- Behavior change occurs in steps. First you become aware of a problem and find new information about it. At this point it's important to identify strengths and weaknesses regarding the intended behavior change.
- A strong commitment to achieving the goals is important for behavior change. No matter how skillfully developed, a plan for behavior change is unlikely to succeed unless you're highly motivated to change.
- You may find it helpful to draw up a contract for the behavior change that lists intended tasks,

the incentive rewards, and the time frame. The contract should first reward positive behaviors and later reward ultimate objectives.
- As you undertake a trial period for the change, controlling your environment can reduce temptations to deviate from the plan. Then, if an initial trial is successful, you may permanently adopt new behaviors.
- It's important to plan for the possibility of relapse. Most people revert to old behaviors during periods of stress or interpersonal conflict. Try to anticipate problem behaviors and devise ways to substitute better options.

The Behavior Change Process—One Step at a Time

Behavior patterns that have evolved throughout a lifetime don't change or disappear overnight. Planned behavior changes occur gradually and with some effort. First, you must become aware that a problem exists[18] (Figure 12-1). For someone who is quite inactive, this might mean becoming more aware of health risks, recognizing a lack of physical stamina, or resisting the impulse to expand one's wardrobe because of creeping weight gain.

After recognizing that a problem indeed exists, you should then develop a **receptive framework for learning** more about the problem. This might involve weighing the costs and benefits of changing behaviors; for example, balancing the time and effort required for greater physical activity and sacrificing some favorite foods against the benefits of weight maintenance, decreasing health risks, and feeling and looking better (Figure 12-2).

Receptive framework for learning

The process by which a person opens and responds to learning more about a problem. It usually involves seeking more information about an issue from books and people.

Are there parts of your health lifestyle that need improvement?

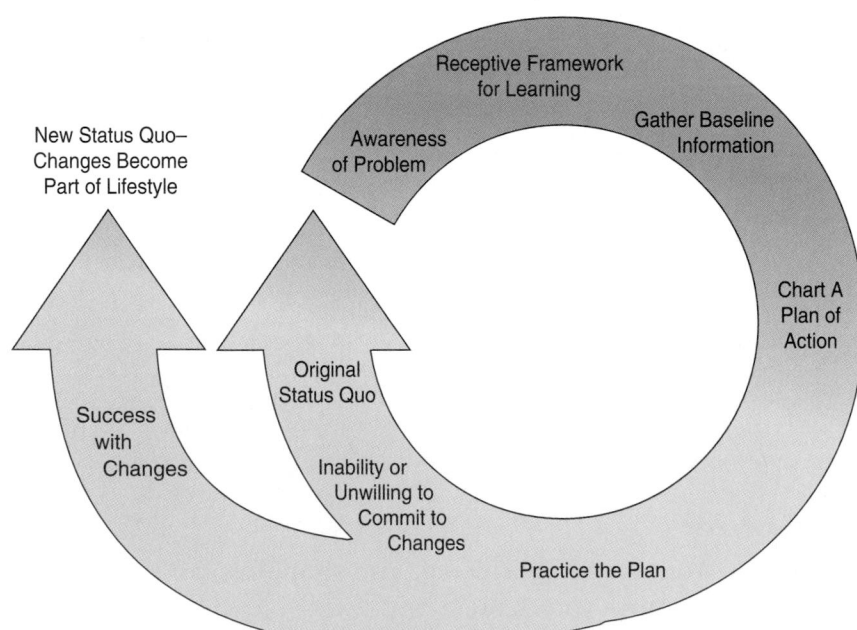

Figure 12-1 *A model for behavior change. It starts with awareness of the problem and ends with the incorporation of new behaviors intended to address the problem.*[3,18]

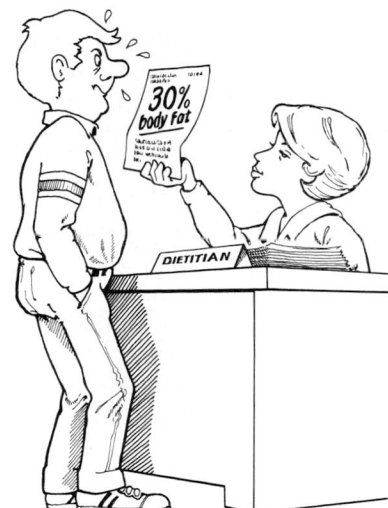

Alan is a 22-year-old college student who has been steadily gaining weight since high school. At the YMCA a registered dietitian calculates that Alan stores about 50% more fat than is desirable. Alan is concerned about his long-term health and wants to correct his overfat condition before it leads to other health problems. Having seen his father change his diet and lose weight after a heart attack, Alan thinks that he too can successfully make dietary changes.

Having decided that the change is sufficiently beneficial, you must then ask: "Can I do it?" You know yourself best. Can you continue the new behaviors for years? Long-term commitment is a key part of any behavior change plan.[10] You may find it helpful to speak with others who have worked on similar health problems and to read about others' experiences. Making changes may then seem less threatening and more realistic. A health professional can also often provide the information and encouragement you need to start (and even persist in) the change process.[7]

BENEFITS AND COSTS ANALYSIS

1 Benefits of increasing physical activity?

What do you expect to get, now or later, that you want? What do you get to avoid that would be unpleasant?

— more stamina

— Feel better physically and psychologically
— look better

— people pay more attention to me

3 Costs involved in increasing physical activity?

What do you have to do that you don't want to do? What do you have to stop doing that you would rather continue doing?

— take time to walk more
— less time to watch TV

— better athletic shoes

2 Benefits of not increasing physical activity?

What do you get to do that you enjoy doing? What do you avoid having to do?

— more free time

— little or no risk of muscle soreness or related injury

4 Costs of not increasing physical activity?

What unpleasant or undesirable effects are you likely to experience now or in the future? What are you likely to lose?

— creeping weight gain

— low self esteem

— poor fitness and health

Figure 12-2 *Benefits and costs analysis applied to increasing physical activity. This process helps put behavior change into the context of total lifestyle.*

Starting on a New Path

Having decided to attempt a change, you begin a trial run. Ideally, you change unwanted patterns one step at a time, beginning with the easiest habit to discard. Changing too many habits too soon can be overwhelming, making it hard to adhere to a plan. As you try new behaviors, you experience both difficulties and rewards: some muscle soreness and loss of free time in exchange for compliments and greater self-esteem. You may perceive some new experiences as positive, but others you'll see as negative—otherwise you wouldn't have cherished the old practices. Giving up sedentary activities and familiar foods may leave a void (Figure 12-3).

To deal with diet difficulties, positive **reinforcement** is critical.[1] A system of rewards should be built into a diet plan. You deserve credit for attempting difficult tasks; you need rewards for hard work—perhaps a night at the movies, a new compact disc, an outing with friends, or a chance to sleep late. During any trial period, it's important to capitalize on success and learn how to derive psychological nourishment from conquering "problem" habits.[5]

Finally, you adopt and integrate the new behaviors into your overall lifestyle. Now you can investigate the possibilities for other improvements, and you can repeat the cycle.[3] In the progression from becoming aware of a problem to adopting new behaviors, you can take charge of your health.

Reinforcement

A reaction by others in response to a person's behavior. Positive reinforcement entails encouragement; negative reinforcement entails criticism or penalty.

THE MIDDLETONS

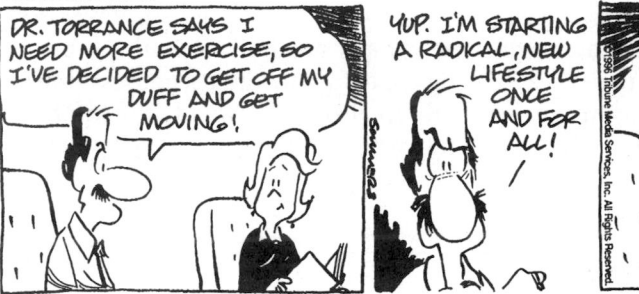

Figure 12-3   *The Middletons.*

Charting a Plan for Change Requires Active Participation

A good plan evolves over time. It is based on rational, deliberate decisions, coupled with trial and error experiences. Because you can't know all possible strategies and tactics before beginning, a good plan incorporates all information readily at hand. Revisions will be necessary and should be expected.

If your goal is to reduce or control your weight, you should know that the typical restrictive diet not only fails to produce the desired results for most people but can also produce undesired results, such as fatigue and depression. As discussed in Chapter 10, effective, long-range weight control programs encourage people to increase physical activity and eat somewhat less, especially fat, rather than severely restrict their eating. To discover the most effective options available, you can investigate some clinic programs and speak with registered dietitians.[4]

Gathering Baseline Data Is Important

Food diary

A written record of sequential food intake for a period of time. Details associated with the food intake are often recorded as well.

The next step in developing a personal plan for change is to monitor behaviors, noting strengths and weaknesses. For example, recording meals and snacks in a **food diary** may expose eating patterns previously unnoticed.[1] An activity diary will provide a similar view of that part of your lifestyle.[17]

Let's assume you want to lower fat intake to help control your weight. You'll have to adjust some habits, but which ones? In a diary, list any relevant factors, such as foods eaten, portion sizes, and amount of fat in the food eaten (Appendix B will help). Also, as you did in Chapter 1, record the intensity of hunger; the time and location of the meal or snack; any other activity performed, such as watching TV; whether others were present; and your reasons for choosing that particular food. A blank form for recording this information is included in Chapter 1 and Appendix B.

Time	Minutes spent eating	M or S*	H†	Activity while eating	Place of eating	Food and quantity	Others present	Reason for choice
7:10 a.m.	15	M	2	Standing, Fixing lunch	Kitchen	1 cup orange juice 1 cup corn flakes ½ cup 1% milk 2 teaspoons sugar black coffee	—	Health Habit Health Taste Habit
10:00 a.m.	4	S	1	Sitting, taking notes	Classroom	12 ounces diet cola	Class	Weight control
12:15 p.m.	40	M	2	Sitting, talking	Union	1 chicken sandwich 1 pear	Friends	Taste Health
2:30 p.m.	10	S	1	Sitting, studying	Library	12 ounces regular cola 6 crackers	Friend	Hunger Hunger
6:30 p.m.	35	M	3	Sitting, talking	Kitchen	1 pork chop 1 baked potato 2 tablespoons margarine ½ cup green beans lettuce ¼ tomato 1 ounce ranch dressing 1 cup whole milk 1 piece cherry pie	Boyfriend	Convenience Health Taste Health Health Health Taste Habit Taste
9:10 p.m.	10	S	2	Sitting, studying	Living room	½ cup nonfat yogurt Toasted whole english muffin with jam	—	Weight control Taste

*M or S: Meal or snack.

†H: Degree of hunger (0 = none; 3 = maximum).

Figure 12-4 *One day's food record. This activity can help you learn more about food habits.*

A review of the food diary might reveal how both your outside environment and internal cues influence your nutrition and health habits. This is the time to look for patterns—identify both positive behaviors and ones that need change. The patterns might suggest which food habits would be easy to change and which might be more difficult to alter. Consider classifying food choices as "ones you can't give up" versus "ones you can live without." See if certain eating habits are paired with other activities. For example, you may find that you often eat while visiting with friends, in response to an angry mood, or perhaps after 6 PM. Subtle associations that influence eating habits can provide a good starting point for behavior changes. [11]

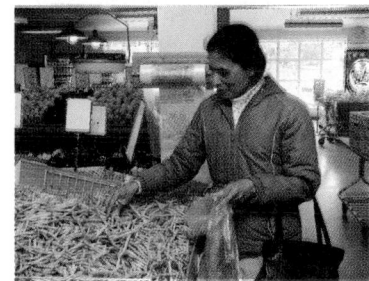

Asking yourself if you eat enough fruits and vegetables is a good first step when considering a diet change.

ANOTHER Bite

Let's assume that information from your food diary, coupled with an evaluation of your current health status, reveals behaviors you need to change to establish better nutrition and health practices. You would like to take the next step, but are unsure how to proceed. At this point a discussion with a physician or registered dietitian would be appropriate.

As mentioned in Chapter 1, habit and sensory appeal—flavor, appearance, texture, and odor—usually determine both our intended and actual food choices. Of lesser importance in choosing foods to eat are health value, time constraints, social influence, energy value, and cost. After reevaluating your food diary from Chapter 1, decide whether this is true for you.

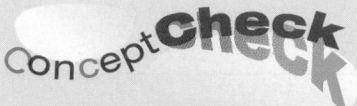

Concept Check

In the process of changing behavior, you first become aware of a problem. Then you study the problem and develop a receptive frame of mind for making a change. You initiate a trial change. If you receive positive reinforcement, you may eventually incorporate the change into your lifestyle—you adopt it. Behavior change is most successful when tailored to specific personal needs. By carefully studying your own behaviors, you can more effectively change problem habits.

Setting Attainable Goals Aids in Success

What can we accomplish, and how long will it take? Setting a realistic goal and allowing a reasonable amount of time to pursue it increase the likelihood of success.[15] For example, if one goal is to improve iron status, planning an iron-rich diet and taking iron supplements can show increased blood iron within just a few months. Progress toward other kinds of goals, such as weight loss and greater strength, might be apparent within a week and then progress from week to week. Seeing week-to-week progress can be the spark needed to continue moving ahead with a program.[9]

When you're aiming to control a chronic disease, such as high blood pressure, diabetes, or heart disease, health professionals can supply specific behavior goals. A clinical examination will confirm your degree of success. If the goal is broader, for example, to maintain or improve overall nutritional health, the path is not as well defined. Chapter 2 offers some suggestions.

It's best to change only a few specific behaviors at first—walking briskly for 30 minutes 5 times a week, lowering fat intake, using more whole-grain products, and not eating after 7 PM. Attempting small and perhaps easier dietary changes first reduces the scope of the problem and increases the likelihood of success.[1]

If you're eating every dinner in quick-service restaurants and you want to change this habit, try fixing one dinner at home each week for a month. Consider this an experiment. Will it work for you?

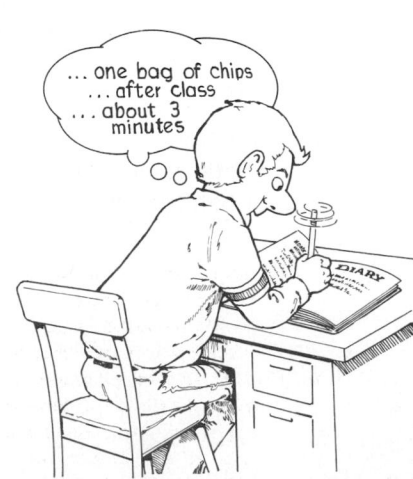

... one bag of chips ... after class ... about 3 minutes

Baseline

To better understand his eating habits, Alan keeps a food diary. In it he tracks what and how much he eats, how quickly he eats, the time, the environment, and his feelings at the time of eating. From this record he finds a previously unnoticed pattern—he starts snacking after his 2 PM class and doesn't stop until dinner. He is alarmed that he consumes so many calories almost unconsciously. In addition, Alan notes that his lunches usually are high in fat and his days contain little physical activity.

Measuring Commitment

The greater the personal commitment, the greater the chance of success. We need to examine the goals we set.[12] Are they worth pursuing? Are health benefits greater than the sacrifices to be made? Some people can ignore persistent **arthritis** in the knees, which is magnified by being overweight, because they derive great pleasure from eating. Others may love eating ice cream and chips and dips but finally decide that the price is too high. They realize that the benefit of keeping off unwanted pounds is greater than the momentary pleasure of immoderate snacking. They see that by changing eating habits, they feel better about themselves, move around more easily, feel less anxious in public, and most likely limit some future health problems.

People who are not strongly committed to changing a behavior often fail and become further discouraged. The more profound benefits from changing health and nutrition behaviors usually take time to achieve. This delayed success makes it difficult to work toward long-term goals: improving fitness, lowering elevated blood pressure, and losing weight. As already noted, many long-term goals require a life-long commitment. Only the person who contemplates the change can determine whether the value of good nutrition and good health is worth the effort.[6]

Working Out the Details

Once you establish goals and discover personal strengths and weaknesses in pursuing them, it's time to work out the details of the plan. To do this, you need to know something about the problem and possible solutions. The information in this book is a good place to start. Again, if you're unable to work out a plan, it's wise to seek professional help from a registered dietitian or physician.

One of your goals may be to reduce fat intake. There are several ways to do this: eat less high-fat meat either by cutting portion sizes or eating this kind of meat less frequently, as well as searching for new recipes and methods of preparation that yield leaner products and use less meat—for example, broiling or stir frying. You can learn many other techniques for managing eating behavior (Table 12-1).

Arthritis
Inflammation at a point where bones join together. The disease has many possible causes.

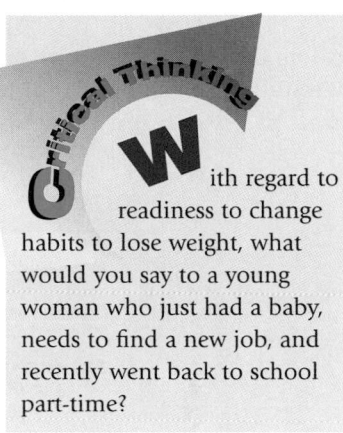

Critical Thinking

With regard to readiness to change habits to lose weight, what would you say to a young woman who just had a baby, needs to find a new job, and recently went back to school part-time?

Planning the details

Alan addresses his overall weight problem in small steps. He plans to eat a more healthful breakfast and lunch every day so he won't feel ravenous by midafternoon. He'll keep low-fat snack foods, such as oranges, handy in the apartment—instead of the usual bag of chips or cookies. He'll start packing his lunch and limit visits to quick service restaurants to twice a week. In addition, at these restaurants he'll make wiser selections from the menu, such as opting for chili rather than his usual double cheeseburger and fries. Finally, he plans to increase activity by walking to class instead of driving and by purchasing an exercise bike to ride each night for 30 minutes while watching television.

these food outlets serve a need in our fast-paced society, they are probably a permanent part of the lifestyle of many Americans. What follows is a list of suggestions for making good nutritional choices in quick-service restaurants.

Breakfast

Before entering a local quick-service restaurant for breakfast, decide whether you can fix this meal at home. Can breakfast be prepared the night before so it's ready for the next morning? The effort might be as simple as putting bread next to the toaster or cereal on the counter with a bowl. Breakfast can be a relaxing time, and many of us need time away from the fast pace of daily life. If you've abandoned breakfast at home, think again. Breakfast at home is usually faster than a visit to a quick-service restaurant.

If you still prefer breakfast out, consider hot or cold cereal with milk. Another option is a plain scrambled egg or an English muffin with no more than 1 teaspoon of margarine. Add orange juice to round out a tasty breakfast. Substitute pancakes without the butter and minimal syrup instead of the egg and English muffin. Either way, you consume a lot less fat and energy than if you choose the typical meat, egg, and cheese-laden muffin or croissant. Be especially wary of croissants: they are loaded with fat. If you still want meat, consider Canadian bacon, a leaner breakfast meat than regular bacon.

Lunch and Dinner

A good choice for lunch or dinner is a sandwich made of whole-wheat bread and some lean meat or tuna. Pizza is a good idea once or twice a week. If ordered with vegetable toppings—mushrooms, green peppers, and onions—pizza provides a very nutritious meal for a moderate number of calories. The cheese most commonly used in pizza is a low-fat variety. The next best choice is probably a hamburger, but not the king-size model. Consider buying the basic hamburger. Be especially wary of mayonnaise, sauces, melted cheese, fried onions, and other sources of added fat. Chili is another alternative. It's lower in fat than a king-size hamburger, and the beans supply dietary fiber. Finally, ordering soup

and a salad is another lower-fat option. Burritos with beans or chicken also are often low in fat, if added cheese is kept to a minimum.

Bite-size pieces of chicken should be made from chicken breast only and not from processed chicken that can include ground chicken skin. Ask the restaurant manager from which parts of the chicken the entrée is made. Let him or her know your nutrition and health interests and see to what extent your needs can be accommodated. Broiled or baked chicken is the most healthful. If the chicken is fried, remove the coating. The same applies to fish: remove the coating. Actually, chicken and fish start out as low-fat protein sources, but by the time they're deep-fat fried, their protein:fat ratio resembles that of a typical hamburger sandwich.

For side dishes, consider portion sizes. Order a small rather than a large portion of french fries. Order a baked potato, and to spice it up, put on plenty of chives but not more than a pat of margarine. Stay away from sour cream, cheese, and other toppings—you can save 300 kcal. Minimize the fats you add to vegetables.

At the salad bar, watch the addition of cheese, bacon bits, and dressing. Mayonnaise-based salads, such as macaroni and potato salad, are relatively high in calories. To minimize saturated fat intake, try the oil and vinegar and French dressings rather than the creamy types such as bleu cheese dressing. Some people find fresh-squeezed lemon juice is a satisfying alternative to dressing. Some restaurants do supply low-calorie dressings. Try these, or otherwise add as little regular dressing as possible. Salad bars also offer fresh fruits and vegetables, which can contribute to a healthful meal.

For beverages, consider low-fat or nonfat milk, water, diet soft drinks, or iced tea. A typical milk shake contains about 350 to 400 kcal. In contrast, a cup of 2% milk has only 120 kcal.

Above all, focus on fat. Its 9 kcal per gram add up fast. By all means, however, enjoy eating out. Look at your total diet, not at whether one food or another is going to ruin your health. For example, if you know you're going to have a high-fat lunch, plan to have a leaner dinner to compensate. We should think of eating as a pleasurable experience. There are some hurdles to clear, but once you learn these tips for eating on the run, you can make choices that fit into a healthful diet even at quick-service restaurants.[19]

Making It Official With a Contract

Drawing up a **behavior contract** often adds incentive to follow through with a plan. The contract could list goal behaviors and objectives, milestones for measuring progress, and regular rewards for meeting the terms of the contract. After finishing a contract, you should sign it in the presence of some friends (Figure 12-4). This encourages commitment.[1]

We need to remember that positive reinforcement for following the contract contributes more to successful behavior change than negative reinforcement for not following it. Initially plans should reward positive behaviors, and then they should focus on positive results. Positive behaviors, such as regular physical activity, eventually lead to positive outcomes, such as increased stamina.

Behavior contract
A written agreement that outlines intended behavior changes, plans for reinforcement, and witnesses to monitor progress.

Name *Alan Young*

Goal
I agree to *ride my exercise bike*
(specify behavior)

under the following circumstances *for 30 minutes, 4 times per week*
in the evening
(specify where, when, how much, etc.)

Substitute behavior and/or reinforcement schedule *I will reinforce myself if I've achieved my goal after a month with a weekend off campus with my roommate.*

Environmental planning
In order to help me do this, I am going to (1) arrange my physical and social environment by *buying a new jogging suit at the local sporting goods store*

and (2) control my internal environment (thoughts, images) by *coordinating riding the bike with the first T.V. watching I do in the evening*

Reinforcements
Reinforcements provided by me daily or weekly (if contract is kept):
I will buy myself a new piece of clothing for off campus trip

Reinforcements provided by others daily or weekly (if contract is kept):
at the end of a month if I've completed my goal my parents will buy me a fitness club membership for winter.

Social support
Behavior change is more likely to take place when other people support you. During the quarter/semester please meet with the other person at least three times to discuss your progress.
The name of my "significant helper" is: *Mr. and Mrs. Young*

This contract should include:
1. Baseline data (one week)
2. Well-defined goal
3. Simple method for charting progress (diary, counter, charts, etc.)
4. Reinforcements (immediate and long-term)
5. Evaluation method (summary of experiences, success, and/or new learnings about self).

Figure 12-5 *Alan's behavior contract. Completing such a contract can help generate commitment to behavior change. What would your contract look like? You'll have a chance to develop one in the Rate Your Plate section later in the chapter.*

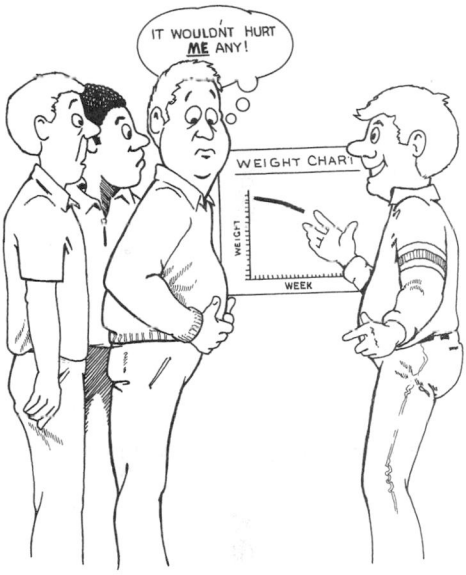

Drafting a contract

To motivate himself, Alan drafts his plan into contract form. In the contract, he outlines his behavior changes and his choice of positive reinforcement for carrying out the plan: a weekend off campus with his roommates. He introduces his roommates to the plan, and one of them even wants to join him, knowing that he too will benefit from more activity and weight loss. Alan posts a chart on the refrigerator to record the amount of time he spends on the exercise bike each night and his weekly body weight.

Psyching Yourself Up

While changing habits, we're likely to get support from some friends, but others may prefer us the way we are. They may try to dissuade us from our plan. Even we may have moments when we want to abandon the plan. We all respond to others' opinions, especially about ourselves. We tend to like approval and are influenced by others to behave in certain ways. No matter how committed we are to changing behaviors, we may need to mentally prepare ourselves to resist when others encourage behavior that defeats our desired goal.[8]

"Psyching yourself up" may enable you to progress toward your goals in spite of others' attitudes and opinions. Almost everyone benefits from some assertiveness training when it comes to changing behaviors. Here are a few suggestions:[14]

- No one's feelings should be hurt if you say, "No, thank you," firmly and repeatedly when others try to dissuade you from a plan. Rather, ask them—and yourself—why they want you to eat their way. Your needs are as important as anyone else's.
- You don't have to eat a lot to accommodate anyone—your mother, business clients, or the chef. For example, at a party with friends you may feel you have to eat a lot to participate, but you don't. Another trap is ordering a lot just because someone else is paying for the meal.
- When entertaining, serve lighter, more healthful low-fat meals. Try some new recipes. This can be a useful step en route to changing your overall approach to cooking.
- Dealing with parties and social occasions built around food is difficult but possible. You can plan celebrations around a hike or a tennis match, rather than around chips, beer, and television. When you attend parties where food is everywhere, eat a low-fat salad (such as fruit salad) before you go, opt for pretzels or plain crackers, converse far from the food table, and don't wear clothes that make it easy to overeat.[16]
- Learn ways to handle "put-downs"—inadvertent or conscious. An effective response can be to communicate feelings honestly, without hostility. Tell criticizers that they have annoyed or offended you; that you are working to change your habits and would really like understanding and support from them.
- Fostering feelings of self-worth can empower you to change behavior. Ridding yourself of the habit of self-criticism requires strong self-restraint and retraining. Create and memorize lists of strengths, giving credit where it's deserved. Practice forgiving yourself. Instead of saying, "I failed," practice saying, "It didn't work out." Lower unrealistic expectations. Stop thinking negative thoughts about yourself; purposely switch to positive thoughts.
- If appropriate, persuade the cook to change the family or group diet. The cook can strongly influence healthful eating. The ideal situation exists when everyone wants to eat healthfully. It takes extra effort to find and develop new recipes and learn shortcuts and substitutions to cut fat and/or calories. However, the information can be found in cookbooks and newspaper recipes. Also, friends may have healthful recipes and food preparation tips.

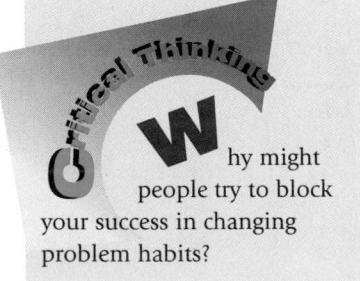

Critical Thinking

Why might people try to block your success in changing problem habits?

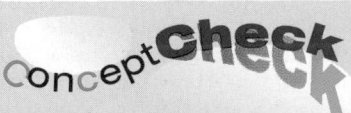

Concept Check

To successfully change habits, you should start by making small changes and providing rewards for sticking with the plan. At first, it's important to reward positive behaviors. Later, the focus switches to positive results, such as a loss of body weight or lower blood cholesterol. Before beginning a plan, determine your degree of commitment to it. Without commitment, your attempt to change habits will likely end up in failure.

Practicing the Plan

Once you've set up a nutrition and health plan, the next step is to implement it. Start with a trial of at least 6 to 8 weeks. Thinking of a lifetime commitment can be overwhelming. Remember that we win the game one point at a time. Aim for a total duration of 6 months of new activities before giving up. It's difficult to overcome the habits of 5, 10, or 20 or more years.[10] More than once we may have to persuade ourselves of the value of continuing the behavior-change program. We may even backslide. That isn't totally disastrous if we can learn to manage our thinking. Here are some suggestions to help keep a plan on track:

- **Focus on reducing, but not necessarily extinguishing, undesirable behaviors.** For example, it's usually unrealistic to say "I'll never eat a certain food again." Better to say "I won't eat that *problem* food as regularly as before."
- **Monitor progress.** Note your progress in a diary and reward yourself according to your contract. Make sure to prove to yourself regularly that you're following the plan. While conquering some habits and seeing improvement, you may find yourself quite encouraged, even enthusiastic, about your plan of action. That can give you the impetus to move ahead with the program.
- **Control environments.** In the early phases of behavior change, try to avoid problem situations, such as parties, coffee breaks, and favorite restaurants. Once new habits are firmly established, you can probably more successfully resist the temptations in these environments (Figure 12-6).

> Practicing new behaviors is much like learning to play a musical instrument: you must practice before you become proficient.

cathy®   **by Cathy Guisewite**

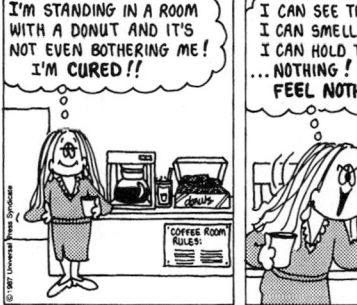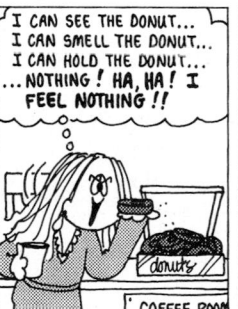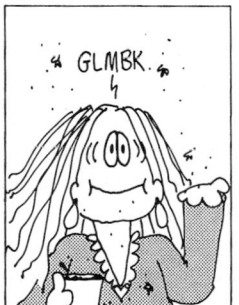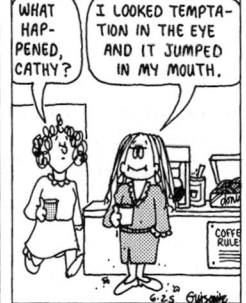

Figure 12-6
Cathy.

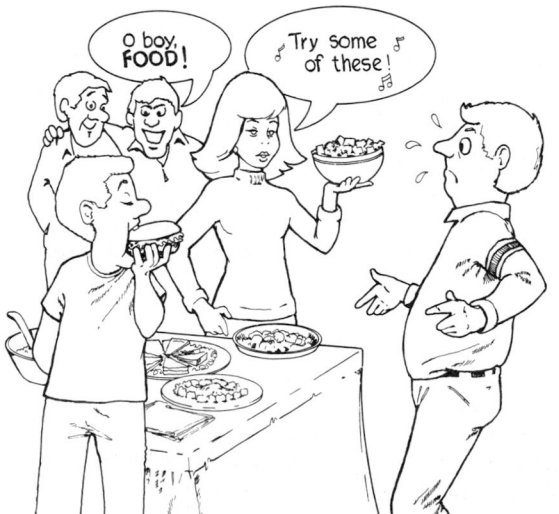

Implementation

As Alan pursues his new practices, unexpected obstacles arise. Friday night parties are a challenge, with their abundance of "munchies" and alcoholic beverages. Alan doesn't enjoy waking up earlier in the morning to pack his lunch, and he has to shop at the grocery store every few days for things he needs.

- **Break problem behavior chains.** A behavior chain is a series of interconnected habitual activities.[8] The way to break the chain is to first identify the activities, pinpoint the weak links, break those links, and substitute other behaviors. If the behavior chain is broken at any point, it probably won't continue. Figure 12-7 shows you how to use a behavior chain diagram to identify the links and break them. It also shows substitute activities you can use instead of the weak links in the chain.

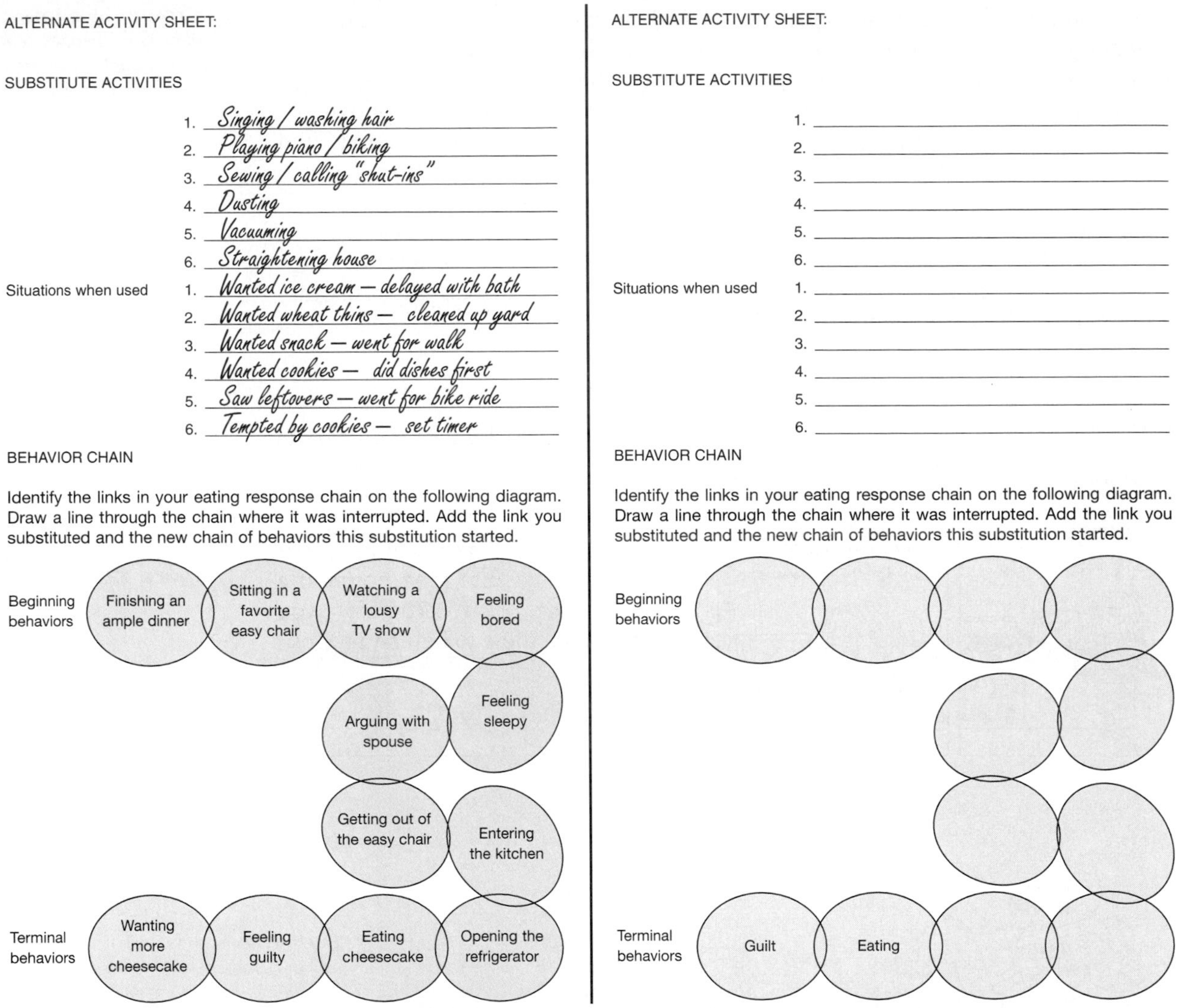

ALTERNATE ACTIVITY SHEET:

SUBSTITUTE ACTIVITIES

1. _Singing / washing hair_
2. _Playing piano / biking_
3. _Sewing / calling "shut-ins"_
4. _Dusting_
5. _Vacuuming_
6. _Straightening house_

Situations when used
1. _Wanted ice cream — delayed with bath_
2. _Wanted wheat thins — cleaned up yard_
3. _Wanted snack — went for walk_
4. _Wanted cookies — did dishes first_
5. _Saw leftovers — went for bike ride_
6. _Tempted by cookies — set timer_

BEHAVIOR CHAIN

Identify the links in your eating response chain on the following diagram. Draw a line through the chain where it was interrupted. Add the link you substituted and the new chain of behaviors this substitution started.

ALTERNATE ACTIVITY SHEET:

SUBSTITUTE ACTIVITIES

1. _____
2. _____
3. _____
4. _____
5. _____
6. _____

Situations when used
1. _____
2. _____
3. _____
4. _____
5. _____
6. _____

BEHAVIOR CHAIN

Identify the links in your eating response chain on the following diagram. Draw a line through the chain where it was interrupted. Add the link you substituted and the new chain of behaviors this substitution started.

Figure 12-7 *Identifying behavior chains. This is a good tool for understanding more about your habits and pinpointing ways to change unwanted habits. The earlier in the chain you substitute a nonfood link, the easier it is to intervene. Four types of behaviors can be substituted in an ongoing behavior chain:*

1. Fun activities (taking a walk, reading a book)
2. Necessary activities (cleaning a room, balancing your checkbook)
3. Incompatible activities (taking a shower)
4. Urge-delaying activities (setting a kitchen timer for 20 minutes before allowing yourself to eat)

Using activities to interrupt behavior patterns that lead to inappropriate eating (or inactivity) can be a powerful means of changing eating habits.

- **Plan for failures.** When faced with a situation or mood that may disrupt your plan, decide in advance what to do. If all else fails. . .
- **Forgive and forget.** Cultivate a long-term vision for a nutrition and health plan. Forgive occasional indiscretions. Focus on behaviors you've established and performed day after day. Assume there will be setbacks, and work your way through them. An occasional lapse doesn't justify a relapse, and certainly not a collapse.
- **Recruit support from others.** Have some family members, roommates, or friends witness your contract; educate them about the program and your needs. They can help prevent probelm situations that encourage you to deviate from the plan.
- **Watch for rationalization, the attempt to fool yourself.** Distorting information and denying facts to support wishful thinking are ways we rationalize. Trying to justify backsliding by saying, "I can't do it," when you've already done it for 4 months, is rationalizing. You won't fool even yourself.
- **Be realistic.** You can't control every facet of your overall health. Genetic makeup and environment influence health, including body weight. If you yearn for the body build of a sports hero or a movie star but have inherited other tendencies, reconsider. You may not achieve the shape you want, but you can maintain a healthy body weight. Accept and like yourself for who you are.

Reevaluating a Plan: Were the Correct Decisions Made?

After practicing a program for several months, reevaluate it to clarify any issues. Does your plan of action actually lead to the goals you set? Are the goals in line with an overall nutrition and health plan? Reevaluation is particularly in order if your general lifestyle changes.

For example, as you switch from a student lifestyle to that of a full-time worker, your level of physical activity may change drastically. A student may walk to classes and participate in intramural sports, whereas, a job may require long hours at a desk. Though lifestyles change, the need for physical activity doesn't. Therefore you may need to reevaluate plans for physical activity and adapt these to new situations.[3]

Reevaluation

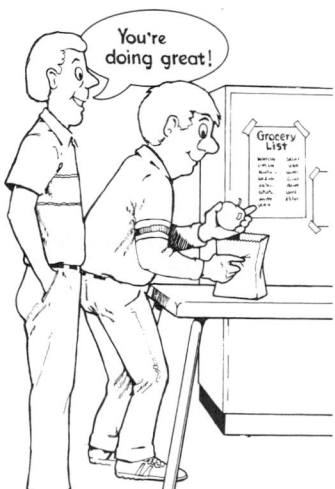

Alan evaluates the obstacles he has encountered and brainstorms with his roommates to find ways to overcome them. He decides to cut back slightly on calories during the day on Fridays so at parties he can allow himself a limited number of snacks. He begins packing his lunch at night so he can grab it on the way to class, and he writes a more complete grocery list that enables him to shop once each week.

Alan begins to notice how much more energy he has and so plans to continue on the exercise bike. In fact, he's really beginning to enjoy it. He also realizes he should move beyond his current food list so he doesn't get bored with his cooking and revert to relying on quick-service restaurants. After a month, he hasn't reached his body weight goal, but friends are commenting on changes they see in him. This encouragement helps him remain patient with his progress and focus on the ultimate goal, rather than on the time needed to achieve it.

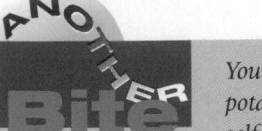

Your friend with whom you often study makes a habit of eating potato chips during your study sessions. You frequently indulge yourself when offered the tempting snack. To stop this, think about buying an electric airpopper for a quick, almost-no-fat popcorn snack. This is a good alternative to high-fat, high-sodium chips.

Changing some habits for a few days or even a few months may be easy. Changing them forever is tough, unless we learn to enjoy the changes and success and identify the new habits as our own. But a lifetime change can pay off. Many who trim fat from their waistlines report greater self-esteem. Having extra energy, feeling good, and looking better provide further motivation to continue to follow the new habits. For many people these assets are much stronger incentives than the less tangible goal of preventing disease.

Preventing Relapse Deserves Attention

Relapse often starts with a high-risk situation. Most people at first don't recognize the conditions that promote a relapse. One slip sometimes snowballs into a series of lapses that lead to complete reversion to old behaviors. The first lapse could be caused by stress, interpersonal conflicts, or inability to cope adequately with everyday events. These factors signal a high-risk situation. One or two slips are not fatal. You can return to healthful behavior if you plan in advance for the possibility of relapse and even expect it. Here are some suggestions[9]:

- **Identify high-risk situations.** As a backslide begins, determine the factors that contributed to the slide and analyze what provoked the high-risk situation. By focusing on the risks inherent in a situation, you can both plan to avoid them in the future and avoid the trap of dwelling on self-defeating guilt feelings.
- **Mentally rehearse a response to a backsliding behavior.** Imagine backsliding and seeing yourself taking positive action to recover. Rehearse responses to as many potential lapses as you can think of.
- **Remember your goals.** Keep in mind your reasons for making the commitment to change behaviors and the hard work it took to achieve them.

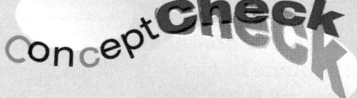

To implement a behavior-change plan, you can write a contract that identifies behaviors to practice, behavior rewards, and the time frame for accomplishing the plan. While trying to change behaviors, it's important to control your environment (to discourage deviation from the plan) and to get support from others. A plan for problems is needed; problems should not be an excuse for a relapse. You need to devise a strategy that will allow you to move ahead despite a few failures along the way. Problems may require you to reconsider your action plan; this is to be expected.

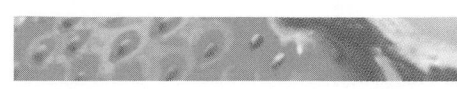

Summary

➤ Behavior change occurs in steps. First you become aware of a problem. Then you openly receive new information about it, evolving a receptive framework for learning. You then undertake a trial period for the change, during which time positive reinforcement is critical. If an initial trial is successful, you may permanently adopt new behaviors.

➤ Before charting a behavior-change plan, it's important to identify your strengths and weaknesses regarding the intended behavior. Keeping a food diary for at least a week may show eating patterns and other behaviors that either contribute to or discourage new behaviors. This and other types of diaries can reveal areas of your outside environment that need to be altered to reduce temptation.

➤ When setting goals for a behavior plan, a key is to plan small steps that lead to the intended result and build in rewards to capitalize on achievements and maintain momentum.

➤ After setting a plan of action, the next step can be to draw up a contract that lists intended tasks, the incentive rewards, and the time frame for the behavior change. The contract should at first reward positive behaviors and later reward ultimate objectives.

➤ Before embarking on the behavior-change program, evaluate your personal commitment. A plan, no matter how skilfully developed, is unlikely to succeed unless you have a strong-commitment to achieving the goals.

➤ When implementing a plan, you need to monitor progress and provide rewards. Controlling your environment can reduce temptations to deviate from the plan. For example, it's helpful to decide in advance to choose low-fat foods at a quick-service restaurant. You should expect small failures and not consider them an excuse to abandon change. A forgive-and-forget attitude can prevent collapse of your whole strategy.

➤ You need to plan for the possibility of relapse. Most people revert to old behaviors during periods of stress or interpersonal conflict. Identify problem behavior chains and devise ways to substitute stronger for weaker links. Strategies to recover from relapse include identifying high-risk situations in advance and mentally rehearsing a response.

Study Questions

1 Why does measuring commitment play a key part in any plan to change behavior?

2 What three elements should a behavior contract contain?

3 Describe one behavior strategy to avoid overeating at a party.

4 At what stages in the behavior change process might professional assistance be of particular value?

5 Why is positive reinforcement a key part of a plan for behavior change?

6 Discuss two strategies for "psyching oneself up" for change.

7 What is a behavior chain? How can this concept be used to aid behavior change?

8 Discuss two strategies for avoiding a relapse into old habits.

9 Describe an incident in your life when you implemented the behavior change process, despite a lack of formal recognition of the steps in the process.

References

1 Brownell KD: *The LEARN program for weight control,* Philadelphia, 1989, KD Brownell.

2 Campbell TC and others: Diet and chronic degenerative diseases: perspectives from China, *American Journal of Clinical Nutrition* 59:1153S, 1994.

3 Christie-Seely J: Counseling tips, techniques, and caveats, *Canadian Family Physician* 41:817, 1995.

4 Committee to Develop Criteria for Evaluating the Outcomes of Approaches to Prevent and Treat Obesity: Weighing the options, Washington, D.C., 1995, National Academy Press.

5 Crawford S: Promoting dietary change, *Canadian Journal of Cardiology* 11(Suppl A):14A, 1995.

6 DuPue JD and others: Maintenance of weight loss: a needs assessment, *Obesity Research* 3:241, 1995.

7 Elford RW and others: A practical approach to lifestyle change counselling in primary care, *Patient Education & Counseling* 24:175, 1994.

8 Ferguson J: *Habits, not diets: the secret to lifetime weight control,* Palo Alto, Calif, 1988, Bull Publishing.

9 Fletcher AM: *Thin for life,* Shelburne, Vt, 1994, Chapters Publishing.

10 Foreyt JP, Goodrick GK: Evidence for success of behavior modification in weight loss and control, *Annals of Internal Medicine* 119:698, 1993.

11 Frankle RT, Yang M: *Obesity and weight control,* Rockville, Md, 1988, Aspen Publishers.

12 Johnson CC, Nicklas TA: Health ahead—the heart smart family approach to prevention of cardiovascular disease, *American Journal of Medical Sciences* 310(Dec Suppl):S127, 1995.

13 McBean LD: Nutritional implications of ethnic and cultural diversity, *Dairy Council Digest* 66:25, 1995.

14 Nash JD: *Maximize your body potential,* Palo Alto, Calif, 1986, Bull Publishing.

15 Nolan RP: How can we help patients to initiate change? *Canadian Journal of Cardiology* 11(Suppl A):16A, 1995.

16 Papazian R: Healthful snacks for the chip & dip crowd, *FDA Consumer,* April 1996, p. 8.

17 Pastors JG and others: Facilitating lifestyle change: a resource manual, *American Dietetic Association,* Chicago, 1996.

18 Thompson B: Implementation aspects of the Seattle "5 a Day" intervention project: strategies to help employees make dietary changes, *Topics in Clinical Nutrition* 11:58, 1995.

19 Warshaw HS: America eats out: nutrition in the chain and family restaurant industry, *Journal of the American Dietetic Association* 93:17, 1993.

20 Willett WC: Diet and health: what should we eat? *Science* 264:532, 1994.

RATE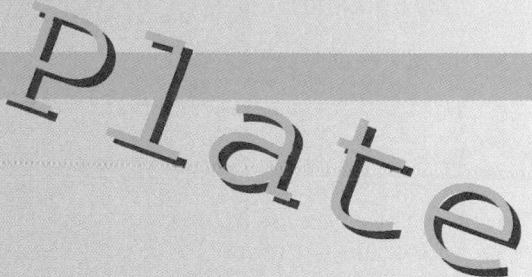

Consider practicing the behavior change strategy described in this chapter. Pick a goal you've been thinking about, such as increasing fruit and vegetable intake. Use the contract below to establish your game plan. Now implement the plan and try your best to succeed. Turn what's in your mind's eye into reality.

Name _____

Goal
I agree to _____
(specify behavior)

_____

under the following circumstances _____
(specify where, when, how much, etc.)

Substitute behavior and/or reinforcement schedule _____

_____

Environmental planning
To help me do this, I will (1) arrange my physical and social environment by _____

_____

and (2) control my internal environment (thoughts, images) by _____

_____

Reinforcements
Reinforcements provided by me daily or weekly (if contract is kept):

_____

_____

Reinforcements provided by others daily or weekly (if contract is kept):

_____

_____

Social support
Behavior change is more likely to take place when other people support you. During the quarter/ semester please meet with the other person at least three times to discuss your progress.

The name of my "significant helper" is: _____

This contract should include:
1. Baseline data (one week)
2. Well-defined goal
3. Simple method for charting progress (diary, counter, charts, etc.)
4. Reinforcements (immediate and long-term)
5. Evaluation method (summary of experiences, success, and/or new discoveries about self).

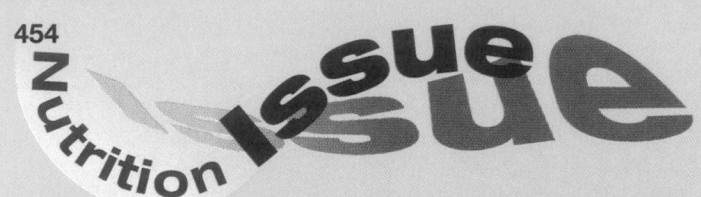

Ethnic Influences on the American Diet

Over the centuries, peoples of various cultures have migrated to new locations. Typical migrants keep some traditional dietary habits, or *foodways*, change some habits, and abandon others. As people migrate and mingle with those of other cultures, their cuisines tend to mingle as well. Changes in affluence and technology also affect dietary habits, some for better and some for worse.

This Nutrition Issue examines how the cuisines of various cultures have affected the American diet. Examining the nutrition attributes of a number of ethnic diets will help you understand that no single cuisine is either completely healthful or unhealthful. The trick to finding healthful food is to evaluate individual dishes carefully. Let's look at six cuisines that contribute to food "American style."

NATIVE AMERICANS

The size and varied geography of the American continent meant that different foods were available to people living in different locations. Some of these people were hunter-gatherers, relying for subsistence on wild vegetation and wild game. Others learned to grow vegetable crops. Depending on where they lived, Native American groups cultivated early forms of such plant foods as tomatoes, sweet potatoes, squash, vanilla, and cocoa. They also hunted whatever wild game was available. Their diets tended to be low in sodium and fat and high in dietary fiber. In the far north, populations subsisted on fish, sea mammals, other game, and a few plants, such as seaweed, willow leaves, and berries.

Recent studies have shown that the diseases that affected these societies differed significantly from the diseases common in American society. For example, Alaska natives who still eat the traditional diet have heart disease rates lower than those in the general U.S. population. Younger generations of Alaska natives, however, who usually do not eat the traditional diet, have developed heart disease at rates similar to those in the overall U.S. population. These and other studies indicate that as societies become more uniform, so too do disease patterns.

MEXICAN-AMERICANS

When Spanish colonists arrived in what is now called Latin America, they brought foods, flavors, and cooking techniques that were then combined with locally available foods. Several cuisines developed from those combinations, influenced also by the arrival of other groups.

Thus the Cuban cuisine combined native foods with those of both Spanish and Chinese immigrants, whereas the Puerto Rican cuisine combined native foods with Spanish and African contributions. In Mexico, the Spanish influence mingled with that of local Native American cuisines.

The Mayans, Aztecs, and other populations in Mexico grew corn, beans, and chili peppers; these were the basis of Mexican cuisine. They also grew such fruits as avocados, papayas, and pineapples. By the end of the fifteenth century, wheat, chickpeas, melons, radishes, grapes, and sugar cane had been brought to the New World. Rice, citrus fruits, and some kinds of nuts came soon afterward. The Spanish also introduced beef, lamb, and chicken. Native inhabitants had previously eaten mostly fish and wild game. Spices such as cinnamon, black pepper, cloves, thyme, marjoram, and bay leaves were introduced and also became part of the cuisine.

Mexican cuisine today shows considerable regional variety. In southern Mexico, savory sauces and stews and corn tortillas reflect the native heritage. The Gulf states are renowned for delicious seafood dishes prepared with tomatoes, herbs, and olives, whereas Yucatan cuisine follows Mayan tradition, with such specialties as wild turkey and fish flavored with lime juice. Fresh produce adds color, flavor, and nutrition to authentic Mexican dining. Markets in the United States are now beginning to offer some of these plant foods, such as chayote, squash, jicama root, plantains, and cactus leaves and fruit.

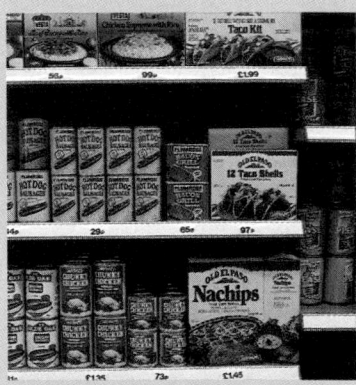

Adaptations of traditional Mexican foods are available in most local supermarkets.

True Mexican cooking bears little resemblance to the dishes usually found in "Mexican" restaurants. Usually it is neither oily nor heavy and is based primarily on rice and beans.[13] Mexican-American restaurants tend to use larger portions of meat, as well as adding portions of high-fat sour cream, guacamole, and cheese to many dishes. To lower fat intake in such a restaurant, order a bean burrito without cheese, or have a bean or meat taco with a soft (unfried) shell. Fajitas also can be made with low-fat ingredients. Many restaurants offer "lite" options. Avoid ordering such fried dishes as tortilla chips, chimichangas, or enchiladas except infrequently.

EUROPEAN-AMERICANS

Immigrants from western Europe are responsible for the "meat-and-potatoes" presentation of traditional American home cooking. The first large group of settlers from Europe—the English, French, and Germans—brought their traditional foodways with them. As all cooks and cultures must do, these immigrants adapted to the foods available in the regions in which they settled. Native Americans shared new foods that are now staples of the American diet: corn and corn products such as popcorn and hominy, some kinds of squash, and tomatoes.

However, because the new immigrants often settled in regions of the "new land" that most closely resembled their homes in Europe, they were able to grow many familiar foods and retain many of their traditional foodways. One of these foodways involved the way food is presented.

A sizable portion of meat arranged with vegetables and potatoes in separate portions on a plate is the European pattern, compared with other cuisines in which a mixture of starch, vegetables, and a much smaller portion of protein (such as a stir-fry) is more typical. The meat on the "American" dinner plate may be, for example, sausage or roast beef, the potatoes may be boiled or mashed, and the vegetable may be sauerkraut or green peas. Whatever the choices, the western European pattern is still followed by many Americans.

This traditional pattern provides abundant protein and nutrients from dairy and meat products. However, the protein also contains saturated fat, and the large portions of protein and starch may mean that insufficient amounts of whole grains, vegetables, and fruits are eaten. One alternative is to try a smaller portion of skinless chicken breast, accompanied by a plain baked potato with the skin and a hearty portion of green beans or broccoli. This combination of foods follows the traditional pattern while allowing for more healthful food choices.

AFRICAN-AMERICANS

Involuntary immigrants to the New World, people from West Africa struggled to survive under harsh conditions. Their ability to adapt familiar foodways to new conditions has had a lasting influence on today's American cuisine.

The "soul food" of African-Americans is the basis of the regional cuisines of the American South. Many understand "soul food" to consist mainly of barbecued meat, fried chicken, sweet potatoes, and chitterlings. In fact, true soul food includes a wide range of dishes created by African-American cooks. They used traditional methods and foods brought from Africa, such as yams, okra, and peanuts, as well as what was available in the New World. African-American women, cooking for their families, created dishes that they often adapted for the plantation owner's table as well, creating the basis of southern cuisine. The combination of these African-American foodways with Native American, Spanish, and French traditions produced the Cajun and Creole cuisines enjoyed today not only in Louisiana but throughout the nation.

Pork and corn products were the basis of soul food. The plantation owner ate the better parts of the pig. As with other foods, slaves learned to make palatable the less desirable parts of the pig, such as entrails, feet, ears, and head. Corn was ground for cornbread. Unrefined yellow cornmeal was mixed with water and lard to make "hoecake," baked on a hoe blade by cooks who had neither ovens nor cooking utensils for their own use. The plantation owner probably ate white cornbread made from refined cornmeal.

Among other dishes still considered soul food staples are greens, usually cooked with a small portion of smoked pork. The greens used include collards, mustard, turnip or dandelion leaves, and kale. Black-eyes peas, first brought to the New World by slaves, are also cooked with pork. Sweet potatoes and yams were and remain basic soul foods; sweet potato pie is the soul food equivalent of pumpkin pie.

Today's traditional African-American cuisine has both nutritional benefits and deficits. The variety of fruits, vegetables, and grain products used provides ample vitamins, minerals, and dietary fiber. For instance, African-Americans in general consume more cruciferous vegetables, and fruits and vegetables containing vitamin A and C, than do Caucasian Americans. However, cured pork products contribute undesirable levels of sodium as well as saturated fat. Traditional reliance on frying, especially with lard, also adds much saturated fat to the diet. Boiling vegetables for long periods depletes water-soluble vitamins. Dairy products may not be used enough, especially by older people who follow traditional dietary customs. This avoidance is based in part on the difficulty many African-American adults experience in digesting lactose; see Chapter 5 for details.[13]

CHINESE-AMERICANS

Known for its variety, the average Chinese diet provides about 70% of energy as carbohydrate, 15% as protein, and 15% as fat.[2] This is similar to the proportions recommended by some Western nutritionists and cancer experts. Over 200 different vegetables are used in Chinese cuisine; bok choy and other forms of Chinese cabbage are perhaps the most widely eaten vegetables in the world. In the southeastern coastal region of China, home

Continued.

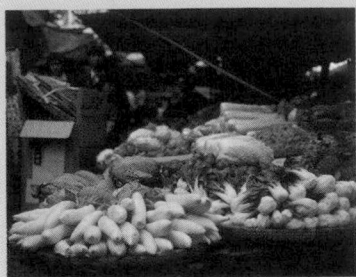

The Chinese diet is known for its variety—over 200 different vegetables are used in Chinese cuisine.

of the Cantonese cuisine, the number of dishes may be as high as 50,000.

China is a huge country, with varying climates and many regional cuisines. Rice is the core of the diet in southern China, whereas in the temperate north, wheat is used in noodles (China is the original home of pasta), bread, and dumplings. Popular dishes include hot pots (stews containing many ingredients) and stir-fried mixtures of vegetables and small amounts of meat or fish cooked in a lightly oiled, very hot pan.

Chinese immigration to America began with the California gold rush in the middle of the nineteenth century. Chinese workers brought with them food preparation methods that tend to preserve nutrients, as well as a variety of sauces and seasonings, such as ginger root, garlic, rice wine, scallions, and sesame seeds and oil. Although many of the traditional foodways have been preserved, North American restaurant versions of Chinese cuisine, whether Cantonese, Szechuan, or Mandarin, are usually not authentic. Chinese-American restaurant food is often prepared with far more fat than in true Chinese cooking, which tends to use flavorful but fat-free sauces and seasoning. The restaurant versions of Chinese dishes also contain much larger proportions of protein.

However, it's still possible to choose a healthful meal in a Chinese-American restaurant. Select dishes that are not deep-fat fried (such as egg rolls or batter-coated meats or seafood). Choose at least one vegetable dish instead of a meat entrée. Leave most of the sauce behind by eating Chinese style: lift the food from the sauce and place it on top of a mouthful of rice, which in China is the basis of the meal. Limit the amount of soy sauce you sprinkle on the rice. (Even in China, health authorities are now calling for a cut in salt intake and a switch from saturated to unsaturated fats.)

ITALIAN-AMERICANS

Authentic Italian cuisine, like Chinese cuisine, is more diverse than most Americans realize. Foods of different regions reflect Italy's varied geography and climate.

Northern Italy, the more affluent part of the country, is the principal producer of meat and dairy products like butter and cheese. Rice dishes such as risotto are popular there. Fish is more important in regions near the sea, and lighter foods, such as fresh vegetables prepared with herbs, garlic, and olive oil, are characteristic. The poorer regions south of Rome, as well as the island of Sicily, have a diet rich in grains, vegetables, dried beans, and fish, with little meat or oil. Compared with northern Italians of the same class, southern Italians eat less beef, veal, chicken, and butter, and more bread, pasta, vegetables, fruit, and fish.

Pasta is the heart of the Italian diet. Italians eat six times more of this simple wheat and water product than do Americans, although Americans have also learned to love this nutritious dish. Pasta in America, however, often means spaghetti with a tomato-based sauce that includes meatballs or sausage. In contrast, Italians eat pasta in a variety of shapes and with a variety of sauces, often excluding meat.

Most of the Italian-American cuisine found in restaurants offers foods more common to the north of Italy, including veal, cheese, and cream and pesto sauces for pasta. Pizza, a southern Italian dish, is the exception, and it is fast becoming the most frequently consumed food in the United States. Pizza in this country is served

> Chapter 6 described the recent interest in the "Mediterranean Diet," a cuisine based on food choices like those traditionally found in the simple cuisines of Greece and southern Italy.

on a variety of flour crusts topped with anything from high-fat meats such as pepperoni to vegetables or even fruit, combined with a variety of cheeses, tomatoes, and oregano for seasoning. Purists in Naples, however, insist that classic pizza consists only of a thin crust, tomato, basil, and mozzarella cheese.

Although some components of the Italian diet contain substantial amounts of saturated fat, nutritionists now know that other compounds, such as pasta, olive oil, and vegetables, contribute to good health.[20] Healthy choices in an Italian-American restaurant might include a pasta dish with fresh tomato sauce and sautéed shrimp rather than cheese-laden Alfredo sauce, or an entrée of fish and vegetables cooked with wine, olive oil, and herbs. Limiting the cheeses and meats offered on the antipasto tray and avoiding fried foods such as veal parmigiana are also wise moves.

ETHNIC DIETS AND PRESENT TRENDS

Only six ethnic diets have been described here; see Table 12-3 for a summary of their advantages and disadvantages. Many other cuisines have also influenced the American diet, and new arrivals continue to bring their traditions and foodways to this country. For example, recent social upheavals have increased the immigration of Russians and other eastern European peoples to the United States. On the other side of the world, continuing unrest in southeast

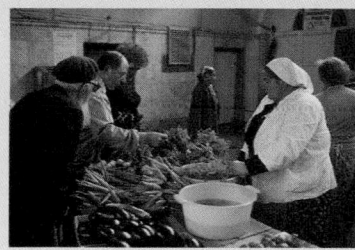

A Russian produce market. Russian immigrants have brought their traditional foodways with them to America.

Asia has brought peoples from that area here. Restaurants serving traditional Russian or Thai fare, for instance, are now offering new foodways to those willing to experiment.

Using research begun many years ago, some scientists suggest that a healthful diet consists of the inexpensive traditional dishes based on grains, fruits, and vegetables that form the backbone of a number of ethnic cuisines. These are precisely the dishes that people abandon as they become affluent and seek convenience.[20] Simple foods prepared in simple ways have fed most of humanity for virtually its entire existence. As we turn toward a new century, some Americans are rediscovering the simple foods of their respective pasts, learning to enjoy a variety of cuisines, and discovering how each cuisine can contribute to a healthier American diet.

TABLE 12-3

The World's Fare Has Influenced the American Diet[13]

Below is a brief summary of healthful attributes and shortcomings of the ethnic diet influences covered in this Nutrition Issue.

	Advantages	Shortcomings
Native American; Alaskan Native	Variety of seafood, lean wild game; early Native Americans ate variety of vegetables, berries, leaves	High fat content of some meat/seafood; low in calcium
Hispanic-American	Excellent variety of vegetables, legumes, fruits; high in dietary fiber	Traditional Hispanic diet may fall short in calcium; Mexican-American restaurants serve much high-fat fare, rich in sour cream, cheese, and guacamole
European-American	Abundant sources of protein, iron, calcium from meat and dairy groups	Less variety from vegetables, fruits, legumes; high in fat
African-American	Good variety of carotenoid-containing vegetables; high dietary fiber. Many variations including Cajun, Creole dishes	Traditional meals high in fat; may fall short in calcium
Chinese-American	Excellent variety of vegetables, grains; cooking methods retain nutrients in foods	Some sauces are high in salt and fat; may fall short in calcium
Italian-American	Varies regionally—some regions provide excellent variety of seafood; overall high grain intake, good vegetable and fruit variety	Italian-American restaurants often serve many foods made with high-fat cheese, sauces, and meats; likely low in calcium

Anorexia Nervosa and Bulimia Nervosa

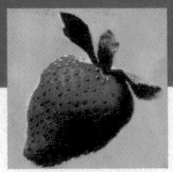

Most of us occasionally

eat until we're stuffed and uncomfortable. Faced with savory and tempting foods, we find that we can't easily stop eating. Usually we forgive ourselves, vowing not to overeat the next time. Nevertheless, many of us have problems controlling our weight. Although creeping weight gain might eventually lead to medical problems, it is usually associated with simple overeating, coupled with too little physical activity.

In stark contrast, the eating disorders explored in this chapter involve severe distortions of the eating process.[1] Dieting for a week on mostly grapefruit in order to fit into a bikini at spring break does not amount to an eating disorder. Rather, the eating disorders discussed here can develop into life-threatening conditions. What's most alarming about these disorders—anorexia nervosa, bulimia nervosa, binge-eating disorder, and baryophobia—is the increasing number of cases reported each year.[4]

Some people are more receptive and vulnerable to these disorders than other people are, for both psychological and physical reasons. Let's examine the causes and treatments of these conditions in detail, because eating disorders touch many of our lives.

CHAPTER 13

ASSESS Yourself

How Restrained Are You?

This brief assessment quiz is not designed to diagnose an eating disorder, but it can help raise your awareness of behaviors associated with eating disorders. It is normal to have some thoughts about food, diet, and weight, but such thoughts should not dominate your daily activities. Complete the following quiz, circling the number of the answer that best completes the question.

1. How often do you diet?
   - 0 never
   - 1 rarely
   - 2 sometimes
   - 3 often
   - 4 always

2. What is the most weight (pounds) you have ever lost within 1 month?
   - 0 0 to 4
   - 1 5 to 9
   - 2 10 to 14
   - 3 15 to 19
   - 4 20+

3. What is the most weight (pounds) you have ever gained within 1 week?
   - 0 0 to 1
   - 1 1.1 to 2
   - 2 2.1 to 3
   - 3 3.1 to 5
   - 4 5.1+

4. In a typical week, how much does your weight (pounds) fluctuate?
   - 0 0 to 1
   - 1 1.1 to 2
   - 2 1 to 3
   - 3 3.1 to 5
   - 4 5.1 or more

5. Would a weight fluctuation of 5 pounds affect the way you live your life?
   - 0 not at all
   - 1 slightly
   - 2 moderately
   - 3 very much

6. Do you eat sensibly in front of others and splurge alone?
   - 0 never
   - 1 rarely
   - 2 often
   - 3 always

7. Do you give too much time and thought to food?
   - 0 never
   - 1 rarely
   - 2 often
   - 3 always

8. Do you feel guilty after overeating?
   - 0 never
   - 1 rarely
   - 2 often
   - 3 always

9. How conscious are you of what you are eating?
   - 0 not at all
   - 1 slightly
   - 2 moderately
   - 3 extremely

10. How many pounds over your desired weight were you at your maximum weight?
    - 0 0
    - 1 1 to 5
    - 2 6 to 10
    - 3 11 to 20
    - 4 21+

Now add together all the numbers you circled. You could have a minimum score of 0 or a maximum of 35. Write your score in the blank here: _____

People with eating disorders often exhibit what is called *restraint*. This means that they regularly worry about what they are eating and their body weight. They often feel like failures if they lapse once by eating something that doesn't appear to help them control their weight. They try to eat "good" things like broccoli and avoid letting people see them eat "bad" things like candy bars. They may feel an intense fear or hatred of "bad" foods because such foods signify lack of self-control. When feeling stressed, a highly restrained person may eat a "bad" food, which can open the floodgate for self-punishing behavior. This behavior may take the form of a secretive binge or relentless exercise for an extended period. Restrained eating can be a sign of depression or other psychological problems.[20]

When people are highly restrained, their self-denial sets them up for a pattern of disordered eating behaviors. The assessment you completed earlier encourages you to examine the degree of dietary restraint you practice in your life. Pick out the appropriate category below based on your score:

0-15   Relatively unrestrained
16-23   Moderately restrained
24-35   Highly restrained

If you fall into the moderately or highly restrained category, you might look at how you can change your beliefs about food, dieting, and your weight. Thinking about food, diet, and weight is normal, but practicing undue restraint in food choices, diet planning, or healthy weight maintenance is not. Solving such problems now will help you achieve physical and emotional well-being for the future.

This assessment is modified from Frankle RT, Yang MU: The revised restraint scale. In Frankle RT, Yang MU, editors: *Obesity and weight control*, Rockville, Md, 1988, Aspen Publications.

Key Chapter Concepts

- Eating serves an extraordinary number of psychological, social, and cultural purposes for humans.
- Our culture bombards us everyday with images of the "ideal" body. It is hard not to compare the media images with our own, seemingly less than perfect bodies.
- Anorexia nervosa usually begins around the age of puberty in girls who begin to diet and then find it difficult to stop. Warning signs include abnormal food habits, such as cooking a large meal and then only watching others eat.
- Physical effects of anorexia nervosa are serious. Treatment requires professional help.

- Bulimia nervosa is characterized by bingeing on a large amount of food at one sitting and then purging by vomiting, using laxatives for weight loss, exercising excessively, and other means. Deliberate vomiting is especially destructive to the body.
- Treatment of bulimia nervosa includes psychological as well as nutritional counseling that focuses on establishing regular eating patterns.
- Binge-eating disorder includes grazing and food bingeing without purging. Emotional disturbances are often at the root of this eating disorder. Treatment primarily addresses deeper emotional issues.

From Ordered to Disordered Eating Habits

Eating—a completely instinctive behavior for animals—serves an extraordinary number of psychological, social, and cultural purposes for humans. As mentioned in Chapter 1, eating practices may take on religious meanings; signify bonds among cultural, ethnic, and family groups; and be a means to express hostility and affection, prestige, and class values. Similarly, providing, preparing, and distributing food may be a means of expressing love or hatred, or even power, in family relationships.

In our society we are bombarded daily with images of the "ideal" body. Dieting is promoted to achieve this ideal body—eternally young and acceptable to those around us. Television programs, billboard advertisements, magazine pictures, movies, and newspapers tell us that an ultra-slim body will bring happiness, love, and even success. Not comparing the media images with our own is hard. People who are overly susceptible to these messages, for both psychological and physical reasons, may be more likely than others to develop eating disorders.[3,24,25]

Given the multiple functions associated with normal eating and the media bombardment about ideal body image, it is not surprising that some people progress from typical responses to hunger and satiety cues, to obsessive weight loss, and then to a full-blown eating disorder, often associated with unusual and strange rituals.[18]

Progression from ordered to disordered eating

Attention to hunger and satiety signals; limitation of energy intake to restore weight to a healthful level
↓
Some "disordered" eating habits begin as weight loss is attempted, such as very restricted eating
↓
Clinically evident eating disorder can be recogized

Food: More Than Just a Source of Nutrients

From birth we link food with personal and emotional experiences. As infants we associate milk with security and warmth, so the bottle or breast becomes a source of comfort as well as food. Even when older, some people continue to derive comfort and great pleasure from food. This is both a biological and a psychological phenomenon. Food can be a symbol of comfort, but eating can also stimulate release of substances called *natural opioids*, which produce a sense of calm and euphoria in the human body. Thus in times of great stress some people will turn to food for a drug-like, calming effect.[12]

Food is also used as a reward or a bribe. Haven't you heard or spoken something like the following comments?

You can't play until you clean up your plate.

I'll eat the broccoli if you let me watch TV.

If you love me, you'll eat what I fixed for dinner.

On the surface, using food as a reward or bribe seems harmless enough. Eventually, however, this practice encourages both caregivers and children to use food to achieve unstated goals. Food may then become much more than a source of nutrients. Regularly using food as a bargaining chip can contribute to abnormal eating patterns. Carried to the extreme, these patterns can lead to disordered eating behavior.[3]

Overview of Two Common Eating Disorders

Anorexia nervosa

An eating disorder involving a psychological loss or denial of appetite and self-starvation, related in part to a distorted body image and to various social pressures commonly associated with puberty.

Bulimia nervosa

An eating disorder in which large quantities of food are eaten at one time (binge eating) and then purged from the body by vomiting, use of laxatives, or other means.

The two most common eating disorders—**anorexia nervosa** and **bulimia nervosa**—have been described since the time of the ancient Greeks.

Both disorders are psychological problems expressed in part by food practices. Both erode medical, social, and psychological well-being.[27] This section provides a brief description of the characteristics and diagnoses of these disorders. Detailed discussion of these disorders, including their treatment, follows.

Anorexia nervosa is characterized by extreme weight loss, distorted body image, and an irrational, almost morbid fear of obesity and weight gain. People with anorexia nervosa typically see themselves as fat even though they are extremely thin (Figure 13-1). The discrepancy between actual and perceived body shape is an important gauge of the severity of the disease.[27]

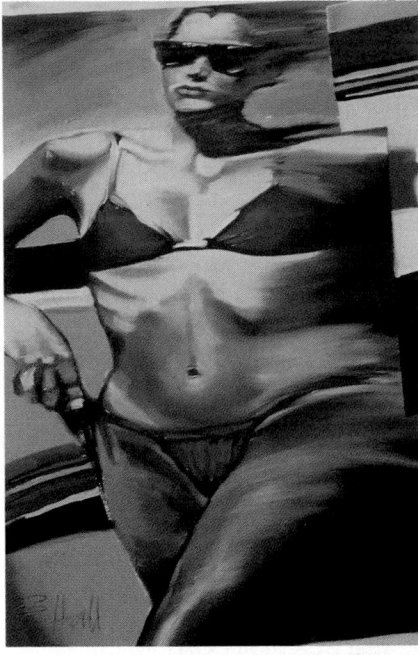

Figure 13-1 *Self-image can be ever changing and deceiving. For people with eating disorders, the difference between the real and desired body image may be too difficult to accept.*

Hypergymnasia

Exercising more than is required for good physical fitness or maximal performance in a sport; excessive exercise.

The term *anorexia* implies a loss of appetite; however, denying one's appetite more accurately describes anorexic behavior. By rough estimate, approximately 1 in 100 girls between the ages of 12 and 18 years suffers from anorexia nervosa. Peak occurrence for the disorder occurs among 14- to 19-year-old girls.[14] It happens less commonly among adult women and African-American women. Men account for only about 5% to 10% of the cases of anorexia nervosa, partly because the ideal image conveyed for men is big and muscular.[27]

Bulimia nervosa (*bulimia* means "great hunger") is characterized by episodes of binge eating followed by attempts to purge the excess energy taken up by the body, usually by vomiting, strict dieting, taking diuretics, **hypergymnasia**, or using laxatives.[3] People with this disorder may be difficult to identify because they keep their binge-purge behaviors secret and their symptoms are not obvious.[9] Between 5% and 17% of adolescent and college-age women suffer from bulimia nervosa.[27] A growing number of male athletes also report these practices, especially those who participate in sports that require achieving weights to fit weight classes, such as boxers, wrestlers, and jockeys.[19] These athletes will vomit and dehydrate to "make weight." "Get thin and win" is a common slogan heard around gyms.

The *Diagnostic and Statistical Manual of Mental Disorders* lists specific criteria for diagnosing eating disorders (Table 13-1).[3] People may exhibit some symptoms of an eating disorder but not enough to enable a medical worker to diagnose the disease. As suggested in the diagnostic criteria, some people show characteristics of both anorexia nervosa and bulimia nervosa, because the diseases overlap considerably (Figure 13-2). About half of the women diagnosed as having anorexia nervosa eventually develop bulimic symptoms. As shown in Table 13-1, bulimic characteristics are included as part of one type of anorexia nervosa, which blurs the distinction. Still, appreciating the differences between the disorders helps in understanding various approaches to prevention and treatment.

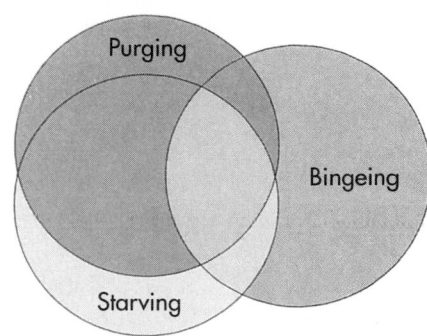

Figure 13-2
The overlap of eating disorders. A combination of binge eating, purging, and/or starving can be found in both anorexia nervosa and bulimia nervosa.

TABLE 13-1

Diagnostic Criteria for Anorexia Nervosa and Bulimia Nervosa

ANOREXIA NERVOSA

A. Refusal to maintain body weight at or above a minimally normal weight for age and height (for example, weight loss leading to maintenance of body weight less than 85% of that expected; or failure to make expected weight gain during periods of growth, leading to body weight less than 85% of that expected).

B. Intense fear of gaining weight or becoming fat, even though underweight.

C. Disturbance in the way in which one's body weight or shape is experienced, undue influence of body weight or shape on self-evaluation, or denial of the seriousness of the current low body weight.

D. In postmenarcheal females, **amenorrhea** (that is, the absence of at least three consecutive menstrual cycles). (A woman is considered to have amenorrhea if her periods occur only following hormone [for example, estrogen] administration)

Specify type:

Restricting type: during the current episode of anorexia nervosa, the person has not regularly engaged in binge-eating or purging behavior (such as, self-induced vomiting and the misuse of laxatives, diuretics, or enemas)

Binge-eating/purging type: during the current episode of anorexia nervosa, the person has regularly engaged in binge-eating or purging behavior (such as, self-induced vomiting and the misuse of laxatives, diuretics, or enemas)

BULIMIA NERVOSA

A. Recurrent episodes of binge eating. An episode of binge eating is characterized by both of the following:

(1) eating, in a discrete period of time (for example, within any 2-hour period), an amount of food that is definitely larger than most people would eat during a similar period of time and under similar circumstances

(2) a sense of lack of control over eating during the episode (for example, a feeling that one cannot stop eating or control what or how much one is eating)

B. Recurrent inappropriate compensatory behavior in order to prevent weight gain, such as self-induced vomiting; misuse of laxatives, diuretics, enemas, or other medications; fasting; or excessive exercise.

C. The binge eating and inappropriate compensatory behaviors both occur, on average, at least twice a week for 3 months.

D. Self-evaluation is unduly influenced by both body shape and weight.

E. The disturbance does not occur exclusively during episodes of anorexia nervosa.

Specify type:

Purging type: during the current episode of bulimia nervosa, the person has regularly engaged in self-induced vomiting or the misuse of laxatives, diuretics, or enemas

Nonpurging type: during the current episode of bulimia nervosa, the person has used other inappropriate compensatory behaviors, such as fasting or excessive exercise, but has not regularly engaged in self-induced vomiting or the misuse of laxatives, diuretics, or enemas

From *Diagnostic and Statistical Manual of Mental Disorders (DSM-IV)*, Washington, DC, 1994, American Psychiatric Association.
This table will help you understand the characteristics of anorexia nervosa and bulimia nervosa. However, please do not attempt to diagnose these disorders in yourself or others. Instead, use this information to determine whether professional help is needed. Note also that for each disorder, all characteristics (A-D or A-E, respectively) must be present to make the diagnosis.

Many people in professions that require ultra-slim bodies have longstanding histories of anorexia nervosa. These include models, actresses, ballet dancers, figure skaters, and gymnasts.

TABLE 13-2

Typical Characteristics of Anorexic and Bulimic Persons

Anorexia nervosa	Bulimia nervosa
• Rigid dieting causing dramatic weight loss	• Secretive binge eating; never overeating in front of others
• False body perception—thinking "I'm too fat," even when emaciated; relentless pursuit of thinness	• Eating when depressed or under stress
• Rituals involving food, excessive exercise, and other aspects of life	• Bingeing followed by fasting, laxative abuse, self-induced vomiting, or excessive exercise
• Maintenance of rigid control in lifestyle; security found in control and order	• Shame, embarrassment, deceit, and depression; low self-esteem and guilt (especially after a binge)
• Feeling of panic after a small weight gain; intense fear of gaining weight	• Fluctuating weight resulting from alternate bingeing and fasting (±10 pounds or 5 kilograms)
• Feelings of purity, power, and superiority through maintenance of strict discipline and self-denial	• Loss of control; fear of not being able to stop eating
• Preoccupation with food, its preparation, and observing another person eat	• Perfectionism, "people pleaser"; food as the only comfort/escape in an otherwise carefully controlled and regulated life
• Helplessness in the presence of food	• Erosion of teeth, swollen glands
• Lack of menses after what should be the age of puberty	• Purchase of syrup of ipecac

This listing can be used in a group discussion to help people assess their risk for developing an eating disorder. Those who exhibit only one or a few of these characteristics may be at risk but probably do not have either disorder. They should, however, reflect on their eating habits and related concerns and take appropriate action.

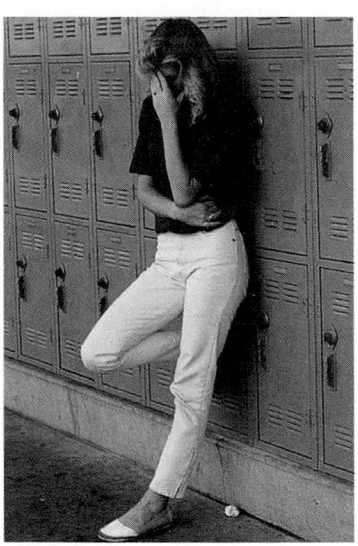

Figure 13-3
The stress of crossing from childhood into adulthood may trigger anorexia nervosa.

Table 13-2 lists some characteristics of people with anorexia nervosa and bulimia nervosa. Do you know someone who is at risk? If so, suggest that the person seek a professional evaluation, because the sooner treatment begins, the better. However, do not try to diagnose eating disorders in your friends or family members. Only a professional can exclude other possible diseases and correctly evaluate the diagnostic criteria required to make a diagnosis of anorexia nervosa or bulimia nervosa.[27] Once an eating disorder is diagnosed, immediate treatment is advisable. As a friend, the best you can do is encourage an affected person to seek professional help. Such help is commonly available at student health centers and student guidance/counseling facilities on college campuses.

There are no simple causes of eating disorders, and there are no simple treatments. The causes are rooted in multiple determinants—biological, psychological, and social. Stress may have an especially strong role in the development of eating disorders.[3,6] An underlying commonality seems to be the lack of appropriate coping mechanisms as individuals begin to reach adolescence and young adulthood, coupled with dysfunctional family relationships[11,14,24] (Figure 13-3).

The Nutrition Issue at the end of this chapter reviews some sociological aspects of these disorders and may help you understand how the disorders develop and why some people are more susceptible than others. As is true for many health problems, both nature and nurture play a role. The increase in the number of cases in recent years supports this premise.

Anorexia Nervosa

Anorexia nervosa evolves from a dangerous mental state to an often life-threatening physical condition. As noted earlier, people suffering from this disorder think they are fat and intensely fear obesity and weight gain. They lose much more weight than is healthful. Although food is entwined in this disease, it stems from psychological conflict.[3]

About 3% to 8% of people with anorexia die prematurely—from suicide, heart ailments, and infections. About half of those with anorexia nervosa recover within 6 years; the rest simply exist with the disease. The longer someone suffers from this eating disorder, the poorer the chances for complete recovery. A young patient with a brief episode and a cooperative family has a better outlook than those without these factors. Prompt and vigorous treatment with close follow-up improves the chances for success.[17]

Anorexia nervosa may begin as a simple attempt to lose weight. A comment from a well-meaning friend, relative, or coach suggesting that the person seems to be gaining weight or is too fat may be all that is needed.[14] The stress of having to maintain a certain weight to look attractive or competent on a job can also lead to disordered eating. Physical changes associated with puberty, the stress of leaving childhood, or loss of a friend may serve as another trigger for extreme dieting. Leaving home for boarding school or college or starting a job can reinforce the desire to appear more "socially acceptable." Still, looking "good" does not necessarily help people deal with anger, depression, low self-esteem, or past experiences with sexual abuse. If these issues are behind the disorder and are not resolved as weight is lost, the individual may intensify efforts to lose weight "to look even better" rather than work through unresolved psychological concerns.[27]

During adolescence, a period of turbulent sexual and social tensions, teenagers seek—and are often expected—to establish separate and independent lives. While declaring independence, they seek acceptance and support from peers and parents and react intensely to how they think others perceive them. At the same time, their bodies are changing, and much of the change is beyond their control (Figure 13-4). Adolescents often lack appropriate coping mechanisms for the stresses of the teen years. In the attempt to take charge of their lives, some teenagers try to maintain extreme control over their bodies, which promotes anorexia nervosa. Genetic factors also appear to increase the risk for anorexia nervosa: often *both* identical twins—rather than only one—develop the disorder.[17]

Once dieting begins, a person developing anorexia nervosa does not stop. The result is long periods of rigidly self-enforced semistarvation, practiced almost with a vengeance, in a relentless pursuit of thinness. Anorexia nervosa may eventually lead to bingeing on large amounts of food in a short time, then purging. Purging occurs primarily through vomiting, but laxatives, diuretics, and exercise are also used. Thus a person with anorexia nervosa may exist in a state of semistarvation or may alternate periods of starvation with periods of bingeing and purging.[3]

For Better or For Worse   by Lynn Johnston

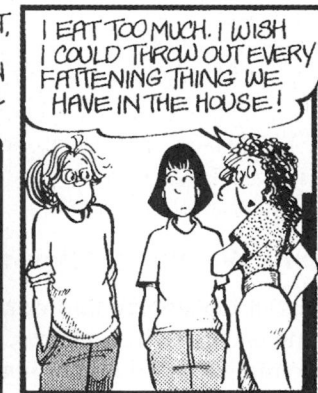
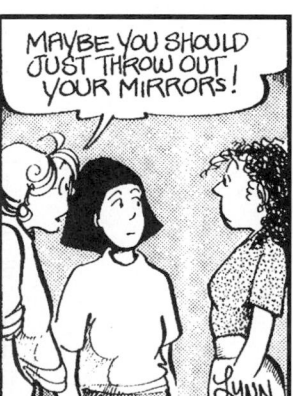

Figure 13-4 *For Better or For Worse.*

Profile of the Typical Person with Anorexia Nervosa

A person with anorexia nervosa refuses to eat enough. This refusal is the hallmark of the disease, whether or not other practices, such as binge-purge cycles, appear. The most typical anorexic person is a white girl from the middle or upper socioeconomic class. Perhaps her mother also has distorted views of desirable body shape and acceptable food habits. The girl is often described by parents and teachers as "the best little girl in the world."[27]

She is competitive and often obsessive. Her parents set high standards for her. At home, she may not allow clutter in her bedroom. Physicians note that after a physical examination, she may fold her examination gown very carefully and clean up the examination room before leaving. Even though such behavior may seem obvious, only a skilled professional can tell the difference between anorexia nervosa and other common adolescent complaints, such as delayed puberty, fatigue, and depression.[27]

A common thread underlying many—but not all—cases of anorexia nervosa is conflict within the family structure, typically manifested by an overbearing mother and an emotionally absent father. When family expectations are always too high, resulting frustration leads to fighting. Overinvolvement, rigidity, overprotection, and denial are typical daily transactions of such families.[17]

Often the eating disorder allows an anorexic person to exercise control over an otherwise powerless existence. Losing weight may be the first independent success the person has had. People with anorexia evaluate their self-worth almost entirely in terms of self-control. Issues of control are central to the development of anorexia nervosa. Some sexually abused children develop anorexia nervosa, believing that if they control their appetite for food, sexual relations, and human contact, they will feel in control and competent and eliminate shameful feelings. Moreover, food restriction, which will arrest development and shut down sexual impulses, may be a strategy to prevent future victimization and guilt feelings in such cases. Often anorexic persons feel hopeless about human relationships and socially isolated because of their dysfunctional families. They substitute the world of food, eating, and weight for the world of human relationships.[3]

> A person with anorexia nervosa may use the disorder to gain attention from the family, sometimes in hopes of holding the family together.

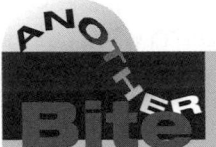

As noted at the outset, some Americans feel that a thin body might make life perfect. Losing weight appeals especially to young people. Most vulnerable are young women who feel alienated from or suffocated by their parents. Parents may not consider a teenager mature enough to make decisions, for instance. She disagrees, and if the situation is very tense, she may turn to purging or starving as a way to show her power. "You may try to control my life, but I can do anything I want with my body."

In the words of one young woman: "I couldn't get angry, because it would be like destroying someone else, like my mother. It felt like she would hate me forever. I got angry through anorexia nervosa. It was my last hope. It's my own body and this was my last-ditch effort."

Early Warning Signs

A person developing anorexia nervosa exhibits important warning signs. At first, dieting becomes the life focus. The person may think, "The only thing I am good at is dieting. I can't do anything else." This innocent beginning often leads to very abnormal self-perceptions and eating habits, such as cutting a pea in half before eating it. An anorexic person may cook a large meal and watch others eat it while refusing to eat anything.[22]

As the disorder progresses, the range of foods may narrow and be rigidly divided into safe and unsafe ones, with the list of safe foods becoming progressively shorter. For people developing anorexia nervosa, these practices say, "I am in control." These people may be hungry, but they deny it, driven by the belief that good things will happen by just becoming thin enough. It becomes a question of willpower.

Soon people with anorexia become irritable and hostile and begin to withdraw from family and friends. School performance generally crumbles. They refuse to eat out with family and friends, thinking, "I won't be able to have the foods I want to eat," or "I won't be able to throw up afterward." They also tend to be excessively critical of themselves and others. Nothing is good enough. Because it cannot be perfect, life appears meaningless and hopeless. A sense of joylessness colors everthing.

As stress increases in the person's life, sleep disturbances and depression are common.[3] Many of the psychological and physical problems associated with anorexia nervosa arise from deficiencies of nutrients, such as thiamin and vitamin B-6, and semistarvation. For this reason a multivitamin and mineral supplement is typically prescribed in therapy.[27] For a female the combination of problems—coupled with lower and lower body weight and fat stores—causes menstrual periods to cease, which is called amenorrhea. This may be the first sign of the disease that a parent notices.

Ultimately an anorexic person eats very little food; 300 to 600 kcal daily is not unusual. In place of food the person may consume up to 20 cans of diet soft drinks and chew many pieces of gum each day.[27]

Physical Effects of Anorexia Nervosa

Rooted in the emotional state of the victim, anorexia nervosa produces profound physical effects. The anorexic person often appears to be skin and bones. This state of semistarvation disturbs many body systems as it forces the body to conserve as much energy as possible. Hormonal responses to semistarvation then cause an array of predictable effects[3]:

- Lowered body temperature caused by loss of fat insulation.
- Slower metabolic rate caused by decreased synthesis of thyroid hormone.
- Decreased heart rate as metabolism slows, leading to easy fatigue, fainting, and an overwhelming need for sleep. Other changes in heart function may also occur, including loss of heart tissue itself.
- Iron-deficiency anemia from a deficient nutrient intake, which leads to further weakness.
- Rough, dry, scaly, and cold skin from a deficient nutrient intake and related anemia. The skin may also show multiple bruises because of the loss of protection from the fat layer normally present under the skin.
- Low white blood cell count caused by a deficient nutrient intake. This condition increases the risk of infection, one cause of death in people with anorexia nervosa.
- Loss of hair caused by a deficient nutrient intake.
- Appearance of **lanugo**, downy hairs on the body that trap air, reducing heat loss and in turn replacing some insulation lost with the fat layer.
- Constipation from semistarvation and laxative abuse.
- Low blood potassium caused by a deficient nutrient intake, loss of potassium from vomiting, and use of some types of diuretics. This increases the risk of heart rhythm disturbances, another leading cause of death in anorexic people.
- Loss of menstrual periods because of low body weight, low body fat content, and the stress of the disease. Accompanying hormonal changes cause a loss of bone mass and increase the risk of osteoporosis later in life.

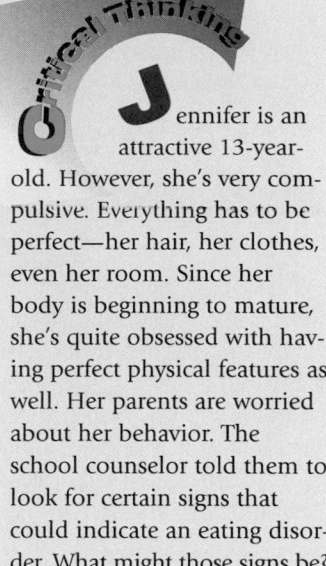

Critical Thinking

Jennifer is an attractive 13-year-old. However, she's very compulsive. Everything has to be perfect—her hair, her clothes, even her room. Since her body is beginning to mature, she's quite obsessed with having perfect physical features as well. Her parents are worried about her behavior. The school counselor told them to look for certain signs that could indicate an eating disorder. What might those signs be?

Lanugo
Downlike hair that appears after a person has lost much body fat through semistarvation. The hair stands erect and traps air, acting as insulation for the body to compensate for the relative lack of body fat, which usually functions as insulation.

Anorexia Nervosa: a Case Study

Jill was 17 years old when she was seen at a sports medicine clinic for stress fractures in her feet and lower left leg. At 5'4" tall and 89 pounds, she was frail and seemed more like a little girl than a blossoming adolescent. A gymnast with a promising future, this young woman had experienced a number of muscle and skeletal injuries in the previous 6 months. She had stopped having menstrual cycles at age 15, when she weighed about 100 pounds. When asked why she started eating a modest diet consisting of a frozen yogurt banana shake for breakfast, fruit or salad for lunch, and a baked potato with nonfat cottage cheese for dinner, she replied, "Because my coach said that I could fly through the roof on my routines if I lost some weight." That was back when she weighed 113 pounds. Jill's coach called the gymnasts with larger bodies "sows."

Her mother reported that Jill was the type of girl who could never sit still. In addition to her daily routine of an hour run, 30 minutes on the stationary bike, and 2 hours of gymnastics practice, she would do deep knee bends while brushing her teeth and bounce on a minitrampoline while watching TV.

Jill's mother and father had been divorced for 2 years. Although rarely at home because of his sales job, her father was critical of her behavior when he was home and would sometimes slap her across the face, frustrated by her imperfection. Jill's mother had multiple sclerosis, and Jill often had to care for her. Despite being popular and well-liked by both teachers and students, Jill felt disconnected from people. Jill stated with great pride, "When I strive for perfection and deprive myself of food, I feel strong, secure, and in control." As she sat in the warm clinic with a bulky sweater and baggy slacks, she proclaimed, "The thinner I get, the greater my chances of competing in the Olympics."

The sports medicine staff who saw Jill referred her immediately to the eating-disorder clinic at the local university medical center. Jill's response was to smile, mumble "OK," and quickly leave. Jill's mother doubted that Jill would be willing to go to the clinic.

- Eventual loss of teeth caused by frequent vomiting. Until vomiting ceases, one way to reduce this effect on teeth is to rinse the mouth with water right away and brushing teeth as soon as possible. Loss of teeth and bone mass can be lasting signs of the disease, even if the other physical and mental problems are resolved.[5]
- Muscle tears and stress fractures in athletes because of decreased bone and muscle mass.

A person with this disorder is psychologically and physically ill and needs help.

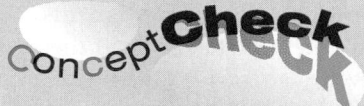

Anorexia nervosa is an eating disorder characterized by semistarvation. It is found primarily—but not exclusively—in adolesent girls, starting at or around puberty. People with anorexia dwindle essentially to "skin and bones" but often believe they are fat. Semistarvation produces hormonal and other changes that lower body temperature, slow the heart rate, decrease immune response, stop menstrual periods, and contribute to hair, muscle, and bone loss. It is a very serious disease that often produces lifelong consequences and may be fatal.

Treatment of Anorexia Nervosa

People with anorexia often sink into shells of isolation and fear. They deny that a problem exists. Frequently, their friends and family members meet with them to confront the problem in a loving way. This is called an *intervention*. They present evidence of the problem and encourage immediate treatment. Treatment then requires a team of experienced physicians, registered dietitians, psychologists, and other health professionals working together. An ideal setting is an eating disorders clinic in a medical center with inpatient facilities. Hospitalization is generally necessary once a person falls below 70% of healthy weight. Still, even in the most skilled hands and using the finest facilities, efforts may fail. This tells us that prevention of anorexia nervosa is of utmost importance.[27]

Once the medical team has gained the cooperation of the patient, the team attempts to work together to restore a sense of balance, purpose, and future possibilities. As previously stated, anorexia nervosa is usually rooted in psychological conflict. However, a person who has been barely existing in a state of semistarvation cannot focus on much besides food. Dreams and even morbid thoughts about food will interfere with therapy until sufficient weight is regained.

Nutrition therapy. The first goal of therapy, then, is to increase food intake, but the therapist must have the patient's cooperation. Otherwise, no long-term benefit will be realized. Ideally, weight gain must be enough to raise the metabolic rate to normal and reverse as many physical signs of the disease as possible. Food intake is designed first to minimize or stop any further weight loss. Then the focus shifts to restoring appropriate food habits. After this, the expectation can be switched to slow weight gain. The initial goal is at least 70% of healthy body weight.[17]

Patients need considerable reassurance during the refeeding process because of uncomfortable effects such as bloating, increase in body heat, and increase in body fat. This is a frightening process, because these changes can lead to feeling out of control. Weight gain is not the only goal of treatment but rather a prelude to fuller engagement in psychological issues. The medical team should assure patients that they will not be abandoned after gaining weight. Because excessive energy expenditure prevents weight gain, professionals must work with anorexic patients to help them moderate their activity. At many treatment centers, patients are placed on moderate bed rest in the early stages of treatment to help promote weight gain.[17]

Experienced professional help is the key. An anorexic patient may be on the verge of suicide and near starvation. Today, suicide is the most common cause of death in people with anorexia nervosa. In addition, anorexic people are often very clever and resistant. They may try to hide weight loss by wearing many layers of clothes, putting coins in their pockets, and drinking numerous glasses of water.[27]

Psychological therapy. Once the physical problems of anorexic patients are addressed, the treatment focus shifts to the underlying emotional problems that led to excessive dieting and other symptoms of the disorder. To heal, these patients must reject the sense of accomplishment associated with an emaciated body. If therapists can discover reasons for the disorder, they can develop strategies for restoring normal weight and eating habits by resolving psychological conflicts. Education about the medical consequences of semistarvation is also helpful.[27] A key aspect of psychological treatment is showing affected individuals how to regain control of some facets of their lives and cope with tough situations. As eating evolves into a normal routine, they then can turn to previously neglected activities.

Therapists may use cognitive therapy, which involves helping the person confront and change irrational beliefs about body image, eating, relationships, and weight.[17] Obviously, issues of sexual abuse need to be addressed as well.

Family therapy is important in treating anorexia nervosa. It focuses on the role of the illness among family members, reactions of individual family members, and ways in which their subconscious behavior might contribute to the abnormal eating patterns. Therapy includes all family members involved with the behavior problem. Frequently a therapist finds family struggles at the heart of the problem. As the disorder resolves, patients must relate to family members in new ways to gain the attention previously tied to the disease. The family needs to help the young person ease into adulthood and accept its responsibilities as well as its advantages.

Self-help groups for anorexic and bulimic people, as well as their families and friends, represent nonthreatening first steps into treatment. People can also attend to get a sense of whether they really do have an eating disorder.

With professional help, many people with anorexia nervosa can lead normal lives. They then do not have to depend on unusual eating habits to cope with daily problems. Although they may not be totally cured, they do recover a sense of normality in their lives. No set answers or approaches exist, because each case is different. Furthermore, there is no specific pharmacological agent used to treat anorexia nervosa. Increasing intake of food is considered the therapy of choice. Establishing a strong relationship with either a therapist or another supportive person is an important key to recovery. Once anorexic patients feel understood and accepted by another person, they can begin to build a sense of self and exercise some autonomy. Then they can progress to substituting healthy relationships with others for a relationship with food, emphasizing alternative coping mechanisms.[20]

A young woman in a self-help group for those with anorexia nervosa explained her feelings to the other group members: "I have lost a specialness that I thought it gave me. I was different from everyone else. Now I know that I'm somebody who's overcome it, which not everybody does."

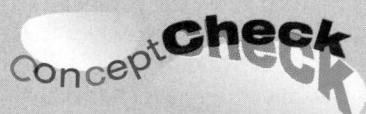

Concept**Check**

To relieve the semistarved condition of most anorexic patients, the initial treatment focuses on moderately increased food intake and slow weight gain. Once this is accomplished, psychotherapy can begin to uncover the causes of the disease and help patients develop skills needed to return to a healthy life. Family therapy is an important tool in treatment.

Bulimia Nervosa

Bulimia nervosa involves episodes of binge eating followed by attempts to purge the food (energy intake). This eating disorder was first classified as a clinical psychiatric disorder in 1980.[3] It is most common among young adults of college age, although some high school students are also at risk. Susceptible people often have biological factors and lifestyle patterns that predispose them to becoming overweight, and many try frequent weight-reduction diets as teenagers.[25] Like people with anorexia nervosa, those with bulimia nervosa are usually female and successful. Unlike anorexics, however, they are usually at or slightly above a normal weight. Females with bulimia nervosa are also more likely to be sexually active than those with anorexia nervosa.

The person with bulimia nervosa may think of food constantly. In contrast to the anorexic person, who turns away from food when faced with problems, the bulimic person turns toward food in critical situations. Also, unlike those with anorexia nervosa, people with bulimia nervosa recognize their behavior as abnormal. These people often have very low self-esteem and are depressed. Approximately half of people with bulimia nervosa have major depression. Lingering effects of child abuse may be one reason for these feelings. Many bulimic persons report that they have been sexually abused. The world sees their competence, while inside they feel out of control, ashamed, and frustrated.[27]

Bulimic people tend to be impulsive, which may be expressed as stealing, drug and alcohol abuse, self-mutilation, or attempted suicide. Some experts have suggested that part of the problem may actually arise from an inability to control responses to impulse and desire. Some studies have demonstrated that bulimic people tend to come from disengaged families, ones that are loosely organized.[6] Roles for family members are not clearly defined. Too little protection is provided for family members, rules are very loose, and a great deal of conflict exists. Anorexic people tend to have families so actively engaged that roles may be too well defined.[17]

Typical Behavior in Bulimia Nervosa

Many people with bulimic behavior are probably never diagnosed. The strict diagnostic criteria specify that to be diagnosed with bulimia nervosa a person must binge at least twice a week for 3 months (see Table 13-1). People with bulimia nervosa lead secret lives, hiding their abnormal eating habits.[9] Moreover, it is impossible to recognize people with bulimia nervosa simply from their appearance. Because most diagnoses of bulimia nervosa are based on self-reports, current estimates of the number of cases are probably low. The disorder, especially in its milder forms, may be much more widespread than commonly thought.

Among sufferers of bulimia nervosa, bingeing often alternates with attempts to rigidly restrict food intake. Elaborate "food rules" are common, such as avoiding all sweets. Thus eating just one cookie or donut may cause bulimic persons to feel they have broken a rule. Then the objectionable food must be eliminated. Usually this leads to further overeating, partly because it is easier to regurgitate a large amount of food than a small amount. For intake to qualify as a binge, an atypically large amount of food must be consumed in a short period of time and the person must exhibit a lack of control over this behavior.

Binge-purge cycles may be practiced daily, weekly, or at longer intervals. A special time is often set aside. Most binge eating occurs at night, when other people are less likely to interrupt, and usually lasts from $1/2$ to 2 hours. A binge can be triggered by a combination of hunger from recent dieting, stress, boredom, loneliness, and depression.[2] It often follows a period of strict dieting and thus can be linked to intense hunger. The binge is not at all like normal eating; once begun, it seems to propel itself. The person not only loses control but generally doesn't even taste or enjoy the food that is eaten during a binge (Figure 13-5).

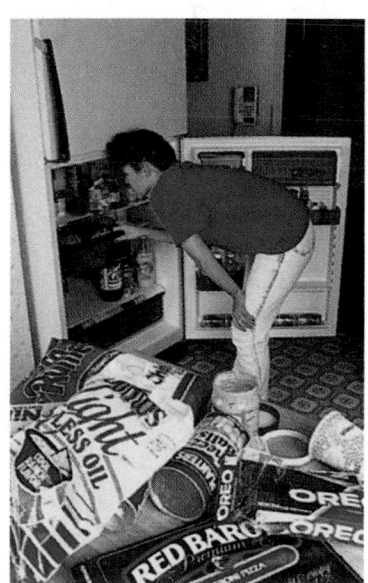

Figure 13-5
The binge-purge cycle. It can lead to a sense of helplessness.

Frequent binges can lead to enormous food bills for a bulimic person.

Most commonly, bulimic people consume cakes, cookies, ice cream, and similar high-carbohydrate convenience foods during binges, because these foods can be purged relatively easily and comfortably by vomiting. In a single binge, foods supplying 10,000 to 15,000 kcal or more may be eaten.[12] Purging follows in hopes that no weight will be gained. However, even when vomiting follows the binge 33% to 75% of the food energy taken in is still absorbed, which causes some weight gain. When laxatives are used, about 90% of the energy is absorbed.[17] The common belief of bulimic persons that purging soon after bingeing will prevent excessive energy absorption and weight gain is clearly a misperception.

Early in the onset of bulimia nervosa, sufferers often induce vomiting by placing their fingers deep into the mouth. They may inadvertently bite down on these fingers. The resulting bite marks around the knuckles are a characteristic sign of this disorder. Once the disease is established, however, a person can often vomit simply by contracting the abdominal muscles. Vomiting may also occur spontaneously.[3]

Another way bulimic people attempt to compensate for a binge is by engaging in hypergymnasia—excessive exercise—to expend a large amount of energy. Some bulimic people try to estimate the amount of energy eaten in a binge and then exercise to counteract this energy intake. This practice, referred to as "debting," represents an effort to control their weight.

People with bulimia nervosa are not proud of their behavior. After a binge they usually feel guilty and depressed. Over time they experience low self-esteem and feel hopeless about their situation (Figure 13-6). Compulsive lying and drug abuse can

Figure 13-6
Bulimia nervosa's vicious cycle of obsession.

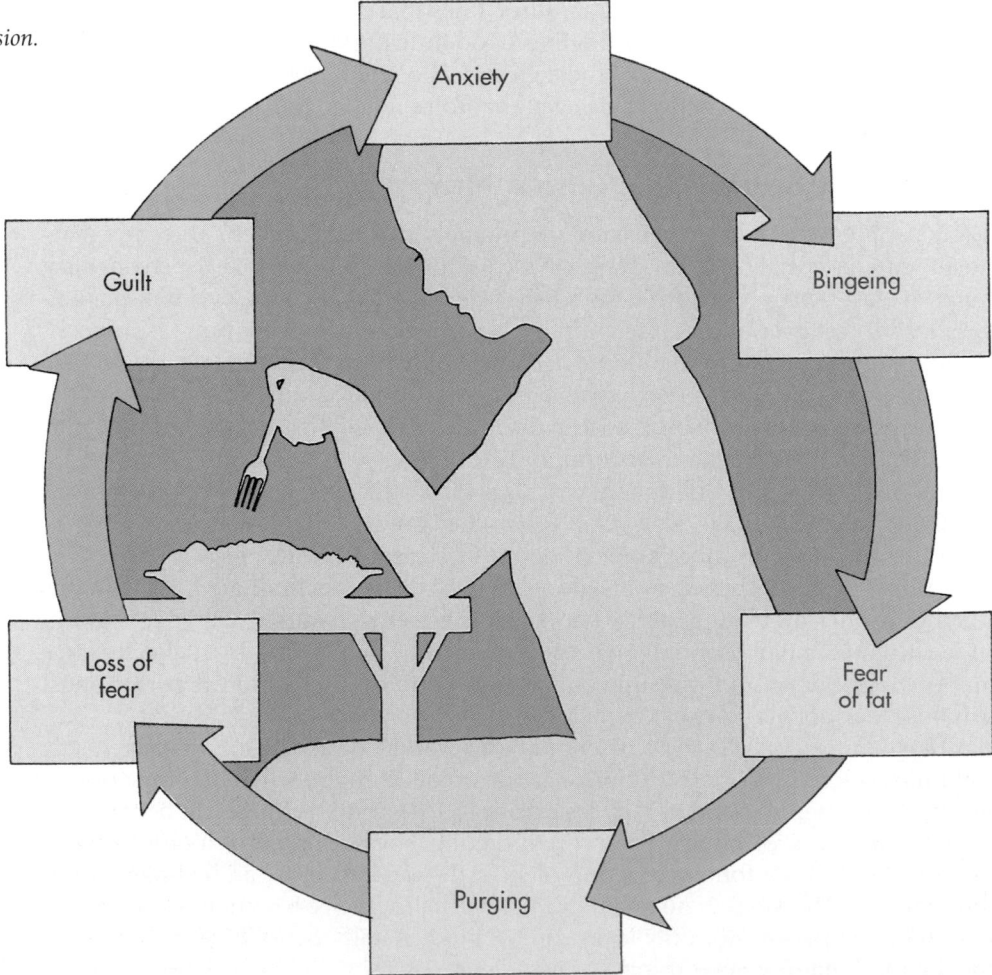

further intensity these feelings.[2] Bulimic people caught in the act of bingeing by a friend or family member may order the intruder to "get out" and "go away." Sufferers gradually distance themselves from others, spending more and more time preoccupied by and engaging in bingeing and purging.

Health Problems Stemming from Bulimia Nervosa

The vomiting that many bulimic sufferers induce is the most physically destructive method of purging. Indeed the majority of health problems associated with bulimia nervosa arise from vomiting.[3,17]

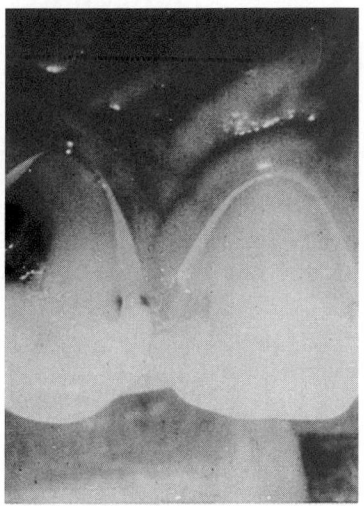

Figure 13-7
Excessive tooth decay is common in bulimic patients.

- Repeated exposure of teeth to the acid in vomit causes demineralization, making the teeth painful and sensitive to heat, cold, and acids. Eventually the teeth may severely decay, erode away from fillings, and finally fall out. Dental professionals are sometimes the first health professionals to notice signs of bulimia nervosa (Figure 13-7). As noted earlier, until vomiting ceases it is important to rinse the mouth with water after a vomiting episode, especially before brushing the teeth.[5]
- Blood potassium can drop significantly with regular vomiting or use of certain diuretics. This can disturb the heart's rhythm and even produce sudden death.
- Salivary glands may swell as a result of infection and irritation from persistent vomiting.
- Stomach ulcers and bleeding and tears in the esophagus develop in some cases.
- Constipation may result from frequent laxative use.[16]
- Ipecac syrup, sometimes used to induce vomiting, is poisonous to the heart, liver, and kidneys. It has caused accidental poisoning when taken repeatedly.

Overall, bulimia nervosa is a potentially debilitating disorder that can lead to death, usually from suicide, low blood potassium, or overwhelming infections.[15]

Treatment of Bulimia Nervosa

Therapy for bulimia nervosa, as for anorexia nervosa, requires a team of experienced clinicians. These patients are less likely than those with anorexia to enter treatment in a state of semistarvation. However, if a bulimic patient has lost significant weight, this must be treated before psychological treatment begins. Although clinicians have yet to agree on the best therapy for bulimia nervosa, they generally agree that treatment should last at least 16 weeks. Hospitalization may be indicated in cases of extreme laxative abuse, regular vomiting, and substance abuse.

The primary aim of psychotherapy is to improve patients' self-acceptance and help them to be less concerned about body weight. To correct the "all-or-none" thinking typical of bulimic persons—if I eat one cookie, I'm a failure and might as well binge—a patient may be asked to role play a scientist testing assumptions and beliefs about food and weight. Patient and therapist together examine the validity of such beliefs. The premise of this therapy is that if abnormal attitudes and beliefs can be altered, normal eating will follow.[17] In addition, the therapist guides the person in establishing food habits that will minimize bingeing: avoiding fasting, eating regular meals, and using alternative methods—other than eating—to cope with stressful situations. Group therapy is often useful to foster strong social support.

One goal of therapy is to help bulimic persons accept as normal some depression and self-doubt. Therapists may prescribe antidepressants and other medications to combat some depression and cravings associated with bulimia nervosa.

Nutritional counseling has two main goals: correcting misconceptions about food and reestablishing regular eating habits. Patients are given information about bulimia nervosa and its consequences. Avoiding binge foods and not constantly stepping on a scale may be recommended early in treatment. The primary goal, however, is to develop a normal eating pattern.[22] To achieve this goal, some specialists

Thoughts of a Bulimic Woman

I am wide awake and immediately out of bed. I think back to the night before, when I made a new list of what I wanted to get done and how I wanted to be. My husband is not far behind me on his way into the bathroom to get ready for work. Maybe I can sneak onto the scale to see what I weigh this morning before he notices me. I am already in my private world. I feel overjoyed when the scale says that I stayed the same weight as I was the night before, and I can feel that slightly hungry feeling. Maybe it will stop today; maybe today everything will change. What were the projects I was going to get done?

We eat the same breakfast, except that I take no butter on my toast, no cream in my coffee, and never take seconds (until Doug gets out the door). Today I am going to be really good, and that means eating certain predetermined portions of food and not taking one more bite than I think I am allowed. I am very careful to see that I don't take more than Doug. I judge myself by his body. I can feel the tension building. I wish Doug would hurry up and leave so I can get going!

As soon as he shuts the door, I try to get involved with one of the myriad responsibilities on my list. I hate them all! I just want to crawl into a hole. I don't want to do anything. I'd rather eat. I am alone; I am nervous; I am no good; I always do everything wrong anyway; I am not in control; I can't make it through the day, I know it. It has been the same for so long. I remember the starchy cereal I ate for breakfast. I am into the bathroom and onto the scale. It measures the same, but I don't want to stay the same! I want to be thinner! I look in the mirror. I think my thighs are ugly and deformed looking. I see a lumpy, clumsy, pear-shaped wimp. There is always something wrong with what I see. I feel frustrated, trapped in this body, and I don't know what to do about it.

I float to the refrigerator knowing exactly what is there. I begin with last night's brownies. I always begin with the sweets. At first I try to make it look like nothing is missing, but my appetite is huge and I resolve to make another batch of brownies. I know there is half of a bag of cookies in the bathroom, thrown out the night before, and I polish them off immediately. I take some milk so my vomiting will be smoother. I like the full feeling I get after downing a big glass. I get out six pieces of bread and toast one side of each in the broiler, turn them over and load them with pats of butter, and put them under the broiler again until they are bubbling. I take all six pieces on a plate to the television and go back for a bowl of cereal and a banana to have along with them. Before the last piece of toast is finished, I am already preparing the next batch of six more pieces. Maybe another brownie or five, and a couple of large bowls full of ice cream, yogurt, or cottage cheese.

My stomach is stretched into a huge ball below my rib cage. I know I'll have to go into the bathroom soon, but I want to postpone it. I am in never-never land. I am waiting, feeling the pressure, pacing the floor in and out of the rooms. Time is passing. Time is passing. It is getting to be time. I wander aimlessly through each of the rooms again, tidying, making the whole house neat and put back together. I finally make the turn into the bathroom. I brace my feet, pull my hair back and stick my finger down my throat, stroking twice, and get up a huge pile of food. Three times, four times, and another pile of food. I can see everything come back. I am so glad to see those brownies because they are so fattening. The rhythm of the emptying is broken and my head is beginning to hurt. I stand up feeling dizzy, empty, and weak. The whole episode has taken about an hour.

From Hall L, Cohn L: *Bulimia—a guide to recovery*, Carlsbad, Calif, 1992, Gurze Books.

encourage patients to develop daily meal plans and keep a food diary in which they record food intake, internal sensations of hunger, environmental factors that precipitate binges, and thoughts and feelings that accompany binge-purge cycles. Keeping a food diary not only is an accurate way to monitor food intake but also may help identify situations that seem to trigger binge episodes. With the help of a therapist, patients can develop alternative coping strategies.[27]

In general, the focus is not on stopping bingeing and purging per se but on developing regular eating habits. Once this is achieved, the binge-purge cycle should stop by itself. Patients are discouraged from following strict rules about healthy food choices, because this simply mimics the typical obsessive attitudes associated with bulimia nervosa. Rather, encouraging a mature perspective on nutrient intake helps patients overcome this disorder—that is, regular consumption of moderate amounts of a variety of foods balanced among the food groups.[1]

People with bulimia nervosa must recognize that it is a serious disorder that can have grave medical complications if not treated. Because relapse is likely, therapy should be long term, as mentioned before. Note that those with bulimia nervosa do need professional help because they can be very depressed and are at a high risk for suicide.[3] About 30% of people with bulimia nervosa recover completely from the disorder. Others continue to struggle with it to varying degrees. This fact underscores the need for prevention, because treatment is difficult.[17]

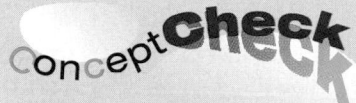

Bulimia nervosa is characterized by episodes of binge eating followed by purging, usually by vomiting. Vomiting is very destructive to the body, often causing severe dental decay, stomach ulcers, irritation of the esophagus, and blood potassium imbalances. Treatment using nutrition counseling and psychotherapy attempts to restore normal eating habits, help the person correct distorted beliefs about diet and lifestyle, and find tools to cope with the stresses of life.

OTHER DISORDERED EATING PATTERNS

In recent years, three other eating disorders—**female athlete triad, binge-eating disorder** and **baryophobia**—have been recognized as requiring professional treatment. Although these disordered eating patterns share some characteristics with anorexia nervosa and bulimia nervosa, they have some distinctive qualities.

Female athlete triad
A condition characterized by disordered eating, lack of menstrual periods, and low age-adjusted bone density.

Female Athlete Triad

As mentioned previously, women participating in appearance-based and endurance sports are at risk of developing an eating disorder.[7,26] A recent study of college-age female athletes found that 15% of swimmers, 62% of gymnasts, and 32% of all varsity athletes exhibited disordered eating patterns.[21] Estimates of eating disorders for college women not involved in competitive sports are much lower.

In addition to disordered eating, college women athletes tend to experience irregular menstruation more frequently than other college women. Disordered eating, particularly food restriction and stress, can precipitate this, causing women to have less dense and weaker bones than normal because of lower estrogen and higher cortisol concentrations in the blood. Some of these young women have bones equivalent to those of 50- to 60-year-olds, making them overly susceptible to fractures during both sports and general activities. Much of the bone loss is irreversible.

The American College of Sports Medicine (ACSM) has named the syndrome consisting of disordered eating, lack of menstrual periods, and compromised bone density *the female athlete triad.*[21] The ACSM has issued a call to teachers, coaches, health professionals, and parents to educate female athletes about the triad and its consequences. Those exhibiting the symptoms should get treatment. One treatment plan has the following goals:

• Reduce preoccupation with food, weight, and body fat.
• Gradually increase meals and snacks to an appropriate amount.
• Rebuild the body to a more appropriate weight.
• Establish regular menstrual periods.

The tragic case of Christy Henrich illustrates why anyone at risk for the female athlete triad should seek professional help. As a young teenager Christy weighed 95 pounds and was 4 feet 11 inches. She showed promise as a gymnast but was told that she was too fat to excel in gymnastics. Christy continued her training but often starved herself, some days consuming just an apple and frequently purging by vomiting. Her success in gymnastics continued, but at age 22 her weight had fallen to 52 pounds, and she died in August 1994 of the effects of long-term semistarvation.

Binge-Eating Disorder

In 1994 binge-eating disorder, commonly called *compulsive overeating,* was formally recognized by the American Psychiatric Association.[3] The diagnostic criteria for this disorder are listed in Table 13-3. Generally it can be defined as binge-eating episodes not accompanied by purging (as typifies bulimia nervosa) at least 2 times per week. In the past the catchall term *compulsive overeating* described a range of habitual excessive eating. Today, health-care professionals recognize this condition as complex and serious, as disturbing a problem as anorexia nervosa or bulimia nervosa.

Binge-eating disorder
An eating disorder characterized by recurrent binge eating and feelings of loss of control over eating. Binge episodes can be triggered by frustration, anger, depression, anxiety, permission to eat forbidden foods, and excessive hunger.

TABLE 13-3

Research Criteria for Binge-Eating Disorder

A. Recurrent episodes of binge eating, an episode being characterized by both of the following:

  (1) Eating, in a discrete period of time (for example, within any 2-hour period), an amount of food that is definitely larger than most people would eat during a similar period of time in similar circumstances.

  (2) A sense of lack of control during the episodes (for example, a feeling that one can't stop eating or control what or how much one is eating).

B. During most binge episodes, at least three of the following occur:

  (1) Eating much more rapidly than usual.

  (2) Eating until feeling uncomfortably full.

  (3) Eating large amounts of food when not feeling physically hungry.

  (4) Eating alone because of being embarrassed by how much one is eating.

  (5) Feeling disgusted with oneself, depressed, or very guilty after overeating.

C. Marked distress regarding binge eating.

D. The binge eating occurs, on average, at least 2 days a week for 6 months.

E. The behavior does not occur only during the course of bulimia nervosa or anorexia nervosa.

From American Psychiatric Association: *Diagnostic and statistical manual of mental disorders (DSM-IV),* Washington, DC, 1994, The Association.

Approximately 30% of subjects in organized weight-control programs have binge-eating disorder, whereas among the general population only 2% to 5% have this disorder.[3] However, many more people in the general population are likely to have less severe forms of the disorder that do not meet the formal criteria for diagnosis. The number of cases of binge-eating disorder is far greater than that of either anorexia nervosa or bulimia nervosa. This disorder is also more common among the severely obese and those with a long history of frequent restrictive dieting.[3]

Development and Characteristics of Binge Eating

Individuals with binge-eating disorder often perceive themselves as hungry more often than normal. They usually started dieting at a young age, began bingeing during adolescence or in their early 20s, and did not succeed in commercial weight-control programs. Almost half of those with severe binge-eating disorder exhibit clinical depression.[23]

Typical binge eaters isolate themselves and eat large quantities of a favorite food. Stressful events and feelings of depression or anxiety can trigger this behavior. Giving themselves permission to eat a forbidden food can also precipitate a binge. They sometimes binge on whatever is easy to eat in large amounts—noodles, rice, bread, leftovers. Characteristically, however, binge eaters consume foods that carry the social stigma of "junk" or "bad" foods—ice cream, cookies, sweets, potato chips, and similar snack foods.

In general, people engage in binge eating to induce a sense of well-being and perhaps even numbness, usually in an attempt to avoid feeling and dealing with emotional pain and anxiety. They eat without regard to biological need and often in a recurrent, ritualized fashion. Some people with this disorder eat food continually over an extended period, called *grazing;* others cycle episodes of bingeing with normal eating. For example, someone with a stressful or frustrating job might come home every night and graze until bedtime. Another person might eat normally most of the time but find comfort in consuming large quantities of food when an emotional setback occurs.[3]

Although people with anorexia nervosa and bulimia nervosa exhibit persistent preoccupation with body shape, weight, and thinness, binge eaters do not necessarily share these concerns. Thus neither purging nor prolonged food restriction is characteristic of binge-eating disorder. Some physicians classify binge-eating disorder as an addiction to food, involving psychological dependence. The person becomes attached to the behavior itself and has a drive to continue it, senses only limited control over it, and needs to persist at it despite negative consequences. Food is used to reduce stress, produce feelings of power and well-being, avoid feelings of intimacy with others, and avoid life problems.[3] Note that obesity and binge eating are not necessarily linked. Not all obese people are binge eaters, and although obesity may result from trying to numb emotional pain with food, it is not necessarily an outcome.

Binge-eating disorder is most likely to develop in people who never learned to appropriately express and deal with their feelings. Rather than face their problems, they turn to food instead. They continue to do the things that perpetuate the experiences or frustration, anger, and pain. For example, people who regularly become frustrated because they don't assert themselves when necessary may eat to forget their frustration rather than learn to deal with this inhibition and practice assertiveness. The frustration will continue because they never attack the basic problem. Binge eating makes them feel they cannot control the behavior pattern and therefore cannot control their lives. Worse, the binge eating usually increases feelings of guilt, embarrassment, and shame.

Often, people who practice binge eating have been shaped by families who do not address and express feelings in healthful ways. The parents nurture and comfort

People with binge-eating disorder may come from families with alcoholism or may have suffered sexual abuse. Members of such dysfunctional families do not know how to deal effectively with emotions. They cope by turning to substances. Family members learn to cover up dysfunctional patterns for the alcoholic person and to nurture him or her at the expense of each other and their own needs.

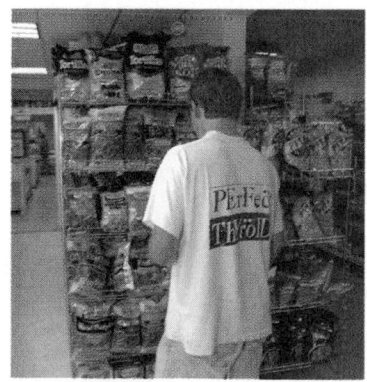

We are all faced with choices related to food. For some people, these choices are more troubling than they are for others.

their children with food rather than engage in healthy exchanges of self-disclosure of feelings and potential solutions. Members of such families learn to eat in response to emotional needs and pain instead of hunger. Those who regularly practice binge eating may grow up nurturing others instead of themselves, avoiding their own feelings and taking little time for themselves. Not knowing how to satisfy their personal and emotional needs in more healthful ways, people in these families turn to food.

For some people, frequent dieting beginning in childhood or adolescence is a precursor to binge-eating disorder.[18] During periods when little food is eaten, they get very hungry and obsessive about food. When allowed to eat more food or given permission to go off the diet, they feel driven to eat in a compulsive, uncontrolled way. The pattern of periods of strict dieting alternating with binge eating may continue over time.

Help for the Binge Eater

Those with binge-eating disorder must learn to eat in response to hunger—a biological signal—rather than in response to emotional needs or external factors (such as the time of day or the simple presence of food). Counselors often direct binge eaters to record their perceptions of physical hunger throughout the day and at the beginning and end of every meal. These people must learn to respond to a prescribed amount of fullness at each meal. They should initially avoid slimming diets because feelings of food deprivation can lead to more disruptive emotions and a greater sense of unmet needs. Diets are likely to encourage more intense problems with binge eating. Many people with this disorder may experience difficulty in identifying personal emotional needs and expressing emotions. Because this problem is a common predisposing factor in binge eating, communication issue should be addressed during treatment.[2] Binge eaters often must be helped to recognize their own buried emotions in anxiety-producing situations and then encouraged to share them. Learning simple but appropriate phrases to say to oneself can help stop bingeing when the desire is strong.[10]

Self-help groups such as Overeaters Anonymous aim to help recovery from binge-eating disorder. The treatment philosophy parallels that of Alcoholics Anonymous. Overeaters Anonymous attempts to create an environment of encouragement and accountability to overcome this eating disorder. Dietary goals typically range from avoiding restraint in eating to limiting binge foods. Some experts feel that learning to eat all foods—but in moderation—is an effective goal for binge eaters. This practice can prevent the feelings of desperation and deprivation that come from limiting particular foods. There is no set answer, but diet extremism is not needed. Antidepressants and other types of medications have been found to help reduce binge eating in these individuals by decreasing depression.[8] Overall, people who have this disorder are usually unsuccessful in controlling it on their own. Professional help is advised.[3]

Baryophobia

A disorder of young children and young adults characterized by stunted growth. It results from parental underfeeding in an attempt to prevent development of obesity and heart disease.

Baryophobia

Some children and young adults who grow more slowly and have a shorter stature than normal may suffer from baryophobia (literally, "the fear of becoming heavy"). Decreased growth in children usually results from disease—commonly a hormonal or other metabolic abnormality. In the absence of a recognized disease in such children, the possibility of baryophobia should be investigated.

This disorder occurs when children are given the same low-fat, high-carbohydrate diet that adults follow.[13] Adults do this in an attempt to prevent children from developing obesity or heart disease later in life. Today's parents and caregivers, themselves frequently harassed by weight problems, may be determined that the children in their care will avoid such ordeals. Although well-intended, such severely restricted diets are detrimental to children because they don't supply enough energy to sustain an adequate growth rate.[27] In young adults, low-energy diets may be self-imposed to avoid a perceived risk of obesity.

Because this disorder results largely from lack of appropriate nutrition information leading to poor food choices, nutritional counseling of caregivers and young adults is the most effective response. They need to be informed about the nutrient requirements and normal weight-gain patterns for the relevant age group. This counseling will show caregivers that including some sweets and medium-fat foods in a child's diet is appropriate (see Chapter 15). The diet can still minimize saturated fat and cholesterol intake, a more important focus in a diet designed to reduce the risk of heart disease. Supplying adequate carbohydrate, protein, and other nutrients is the key to promoting growth in both height and weight during childhood and the young-adult years, and it can be done in a healthful manner.[13]

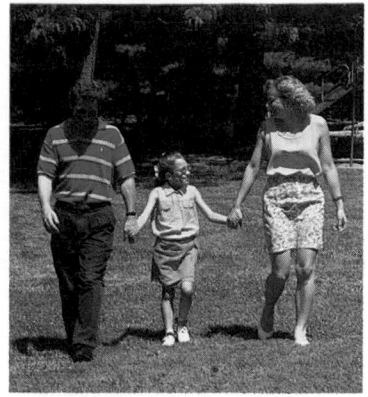

Adults need to be cautious when making weight-related comments to children.

PREVENTING EATING DISORDERS

A key to developing and maintaining healthful eating behavior is to realize that some concern about diet, health, and weight is normal. It is also normal to experience variation in what we eat, how we feel, and even how much we weigh. For example, it is not abnormal to experience some minimal weight change (up to 2 to 3 pounds) throughout the day and even more over the course of a week. A large weight fluctuation or ongoing weight gain or weight loss is a more likely indicator that a problem is present. If you notice a large change in your diet, how you feel, or your body weight, it is a good idea to consult with your personal physician. Treating physical and emotional problems early helps lead you to peace of mind and good health.

With a view to society as a whole, many people begin to form opinions about food, nutrition, health, weight, and body image especially during puberty. Parents, friends, and professionals working with young adults should consider the following advice for preventing eating disorders:

- Discourage restrictive dieting, meal skipping, and fasting.
- Provide information about normal changes that occur during puberty.
- Correct misconceptions about nutrition, healthy body weight, and approaches to weight loss.
- Carefully phrase weight-related recommendations and comments.
- Don't overemphasize numbers on a scale. Instead, primarily promote healthful behavior.
- Encourage normal expression of disruptive emotions.
- Encourage children to eat only when they're hungry.
- Teach the basics of proper nutrition and exercise in school and at home.
- Provide adolescents with an appropriate but not unlimited degree of independence, choice, responsibility, and self-accountability for their actions.
- Encourage coaches to be sensitive to weight and body-image issues among athletes.
- Emphasize that thinness is not necessarily associated with better athletic performance.

Our society as a whole can benefit from a fresh focus on healthful food practices and a healthful outlook toward food and weight.[18]

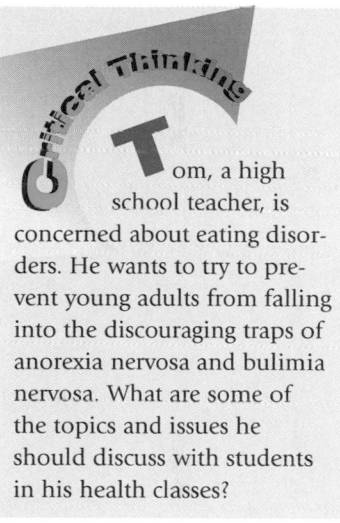

Critical Thinking

Tom, a high school teacher, is concerned about eating disorders. He wants to try to prevent young adults from falling into the discouraging traps of anorexia nervosa and bulimia nervosa. What are some of the topics and issues he should discuss with students in his health classes?

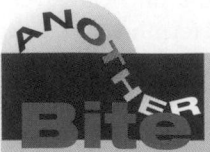

Along with the technical articles in the references, you can gain more insight into eating disorders from the following sources designed for the lay public.

BOOKS

Arenson S: A substitute called food, *ed 2, Blue Ridge Summit, PA, 1989, Tab Books.*

Eades MD: Freeing someone you love from eating disorders, *New York, 1993, Perigee Books/Putnam.*

Freedman R: Body love: learning to like our looks and ourselves, *Carlsbad, Calif, 1989, Gurze Books.*

Hall L, Cohn L: Bulimia: a guide to recovery, *Carlsbad, Calif, 1992, Gurze Books.*

Kano S: Making peace with food, *New York, 1989, Harper & Row.*

Siegel M, Brisman J, Weinshel M: Surviving an eating disorder: perspectives and strategies for family and friends, *Carlsbad, Calif, 1988, Gurze Books.*

Tannehaus N: What you can do about eating disorders, *New York, 1992, Lyn Sonberg Book Services.*

Way K: Anorexia nervosa and recovery: a hunger for meaning, *Binghamton, NY, 1993, Harrington Park Press.*

ORGANIZATIONS AND SELF-HELP GROUPS

American Anorexia/Bulimia Association, Inc., 418 East 76th Street, New York, NY 10021, phone: (212) 501-8351.

Anorexia Nervosa and Related Eating Disorders, Inc., P.O. Box 5102, Eugene, OR 97405, phone: (503) 344-1144.

Anorexia Nervosa and Associated Disorders, Inc., P.O. Box 7, Highland Park, IL 60035, phone: (847) 831-3438.

National Eating Disorders Association (NEDO) at Laureatte Psychiatric Hospital, P.O. Box 470207, Tulsa, OK 74147, phone: (918) 481-4092.

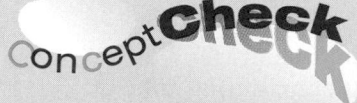

The female athlete triad consists of disordered eating, lack of menstrual periods, and abnormally low bone density associated with female athletes, particularly those in appearance-related and endurance sports. Parents, coaches, teachers, and health professionals need to initiate efforts to prevent and treat this problem. Grazing and food bingeing without purging are two behaviors characteristic of binge-eating disorder. Emotional disturbances are often at the root of this disordered form of eating. Treatment addresses deeper emotional issues, and endorses avoiding food deprivation and restrictive diets, while restoring normal eating behaviors. Baryophobia describes a condition in which children are underfed by parents in an attempt to limit risk of future disease, such as obesity or heart disease. Growth failure—lack of expected weight and height gains—can result if nutrient intake is not increased to an appropriate amount.

Summary

➤ Anorexia nervosa is most common among high-achieving perfectionist girls from middle- and upper-class families marked by conflict, high expectations, rigidity, and denial. The disorder usually starts with dieting in early puberty and proceeds to the near-total refusal to eat. Early warning signs include intense concern about weight gain and dieting as well as abnormal food habits, such as cooking food that they won't allow themselves to eat and classifying foods as safe and unsafe. Anorexic persons become irritable, hostile, overly critical, and joyless; they tend to withdraw from family and friends. Eventually anorexia nervosa can lead to numerous physical effects, including a profound decrease in body weight and body fat, a fall in body temperature and heart rate, iron-deficiency anemia, a low white blood cell count, hair loss, constipation, low blood potassium, and the cessation of menstrual periods. Those with anorexia nervosa are physically very ill.

➤ Treatment of anorexia nervosa includes increasing food intake to support slow weight gain. Psychological counseling attempts to help patients establish regular food habits and to find means of coping with the life stresses that led to the disorder. Hospitalization may be necessary.

➤ Bulimia nervosa is characterized by bingeing on large amounts of food at one sitting and then purging by vomiting, laxative use, exercise, or other means. Both men and women are at risk. Vomiting as a means of purging is especially destructive to the body; it can cause severe tooth decay, stomach ulcers, irritation of the esophagus, low blood potassium, and other problems. Bulimia nervosa poses a serious health problem and is associated with significant risk of suicide.

➤ Treatment of bulimia nervosa includes psychological as well as nutritional counseling. During treatment, bulimic persons learn to accept themselves and to cope with problems in ways that do not involve food. Regular eating patterns are developed as these patients begin to plan meals in an informed, healthful manner.

➤ The female athlete triad consists of disordered eating, amenorrhea, and abnormally low bone density and is particularly common in appearance-related and endurance sports. If not corrected, this disorder will eventually lead to decreased athletic performance and general health problems.

➤ Binge-eating disorder, which is more widespread than either anorexia nervosa or bulimia nervosa, is most common among people with a history of frequent, unsuccessful dieting. Binge eaters typically either practice grazing (i.e., eating continually over extended periods) or bingeing without purging. Emotional disturbances are often at the root of this disordered form of eating. Treatment addresses deeper emotional issues, discourages food deprivation and restrictive diets, and helps to restore normal eating behaviors.

➤ Baryophobia describes a condition in which children are underfed by caregivers in an attempt to limit risk of future disease, such as obesity or heart disease. Growth failure—in weight and height gains—can result if nutrient intake is not increased to appropriate amounts.

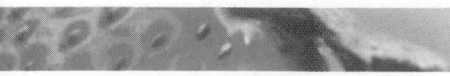

Study Questions

1 What are the typical characteristics of a person with anorexia nervosa? What may influence a person to begin rigid, self-imposed dietary patterns?

2 List the detrimental physical and psychological side effects of bulimia nervosa. Describe important goals of the psychological and nutrition therapy used to treat bulimic patients.

3 How might parents significantly contribute to the development of an eating disorder? Suggest an attitude that a parent or adult friend of yours displayed that may not have been conducive to developing a normal relationship to food.

4 Based on your knowledge of good nutrition and sound dietary habits, answer the following questions:

a How can repeated bingeing and purging lead to significant nutrient deficiencies?

b How can significant nutrient deficits contribute to major health problems in later life?

c A friend asks you, the nutrition expert, if it is okay to "cleanse" the body by eating only grapefruit for a week. What is your response?

5 How, in your opinion, has society contributed to the development of various forms of disordered eating? Provide an example.

6 List the three symptoms that compose the female athlete triad. What is the major health risk associated with amenorrhea in the female athlete?

7 How does binge-eating disorder differ from bulimia nervosa? Describe factors that contribute to the development and treatment of binge-eating disorder.

References

1 ADA Reports: Position of the American Dietetic Association: Nutrition intervention in the treatment of anorexia nervosa, bulimia nervosa, and binge eating, *Journal of the American Dietetic Association* 94:902,1994.

2 Agras WS and others: Does interpersonal therapy help patients with binge eating disorder who fail to respond to cognitive-behavioral therapy? *Journal of Consulting and Clinical Psychology* 63:356, 1995.

3 American Psychiatric Association: *Diagnostic and statistical manual of mental disorders (DSM-IV)*, Washington, DC, 1994, The Association.

4 Ash JB, Piazza E: Changing symptomatology in eating disorders, *International Journal of Eating Disorders* 18:27, 1995.

5 Barlett DW, Smith BG: The dental impact of eating disorders, *Dental Update* 21:404, 1994.

6 Chandy JM and others: Female adolescents of alcohol misusers: disordered eating features, *International Journal of Eating Disorders* 17:283, 1995.

7 Clark N: Counseling the athlete with an eating disorder: a case study, *Journal of the American Dietetic Association* 94:656, 1994.

8 Drewnowski A and others: Naloxone, an opiate blocker, reduces the consumption of sweet high-fat foods in obese and lean female binge eaters, *American Journal of Clinical Nutrition* 61:1206, 1995.

9 Eilers GM: Bulimia: my secret no more, *Journal of the American Medical Association* 275:83, 1996.

10 Fairburn CG and others: Cognitive-behavioral therapy for binge eating and bulimia nervosa. In Fairburn CG, Wilson GT, editors: *Binge eating*, New York, 1994, Guilford Press.

11 Gleaves DH, Eberenz KP: Sexual abuse histories among treatment-resistant bulimia nervosa patients, *International Journal of Eating Disorders* 15:227, 1994.

12 Hetherington MM and others: Eating behavior in bulimia nervosa: multiple meal analyses, *American Journal of Clinical Nutrition* 60:864, 1994.

13 Lifshitz F: Children on adult diets: Is it harmful? Is it helpful? *Journal of the American College of Nutrition* 11:84S, 1992.

14 Lucas AR, Huse DM: Behavioral disorders affecting food intake: anorexia nervosa and bulimia nervosa. In Shils ME and others, editors: *Modern nutrition in health and disease*, Philadelphia, 1994, Lea & Febiger.

15 Marcos A and others: Evaluation of immunocompetence and nutrition in patients with bulimia nervosa, *American Journal of Clinical Nutrition* 57:65, 1993.

16 McClain CJ and others: Gastrointestinal and nutritional aspects of eating disorders, *Journal of the American College of Nutrition* 12:466, 1993.

17 McDuffe JR, Kirkley BG: Eating disorders. In Krummel DA, Kris-Etherton PM, editors: *Nutrition in women's health*, Gaithersburg, Md., 1996, Aspen Publishers.

18 Neumark-Sztainer D: Excessive weight preoccupation, *Nutrition Today* 30:68, 1995.

19 Olivardia R and others: Eating disorders in college men; *American Journal of Psychiatry* 152:1279, 1995.

20 Polivy J: Psychological consequences of food restriction, *Journal of the American Dietetic Association* 96:589, 1996.

21 Skolnick AA: Female athlete triad risk for women, *Journal of the American Medical Association* 270:921, 1993.

22 Strubbe JH: Anorexia and bulimia nervosa. In Westerterp-Plantenga MS and others, editors: *Food intake and energy expenditure*, Boca Raton, Fla., 1994, CRC Press.

23 Telch CF and others: Obesity, binge eating, and psychopathology: are they related? *International Journal of Eating Disorders* 15:53, 1994.

24 Varner LM: Dual diagnosis: patients with eating and substance-related disorders, *Journal of the American Dietetic Association* 95:224, 1995.

25 Weltzin TE and others: Serotonin and bulimia nervosa, *Nutrition Reviews* 52:399, 1994.

26 Williamson DA and others: Structural equation modeling of risk factors for the development of eating disorder symptoms in female athletes, *International Journal of Eating Disorders* 17:387, 1995.

27 Zerbe KJ: Anorexia nervosa and bulimia nervosa, *Postgraduate Medicine* 99:161, 1996.

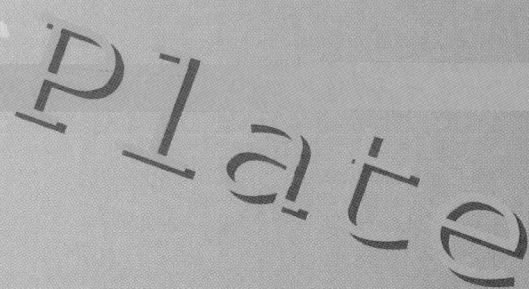

R A T E

Assessing Your Risk of Developing an Eating Disorder

The statements below are based on the primary diagnostic criteria for anorexia nervosa and bulimia nervosa listed in Table 13-1. Put an "X" in the space before statements that describe your characteristics and lifestyle. Respond as honestly as possible.

_____ 1. You refuse to keep your body weight over a minimal normal weight for age and height.
_____ 2. You intensely fear gaining weight or becoming fat, even though you are underweight.
_____ 3. You feel fat even though you are quite thin.
_____ 4. If you are female, you have missed at least three consecutive menstrual cycles.
_____ 5. You have recurrent episodes of binge eating.
_____ 6. You can't control your eating behavior during food binges.
_____ 7. You regularly self-induce vomiting, use laxatives or diuretics, diet strictly or fast, or vigorously exercise for long periods to prevent weight gain.
_____ 8. You engage in a minimum average of two binge-eating episodes a week.
_____ 9. You are persistently and excessively concerned with your body shape and weight.

Questions 1 through 4 pertain to anorexia nervosa and 5 through 9 to bulimia nervosa. Complete this activity by answering the following questions:

1. After having completed this checklist, do you feel that you might have an eating disorder or the potential to develop one?
   _____
   _____

2. Do you think some of your friends might have an eating disorder?
   _____
   _____

3. What counseling and education resources exist in your area or on your campus to help with a potential eating disorder?
   _____
   _____

4. If a friend had an eating disorder, what do you think would be the best way to assist him or her in getting help?
   _____
   _____

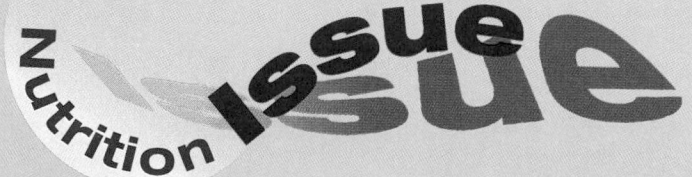

Eating Disorders: A Sociological Perspective

One of the many criteria we use to evaluate ourselves is body image. We identify our body with our self and judge it as we think others see us, knowing that our appearance affects their opinions of us.

Early in life, we develop images of "acceptable" and "unacceptable" body types. Of all the attributes that constitute attractiveness, many people view body weight as the most important, partly because we can control our weight somewhat. Fatness is the most dreaded deviation from our cultural ideals of body image, the one most derided and shunned, even among school children.[18]

Women in particular are likely to diet because they feel strongly about what is acceptable in both size and weight[3] (Figure 13-8). In general, though, most dieting women aren't technically obese. Rather, they diet to correct some perceived flaw or because they simply feel they should weigh less than they do now. Their impulse "to please" fosters this desire to look socially acceptable.

A *Glamour* magazine survey indicated that 80% of the 30,000 respondents were ashamed of their bodies. Those who were dissatisfied primarily wanted to weigh less and have smaller thighs, hips, buttocks, and waists, typical sites of greatest fat deposition in sexually mature women.

CHANGING TIMES

The cultural ideal of the "full-bodied" woman did not survive into the twentieth century in Western society, though it is still in fashion in many nonindustrialized countries, where a large body is a sign of wealth. Over the course of this century the "ideal" female body form in the United States has become progressively thinner. A thin waist with modest hips is the overriding cultural "gold standard," at least as exemplified by models. Our passion for thinness may have its roots in the Victorian era, which specialized in denying "unpleasant" physical realities, such as appetite and sexual desire. Flappers of the 1920s cemented a trend for thinness (Figure 13-9). Even as the ideal gradually moved toward a thinner, more angular body shape, the average weight among the general female population increased.

Researchers have linked this preference for a lean body type to the recent surge in eating disorders.[18] As the more full-figured woman (earth mother) was displaced by the ultra-thin woman, the number of eating disorders increased, along with our society's preoccupation with obesity. The cultural pressures toward thinness seem to be stretching the physiological capabilities of many women (and men). For example, researchers surmise that the theoretical body fat content of the "Barbie doll" would not allow for menstruation. Given the natural variability in human basal metabolism and genetic makeup, as well as American's easy access to food and increasingly sedentary lifestyles, it is no surprise that some of us gain weight. People predisposed to eating disorders for either biological or emotional reasons may be nudged "over the edge" by these social changes.

CATHY

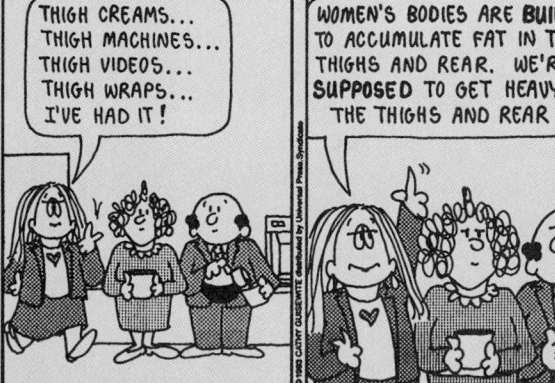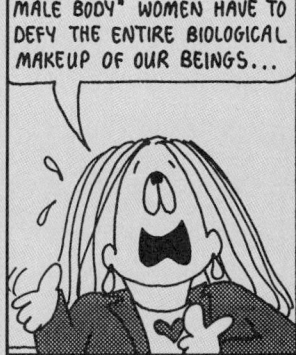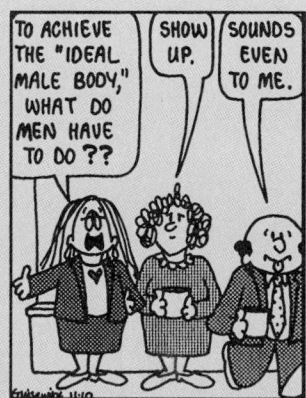

Figure 13-8 *Cathy*

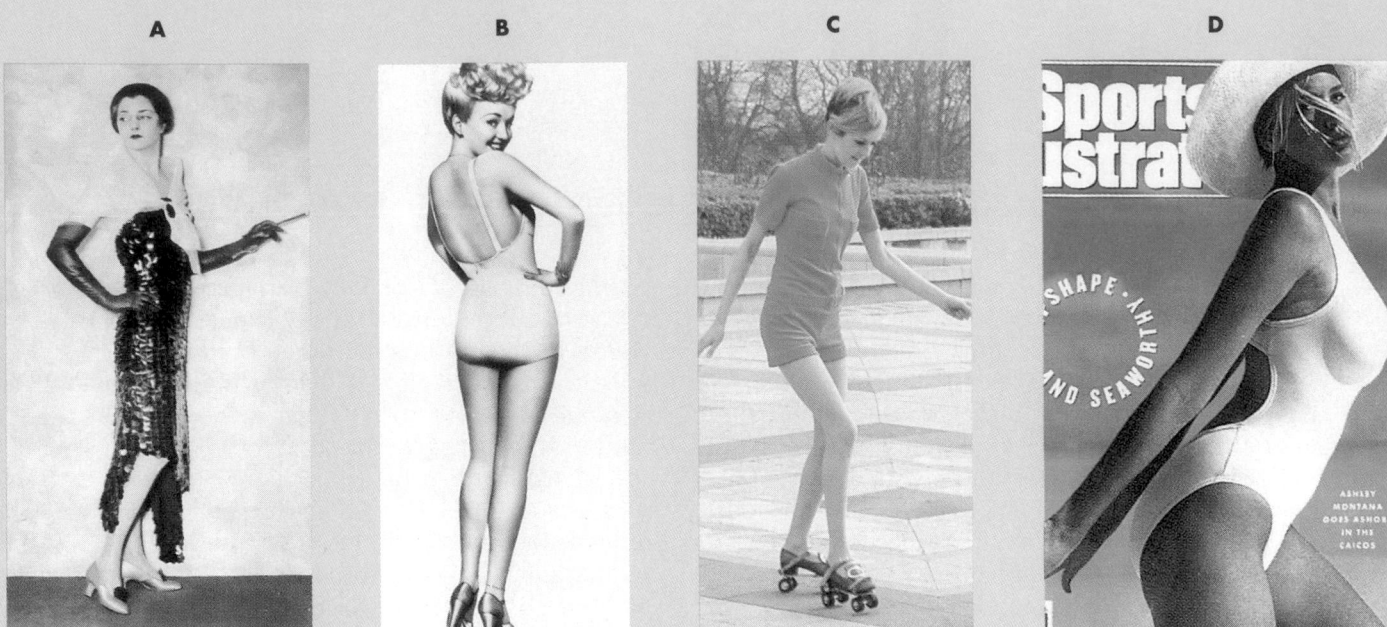

Figure 13-9 *The changing views of body weight. American society has imposed varying stereo-types for body weight, especially for women. **A,** The svelte flapper of the 1920s. **B,** The "thin but curvaceous" look of the 1940s. **C,** Ultra-thin was in during the 1960s. **D,** Lean and well-toned physiques grace magazine covers of the 1980s and 1990s.*

THINNESS AS AN INDICATOR OF COMPETENCE

Unfortunately, many Americans today view obesity as a failure of control, willpower, competence, and productivity. At stake are social acceptance and even access to scarce resources, such as good jobs and an attractive spouse. Whether we like it or not, in today's society our appearance says a lot about us, even though the way we were raised and our genetic background are beyond our control. Some people are simply much more likely to become obese than others. Implicit in our societal attitudes is the notion that those who can't control themselves enough to stay slim are unlikely to be good at supervising employees, organizing their work day, and shoulder-

ing heavy responsibilities. Clearly, fat is out! A prevailing myth is that thin people are more competent, energetic, and forceful than obese people.

MIXED MESSAGES AND SOCIAL TRENDS

Despite the pressure for thinness, our society is filled with mixed messages. Half the advertisements in women's magazines may describe diets or feature emaciated models; the other half displays tasty foods. Movie and television stars are almost always perfect physical specimens. Nevertheless, television advertisements encourage us to visit our local quick-service restaurant. There you can buy a hamburger, french fries, and milk shake, totaling approximately 1200 kcal—about the amount of energy our daily basal metabolism uses—without even leaving the car.

In the past several decades, divorce, alcoholism in families, child abuse, school- and work-related stress, socioeconomic changes, and crowded urban conditions have all increased. These changes in our family and social environments encourage children, adolescents, and adults alike to find a release from the pressure. Many find relief in food, which sets the stage for development of an eating disorder.

INTERNALIZING THE THINNESS IDEAL

Eating disorders are usually only a symptom of significant emotional trauma or psychological stress in a person's life. When psychiatrists are able to dig deeper, they find that eating disorders mask serious questions of self-worth, family struggles, and sometimes fears of puberty and the future. The real illnesses are not the eating disorders—though they eventually contribute to poor health—but, rather, the way people feel about themselves. When people internalize the social value favoring thinness and can't meet that goal, their negative self-image is reinforced.[3]

GLIMMERS OF HOPE

Because eating disorders stem in part from certain cultural values, changing these values might reduce the pressures predisposing some people to various types of disordered eating behavior. Feminists, for example, assert that true liberation means being free to find one's natural weight. Women who combine careers and motherhood are saying that they have more important things to worry about; some fashion leaders are tolerating more curves; exercise programs are encouraging regular brisk walking, rather than mostly jogging and working out. Writers, therapists, and some registered dietitians are working to help women accept their bodies.

What is the difference between people who can accept themselves—even with a few more pounds than the glamorous people have—and those who chronically diet and feel dissatisfied? Perhaps it is the willingness to recognize that satisfaction comes from within, not from the mirror or the approval of others. The challenge facing many Americans is achieving a healthy body weight without excessive dieting. This means adopting and maintaining sensible eating habits, a physically active lifestyle, and realistic and positive attitudes and emotions while practicing creative ways to handle stress.[20]

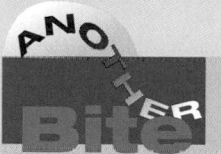

By severely restricting energy intake for long periods, adolescent girls and young adult women greatly compromise their nutritional status, impair their reproductive systems, and retard growth. The harm produced by milder, shorter periods of diet restriction is not clear. Evidence, however, suggests that even moderate diet restriction, if continued, contributes to the risks for various anemias, later pregnancy complications and low-birth-weight infants, and permanently reduced bone density. The percentage of adolescents and young adults who significantly restrict food intake is not known. However, at least two problems, iron-deficiency anemia and pregnancy complications, affect this age-group to a significant degree.

NUTRITION

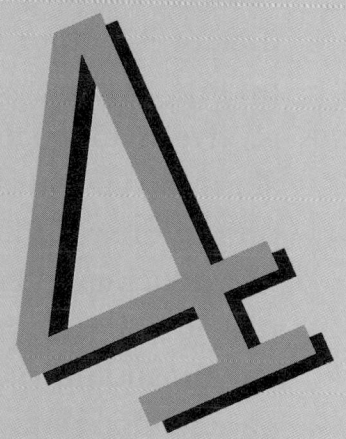

A Focus on Life Stages

PART 4

Pregnancy and Breastfeeding

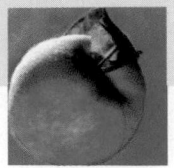

PREGNANCY CAN BE A VERY

special time for a couple. Along with the responsibility of shaping a child's health and personality comes the prospective exhilaration of watching the child develop and grow. Prospective parents often feel an overriding desire to produce a healthy baby, which opens them up to new nutrition and health information. The parents-to-be usually want to do everything possible to maximize their chances of having a robust, lively newborn.[29]

Despite these possibilities, the infant mortality rate in the United States is higher than that of 23 other industrialized nations. In the United States about 8.5 of every 1000 infants per year die before their first birthday, and about 20% of pregnant women receive inadequate prenatal care. Teenage mothers are at the highest risk.[24] These are alarming statistics for the country that has the highest per capita expenditure for health care in the world.

Producing a healthy baby is not just a matter of luck. True, some aspects of fetal and newborn health are beyond a parent's control. Still, conscious decisions about social, health, and nutritional factors significantly affect the baby's health and future.[9] What the parents do relates directly to the likelihood of having a healthy newborn. Let's examine the practices that build toward a healthy baby.

CHAPTER 14

ASSESS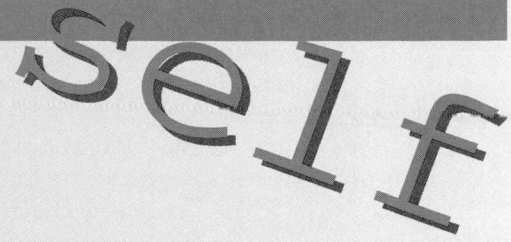

The Right Start for a Healthy Life

Preterm (also called *premature*) and low–birth-weight infants are commonplace in the United States today. Do you know the risk factors for these outcomes of pregnancy?

Find out by indicating whether the following statements are true or false.

T F 1. A pregnancy duration of less than 37 weeks does not cause concern with respect to an infant's birth weight.

T F 2. Women younger than 18 years of age have an increased risk of having a low–birth-weight infant.

T F 3. Weight gain during pregnancy is an important factor in determining the infant's birth weight.

T F 4. The greater the number of previous offspring, the less the risk of a preterm infant.

T F 5. Risk of having a low–birth-weight infant increases as time between pregnancies decreases.

T F 6. Prenatal education and prenatal care do not significantly increase the chance of having a healthy infant.

T F 7. Financial education and educational level generally affect the outcome of pregnancy.

T F 8. Extreme food faddisms or crash diets can have a detrimental effect on the infant's birth weight.

T F 9. Drug and alcohol use during pregnancy is a major risk factor in delivering a preterm or underweight infant.

T F 10. A woman carrying more than one fetus does not run a greater risk for having a low–birth-weight infant than does a woman carrying a single fetus.

Answers:

True: 2, 3, 5, 7, 8, 9.
False: 1, 4, 6, 10.

How Did You Do?

Perhaps you would like to learn more about nutrition and pregnancy. This chapter reviews the guidelines to maximize the chances of having a healthy infant. Knowing the risk factors to avoid and the health habits to foster is vital information for all parents-to-be.

Key Chapter Concepts

- Pregnancy should be planned because many practices of the mother that can harm the developing offspring are modifiable, such as use of alcohol and certain medications, megadose supplements, and illegal drugs; job-related hazards; and smoking.
- Adequate nutrition is vital during pregnancy to ensure the well-being of both the infant and mother. Poor habits, especially during the first trimester, can cause birth defects. Associated growth retardation and altered development can also occur later in pregnancy.
- Infants born preterm (before 37 weeks of gestation) or with low birth weight (less than 5.5 pounds or 2.5 kilograms) usually have more medical problems at and following birth than typical infants.
- A woman generally needs an additional 300 kcal per day during the second and third trimesters of pregnancy to meet her energy needs. Weight gain during pregnancy should occur slowly, reaching a total of 25 to 35 pounds in a woman at healthy body weight.

- Protein, vitamin, and mineral needs increase during pregnancy. Extra servings from the milk, yogurt, and cheese group and the meat, poultry, fish, dry beans, eggs, and nuts group of the Food Guide Pyramid are recommended. Supplements of iron, calcium, and folate, in particular, may be needed, depending on the woman's current diet.
- Pregnant teenagers require very careful prenatal and nutritional care. Complications of pregnancy are more common in teenagers than in more mature women. Ideally, teenagers should avoid pregnancy.
- Almost all women have the ability to breastfeed their infants. The nutrient composition of human milk is very different from unaltered cow's milk and much more desirable. Colostrum, the first fluid produced by the human breast, is very rich in immune factors.
- Advantages of breastfeeding over formula-feeding for the infant include fewer intestinal, respiratory, and ear infections and fewer allergies and food intolerances. Breastfeeding is also less expensive and may be more convenient for the mother than formula-feeding.

Pregnancy Should Be Planned

Pregnancy deserves planning because many practices or conditions of the mother that can harm the developing infant are modifiable, such as the following:

Pregnancy, in particular, is not a time to self-prescribe vitamin and mineral supplements.

- Alcohol consumption
- Use of certain medications
- Use of illegal drugs, such as cocaine
- Job-related hazards and stresses
- Smoking
- Inadequate diet, such as too little folate and iron intake
- Excess vitamin A intake and megadose nutrient supplement use
- Heavy caffeine use
- Lack of medical treatment with HIV-positive status or AIDS
- Ongoing diabetes or high blood pressure

Trimesters

Three 13- to 14-week periods into which the normal pregnancy of 38 to 42 weeks is divided somewhat arbitrarily for purposes of discussion and analysis. Development of the embryo and fetus, however, is continuous throughout pregnancy with no specific physiological markers demarcating the transition from one trimester to the next.

Women need to pay attention to these risks in the months before attempts at conception begin.[25] This precaution is necessary because women often do not suspect they are pregnant during the first few weeks after conception and may not seek medical attention until after about the first 2 to 3 months (first **trimester**).

Still, even without fanfare, the child-to-be grows and develops daily. For that reason the health and nutritional habits of a woman who is trying to become pregnant—or has the potential of becoming pregnant—are particularly important. Although some aspects of fetal and newborn health are beyond our control, a woman's conscious decisions about social, health, and nutritional factors affect her infant's health and future. A great deal of research suggests that an adequate vitamin and mineral intake in the months before conception and during pregnancy may help prevent birth defects such as neural tube defects. This problem has been linked to folate deficiency[23] (see Chapter 8). For these reasons, parents should be aware of the role nutrition plays in the development of a healthy infant both before and during pregnancy.

Prenatal Growth and Development

For 8 weeks after its conception, a human **embryo** develops from an **ovum** into a fetus. For about another 32 weeks the incomplete fetus continues to develop. When its body finally matures enough, the infant is born. Until birth, the mother nourishes it via a **placenta,** an organ that forms in her uterus to accommodate the growth and development of the fetus (Figure 14-1).

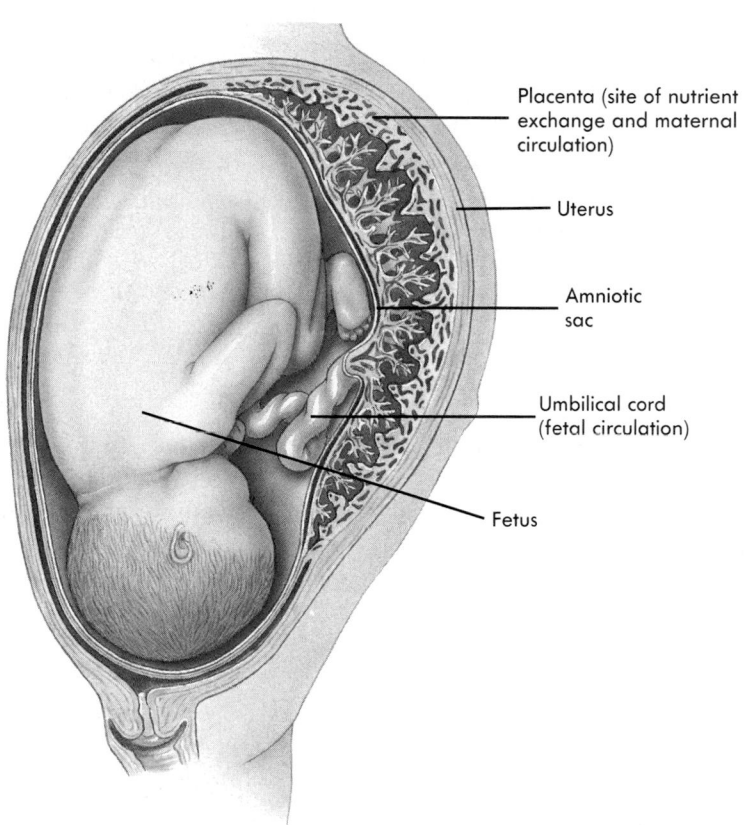

Placenta (site of nutrient exchange and maternal circulation)

Uterus

Amniotic sac

Umbilical cord (fetal circulation)

Fetus

Figure 14-1 *The fetus in relationship to the placenta. The placenta is the organ through which nourishment flows to the fetus.*

Early Growth—The First Trimester Is A Most Critical Time

Embryo growth begins with a rapid increase in cell number (called *hyperplasia*). This type of growth also dominates fetal development. Newly formed cells then grow larger (called *hypertrophy*). Further growth and development combined increase the cell number and size. At about 3 weeks, cells begin to form specialized organs and body parts. By the end of 15 weeks the heart is complete and beating, most organs have formed, and the fetus can move[29] (Figure 14-2).

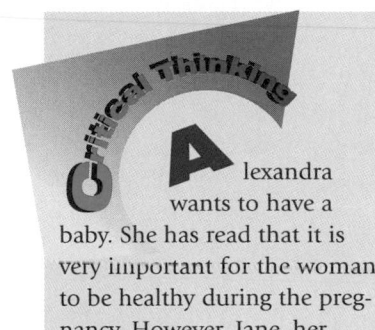

Critical Thinking

Alexandra wants to have a baby. She has read that it is very important for the woman to be healthy during the pregnancy. However, Jane, her sister, tells her that actually before she becomes pregnant is the time to begin to assess her nutritional and health status. What information should Jane have given Alexandra?

Embryo
In humans, the developing in utero offspring from about the beginning of the third week to the end of the eighth week after conception.

Ovum
The egg cell from which a fetus eventually develops if the egg is fertilized by a sperm cell.

Placenta
An organ that forms in pregnant women. Through this organ oxygen and nutrients from the mother's blood are transferred to the fetus and fetal wastes are removed. The placenta also releases hormones that maintain the pregnant state.

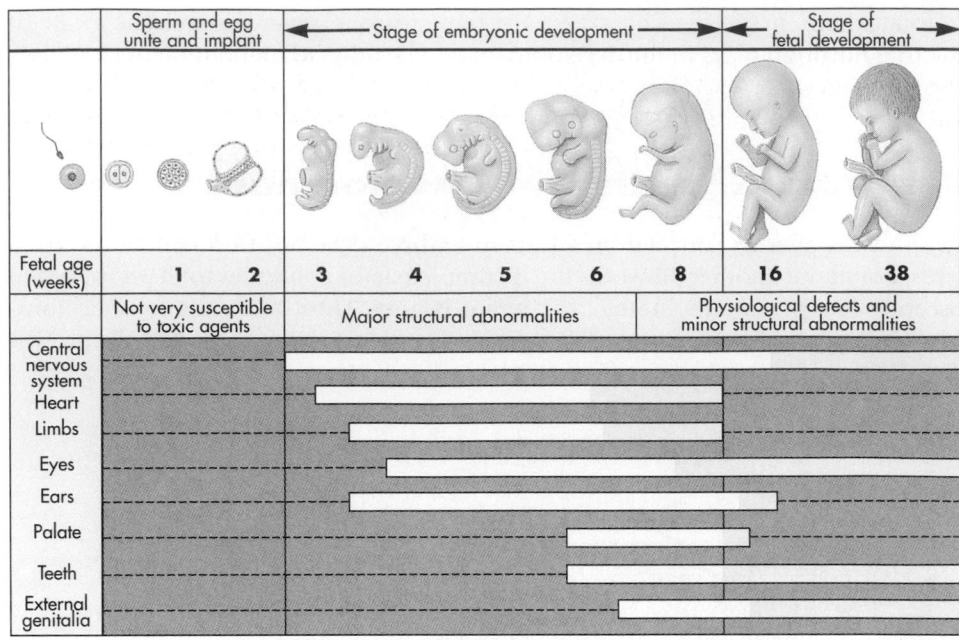

Figure 14-2 *Vulnerable periods of fetal development are indicated with yellow bars. The yellow shading indicates the time of greatest risk to the organ. The most serious damage to the fetus from exposure to toxins is likely to occur during the first 8 weeks after conception. As the chart shows, however, damage to vital parts of the body—including the eyes, brain, and genitals—can also occur during the last months of pregnancy.*

Spontaneous abortion
Any cessation of pregnancy and expulsion of the embryo or nonviable fetus as the result of natural causes, such as a genetic defect or developmental problem; also called miscarriage.

Although a mother's decisions, practices, and precautions during pregnancy contribute to the health of her fetus, she cannot guarantee fetal good health because some genetic and environmental factors are beyond her control. Parents should not hold an unrealistic illusion of control.

Nutritional deficiencies and other insults transmitted through the mother to the embryo or fetus—for example, injuries caused by medications and other drugs, high intakes of vitamin A, radiation, or trauma—can alter or arrest the progressing phase of development. The effects may last a lifetime. The most critical time for these problems to happen is during the first trimester. Most **spontaneous abortions**—premature termination of a pregnancy—occur at this time. Currently, about one third of all pregnancies miscarry, often so early that a woman does not realize she was indeed pregnant. Early miscarriages usually result from a genetic defect or fatal error in fetal development.[12]

A woman should avoid substances that may harm the developing fetus, especially during the first trimester. This holds true for the time when a woman is trying to become pregnant. As previously mentioned, she is unlikely to be aware of her pregnancy for at least a few weeks. In addition, the fetus develops so rapidly during the first trimester that if an essential nutrient is not available, the fetus may be affected even before evidence of the deficiency appears in the mother. Though some women lose their appetite and feel nausea during the first trimester, they must be careful to obtain adequate nutrition.[19]

The Second Trimester

By the beginning of the second trimester a fetus weighs about 1 ounce. Arms, hands, fingers, legs, feet, and toes are fully formed. The fetus has ears and begins to form tooth sockets in its jawbone. Organs continue to grow and mature, and with a stethoscope, physicians can detect the fetus' heartbeat. Most bones are distinctly evident through the body. Eventually the fetus begins to look more like an infant. It may suck its thumb and kick strongly enough to be felt by the mother.

The Third Trimester

By the beginning of the third trimester a fetus weighs about 2 to 3 pounds. An infant that is born after about 26 weeks of **gestation** has a good chance of survival if it is cared for in a nursery for high-risk newborns. However, the infant will not contain the mineral and fat stores normally accumulated during the last month of gestation. This and other medical problems, such as a poor ability to suck and swallow, complicate nutritional care for preterm infants.[29]

At 9 months the fetus weighs about 7 to 9 pounds (3 to 4 kilograms) and is about 20 inches (50 centimeters) long (Figure 14-3). A soft spot in the forehead indicates where the skull bones (fontanels) are growing together. The bones finally close by the time the baby is about 12 to 18 months of age.

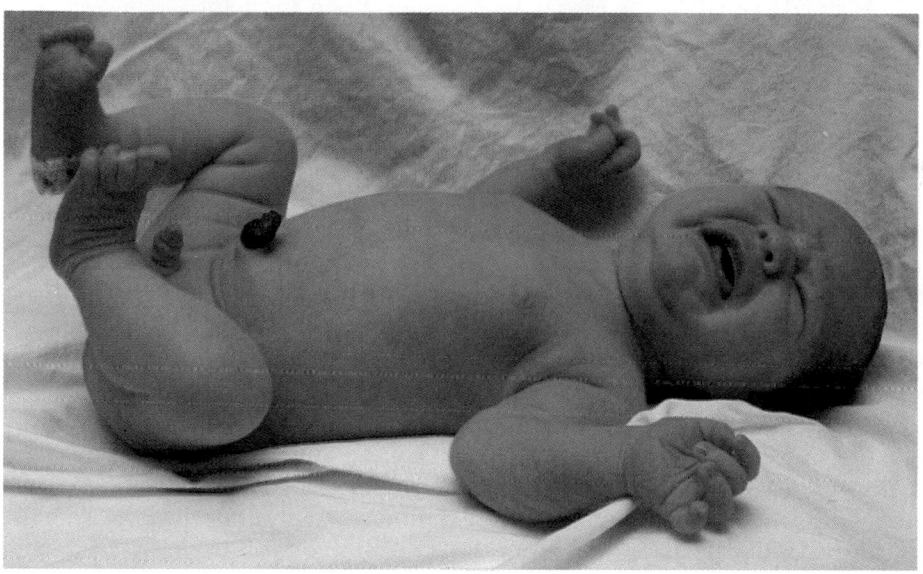

Figure 14-3 *A healthy 1-week-old baby. At birth the baby usually weighs about 7.5 pounds and is 20 inches long.*

Defining a Successful Pregnancy

No generally accepted standards have been adopted by medical organizations to define a successful pregnancy. However, one common criterion is protection of the mother's physical and emotional health so that she can return to her prepregnancy health status. As for the infant, two widely accepted criteria are (1) a gestation period longer than 37 weeks and (2) a birthweight greater than 5.5 pounds (2.5 kilograms). Sufficient lung development, which is likely to have occurred by 37 weeks' gestation, is critical to survival of a newborn. The longer the gestation, the greater the ultimate birthweight and maturation, and hence fewer medical problems are likely to occur.[27]

Low–birth-weight (LBW) infants are those weighing less than 5.5 pounds (2.5 kilograms) at birth. Most commonly LBW is associated with preterm birth. Full-term and preterm infants who weigh less than the expected weight for their duration of gestation, the result of insufficient growth, are described as **small for gestational age (SGA).** Thus a full-term infant weighing less than 5.5 pounds at birth is SGA but not **preterm,** whereas a preterm infant born at 30 weeks' gestation will probably be LBW without SGA. Infants who are SGA are more likely than normal-weight infants to

Gestation
The period of development of the offspring from conception to birth; in humans, gestation lasts for about 40 weeks after the woman's last menstrual period.

Low birth weight (LBW)
Referring to any infant weighing less than 5.5 pounds (2.5 kilograms) at birth; most commonly results from preterm birth.

Small for gestational age (SGA)
Referring to any infant whose birth weight is less than the expected weight corresponding to the duration of gestation. A full-term newborn weighing less than 5.5 pounds (2.5 kilograms) is SGA. A preterm infant who is also SGA will most likely develop some medical complications.

Preterm
An infant born before 37 weeks of gestation; also referred to as premature.

For Better or For Worse®   by Lynn Johnston

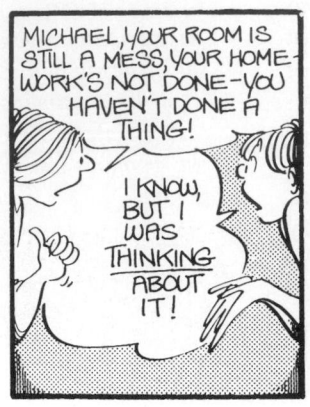 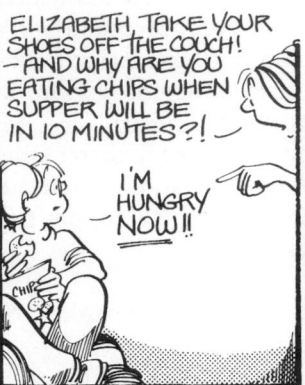 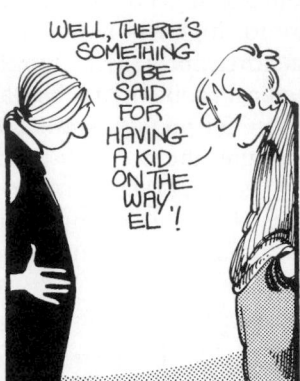 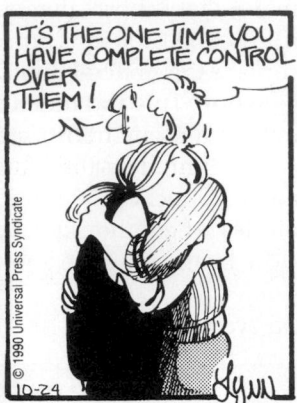

Figure 14-4 *For Better or For Worse.*

Studies from Britain suggest that low–birth-weight infants are likely to develop high blood cholesterol during later adult years. Reduced growth of the liver during gestation is one possible reason. Recall that the liver is a major site in the body for blood cholesterol regulation.[2]

have medical complications, including problems with blood glucose control, temperature regulation, and growth and development in the early weeks after birth.[29]

The newborn's quality of life must also be considered in rating the success of a pregnancy. Overall, prospective parents should strive toward producing a baby who is born healthy, on time, and with the mental, physical, and physiological capabilities to take advantage of whatever life offers, while also protecting the mother's health (Figure 14-4).

Nutrition is one key to a successful pregnancy. Eating healthfully is vital during pregnancy to ensure the health of both the offspring and the mother. Fetal organs and body parts begin to develop very soon after conception. Again, the first trimester (13 weeks) is an especially critical period when poor nutrition or drug use can result in birth defects.

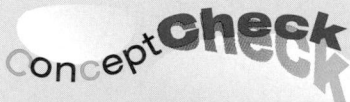

Adequate nutrition is vital both before and during pregnancy to help ensure optimal health of both the mother and her offspring. Organs and body parts in the offspring begin to develop very soon after conception. The first trimester is a critical period when inadequate nutrient intake or alcohol and drug use can result in birth defects.

Infants born after 37 weeks of gestation who weigh more than 5.5 pounds (2.5 kilograms) have the fewest medical problems at birth. To reduce infant and maternal medical problems or death, those involved should take the steps necessary to allow the mother to carry the baby in her uterus for the entire 9 months and contribute to adequate growth. Good nutrition and health practices aid in this goal.

Meeting Increased Nutrient Needs to Support Pregnancy

Over the past century the medical community has changed nutritional advice to pregnant women. In the 1950s, doctors commonly recommended that women restrict weight gain to between 15 and 18 pounds. At times they also recommended severe energy and sodium restrictions to keep the baby small, in hopes of easing labor and avoiding complications. Few of these practices were based on sound research. Scientists know now that many of these recommendations can actually harm the mother and fetus.

The first comprehensive scientific report about nutrition and pregnancy was issued in 1970 by the National Academy of Sciences and updated in 1990. Both documents emphasize an increase in nutritional requirements during pregnancy (not restrictions) and the importance of individually assessing and counseling mothers-to-be.[19]

Increased Energy Needs

An average pregnancy requires approximately 300 extra kcal daily during the second and third trimester. Energy needs during the first trimester are essentially the same as for the nonpregnant woman.[19] Just 2 cups of low-fat milk and a piece of bread, for example, can provide 300 kcal. Though she may "eat for two," the pregnant woman must not double her normal energy intake. She cannot afford a cheeseburger for herself and another for the fetus. She will want to seek the best quality foods to ensure the best possible health for her child. Note that many vitamin and mineral needs are increased by 20% to more than 100% during pregnancy, whereas energy needs during the second and third trimesters represent only about a 15% increase, based on an intake of 2000 kcal per day by nonpregnant women (Figure 14-5). Thus, in order to obtain the necessary vitamins and minerals without increasing her energy intake too much, a pregnant woman needs to seek high-quality, nutrient-dense foods.

If a woman is active during pregnancy, she can add the extra energy she uses to the energy allowance for pregnancy. Her greater body weight requires more energy for activity. Physicians strongly encourage women to continue most activities during pregnancy, except certain calisthenics such as deep knee bends, scuba diving, downhill skiing, weight lifting, and contact sports (such as hockey). Walking, cycling, swimming, and light aerobics are generally advised. However, because many women find that they are inactive during the later months, partly because of their increased size, an extra 300 kcal daily is usually enough.

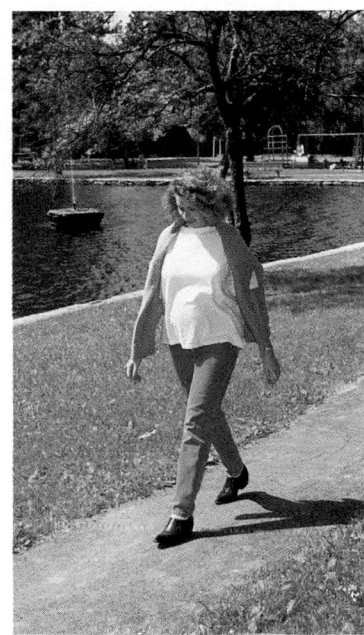

Walking, cycling, swimming, and light aerobics are all suitable exercises during pregnancy.

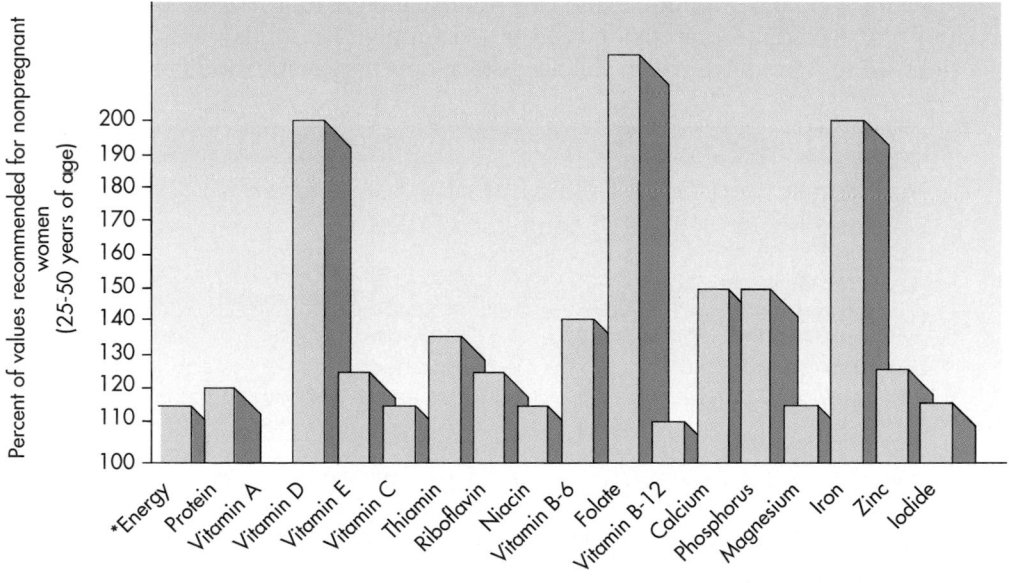

*Second and third trimesters only

Figure 14-5 *Nutrient needs of pregnant women, expressed as percentage of the RDA for adult nonpregnant women. During pregnancy, women need higher amounts of most nutrients, with the exception of vitamin A, than at other times.*

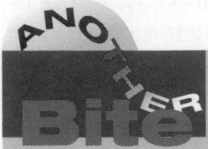

The American College of Obstetrics and Gynecology suggests the following guidelines for physical activity during pregnancy.

1. Do not allow heart rate to exceed 140 beats per minute.
2. Avoid exercising in hot, humid weather.
3. Discontinue exercise that causes discomfort or overheating.
4. Drink plenty of liquids to avoid dehydration and overheating.
5. After about the fourth month, don't exercise while lying on your back.
6. Avoid an abrupt decrease in exertion. In other words, don't just stop and stand around after a hard workout; rather, continue exercising but at a slow pace, gradually reducing pulse rate.

Women with high-risk pregnancies may need to restrict their physical activity. To ensure optimal health for both herself and her infant, a pregnant woman should first consult her physician about physical activity and possible limitations.

Recommended weight gain. Adequate weight gain for a mother is one of the best predictors of pregnancy outcome. Her diet should allow for approximately 2 to 4 pounds (0.9 to 1.8 kilograms) of weight gain during the first trimester and then a subsequent weight gain of 0.75 to 1 pound (0.3 to 0.5 kilogram) weekly during the second and third trimesters. Total weight gain goal normally averages about 25 to 35 pounds (11.5 to 16 kilograms).[19] Adolescents and African-American women, who often have smaller babies, are strongly advised to aim for the greater amount. Women carrying twins should gain 35 to 45 pounds.[14]

For underweight women the goal increases to 28 to 40 pounds (12.5 to 18 kilograms). Body mass index (BMI) is currently the preferred means of establishing this weight status (Table 14-1). The goal decreases to 15 to 25 pounds (7 to 11.5 kilograms) for obese women. Figure 14-6 shows why the typical recommendation begins at 25 pounds. This weight accounts for the total weight of the baby (8 pounds), placenta (1 pound), amniotic fluid (2 pounds), and the mother's increases in uterus and breast tissue (6 pounds), greater blood supply (4 pounds), and increased fat stores (4 to 8 pounds), which she needs to support pregnancy and lactation.

TABLE 14-1

Recommended Weight Gain in Pregnancy Based on Prepregnancy Body Mass Index (BMI)

BMI category*	Total weight gain†	
	(pounds)	(kilograms)
Low (BMI < 19.8)	28-40	12.5-18
Normal (BMI 19.8 to 26)	25-35	11.5-16
High (BMI 26 to 29)	15-25	7-11.5
Obese (BMI > 29)	≤15	≤7

From National Academy of Sciences–Institute of Medicine: *Nutrition during pregnancy*, Washington, DC, 1990, National Academy of Sciences Press.
*See Chapter 10 to review the concept of body mass index (BMI).
†The listed values are for singleton pregnancies. For women of normal BMI who are carrying twins, the range is 35 to 45 pounds (16 to 20 kilograms). Adolescents within 2 years of menarche and African-American women should strive for gains at the upper end of the ranges; short women (<62 inches) should strive for gains at the lower end of the ranges.

A weight gain of between 25 and 35 pounds has repeatedly been shown to yield optimal health for both mother and fetus if gestation lasts at least 38 weeks.[19] The weight gain should yield a birth weight of 7.5 pounds (3.5 kilograms). Although some extra weight gain during pregnancy is usually not harmful, it can set the stage for creeping obesity during the childbearing years if the mother does not return to about her prepregnancy weight. This is especially true if the woman intends to have more than one child.

Weight gain during pregnancy, especially in the teenage years, requires regular monitoring that approximately follows the pattern in Figure 14-6.[11] Infant birth weights improve if the mother's weight gain meets the ranges previously mentioned. Keeping weekly records of a pregnant woman's weight gain can help assess how much to adjust her food intake. Weight gain is a key issue in prenatal care and a concern of many mothers. Inadequate weight gain can cause many problems. If a woman deviates from the desirable pattern, she should be warned of this and counseled on how to make the appropriate adjustment.[29]

For example, if a woman begins to gain too much weight during her pregnancy, she should not be encouraged to lose weight to get back on track. She should simply slow the increase in weight to parallel the rise on the prenatal weight gain chart. In other words, the sources of the unnecessary food energy should be found and then minimized. Alternately if a woman has not gained the desired weight by a given point in pregnancy, she shouldn't be encouraged to gain the needed weight rapidly. Instead, she should slowly gain a little more weight than the typical pattern to meet the goal by the end of the pregnancy.

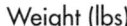

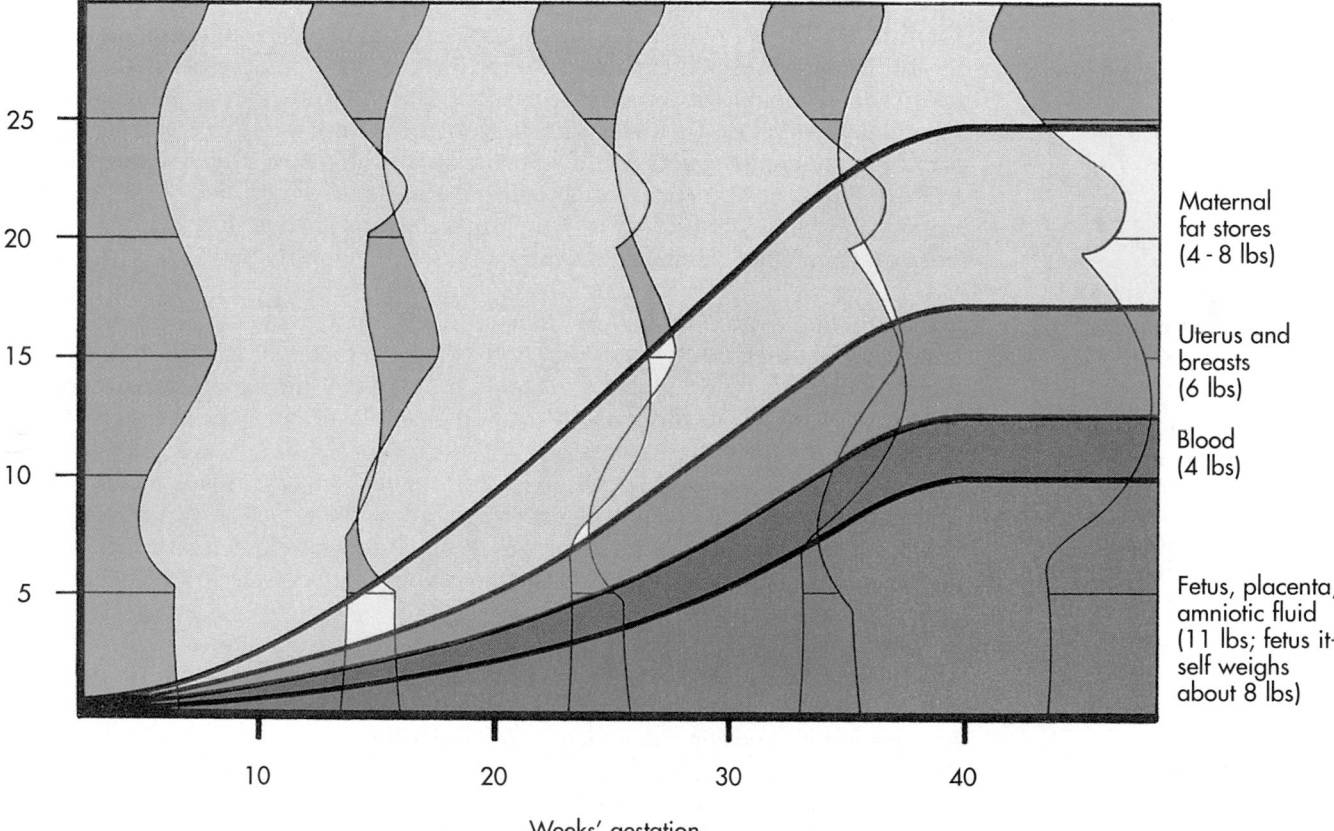

Figure 14-6 *The components of weight gain in pregnancy. A weight gain of 25 to 35 pounds is recommended for most women. Note that the various components total about 25 pounds.*

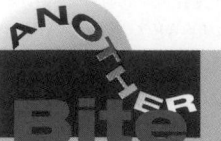

Increased Protein and Carbohydrate Needs

The RDA for protein increases by 10 to 15 grams daily, depending on age. A glass of milk alone contains 8 grams. Many nonpregnant women already eat the recommended 60 grams of protein per day and therefore don't need to increase protein intake. However, all women should check to make sure they are actually eating enough protein. Carbohydrate needs are at least 100 grams daily. This amount prevents ketosis, which can harm the fetus (see later section). Most women already consume almost twice this amount.

Increased Vitamin Needs

Vitamin needs generally increase, especially the need for vitamin D and folate (see Figure 14-5).

Vitamin D. The woman's body increases its calcium metabolism during pregnancy to absorb and distribute extra calcium for forming fetal bones. The mother's need for vitamin D doubles to aid the calcium absorption. To provide it, pregnant women should get regular sunlight exposure. If exposure is impossible or insufficient, they can drink vitamin D–fortified milk to make up the difference. A quart (liter) per day suffices. Pregnant women, especially African-Americans, could also consider a vitamin D supplement that contains 5 to 10 micrograms (200 to 400 IU). The typical prenatal supplement contains this extra amount of vitamin D.

As noted in Chapter 8, in an effort to ensure that folate status is adequate in most women at the time of conception, the FDA has mandated the addition of folate to enriched flours, breads, rolls, buns, corn grits, corn meal, farina, rice, macaroni, and noodle products by 1998.

Folate. Because the synthesis of DNA requires folate, this nutrient is especially crucial during pregnancy. Ultimately both fetal and maternal growth in pregnancy depends on an ample supply of folate. Red blood cell formation, which requires folate, increases during pregnancy. Serious megaloblastic anemia can result if folate intake is inadequate during pregnancy (see Chapter 8). The RDA for folate more than doubles during pregnancy to 400 micrograms per day. This is a critical goal in the nutritional care of a pregnant woman and is advocated for women who have the potential to become pregnant as well. As mentioned before, folate deficiency at conception and after has been associated with birth defects, specifically neural tube defects such as spina bifida.[23]

Some women have difficulty consuming sufficient folate from foods alone to satisfy their pregnancy needs. Recent studies show that some pregnant women consume only about the RDA for nonpregnant women. However, a woman can meet her needs by choosing folate-rich fruits and vegetables as outlined in the Food Guide Pyramid (see later section). Most breakfast cereals provide folate via the fortification process. A prenatal vitamin and mineral supplement may also be used to meet the RDA for folate, especially for women with histories of inadequate folate intake, frequent or multiple births, folate-related anemia, or use of medications that increase folate needs. Normally, however, wise diet choices alone can suffice.

Women who have previously given birth to an infant with a neural tube defect should consult their physician about the need for folate supplementation; an intake of 4 milligrams per day is advocated but must be taken under a physician's supervision.[23]

Meeting folate needs during pregnancy may be problematic for women who have taken oral contraceptives for extended periods, because this can inhibit folate absorption. A recent history of oral contraceptive use necessitates careful attention to folate intake during pregnancy. Ideally the woman would begin a folate-rich diet (or take folate supplements) 4 to 5 weeks before conception.

Increased Mineral Needs

Mineral needs generally increase during pregnancy, especially the need for iron, calcium, and zinc (Figure 14-5).

Iron. Pregnant women need extra iron (twice the RDA for nonpregnant women) to synthesize the greater amount of hemoglobin needed during pregnancy and provide iron stores for the fetus. The greatest need occurs during the last two trimesters. Women often need an iron supplement, especially if they don't consume iron-fortified foods, such as breakfast cereals. Because iron supplements decrease appetite and can cause nausea and constipation, taking them between meals or just before going to bed is best. Milk, coffee, or tea should not be consumed with an iron supplement because these have substances that interfere with iron absorption.[19] Pregnant women may also wait until the second trimester, when pregnancy-related nausea generally lessens, to start iron supplementation. Severe iron-deficiency anemia in pregnancy may lead to preterm delivery, low birth weight, and increased risk for fetal death in the first weeks after birth.[13]

Calcium. Calcium is needed during pregnancy to promote adequate mineralization of the fetal skeleton and teeth. Most calcium is required during the third trimester, when skeletal bones are growing most rapidly and teeth are forming. However, extra calcium intake should start immediately after conception. The current RDA for calcium in pregnancy is the same as for women ages 11 to 24 years (1200 milligrams) and one and a half times the RDA for women over age 24 years. A recent NIH Consensus Conference on Optimal Calcium Intake, however, recommended that calcium intake for pregnant women be increased to 1500 milligrams per day. The only practical food sources of calcium are foods in the milk, yogurt, and cheese group of the Food Guide Pyramid, calcium-fortified orange juice and other beverages, and various calcium-fortified snacks. Calcium supplements are advised if these options are not chosen. A prenatal supplement generally contains 200 milligrams of calcium.

Zinc. Zinc is a mineral important for supporting growth and development. The RDA increases 25% for pregnant women. The protein foods in the diet of a pregnant woman should supply this much zinc. Poor zinc status in pregnancy increases the risk for having a low-birth-weight infant.[7]

Is There an Instinctive Drive in Pregnancy to Eat More Nutrients?

Extra needs in pregnancy for folate, iron, and calcium are the most difficult for women to satisfy. These, then, should be the focus of diet planning for pregnant women. Before diet planning is discussed, however, one important misconception about pregnancy needs to be dispelled. You may have heard that mothers instinctively know what to eat and that their craving for pickles and ice cream is dictated

Iron supplementation is routine during pregnancy in the United States, but its usefulness is under debate.[30] This is partly because prepregnancy iron status varies considerably among women and because iron absorption increases during pregnancy. Individual assessment of iron status is instead advocated by some experts, with treatment using medicinal iron only in women who show iron deficiency.

by a natural desire to consume needed nutrients. These cravings are most common during the last two trimesters and could be related to hormonal changes in the mother or just family traditions.

It remains an even greater mystery why some women crave nonfood items during pregnancy. The craving for and eating of items such as starch, ice, chalk, burnt matchsticks, soap, plaster, and clay, especially noted during pregnancy, is called *pica*. This practice occurs more frequently among African-American women in the United States and probably results more from cultural influences and learned behaviors than from a need for specific nutrients like iron and zinc. It also poses some health risks. Eating soil raises the risk of infections from parasites or lead toxicity and can cause anemia as well as life-threatening blockages of the intestinal tract. Eating laundry starch should be discouraged because it contains toxic compounds, as do the wall plaster, mothballs, and toilet air fresheners consumed by some. Eating ice can break teeth.

Overall, although women may have a natural instinct to consume the right foods in pregnancy, humans are so far removed from living by instinct that relying on our desires is risky. Good nutritional counseling can focus food choices more reliably.[29]

Pica

The practice of eating nonfood items such as dirt, laundry starch, or clay.

If a woman finds herself with no desire at all for pickles and ice cream or frijoles and hot fudge, there is no need to panic: about a third of pregnant women experience no strong food cravings.

A Food Plan for Pregnant Women

One approach to a diet that supports a successful pregnancy is based on the Food Guide Pyramid. It includes at least the following:

- 3 servings from the milk, yogurt, and cheese group
- 3 servings from the meat, poultry, fish, dry beans, eggs, and nuts group
- 3 servings from the vegetable group
- 2 servings from the fruit group
- 6 servings from the bread, cereal, rice, and pasta group

Specifically the servings from the milk, yogurt, and cheese group could include low-fat or nonfat versions of milk, yogurt, and cheese. These foods supply extra protein, calcium, riboflavin, and magnesium. Servings from the meat, poultry, fish, dry beans, eggs, and nuts group should include both animal and vegetable sources. Besides protein, the animal sources help provide the extra iron and zinc needed, and the vegetable sources help provide much of the extra magnesium needed during pregnancy.

The vegetable and fruit group servings provide a variety of vitamins and minerals. One serving from this combination should be a good vitamin C source, and one serving should be a green vegetable or other rich source of folate, such as spinach or orange juice. Selections from the bread, cereal, rice, and pasta group should focus on whole-grain and enriched foods.

Table 14-2 illustrates one daily menu based on the basic diet plan shown. This daily menu supplies about 1800 kcal but still meets the extra nutrient needs associated with pregnancy. Women who need to consume more than this—and some do for various reasons—should add more servings from the fruit and vegetable groups and the bread, cereal, rice, and pasta group to the basic plan above.

Use of Vitamin and Mineral Supplements by Pregnant Women

The National Academy of Sciences supports the use of iron supplements but no other vitamin or mineral supplements during a routine pregnancy.[19] To meet the higher calcium intake recommended by a recent NIH Consensus panel, however, some pregnant women may need to take a calcium supplement.

TABLE 14-2

Sample 1800 Kcal Daily Menu That Meets Nutritional Needs of Most Pregnant and Breastfeeding Women

	Vitamin D	Folate	Calcium	Iron	Zinc
BREAKFAST					
1 hard-cooked egg				✓	✓
1 cup raisin bran cereal	✓	✓		✓	✓
½ cup orange juice		✓			
½ cup 1% milk	✓		✓		
SNACK					
2 tablespoons peanut butter		✓		✓	✓
1 slice whole-wheat toast		✓		✓	✓
½ cup plain low-fat yogurt			✓		
½ cup strawberries					
LUNCH					
1½ cups spinach salad with 1 tablespoon oil and vinegar dressing		✓			
½ tomato					
1 slice whole-wheat toast		✓		✓	✓
1½ oz provolone cheese			✓		
SNACK					
4 whole-wheat crackers				✓	✓
1 cup 1% milk	✓		✓		
DINNER					
3 ounces lean hamburger, broiled				✓	✓
½ cup baked beans		✓		✓	✓
1 hamburger bun				✓	
¾ cup cooked broccoli		✓			
1 teaspoon soft margarine	✓				
Iced tea (milk if a teenager)					

*This diet meets the RDAs for pregnancy and lactation and supplies 24 milligrams of iron. The vitamin-and-mineral–fortified cereal makes an important contribution to meeting nutrient needs.

Although not necessarily recommended by these scientific organizations, specially formulated supplements for pregnant women are prescribed routinely by most physicians. These are dispensed by prescription because of their high folate content, which could pose problems for others, such as older people (see Chapter 8). This routine may exist because it is easier to prescribe supplements than to discuss diet changes. Also, some pregnant women are just not willing to change their diets to meet their increased nutrient needs, or they simply expect (or demand) this treatment. These prenatal supplements typically include the critical nutrients for pregnancy—that is, iron, folate, vitamin D, and calcium—and many others as well.

There is no evidence that potential supplements cause significant health problems in pregnancy, aside perhaps from the combined amounts of supplementary and dietary vitamin A (mainly during the first trimester). While generally unnecessary, prenatal supplements may contribute to a successful pregnancy for certain pregnant women, particularly poor women, teenagers, those with a generally deficient diet, and women carrying multiple fetuses.[19]

Pregnant Vegetarians

Women who practice either lacto-ovo vegetarianism or lacto vegetarianism generally do not face special difficulties in meeting their nutritional needs during pregnancy. Like nonvegetarian women, they should be concerned primarily with meeting iron needs.

On the other hand, when a total vegetarian (vegan) becomes pregnant, she must carefully plan a diet that includes sufficient protein, vitamin D (or sufficient sun exposure), vitamin B-6, iron, calcium, and zinc and also use a vitamin B-12 supplement. The basic vegan diet listed in Table 7-4 in Chapter 7 should be modified to include more grains, beans, nuts, and seeds to supply the necessary extra amounts of some of these nutrients. Because iron and calcium are poorly absorbed from most plant foods, iron and calcium supplements are probably necessary but should not be taken together to avoid competition for absorption. The amounts provided by typical prenatal supplements should suffice to meet iron needs but not calcium needs. The prenatal supplement will also fulfill vitamin D needs if sufficient sun exposure does not take place.

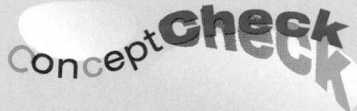

Concept Check

Energy needs increase by an average of about 300 kcal per day during the second and third trimesters of pregnancy. Weight gain should be slow and steady up to a total of 25 to 35 pounds for a woman of healthy weight. Protein, vitamin, and mineral needs all increase during pregnancy. Vitamin D, folate, iron, calcium, and zinc are nutrients of particular concern. A pregnant woman's diet should be varied and generally include more milk products and more specified fruits and vegetables (e.g., those rich in folate) than a prepregnancy diet. Prenatal supplemental vitamins and minerals are commonly prescribed but are often unnecessary, aside from the folate and iron they supply. Taking too many supplements—especially vitamin A—can be hazardous to the fetus.

The Effect of Nutrition on the Success of Pregnancy

Is this attention to nutrition worth the effort? Yes, evidence shows that the effort is justified. Extra nutrients and energy are used for fetal growth, as well as the changes in the mother's body to accommodate the fetus. Her uterus and breasts grow, the placenta develops, her total blood volume increases, the heart and kidneys work harder, and stores of body fat increase. All these changes prepare a woman's body for birth and production of milk. The nutrients needed for these support-system changes are added to the nutrient needs of both the growing fetus and the mother's own normal body functions.[29]

It is difficult to pinpoint the specific harm to fetal development if a mother either gets too little energy and nutrients during pregnancy or begins pregnancy with only minimal nutritional stores. A daily diet containing only 1000 kcal has been shown to greatly retard fetal growth and development. Increased maternal and infant death rates recently seen in famine-stricken areas of Africa supply further evidence (see Chapter 18). For some nutrients, however, such as iron and calcium, the fetus may also use—and deplete—the mother's stores if the mother doesn't get enough in her diet. Moreover, a successful pregnancy is one that not only results in a healthy infant but also maintains the health of the mother.[19]

Research shows that genetic background can explain very little of the observed differences in birth weight. Both environmental factors and nutritional factors, such as the length of gestation and mother's weight gain, are more important.[29] The worse the nutritional condition of the mother at the beginning of pregnancy, the

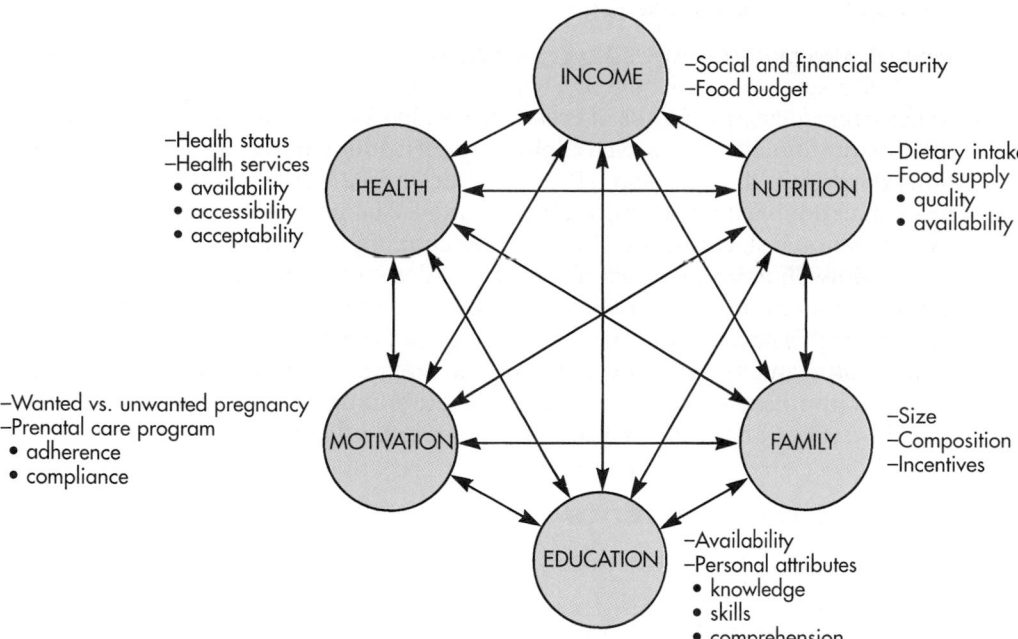

Figure 14-7 *The seamless web of influences that can affect the outcome of pregnancy. Choices concerning a number of factors influence the chances of having a healthy infant.*

more valuable a good prenatal diet and/or use of prenatal supplements will be in improving the course and outcome of her pregnancy. Figure 14-7 depicts many factors that influence the quality of pregnancy.

Much Evidence Supports the Importance of Good Nutrition in Pregnancy

During World War II, parts of Russia and much of Holland were blockaded. Food supplies were quickly exhausted. The resulting undernutrition greatly affected birth weights of infants developing in the second or third trimester. Birth defects also occurred more commonly, and the number of new pregnancies fell. After the blockades were lifted, birth weights, subsequent infant health, and the numbers of new pregnancies quickly returned to prewar levels.[29]

At the same time, researchers working in Boston noticed that a good protein intake was associated with a greater success of pregnancy. It appeared that the mother's diet—not only during pregnancy but also preceding conception—affected the health of both mother and infant. Studies in Toronto then showed that dietary supplements and nutritional counseling improved the health of the pregnant mother and yielded a healthier baby. As health improved, complication rates also dwindled. Researchers in Great Britain took this one step further. They showed that height and social class were better predictors of pregnancy outcome than dietary intake during pregnancy. Supporting this is a recent study of middle-class African-American women in Chicago. Even with nutritional supplements, their risk of having low–birth-weight infants still exceeded that of middle-class whites, possibly reflecting the effects of poverty on previous generations. This finding suggests that long-term nutritional intake may be critical to pregnancy outcome.[19]

Laboratory animal studies have supported the importance of diet during pregnancy. Food deprivation during animal pregnancy led to smaller organ size in the offspring, affecting even the brain, which usually resists nutritional insults. In addition, placentas weighed less, and fewer healthy offspring survived the first weeks of life.

Effects of Nutritional and Other Factors on Pregnancy Outcome

In the United States, about 12 of every 100,000 live births end in the mother's death. The infant mortality rate is even higher: for each 100,000 live births, about 840 infants die within the first year.[5] The infant death rate among African-Americans is more than double the rates among Whites and Hispanics in the United States. Based on the national statistics, the United States currently ranks 24th among industrialized nations in terms of maternal and infant death rates. Such grim and discomfiting statistics can be attributed largely to the current high number of teenage pregnancies in this country and to inadequate prenatal care, as well as marginal nutritional status among poor pregnant woman. Health professionals are working to reduce both infant and maternal deaths by promoting good health care and nutritional practices. These efforts also benefit pregnant women over age 35.

Beyond the Nutrients

Many nutrition-related factors also affect the health of mother and fetus.

Low socioeconomic status. A constellation of characteristics that lead to poverty, inadequate health care, poor health practices, lack of education, and unmarried status is associated with problems in pregnancy. Currently in the United States about 25% of all births are to unwed mothers, with a range of 17% to 67% for various racial groups.

Closely spaced births. Siblings born in succession with less than a year between them are more likely to be born with low birth weights than are those further apart in age. This danger is especially prevalent among African-American women.[22]

Age younger than 18. Young women continue maturing into physical adulthood for 5 years after **menarche.** Because the average age of menarche is 13 years in the United States, a woman younger than 18 years is not as physically ready to be pregnant as she will be later. Pregnancies that occur when the mother is younger than 18 are high risk and necessitate special monitoring (see the Nutrition Insight). Overall, mothers who are between 25 and 34 have the best pregnancy outcomes.

Prenatal care. Inadequate, absent, or delayed prenatal care can allow maternal nutritional deficiencies to deprive a fetus of needed nutrients. Chronic diseases, such as high blood pressure or diabetes, increase the risk of fetal damage. Without prenatal care, a woman is three times more likely to give birth to a low–birth-weight baby—one who will be 40 times more likely to die during the first 4 weeks of life than a normal-birth-weight infant. As noted earlier, the ideal time to start prenatal care is before conception.[16] Still, about 20% of women in the United States receive no prenatal care in the first trimester—a critical time to change habits.

Lifestyle. Smoking, alcohol consumption, use of some medications, and illegal drug use in pregnancy all lead to harmful effects. The Nutrition Issue in this chapter reviews one effect of alcohol—**fetal alcohol syndrome.** Smoking is linked to preterm birth and low birth weight and appears to increase the risk of birth defects, sudden infant death, and childhood cancer. These problems are associated with the effect of nicotine, which constricts arteries and may then reduce fetal oxygen flow; carbon monoxide; and other compounds in cigarette smoke. Problem drugs include aspirin (when used heavily), hormone ointments, nose drops, rectal suppositories, weight-control pills, and medications that were prescribed for previous illnesses.

The risks of low birth weight and preterm delivery increase modestly, but progessively, with maternal age. Given close monitoring, however, a woman older than 35 has an excellent chance of producing a healthy infant. Most women in this age group exhibit typical pregnancy-related problems, which usually are manageable.

Menarche
The onset of menstruation. Menarche usually occurs around age 13, 2 or 3 years after the first signs of puberty start to appear.

Fetal alcohol syndrome (FAS)
A group of physical and mental abnormalities in the infant that result from the mother's consumption of alcohol during pregnancy.

Of the illegal drugs, cocaine has the most troubling consequences for the developing fetuses. As cocaine use has become more common in recent years, the number of infants born to cocaine-using women has increased. Maternal use of cocaine during pregnancy has been linked to preterm birth, as well as to an undersized head and body and several other physical malformations in the newborn. Exposure of the fetus to cocaine appears to disrupt development of the brain and nervous system and may reduce interactive behaviors and responses to environmental stimuli in the infant. Further studies and improved testing procedures are needed to assess the long-term developmental abnormalities in infants exposed to cocaine during gestation.

Various surveys in recent years report the number of pregnant women using substances potentially harmful to the fetus. For instance, a 1989 study at a major Philadelphia hospital revealed that 15% of 852 pregnant women tested positive for cocaine or combinations of cocaine, marijuana, and narcotics. The percentage of drug users was about the same among private and publicly subsidized patients. Another study involving 36 hospitals located throughout the United States found that, on average, 11% of women used illegal drugs during pregnancy; the percentage reported from individual hospitals ranged from 1% to 27%. According to a 1992 survey of approximately 67,000 maternity patients at California hospitals, an estimated 11% were found to have consumed alcohol and/or used an illegal drug within hours or days of delivery. These estimates of alcohol and illegal drug use are probably quite conservative because the urine tests in these studies detect only recent substance abuse. About 9% of the patients in the California study reported that they had recently smoked cigarettes.

Prenatal ketosis. Ketosis is not desirable for the growing fetus. Ketone bodies are thought to be poorly used by the fetal brain. This suggests that they could slow fetal brain development. Researchers stress the need for a pregnant woman not to "crash" diet or fast for more than 12 hours. A pregnant woman can develop significant ketosis after only 20 hours of fasting. Eating about 100 grams of carbohydrate every day prevents ketosis. As noted earlier, even nonpregnant women usually eat twice this amount.

Body weight and weight gain. Obesity leads to an increased rate of high blood pressure and diabetes during pregnancy. The need for surgery and other complications during delivery likewise increase, largely because the baby can be very large. These pregnancies require intense monitoring, and are linked to increase in risk of birth defects in the infant.

Inadequate weight gain, especially among underweight women, often produces infants of low birth weight. Undernourished women often have borderline vitamin and mineral intakes and need to build up body stores. They should try to reach healthy weight by the end of the first trimester. As mentioned previously, the recommendation for underweight women is to gain more weight (28 to 40 pounds total) than a woman at healthy weight. Overweight women who try to avoid weight gain during pregnancy may rob both themselves and their infants of essential nutrients. Also, for effcient protein metabolism during pregnancy, enough carbohydrate and fat are needed to meet energy needs.

In the United States, about 7% of infants are born with low birth weight—that is, they weigh less than 5.5 pounds (2.5 kilograms). Low–birth-weight infants are more susceptible to infections, illnesses, and disabilities and are more likely to die than normal-weight infants. Preterm birth, poor diet during pregnancy, some medical conditions in the mother, and the factors highlighted previously influence an infant's birth weight. Reducing the number of low–birth-weight infants will help reduce infant deaths.

Hospital-related costs of caring for low–birth-weight newborns total more than $2 billion per year in the United States, an average of $21,000 per child. Compare this with an average hospital-related cost of $2842 for a normal delivery and an average of $500 for preventive prenatal care.

Caffeine consumption. Research on the effects of caffeine consumption by pregnant women has yielded some provocative findings. Caffeine decreases absorption of iron, a key nutrient during pregnancy (as discussed earlier) and may reduce blood flow through the placenta. The risk of spontaneous abortion has been shown to increase in the first trimester and early in the second trimester with heavy caffeine consumption (>300 milligrams per day).[8] About 2 to 3 cups of coffee per day contain this amount of caffeine (see Appendix J). In addition, as caffeine intake increases, so does the risk of delivering a low–birth-weight infant. Heavy caffeine use during pregnancy may also lead to caffeine withdrawal symptoms in the newborn. Although more research is needed, it is advisable to limit intake. Drinking no more than 2 cups of coffee and no more than 4 cups of caffeinated soft drinks per day during pregnancy, or when pregnancy is possible, is advocated. Limiting intake from tea, over-the-counter medicines, and chocolate is also important. Some researchers advocate complete avoidance of caffeine during pregnancy.

Aspartame use. Phenylalanine, a component of aspartame (Nutrasweet and Equal), causes problems for some pregnant women. High amounts of phenylalanine in maternal blood disrupt fetal brain development if the mother has a disease known as *phenylketonuria* (see Chapter 7). If the mother does not have this condition, however, it is unlikely that the baby will be affected by aspartame use. Some experts still recommend caution with regard to aspartame, but total abstinence is hardly warranted, based on our current knowledge.

Listeria infection. Infection by the bacterium *Listeria monocytogenes* causes mild flulike symptoms, such as fever, headache, and vomiting, about 7 to 30 days after exposure. However, pregnant women, newborn infants, and people with depressed immune function may suffer more severe symptoms, including spontaneous abortion and serious blood infections. In these high-risk people, 25% of infections may be fatal.

Because unpasteurized milk, soft cheeses made from raw milk, and cabbage can be sources of listeria organisms, it is especially important that pregnant women and other people at high risk avoid these products. Experts advise consuming only pasteurized milk products and cooking meat, poultry, and seafood thoroughly to kill this organism. It is unsafe in pregnancy to eat any raw meats or other raw animal products. Chapter 17 covers food-borne illness, such as listeria infections, in more detail.

Prenatal Care and Counseling

Education, an adequate diet, and early and consistent prenatal medical care maximize the chances of producing a healthy baby and avoiding the risks just covered, such as x-ray exposure, smoking, vitamin A supplements, medicines, illegal drugs, and alcohol use. If diabetes or high blood pressure is present or developing, it must be carefully controlled to minimize complications in the pregnancy.

Again, women should receive these examinations and counseling strategies before becoming pregnant. Certainly they should begin early in pregnancy. Many potential problems that develop during pregnancy can be diagnosed and quickly treated medically.

Almost all women need prenatal nutritional counseling because nutrition needs are unique during pregnancy.[19] Food habits cannot be predicted from income, education, or lifestyle. Although some women already have good nutritional habits, most can benefit from nutritional advice. All should be reminded of habits that may harm the growing fetus, such as severe dieting or fasting. By focusing on appropriate prenatal care, good nutritional intake, and proper health habits, as well as using common sense, parents give their fetus—and later infant—the very best chance of thriving.

Toxoplasmosis is another infection that causes birth defects. Pregnant women can avoid exposure to the organism that causes toxoplasmosis by having someone else clean the cat's litter box, by avoiding contact with kittens or garden soil, and by not eating raw or undercooked meat.

Several U.S. government programs exist to reduce infant mortality by providing high-quality health care and foods. These are designed to alleviate the effects of poverty and insufficient education. An example of such a program is the Special Supplemental Food Program for Women, Infants, and Children (WIC). This program offers health assessments and foods (or vouchers for foods) that supply high-quality protein, calcium, iron, and vitamins A and C to pregnant women, infants, and children (to age 5 years) from low-income populations.

On the WIC program, participants' diets have improved markedly, as has the likelihood that women will have a healthy baby. This program is credited with decreasing the cases of iron-deficiency anemia and low–birth-weight infants within the population it serves. Studies have estimated that every dollar spent on the prenatal component of WIC saves up to three dollars in public health expenditures for the care of low–birth-weight babies.

The WIC program is available in all areas of the United States and has a staff trained to help women have healthy babies. More than 6 million women, infants, and young children are currently enrolled in the program. Pregnant women are a priority for this program. Budget constraints force some programs to discontinue serving children to make more money available for serving pregnant women.

Women with acquired immune deficiency syndrome (AIDS) may pass the virus that causes this disease to the fetus during pregnancy or the birth process. About 1 in 3 infected newborns will develop AIDS symptoms and die within just a few years. Recent studies show that these odds of mother-infant transmission can be cut significantly if the woman begins taking the drug zidovudine (AZT) by the fourteenth week of pregnancy. Thus screening pregnant women for AIDS and treating those infected with AZT are currently advocated.

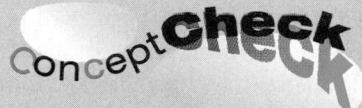

Infants born after 37 weeks of gestation and weighing more than 5.5 pounds (2.5 kilograms) have the fewest medical problems at birth. Individual mothers and whole societies can attempt to reduce infant and maternal death and medical problems by limiting factors that increase the risk of having a preterm or small-for-gestational-age infant. Such contributing factors, besides an inadequate diet in general, include low socioeconomic status; closely-spaced births; obesity; inadequate or absent prenatal care; cigarette smoking; alcohol consumption; illegal drug use; teenage pregnancy; inadequate prenatal weight gain; and prenatal ketosis. Adequate nutrition can reduce the risk of many medical problems in pregnancy.

Physiological Changes Can Cause Discomfort in Pregnancy

During pregnancy, the fetus' needs for oxygen, nutrients, and excretion increase the burden on the mother's lungs, heart, and kidneys. Although a mother's digestive and metabolic systems work very efficiently, some discomfort accompanies the changes her body undergoes to accommodate the fetus.

Heartburn, Constipation, and Hemorrhoids

Hormones produced by the placenta relax muscles in both the uterus and the intestinal tract. This often causes heartburn as stomach acid slips up into the esophagus (see Chapter 4). When this occurs, the woman should avoid lying down after eating, eat less fat so that foods pass more quickly from the stomach into the small intestine, and avoid spicy foods she can't tolerate. She should also consume liquids between meals to decrease stomach volume and pressure. Women with more severe cases may need antacids or related medications.

Constipation often results as the intestinal muscles relax during pregnancy. It is especially likely to develop late in pregnancy, as the fetus competes with the GI tract

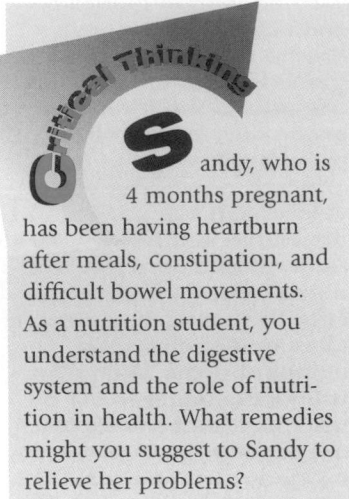

for space in the abdominal cavity. To offset these discomforts, a woman should perform regular exercise and consume more fluid, dietary fiber, and dried fruits, such as prunes. These practices can help prevent constipation and a problem that frequently accompanies it, hemorrhoids. Straining during elimination can lead to hemorrhoids, which are already more likely to occur during pregnancy because of other bodily changes.

Edema

Placental hormones cause various body tissues to retain fluid during pregnancy.[29] Blood volume also greatly expands during pregnancy. The extra fluid normally causes some swelling (edema). There is no reason to severely restrict salt or use diuretics to limit mild edema. However, the edema may limit physical activity late in pregnancy and occasionally require a woman to elevate her feet to control the symptoms. Overall, edema generally spells trouble only if high blood pressure and the appearance of much protein in the urine accompany fluid retention (see later section).

Morning Sickness

About 50% of pregnant women experience nausea during the early stages of pregnancy. This nausea may be related to the increased sense of smell induced by pregnancy-related hormones circulating in the bloodstream. Although commonly called "morning sickness," pregnancy-related nausea may occur at any time and persist all day. It is often the first signal to a woman that she is pregnant. To help control mild nausea, pregnant women can try the following: avoiding nauseating foods, such as fried or greasy foods; cooking with open windows to dissipate nauseating smells; eating soda crackers, potato chips, or dry cereal before getting out of bed; avoiding large fluid intakes early in the morning; and eating smaller, more frequent meals. Because the iron in prenatal supplements triggers nausea in some women, changing the type of supplement used may provide relief in some cases. If a woman thinks her prenatal supplement is related to morning sickness, she should discuss switching to another supplement with her physician.

Overall, whether it is broccoli or potato chips, if a food sounds good to a pregnant woman with morning sickness, she should eat it and eat when she can while also striving to follow her prenatal diet.[6] If she has a great deal of difficulty in following her diet, she should alert her physician of this and follow the advice given. Usually nausea stops after the first trimester, but in about 10% to 20% of cases it can continue throughout the entire pregnancy. In cases of serious nausea the preceding practices offer little relief. Vitamin B-6 in amounts about 7.5 times the RDA may be helpful, under a physician's supervision. When appetite is severely reduced or vomiting persists, additional medical guidance is warranted. Hospitalization may be needed if the mother exhibits significant dehydration or weight loss.

Anemia

Physiological anemia
The normal increase in blood volume in pregnancy that dilutes the concentration of red blood cells, resulting in anemia; also called hemodilution.

To supply fetal needs, the mother's blood volume expands up to approximately 150% of normal. The amount of red blood cells expands only 20% to 30% above normal and occurs more gradually. This leaves proportionately fewer red blood cells in a pregnant woman's bloodstream. The lower ratio of red blood cells to total blood volume is a condition known as *physiological anemia.* It is a normal response to pregnancy rather than the result of inadequate nutrient intake. If during pregnancy, however, iron stores and/or dietary iron intake are not sufficient to meet needs, any resulting iron-deficiency anemia requires medical attention.[30]

Pregnancy-Induced Hypertension

Pregnancy-induced hypertension is a high-risk disorder. In its mild forms it is known as *preeclampsia* and in severe forms as *eclampsia*. The problem resolves once the pregnancy ends. Early symptoms include a rise in blood pressure, excess protein in the urine, edema, changes in blood clotting, and nervous system disorders. Very severe effects, including convulsions, can occur in the second and third trimesters. An adequate calcium intake (1200 to 1500 milligrams per day) may prevent or lessen the symptoms.[4] Mild effects can be lessened by bed rest and low-dose aspirin therapy. If not controlled, eclampsia eventually damages the liver and kidneys, and mother and fetus may both die. Careful medical attention is needed.

Although pregnancy brings with it some physical discomforts for the mother, the inconvenience is temporary and many potential discomforts can be diffused through good eating and health habits. More than that, the good habits bring double benefits, because they are the basis of good health for both mother and infant.

Pregnancy-induced hypertension

A serious disorder that can include high blood pressure, kidney failure, convulsions, and even death of the mother and fetus. Although its exact cause is not known, good nutrition (especially adequate calcium intake) and prenatal care may prevent or limit its severity. Mild cases are known as preeclampsia; *more severe cases are called* eclampsia *(formerly called* toxemia*).*

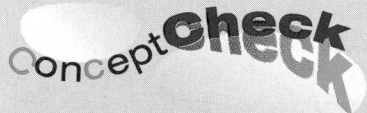

Heartburn, constipation, nausea and vomiting, edema, and anemia are possible discomforts and complications of pregnancy. Changes in food habits can often ease these problems. Pregnancy-induced hypertension, with high blood pressure and kidney failure, can lead to severe complications or even death of both the mother and fetus, if not treated. Adequate calcium intake is linked to a reduced risk for pregnancy-induced hypertension.

Breastfeeding

Before the 1900s, if a mother didn't breastfeed (nurse) her infant, a substitute "wet-nurse" was hired to do it. Formula-feeding was fraught with complications, primarily because people did not know the importance of sterilizing formulas against bacteria. Nor did people know much about the nutritional needs of infants. During the early 1900s, the technology of formulas based on cow's milk and methods of feeding improved. From the 1920s and especially in the 1940s when women worked in armament factories during World War II, more and more babies were fed formula. Throughout the 1950s and early 1960s, interest in breastfeeding further waned. In the 1970s, breastfeeding enjoyed a resurgence, which has since leveled off.

Healthy People 2000, a federally sponsored program, has set a goal of 75% of women nursing their infants at time of hospital discharge, and 50% still nursing 6 months later. Recent surveys show, however, that only about 55% of American mothers now nurse their infants in the hospital, and at 6 months only 20% are still breastfeeding their infants. Clearly, American women have far to go to meet the Healthy People 2000 goal.[28]

Women who choose to breastfeed usually find it an enjoyable and special time in their lives and their relationship with their new infant. Bottle-feeding with an infant formula is also safe for infants, as discussed in the next chapter, but does not equal the benefits derived from human milk in all aspects.[15,20] Note that if a woman doesn't nurse her child, breast weight returns to normal very soon after birth.

Teenage Pregnancy

Surveys indicate that between about 10% and 13% of teenage girls become pregnant at least once by the age of 18, giving the United States the highest teenage pregnancy rate in the Western World—more than twice that of England, France, or Canada.[24] About 95% of these pregnancies are unintended. According to one survey, 33% of teenage girls do not use any form of contraception during their first act of sexual intercourse.

About half a million teenagers give birth in the United States each year, accounting for about 13% of all births. Historically the teenage birth rate has been highest among African-Americans. In 1970 the birth rate for African-Americans age 15 to 19 was 141 per 1000, compared with 57 per 1000 Caucasians. In 1991, this disparity remained, with birth rates for Africa-American adolescents at 118 per 1000, compared with 43 per 1000 for Caucasian adolescents. Overall, minority teenagers with below-average academic skills from families with below-poverty incomes are considerably more likely to become pregnant than other adolescent girls. Often these young mothers are themselves the daughters of teenage mothers.

Teenage pregnancy poses special health problems for both the mother and child. To accommodate their normal growth even when not pregnant, teenagers need an extraordinary nutrient supply. Adolescent girls normally continue to grow taller for 2 years after they begin menstruating and to mature physically for 5 years. Teenage pregnancy adds the needs of the growing fetus to those of the growing mother. They both need considerable amounts of nutrients for their growing bodies.[31]

Diets of teenagers—including those who are pregnant—vary greatly in nutritional adequacy. Many teenagers eat irregularly, skip meals, snack on foods with low nutrient density, and frequently follow restrictive diets. Many of them eat less than two thirds of the RDA for various vitamins and minerals.

Pregnant teenagers frequently exhibit a variety of risk factors that can complicate pregnancy and pose a risk to the fetus (Table 14-3). For instance, teenagers are more likely than older women to be underweight at the beginning of pregnancy and to gain fewer than 16 pounds during pregnancy. In addition, their bodies generally lack the maturity needed to safely carry a pregnancy. Teenagers frequently give birth to preterm or low–birth weight infants; about 16% of low–birth weight infants are born to teenagers.[9] This occurs even despite adequate prenatal care. Additional complications, such as infant illness or even death, are tied to the teenage mother's day-to-day health practices.

The specific needs of pregnant teenagers vary according to their own growth patterns, body build, and physical activity habits. This makes it difficult to predict their nutrient needs. Clinicians can evaluate the adequacy of their diet by checking for appropriate weight gain during pregnancy and for appropriate food choices. Teenagers should be regularly counseled on nutrition during their prenatal care.[24] They need information about basic nutritional guidelines: the relationship between food and health, the kind and amount of food energy needed to support appropriate weight gain, how to select nutrient-rich foods, appropriate use of prenatal supplements, and preparation for breastfeeding or using infant formulas. They also need to be aware of the risks involved with smoking, drinking alcohol, and using drugs and medications not approved by their physicians.

TABLE 14-3

Nutrition-Related Risk Factors in Teenage Pregnancy

- Low pregnancy weight gain

- Low prepregnancy weight for height (or other evidence of inadequate nutrition)

- Smoking (mothers 18 to 19 years of age smoke more than do any other group of mothers)

- Excessive prepregnancy weight for height

- Anemia

OTHER RISK FACTORS SUGGESTED BY HEALTH HISTORIES

- Unhealthy lifestyle (such as the use of drugs and alcohol)

- Unfavorable reproductive history

- Chronic diseases

- History of an eating disorder or excessive worry about maintaining a thin appearance

From ADA Reports: *Journal of the American Dietetic Association* 89:106, 1989.

Programs specifically designed for pregnant teenagers are available in many communities. These typically provide information about community resources; many also offer clothing and supplies for the infant, food resources, transportation for prenatal checkups, and a supportive environment. Nonetheless, even when a teenager successfully delivers a healthy baby, the subsequent impact of parenthood on the mother's education and economic future is often devastating. Some teenage girls view early pregnancy as a quick route to a meaningful adult role. The reality of this adult role, however, may shock them. Few teenaged mothers can successfully care for and support themselves and their children. Many young mothers end up forgoing the very education that would qualify them for better jobs, which might permit them to adequately care for and support themselves and their children. Moreover, the vast majority of pregnant teenagers are unmarried and don't get married before the birth of their child, further compounding the economic and social difficulties of the young mother and child.[26]

Given all the problems associated with teenage pregnancy and the subsequent situation of the young, often unmarried mother and her infant, many efforts are under way to reduce the rate of teenage pregnancy. Prevention is the best medicine. This approach is currently receiving high priority by the federal government, especially as part of an overhaul of our nation's welfare programs. A few broad strategies for public interventions that are designed to reduce the problems associated with teenage pregnancy have been advocated: less acceptance of teenage pregnancy by society in general, an emphasis on abstinence, more sex education and contraceptive services, and better support services for those teenagers who become pregnant. Some politicians also advocate the idea of denying the teenager welfare payments and essentially requiring her to remain with her parents rather than set up her own household. Ideally some solution will arise as an effective measure, because the current outlook for teenage mothers and their infants is often so bleak.[26]

Ability to Breastfeed

In most cases, problems encountered in breastfeeding are due to a lack of appropriate information, because almost all women are physically capable of nursing their children.[18] Anatomical problems in breasts, such as inverted nipples, can be corrected during pregnancy. Breast size is no indication of success in breastfeeding and generally increases during pregnancy. Most women notice a dramatic increase in the size and weight of their breasts by the third or fourth day of breastfeeding. If these changes don't occur, a woman needs to speak with her physician.

Breastfed infants must be followed closely over the first days of life to ensure that the process is proceeding normally. Monitoring is especially important with a mother's first child, because the mother will be inexperienced with the process of breastfeeding. Nowadays, mothers and healthy infants are commonly discharged from the hospital 1 to 2 days after delivery, whereas 20 years ago they stayed in the hospital for 3 to 4 days or longer. One result of such rapid discharge is a decreased period of infant monitoring by health-care professionals. Incidents have been reported of infants developing dehydration and blood clots soon after hospital discharge when breastfeeding did not proceed smoothly.[2]

New parents generally need guidance about their infant's nutritional and other health-related needs by appropriate professionals for several weeks after hospital discharge. First-time mothers who plan to breastfeed should learn as much as they can about the process early in their pregnancy. Interested women should learn the proper technique, what problems to expect, and how to respond to them. Overall, breastfeeding is a learned skill, and mothers need knowledge to nurse safely, especially the first time.

Producing Human Milk

During pregnancy, cells in the breast form milk-producing **lobules** (Figure 14-8). Hormones from the placenta stimulate these changes in the breast. After birth the mother produces more **prolactin** hormone to maintain the changes in the breast and therefore the ability to produce milk. During pregnancy, breast weight increases by 1 to 2 pounds.

The hormone prolactin also stimulates the synthesis of milk. Suckling stimulates prolactin release. Milk synthesis then occurs as an infant nurses. The more the infant suckles, the more milk is produced. Milk production closely parallels infant demand. Because of this fact, even twins can be nursed. Demand is the driving force for milk production.[29]

Most protein found in human milk is synthesized by breast tissue. Some proteins also enter the milk directly from the mother's bloodstream. These proteins include immune factors and enzymes.[20] Fats in human milk come from the mother's diet, and some are also synthesized by breast tissue. The sugar galactose is synthesized in the breast, while glucose enters from the mother's bloodstream. Together these sugars form lactose, the main carbohydrate in human milk.

The Let-Down Reflex

An important brain-breast connection—the **let-down reflex**—is necessary for breastfeeding. The brain releases the hormone oxytocin to allow the breast tissues to let down (release) the milk from storage sites. It travels to the nipple area. A tingling sensation signals the let-down reflex shortly before milk flow begins. If the let-down reflex doesn't operate, little milk is available to the infant. The infant then gets frustrated, and this can frustrate the mother.

The let-down reflex is easily inhibited by nervous tension, a lack of confidence, and fatigue. Mothers should be especially aware of the link between tension and a weak let-down reflex. They need to find a relaxed environment where they can breastfeed.

Currently Congress is debating whether to pass legislation that guarantees a mother at least 48 hours of hospital recuperation after a vaginal delivery, and up to 96 hours for a cesarean delivery. This is most important for first-time mothers, especially if good follow-up care at home is not available.

Lobules
Saclike structures in the breast that store milk.

Prolactin
A hormone secreted by the mother that stimulates the synthesis of milk.

Let-down reflex
A reflex stimulated by infant suckling that causes the release (ejection) of milk from milk ducts in the mother's breasts.

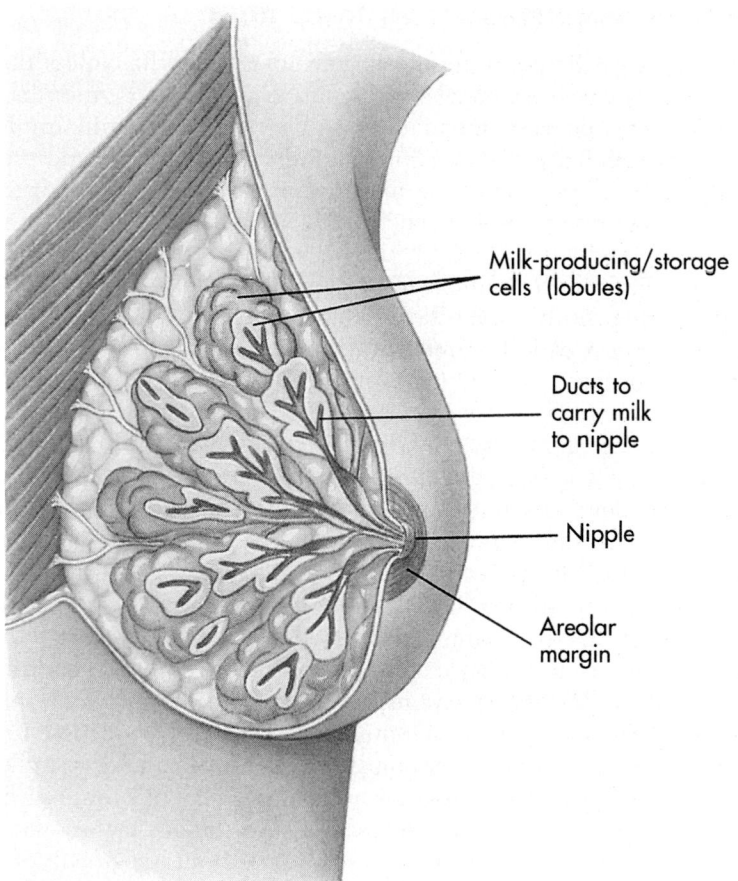

Milk-producing/storage cells (lobules)

Ducts to carry milk to nipple

Nipple

Areolar margin

Figure 14-8 *The anatomy of the breast. Many types of cells form a coordinated network to produce and secrete human milk.*

After a few weeks, the let-down reflex becomes automatic. The mother's response can be triggered just by thinking about her infant or seeing or hearing another one. At first, however, the process can be a bit bewildering. Because she cannot measure the amount of milk the infant takes in, a mother may fear that she is not adequately nourishing the infant.

As a general rule, a well-nourished breastfed infant should (1) have six or more wet diapers per day after the second day of life, (2) show a normal weight gain, and (3) pass one or two stools per day that look like lumpy mustard. In addition, softening of the breast during the feeding helps indicate that enough milk is being consumed. Parents who sense their infant is not consuming enough milk should consult a physician immediately because dehydration can develop rapidly.

It generally takes 2 to 3 weeks to fully establish the feeding routine: infant and mother both feel comfortable, the milk supply meets infant demand, and initial nipple soreness disappears. Establishing the breastfeeding routine requires patience, but the rewards are great. The adjustments are easier if supplemental formula feedings are not introduced until breastfeeding is well established, after at least 3 weeks but preferably not until after 2 to 3 months. Then a supplemental bottle or two of infant formula per day is fine.

Parents need not be concerned that breastfed infants grow a bit more slowly after about 3 months of age than formula-fed infants, based on increases in body weight. The infant's physician is the best judge of whether the rate of growth of the breastfed infant is satisfactory. Essentially the difference is of no consequence, in part because some of it is related to increased fat deposition.

Disposable diapers can absorb so much urine that it is difficult to judge when they are wet. A strip of paper towel laid inside a disposable diaper makes a good wetness indicator. Or cloth diapers may be used for a day or two to assess whether nursing is supplying sufficient milk.

Nutritional Qualities of Human Milk

Human milk is very different in composition from cow's milk. Unless altered, cow's milk should not be used in infant feeding until the infant is 12 months old. Many authorities support this recommendation against using cow's milk until the infant is at least 1 year old, because cow's milk is too high in minerals and protein, does not contain enough carbohydrate to meet infant needs, and may trigger development of diabetes in infants with a genetic predisposition to the disorder.[10] In addition, the major protein in cow's milk, casein, is harder for an infant to digest than the major protein found in human milk.[29] Finally, certain compounds in human milk presently under study show other possible benefits for the infant. These factors, such as the fatty acids typically found in fish (see below), are not present in cow's milk or infant formulas.

Colostrum. The first fluid made by the human breast is **colostrum.** This thick, yellowish fluid may leak from the breast during late pregnancy and is produced in earnest for a few days to a week after birth. Colostrum contains **antibodies** and immune-system cells, some of which pass unaltered through the immature GI tract of the infant into the bloodstream. These immune factors and cells protect the infant from some gastrointestinal diseases and other infectious disorders, compensating for its own immature immune system during the first few months of life.[20] Various growth factors and other compounds in breast milk also contribute to the health of the infant. One likely reason breastfed infants have fewer respiratory and intestinal infections than formula-fed infants is the presence of these immune factors, growth factors, and other compounds in colostrum and breast milk.

Colostrum facilitates the passage of **meconium,** a stool produced during fetal life. One component of colostrum, the *Lactobacillus bifidus* **factor,** encourages the growth of *Lactobacillus bifidus* bacteria. These bacteria limit the growth of potentially toxic bacteria in the intestine. Overall, breastfeeding promotes the intestinal health of the breastfed infant in this way and in other ways.[20]

Mature milk. Human milk composition gradually changes until several days after delivery, when it achieves the normal composition of mature milk. Human milk looks very different from cow's milk. (Table 15-1 in the next chapter provides a direct comparison.) Human milk is thin and almost watery in appearance and often has a slight bluish tinge. Its nutritional qualities are impressive.

Human milk's main protein forms a soft, light curd in the infant's stomach, easing digestion. Other proteins bind iron, reducing the growth of iron-requiring bacteria. Many of these types of bacteria cause diarrhea. Still other proteins offer the important immune protection already noted.

The lipids in human breast milk are high in linoleic acid and cholesterol, which are needed for brain development. Breast milk also contains long-chain omega-3 fatty acids, such as docosahexaenoic acid (DHA). This unsaturated fatty acid is used for synthesis of tissues in the brain, rest of the central nervous system, and eyes. Some evidence indicates that breastfed infants show greater visual acuity and better nervous system development than infants fed formulas, none of which currently contain DHA. Breastfeeding for at least 4 months is advocated to obtain this benefit.

Researchers are currently determining the potential benefits of adding DHA to infant formulas.[15] The long-term safety of this addition is under study. Eventually, manufacturers may produce formulas for preterm and full-term infants with a fatty-acid composition equivalent to that of human milk, just as they have done for the protein and mineral content.

Human milk changes in fat composition during each feeding. The consistency of milk released initially (about 60% of the volume) resembles that of skim milk. The next amount (about 35% of the total volume) has a greater fat proportion, similar to whole milk. Finally, the hindmilk (about 5% of the total) is essentially like cream and usually released 10 to 20 minutes into the feeding. Babies need to nurse

Colostrum

The first fluid secreted by the breast during late pregnancy and the first few days after birth. This thick fluid is rich in immune factors and protein.

Meconium

The first thick mucuslike stool passed by the infant after birth.

***Lactobacillus bifidus* factor**

A protective factor secreted in the colostrum that encourages growth of beneficial bacteria in the newborn's intestines.

long enough (for example a total of 20 or more minutes) to get the energy in the rich hindmilk to be satisfied between feedings and grow well.

Human milk also allows for adequate hydration of the infant, provided the baby is exclusively breastfed. A question commonly asked is whether the infant needs additional water, if stressed by hot weather, diarrhea, vomiting, or fever. Providing up to 4 ounces of water a day from a bottle to young breastfed infants is fine. Note, however, that greater amounts of supplemental water can lead to brain disorders, low blood sodium, and other problems, as discussed in Chapter 15. Thus extra water may be given, but only with a physician's guidance.

A Food Plan for Women Who Breastfeed

Nutrient needs for a breastfeeding mother change slightly if at all from those of the pregnant woman. Exceptions are decreases in folate and iron needs and an increase in the need for energy, vitamins A and C, niacin, and zinc. The diet for breast-feeding women can be the same as that for pregnant women, except teenagers should add an additional serving from the milk, yogurt, and cheese group. Some researchers recommend eating fish at least twice a week, because the omega-3 fatty acids present in fish are thought to be important for brain development.

A reasonable approach for a breastfeeding woman is to eat a balanced diet that supplies at least 1800 kcal per day, has a moderate fat content, and includes a variety of dairy products, fruits, vegetables, and grains. The woman should drink fluids every time the infant nurses, because drinking to quench thirst encourages ample milk production. If a woman restricts her energy intake too severely, the quantity of milk also decreases. This is not a time to crash diet. Research also shows that more than two alcoholic drinks a day decreases milk output, as does smoking.[29]

Milk production requires approximately 800 kcal every day. The RDA for energy during lactation is an extra 500 kcal daily above prepregnancy recommendations. The difference between energy needs and intake—about 300 kcal—should contribute to gradual loss of the extra body fat accumulated during pregnancy, especially if breastfeeding is continued for 6 months or more and the woman performs some physical activity. This shows how practical the link is between pregnancy and breastfeeding.[18] Breastfeeding also encourages rapid return of the uterus to normal size and may reduce risk of breast cancer in the mother if breastfeeding continues for at least 3 months. Weight loss of 1 to 4 pounds per month in the nursing mother is appropriate. Milk output decreases at significantly greater rates of weight loss, as occur with severe dieting when energy intake is less than about 1500 kcal per day.

Breastfeeding mothers should get their physician's permission before embarking on an exercise program. Breastfeeding women must also take care to drink plenty of fluids before and after workouts and should avoid exercising when fatigued.

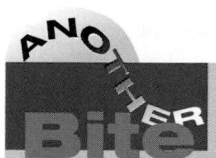

Most substances the mother ingests are secreted into her milk. For this reason she should limit intake of or avoid all alcohol and caffeine and check all medications with a pediatrician. Some mothers believe that some foods, such as garlic and chocolate, flavor the breast milk and upset the infant. If a woman notices a connection between a food she eats and the infant's later fussiness, she could consider avoiding that food. However, she might want to experiment again with it later. Infants become fussy for many reasons, and the suspected ingredient may not be the cause. Some researchers, on the other hand, feel that the passage of flavors from the mother's diet into her milk affords an opportunity for the infant to learn about the flavor of the foods of its family long before solids are introduced. These researchers suspect that bottle-fed infants are missing significant sensory experiences that until recent times in human history were common to all infants.[17]

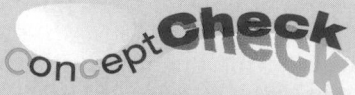

Recognition of the importance of breastfeeding has contributed to its greater popularity during the last 20 years. Almost all women have the ability to breast-feed. The hormone prolactin stimulates breast tissue to synthesize milk. Some components of human milk come directly from the mother's bloodstream. Infant suckling triggers a let-down reflex that releases the milk. The more an infant nurses, the more milk is synthesized. The nutrient composition of human milk is very different from that of cow's milk and changes as the infant matures. The first fluid produced, colostrum, is rich in immune factors. The diet for breast-feeding is generally similar to that for pregnancy, except for additional fluids, as well as an extra serving from the milk, yogurt, and cheese group for a teenage pregnancy.

Pros and Cons of Breastfeeding

As noted already, the vast majority of women are capable of breastfeeding, and infants benefit from it. Nonetheless, a woman's decision to nurse depends on a variety of factors, some of which may make breastfeeding impractical or undesirable for a woman. Mothers who don't want to breastfeed their infant should not feel compelled to do so. Breastfeeding provides distinct advantages, but none so great that a woman who decides to bottle-feed should feel she is significantly penalizing her infant.

Advantages of Breastfeeding

Human milk is tailored to meet infant nutrient needs for the first 4 to 6 months of life. The possible exceptions are the relative lack of fluoride, iron, and vitamin D. Infant supplements, used under the guidance of a pediatrician, can supply these and are often recommended. Sun exposure also helps compensate for the gap in vitamin D nutriture. Fluoride may be found in the household water supply. If it is not present in adequate amounts or the child is not receiving tap water, a fluoride supplement should be considered and a dentist consulted. Vitamin B-12 supplements are recommended for the breastfed infant whose mother is a complete vegetarian (vegan).

Fewer infections. Breastfeeding reduces the general risk of infections to the infant. This is partially because of the antibodies in human milk that an infant can use. As already mentioned, these reduce the risk of respiratory and intestinal infections. Breastfed infants also have fewer ear infections because they do not sleep with a bottle in the mouth. Experts strongly discourage allowing infants to sleep with a bottle in their mouths because when that happens, milk pools there, backs up through the throat, and eventually settles in the ears, creating a growth medium for bacteria. Infant ear infections are a common problem. By avoiding them, parents can decrease discomfort for the infant, avoid trips to the doctor, and prevent possible hearing loss. Tooth decay from nighttime bottles is another likely consequence (see Chapter 15).

Fewer allergies and intolerances. Breastfeeding also reduces the chances of allergies, especially in allergy-prone infants (see the Nutrition Issue in Chapter 15). The key time to attain this benefit from breastfeeding is during the first 2 to 3 months of an infant's life. Breastfeeding for even just the first few weeks is beneficial. A

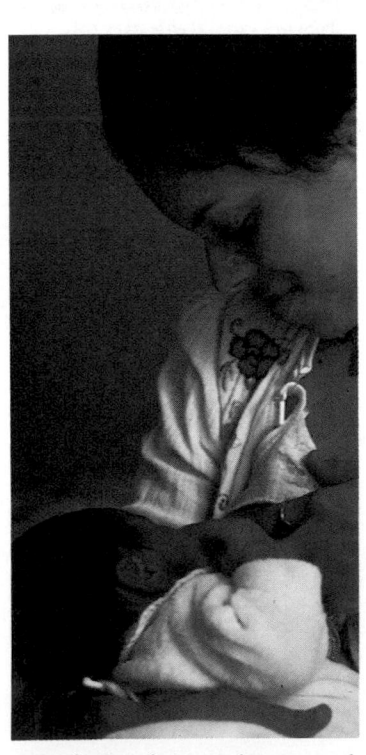

Breastfeeding fosters a closeness and bonding between the mother and the infant.

longer commitment than 2 to 3 months is better, but the first few months are most critical. Cow's milk contains a number of potential allergy-causing proteins absent in human milk. Furthermore, certain factors in human milk speed maturation of the GI tract, another mechanism that decreases allergy risk. Another benefit of breastfeeding is that infants are better able to tolerate human milk than formulas. Formulas must occasionally be switched several times until caregivers find the best one for the infant.

Convenience and cost. Breastfeeding frees the mother from the time and expense involved in buying and preparing formula and washing bottles. Human milk is ready to go and sterile. This allows the mother to spend more time with her baby. On the other hand, if the child is bottle-fed, the mother may be free to do other things while others feed the baby. This trade-off needs to be considered.

Barriers to Breastfeeding

A lack of role models, widespread misinformation, fear of appearing immodest, and workplaces outside the home all serve as barriers to breastfeeding.

Misinformation. Probably the major barriers to breastfeeding are misinformation and lack of role models. If a woman is interested in breastfeeding, she should talk to women who have done it successfully. Experienced mothers can be an enormous help to the first-time mother. The first-time mother should find a friend she can call on for advice. In almost every community, a group called La Leche League offers classes in breastfeeding and advises women who have problems with it (1 [800] LALECHE).

Returning to an outside job. Working outside the home can complicate plans to breastfeed. One possibility after a month or two of breastfeeding is for the mother to regularly express and save her own milk. She can express milk by breast pump or manually into a sterile plastic bottle or nursing bag (used in a disposable bottle system). Saving human milk requires careful sanitation and rapid chilling. It can be stored in the refrigerator for 1 day and be frozen for 1 month. There is a knack to learning how to express milk, but the freedom can be worth it, because it allows others to feed the infant the mother's milk.

Some women can juggle both a job and breastfeeding, but others find it too cumbersome and decide to formula-feed. A compromise—balancing some breastfeedings, perhaps early morning and night, with formula-feedings during the day—is possible. However, too many supplemental feedings decrease milk production.

Frozen human milk should not be thawed in a microwave. The heat can destroy immune factors in the milk and create hot spots that may scald the infant's tongue.

ANOTHER Bite

A schedule of expressing milk and using supplemental formula feedings is most successful if begun after 1 to 2 months of exclusive breast-feeding. After 2 months the baby is well-adapted to breastfeeding and probably feels enough emotional security and other benefits from nursing to drink both ways.

Overall, the American Academy of Pediatrics recommends breastfeeding an infant exclusively for the first 4 to 6 months when possible and as a supplement with solid food for the second 6 months of life. Again, the first few months are the most important ones.

Social reticence. Another barrier for some women is embarrassment about nursing a child in public. Historically our society has stressed modesty and discouraged public displays of breasts—even for as good a cause as nourishing babies. Women who feel reticent should be reassured that with appropriate clothing, they can nurse quite discreetly.

Medical conditions precluding breastfeeding. Breastfeeding may be ruled out by certain medical conditions in either the infant or mother. For example, infants with the disease galactosemia can't break down galactose, the major sugar in breast milk. These infants do not grow well if nursed and often suffer from vomiting and diarrhea. If left untreated, the infants ultimately develop liver disease, cataracts, and mental retardation. A special infant formula free of galactose must be used. Breastfeeding may also be detrimental to infants with phenylketonuria; the high concentration of phenylalanine in breast milk may overwhelm the impaired ability of these infants to metabolize this amino acid, leading to production of toxic products.

Mothers who take certain medications that pass into the milk and adversely affect the nursing infant may be advised to avoid breastfeeding. In addition, a woman who has a serious chronic disease (such as tuberculosis, AIDS or HIV-positive status, and hepatitis) or who is being treated with chemotherapy medications should not breastfeed.[21]

What About Environmental Contaminants in Human Milk?

Some women wonder whether breastfeeding is safe. There is some legitimate concern over the levels of various environmental contaminants in human milk. However, the benefits from human milk are very well established, and the risks from environmental contaminants are still largely theoretical. Thus it is probably best to continue with what has been shown to work until sufficiently strong research data contradicts it.

A few measures a woman could take to counteract some known contaminants are to (1) avoid freshwater fish from polluted waters, (2) carefully wash and peel fruits and vegetables, and (3) remove the fatty edges of meat. In addition, a woman should not try to lose weight rapidly while nursing, because contaminants stored in fat tissue might then enter her bloodstream and affect her milk. If a woman questions whether her milk is safe, especially if she has lived in an area known to have a high concentration of toxic wastes or environmental pollutants, she should consult her local health department.

Can a Preterm Infant Be Breastfed?

There is no clear-cut answer to whether a woman can breastfeed a preterm infant. In some cases, human milk is the most desirable form of nourishment, depending on weight and length of gestation. If so, it must usually be expressed from the breast and fed through a tube. This type of feeding demands great maternal dedication. Fortification of the milk with such nutrients as calcium, phosphorus, sodium, and protein is often necessary to match an infant's rapid growth.[29] In other cases, special feeding problems may prevent the use of human milk or necessitate supplementing it with formula. Sometimes intravenous nutrition is the only option. Working as a team, the pediatrician, neonatal nurses, and registered dietitian must guide the parents in this decision.

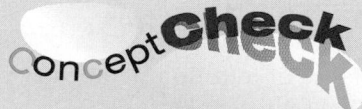

Human milk supplies most of an infant's nutritional needs for the first 6 months, although supplementation with vitamin D, iron, and fluoride may be needed. Breastfeeding is less expensive and often more convenient than formula-feeding. Compared with formula-fed infants, breastfed infants have fewer intestinal, respiratory, and ear infections and are less susceptible to allergies and food intolerances. Despite the advantages of breastfeeding, a lack of role models, misinformation, and social reticence may dissuade a mother from breastfeeding. A combination of breastfeeding and formula-feeding may be possible when a mother is regularly away from the infant. Breastfeeding is not desirable if a mother has certain diseases or must take medication potentially harmful to the infant. The preterm infant, depending on its condition, may benefit from consuming human milk.

Summary

➤ Adequate nutrition is vital during pregnancy to ensure the well-being of both the infant and mother. Poor maternal nutrition and use of some medications, especially during the first trimester, can cause birth defects. Growth retardation and altered development can also occur if these insults happen later in pregnancy.

➤ Infants born preterm (less than 2.5 kilograms, or 5.5 pounds) usually have more medical problems at and following birth than normal infants.

➤ A woman typically needs an additional 300 kcal per day during the second and third trimesters of pregnancy to meet her energy needs. Weight gain should occur slowly, reaching a total of 25 to 35 pounds in a woman of healthy weight.

➤ Protein, vitamin, and mineral needs increase during pregnancy. Extra servings from the milk, yogurt, and cheese group and the meat, poultry, fish, dry beans, eggs, and nuts group of the Food Guide Pyramid are recommended. Supplements of iron, in particular, may be needed. Folate nutriture should be adequate at the time of conception.

➤ Pregnant teenagers require very careful prenatal and nutritional care. Complications of pregnancy are more common in teenagers than in more mature women because the teenagers have very high physiological demands and often compromised social and economic support.

➤ Pregnancy-induced hypertension, heartburn, constipation, nausea, vomiting, edema, and anemia are all possible discomforts and complications of pregnancy. Often, nutrition therapy can help minimize these problems.

➤ Almost all women are able to nurse their infants. The nutrient composition of human milk is very different from unaltered cow's milk and much more desirable. Colostrum, the first fluid produced by the human breast, is very rich in immune factors. Mature milk is rich in the protein lactalbumin and in lactose.

➤ For the infant the advantages of breastfeeding over formula-feeding are numerous, including fewer intestinal, respiratory, and ear infections and fewer allergies and food intolerances. Moreover, breastfeeding is also less expensive and possibly more convenient for the mother than formula-feeding. However, an infant can be adequately nourished with formula if the mother chooses not to breastfeed. Breastfeeding is not desirable if the mother has certain diseases or must take medication potentially harmful to the infant. Likewise, breastfeeding is not advised for infants with certain medical conditions, including some preterm infants.

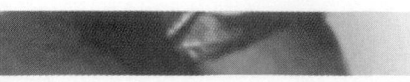

Study Questions

1 What historical evidence established the importance of nutrition in pregnancy outcome?

2 Provide three key pieces of advice for parents seeking to maximize their chances of having a healthy infant. Why did you identify those specific factors?

3 Outline current weight-gain recommendations for pregnancy. What is the basis for these recommendations?

4 How is the Food Guide Pyramid adapted to meet increased nutrient needs of pregnancy?

5 Why does teenage pregnancy receive so much attention these days? At what age do you think pregnancy would be ideal? Why?

6 Give three reasons that a woman should give serious consideration to breast-feeding her infant.

7 Describe the physiological mechanisms that stimulate milk production and release. How can knowing about these help mothers to nurse successfully?

8 What guidelines can a woman use to determine whether her breastfed infant is receiving sufficient nourishment?

9 How should the basic food plan suitable for pregnancy be modified during breastfeeding?

References

1 Annas GJ: Women and children first, *The New England Journal of Medicine* 333:1647, 1995.

2 Barker DJP: Growth in utero and coronary heart disease, *Nutrition Reviews* 54(2):S1, 1996.

3 Bratton RL: Fetal alcohol syndrome, *Postgraduate Medicine* 98(5):197, 1995.

4 Bucher HC and others: Effect of calcium supplementation on pregnancy-induced hypertension and preeclampsia, *Journal of the American Medical Association* 275:1113, 1996.

5 Centers for Disease Control: Infant mortality: United States, 1992, *Journal of the American Medical Association* 273:101, 1995.

6 Erick M: Hyperolfaction and hyperemesis gravidarum: what is the relationship? *Nutrition Reviews* 53:289, 1995.

7 Goldenberg RL and others: The effect of zinc supplementation on pregnancy outcome, *Journal of the American Medical Association* 274:463, 1995.

8 Golding J: Reproduction and caffeine consumption: a literature review, *Early Human Development* 43:1, 1995.

9 Hack M, Merkatz IR: Preterm delivery and low birth weights—a dire legacy, *The New England Journal of Medicine* 333:1772, 1995.

10 Levy-Marchal C and others: Antibodies against bovine albumin and other diabetes markers in French children, *Diabetes Care* 18:1089, 1995.

11 Lovelady C: Nutritional concerns during pregnancy and lactation. In Krummel DA, Kris-Etherton PM, editors: *Nutrition in women's health*, Gaithersburg, Md., 1996, Aspen Publishers.

12 Lie RT and others: A population-based study of the risk of recurrence of birth defects, *The New England Journal of Medicine* 331:1, 1994.

13 Lops VR and others: Anemia in pregnancy, *American Family Physician* 51:1189, 1995.

14 Luke B, Leurgans S: Maternal weight gains in ideal twin outcomes, *Journal of the American Dietetic Association* 96:178, 1996.

15 Makrides M and others: Are long-chain polyunsaturated fatty acids essential nutrients in infancy? *Lancet* 345:1463, 1995.

16 McGanity WJ and others: Embryonic development, pregnancy, and lactation. In Shils ME and others, editors: *Modern nutrition in health and disease*, ed 8, Philadelphia, 1994, Lea & Febiger.

17 Mennella JA, Beauchamp GK: Early flavor experiences: when do they start? *Nutrition Today* 29:25, 1994.

18 National Academy of Sciences–Institute of Medicine: *Nutrition during lactation*, Washington, DC, 1991, National Academy of Sciences Press.

19 National Academy of Sciences–Institute of Medicine: *Nutrition during pregnancy*, Washington, DC, 1990, National Academy of Sciences Press.

20 Newman J: How breast milk protects newborns, *Scientific American*, p 76, December 1995.

21 Peckham C, Gibb D: Mother-to-child transmission of the human immunodeficiency virus, *The New England Journal of Medicine* 333:298, 1995.

22 Rawlings JS and others: Prevalence of low birthweight and preterm delivery in relation to the interval between pregnancies among white and black women, *The New England Journal of Medicine* 332:69, 1995.

23 Rayburn WF and others: Periconceptional folate intake and neural tube defects, *Journal of the American College of Nutrition* 15:121, 1996.

24 Story M, Alton I: Nutrition issues and adolescent pregnancy, *Nutrition Today* 30:142, 1995.

25 Swan LL, Apgar BS: Preconceptual obstetric risk assessment and health promotion, *American Family Physician* 51:1875, 1995.

26 U.S. Public Health Service: Reducing teenage pregnancy increases life options for youth, *Prevention Report*, April/May 1994.

27 Wilcox A and others: Birth weight and perinatal mortality, *Journal of the American Medical Association*, 273:709, 1995.

28 Williams RD: Breast-feeding best bet for babies, *FDA Consumer*, p 19, October 1995.

29 Worthington-Roberts B and others: *Nutrition in pregnancy and lactation*, St Louis, 1993, Mosby.

30 Yip R: Iron supplementation during pregnancy: is it effective? *American Journal of Clinical Nutrition* 63:853, 1996.

31 Zemel PC, Levi B: Adolescent pregnancy: implications for nutritional care. In Krummel DA, Kris-Etherton PM, editors: *Nutrition in women's health*, Gaithersburg, Md., 1996, Aspen Publishers.

R A T E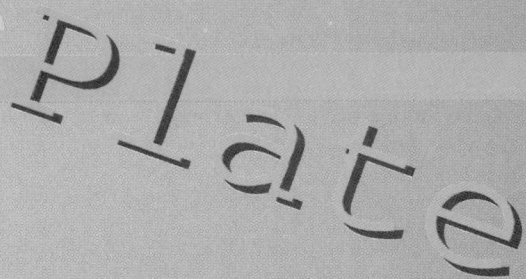

Targeting Nutrients Necessary for Pregnant Women

This chapter mentioned that pregnant women may have difficulty meeting their increased needs for folate, vitamin D, iron, calcium, and zinc. List five foods rich in each of these nutrients next to the appropriate heading below. Refer to Chapters 8 and 9 if necessary.

Nutrient	**Foods**	**Nutrient**	**Foods**
Folate	_____	Calcium	_____
	_____		_____
	_____		_____
	_____		_____
	_____		_____
Vitamin D	_____	Zinc	_____
	_____		_____
	_____		_____
	_____		_____
	_____		_____
Iron	_____		
	_____		
	_____		
	_____		
	_____		

1. Foods rich in more than one of these nutrients would be especially valuable for pregnant women. Write on the line below any foods you listed above that are good sources of more than one of these critical nutrients.

   _____

2. The RDAs for folate, vitamin D, iron, calcium, and zinc all increase considerably during pregnancy. For which of these nutrients can pregnant women usually obtain adequate intakes from dietary sources?

   _____

   Which of these nutrients are commonly taken in supplement form during pregnancy? Why might it be hard for pregnant women to meet their increased needs for these nutrients from foods alone?

   _____

   _____

3. Now design a diet you would like to follow that meets prenatal nutrient recommendations. Use the foods you selected in the above exercise to plan these meals. Try to show it to a pregnant woman. What insights have you gained?

   BREAKFAST: _____

   LUNCH: _____

   SNACK: _____

   DINNER: _____

   SNACK: _____

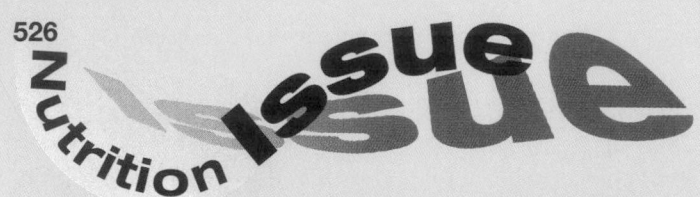

Fetal Alcohol Syndrome

Although much is known about diagnosing and treating some learning problems in children, many causes remain elusive. One particular question haunts many mothers: Did something happen while I was pregnant that created a learning disability in my child? This question leads directly to the topic of alcohol use during pregnancy, since alcohol is the most common damaging substance to which fetuses are exposed.

Conclusive evidence shows that large amounts of alcohol harm the fetus, especially when associated with binge drinking (consumption of five or more alcoholic drinks at one sitting). Binge drinking is especially perilous during the first 12 weeks of pregnancy as this is when critical early developmental events take place in the womb. Scientists don't know whether pregnant women must eliminate alcohol use entirely to avoid risk of damage to the fetus, but until a safe level can be established, women are advised not to drink any alcohol during pregnancy or when there is a chance pregnancy might occur.[3]

When a pregnant woman drinks more alcohol than she can metabolize, the excess reaches the embryo (and at later stages the fetus), which has no means of detoxifying it. Women with chronic alcoholism produce children with a recognizable pattern of malformations called fetal alcohol syndrome (FAS). A diagnosis of FAS is based mainly on poor fetal and infant growth, physical deformities (especially of facial features), and mental retardation (Figure 14-9). The infant is frequently irritable and may develop hyperactivity and a short attention span. Limited hand-eye coordination is common. Defects in sight, hearing, and mental processing often then develop over time.

The range of abnormalities from alcohol exposure varies from the severe effects associated with FAS to reduced birthweight, behavioral effects, growth retardation, and hampered learning ability in infants born to women who report only social drinking. The latter condition, termed *fetal alcohol effects (FAE)*, is not marked by telltale facial abnormalities. For this reason, parents may not suspect the presence of subtle defects caused by alcohol, even when they exist. FAE can devastate learning potential.

An estimated 3.3 per 10,000 infants born each year exhibit FAS; the incidence of FAS also has increased since the late 1970s. Many more infants are born annually with FAE. Alcohol use is in fact the leading cause of preventable birth defects and mental retardation in the United States and in the Western World as a whole.[3]

Exactly how alcohol causes these defects is not known. One line of research suggests that alcohol, or products produced by metabolism of alcohol, causes faulty migration of cells in the brain during early stages of development. In addition, inadequate nutrient intake, reduced nutrient and oxygen transfer across the placenta, cigarette smoking commonly linked to alcohol intake, drug use, and possibly other factors contribute to the overall result. Furthermore, we do not know how much alcohol it takes to produce these adverse effects. Again, for this reason many authorities—including the U.S. Surgeon General and the American Medical Association—believe it is best that mothers-to-be avoid alcohol altogether.

Abstinence is especially important during the first trimester, when key growth and development occur. Alcohol reaches the fetal blood at the same concentration as the mother's blood within 15 minutes of her drinking. How-

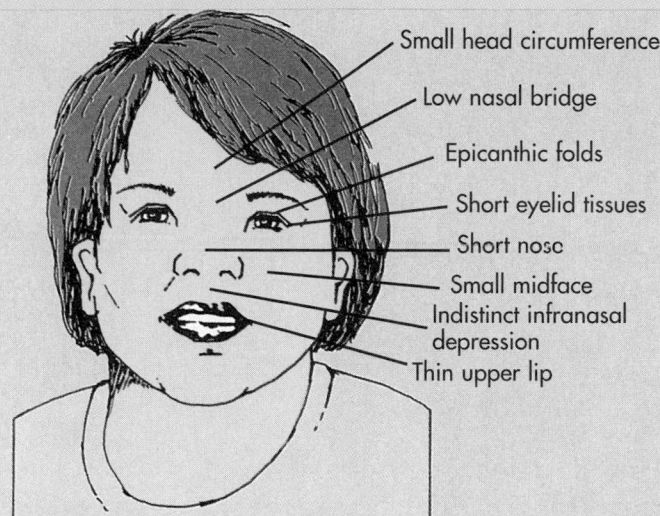

- Small head circumference
- Low nasal bridge
- Epicanthic folds
- Short eyelid tissues
- Short nose
- Small midface
- Indistinct infranasal depression
- Thin upper lip

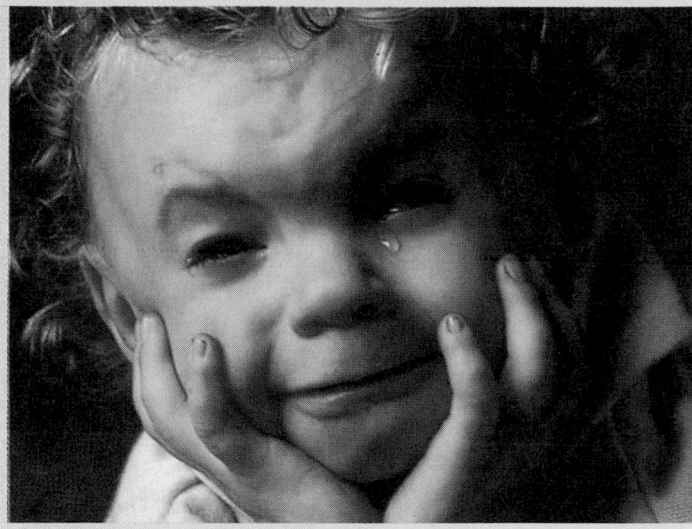

Figure 14-9 *Fetal alcohol syndrome. Milder forms of alcohol-induced changes in the fetus and the infant are known as fetal alcohol effects. The facial features shown are typical of affected children. Additional abnormalities in the brain and other internal organs accompany fetal alcohol syndrome but are not immediately apparent by simply looking at the child.*

ever, the effect on the fetus may be up to 10 times greater. For example, just one bout of binge drinking can arrest and alter cell division during critical phases of fetal development. The fetus then may develop an irreversible defect.

Physical damage to the embryo (and later the fetus) results more from first-trimester drinking because the basic structures of tissues and organs develop during this period. Emotional and learning problems stem more from third-trimester drinking because this is when critical further development of the brain occurs. And throughout the pregnancy alcohol interferes with growth. Overall, mothers who drink at least one to two drinks a day throughout pregnancy are much more likely to have growth-retarded infants, and mothers who drink only in late pregnancy are more likely to give birth to preterm infants.

Because alcohol has the capacity to adversely affect each stage of fetal development, the earlier in pregnancy that drinking ceases, the greater the potential for improved outcome. The best course is to consider alcohol an indulgence that must be eliminated from the time of conception until after pregnancy. Currently about half of all women are drinking at the time of conception (that is, before learning they were pregnant). One step in the right direction is the new congressionally mandated warnings about drinking during pregnancy that appear on all alcoholic beverage containers.

Pregnancy lasts only 9 months. In contrast, parents may spend a lifetime caring, often at great expense (estimated at $1.4 million in the United States), for their offspring needlessly handicapped by FAS or FAE.[3]

> Pregnant women should recognize that many cough syrups contain alcohol. Cases have been reported of infants with FAS born to mothers who consumed generous amounts of such cough syrups but no other alcoholic beverages.[29]

Nutrition from Infancy through Adolescence

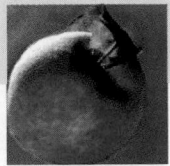

AS WE GROW THROUGH EARLY years into adulthood, our needs for energy and nutrients change. Infants need more energy, protein, vitamins, and minerals per pound of body weight than do adults to support their tremendous growth and development. As growth tapers, children need and eat proportionately less.[25] The erratic eating behaviors of young children pose major challenges for parents and other caregivers. In turn, childhood becomes an important time to establish healthful habits, including those related to food choice and physical activity.

The family wields a subtle but important influence over the child. Thus education designed to change eating behaviors of children must be directed simultaneously at the main caregivers. They usually determine what foods are purchased and how they are prepared. By stocking a variety of foods at home, introducing different foods regularly, and making mealtimes fun for the whole family, parents and other caregivers can steer children toward lifelong healthful eating patterns.[26] Maintaining a healthful eating pattern should continue as children grow into teenagers. In exploring all these stages of life, this chapter looks at the key role nutrients play and how food choices should be tailored to meet those needs.

ASSESS *Yourself*

Avoiding Table Wars

If you have children or have ever worked as a babysitter, you probably know how difficult it can be to get kids to eat on command. The problem doesn't go away—parents and other caregivers also worry later about the eating habits of their teenagers. During adolescence, teenagers establish their own identities and their busy lifestyles often leave little time for structured eating.

How can household wars about eating be avoided? Listed below are some statements about children and adolescents and their eating habits. Which are true? Place a "T" in the blank to the left if you think the statement is true, or an "F" if false. If caregivers know the truths, they may be able to avoid table wars.

_____ 1. Around 9 to 10 months of age, infants explore, test, and play with food. Unless they are disciplined to eat neatly and treat food seriously, they will be undisciplined eaters in the future.

_____ 2. Expect babies to take only two or three bites of solid food at first meals.

_____ 3. Infants enjoy bland foods much more than do adults.

_____ 4. Infants should be encouraged to consume a lot of apple juice because it's rich in so many nutrients.

_____ 5. Honey is a good sweetener for infants because it has a high nutrient content.

_____ 6. Toddlers typically have less appetite than they had during the first year of life.

_____ 7. You can normally expect children to avoid vegetables and whole grains.

_____ 8. Adult modeling of healthful eating habits influences a child's behavior.

_____ 9. A good policy for toddlers is the one-bite rule, which asks them to take at least one bite of the foods presented to them.

_____ 10. Children like foods with soft textures and strong flavors.

_____ 11. Children should be made to eat three meals a day, rather than many small meals.

_____ 12. Children often object to having foods mixed, as in stews and casseroles.

_____ 13. Using one food as a reward for eating another food—for example, cookies for vegetables—is a good strategy for promoting healthful eating patterns.

_____ 14. Infants and children of all ages should eat low-fat diets to decrease their risk of future heart disease.

_____ 15. Teenagers are more likely to try healthful foods when immediate positive outcomes are emphasized—such as their contributions to a better appearance and physique—as opposed to when potential future health hazards from a poor diet are stressed.

_____ 16. Involving teenagers in cooking and purchasing food helps promote healthful eating habits.

True: 2, 3, 6, 8, 9, 12, 15, 16
False: 1, 4, 5, 7, 10, 11, 13, 14

Key Chapter Concepts

- Growth is very rapid during infancy. An adequate diet, especially in terms of energy, protein, and zinc intake, is very important to support this growth.
- Nutrient needs in the first 6 months can be met by human milk or infant formula (generally based on cow's milk). Supplementary vitamin D and iron may be needed in the first 6 months for breastfed infants, and many infants benefit from supplemental fluoride.
- Infant formulas may or may not be fortified with iron. Sanitation is very important when preparing and storing formula.
- Most infants don't need solid foods before about 4 to 6 months of age. This practice reduces the risk that the infant will develop food allergies.
- The first solid food given generally should be iron-fortified infant cereals. Other single foods, such as ground meats, can be added gradually, at the rate of about one each week.
- Some foods to avoid giving infants in the first year are honey, cow's milk, very salty or sweet foods, or foods that may cause choking.
- A slower growth rate typifies the preschool years and underlies the importance of children's eating nutrient-dense foods and reducing their food serving sizes. A good rule of thumb is to serve portion sizes at meals of 1 tablespoon of each food for each year of life.
- Teens and young adults, especially girls, particularly need adequate iron and calcium in the diet, and should generally strive to moderate high-fat food choices, as shown in the Food Guide Pyramid.

Infant Growth and Physiological Development

For convenience, we often use the term *parents* in this chapter to refer generally to those who are raising children, including both single parents and adults who are not a child's biological parents.

During infancy a child's attitudes toward foods and the whole eating process begin to take shape. If parents and other caregivers practice good nutrition and are flexible, they can lead a child into lifelong healthful food habits. Such an infant has a good chance of starting life with the nutrients needed to support brain and body growth spurts and of developing a willingness to try new foods. However, these physical and psychological advantages alone don't guarantee that a child will thrive.

Children also need specific attention focused on them; they need to grow in a stimulating environment, and they need a sense of security.[25] Children hospitalized for growth failure tend to gain weight more quickly when loving care accompanies needed nutrients.

The Growing Infant

All babies seem to do is eat and sleep. There's a good reason for this. An infant's birth weight doubles in the first 4 to 6 months and triples within the first year. Such rapid growth requires a lot of both nourishment and sleep. Beyond the first year, growth is slower; it takes 5 more years to double the weight seen at 1 year. An infant also increases in length in the first year by 50% and then continues to gain height throughout preschool and teen years.[25] These gains are not necessarily continuous— spurts of growth alternate with plateaus. Height is essentially complete by age 19, though increases of several inches may occur in the early 20s (Figure 15-1). Head size in proportion to total height shrinks from one fourth to one eighth during the climb from infancy to adulthood.

The human body needs a lot more food to support growth and development than to merely maintain itself once growth ceases. In some populations, food is not regularly available. When nutrients are missing at critical phases of growth and development, growth slows and may even stop. From observations of Egyptian mummies, we see that infants were about the same size in 300 BC as they are today. However, adult mummies are much smaller than adults today. Furthermore, the suits of armor in museum collections of the Middle Ages typically would not fit modern

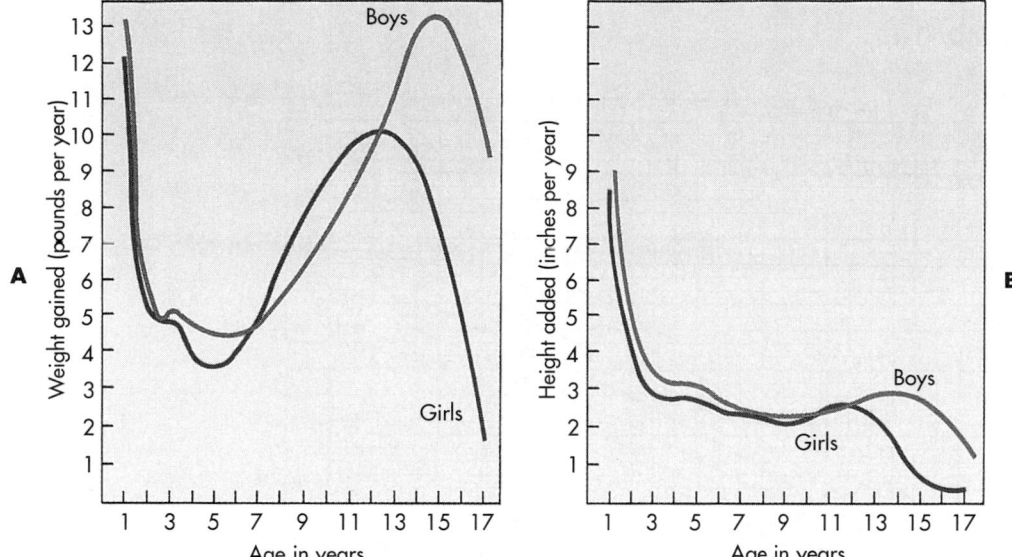

Figure 15-1 *Growth rates.* **A,** *Average gains in weight for girls and boys.* **B,** *Average additions to height for girls and boys. The higher the line in any one year, the greater the amount of annual gain compared with that in other years. Large gains in weight occur in both infancy and puberty, whereas the very high length gain in infancy is never reached again. If graphs such as these were plotted in smaller time segments, they would appear as zigzag lines rather than smooth lines, reflecting short, periodic spurts in growth during the course of each year.*

adults. This suggests that people of that time generally ate nutrient-poor diets that did not support the growth we typically experience today.

In countries of the developing world today, about half the children are short and underweight for their ages. Poor nutrition—called *undernutrition*—is at the heart of the problem. This occurs to a lesser extent in the United States. The undernourished children are simply smaller versions of nutritionally fit children. In poorer countries, when breastfeeding ceases, children are often fed a high-carbohydrate, low-protein diet. This diet supports some growth but does not allow children to attain their full genetic potential. To grow, children must consume adequate amounts of energy, protein, zinc, and other nutrients.

Infant development follows a pattern in which body water reduces from about 75% at birth to 60% at 1 year. The latter is also the proportion typical in adults. By age 1 an infant's body nitrogen content (and thus protein content) has increased from 2% of body weight at birth to 3%, indicating the infant has synthesized much new lean tissue.[25]

The Effect of Undernutrition on Growth

As with the fetus **in utero,** the long-term effects of nutritional problems in infancy and childhood depend on the severity, timing, and duration of the nutritional insult to cell processes.

Probably the single best indicator of a child's nutritional status is growth. Mild zinc deficiencies in American children have been linked to poor growth. Improving the diets of these children then leads to improved growth. Overall, eating a poor diet as an infant or child hampers cell division that occurs at that critical stage. Getting an adequate diet later usually won't compensate for lost growth, because high amounts of key hormones are then missing from the bloodstream, although they were present during the critical time when cells should have been dividing. In addition, the size of the skeleton is for the most part set. For example, a 17-year-old Central American girl

In utero
In the uterus; in other words, during pregnancy.

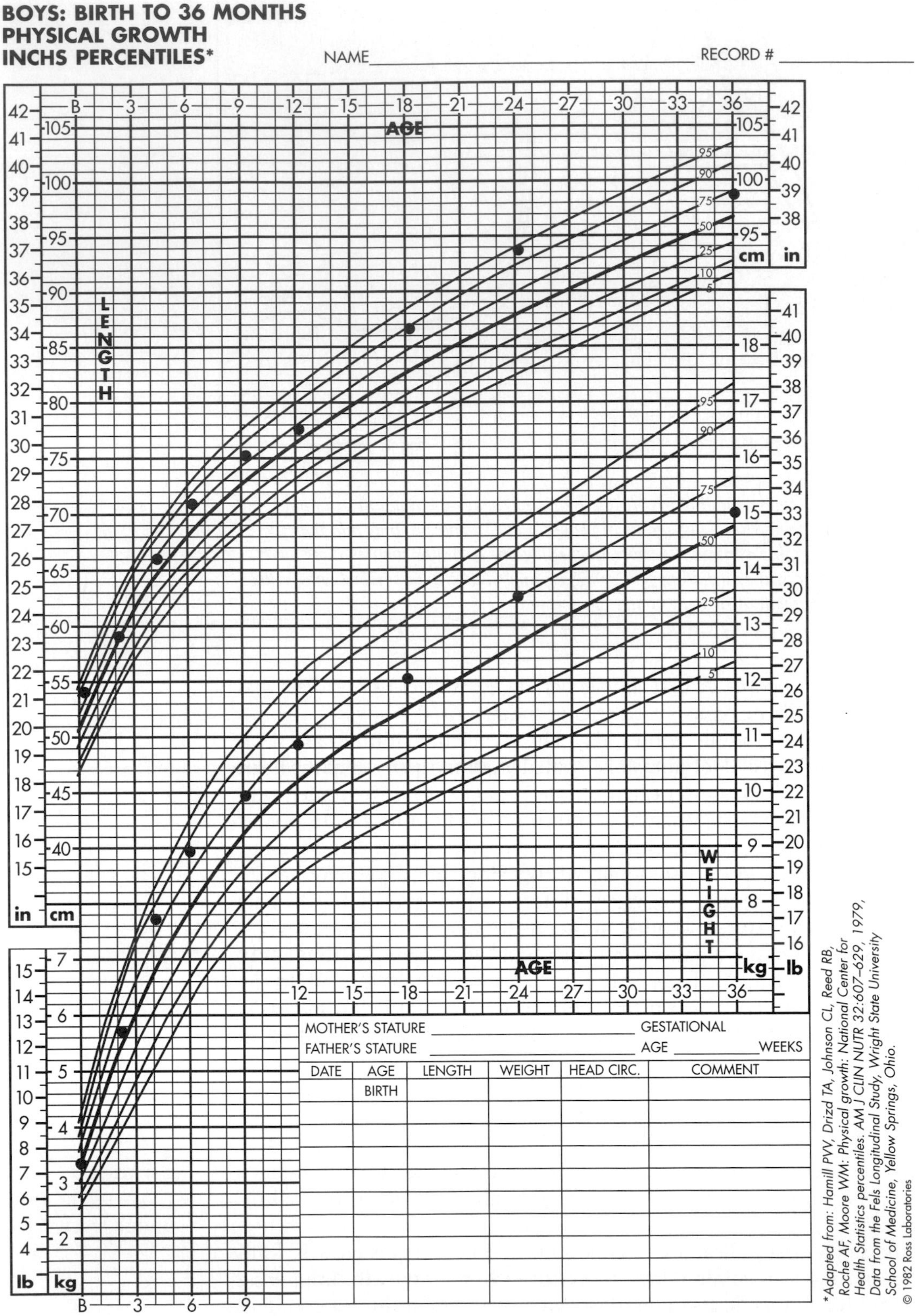

Figure 15-2 *Growth charts used to assess length (height) and weight in young boys. A certain weight and length (height) correspond to a percentile value, which is a ranking of the person among 100 peers. The growth pattern of Dr. Wardlaw's son is plotted to illustrate how this tool is used in medical practice.*

who is 4 feet 8 inches tall cannot attain the adult height of a typical American girl simply by now eating better. Girls experience their peak rate of growth before the onset of the menses. Once the time for growth ceases (in women this is about 2 years after they start menstruating), a good nutrient intake will help maintain health and weight but will not make up for all lost growth.[25]

Assessing Infant Growth and Development

Health professionals assess a child's increases in height and weight by comparing these with typical growth patterns recorded on charts. The typical charts contain seven percentile divisions, which represent 90% of children (Figure 15-2). A percentile simply represents the rank of the person among 100 peers matched for age and gender. Tony, for example, is at the ninetieth percentile height for age, meaning that of 100 boys of that age, he is shorter than 10 and taller than 89. A child at the fiftieth percentile is considered average. Fifty children will be taller than this child; 49 will be shorter.

Individual growth charts are available for both males and females, for ages ranging from 0 to 36 months and 2 to 18 years. Height for age, weight for age, and weight for height can be plotted. Infants and children should have their growth assessed during regular health checkups. It takes 1 to 3 years for an infant to establish his or her own genetic percentile. Once this figure is established, such as length (height) for age, the child's measurement should then track along that percentile. If the child's growth doesn't keep up with its length-for-age percentile, the physician needs to investigate whether a medical or nutritional problem is impeding the predicted growth. Inappropriate weight gain—too little or too much—should also be investigated.

Infants born preterm may catch up in growth in 2 to 3 years. This requires that the child jump up in the percentiles. If this occurs—especially in length for age—it is usually no cause for alarm. On the other hand, jumping percentiles in weight for height can be disturbing if the child approaches the eightieth to ninetieth percentiles. Generally a child at the 85th percentile for weight for height is considered overweight. Above the 95th percentile, the child is considered obese.[22]

Brain Growth

The brain grows faster in infancy than at any other time of life. To accommodate the growth, an infant's head must be very large in proportion to the rest of the body. The rapid growth stops at about 18 months of age. The rest of the body eventually grows to reach a typical proportion to head size. In early physical checkups, a health professional usually measures the head circumference as another means of assessing growth, especially brain growth. How nutritional status affects brain development and intelligence quotient (IQ) is difficult to measure because scientists haven't figured out how to separate the effects of nature from nurture. However, studies from Central America suggest that IQ after age 5 years relates more closely to the amount of schooling a child receives than to nutritional intake during childhood.

Adipose (Fat) Tissue Growth

Since 1970 researchers have speculated that overfeeding during infancy may increase adipose (fat) tissue cell numbers. Today we know that adipose cells can also increase as adulthood obesity develops (see Chapter 10). Still, if energy intake is limited during infancy to keep down the number of adipose cells, the growth of other organ systems may also be severely retarded. Special concern revolves especially around proper brain and nervous system development. In addition, most obese infants become normal-weight preschoolers without excessive diet restrictions. For these reasons it's

Weight primarily reflects current nutrient intake. Height is a measure of long-term nutrient intake.

Children under 2 to 3 years of age are measured with knees unflexed and while lying on their backs, so the term length is used rather than height.

unwise to restrict diet, and especially fat intake, before 2 years of age. About 40% of energy intake from fat is recommended.[10] As mentioned earlier, without adequate nutrients, infants are unlikely to eventually attain their potential adult height.

Failure to Thrive

Occasionally an infant doesn't grow much in the first few months. Physical problems that may contribute to retarded growth range from poor oral cavity development, infections, and heart irregularities to constant diarrhea associated with intestinal problems. However, more than half the infants who fail to thrive have no apparent disease. Instead the usual cause is poor infant-parent interaction.[2] This stems from misinformation, lack of a parent role model, or apathy about the child's welfare. In general, the problems often arise from the parents' inexperience, rather than intentional negligence.

Infants not only need cuddling; they also respond to voices and eye contact, especially at feeding times. New parents need to appreciate the importance of these practices to their infant's well-being. Some parents also may be overcommitted to maintaining a lean child in the hope of preventing future obesity, as discussed in Chapter 13. The result, even though the intention was good, can be failure to thrive.

When clinicians encounter an infant who is failing to thrive from a nutritional standpoint, they must first determine whether the child is consuming enough energy. For infants, approximately 45 kcal per pound (95 kcal per kilogram) of body weight daily is adequate in early infancy. By 6 months of age, closer to 40 kcal per pound (85 kcal per kilogram) is recommended. For a breastfed infant, the clinician needs to make sure that sufficient milk is being consumed. The child should be nursing about 6 to 8 times a day for about 20 minutes a session and have six to eight wet diapers each day. The mother should consume adequate food and fluid (see Chapter 14). Children older than 2 years are less likely to experience failure to thrive because they can often get food for themselves. Younger children, for the most part, are limited to what the caregivers provide.

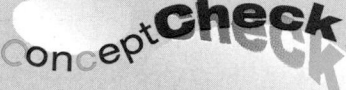

Growth occurs rapidly during infancy: birth weight doubles in about 4 to 6 months and triples within the first year. Lean tissue increases and the percentage of body water falls during the first year. Undernutrition in childhood can irreversibly inhibit growth and maturation so that an individual never attains his or her full genetic potential. Infant and child growth is assessed by tracking body weight, length (height), and head circumference over time. It is not desirable for infants to become obese, although no evidence strongly indicates that obese infants become obese adults. However, severe restriction of energy intake is not recommended for infants because it may slow the growth of organ systems. When infants do not grow properly, their failure to thrive may stem from physical disorders or inadequate care, including inappropriate feeding practices.

Infant Nutritional Needs

Infants' nutritional needs vary as they grow, and these differ from adult needs in both amount and proportion (Figure 15-3). Initially, human milk or infant formula (generally using heat-treated cow's milk as a base) supplies needed nutrients. Solid foods are usually not needed until after 4 to 6 months.[25] Even after solid foods are added, the basis of an infant's diet for the first year is still human milk or infant formula. Because of the critical importance of adequate nutrition in infancy and the difficulties encountered in feeding some infants, more time is spent in this chapter on this developmental period than on the later periods of childhood.

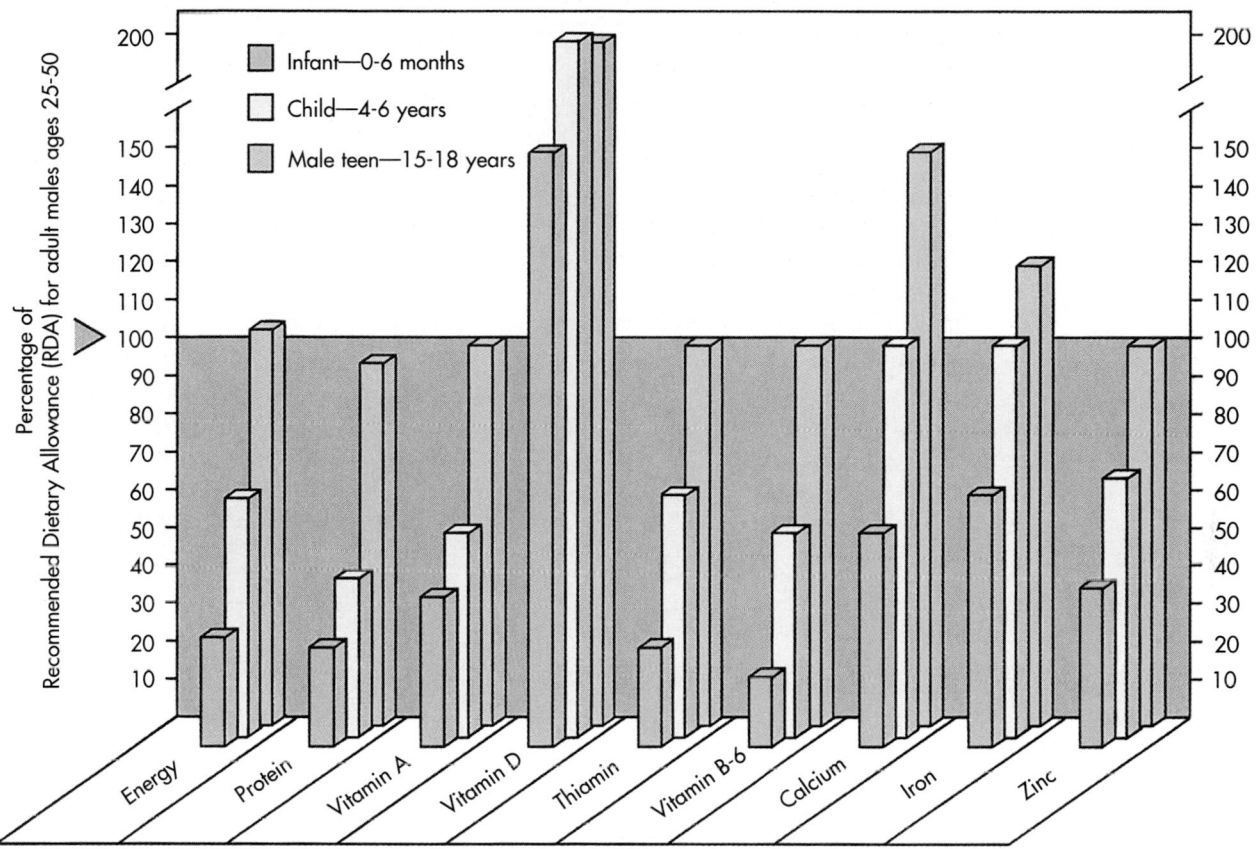

Figure 15-3 *RDAs for infants, children, and teenagers as percentages of RDAs for adult males. Compared with adults, infants' relative energy needs are lower than are their needs for other nutrients, as illustrated by the different heights of the green bars. Thus infants need to obtain relatively larger amounts of nutrients from a smaller intake of food than do adults. This is also true of young children (yellow bars), but to a lesser extent.*

Energy

As mentioned earlier, infants need about 40 to 45 kcal per pound of body weight daily (85 to 95 kcal per kilogram) to supply them with adequate energy. At 6 months of age this amounts to about 700 kcal daily. Based on body weight, this amounts to two to four times more energy than adults need. Infants need an easy way to get this amount of energy. Either human milk or infant formula is ideal for the first few months. Both are high in fat and supply about 650 kcal per quart of fluid (700 kcal per liter; Table 15-1). Later, human milk or infant formula, supplemented by solid foods, can provide even more energy.

The infant's high energy needs are primarily driven by its rapid growth and high metabolic rate. The high metabolic rate is caused in part by the ratio of the infant's body surface to its weight. More body surface allows more heat loss from the skin; the body must use extra energy to replace that heat.[2]

TABLE 15-1

Composition of Human and Cow's Milk and Infant Formulas Per Liter (L)

Milk or formula	Energy (kcal/L)	Protein (gram/L)	Fat (gram/L)	Carbohydrate (gram/L)	Minerals* (gram/L)
MILK					
Human milk	750	11	45	70	2
Cow's milk, whole	670	36	36	49	7
Cow's milk, skim	360	36	1	51	7
CASEIN/WHEY-BASED FORMULAS					
Similac	680	14	36	71	3
Enfamil	670	15	37	69	3
Carnation	670	16	34	73	3
SOYBEAN PROTEIN-BASED FORMULAS					
ProSobee	670	20	35	67	4
Isomil	680	16	36	68	4
PREDIGESTED PROTEIN					
Nutramigen	670	19	26	89	1
Alimentum	680	18	37	68	1
TRANSITION FORMULAS/BEVERAGES†					
Similac Toddler's Best	670	25	33	75	3
Enfamil Next Step	670	17	33	74	3
Carnation Follow-Up	670	17	27	88	3

*Calcium, phosphorus, and other minerals.
†For use after 6 months of age or later (see label).

Protein

Daily protein needs vary in infancy from 0.7 to 1 gram of protein for each pound of body weight (1.6 to 2.2 grams per kilogram). About 40% of total protein intake should come from essential amino acids. Both goals are satisfied by either human milk or infant formula. Total protein intake should not exceed 20% of energy needs. Excess nitrogen and minerals supplied by high-protein diets would exceed the ability of an infant's kidneys to excrete the resulting metabolic waste products.

In the United States, infant protein deficiency is unlikely, except in cases of mistaken feeding practices, such as when an infant's formula is excessively watered down. Protein deficiency may also be induced by elimination diets used to detect food **allergies.** As foods are eliminated from the diet, infants may not be offered enough protein to compensate for the high-protein sources no longer present (see the Nutrition Issue at the end of the chapter).

Fat

Infants and children up to 2 years of age should get about 40% of their energy from fat. More than 50% may lead to poor fat digestion. About half the energy supplied by both human milk and infant formula comes from fat. Essential fatty acids should make up at least 3% of total energy. Fats are an important part of the infant's diet because they are energy-dense and vital to the development of the nervous system. As a concentrated energy source, fat helps resolve the potential problem of the infant's high energy needs and small stomach capacity. This is not an age to greatly restrict fat (or cholesterol) intake.[10]

Allergy

A hypersensitive immune response that is triggered by foreign proteins (allergens) and is associated with various adverse physical effects.

Vitamins of Special Interest

Vitamin K is routinely given by injection to all infants at birth. This dose lasts until the infant's intestinal bacteria are established and begin to synthesize vitamin K. Formula-fed infants receive the rest of the vitamins they need from the formula. Breastfed infants, especially dark-skinned ones, may require a vitamin D supplement if they are not exposed to much sunlight. (Sunlight exposure on human skin activates synthesis of vitamin D; see Chapter 8.) Breastfed infants whose mothers are total vegetarians (vegans) should receive a vitamin B-12 supplement.

Minerals of Special Interest

The iron stores with which children are born are generally depleted by the time birth weight doubles, in 4 to 6 months. The American Academy of Pediatrics recommends that to maintain a desirable iron status, formula-fed infants should be given an iron-fortified formula from birth. Breastfed infants need solid foods to supply extra iron at about 6 months of age. The need for iron is a major consideration in deciding when to introduce solid foods. Some researchers recommend liquid iron supplements from birth or by 1 month of age for breastfed infants.

Infants need adequate amounts of zinc and iodide to support growth. Human milk and infant formula adequately supply these needs when they supply enough energy to meet needs. In addition, some clinicians recommend fluoride supplements to aid tooth development for breast-fed infants if the water supply used in home formula preparation—either tap or bottled water—doesn't contain fluoride. Note that formula manufacturers use fluoride-free water in formula preparation. Parents should consult their dentist for advice on the infant's need for fluoride.[14]

Water

An infant needs about 2 ounces of water and other fluids combined per pound of body weight (about 150 milliliters per kilogram). Infants typically consume enough human milk or formula to supply this amount. In hot climates, however, supplemental water may be necessary. Furthermore, any conditions that lead to water loss—diarrhea, vomiting, fever, and too much sun—can call for supplemental water.

Infants are easily dehydrated, a condition that has serious effects if not remedied. Dehydration can result in rapidly decreasing kidney function, and the infant may then require hospitalization for rehydration. Special fluid replacement formulas are available to treat dehydration.[21] A physician should guide any use of these products. It's important to remember that excessive fluid can also be harmful, especially to the brain. Overall, it's best to limit supplemental fluids to about 4 ounces per day, unless the physician thinks that a greater need exists because of disease or other conditions. In sum, extremes in fluid intake—either too little or too much—can lead to health problems.

Critical Thinking

Tatiana has been breastfeeding her baby since he was born 7 months ago. When she and her husband took the baby for his checkup, they were told that he was anemic. They were very surprised, because they thought human milk contained all the nutrients the baby needed for the first year of life. How can you explain the baby's anemia?

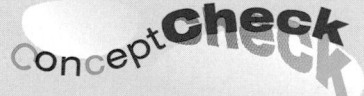

Concept Check

Most nutrient needs in the first 6 months are met by human milk or infant formula. Breastfed infants may need vitamin D, fluoride, and iron supplements, and formula-fed infants may need fluoride supplements. Infants usually receive enough water from the human milk or formula they drink.

Formula Feeding for Infants

Breastfeeding was covered in detail in Chapter 14. Let's now focus on formula-feeding. You'll recall that a major advantage of breastfeeding is provision of antibodies that impart immune protection to the infant. That advantage is very important in the context of poverty and poor hygiene. It's less important in America, where high standards for water purity and cleanliness in most communities make formula feeding a safe alternative for infants.

Formula Composition

Infants cannot tolerate cow's milk as such because of its high protein and mineral content. Cow's milk reflects the greater growth needs of calves. Thus cow's milk must be altered to be safe for infant feeding. The altered forms, known as infant formulas, were first available commercially in 1931. Since 1980 they have been required to conform to strict guidelines for nutrient composition and quality set by federal law. Formulas generally contain lactose and/or sucrose for carbohydrate, heat-treated proteins from cow's milk, and vegetable oils for fat (see Table 15-1). Soy protein-based formulas are available for infants who can't tolerate lactose or the types of proteins found in cow's milk. If the soybean-based formula is not tolerated, the next step is to try a predigested (hydrolyzed) protein formula, such as Nutramigen or Alimentum. A variety of other specialized formulas also are available for specific medical conditions.[28]

Some new transition formulas/beverages recently have been introduced for older infants and toddlers (see Table 15-1). Some of these products are intended for use after 6 months of age if the infant is consuming solid foods, whereas others are intended for use only by toddlers. These transition products are lower in fat than human milk or standard infant formulas; their iron content is higher than that of cow's milk, and their overall mineral content is generally more like that of human milk than cow's milk. According to the manufacturers, the advantages of these transition formulas/beverages over standard formulas for older infants and toddlers include reduced cost and better flavor. Parents should consult their pediatrician with regard to use of these products, which to date have seen little use.

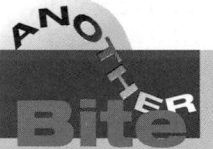

Note that health food stores often sell formula-type products that can lead unsuspecting parents into thinking they are providing their infants with a complete nutritional formula. Soy Moo, for example, a soy beverage sold in health food stores, should not be confused with soy-based infant formulas. Unlike nutritionally complete infant formulas, this product and others like it lack some essential nutrients and can lead to severe nutritional deficiencies in infants. For example, a severely undernourished 5-month-old infant was admitted to Arkansas Children's Hospital in Little Rock with symptoms of heart failure, rickets, inflamed blood vessels, and possible nerve damage. The infant girl had been fed nothing but Soy Moo since she was 3 days old. Because of cases such as this one, parents should consult their physician for advice in choosing an appropriate infant formula.

Preparation of Formula

In the 1950s it was common to prepare a day's supply of bottles and then sterilize them in boiling water for about 30 minutes. Today bottles are often prepared one at a time. Some infant formulas even come in a ready-to-feed form. These simply are poured into a clean bottle and fed immediately. Room-temperature formula is

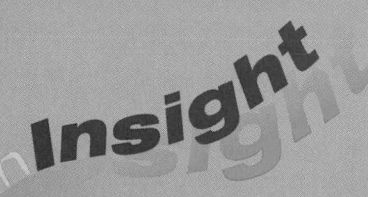

Dietary Guidelines for Infant Feeding

In response to various controversies surrounding infant feeding, the American Academy of Pediatrics has issued a number of statements concerning infant diets. The following guidelines are based on these statements[6]:

- **Build to a variety of foods.**
  For the first months of life, human milk is all an infant needs. When the infant is ready, start adding new foods one at a time. During the first year, the goal is to teach an infant to enjoy a variety of nutritious foods. A lifetime of healthy eating habits begins with this important first step.
- **Pay attention to your infant's appetite to avoid overfeeding or underfeeding.**
  Feed infants when hungry. Never force an infant to finish an unwanted serving of food. Watch for signs that indicate hunger or fullness.
- **Infants need fat.**
  Although fat is the cause of many adult health problems, it's an essential source of energy for growing infants. Fat also helps the brain and nervous system develop.
- **Choose fruits, vegetables, and grains, but don't overdo high-fiber foods.**
  Although many adults benefit from higher-fiber diets, they are not good for infants. They are bulky, filling, and often low in energy. The natural amounts of fiber and nutrients in fruits, vegetables, and grains are appropriate as part of a healthy infant diet.
- **Infants need sugars in moderation.**
  Sugars are an additional source of energy for active, rapidly growing infants. Foods such as human milk, fruits, and juices are natural sources of sugars and other nutrients as well. Foods that contain artificial sweeteners should be avoided; they don't provide the energy growing infants need.
- **Infants need sodium in moderation.**
  Sodium is a necessary mineral found naturally in almost all foods. As part of a healthy diet, infants need sodium for their bodies to work properly.
- **Choose foods containing iron, zinc, and calcium.**
  Infants need good sources of iron, zinc, and calcium for optimum growth in the first 2 years. These minerals are important for healthy blood, proper growth, and strong bones.

The recommendations in this chapter are consistent with these guidelines. In essence, there is no evidence that very restrictive diets during infancy have positive effects, whereas their hazards are well documented.

acceptable in many infants. Otherwise, to warm a bottle of formula, a caregiver can run hot water over it or place it briefly in a pan of simmering water. Note that infant formulas should not be heated in a microwave oven because hot spots may develop that can burn the infant's mouth and esophagus.

Powdered and concentrated fluid formula preparations are more commonly used than ready-to-feed varieties. All utensils used in preparing formula from these preparations should be washed and thoroughly rinsed. Powdered or concentrated formulas are poured into a bottle to which clean, cold water is added (following label directions) and then mixed. The formula is then warmed, if desired, and fed immediately to the infant. Hot water from the faucet should not be used to make formula, since it poses a risk for high lead content (see Chapter 17).

A convenient practice when using powdered formula is to measure out the correct amount of dry formula into a series of bottles to have on hand. When a bottle is needed, cold or warmed water is added and mixed; the formula is then ready for immediate use. Likewise, a whole can of concentrated formula (13 ounces of formula plus 13 ounces of water) can be made up and stored in the refrigerator in a clean, covered jar or pitcher. When feeding time comes, a caregiver need only fill a bottle with the diluted formula.

Refrigerating diluted formula for 1 day is safe. However, formula left over from a feeding should be discarded because it will be contaminated by bacteria and enzymes in the infant's saliva. If well water is used, it should be boiled before making formula for at least the infant's first 3 months of life and also be analyzed for excessive concentration of naturally occurring nitrates, which can lead to a severe form of anemia. Boiling tapwater is also advised by some groups, based on recent evidence that even municipal water may contain microbes that can harm the vulnerable, such as infants[28] (see Chapter 9).

Feeding Technique

Because infants swallow a lot of air along with either formula or human milk, it's important to burp an infant after either 10 minutes of feeding or 1 to 2 ounces (30 to 60 milliliters) from a bottle, and again at the end of feeding. Spitting up a bit of milk is normal at this time. Once fed, infants should be placed on their side, with a rolled-up blanket placed behind their back to support that position. In this position, infants have the least chance of choking on any milk they spit up. Infants should not be placed on their stomachs, because this sleeping position has been linked to sudden infant death syndrome.[2]

When the infant begins acting full, bottle feeding should be stopped, even if some milk is left in the bottle. Common cues that signal that an infant has had enough include turning the head away, inattention, falling asleep, and becoming playful (Figure 15-4). Generally the infant's appetite is a better guide than standardized recommendations concerning feeding amounts. As noted earlier, breastfeeding infants usually have had enough to eat after about 20 minutes. Although it's difficult to tell how much milk breastfed infants are getting, they also give signs when full. By carefully observing bottle-feeding or nursing infants and responding to their cues appropriately, caregivers not only can be assured that the infants' energy needs are being met but also can foster a climate of trust and responsiveness.

Development of Feeding Skills in the Older Infant

By 6 to 7 months the infant has learned to grab and transfer objects from one hand to the other (Table 15-2). At about this time teeth begin to appear, and the infant begins to handle finger foods with some dexterity. Dry toast, sliced in strips, offers hours of enjoyment.

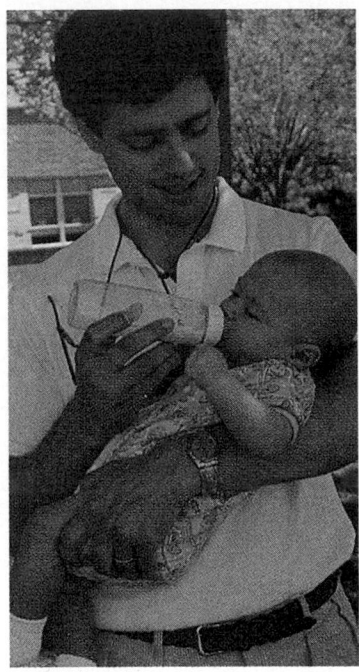

Figure 15-4
Careful attention during feeding allows the caregiver to pick up on the infant's signal as to when the feeding should cease.

TABLE 15-2

Typical Progression of Infant Eating Skills and Solid-Food Introduction*

Age	Feeding skills	Oral motor skills	Types of food	Suggested activities
Birth–4 months		Rooting reflex Sucking reflex Swallowing reflex Extrusion reflex	Human milk Infant formula	Breastfed or bottle-feed
5 months	Able to grasp objects voluntarily Learning to reach mouth with hands	Disappearance of extrusion reflex		Possible introduction of thinned cereal if baby not satisfied by breast-feeding or bottle-feeding
6 months	Sits with balance while using hands	Transfers food from front of tongue to back	Infant cereal Strained fruit Strained vegetables Egg yolk (if no family history of egg allergy)	Prepare cereal with formula or human milk to a semiliquid texture Use spoon Feed from a dish Advance to ⅓-½ cup cereal before adding fruits or vegetables
7 months	Improved grasp Can transfer objects from hand to hand	Mashes food with lateral movements of jaw Learns side-to-side or "rotary" chewing Tooth eruption	Infant cereal Strained to junior texture of fruits, vegetables, and meats	Thicken cereal to lumpier texture Sit in highchair with feet supported Introduce cup
8-10 months	Holds bottle without help Drinks from cup Decreases fluid intake and increases solids Coordinates hand-to-mouth movement		Juices (small amounts) Soft, mashed, or minced table foods	Begin finger foods like toast or crackers Do not add salt, sugar, or fats to food Present soft foods in chunks ready for finger-feeding
10-12 months	Feeds self Holds cup without help	Improved ability to bite and chew	Soft, chopped table foods Whole egg and whole milk (at 1 year of age)	Provide meals in pattern similar to rest of family Use cup at meals

Modified from Queen P, Lang C: *Handbook of pediatric nutrition*, Rockville, Md, 1993, Aspen.
*This timeline is just an estimate, and individual infants may vary by several months from the ages given. A pediatrician should be consulted if caregivers are concerned about an infant's developmental progress. In general, there is no nutritional reason to begin introduction of solid foods before 4 to 6 months of age.

By age 7 to 8 months, infants can push food around on a plate and play with a drinking cup. They can hold a bottle and self-feed a cracker or piece of toast. In mastering these manipulations, infants develop self-confidence and self-esteem. It's important that parents be patient and support these early feeding attempts, even though they appear inefficient.

At around 10 months of age, infants practice in earnest self-feeding finger foods and drinking from a cup. Feeding time is often very messy. Food is used as a means to explore the environment. By the first birthday, their bodies have developed sufficiently to accommodate crawling, probably walking, and self-feeding. Although attempts at feeding are still erratic, developing children take great pride in doing more things independently. As children drink from a cup more frequently, fewer bottle feedings and/or breastfeedings are necessary. The added mobility of walking should naturally lead to gradual weaning from the bottle or breast.[2]

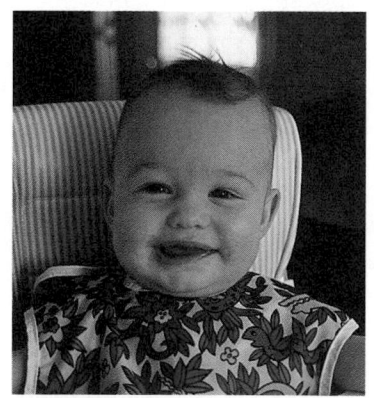

Early self-feeding attempts should be encouraged, even though they're messy.

Introducing Solid Foods

The time to introduce solid foods into an infant's diet hinges on a few important factors[9]:

Nutritional need—As noted, iron stores are exhausted by about 6 months of age. Either solid foods or iron supplements are then needed to supply iron if the child is breastfed or fed a formula not supplemented with iron. Iron, however, is not the only nutrient missing from human milk and unfortified infant formulas. Vitamin D and fluoride may also deserve attention. Still, before 4 to 6 months, it's unnecessary to add solid foods for any nutrients other than iron.

Physiological capabilities—Infants cannot readily digest starch before 3 months. As they age, their digestive capacilities increase. Kidney function likewise is quite limited until about 4 to 6 weeks of age. Until then, waste products from high amounts of dietary protein or minerals are difficult to excrete.

Physical ability—Three markers indicate that a child is ready for solid foods: (1) the disappearance of the extrusion reflex (thrusting the tongue forward and pushing food out), (2) head and neck control, and (3) the ability to sit up with support. These usually occur around 4 to 6 months of age, but they vary with each infant.

Preventing allergies—An infant's intestinal tract can readily absorb whole proteins from birth until 4 to 5 months of age. Thus early exposure to many types of proteins—particularly proteins in cow's milk and egg whites—may predispose a child to future allergies and other health problems, because some types of these proteins may be absorbed intact. For this reason, it's best to minimize the number of different types of proteins in a child's diet, especially during the first 3 months.[2]

With these considerations in mind—nutritional need, physiological and physical readiness, and allergy prevention—the American Academy of Pediatrics recommends that solid foods not be introduced until about 6 months of age (see Table 15-2). In general, a child starting solid foods should weigh at least 13 pounds (6 kilograms) and should be drinking more than 32 ounces (1 liter) of formula daily or breastfeeding more than 8 to 10 times within 24 hours. This description generally applies to 6-month-old infants and to some 4-month-old infants.

Before 4 to 6 months, infants are not physically mature enough to consume much solid food. Attempts to push down solid foods have sometimes led to force-feeding with a feeder (a giant syringe) or mixing infant cereal with milk and putting it in a bottle. Even if these are traditional alternatives in your family, there is no reason to carry on these practices. The inconvenience alone should make one consider whether all the effort is worth it. This practice is unnecessary nutritionally, tedious, and possibly dangerous for the infant because it increases the risk of allergies and choking or inhaling food when crying. Even so, many children are already eating solids by 2 months of age.[9] Only occasionally does a rapidly growing infant—one who consumes more than 32 ounces (1 liter) of formula daily—need solid foods at 4 months to meet high energy needs.

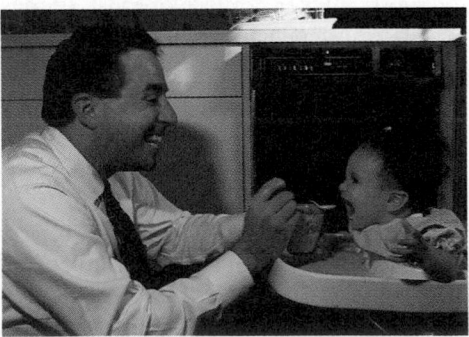

By 6 months of age, a baby is ready for more than just infant formula or human milk.

A common reason offered for introducing solid foods early—before 4 to 6 months of age—is the belief that it helps the infant sleep through the night. However, many studies show that sleeping through the night is a developmental milestone for the infant. It has nothing to do with how much food the infant eats. Infants naturally begin sleeping through the night between the ages of 1 and 3 months. Girls reach this stage before boys. Filling them with cereal won't influence that process.

Which Solid Foods Should Be Fed First?

Before 6 months of age the first solid foods should be iron-fortified cereals. A good idea is to offer foods after some breastfeeding or formula-feeding, when the edge has been taken off the infant's hunger. This practice aids in early spoon-feeding. Rice cereal is the best cereal to begin with because it's least likely to cause allergies. After the age of 6 months the first food is not such an important issue. Some pediatricians may recommend lean ground (strained) meats for more absorbable forms of iron. Although yogurt and cottage cheese are also well tolerated and their consistencies make them good candidates for early foods, they are not good sources of iron.

Typical solid food progression starting at 6 months*	
Week 1	rice cereal
Week 2	add strained carrots
Week 3	add applesauce
Week 4	add oat cereal
Week 5	add cooked egg yolk
Week 6	add strained chicken
Week 7	add strained peas
Week 8	add plums

*If signs of allergy or intolerance develop, substitute another similar food item.

It's best to start with teaspoon amounts of a single food item, such as rice cereal, and increase the serving size gradually. Once the new food has been fed for about a week without ill effects, another food can be added to the infant's diet. At first this can be another type of cereal or perhaps a cooked and strained (blended) vegetable, meat, fruit, or egg yolk. Each feeding step builds on the last.

Waiting about 7 days between new foods is important, because it can take that long for evidence of an allergy or intolerance to develop. Symptoms to look for are diarrhea, vomiting, a rash, or wheezing. If one or more of these symptoms appear, the suspected problem food should be avoided for several weeks and then reintroduced in a small quantity. If the problem continues, a doctor should be consulted.[8]

It's important not to introduce mixed foods until each component of the mixed food has been given separately. Otherwise, if an allergy or intolerance develops, it will be difficult to identify the offending food. Note that many babies outgrow food sensitivities in childhood.

Some foods that commonly cause an allergic response in infants are egg whites, chocolate, nuts, and cow's milk.[8] It's best not to introduce these foods early in infancy. The American Academy of Pediatrics discourages the use of cow's milk during the first year of life.

A variety of strained foods is available for infant feeding. Investigate these and other foods intended for infants the next time you're in a supermarket (Figure 15-5). Single-food items are more desirable than mixed dinners and desserts, which are less nutrient-dense. Most brands have no added salt, but some fruit desserts contain a lot of added sugar.

As an alternative, plain foods from the table—vegetables, fruits, and meats (no seasoning added)—can be ground up in an inexpensive plastic baby food grinder/mill. Another option is to pureé a larger amount of food in a blender, freeze it in ice-cube portions, store in plastic bags, and defrost and warm as needed. Careful attention to cleanliness is necessary. Infant foods made at home should be ground before seasonings are added to please the rest of the family. The infant doesn't notice the difference if salt, sugar, or spices are omitted. It's best to introduce infants to a variety of foods, so that by the end of the first year the infant is consuming many foods—milk, meats, fruits, vegetables, and grains.

As early as possible, by about 8 months or so, juices and formulas should be offered in a cup. A heavy cup with a wide, flat bottom aids success. Drinking from a cup helps prevent nursing bottle syndrome (Figure 15-6). As an infant plays with a bottle, the carbohydrate-rich fluid bathes the teeth, providing an ideal growth medium for bacteria. Bacteria on the teeth then make acids that dissolve tooth

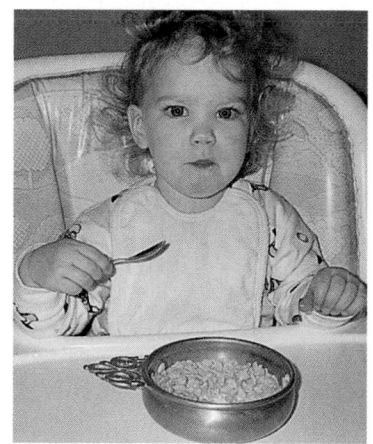

Childhood is the ideal time to begin to enjoy healthy foods.

RICE
CEREAL FOR BABY

Nutrition Facts
Serving Size 1/4 cup (15g)
Servings Per Container About 15

Amount Per Serving

Calories 60

Total Fat	0.5mg
Sodium	0mg
Potassium	20mg
Total Carbohydrate	12g
Fiber	0g
Sugars	0g
Protein	1g

% Daily Value	Infants 0-1	Children 1-4
Protein	4%	4%
Vitamin A	0%	0%
Vitamin C	0%	0%
Calcium	15%	10%
Iron	45%	60%
Thiamin	45%	30%
Riboflavin	45%	30%
Niacin	25%	20%
Phosphorus	10%	6%

INGREDIENTS: RICE FLOUR, SOY OIL-LECITHIN, TRI- AND DICALCIUM PHOSPHATE, ELECTROLYTIC IRON, NIACINAMIDE, RIBOFLAVIN (VITAMIN B-2), THIAMIN (VITAMIN B-1).

Serving size

Serving sizes for infant foods are based on the average amount eaten at one time by a child under 2 years.

Total fat

Shows the amount of total fat in a serving of the food. Unlike labels on adult foods, labels on infant foods do not list calories from fat, saturated fat, or cholesterol. Since infants and toddlers under 2 years need fat, the labels do not include details on fat content. Parents should not attempt to limit their infant's fat intake.

Daily Values

Food labels for infants and children under 4 years list the Daily Value percentages for protein, vitamins, and minerals. Unlike labels on adult foods, Daily Values for fat, cholesterol, sodium, potassium, carbohydrate, and fiber are not listed because these values have not been set for children under 4 years.

Figure 15-5

The labels on infant foods, like those on adult foods, contain a Nutrition Facts panel. However, the information provided on infant food labels differs from that on adult food labels, especially with respect to saturated fat and cholesterol intake (see Figure 2-7 for a comparison).

enamel. Infants should never be put to bed with a bottle or placed in an infant seat with a bottle propped up. When children are allowed to do this, fluid (even milk) pools around the teeth, increasing the likelihood of dental caries. Again, infants need careful attention when being fed. Propping bottles does not constitute careful attention.

Getting a baby out of the bedtime-bottle habit is difficult. Determined caregivers can either wince through a few nights of their baby's crying or slowly wean the baby away from the bottle with either a pacifier or water (for a week or so).

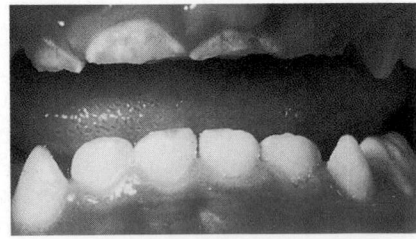

Figure 15-6 *Nursing bottle syndrome. An extreme example of tooth decay caused by nursing-bottle syndrome. This child was probably often put to bed with a bottle. The upper teeth have decayed almost all the way to the gum line.*

In the first attempts to introduce solid foods, just getting the food into the infant's mouth proves to be a challenge. The caregiver must proceed slowly. Initially, table foods supplement—rather than replace—formula or human milk. These infants control the situation by signaling when they are hungry and when they have had enough to eat. Self-feeding skills require coordination and can develop only if the infant is allowed to practice and experiment. By 9 to 10 months the infant's desire to explore, experience, and play with food can also hinder feeding. Caregivers need to relax and take this phase of infant development in stride. Sloppy, friendly mealtimes actually make for good memories.

To ease efforts in feeding solid foods, consider the following tips:

- Use a baby-sized spoon; a small spoon with a long handle is best.
- Hold the infant comfortably on the lap, as for breastfeeding or bottle-feeding, but a little more upright to ease swallowing. When in this position, the infant expects food.
- Put a small dab of food on the spoon tip and gently place it on the infant's tongue.
- Convey a calm and casual approach to the infant, who needs time to get used to food.
- Expect the infant to take only two or three bites of the first meals. Anything more than that is real success.

By the end of the first year, finger-feeding becomes more efficient, drinking from a cup improves, and chewing is easier as more teeth erupt. Still, experimentation and unpredictability are to be expected (Figure 15-7).

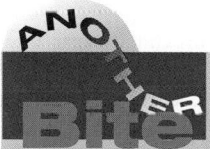

A SUMMARY OF INFANT FEEDING RECOMMENDATIONS:

Breastfed Infants
- *Breastfeed for 6 months or longer if possible. Then introduce infant formula if and when breastfeeding declines or ceases.*
- *Add iron-fortified cereal at about 6 months of age.*
- *Investigate the need for fluoride, iron, and vitamin D supplements.*
- *Provide a variety of basic, soft foods after 6 months of age, advancing to a varied diet (Table 15-3).*

Formula-Fed Infants
- *Use infant formula for the first year of life, preferably an iron-fortified type.*
- *Add iron-fortified cereal at about 6 months of age.*
- *Investigate the need for a fluoride supplement if the water supply is not fluoridated.*
- *Provide a variety of basic, soft foods after 6 months, advancing to a varied diet (Table 15-3).*

MARVIN

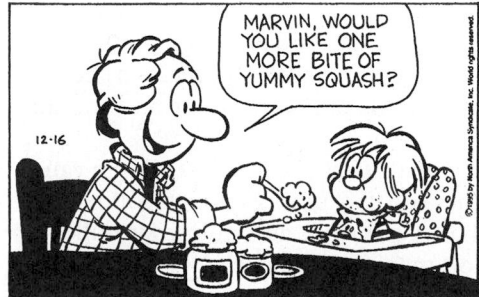
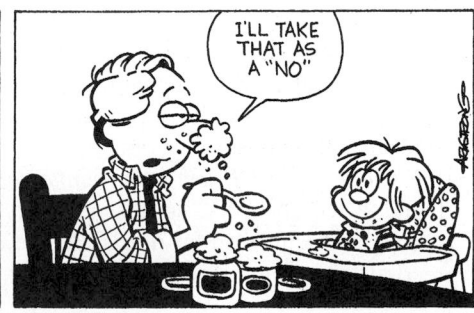

Figure 15-7
Marvin.

TABLE 15-3

Sample Daily Menu for a 1-Year-Old Child*

BREAKFAST

1-2 tbsp applesauce
¼ cup Cheerios
½ cup whole milk

SNACK

½ hard-cooked egg
½ slice wheat toast with ½ tsp margarine
½ cup orange juice

LUNCH

1 oz roasted chicken, minced
1-2 tbsp rice with ½ tsp margarine
1-2 tbsp cooked peas
½ cup whole milk

SNACK

½ ounce cheese
4 wheat crackers
½ cup whole milk

DINNER

1 ounce hamburger (crumbled)
1-2 tbsp mashed potatoes with ½ tsp margarine
1-2 tbsp cooked carrots (cut in strips, NOT coins)
½ cup whole milk

SNACK

½ banana
2 oatmeal cookies (no raisins)
½ cup whole milk

Nutritional analysis

Total energy (kcal)	1100
% energy from:	
Carbohydrate	40%
Protein	19%
Fat	41%

*This diet plan is just a start. A 1-year-old may need more or less food. In those cases, serving sizes should be adjusted. The milk can be fed by cup; some can be put into a bottle if the child has not been fully weaned from the bottle. The juice should be fed in a cup.

What Not to Feed an Infant

Following are several foods and practices to avoid when feeding an infant:

- *Honey and corn syrup*—These products may contain spores of *Clostridium botulinum*. The spores can eventually develop into bacteria in the stomach and lead to a food-borne illness known as *botulism*. This can be fatal in children under 1 year old (see Chapter 17).
- *Very salty and very sweet foods*—Infants don't need a lot of sugar or salt added to their foods. They enjoy bland foods much more than do adults.
- *Excessive infant formula or human milk*—After 6 to 8 months, solids foods should play a greater role in satisfying an infant's increasing appetite. The main reason to switch is that solid foods contain considerably more iron than do human milk, cow's milk, and low-iron formulas. About 24 to 32 ounces (³/₄ to 1 liter) of human milk or formula daily is ideal after 6 months, with food supplying the rest of the infant's energy needs.
- *Foods that tend to cause choking*—These foods include hot dogs (unless finely cut into sticks, not coin shapes), candy, whole nuts, grapes, coarsely cut meats, raw carrots, and popcorn. Most choking deaths are caused by hot dogs, grapes, chunks of meat, carrots, peanuts, popcorn, or peanut butter. Caregivers should not allow younger children to gobble snack foods during playtime and should supervise all meals.
- *Cow's milk, especially low-fat or nonfat cow's milk*—Beyond 2 years, children can drink 1% or 2% milk, because by then they are consuming enough solid foods to supply energy and fat needs. Before that age, the amount of low-fat milk needed for energy needs would supply too many minerals. That could over-

whelm the kidneys' ability to excrete the excess. The lower fat intake might also harm nervous system development. The American Academy of Pediatrics strongly urges parents not to give children under age 1 cow's milk, and children under age 2 low-fat or nonfat milk.

- *Feeding excessive amounts of apple or pear juice*—The fructose and sorbitol (a form of carbohydrate) contained in these juices can lead to diarrhea, because they are slowly absorbed. Diluting juices with an equal part of water is a good idea, but it should be begun early, before the infant becomes accustomed to full-strength juices. Infants can usually safely consume 4 to 8 ounces of juice in the course of a day, with no more than 2 to 4 ounces given at a time.

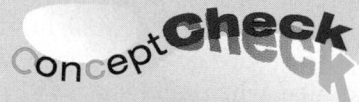

Infant formulas generally contain lactose or sucrose, heat-treated proteins from cow's milk, and vegetable oil. Formulas may or may not be fortified with iron. Sanitation is very important in preparing and storing formula. Solid foods should not be added to an infant's diet until the child is both ready for and needs solid food, usually at about 4 to 6 months of age. The first solid food can be iron-fortified infant cereals, with very gradual additions of other foods—one at a time each week. Some foods to avoid giving infants in the first year are honey, cow's milk (particularly low-fat and nonfat milk), very salty or sweet foods, and foods that may cause the child to choke.

Health Problems Related to Infant Nutrition

Parents, other caregivers, and clinicians should be alert for a variety of potential health problems related to infant nutrition so corrective action can be taken quickly. In some cases such problems stem from inappropriate feeding practices or inadequate nutrient intakes, including the following[11, 25]:

- Diet providing insufficient iron
- Absence from the diet of an entire food group of the Food Guide Pyramid as solid foods are introduced and become the main source of nutrients
- Drinking raw (unpasteurized) milk, which may be contaminated with bacteria or viruses
- Drinking goat's milk, which is low in folate; if used, it must be pasteurized and given in conjunction with a folate supplement
- Failure to begin drinking from a cup by 1 year of age
- Continuing to feed from a bottle past 18 months of age
- Intake of supplemental vitamins or minerals above 150% of the appropriate RDA
- Drinking much fruit juice before 6 months of age as a substitute for infant formula or human milk

Now let's look more closely at four common infant health problems that cause concern for caregivers. Parents and other caregivers usually need to consult with a physician in dealing with these conditions.

Colic

The first time an otherwise healthy, well-fed infant has a lengthy, unexplained crying spell, most parents panic. Repeated crying episodes lasting 3 or more hours that don't respond to typical remedies—such as feeding, holding, or diaper changes—are

Colic

Sharp abdominal pain that generally occurs in otherwise healthy infants and is associated with periodic inconsolable crying spells.

characteristic of infants who develop **colic.** Colic affects about 10% to 40% of all infants, so it is neither uncommon nor abnormal. Colicky infants typically cry during the late afternoon and early evening, and their nighttime sleeping is almost always disturbed by crying spells. The only good news is that colic usually goes away after a few months.[3]

Colic generally occurs in the absence of any physical problem in the infant. It tends to be most common in "temperamental" infants—those who are more sensitive, more irritable, more intense, less adaptable, and less soothable than average for their age. In addition, a lack of harmonious interaction between parents and the infant may contribute to the problem. Some researchers have speculated that colic may be caused by immaturity of the central nervous system mechanisms.

Parents state that colicky infants frequently pass gas rectally, clench their fists, draw up their legs, cry in the late afternoon and evening, hold the body straight, and want to be held. Parents can do several things to help reduce excessive crying. For instance, many infants tend to become quiet and alert when held snugly to the shoulder. Others can be settled down with movement, such as walking or rocking in an infant seat. For others, rhythmic sounds and pacifiers can be of some help.

Breastfeeding of colicky infants should continue. A temporary decrease or cessation in consumption of dairy products, chocolate, and vegetables such as broccoli and onions by a breastfeeding mother may help reduce colic in her infant.[16] Formula-fed infants with severe colic are sometimes helped by changing from a standard formula to a soy-based or predigested protein formula (see Table 15-1). In addition, physicians may prescribe certain medications to calm colicky infants and reduce gas build-up.

Caring for an inconsolable, colicky infant is stressful and frustrating for parents. Most parents benefit from the counsel and support of other adults during this trying period, which may last for several months. Sharing with others who have been through similar experiences can help parents improve their tolerance of stress and ability to cope, and increase confidence in their parenting abilities. Furthermore, to optimize their ability to be sensitive and responsive to their infant, parents need to be well rested and set aside some time for themselves.[3]

Diarrhea

Diarrhea in infants, characterized by numerous loose stools in a day, results from various causes, including bacterial and viral infections. In the United States, about 500 infants die each year of simple dehydration resulting from diarrhea, and about 210,000 are hospitalized for this reason. For prevention of dehydration, infants with diarrhea should be given plenty of fluids, as advised by a physician.[21] Specialized electrolyte-replacement fluids, such as Pedialyte, may be recommended. These contain glucose, sodium, potassium, chloride, and water.[31]

Once diarrhea subsides, a bottle-fed infant may be switched to a soy-based, lactose-free formula for a few days. This allows time for the intestine to produce sufficient lactase enzyme to digest the large amount of lactose typically found in formulas. A breastfed infant should continue at the breast for the duration of the diarrhea. If solid foods are consumed, the physician may also prescribe a BRAT diet (bananas, rice, applesauce, toast) for short-term use.

Milk Allergy

Cow's milk contains more than 25 proteins that can cause allergic reactions in infants.[13] Although some of these proteins are inactivated by heating (scalding) milk, others are very heat stable. A "true" milk allergy develops in about 1% to 4% of formula-fed infants. Such infants may experience vomiting, diarrhea, blood in the stool, constipation, and other symptoms. If milk allergy is suspected, a formula-fed infant can be switched to a soy-based formula. In 20% to 50% of cases, however, use of soy formula provides only temporary relief because the soy protein eventually triggers an allergic reaction in some infants. In such cases a predigested-protein formula will be necessary[15] (see Table 15-1). If the child is breastfeeding, the mother may experiment with eliminating cow's milk from her diet.

Iron-Deficiency Anemia

Iron-deficiency anemia typically occurs in older infants who consume few solid foods and whose diets are dominated by cow's milk, which contains little iron. Iron stores are then quickly depleted by the daily need to synthesize new red blood cells. The best way to prevent iron-deficiency anemia is to start an infant on iron-fortified cereals and meats at about 6 months and limit formula to 16 to 25 ounces (500 to 750 milliliters) daily at this time. Not only is cow's milk low in iron, but it can also cause intestinal bleeding in young infants. As mentioned earlier, cow's milk is not recommended during the first year of life; it's especially important that infants not consume cow's milk during the first 3 months. If anemia does develop, medicinal iron is used under a physician's guidance.[24]

Feeding Preterm Infants

Preterm infants are fed either a specially designed formula or human milk. As noted in Chapter 14, nutrients may be added to human milk to increase its protein, mineral, and energy content. Preterm infants must be fed immediately because their bodies store little fat or carbohydrate. The body composition of a full-term infant includes about 12% fat, whereas the composition of a very preterm infant can include as little as 2% fat.[2]

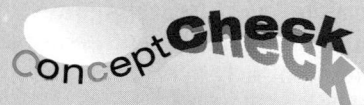

Colic is commonly associated with inconsolable crying. Switching to an infant formula made with soy or predigested proteins may reduce colic. It may also be helpful for breastfeeding mothers to decrease or avoid intake of dairy products, chocolate, and certain vegetables, under a physician's guidance. Diarrhea requires additional fluids to prevent dehydration. Infants allergic to proteins in standard cow's milk formula can be switched to an infant formula containing soy protein or predigested protein. Introducing iron-containing solid foods at an appropriate time and avoiding use of cow's milk during the first year can generally prevent iron-deficiency anemia in infants.

Childhood

The rapid growth rate that characterizes infancy tapers off quickly during the subsequent few years. The average annual weight gain is only 4.5 to 6.6 pounds (2 to 3 kilograms), and the average annual height gain is only 3 to 4 inches (7.5 to 10 centimeters) between the ages of 2 and 5 (see Figure 15-1). As a toddler's growth rate tapers off, eating behavior changes. For example, the decreased growth rate leads to a decreased appetite compared with infants.[25]

Because of the reduced appetite of preschool children, planning a diet that meets their nutrient needs poses a challenge to caregivers. Choosing nutrient-dense foods is particularly important with children who eat relatively little. This is a good time to emphasize whole grains, fruits, and vegetables without increasing fat intake.[12] A whole-grain breakfast cereal with limited fat and sugar is an excellent choice. There is no need to decrease fat intake severely, but fatty food choices should not overwhelm more nutritious ones.

The preschool years are the best time for a child to start a healthful pattern of living and eating, focusing on regular physical activity and nutritious foods. Parents and other caregivers are role models: if they eat a variety of foods, the children will eat a variety of foods. One possible policy is the one-bite rule: within reason, children should take at least one bite or taste of the foods presented to them. For snacks, parents should select several possibilities and allow children to choose one; responsibility for food choice ideally should start early.[26]

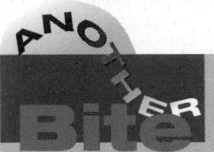

Surprisingly, children generally eat what they are offered. If given whole-grain breakfast cereals, whole-wheat bread, vegetables, salad, and fresh fruits regularly, young children accept most of these foods and eat them. Only a lack of imagination limits—and possibly deprives—a child's diet. If caregivers don't like a particular food, they should still offer it to the child.

In the early school years, regular meals—especially breakfast—become increasingly important. Some research suggests that eating a healthful breakfast helps children learn better in the subsequent hours they spend in school. The energy and nutrients consumed can stimulate attention, energy level, and motivation, yielding better test scores.[17] Sports performance also can be improved. This makes sense, because breakfast can replenish depleted carbohydrate stores in the liver. Still, some researchers dispute the importance of breakfast as it relates to learning. They claim that it's the more motivated students who eat breakfast, not that eating breakfast motivates students. Still, it's a good idea to give breakfast to all students, especially to otherwise sluggish ones, because it can give a nutrient-rich start to the day's intake.

Breakfasts can be imaginative. Instead of conventional breakfast foods, caregivers can offer choices like pizza, spaghetti, soups, yogurt with trail mix on top, chili, sandwiches, or shish kabob.

How to Help a Child Choose Nutritious Foods

One way adults can encourage young children to eat nutritious, well-balanced meals is to serve new foods and repeat exposure to them. If a child observes adults and older children eating and enjoying a food, there's a good chance he or she will eventually accept it. The dinner hour is a good time for children to experience new foods and to develop their own likes and dislikes. Preschool children especially tend to be wary of new foods. One reason is that their taste buds are more sensitive than those of adults. In addition, they have a general distrust of unfamiliar foods. If adults can be patient and persevere, children will build good food habits. Above all, the dinner table should not become a battleground, and using one food as a bribe to eat another—a piece of pie for peas—is strongly discouraged.

Perseverance with children is critical, because it takes effort and commitment to guide them into liking a variety of foods. Be ready for some surprises. Note also that if left to their own devices, preschool children would find a few foods they like and eat them every day. But by constantly being introduced to new foods, children at this age can expand their nutritional choices, develop an experimental approach, and learn to appreciate a variety of foods. It may take 10 to 15 exposures, but eventually children will accept most foods. A positive outlook by the caregivers helps a lot.

Critical Thinking

Tim refuses to eat breakfast before school. He doesn't like cereal, toast, or any of the other usual breakfast foods. What can Tim's parents do to ensure that he eats nutritious foods before leaving for school?

TABLE 15-4

Observed Emotional Traits, Eating Behavior, and Food-Related Skills of Preschoolers

Age (years)	Emotional traits	Eating behavior	Food-related skills
1-2	• Fears new things • Sharing is difficult • Requires constant supervision • Enjoys helping but can't be left alone • Curious • Often defiant • Eager for attention	• "Finicky" eater • Holds food in mouth without swallowing • May insist on eating the same food at meal after meal (called a food jag)	• Uses spoon with some skill (especially if hungry) • Can begin to tear, break, snap, and dip foods • Has good control of cup—lifts, drinks, sets it down, holds with one hand • Helps self-feed
3	• The "me too" age—wants to be included in everything • Responds well to options rather than demands • Sharing is still difficult • Somewhat rigid about the "right" way to do things	• Eats most foods, except for certain vegetables • Dawdles over food when not hungry • Comments on how foods are served	• Uses spoon in semi-adult fashion; may spear with fork • Medium hand muscle development • Feeds self independently, especially if hungry • Can pour milk and juice and serve individual portions from a serving dish if given instructions
4	• Shares well • Needs adult approval and attention—shows off • Understands; needs limits • Follows rules most of the time • Still rigid about the "right" way to do things	• Eating and talking get in the way—prefers to talk • Strong food likes and dislikes • Refuses to eat, to the point of tears	• Uses all eating utensils • Small-finger muscle development • Can wipe, wash, set table, and pour premeasured ingredients • Can peel, spread, cut, roll, mash foods; cracks eggs
5	• Helpful and cooperative with family chores and routines • Still somewhat rigid about the "right" way to do things • Very attached to mother, home, and family	• Likes familiar foods; prefers most vegetables raw • Latches on to food dislikes of family members and declares these as own	• Fine coordination in fingers and hands • Makes simple breakfast and lunch • Can measure, cut, grind, and grate

Modified from Sigman-Grant M: *Nutrition Today*, p 13, July/Aug 1992.

Research shows that children like certain foods—especially those with crisp textures and mild flavors—and familiar foods. Young children are especially sensitive to hot-temperature foods and tend to reject them.

Parents and other caregivers play a central role in teaching by example. Children more readily learn good table manners alongside others who practice them. The harmony that comes from working at being polite creates a positive environment for learning good nutrition habits. Preschoolers eventually develop skill with spoons and forks and can even use dull knives (Table 15-4). However, it's still a good idea to serve some finger foods. A goal should be to make mealtime a happy, social time. Share enjoyment of healthful foods. A regular family meal daily—whether breakfast, lunch, or dinner—is an appropriate setting for children to learn about healthful eating and to build good eating habits.[26]

Childhood Feeding Problems

Tensions between parents, or between parents and children, often contribute to eating problems. Getting to the root of family problems and creating a more harmonious family atmosphere are important steps toward resolving many childhood feeding problems. In addition, parents must often be educated as to what to expect of a preschool child and what food-related goals to set (see Table 15-4). Let's consider some typical complaints and concerns of parents, the causes of the problems, and suggestions for correcting them.

Two-year-olds commonly prefer particular foods, but parents needn't worry about this. A child may switch from one specific food focus (often called a *jag*) to another with equal intensity. If the caregiver continues to offer choices, the child will soon begin to eat a wider variety of foods again, and the specific food focus will disappear as suddenly as it appeared.

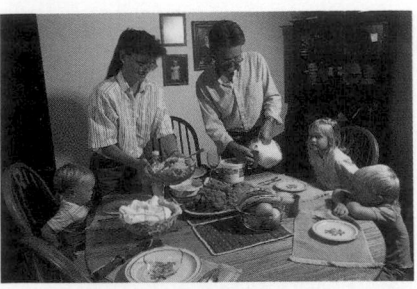

Meals should be a happy, sociable time for sharing enjoyment of healthful foods.

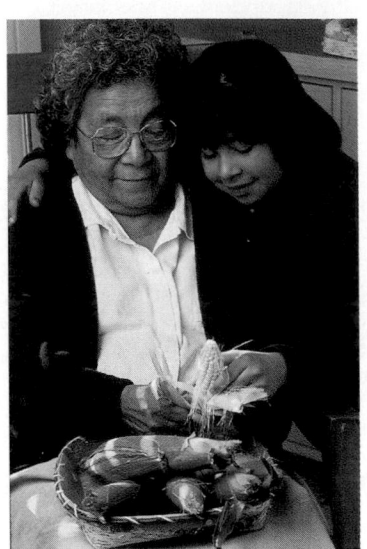

Children master their eating environments when adults provide opportunities to learn.

"My child won't eat as much or as regularly as he did as an infant." This behavior is typical of preschoolers, because their growth rate slows after infancy and thus they don't need as much food. Parents often need reminding that a 3-year-old can't be expected to eat as voraciously as an infant, or to eat adult-size portions. Table 15-5 shows a general food plan, based on the Food Guide Pyramid, that is appropriate for preschool and school-age children. Note that until about 5 years of age, serving sizes in the vegetable group, fruit group, and meat, poultry, fish, dry beans, eggs, and nuts group can be estimated as 1 tablespoon per year of life. Normal-weight children have a built-in feeding mechanism that adjusts hunger to regulate food intake at each stage of growth. If a child is developing and growing normally and the caregiver is providing a variety of healthful foods, all can be confident the child isn't starving. Caregivers should avoid nagging, forcing, and bribing.

Appetite also varies with activity level and general health. An initial symptom of a sick child is poor appetite. Picky eating is also just another indication of a child's striving toward independence and his or her strong desire to establish routines. Asserting himself or herself about food preferences is a relatively easy way for the child to do this.

Parents should also be reminded that food likes and dislikes change rapidly in childhood and are influenced by food temperature, appearance, texture, and taste. Sometimes children object to having foods mixed, as in stews and casseroles, even if they normally like the ingredients separately.

Battling to get a child to eat more is strongly discouraged. Parents should present nutritious food choices, eat some themselves, and let the child decide the serving size. It all boils down to a division of responsibility in feeding. The parents are responsible for what their child is offered to eat and for establishing a pleasant eat-

---

TABLE 15-5

Food Plan for Preschool and School-Age Children Based on the Food Guide Pyramid

Food group	No. of servings	APPROXIMATE SERVING SIZE*			
		Age 1-2	Age 3-4	Age 5-6	Age 7-12
Milk, yogurt, and cheese:	3	½-¾ cup or 1 ounce	¾ cup or 1½ ounces	1 cup or 2 ounces	1 cup or 2 ounces
Meat, poultry, fish, dry beans, eggs, and nuts:	2 or more	1 ounce or 1-2 tbsp	1½ ounce or 3-4 tbsp	1½ ounce or ½ cup	2 ounces or ½ cup
Vegetables:	3 or more	1-2 tbsp	3-4 tbsp	½ cup	½ cup
Fruit:	2 or more	1-2 tbsp or ½ cup juice	3-4 tbsp or ½ cup juice	½ cup or ½ cup juice	½ cup or ½ cup juice
Bread, cereal, rice, and pasta:	6 or more	½ slice or ½ cup	1 slice or ½ cup	1 slice or ¾ cup	1 slice or ¾ cup

Adapted from Food and Nutrition Service, US Department of Agriculture: *Meal pattern requirements and offer versus serve manual*, FNS-265, 1990.
*Use as a starting point. Increase serving size as energy yields dictate, but maintain variety in the diet by making sure all food groups are still appropriately represented.

ing environment. The child is responsible for deciding how much or even whether to eat.[26] In addition, parents should recognize that this is an important age for children to explore the world around them. Even good eaters are sometimes more interested in exploring than eating. There's room for occasional indulgences, a skipped meal or two, or once-in-a-while "less-than-ideal" choices. It's eating and lifestyle habits over the course of a month and lifetime that matter. Children master their eating when adults provide opportunities to learn, give support for exploration, and limit inappropriate behavior.

"My child is always snacking, yet she never finishes her meal." Children have small stomachs. Offering them six or so small meals succeeds better than limiting them to three meals each day. Sticking to three meals a day offers no special nutritional advantages; it's just a social custom. Snacking is fine, as long as good dental habits are practiced. When we eat isn't nearly so important as what we eat. If nutritious snacks are readily available, these would be good to offer at midmorning or midafternoon when the child becomes hungry (Table 15-6). Fruits and vegetables (fresh, frozen, or juice) and whole-grain breads and crackers are good snack choices. Working parents should make sure their children are provided with nutritional snacks to tide them over until dinnertime.

TABLE 15-6

Ideas for Nutritious Snacks and Beverages

Snack	Serving suggestion	Snack	Serving suggestion	Snack	Serving suggestion
Fresh raw vegetables	Serve with a dip of cottage cheese or yogurt blended with dried buttermilk dressing	Flour tortillas	Spread with refried beans or canned chili, sprinkle with grated cheese and broil; top with chili sauce	Parfait	Make with yogurt, fruit, and granola
Celery	Spread with peanut butter and sprinkle on raisins, shredded carrots, or finely chopped nuts	Ready-to-eat cereals	Use brands low in sugar and containing fiber; serve with raisins	Gelatin	Add fruit or vegetable juice, vegetables, fruits, or cottage cheese
		Pita bread	Place sliced meat, cheese, lettuce, and tomato in open pocket	Frozen fruit cubes	Freeze puréed applesauce or fruit juice into cubes
Bananas	Dip in sweetened yogurt or spread with peanut butter and roll in coconut, chopped nuts, or granola	English muffins or pita bread	Top with spaghetti sauce, grated cheese, and meats; broil or bake and cut in fourths	Fruit fizz	Add club soda to juice instead of serving soft drinks
Sliced apples or crackers	Serve with a dip of peanut butter, honey, nuts, raisins, and coconut	Potato skins	Sprinkle with shredded cheese, broil, and top with yogurt and bacon bits	Fruit shake	Blend milk with fresh fruit (bananas, berries, or a peach) and a dash of cinnamon or nutmeg
Bagels	Spread with cream cheese or peanut butter and top with chopped bananas, crushed pineapple, or shredded carrots	Canned chili	Heat and top with onions, lettuce, and tomato; use as dip for Italian or French bread, biscuits, or cornbread	Yogurt frost	Combine fruit juice and yogurt; add fresh fruit if desired
				Hot chocolate	Make hot chocolate or cocoa with milk chocolate and a dash of cinnamon
		Kabobs	Make with any combination of fruit, vegetables, and sliced or cubed cooked meat (remove toothpicks before serving)	Seeds	Shelled sunflower seeds
Quick bread or muffins	Make with carrots, zucchini, pumpkin, bananas, nuts, dates, raisins, lemons, squash, or berries			Fish	Tunafish on crackers
		Popcorn	Serve plain or make 3 quarts and sprinkle with ¼ cup grated cheese and ½ tsp garlic or onion salt	Canned soup	Cup of vegetable or minestrone; nice on a cold winter day

Modified from National Meat and Livestock Board: *A food guide for the first five years,* Chicago.

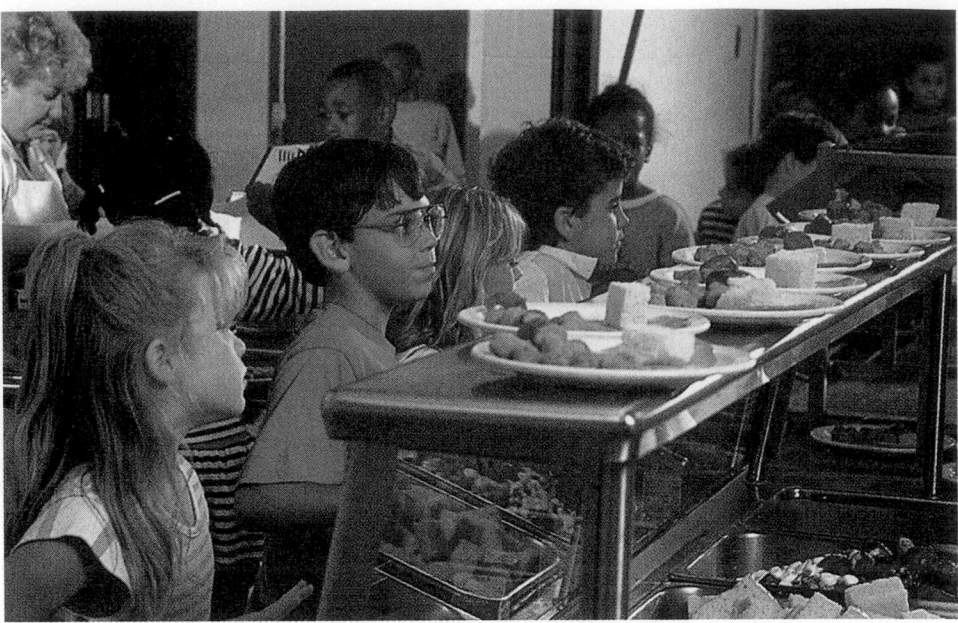

School lunch menus follow federal guidelines in the United States. What is eaten is up to the student.

When a child refuses to eat, it's best not to overreact. Doing so may give the child the idea that eating is a means of getting attention or manipulating a scene. Most children don't starve themselves to any point approaching physical harm. When children refuse to eat, have them sit at the table for a while, and if they still aren't interested in eating, remove the food and wait until the next scheduled meal or snack.

Dental Health Tips for Children
- Begin oral hygiene when an infant receives his or her first tooth.
- Seek early pediatric dental care.
- Drink fluoridated water.
- Use fluoridated toothpaste twice daily.
- Snack in moderation.
- Have your dentist apply tooth sealants if needed.

"My child never eats his vegetables." Everyone dislikes certain foods. Again, the one-bite policy can be encouraged, and guidelines can be set to discourage fussing over unfamiliar foods. Children eventually learn that they can eat some of a food they don't particularly like without first gagging, choking, and yelling, "Oh, gross!" It takes time for a child to become enthusiastic about a new food, but with continual exposure and a positive role model, chances are the child may even grow to like it.

Children cannot and should not be forced to eat. They need to develop independence and identities separate from their parents (Figure 15-8). In other words, children have to choose for themselves—a practice that should be encouraged. No one food is an essential part of a diet. Hunger is still the best means for getting a child to eat. It may be effective to feed children vegetables at the start of a meal, when they are hungriest. Offer new foods with familiar ones. A platter of raw or lightly cooked carrots, broccoli, green and red peppers, cabbage, and mushrooms eaten as a snack with friends can do a lot to remedy a vegetable problem. A 4- or 5-year-old child can safely eat raw vegetables without fear of choking. Recall that children often are more sensitive than adults to strong flavors and odors. Nutritious dips "sell" vegetables to many children. Using heroes as role models may work. Vegetables may acquire more appeal when children help prepare them.

Do Children Need a Vitamin/Mineral Supplement?

Major scientific groups, such as the American Dietetic Association and the American Society for Clinical Nutrition, believe that vitamin and mineral supplements are unnecesary for healthy children; it's better to emphasize good foods. However, a child

Calvin and Hobbes
by Bill Watterson

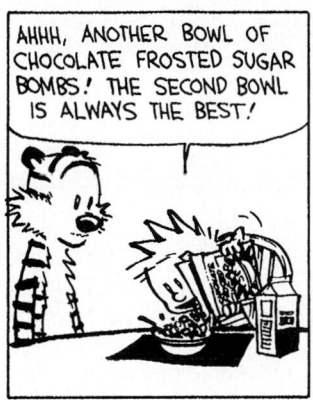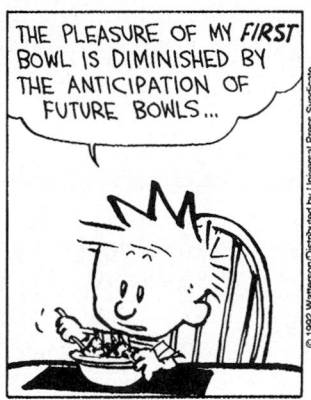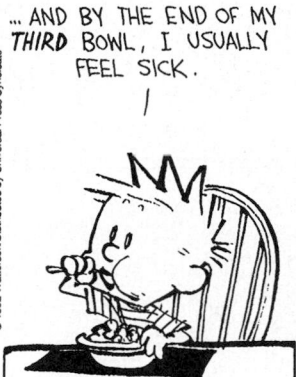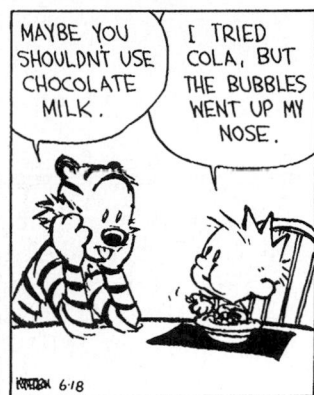

Figure 15-8 *Calvin and Hobbes.*

who is ill may need a nutrient supplement not exceeding 150% of Daily Values on the label, especially if the illness persists. Diets for children who eat totally vegetarian fare should focus especially on protein, vitamin B-12, iron, and zinc. Studies show that many parents offer children conservative amounts of nutrient supplements, so toxicity is unlikely. Still, giving supplements is often unnecessary, especially in light of today's typically highly fortified breakfast cereals, which children often eat.

If current childhood feeding practices are to become more healthful, they should gradually shift away from high-fat diets to diets containing more complex carbohydrates. The bottom half of the Food Guide Pyramid, with its emphasis on starches, fruits, and vegetables, leads to such a pattern.

Children are exposed to high-fat foods in quick-service restaurants. These foods are often both sweet and high in salt. Caregivers can teach and model healthful ways to eat at quick-service restaurants by ordering from the salad bar or ordering french fries only once in a while. Children aren't born with a preference for high-fat or extremely salty foods; they develop this preference through repeated exposure.

Many of us should consider a diet higher in carbohydrate and lower in fat. For children, the idea is not to force them to follow severely restricted diets, such as adults with weight or elevated blood cholesterol problems might follow. Instead children can simply limit the amount of high-fat, nutritionally empty foods they eat each day. Some easy diet changes to begin with are bagels instead of doughnuts, nonfat frozen yogurt instead of ice cream, low-fat milk instead of whole milk, fruit instead of crackers and cheese for snacks, and air-popped popcorn instead of chips.

Nutritional Problems in Childhood

The two most common nutritional problems in childhood are obesity, which is discussed in the second Nutrition Insight, and iron-deficiency anemia.

Iron-Deficiency Anemia

Childhood iron-deficiency anemia is most likely to appear in children between the ages of 6 and 24 months.[24] It can lead to decreases in both stamina and learning ability, because the oxygen supply to cells decreases. Another effect is lowered resistance to disease. Fortunately, childhood anemia is fairly uncommon here,

Chapter 5 noted that it's unlikely that use of sugar is the cause of hyperactivity or antisocial behavior in most children.

Obesity in the Growing Years

In the United States about 22% of school-age children place above the 85th percentile in weight for height and are considered overweight, and the number of cases is currently increasing.[18] In the short run, ridicule and embarrassment are the main consequences of such obesity. Significant health problems associated with obesity, such as heart disease, diabetes, and high blood pressure, usually don't appear until adulthood.[22] Unfortunately, about 40% of obese children (and about 80% of obese adolescents) become obese adults. Significant weight gain generally begins either between ages 5 and 7 or during the teenage years.[5] Childhood obesity should not be ignored, because the chances are great that an obese school-age child will become an obese adult. The sooner corrective measures are taken, the more likely they are to succeed.

Causes of Obesity in Children

Current research points to many potential causes of childhood obesity. Recall the nature versus nurture discussion in Chapter 10. Some infants are born with lower metabolic rates; they use energy more efficiently and in turn can more easily save energy intake for fat storage. Thus childhood obesity is linked to heredity. Obesity in children also has a correlation to sibling and maternal obesity.

Research shows a moderate relationship between obesity and the number of hours a child spends watching television and playing video games. The TV generation now glues itself to the tube for an average of 24 hours a week, including hours of advertisements for high-fat and sugar-laden foods; many children spend another 10 hours or so playing computer and video games. In addition, excessive snacking, overreliance on quick-service restaurants, little physical activity (especially in girls), parental neglect, lack of safe areas to play, latch-key conditions, and high-fat/high-energy food choices most likely contribute to childhood obesity. Fundamentally, obesity results from an imbalance between energy input and output. For many children, a low amount of physical activity, rather than excessive energy intake, may be the primary culprit leading to obesity.[18]

Treating the Obese Child

The initial approach in treating an obese child is to assess how much physical activity he or she engages in. If a child spends much free time in sedentary activities (such as watching television or playing video games), more physical activities should be encouraged. Two good ideas are getting the family together for a brisk walk after dinner and finding an after-school sport the child enjoys. An increase in physical activity won't just happen; parents need to plan for it.

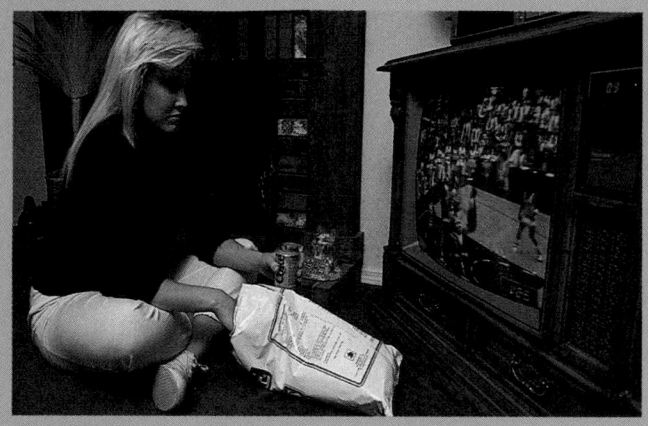

Snacking on foods with little nutrient value is common among teenagers, especially during inactivity..

Moderation in energy intake is important, especially limitation of high-fat and high-energy foods and sugar-laden carbonated beverages. The focus should be on more nutrient-dense foods.

Resorting to a weight-loss diet is usually necessary. In the short run, it's best to emphasize changing habits. Children have an advantage over adults in dealing with obesity; their bodies can use stored energy for growth. Thus if weight gain can be moderated, increases in height and resulting lean body tissue may reduce the percent of body weight accounted for as stored fat, yielding a more healthful weight-to-height ratio. This is one reason it's desirable to treat obesity in childhood. Further growth can contribute to success.

If a child will still be obese after attaining ultimate adult height, a weight-loss regimen may be necessary. This is especially appropriate after the adolescent growth spurt. Weight loss should be gradual, perhaps $\frac{1}{2}$ pound per week. If weight loss is necessary in younger children, the child should be watched closely to ensure that the rate of growth continues to be normal. The child's energy intake shouldn't be so low that gains in height diminish.

Behavior modification is a third important component of treating childhood obesity. One underlying environmental cause of obesity can be parents' attitudes and behaviors toward their child's eating. A heavy parental hand in overly restricting or controlling the child's food intake may lead to struggles around eating that actually interfere with a child's ability to eat sensibly. Obese children often need to find a new way to relate to foods, especially snack foods. An important family rule could be that children are allowed to eat only while sitting at the dining table or in the kitchen. This could stop endless hours of snacking in front of the television and make all family members more conscious of when they are eating. It also might be helpful to put portions of snack foods on plates rather than allow snacking to go on indefinitely, as often happens when children eat directly from a full box of crackers or cookies.

A child's self-esteem is extremely fragile. Obesity itself affects the child's psyche. Humiliation doesn't work; it only makes the child feel worse. Support, admiration, and encouragement of the child's efforts at weight control are more effective and should be emphasized.[25]

probably because of children's use of iron-fortified breakfast cereals. Also deserving of credit is the Special Supplemental Food Program for Women, Infants, and Children (WIC), sponsored by the federal government. This program emphasizes the importance of iron-fortified formulas and cereals and distributes them—along with nutrition education—to low-income parents of infants and preschool children considered to be at nutritional risk.

The best way to prevent iron-deficiency anemia in children is to regularly feed them foods that are adequate sources of iron. Iron-fortified breakfast cereals and a few ounces of lean meat are convenient means of getting more iron into a child's diet. The high proportion of heme iron in many animal foods allows the iron to be more readily absorbed than is iron from plant foods. Consuming a vitamin C source along with the less readily absorbed iron in plants and supplements will aid absorption.

Is Childhood the Time to Start a Diet Designed to Limit the Risk of Heart Disease?

Children in the United States currently derive about 33% of their energy from fat, with about 13% of energy from saturated fat.[20] Today two schools of thought exist with regard to fat intake of children in preschool and later school years. The National Cholesterol Education Program suggests that children 2 years and older consume no more than 30% of energy as fat, 10% of energy as saturated fat, and 300 milligrams of cholesterol. (Note that this is the same recommendation given to adults.) The American Academy of Pediatrics recommends that children eat a similar diet by about age 5 years but cautions against including less than 30% of energy as fat.[18] However, other researchers have recently proposed that fat simply be gradually reduced from about 40% of energy intake in infancy to the 30% figure by the time a child's linear growth ceases (at about age 16 to 18 years).[10] Some studies show that if diets containing about 30% of energy as fat are carefully planned (that is, they follow the Food Guide Pyramid), normal childhood growth can be expected.[32] Parents can choose which path to follow in conjunction with their child's physician. In general it's unnecessary to discourage children from consuming nutrient-dense foods such as milk, meat, and whole grains, just because they contain some fat. The overriding message is moderation in fat intake.[18]

Heart disease starts in childhood. Autopsies of young military men who died in Korea and Vietnam showed the early signs of plaque buildup in their blood vessels. The same holds for teens killed in auto accidents. As a result, many experts recommend screening for blood cholesterol in children whose families have histories of early heart disease, then treating children found to have high blood cholesterol with appropriate diet and drug therapy[29], as discussed in Chapter 6.

Are Low-Sodium Diets Appropriate for Children?

Scientific data neither confirm nor refute the notion that eating less sodium will reduce the risk of future high blood pressure. Moderation in sodium consumption does help build good health habits for the future—especially if the person later develops high blood pressure and needs to eat even less sodium. If children become accustomed to less salt, they'll be less inclined to eat very salty foods as adults.

Are High-Fiber Diets Recommended?

Some children eat too little dietary fiber, especially if they don't regularly consume fruits, vegetables, and whole grains. The current daily dietary fiber goal for children between ages 3 and teen years is the child's age plus 5 grams.[30] More fiber than that can crowd out other foods, providing bulk but insufficient energy content. Fluid recommendations to go along with this fiber intake are 5 cups per day for toddlers and up to 9 cups per day for older children. After about age 18, typical adult recommendations for fiber and fluid are appropriate (see Chapter 5).

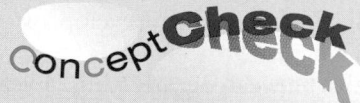

The rapid growth rate of an infant's first year slows during the toddler and preschool years (about ages 1 to 5). As a child's appetite decreases, adults should serve nutrient-dense foods and allow the child to decide how much to eat. Sudden shifts in food preferences are to be expected. Snacking is fine if attention is given to selecting healthful foods and good dental hygiene. Vitamin and mineral supplements are usually unnecessary—a plan following the Food Guide Pyramid should meet nutrient needs. Children should have plenty of iron-rich foods available to prevent iron-deficiency anemia. Developing heart-healthy habits after the age of 2 to 5 years is advocated by some researchers; however, greatly restricted diets are not recommended.

The Teenage Years

Most girls begin a rapid growth spurt between the ages of 10 and 13, and most boys experience rapid growth between the ages of 12 and 15. Nearly every organ in the body grows during these periods. Most noticeable are increases in height and weight and development of secondary sexual characteristics. Girls usually begin menstruating (reach menarche) during this growth spurt, and they grow very little beyond 2 years after menarche. Early-maturing girls may begin their growth spurt as early as age 7 to 8, whereas early-maturing boys may begin growing by age 9 to 10.[2]

During the growth spurt, girls gain about 10 inches (25 centimeters) in height and boys gain about 12 inches (30 centimeters). Girls also tend to accumulate both lean and fat tissue, whereas boys tend to gain mostly lean tissue. This growth spurt provides about 50% of ultimate adult weight and about 15% of ultimate adult height (see Figure 15-1).

As the growth spurt begins, teenagers begin to eat more. If teens choose nutritious food, they can take advantage of their increased hunger and easily satisfy their nutrient needs. As with older age groups, the Food Guide Pyramid provides the basis for meeting these nutrient needs (Table 15-7).

TABLE 15-7

Food Plan for Teenagers Based on the Food Guide Pyramid*

Food category	Minimum number of daily servings†
Milk, yogurt, and cheese (preferably low fat or nonfat)	3
Meat, poultry, fish, dry beans, eggs, and nuts	2-3
Vegetables	3-5
Fruit	2-4
Bread, cereal, rice, and pasta (preferably whole grain; otherwise, enriched or fortified)	6-11
Fats, oils, and sweets	Use sparingly

*Here we define "teenager" as a person who has added height in the past year and is at least 12 years old. This food plan is applicable through age 24 years.
†Use same serving size as for adults (see Table 2-1).

Nutritional Problems and Concerns of Teens

Anorexia nervosa and bulimia nervosa were covered in detail in Chapter 13. Other nutritional problems are more common during the teen years. A major concern is that many teenage girls stop drinking milk, so they may not consume enough calcium to allow for maximal mineralization of bones through their early twenties. Young women who don't consume enough calcium are likely to develop osteoporosis later, as discussed in the Nutrition Issue in Chapter 9.

The RDA for calcium for both males and females between ages 11 and 24 years is 1200 milligrams per day, compared with 800 milligrams per day for younger children. A recent NIH Consensus Conference on Optimal Intake of Calcium increased the calcium goal further in adolescence, to 1500 milligrams per day. Unfortunately, only about 1 in 6 teenage girls consumes the RDA for calcium. Three servings per day from the milk, yogurt, and cheese group are recommended for all teenagers and young adults until age 24.

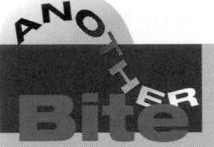

Drinking soft drinks in place of milk causes many teenagers to have inadequate calcium intake. Because soft drinks are rich in phosphorus, this practice produces an imbalance in the intakes of calcium and phosphorus, a pattern that fails to promote optimal bone development.

A second concern is iron deficiency. Iron-deficiency anemia sometimes appears in girls after they start menstruating and in boys during their growth spurt. About 10% of teenagers have low iron stores or related anemia.[24] Teens who strive to forge an identity by adopting dietary patterns unfamiliar to their families—vegetarianism, for example—may not know enough about the alternate diet pattern to keep from developing health problems, such as iron-deficiency anemia. It's important that teenagers choose good food sources of iron, such as lean meats, whole grains, and enriched cereals. Teenage girls, particularly those with heavy menstrual flows, especially need to eat good sources of iron (or regularly consume an iron supplement). Iron-deficiency anemia is a highly undesirable condition for a teen. It can produce increased fatigue and decreased ability to concentrate and learn. School and athletic performance may suffer.

Acne is a common teen concern—about 80% of teens experience it.[23] Although it's popularly believed that eating nuts, chocolate, and pizza can make acne worse, scientific studies have failed to show a strong link between any dietary factor and acne. Teens are simply warned to avoid "trigger foods," assuming that planning a well-balanced diet is still possible. Acne naturally waxes and wanes, so teens fall easy prey to notions about relationships to dietary factors. Acne may be more dormant in summer, because sunlight appears to improve the condition. The effect of artificial ultraviolet light on acne is less pronounced. The main culprit of acne is overactivity by the **sebaceous glands** in the skin. They respond to testosterone, which is mainly a male hormone. This is why men tend to have more serious cases of acne and to a greater extent than do women. Women also secrete testosterone and other **androgen** (testosterone-like) compounds. If these compounds are produced in large amounts, a woman also may experience serious acne.

One medication dermatologists sometimes prescribe for acne is tretinoin, which is sold under various trade names, such as Retin-A. A derivative of vitamin A, tretinoin is rubbed onto the skin once nightly. It is highly effective for treating blackheads and modestly effective for treating pimples, especially when used with benzoyl peroxide. Scientists don't know exactly how tretinoin works, but research suggests that it both pushes out the plugs in the ducts beneath the skin and helps prevent their reformation.

Sebaceous glands
Small glands surrounding hair follicles on the face, ears, back, chest, eyelids, and other areas. Blockage of a duct in a sebaceous gland by small particles can lead to an infection and local pressure, resulting in an acne lesion.

Androgens
A general term for hormones that stimulate development in males sex organs; one example is testosterone.

The most exciting news for serious acne is the introduction of Accutane (13-cis retinoic acid or isotretinoin). This prescription oral medication, another derivative of vitamin A, appears to change the nature of sebaceous gland development. It decreases the production of **sebum** and in turn reduces the number of acne lesions. The medication is especially helpful in treating cases resistant to antibiotic therapy[23] (see Chapter 8 for more information about Accutane). Teens should not self-medicate with vitamin A itself in hopes of curtailing acne. Instead they should rely on advice from their physician. It is the derivatives of vitamin A—not the vitamin itself—that are helpful, and these are available only by prescription. Recall as well that excessive dosages of vitamin A can cause toxicity, so this would likely be a hazardous choice.

Sebum
Secretion of the sebaceous gland consisting of waxes and various triglycerides.

A Closer Look at the Diets of Teenage Girls

Teenagers in general are apt to adopt fad diets, eat away from home or miss meals completely, and snack a lot. Teenage girls especially are very concerned with weight gain, appearance, and social acceptance. Recent government statistics revealed that female students were significantly more likely to report currently trying to lose weight (44%) than were male students (15%). Moreover, 27% of female students who considered themselves the right weight reported they were currently trying to lose weight. In an attempt to reach personal goals, they may eat dangerously little, select just a few items, and frequently skip meals altogether. If their limited food choices then consist of french fries, soft drinks, and pastries, little room is left for foods that are good nutrient sources. It's not only calcium and iron that teenage girls need to be concerned about—they often don't consume enough folate, zinc, and vitamins A and C. Common use of diet pills and the increasing number of bulimia nervosa cases further add to these nutritional problems.[27]

Helping Teens Eat More Nutritious Foods

Teenagers face a variety of challenges. They pursue their independence, experience identity crises, seek peer acceptance, and worry about physical appearance. All of these factors affect food choice. Advertisers take advantage of this by pushing a vast array of products—candy, gum, soda pop, and snacks—targeted toward the teenage market.

Teens often don't think about the long-term benefits of good health. They have a hard time relating today's actions to tomorrow's health outcomes. Many teenagers tend to think they can just change habits later; there's no hurry.

Still, healthful teen food habits don't have to include giving up favorite foods. Small portions of fatty foods can complement larger portions of nonfat and low-fat dairy products, lean meats, vegetable proteins, fruits, vegetables, and grain products. An example is a plain hamburger with a garden salad (minimize the amount of regular dressing or use a low-fat variety) and a small order of french fries or chili.

Overcoming the Teenage Mind-set

One strategy for working with teenage boys is to stress the importance of nutrition and physical activity for physical development—especially muscular development—and for fitness, vigor, and health. With teenage girls, one approach is to help them understand how to choose nutrient-dense foods and activities that lead to better health while maintaining a healthy weight. It can be explained that beauty is based on the glow of health, something that sick people often don't have. For teenagers, it's more effective to focus on the benefits of healthful foods and regular physical activity they can reap right now than to talk about health hazards that may or may not happen at some later time.

Are Teenage Snacking Practices Harmful?

Teens often obtain one fourth to one third of all their energy and major nutrients from snacks (Figure 15-9). Unfortunately, recent studies find just what you might expect—that teens snack mostly on potato and corn chips, cookies, candies, and ice cream.[4] Key reasons for snacking include an opportunity to get out and socialize with friends, accessibility, hunger, and celebrating a special event. Teenagers can obtain many nutrients from snacking. Even quick-service restaurants offer some good food choices. By choosing wisely and eating in moderation, teens can eat at quick-service restaurants and still consume a very healthful diet. Snacks and quick-service restaurants themselves are not the problem; poor food choices are.

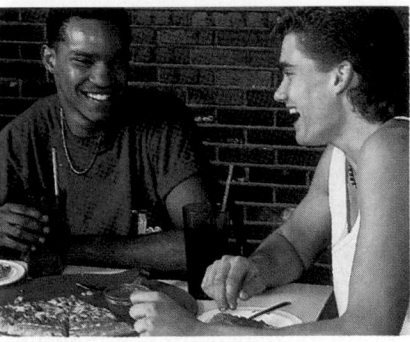

Figure 15-9 *The teenage years are noted for snacking and eating at quick-service restaurants. With appropriate food choices, teenagers can have healthful diets while still enjoying snacks and socializing at their favorite hangouts.*

Poor dietary habits formed during teenage years often continue into adulthood, giving rise to an increased risk of chronic diseases, such as heart disease, osteoporosis, and some types of cancer.[1] Getting this message across to teenagers is an important and challenging task for parents and health professionals.

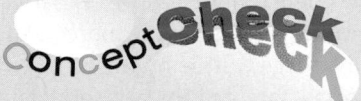

A second period of rapid growth occurs during the teen years. Girls generally start this growth spurt earlier than boys. The Food Guide Pyramid should guide meal planning. Common nutritional problems in these years arise from poor food choices and include inadequate calcium intake in girls, iron-deficiency anemia, and sometimes excessive intake of total fat and saturated fat. Because changes occur so rapidly during these years, and in so many areas—psychological, social, and physical—it may be difficult to stress the importance of nutrition to teenagers. Moderation in fat intake is one goal to consider when choosing snacks.

Summary

➤ Growth is very rapid during infancy; birth weight doubles in 4 to 6 months, and length increases by 50% in the first year. An adequate diet, especially in terms of energy, as well as the nutrients protein and zinc, is essential to support normal growth. Undernutrition can cause irreversible changes in growth and development. Growth in infants and children can be assessed by measuring body weight, height (or length), and head circumference over time.

➤ Nutrient needs in the first 6 months can be met by human milk or infant formula. Supplementary vitamin D and iron may be needed in the first 6 months for breastfed infants, and many infants may need supplemental fluoride.

➤ Infant formulas generally contain lactose or sucrose, heat-treated proteins from cow's milk, and vegetable oil. These formulas may or may not be fortified with iron. Sanitation is very important when preparing and storing formula.

➤ Most infants don't need solid foods before about 4 to 6 months of age. Solid food should not be added to an infant's diet until the nutrients are needed, the GI tract can digest complex foods, the infant has the physical ability to control tongue thrusting, and the risk of developing food allergies has decreased.

➤ The first solid food given should be iron-fortified infant cereals or ground meats. Other single foods can be added gradually, at the rate of about one each week. Some foods to avoid giving infants in the first year include honey, cow's milk (especially fat-reduced varieties), very salty or sweet foods, or foods that may cause choking.

➤ Introducing iron-containing solid food at the appropriate time and not offering cow's milk until 1 year of age can generally prevent iron-deficiency anemia in late infancy.

➤ Obese children and adolescents are more likely to become obese adults and so incur greater health risks. Parents can provide healthful food choices, while children should control portion sizes. When controlled early, a problem of obesity may correct itself as the child continues to grow in height. Obese infants, on the other hand, don't necessarily become obese children.

➤ A slower growth rate in preschool years underlies the importance of children's eating nutrient-dense foods and reducing their food serving sizes. Choosing iron-rich foods, such as lean red meats, is important at this age. Portion sizes at meals of 1 tablespoon of each food for each year of life is a good rule of thumb. Highly restrictive diets designed to reduce the risk of heart disease or high blood pressure are not recommended for preschoolers or older children unless prescribed by a physician.

➤ During the adolescent growth spurt, both boys and girls have increased needs for iron and calcium. Inadequate calcium intake by teenage girls is a major concern because it can set the stage for development of osteoporosis later in life. Teenagers generally should moderate their intake of high-fat foods, especially snacks and quick-service foods, which they often consume in abundance, and perform regular physical activity.

Study Questions

1 List two factors that limit "catch-up" growth in adulthood when a nutrient-deficient diet has been consumed throughout childhood.

2 Outline the procedures for preparing various types of infant formula: powdered, concentrated, and ready-to-feed.

3 Describe how you would assess whether an 8-month-old infant is consuming a healthful diet.

4 Outline three key factors that help determine when to introduce solid foods into an infant's diet.

5 List three reasons why preschoolers are noted for "fussy" eating. For each, describe an appropriate parent response.

6 Why should obesity in childhood be discouraged? What three factors are likely to contribute to this problem in a typical 6-year-old child?

7 Compare the guidelines for infant feeding summarized in the first Nutrition Insight with the Dietary Guidelines for children over 2 and adults discussed in Chapter 2. Which guidelines are similar? Do any contradict each other? If so, why?

8 Describe three pros and cons of snacking. What is the basic advice for healthful snacking from childhood through the teenage years?

9 Which two nutrients are of particular interest in planning diets for teenagers? Why does each deserve to be singled out?

10 In the teenage years, which nutrient generally most deserves a "consume in moderation" warning? Briefly explain why.

References

1 Anding JD and others: Blood lipids, cardiovascular fitness, obesity, and blood pressure: the presence of potential coronary heart disease risk factors in adolescents, *Journal of the American Dietetics Association* 96:238, 1996.

2 Behrman RE, Kliegman RM: *Nelson essentials of pediatrics,* ed 2, Philadelphia, 1994, WB Saunders.

3 Cary WB: The effectiveness of parent counseling in managing colic, *Pediatrics* 94:333, 1994.

4 Cross AT and others: Snacking patterns among 1,800 adults and children, *Journal of the American Dietetic Association* 94:1398, 1994.

5 Dietz WH: Critical periods in childhood for the development of obesity, *American Journal of Clinical Nutrition* 59:955, 1994.

6 Glinsmann WH and others: Dietary guidelines for infants, *Nutrition Reviews* 54:50, 1996.

7 Hamburger RN: Diagnosing food allergy, *Journal of the American College of Nutrition* 14:217, 1995.

8 Hefle SL: The chemistry and biology of food allergens, *Food Technology,* March 1996, p 86.

9 Hendricks KM, Badruddin SM: Weaning recommendations: the scientific basis, *Nutrition Reviews* 50:125, 1992.

10 Joint Working Group of the Canadian Pediatric Society and Health Canada: Nutrition recommendations update: dietary fats and children, *Nutrition Reviews* 53:367, 1995.

11 Kaste LM, Gift HC: Inappropriate infant bottle feeding, *Archives of Pediatric and Adolescent Medicine* 149:786, 1995.

12 Kennedy E, Goldberg J: What are children eating? Implications for public policy, *Nutrition Reviews,* 53:111, 1995.

13 King C: Cow's milk intolerance, *Maternal and Child Health,* p 125, April 1995.

14 Klish WJ and others: Fluoride supplementation for children: interim policy recommendations, *Pediatrics* 95:777, 1995.

15 Lo CW, Kleinman RE: Infant formula, past and future: opportunities for improvement, *American Journal of Clinical Nutrition* 63:646S, 1996.

16 Lust KD and others: Maternal intake of cruciferous vegetables and other foods and colic symptoms in exclusively breast-fed infants, *Journal of the American Dietetic Association* 96:46, 1996.

17 Mathews R: Importance of breakfast to cognitive performance and health, *Perspectives in Applied Nutrition* 3(3):204, 1996.

18 McBean L: New developments related to nutritional requirements for growth, *Dairy Council Digest* 66(6):31, 1995.

19 McBean L: Teens at risk: nutrition issues for the 90's, *Dairy Council Digest* 67(3):13, 1996.

20 McDowell MA and others: Energy and macronutrient intakes of persons ages 2 months and over in the United States: Third National Health and Nutrition Examination Survey, Advanced Data No. 255, Oct 24, 1994.

21 Meyers A: Modern management of acute diarrhea and dehydration in children, *American Family Physician* 51:1103, 1995.

22 Must A: Morbidity and mortality associated with elevated body weight in children and adolescents, *American Journal of Clinical Nutrition* 63(suppl):445S, 1996.

23 Nguyen QH and others: Management of acne vulgaris, *American Family Physician* 50:89, 1994.

24 Oski FA: Iron deficiency in infancy and childhood, *The New England Journal of Medicine* 329:190, 1993.

25 Pipes PL, Trahms CM: *Nutrition in infancy and childhood,* ed 5, St Louis, 1993, Mosby.

26 Satter E: Feeding dynamics: helping children to eat well, *Journal of Pediatric Health Care* 9:178, 1995.

27 Story M, Alton I: Becoming a woman: nutrition in adolescence. In Krummel DA, Kris-Etherton PM, editors: *Nutrition in women's health,* Gaithersburg, Md, 1996, Aspen.

28 Stehlin IB: Infant formula: second best but good enough, *FDA Consumer,* p 6, June 1996.

29 US Public Health Service: Cholesterol screening in children, *American Family Physician* 51:1923, 1995.

30 Williams CL: Importance of dietary fiber in childhood, *Journal of the American Dietetic Association* 95:1140, 1995.

31 Williams RD: Dehydration in children, *FDA Consumer,* p 19, July/Aug, 1996.

32 Writing Group for the DISC Collaborative Research Group: Efficacy and safety of lowering dietary intake of fat and cholesterol in children with elevated low-density lipoprotein cholesterol, *Journal of the American Medical Association* 273:1429, 1995.

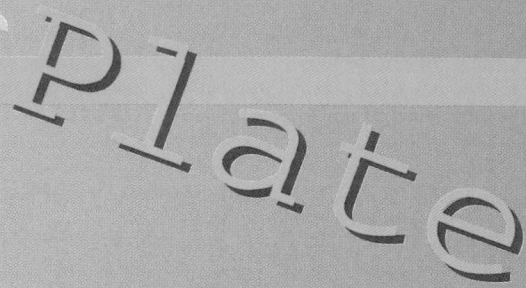

R A T E *Your Plate*

Getting Young Bill to Eat

Bill is 3 years old, and his mother is worried about his eating habits. He absolutely refuses to eat vegetables, meat, and dinner in general. Some days he eats very little food. He wants to eat snacks most of the time. His mother wants him to eat a formal lunch and dinner to make sure he gets all the nutrients he needs. Mealtime is a battle because Bill says he isn't hungry, but his mother wants him to eat everything served on his plate. He drinks five or six glasses of whole milk per day because that is the one food he adores.

When his mother prepares dinner, she makes plenty of vegetables, boiling them until they are soft, hoping this will appeal to Bill. Bill's dad waits to eat his vegetables last, regularly telling the family that he eats them only because he has to. He also regularly complains about how dinner has been prepared. Bill saves his vegetables until last and usually gags when his mother orders him to eat them. Bill has been known to sit at the dinner table for an hour until the war of wills ends. Bill's mother serves casseroles and stews regularly because these are her best dishes. Bill likes to eat breakfast cereal, fruit, and cheese and will regularly request these foods for snacks. However, his mother tries to deny his requests so he will have an appetite for dinner. Bill's mother comes to you and asks you what she should do to get Bill to eat.

ANALYSIS

1. List four mistakes Bill's parents are making that contribute to Bill's poor eating habits.

_____

_____

_____

_____

2. List four strategies they might try to promote good eating habits in Bill.

_____

_____

_____

_____

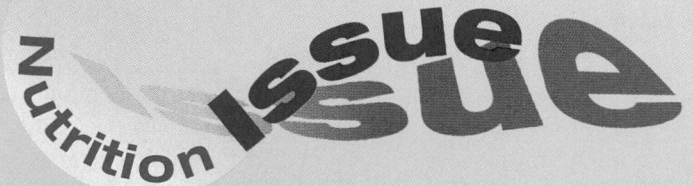

Food Allergies and Intolerances

Adverse reactions to foods—indicated by sneezing, coughing, nausea, vomiting, diarrhea, hives, and other rashes—are broadly classed as food allergies (also called *hypersensitivities)* or **food intolerances.** Allergies involve responses of the immune system designed to eliminate foreign proteins, called **allergens.** The symptoms experienced by susceptible people, such as rapid increase in heart rate and shortness of breath, are the result of this battle. In contrast, the symptoms of food intolerances do not result from a true allergic reaction. Rather food intolerances are caused by an individual's inability to digest certain food components or by the direct effect of a food component or contaminant on the body. Let's examine each process, first allergies and then intolerances, so you can learn how to reduce the risk of becoming a victim of the food you eat.

FOOD ALLERGIES: SYMPTOMS AND MECHANISM

Allergic reactions to foods are quite common and occur more frequently in females than males. Food allergies occur most frequently during infancy and young adulthood. Experts estimate that about 2% of adults and from 2% to 8% of children are allergic to certain foods. Three types of reactions may occur after ingestion of problem foods by susceptible people[8]:

- *Classic*—itching, reddening skin, asthma, swelling, choking, and a runny nose
- *GI tract*—nausea, vomiting, diarrhea, intestinal gas, bloating, pain, constipation, and indigestion
- *General*—headache, skin reactions, tension and fatigue, tremors, and psychological problems

Food intolerance

An adverse reaction to food that does not involve an allergic reaction.

Allergen

A foreign protein, or antigen, that induces excess production of certain immune system antibodies; subsequent exposure to the same protein leads to allergic symptoms. While all allergens are antigens, not all antigens are allergens.

Food sensitivity

A mild reaction to a substance in a food that might be expressed as light itching or redness of the skin.

Any reaction that is milder than these distinct allergic ones is referred to as a **food sensitivity.**

Allergic reactions vary not only in the body system affected but also in their duration, ranging from seconds to a few days. A generalized, all-systems reaction is called **anaphylactic shock.** This severe allergic response results in lowered blood pressure and respiratory and GI tract distress. It can be fatal. A person who is extremely sensitive to a food may not be able to touch the food or even be in the same room where it is being cooked without responding to it. Although any food can trigger anaphylactic shock, the most common culprits are peanuts, tree nuts (walnuts, pecans, etc.), shellfish, milk, eggs, soybeans, wheat, and fish. For a small number of people, avoiding foods like peanuts or shellfish is a matter of life and death.[8]

Anaphylactic shock

A severe allergic response that results in lowered blood pressure and respiratory and GI tract disorders. It can be fatal.

People with a history of serious allergic reactions should carry a self-administered form of epinephrine, such as EpiPen.

About 95% of food allergies are caused by proteins in milk, eggs, nuts (especially peanuts), seafood, soy products, and wheat. Other foods frequently identified with adverse reactions include meat and meat products, corn, fruits, and cheese.

Testing for a food allergy

Diagnosis of a food allergy can often be a difficult task. It requires the advice of a skilled physician.[7] The first step in determining whether a food allergy is present is to record in detail a history of symptoms, time from ingestion to onset of symptoms, most recent reaction, quantity and nature of food needed to produce a reaction, and the food suspected of causing a reaction. A family history of

Continued.

allergic diseases can also help, as allergic reactions tend to run in families. A physical examination may reveal evidence of an allergy, such as skin diseases and asthma. Various diagnostic tests can rule out other conditions.

The next step is to eliminate from the diet for 1 to 2 weeks all tested compounds that appear to cause allergic symptoms, plus all other foods suspected of causing an allergy based on the person's food history. The person generally starts out eating foods to which almost no one reacts, such as rice, vegetables, non-citrus fruits, and fresh meats and poultry. If symptoms are still present, the person can more severely restrict the diet or even use special formula diets that are hypoallergenic.

The American Academy of Allergy and Immunology has a 24-hour toll-free hot-line (800-822-2762) to answer questions about food allergies and to help direct people to specialists who treat the problem. Free information on food allergies is available by writing to The Food Allergy Network, 4744 Holly Ave., Fairfax, VA. 22030.

Once a diet is found that causes no symptoms, called an **elimination diet,** foods that are known not to trigger anaphylactic shock can be added back one at a time. Doses of $1/2$ to 1 teaspoon (2.5 to 5 ml) are given at first. The amount is increased until the dose approximates usual intake. This should be done using a double-blind approach (see Chapter 3), especially when the reaction has a psychological component or when symptoms are vague or ill-defined. Dried foods can be encapsulated and then given to the person. Any reintroduced food that causes significant symptoms to appear is identified as an allergen for the person.

Treatment of food allergies

Once potential allergens are identified, the best treatment is to avoid them, especially for people with zero tolerance. Careful reading of food labels is essential for many allergic people and advisable for all. A major challenge for the clinician treating a person with a food allergy is to make sure that what remains in the diet can still provide essential nutrients. The small food intake of children permits less leeway in removing offending foods that may contain numerous nutrients. A registered dietitian can help guide the diet-planning process to ensure that what remains of the food choices still meets nutrient needs, or to guide supplement use if that is necessary.

If an allergy-prone woman is pregnant or breast-feeding, she should avoid offending foods—like eggs and peanuts—because allergens can cross the placenta during pregnancy. Allergens will also be secreted in her milk. She should work with her physician and registered dietitian to make sure she still consumes an adequate diet. In addition, when food allergies run in the family, women are advised to breastfeed their infants exclusively for 6 months.[15] Human milk contains factors that play a role in maturation of the small intestine. Formula-fed infants, especially those on formulas based on cow's milk, have a greater risk for developing allergies. Breastfeeding thus should continue for as long as possible, preferably to 1 year.

The **prognosis** for food allergies that first appear before 3 years of age is good. About 80% of young children with food allergies outgrow them before 3 years. Parents should be made aware of this and certainly not assume the allergy will necessarily be long-lived. Food allergies diagnosed after 3 years of age, however, are often more long-lived, but not always. In these cases about 33% of people outgrow their food allergies within 3 years. For others, the condition may be prolonged; some food allergies can last a lifetime. Periodic reintroduction of offending foods can be tried every 6 to 12 months or so to see whether the allergic reaction has decreased. If no symptoms appear, tolerance to the food has developed.

Elimination diet
A restrictive diet to systematically test foods that may cause an allergic response by first eliminating them for 1 to 2 weeks and then adding them back one at a time.

Prognosis
A forecast of the course and end of a disease.

FOOD INTOLERANCES

Food intolerances are adverse reactions to food that do not involve allergic mechanisms. Generally, larger amounts of an offending food are required to produce symptoms of an intolerance than to trigger allergic symptoms. Common causes of food intolerances include:

- Constituents of certain foods (e.g., red wine, tomatoes, pineapples) that have a druglike activity, causing physiological effects such as changes in blood pressure
- Certain synthetic compounds added to foods, such as sulfites, food-coloring agents, and monosodium glutamate (MSG)
- Food contaminants, including antibiotics and other chemicals used in the production of livestock and crops, as well as insect parts not removed during processing

- Toxic contaminants resulting from ingestion of improperly handled and prepared foods containing *Clostridium botulinum*, *Salmonella* bacteria, or other food-borne microbes (see Chapter 17)
- Deficiencies in digestive enzymes, such as lactase (see the Nutrition Insight in Chapter 5)

Almost everyone is sensitive to one or more of these causes of food intolerance, many of which produce GI tract symptoms.

Sulfites, which are added to foods and beverages as antioxidants, cause flushing, spasms of the airways, and a loss of blood pressure in susceptible people. Wine, dehydrated potatoes, dried fruits, gravy, soup mixes, and restaurant salad greens commonly contain sulfites. A reaction to MSG may include an increase in blood pressure, numbness, sweating, vomiting, headache and facial pressure. MSG is commonly found in Chinese food and many processed foods (for example, soups). A reaction to tartrazine, a food-coloring additive, includes spasm of the airways, itching, and reddening skin. Tyramine, a derivative of the amino acid tyrosine, is commonly found in "aged" foods, such as cheeses and red wines. This natural food constituent can cause high blood pressure in people taking monoamine-oxidase inhibitor medications, which may be prescribed for mental depression.

The basic treatment for food intolerances is to avoid specific offending components. However, total elimination often is not required because people generally are not as sensitive to compounds causing food intolerances as they would be to allergens. For instance, a slight amount of sulfites in a glass of wine may be tolerable, whereas a large amount from a chef's salad may cause a reaction.

FOOD ADDITIVES AND HYPERACTIVITY IN CHILDREN: A POSSIBLE LINK?

In 1973 Dr. Benjamin Feingold suggested that food additives could cause hyperactivity in some children. This condition is now considered part of attention-deficit hyperactivity disorder (ADHD). Feingold theorized that children who are allergic to aspirin-like medications would also be allergic to certain food additives that have aspirin-like chemical structures. Although this proposal stimulated much research, the results generally have not supported a strong or predictable association between the consumption of food additives and hyperactivity in children.

Today ADHD is seen in up to 9% of school-age children; boys are affected four to six times more frequently than are girls. The initial identification of hyperactive children commonly occurs when they enter nursery or elementary school. Teachers report that these students are uncontrollable, easily distracted, and unable to sit still; fail to finish assignments; act impulsively; bother other children; and especially intrude into other children's activities. Psychological testing can be used to further characterize these behaviors and reasons behind them.[2]

Not only is the diagnosis of ADHD surrounded by some controversy, but research on the association between diet and hyperactive behavior is also confounded by many pitfalls. For example, when parents give a hyperactive child a special additive-free diet, they are likely to pay more attention to the child and his behavior. If the child's disruptive behavior subsequently decreases, it's unclear whether the diet or the extra attention or the combination should get the credit. In addition, an additive-free diet is likely to be more nutrient rich than a typical diet for children because it contains more whole foods and fewer processed foods. Again, it's difficult to know whether behavior changes in a hyperactive child on such a diet result from eliminating additives or adding more nutrients.

The only definitive way to study this relationship is to use a double-blind protocol. A child would be given an additive-free food and then later a food full of additives. Neither the parents, the child, nor the researchers should know what is in the food. After the child has consumed the foods, the researchers score the child's behavior.

This procedure is much too cumbersome to be used in a school system or by a private pediatrician. Thus many suspected cases of food additive–linked hyperactivity are not tested in a definitive scientific manner. This is a real problem because diets used for hyperactive children may eliminate more than just food additives. Some popular approaches eliminate nutrient-rich foods, such as milk, fruits, and some grain products. The more limited the diet, the greater the risk of nutrient deficiencies and poor growth.

If an additive-free diet follows the Food Guide Pyramid and actually improves a child's attention span and behavior, there is no reason not to employ it. Eliminating food colors from the diet has no harmful effect as such. However, a physician should agree that special diet restrictions are worth trying.

Will anything actually help the hyperactive child? Time is a very important therapy; hyperactivity may decrease as a child matures, but it can also linger through adulthood. When hyperactivity contributes to true ADHD, the problem can be treated with behavior therapies (especially to reinforce structure in the child's life), frequent opportunities for physical activity, and stimulant medications (for example, Ritalin). Parents should seek the advice of a pediatrician skilled in the diagnosis and treatment of this disease.[2]

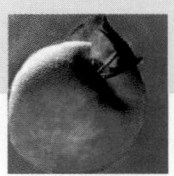

Nutrition During Adulthood

EATING IS ONE OF OUR GREAT pleasures. Guided by common sense and moderation, eating well is also a means to good health. Most of us want a long, productive life, free of illness. Yet, many people from early middle age onward suffer heart disease, strokes, diabetes, osteoporosis, and other chronic diseases. We can slow the development of, and in some cases even prevent, these diseases by pursuing a diet that works against them.[17] This action is most profitable if we begin early and continue throughout adulthood. We serve ourselves best—as individuals and as a nation—by striving to maintain vitality even in the later decades of life. This concept was first explored in Chapter 1 and is discussed again in this chapter, along with the special nutrition needs of older persons.

Keep in mind that present day-to-day health practices can significantly influence health during later life. Although genetics does play a role, as discussed in Chapter 1, many health problems that occur with age are not inevitable; they result from disease processes that influence physical health.[19] Much can be learned from healthy older people whose attention to health and physical activity—along with a little luck—keeps them active and vibrant well beyond typical retirement years. Successful aging is the goal. Age fast or slow—it is partly your choice.

CHAPTER 16

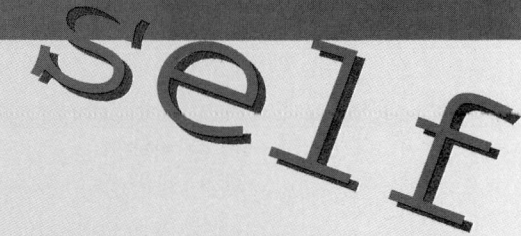

Could You or Someone You Know Have a Problem with Alcohol?

The Nutrition Issue in this chapter discusses ethanol, commonly known as *alcohol*. Problem drinking often has its seeds in the teen years. Significant health consequences of this typically arise in adulthood. A prominent contributor to 5 of the 10 leading causes of death in the United States, misuse of alcohol is one of our most preventable health problems. The social consequences of alcohol dependency include divorce, unemployment, and poverty. The following questionnaire was developed by the National Council on Alcoholism. With this assessment you can examine whether you or someone you know might need help. Answer the following questions by placing an "X" in the appropriate blank.

	Yes	No
1. Do you occasionally drink heavily after disappointment, a quarrel, or when someone gives you a hard time?	_____	_____
2. When you have trouble or feel under pressure, do you drink more heavily than usual?	_____	_____
3. Have you ever noticed that you're able to handle liquor better than you did when you first started drinking?	_____	_____
4. Do you ever wake up the morning after you've been drinking and discover that you can't remember part of the evening before, even though your friends tell you that you didn't pass out?	_____	_____
5. When drinking with other people, do you try to have a few extra drinks when others won't know it?	_____	_____
6. Are there certain occasions when you feel uncomfortable if alcohol isn't available?	_____	_____
7. Have you recently noticed that when you begin drinking, you're in more of a hurry to get the first drink than you used to be?	_____	_____
8. Do you sometimes feel a little guilty about your drinking?	_____	_____
9. Are you secretly irritated when your family or friends discuss your drinking?	_____	_____
10. Have you recently noticed an increase in the frequency of memory blackouts?	_____	_____

Continued.

11. Do you often find that you wish to continue drinking after your friends say they've had enough?   _____   _____

12. Do you usually have a reason for the occasions when you drink heavily?   _____   _____

13. When you're sober, do you often regret things you have done or said while drinking?   _____   _____

14. Have you tried switching brands or following different plans to control your drinking?   _____   _____

15. Have you often failed to keep promises you've made to yourself about controlling or stopping your drinking?   _____   _____

16. Have you ever tried to control your drinking by changing jobs or moving to a new location?   _____   _____

17. Do you try to avoid family or close friends while you're drinking?   _____   _____

18. Are you having an increasing number of financial and work problems?   _____   _____

19. Do more people seem to be treating you unfairly without good reason?   _____   _____

20. Do you eat very little or irregularly when you're drinking?   _____   _____

21. Do you sometimes have the "shakes" in the morning and find that it helps to have a little drink?   _____   _____

22. Have you recently noticed that you can't drink as much as you once did?   _____   _____

23. Do you sometimes stay drunk for several days at a time?   _____   _____

24. Do you sometimes feel very depressed and wonder whether life is worth living?   _____   _____

25. Sometimes after periods of drinking do you see or hear things that aren't there?   _____   _____

26. Do you get terribly frightened after you have been drinking heavily?   _____   _____

Interpretation

These are all symptoms that may indicate alcoholism. "Yes" answers to several of the questions indicate the following stages of alcoholism:

Questions 1-8:	Potential drinking problem
Questions 9-21:	Drinking problem likely
Questions 22-26:	Definite drinking problem

It is vital that people assess themselves honestly. If you or someone you know demonstrates some or a number of these symptoms, it is important that help be pursued. If there is even a question in your mind, go talk to a professional about it. Alcohol abuse is one of many problems adults, including older people, face.[6]

Key Chapter Concepts

- Delaying symptoms of and disabilities from chronic disease for as many years of life as possible is a laudable life goal. Nutrient intake plays a part in this process.
- A basic plan for health promotion and disease prevention includes eating a proper diet that focuses on a variety of foods and moderation in fat intake, performing regular physical activity, maintaining or improving body weight, consuming an adequate amount of fluids, abstaining from smoking, getting adequate sleep, and limiting alcohol intake.
- Scientists disagree as to the best diet recommendations for the general public. Genetic background, medical condition, and other lifestyle practices influence your optimal diet. Most experts agree, however, on the importance of an emphasis on variety in the diet; control of body weight; moderation in total fat and saturated fat intake; consumption of ample fruits, vegetables, and whole grains; and moderation in alcohol intake.
- Although maximum life span hasn't changed, life expectancy has increased dramatically over the past century. Aging probably begins before birth. This aging likely results from automatic cellular changes and environmental influences, such as DNA damage, free-radical reactions, hormonal changes, and alterations in immune function.
- Nutritional problems of older people relate to the presence of chronic disease and typical decreases in organ function that occur with age. These can include loss of teeth, a reduction in the senses of taste and smell, changes in gastrointestinal tract function, and deterioration in heart and bone health.
- Scientists are only now beginning to study specific nutrient requirements for older people. Diet plans should be based on the Food Guide Pyramid, with consideration for present health problems, decreased physical abilities, presence of drug-nutrient interactions, possible depression, and economic constraints.
- Nutrients such as protein, vitamin D, vitamin B-6, folate, vitamin B-12, zinc, and calcium, along with dietary fiber, often deserve special attention in diet planning in later life.

Your Adult Years

Many adults in America today have turned a healthful diet and moderate physical activity into lifetime pursuits. Coupled with avoiding tobacco products, sleeping an adequate amount, and limiting stress, these actions contribute to a healthful, long life.[17]

A Diet for the Adult Years

One diet approach that optimizes long-term nutritional health emphasizes low-fat and nonfat dairy products, some lean meats, plant proteins, a rich variety of fruits and vegetables, and generous amounts of whole-grain breads and cereals. The Food Guide Pyramid in Chapter 2 is a blueprint for this diet (Table 16-1).

To further refine these food choices, recall also from Chapter 2 the latest Dietary Guidelines issued by the USDA/DHHS. The U.S. Surgeon General, the American Heart Association, the American Dietetic Association, the American Medical Association, the National Cancer Institute, the National Academy of Sciences, and the World Health Organization have added recommendations to the framework of the Dietary Guidelines. Following is a summary of the advice provided by the Dietary Guidelines, with additional comments from various health-related organizations.

1. **Eat a variety of foods.** Most groups specifically suggest variety and moderation in food choices. In addition, limit protein intake to no more than twice the RDA and do not take nutrient supplements in quantities greater than 150% of the Daily Values listed on the label in any one day. Everyone, especially women, should also at least meet the RDA for calcium.
2. **Balance the food you eat with physical activity; maintain or improve your weight.** Use the middle ranges of the Metropolitan Life Insurance Table as a

Appendix F reviews diet planning guidelines issued by the Canadian government for Canadians. In addition, Chapter 1 discussed Healthy People 2000, a U.S. federal agenda aimed at disease prevention and health promotion for Americans.

TABLE 16-1

Two Dietary Paths of Adulthood—Which One Looks More Like Your Typical Choices?

Unhealthful	Healthful
BREAKFAST	
1 glazed doughnut Coffee or tea (if desired)	1 cup grapefruit juice 1 bran muffin 1 cup fruited low-fat yogurt Coffee or tea (if desired)
LUNCH	
Cheeseburger sandwich 1 cup french fries 1½ cups cola	Hamburger sandwich Medium salad with tomato, mushrooms, and vinaigrette dressing 1 cup nonfat milk
SNACK	
_____	4 fig bars 1 apple
DINNER	
2 slices pepperoni pizza 1½ cups lemonade 1 Snickers candy bar	3 ounces broiled halibut 1 cup rotini pasta 2 tsp soft margarine ½ cup carrots 1 cup nonfat milk
SNACK	
1 ounce potato chips	2 slices cinnamon toast on whole wheat bread Hot tea with lemon
2150 kcal 32% energy as fat 13% energy as saturated fat 9 grams dietary fiber Below RDA for vitamin A, vitamin C, calcium, and iron	2150 kcal 24% energy as fat 6% energy as saturated fat 27 grams dietary fiber Meets RDA for vitamin A, vitamin C, calcium, and iron

Note that focusing on a pattern of low-fat choices based on the Food Guide Pyramid generally increases nutrient adequacy in your diet and also increases the amount of food you can eat.

standard, Figure 10-6 in Chapter 10, or a Body Mass Index (BMI) of 19 to 25. It is important to balance food intake with regular physical activity to avoid substantial weight gain in adulthood that can frequently lead to obesity (Figure 16-1).

For those trying to lose weight the recommended rate of weight loss is 1 to 2 pounds a week once an interval of weight maintenance has been demonstrated (see Chapter 10). To do this, increase physical activity and eat low-fat, nutrient-rich foods: more fruits, vegetables, and grains; less sugar and fewer alcoholic beverages.

3. **Choose a diet with plenty of grain products, vegetables, and fruits.** Choose at least five or more servings of vegetables and fruits daily. This recommendation enjoys the most overwhelming support of nutrition experts. Note that only about 12% of adults currently meet this goal. Add to that six or more servings of a combination of bread, cereals, rice, and pasta daily, many of which are whole-grain varieties. These food choices should meet the goal of 20 to 35 grams of dietary fiber per day. The current U.S. average for dietary fiber intake is closer to 16 grams per day.

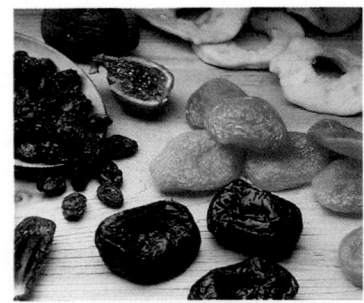

Eating dried fruit is an excellent way to increase your dietary fiber intake.

Because there are several kinds of dietary fiber, each with a different chemical structure and biological effect, it's best to include a variety of fiber-rich foods (see Chapter 5 for details).

4. **Choose a diet low in fat, saturated fat, and cholesterol.** Limit fat intake to 20% to 30% of total energy intake and saturated fat to no more than one third of total fat intake (10% or less of total energy intake). A common dietary cholesterol limit is 200 to 300 milligrams per day. (The average American consumes 12% of total energy as saturated fat and about 300 milligrams of cholesterol per day.) Choose lean meat, fish, poultry, and dry beans and peas as protein sources; use nonfat or low-fat milk and milk products; limit eggs to 3 to 4 per week; limit intake of dairy fats, hydrogenated fats, and other fats and oils high in saturated fat; trim fat off meats; broil, bake, or boil instead of frying; and aim for moderate or scant consumption of breaded or deep-fried foods.

5. **Choose a diet moderate in sugars.** Some authorities recommend that simple sugars supply no more than 10% to 15% of total energy intake. As noted in Chapter 5, 15% of energy intake corresponds to about 75 grams of simple sugars per day, or about 15 teaspoons. American adults eat about 80 grams of simple sugars daily. This 80 grams is made up mostly of simple sugars added during food processing and cooking. This total intake of sugars corresponds to about 18% of total energy intake.

6. **Choose a diet moderate in salt and sodium.** Limit sodium intake to 2.4 to 3 grams per day. This is the amount of sodium contained in 6 grams (3 teaspoons) of salt (40% of salt is sodium). To do this, especially limit the amount of salt in cooking and avoid adding it to food at the table. In addition, only very small amounts of salty, highly processed, salt-preserved, and salt-pickled foods should be eaten. The average person eats 4 to 7 grams of sodium per day. A sodium restriction of 2.4 to 3 grams per day requires a great change in food habits for many of us. It means not eating processed (lunch) meats, salted snack foods, most canned and prepared soups, most types of cheese, and many tomato-based processed foods on more than an occasional basis.

7. **If you drink alcoholic beverages, do so in moderation.** A moderate alcohol intake consists of 2 or fewer servings of 12 ounces of beer, 5 ounces of wine, or 1½ ounces of distilled spirits (80 proof) per day. Women are advised to strive for no more than 1 serving a day, because they are more sensitive than men to alcohol-related cirrhosis of the liver. If you are concerned about excess energy intake and want a nutritious diet, keep in mind that alcoholic beverages are energy-rich and low in or devoid of essential nutrients (see Table 16-8).

Beyond these general recommendations, aim for moderate use of salt-cured, smoked, and **nitrate**-cured foods because they are likely to increase the risk of certain forms of cancer. Obtain adequate fluoride to promote dental health and drink plenty of fluids. Finally, women of childbearing age need to eat iron-rich foods, primarily to avoid developing iron-deficiency anemia.

This group of guidelines provides a good general focus for diet planning. The practices recommended can accommodate many cultural dietary patterns (see Chapter 13). They are broad enough to allow you to include all the foods you enjoy in an eating plan—you just may have to eat some foods less frequently than others or in smaller portions, depending on your health needs and preferences. Moderation, rather than elimination, should be your overriding consideration.

Are Adults Following These Diet Recommendations?

In general, American adults, both young and old, are trying to follow many of the diet recommendations listed. Since the mid-1950s we have consumed less saturated

Recall from the discussion in Chapter 6 that fat-free does not necessarily mean low calorie. It is best to read the Nutrition Facts panel on any product touting fat reduction as you evaluate how it could fit into your diet.

GRIN AND BEAR IT

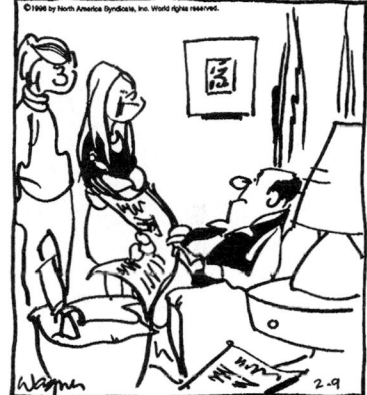

"Daddy, Rodney needs some advice on how not to end up like you."

Figure 16-1
Grin and Bear it.

Nitrate
A nitrogen-containing compound used to cure meats. Its use contributes a pink color to meats and confers some resistance to bacterial growth.

fat as more people substitute nonfat and low-fat milk for cream and whole milk. We eat more cheese, however, which is usually a concentrated form of saturated fat. Since 1963 we have eaten less butter, fewer eggs, less animal fat, and more vegetable fats and oils and fish. These changes generally follow the recommendations to reduce the intake of saturated fat and cholesterol and instead emphasize unsaturated fat. Today, animal breeders are raising much leaner cattle and hogs than in 1950, which helps. Our demand for chicken, a relatively lean source of animal protein, has skyrocketed.

Other aspects of the average U.S. diet are more mixed. Nutrition surveys from the early 1980s (the most comprehensive to date) show that the major contributors of energy to the adult diet are white bread, rolls, and crackers; doughnuts, cakes, and cookies; alcoholic beverages; whole milk and beverages made with whole milk; and hamburgers, cheeseburgers, and meatloaf. If the trend in diets were truly toward decreasing alcohol, sugar, and saturated fat and increasing dietary fiber, these foods could hardly appear at the top of the list.

A list following suggestions for improvement covered in this book would stress low-fat and nonfat milk, whole-wheat bread and whole-grain cereals, lean meat and tuna, peanuts and kidney beans, and oranges, carrots, and broccoli. What would your list look like?

Your task is to identify and change lifestyle practices most likely to cause illness and chronic disease. You began that process in Chapter 1. You can determine whether needed changes include switching to raisin bran cereal, rice, spinach pasta, fish, chicken, asparagus, and bok choy and walking briskly every day. These practices all promote and maintain nutritional and overall health.

A lifestyle that includes at least 30 minutes of moderate physical activity each day, combined with a sensible diet, can reduce the risk of premature development of almost all the chronic diseases adults face, including those that may develop in later life.[17] For physical activity to contribute significantly to longevity, however, it must be fairly vigorous. This might mean walking briskly at 4 to 5 mph for 45 minutes a day, 5 days a week. Jogging or playing tennis at least an hour 3 times a week also qualifies.[14]

The overriding consideration should be quality and length of life and the impact dietary changes might have on them. Now is the time to design and begin to practice this plan. Adulthood, and the sooner the better, is a key time to learn more about your risk factors for chronic diseases and do something about each one where possible.[23]

A Note of Caution

Not all nutrition and health researchers agree with the blanket guidelines set by major health and science institutions, as noted in Chapter 2. Some scientists do not think that general recommendations for the public can be justified for sugar, sodium, and cholesterol. Rather, they believe these recommendations need to be individualized.

Although it can be argued that individualized dietary recommendations for such nutrients as sodium are best, that approach is too costly for the nation and therefore impractical. General recommendations are appropriate if they benefit most people while not hampering the health of others. Not all people will benefit equally from following the general recommendations—for example, a reduction in sodium intake—but no one is likely to be harmed. The dietary change may cause some inconvenience and necessitate the formation of new eating habits for some people. Nevertheless, we should all consider the general dietary recommendations, personalizing the advice when possible under the guidance of our health-care advisors.

Recall from Chapter 1 that nutrition expert Dr. Irwin Rosenberg recently provided his "bottom line" for a healthy lifestyle: "Research has shown no better way to slow or even reverse the progress of aging itself and of all the age-related degenerative conditions than through the combination of aerobic and strength-building exercise and a balanced, nutritious diet."[7]

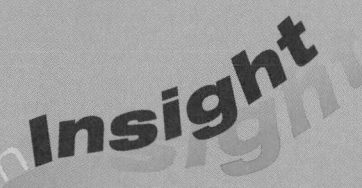

A Prescription for Longevity?

Some of us live longer and enjoy better health than others. Whole communities also show differences in longevity. In the United States, Seventh Day Adventist men live an average of 6 years longer than do other men. They have unusually low death rates from heart disease and cancer.

People who follow seven simple health habits generally live longer than those who do not. Long-lived groups typically have the following habits: (1) they never smoked, (2) they moderated their alcohol consumption, (3) they ate breakfast regularly, (4) they didn't snack, (5) they slept 7 to 8 hours a night, (6) they performed regular physical activity, and (7) they maintained healthy body weights.

As we learned in the chapter on weight control, factors influencing weight—and hence longevity—appear to be related to nature as well as nurture. When researchers closely examine the genetic and lifestyle backgrounds of long-lived people, they surmise that vigorous physical activity, low-fat diets, and the prevention of excessive weight gain may be key factors of longevity. Studies of families, and of twins in particular, also provide evidence for genetic control of human longevity. Identical twins tend to have very similar life spans and causes of death. Because identical twins have exactly the same genetic information, this makes a strong case for the importance of heredity in determining longevity.

What Does Animal Research Tell Us About Longevity?

Animal studies on longevity are quite extensive. By limiting rodents' energy intake to about 70% of usual, researchers have increased their life span by 35%.[11] The same treatment results in at least 50% lower incidence of cancer (see Chapter 8). Only energy should be limited; the rodent diet is supplemented with vitamins and minerals. Some studies have shown that food restriction can be started later in life and still extend the life span of rats. Scientists have found similar results using reduced-energy diets in other species—including mice, hamsters, spiders, fish, and mollusks—and are optimistic that it may work in monkeys. A study of this possibility is cur-

rently under way. Many other hypotheses have been tested in animals, but none is as effective in extending life expectancy as energy restriction (Figure 16-2).

There are many theories to explain how energy restriction increases life expectancy in rodents. A greatly reduced intake may lower the metabolic rate, which in turn reduces wear and tear on the body. Another possibility is that the mechanism may involve the immune system. Fewer calories may mean a delay in the natural aging of the immune system, thereby postponing the onset of diseases more commonly associated with old age. Other theories focus on what happens to hormonal systems under conditions of severe energy restriction. Less insulin release, for example, could reduce cell turnover—a factor associated with aging. Energy intake could also affect the ability of cells to repair damaged DNA. Probably several of these mechanisms come into play when animals are underfed. Other reasons for the longer life expectancy are also possible.[27]

The extended life expectancies gained from reduced feeding may actually be equal to the natural life span of animals in the wild. Perhaps what we see in the laboratory is an acceleration of the aging process caused by **ad libitum** feeding that is typically allowed for laboratory animals. Might well-fed Western humans again look to long-lived rural Asian people in the quest for the fountain of youth?

Pass the Butter?

From animal studies, we can infer that many mammalian species—and maybe humans—might live longer by restricting energy intake. In every species studied so far, being lean has meant living longer. With humans, however, the question is, are people willing to give up cheeseburgers and fries to have an unknown number of additional years of life? For most of us the deferred benefit of a longer, healthier life is overshadowed by the immediate pleasure of a hot fudge sundae. Clearly, we should consider striking a balance between immediate gratification and a pleasant long-term future. Both longevity and quality of life deserve your serious consideration.

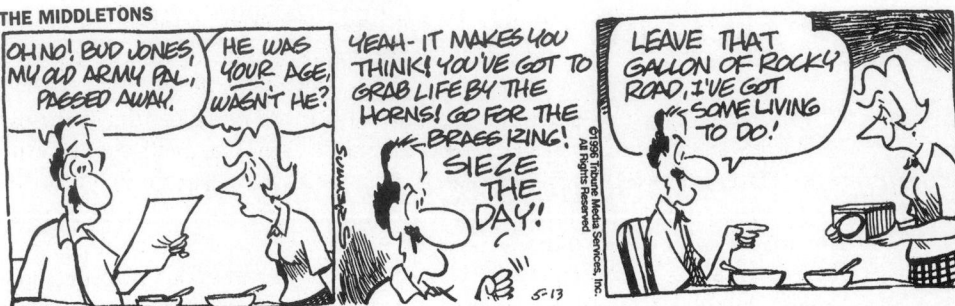

Figure 16-2 *The Middletons.*

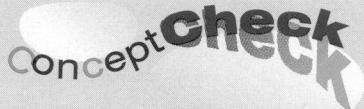

Attempting to delay symptoms of and disabilities from chronic disease for as many years as possible is a worthwhile goal. A basic plan to promote health and prevent disease includes eating a balanced, varied diet, performing regular physical activity, abstaining from smoking, limiting or abstaining from alcohol intake, obtaining adequate fluid and sleep, and limiting or learning ways to deal with stress more effectively. More specific dietary guidelines direct people to eat a variety of foods; maintain healthy weight; choose a diet low in fat, saturated fat, and cholesterol; choose a diet with plenty of vegetables, fruits, and grain products; use sugars only in moderation; use salt and sodium only in moderation; and, if you drink alcoholic beverages, do so in moderation. Women are advised to pay particular attention to iron and calcium intake, with general warnings against abusing nutrient supplements. Some scientists believe that these guidelines do not necessarily constitute an individual "prescription."

A Focus on the Older Years

How long do your family members generally live? Of those who died early in adulthood, can you pinpoint some causes? Do you plan to live longer than your parents did or will? How long will that be? Some basic statistics can help you predict this.

Life Span

Life span refers to the maximal number of years humans live. As far as we know, this hasn't changed in recorded time. The longest human life documented to date is 121 years. In contrast, the domestic dog has a life span of 20 years, and a rat, 5 years.

Life Expectancy

Life expectancy is the time an average person born in a specific year, such as 1996, can expect to live. Currently, life expectancy in America is about 73 years for men and about 80 years for women, with a span of "healthy years" of about 64. Furthermore, if you survive to the age of 80, you can tack on another 7 to 9 years of life expectancy.

Worldwide the highest average life expectancy is 82 years for women and 76 years for men in Japan. Researchers suggest that a diet based on rice, fish, vegetable protein sources, and limited meat contributes to this record longevity. Life expectancy hasn't always been this long; for primitive humans, it was about 20 to 35

Life span

The potential oldest age a person can reach.

Life expectancy

The average length of life for a given group of people born in a specific year (such as this year).

years. It increased to 49 years in Medieval England and remained so until the turn of this century. During the last 80 years, life expectancy for nearly all people has increased, mainly because of changes in the principal causes of death.[5]

At the turn of this century, infectious diseases commonly caused death. Vaccines and antibiotics have tremendously lowered death from disease. The decline in infant and childhood deaths, coupled with better diets and health care, has allowed more people to age first into maturity and then into older years. Now the principal causes of death in Westen societies are related to heart disease and cancer (Table 16-2).

Historically the trend in America has been toward an ever-older population. During colonial times, half the population was over 16 years of age. By 1990, half were over 33. By 2050, half could be over 43, and approximately 20% of the entire U.S population will be 65 years and older, twice as many as reach 65 today. This age—65 years—is arbitrarily listed as a dividing line for the beginning of later life because one can qualify for full Social Security benefits. When old age occurs, however, varies for each of us according to health and independence. Some people are quite healthy and independent at age 65, whereas others are disabled and greatly dependent on assistance for activities of daily living.

Among the older population the group constituting those aged 85+ years is the fastest growing segment. Between 1986 and 2050 the population aged 85+ years is expected to increase from about 1% to more than 5% of the total U.S. population. This is the first time in history our society will need to deal with such a large population of older people. The associated expense will be enormous if a large percentage need special care because of ill health.[4]

Critical Thinking

The "fountain of youth" remains a mystery. Many people believe a source exists that can stop the aging process, allowing youth to remain. However, Neil, a history student, asserts that the fountain of youth is not a place or a particular thing but rather a combination of diet and lifestyle. How can he justify this claim?

TABLE 16-2

Changes in Leading Causes of Death During this Century in the United States

Chronic diseases, rather than infectious diseases, are now the major killers.

Rank	Cause of death	Percentage mortality*
1900		
1	Pneumonia and influenza	12
2	Tuberculosis	11
3	Diarrhea and enteritis	8
4	Heart disease	8
5	Cerebrovascular disease (stroke)	6
6	Nephritis	5
7	Accidents	4
8	Cancer	4
9	Diphtheria	2
10	Meningitis	2
Today		
1	Heart disease	29
2	Cancer	26
3	Cerebrovascular disease (stroke)	5
4	Chronic obstructive pulmonary disease and allied conditions	4
5	Accidents and adverse effects	6
	Motor vehicle accidents	3
	All other accidents and adverse effects	3
6	Pneumonia and influenza	3
7	Diabetes	2
8	Acquired immunodeficiency syndrome (AIDS)	2
9	Suicide	2
10	Homicide and legal intervention	2

*Percentage of all deaths in that year.

The "Graying" of America

The "graying" of America poses some problems. Today, while people older than age 65 account for 13% of the U.S. population, they account for more than 25% of all prescription medications used, 40% of acute care hospital stays, and 50% of the federal health budget. Of older persons, 85% have nutrition-related problems, such as heart problems, diabetes, high blood pressure, osteoporosis, and obesity.

Postponing these chronic diseases for as long as possible will help control health care costs. The more independent, healthy years people live, the better life can be for them and the less they burden the health care system, which will increasingly have to scramble to accommodate a growing elderly population. Keep in mind that aging is not a disease, although the process of aging is still a mystery. It is difficult to design a model that predicts aging because so often disease speeds the process. However, diseases that commonly accompany old age—osteoporosis and atherosclerosis, for example—are not an inevitable part of aging.[23] Many can be prevented or managed, for the most part. Some people do die of old age, not as a direct result of disease.

What Actually Is Aging?

Reserve capacity
The extent to which an organ can preserve essentially normal fucntion despite decreasing cell number or cell activity.

One view of aging describes it as processes of slow cell death beginning soon after fertilization. When we are young, aging is not apparent because the major metabolic activities are geared toward growth and maturation. We produce plenty of active cells to meet physiological needs. During late adolescence and adulthood the body's major task is to maintain cells. Inevitably, though, cells age and die. Eventually, as more cells die, the body can't adjust to meet all physiological demands. Body functioning begins to decrease (Figure 16-3). Still, organs usually retain enough **reserve capacity** so that for a long time the body shows no outward disease. Although no symptoms appear, subclinical disease may develop, and if the disease is allowed to progress unchecked, organ function and then body function eventually deteriorate noticeably.[23]

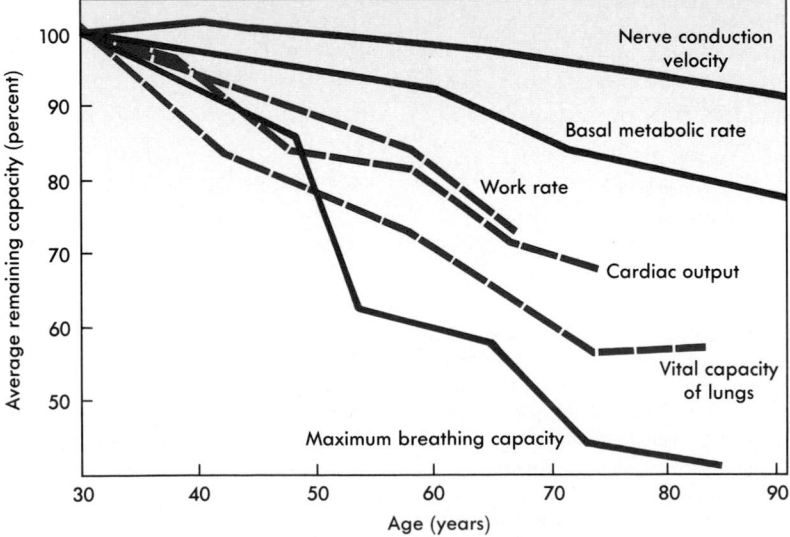

Figure 16-3 *Declines in physiological function seen with aging. The decline in many body functions is especially evident in sedentary people.*

The aging process is clearly illustrated by changes for many people in the function of the enzyme lactase. For some people, lactase activity in the small intestine slows during childhood. Generally, however, clear symptoms of the deficiency—gas and bloating after milk consumption—do not appear until adulthood. Although lactase output decreases in these cases, perhaps from birth, enough enzyme is present to digest the lactose consumed until adulthood.

Cells age probably because of automatic cellular changes and environmental influences.[23] Even in the most supportive of environments, cell structure and function inevitably change. Eventually, cells lose their ability to regenerate the internal parts they need, and they die. As more and more cells in an organ system die, organ function decreases. After age 14 months, human brain cells are continually lost, but we have enough reserve capacity to maintain mental function throughout life. **Kidney nephrons** are also continually lost. In some people this loss leads to eventual kidney failure, but most of us maintain sufficient kidney function. Again, in aging, there is first a reduction in reserve capacity. Only after that is exhausted does actual organ function noticeably decrease.

Hypotheses About the Causes of Aging

Although the causes of aging remain a mystery, many hypotheses have been promoted to explain it.

Errors occur in copying the genetic blueprint (DNA). Some of these errors are spontaneous, and others arise from degradative processes induced by chemicals and radiation, and time alone (recall the discussion of telomeres on DNA in Chapter 8). Once sufficient errors in DNA copying accumulate, a cell can no longer synthesize the major proteins needed to function, and it therefore dies. The ability to combat this type of damage is genetically determined. Gene variants that give rise to unusually efficient resistance to damage could contribute to life span by slowing the rate at which cells experience lethal damage.[27]

Connective tissue stiffens. Parallel collagen protein strands, found mostly in connective tissue, chemically bond and crosslink to each other. The bonding decreases flexibility in key body components, altering organ function. Skin wrinkles, and joints and arteries stiffen. The bonding may also restrict nutrients from entering cells.

Toxic products build up. Breakdown products of lipids called **lipofuscin** may act as intracellular sludge, hampering normal metabolic processes by clogging cells.

Electron-seeking compounds damage cell parts. Electron-seeking free radicals can break down cell membranes and proteins. One way to prevent some damage from these compounds is to consume adequate—not excessive—amounts of vitamins E and C, selenium, and carotenoids. In contrast, it's not effective to consume enzymes designed to break down the damaging compounds, such as **superoxide dismutase.** Ingested enzymes are themselves broken down during digestion before they can act in the body. Despite that, some health food stores sell superoxide dismutase, as noted in Chapter 8.

Hormone function changes. The hormone known as *dehydroepiandrosterone (DHEA)*, produced by the adrenal glands (located on top of the kidneys), circulates at extremely high concentration in young adults and falls after the age of 30. This change has led to speculation that DHEA decline plays a role in aging. However, the physiological function of this steroid hormone is unclear, and long-term effects of using products containing this hormone are also unknown. Research is ongoing. FDA has not approved the use of DHEA for symptoms related to aging, so marketing

Kidney nephrons
Unit of kidney cells that filters wastes from the bloodstream and deposits them into the urine.

Lipofuscin (ceroid pigments)
Lipid breakdown products in cells. Those compounds have fluorescence and can therefore be detected in aged cells, such as those in the eye, heart, and brain.

Superoxide dismutase
An enzyme that can quench (deactivate) a superoxide negative free radical (O_2^-).

it to the public is illegal in the United States. Even if current research on DHEA produces promising results, it will be at least another year or two before it is ready for government evaluation. Then FDA approval could take years.

A fall in growth hormone concentration is also being investigated as a potentially treatable hormonal cause of aging. Growth hormone is secreted by the pituitary gland and stimulates protein synthesis in cells, such as muscle cells, as well as produces various other effects in the body. Replacing growth hormone has wide-ranging, unpredictable effects and is very costly. Studies so far support the hypothesis that growth hormone–related loss of lean body mass plays a role in aging. However, once treatment with growth hormone in adults is stopped, gains in lean body mass are lost. The risks and benefits of this treatment probably will be known within 2 or 3 years, but it could take another 5 to 10 years to determine the best dosage. Growth hormone therapy has also been associated with significant adverse side effects that may limit its clinical usefulness in older people. FDA has not approved growth hormone treatment for prevention of the effects of aging.

Testosterone concentration declines with age. This decline in testosterone is linked to a decline in muscle strength. Animal studies have also suggested that testosterone may improve memory retention. These studies support the concept that a subgroup of older males may benefit from testosterone therapy. Postmenopausal women, especially those who have undergone surgical menopause, may also be candidates for testosterone therapy if estrogen therapy alone does not reduce related symptoms. Note that these are some side effects with use; treatment is still in the experimental phase.

Finally, production of melatonin by the pineal gland (located in the center of the brain) declines after puberty. Melatonin is best known for its ability to induce sleep; laboratory animal studies suggest that it may also slow the aging process. FDA has not yet approved use of melatonin, but there is great interest in its use as a sleeping aid. It is not currently available in a pure form. The melatonin sold in health food stores can be of questionable quality. Leading researchers note that little is known about the long-term effects of melatonin treatment on humans; there is evidence that it reduces ovulation in women. In fact, French, British, and Canadian governments have banned its sale. Overall, it is premature to take melatonin preparations in the hope of slowing the aging process until it is shown to be safe and effective for this purpose. Any use should be supervised by a physician.

The immune system loses some efficiency. The thymus gland (located in the upper part of the chest) is a major component of the immune system. During adolescence the thymus gland reaches its maximal size, and by age 50 it is barely visible. The immune system itself runs a somewhat parallel course. It is most efficient during childhood and young adulthood, but with advancing age it is less able to recognize and counteract foreign substances, such as viruses, that enter the body. As we age, then, the immune system's ability to detect and destroy developing cancer cells decreases, allowing them to multiply autonomously.

Nutrient deficiencies, particularly of protein, vitamin B-6, and zinc, hamper immune function, making matters worse for the aging body. Maintaining an adequate nutrient intake, especially in later life, is crucial for immune function.[3]

Autoimmune

Immune reactions against normal body cells; self against self.

Autoimmunity develops. **Autoimmune** reactions occur when white blood cells and other immune bodies fail to distinguish between substances normally present in the body and invading foreign antigens. White blood cells and other immune bodies then begin to attack body tissues in addition to foreign antigens. Many diseases, including some forms of diabetes and arthritis, involve this autoimmune response.

Death is programmed into the cell. Each human cell can divide only about 50 times. Once this number of divisions occurs, the cell automatically succumbs. This degradation occurs by design, probably as a way for the body to regulate cell number. Programmed cell death plays one of its most important roles in the maturation of cells used for immune function.

Glycosylation of proteins. Blood glucose, especially when chronically elevated—as occurs in poorly controlled diabetes—attaches to various blood and body proteins. This decreases protein function and can encourage immune system attack on such altered proteins. Eventually cell health declines.

Most likely, aging results from an interaction of these events and changes. Even very healthy people have a shortened life expectancy if they are exposed to sufficient environmental stress, such as radiation and certain chemical agents like industrial solvents. Because cell aging and diseases such as cancer are aggravated by environmental factors, it makes good sense to avoid such risks as excessive sunlight exposure and hazardous chemicals. Again, as has been stressed, we have some control over how quickly we age.[19]

With regard to vitamins, some scientists suggest that each day adults should consume from 250 to 500 milligrams of vitamin C, and 100 to 800 IU of vitamin E as an additional means to prevent chronic age-related disease. However, as noted in Chapter 8, agencies including FDA and the National Academy of Sciences consider such a recommendation to the general public premature, based on the available supporting evidence. Furthermore, this emphasis on vitamins certainly doesn't substitute for the practices recommended in the introductory section in this chapter.

As the number of possible cell divisions increases, so does life span. The Galapagos tortoise, whose cells divide about 140 times, has a lifespan of perhaps almost 200 years.

Glycosylation
The process by which glucose attaches to other compounds, such as proteins.

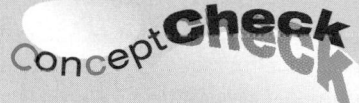

Although life span has not changed, life expectancy has increased dramatically over the past century. In many societies this means an increasing proportion of the population is, and will be, over 65 years of age. Avoiding continually rising healthcare costs and maximizing satisfaction with life require postponing and minimizing chronic illness. Aging begins early in life and probably results from both automatic cellular changes and environmental influences. Some current hypotheses of aging suggest these possible causes: errors in DNA replication accumulate, connective tissue stiffens, lipid by-products build up, electron-seeking free-radical compounds break down cell parts, hormonal and immune systems don't function well, and autoimmune responses and high blood glucose damage key body compounds. Diet can play a role in slowing some of these processes. Medical therapies to do so are also in experimental phases.

The Effects of Aging on the Nutritional Health of Older People

Older adults vary more in health status among themselves than do persons in any other age-group. This means that chronological age is not so useful in predicting physical health status (physiological age). As noted earlier, among people aged 65 and over, some are totally independent, healthy people, whereas others are frail and require almost total care. To predict the nutritional problems of an older person, it is necessary to know the extent of physiological change caused by aging and whether the person shows early warning signs for long-term poor nutrition.[29] As you examine how aging affects body systems and how these changes contribute to nutritional health, note the suggested ways to lessen health risks in your life and adopt changes in diet to counteract problem conditions (Table 16-3).

TABLE 16-3

Typical Physiological Changes Experienced by Older Adults and Recommended Diet/Lifestyle Responses

Change	Response
Decrease in appetite and food intake	Monitor weight and strive to eat enough to maintain healthy weight (see Table 16-6 for ideas)
Decline in sense of taste and smell	Vary the diet and experiment with herbs and spices
Loss of teeth	Work with dentist to maximize chewing ability; modify food consistency as necessary
Decreased sense of thirst	Consume about 8 cups of fluid each day, and watch for evidence of dehydration (for example, minimal urine output)
Constipation	Consume 20 to 35 grams of dietary fiber daily, choosing primarily fruits, vegetables, and whole grains; meet fluid needs (as above)
Decline in lactase production	Limit milk serving size; consume yogurt or cheese; seek other calcium sources (see Chapters 5 and 9 for more ideas)
Iron-deficiency anemia	Include some lean meat in the diet; ask physician to monitor blood iron status
Decline in liver function	Consume alcohol in moderation, if at all
Decline in insulin function	Maintain healthy body weight and perform regular physical activity (see Chapter 5)
Decline in kidney function	Modify protein and other nutrients in diet when advised by physician
Decline in immune function	Meet nutrient needs, especially protein, vitamin B-6, and zinc
Decline in lung function	Don't smoke tobacco products; perform regular physical activity
Decline in vision	Consume fruits and vegetables regularly to gain benefit of carotenoids and vitamin C
Decrease in lean tissue	Meet nutrient needs, and perform regular physical activity, including some resistance activity (see Chapter 11)
Decrease in cardiovascular function	Keep blood lipids and blood pressure within desirable range, using diet and medications when needed (see Chapters 6 and 9); stay physically active.
Decrease in bone mass	Meet nutrient needs, especially calcium and vitamin D, and perform regular physical activity (see Chapter 9)

What we see as the physiological changes associated with aging is the sum of natural processes and lifestyle practices. By adopting practices that minimize a decline in body function in the adult years, we invest in our future health.

Decreased Appetite and Food Intake

Decreases in body weight are common in adults age 65 to 90, who may not eat enough to meet energy needs. This phenomenon is a problem for older people in particular because it increases the risk of nutrition-related illness, especially when the concentration of the blood protein albumin falls below about 4 grams per 100 milliliters.

Many causes of inadequate food intake in older people are possible. Researchers suggest that biological origins, such as changes in neuroendocrine factors that influence feeding, account for some of this (see Chapter 10 for a review of these factors). When older men are underfed in metabolic ward settings, they do not later increase food intake to compensate for reduced food consumption when given the opportunity. Changes in taste and smell may also be important. In addition, social aspects play a role in reduced food intake. Many older people live alone, a circumstance that is associated with less food consumption.

To maintain health, older adults need to address the issue of declining weight.[25] Significant weight loss in older people, sometimes termed the "dwindles," increases risk of death. It may also indicate ongoing illness and reduced tolerance to medication or simple withdrawal from life itself. Even in apparently healthy older individuals, successful weight maintenance may require an increased conscious control over food intake relative to younger individuals.[16] Consuming energy-dense snacks between meals is one strategy, such as cheese, nuts, yogurt, oatmeal cookies, and bananas.

Pharmaceutical companies have recently begun to market liquid meal-replacement formulas to older adults. Previously, these products were primarily used in hospitals and nursing homes. These products are protein rich and have a fat content similar to 2% or whole milk, with added vitamins and minerals. It generally takes 4 cups (1 liter) or more of the product to yield the Daily Values for vitamins and minerals, at an energy cost of about 1000 kcal. Many of these products have an unusual taste because of the vitamins that have been added. Older adults can decide if the convenience, cost, and taste make this a wise diet choice.

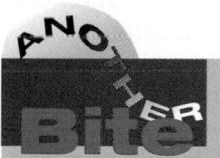

In early adulthood and middle age, significant weight gain is a major problem. Late in life, weight loss is more of a concern. Weight loss in older people often means increased risk of death. It may also indicate increased sickness and poor tolerance of medications. When assessing weight in older people, compare present weight with the previous year's weight.

The Senses of Taste and Smell

Sensitivity to taste and smell often decreases with age, starting at about age 60. Food may require stronger seasonings. Food companies are carving a niche in the marketplace by capitalizing on this change; by using a variety of flavor enhancers, they make foods tastier for older consumers. An inadequate diet and possibly zinc deficiency can also contribute to a loss of taste, however. Therefore a poor appetite should never be dismissed as a characteristic of old age. Many causes can be remedied by measures such as making sure to vary the diet.

Dental Health

About 30% or more older people in the United States have lost all their teeth. Attention to dental hygiene and dental care throughout life greatly lessens this risk. Gum disease commonly causes tooth loss. Replacement dentures enable some to chew normally, but many older adults—especially men—have denture problems. Solving individual dietary needs requires identifying foods that need to be modified in consistency. When people have problems chewing, the nutrient-dense snacks just mentioned can help. Sometimes just allowing extra time for chewing and swallowing encourages more eating.

Incontinence, the inability to control the muscle responsible for retaining urine, affects up to 20% of older adults living at home and about 75% of those in nursing homes. The embarrassment of having to wear diapers causes many to avoid fluids (resulting in dehydration and constipation) and to become socially isolated.

Thirst

Older adults often partially lose their sense of thirst and in turn don't drink enough fluids. They are then more likely to become dehydrated, a condition that leads to confusion and sometimes hospitalization.[26] It is important for them to consume enough fluids, and if necessary, they should be monitored to ensure they do so. About 8 cups of fluid daily is a good goal. An approximate fluid recommendation is the same as for younger adults, 1 milliliter per kcal expended. This amount must be adjusted if diuretics are used or in certain other medical conditions. Some important signs of dehydration, other than confusion, include dry lips, sunken eyes, increased body temperature, decreased blood pressure, constipation, decreased urine output, and nausea.

Gastrointestinal Tract

The main intestinal problem for older people is constipation (see Chapter 4 for a review of this problem). To keep the intestinal tract performing efficiently, older people generally need to consume more dietary fiber than they characteristically did in their youth. The goal is approximately 10 to 13 grams per 1000 kcal in the diet but generally no more than 35 grams on a daily basis. Regular consumption of nuts, fruits, vegetables, beans, and whole grains provides enough dietary fiber. Fiber supplements are generally unnecessary. They should also drink more fluid to move along masses that could form from high fiber intake. Physical activity likewise helps keep things moving smoothly. Because medications can induce constipation, a physician should be consulted if constipation might be related to a medication. If mineral oil is taken as a laxative, it should always be used with caution—and not at mealtimes—because it binds fat-soluble vitamins and limits their absorption.

As noted earlier, lactase production frequently decreases with age. Chapter 5 listed several options for people with lactose intolerance. The stomach slows its acid production as people age, usually limiting, in turn, the synthesis of intrinsic factor. These changes can contribute to poor absorption of vitamin B-12, and eventually, to pernicious anemia.[18]

Less stomach acid may also hamper iron absorption. Other conditions that affect the body's iron status occur with regular use of aspirin, which frequently causes blood loss in the stomach, and use of antacids, which may bind iron. Ulcers and hemorrhoids can also cause blood loss. Careful attention to iron status is necessary in these cases.

Liver, Gallbladder, and Pancreas

With age the liver functions less efficiently. When there is a history of significant alcohol consumption, fat buildup in the liver accounts for some decline. Alcohol abuse is a problem among a small but significant group of older individuals who may continue this pattern from earlier in life or develop heavy drinking patterns and alcoholism later. Later development of this problem sometimes arises from the loneliness and social isolation of retirement or loss of a spouse. Alcohol-related sickness is high in older people, so the health consequences of this excess are considerable. Also, older adults are more likely to take medications that potentiate alcohol's deleterious effects.[6] If cirrhosis then ultimately develops, the liver functions even less efficiently (see the Nutrition Issue at the end of this chapter).

When its function significantly deteriorates, the liver cannot efficiently detoxify many substances. The possibility for vitamin A toxicity in turn increases. Elderly people should be warned not to take excessive amounts of vitamin A, because toxic dosages can cause malaise, headache, bone pain, liver dysfunction, and a decrease in white blood cell count.[4]

The gallbladder also functions less efficiently as we age. Gallstones may dam up the bile to be secreted through the gallbladder, causing it to pool and back up into the liver instead. Gallstones can also interfere with fat digestion by allowing less bile into the small intestine. A low-fat diet or surgery may be necessary.

Although the digestive function of the pancreas may decline with age, the pancreas has a large reserve capacity. A sign of a failing pancreas is high blood glucose, which occurs under several different conditions. Glucose may circulate in the bloodstream, instead of being taken up by cells, because the pancreas secretes less insulin or because cells resist insulin actions—especially adipose (fat) cells in obese people with upper body fat storage.[2] Another cause can be insufficient chromium intake. Where appropriate, improved nutrient intake, regular physical activity, and weight loss can improve insulin action and blood glucose regulation.

Kidney Function

Over time the kidneys filter wastes more slowly as they lose nephrons (filters). As noted in Chapter 7, kidneys deteriorate more often in people who have regularly eaten excessive protein, and in some cases, excess energy (as inferred from studies on laboratory animals). The deterioration significantly decreases the kidneys' ability to excrete the products of protein breakdown. Although an increased protein intake of 1 to 1.25 grams per kilogram of healthy body weight has been recommended for physically active older people, that recommendation does not apply to people whose decreased kidney function causes urea—a main by-product of protein metabolism—to accumulate in the bloodstream.

Immune Function

With age the immune system often operates less efficiently. Consuming adequate protein, the gamut of vitamins, and zinc helps maximize the health of the immune system.[3] Recurrent sicknesses and poor wound healing are warning signs of a diet deficient especially in protein and zinc. Eating too little food in general or too few animal proteins is usually the reason. Older people often eliminate meat from their diet because it's too hard to chew. Recall that animal proteins are an excellent source of zinc. Balanced nutrient supplements can help bridge gaps in vitamin and mineral intake. On the other hand, overnutrition appears to be equally harmful to the immune system. For example, obesity and excessive fat, iron, and zinc can suppress the immune system.

Lung Function

Lung efficiency declines somewhat with age and is especially pronounced in older people who have smoked and continue to smoke tobacco products. Breathing becomes shallower and faster and more difficult as the number of lung air sacs decreases. Smoking often leads to emphysema and lung cancer. The decrease in lung efficiency contributes to a general downward spiral in body function; breathing difficulties limit physical activity and endurance and frequently discourage eating. These changes eventually cancel other efforts to maintain overall health.

Besides not smoking, being physically active helps prevent lung problems. People need not lose their capacity to breathe deeply, as long as sufficient aerobic activity is part of their regular routine. Otherwise, merely walking can demand the "exertion" of a marathon pace. Coupled with poor muscle tone and decreased muscle mass, movement becomes continually more difficult. What is the answer? Stay physically active throughout life.

Hearing and Vision

Hearing and vision both decline in aging. Experts disagree as to when or whether these losses become disabling. Hearing impairment occurs mainly in members of industrial societies with urban traffic and aircraft noise and loud music. Elderly people may also avoid social contacts because they can't hear.

Degenerating eyesight, frequently caused by retinal degeneration, can affect a person's ability to physically get to a grocery store, locate the foods desired, read labels for nutritional content, and prepare the foods at home. Regular consumption of foods rich in carotenoids, in particular dark green, leafy vegetables, such as kale, collard greens, spinach, swiss chard, mustard greens, and romaine lettuce, decreases the risk of developing retinal degeneration. These vegetables are rich in lutein and zeaxanthin, two carotenoids found in the portion of the eye subject to damage from age-related degeneration.[18] Such vision changes may make people afraid to socialize, be active, or take care of important routines of daily life, such as shopping. Recall from Chapter 8 the role vitamin C plays in reducing cataracts in the eye. This benefit serves as another reason adults should have a diet rich in fruits and vegetables.[21]

Decrease in Lean Tissue

Some muscle cells shrink and others are lost as muscles age; some muscles lose their ability to contract as they accumulate fat and collagen protein. Lifestyle greatly determines the rate of muscle mass deterioration. As you might predict, an active lifestyle tends to maintain muscle mass, whereas a very inactive one encourages its loss. Ideally an active lifestyle should include some resistance activity (weight training) throughout life. The latter reduces muscle loss in older people.[9]

Physical activity increases muscle strength and mobility, improves mental outlook, eases daily tasks that require some strength, improves sleep, and slows bone loss. However, according to one study, when older adults stopped their weight-training program, any gains in muscle strength were quickly lost. This illustrates the importance of regular physical activity throughout life.

After obtaining their physician's approval to get started, older people can seek out programs to begin strength and aerobic training at community recreation centers or the local YMCA or YWCA. Most of these organizations have qualified trainers who can help set up a program. Dumbbells are inexpensive and thus ideal for performing weight training at home. Chapter 11 provides some general advice on this topic, including advice for warm-up, stretching, and cool-down activities.

Older adults also benefit from physical activity because it stimulates food intake by raising energy expenditure. By eating more, they increase their chances of consuming adequate amounts of nutrients. Overall, much of what we associate with aging in terms of physical health results from long-standing sedentary lifestyles.[8]

Increases in Fat Stores

As lean tissue decreases with age, the body often takes on more fat. Much of this results from overeating and minimal physical activity.[10] If obesity results, this is not desirable, especially because it can raise blood pressure and blood glucose. Obesity can also make walking and performing daily tasks more difficult. Although a small fat gain in adulthood may not compromise health, large gains are often problematic.

Cardiovascular Health

The heart often pumps blood less efficiently in older people, usually because of insufficient physical activity. Poor heart conditioning allows fatty and connective tissues to infiltrate the heart's muscular wall. This decline in **cardiac output** is not inevitable with aging and does not occur among older people who remain physically active.

Heart attack and stroke, the major causes of death in all adults, are caused primarily by atherosclerosis and high blood pressure. As we age, atherosclerotic plaque

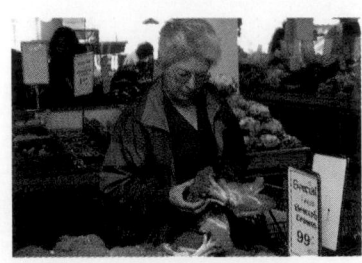

Deteriorating vision can hamper a person's ability to get to a grocery store, purchase nutritious foods, and prepare them at home.

Since 1958 the number of Americans with diabetes has tripled, in part because the population is getting older and more obese. Currently about 16 million Americans have diabetes, an increase of 5 million since just 1983.

accumulates in the arteries, reducing their elasticity, constricting blood flow, and consequently, elevating blood pressure.

You already know the main way to limit the buildup of atherosclerotic plaque: keep your LDL and total cholesterol/HDL ratio in the desirable range (see Chapter 6). New evidence shows that a diet very low in fat can cause some plaques to decrease in size. Other studies use diet and medications or surgery to lower blood cholesterol, which in turn reduces the amount of plaque in the arteries supplying the heart. This suggests that a heart-healthy diet is more important during middle to late adulthood than researchers previously thought. Consuming sufficient vitamin B-6, folate, and vitamin B-12 is also important to avoid elevated blood homocysteine, an additional risk factor for heart disease.[18]

Much controversy surrounds the treatment for elevated LDL in people over the ages of 70 to 75. If these people adhere to extremely restrictive diets limited in fat and energy to the point that they can't keep up their weight, or if their diets lack variety, they may become undernourished. This may be a worse predicament for them than having high LDL. Therefore treating elevated LDL in an older person who has other illnesses, such as chronic lung disease and **dementia**, which are likely to shorten life as well as hamper its quality, is probably inappropriate. But if a healthy 70-year-old who is likely to live another 10 to 15 years has both elevated LDL and evidence of heart disease, an eating and exercise plan is probably in order to reduce the chance of heart attack. Overall, the pros and cons of different treatments to reduce heart disease need to be weighed carefully before they are advocated for an older adult. Discussing the person's health and quality of life should be the first step. Note that the advisability of fat restrictions for the very old (those older than 85 years of age) for the amelioration of chronic disease is questionable. Dietary modifications should be made instead to respond to the current disease state, such as the presence of diabetes or failing kidney function.

High blood pressure is heavily implicated in both stroke and heart attack in older adults. Blood pressure can be lowered in most people by severe sodium restriction. A limit of 2 grams of sodium helps many people with high blood pressure, but that is a difficult diet to plan and follow. Alternatively, a mild sodium restriction (not to exceed 4 grams of sodium daily) may be effective for salt-sensitive people but is not so helpful by itself for those who are not salt sensitive; it does, however, aid the action of medications used to treat high blood pressure. (The Nutrition Insight in Chapter 9 reviews the effects of other nutrients and lifestyle interventions on blood pressure.)

We can do much to prevent heart attack and stroke just by eating a balanced diet, walking briskly and otherwise performing regular physical activity, controlling blood pressure, not smoking, and maintaining healthy weight. Regular physical activity and a diet rich in fruits and vegetables are also associated with fewer strokes as adults age.[18]

Bone Health

Chapter 9 discussed the decline in bone density associated with aging. Recall that bone loss in women occurs primarily after menopause. Bone loss in men is slow and steady from middle age throughout later life. Estrogen replacement at menopause is the most reliable treatment to lessen bone loss in women. For older women not taking estrogen, increasing calcium intake to 1500 milligrams per day helps maintain bone density in some types of bones, such as the hip. The recent NIH Consensus Report on Optimal Calcium Intake made a similar recommendation for older men. Currently many older people fail to meet this recommendation.

Other measures to prevent bone loss can be started earlier and continued throughout life—maintaining adequate vitamin D nutriture, not smoking, and

Cardiac output
The amount of blood pumped by the heart.

Dementia
General persistent loss or decrease in mental function.

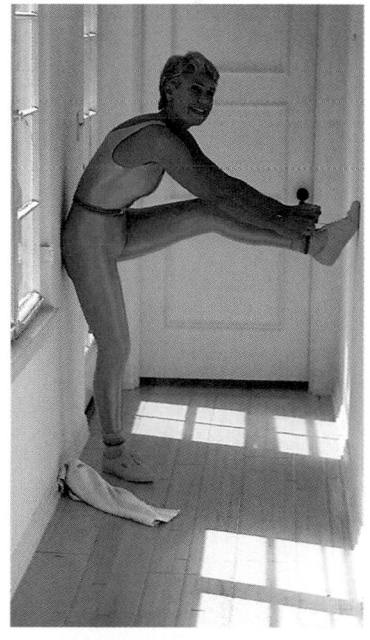

Age is no reason to stop exercising.

drinking alcohol moderately or not at all (refer to the Dietary Guidelines). Underweight women are at especially high risk for developing osteoporosis. Performing weight-bearing activity, such as walking, also helps sustain bone.

For menopausal women who are at high risk for or who may have osteoporosis, medical treatment should be considered—estrogen replacement therapy, active vitamin D hormone (calcitrol) therapy, bisphosphonate or calcitonin therapy—administered under the supervision of a physician (see Chapter 9).

Very severe osteoporosis limits the ability of older people to move about, shop, prepare food, and live normally. They eat less and get fewer nutrients.

Older people should also work with their physicians to develop a plan for limiting falls. Falls may be caused by the side effects of medication, gait and balance disorders, impaired vision, and environmental hazards. Protective hip padding can reduce the risk of fracture in individuals who tend to fall. Typical measures to reduce the risk of falling include the following:

- Remain as physically active as possible
- Remove clutter and clear pathways
- Secure carpets and stair treads
- Remove loose electrical cords
- Replace or repair unstable furniture
- Do not wax floors
- Increase lighting, especially at night
- Use a cane, walking stick, or walker if needed to maintain balance
- Install grab bars in bathroom (tub, shower, toilet)
- Use nonskid bathmats
- Store personal items and frequently used items at eye level or below
- Do not rise quickly after eating or sitting for a period of time; if you tend to feel dizzy, begin instead to rise up slowly

Many older people may suffer from hidden osteomalacia, a condition primarily caused by not enough sun exposure and therefore lessened vitamin D synthesis in the skin. When they can't get regular sun exposure—during the winter or when they are homebound—older people need a source for 10 to 20 micrograms (400 to 800 IU) of vitamin D per day. Both fortified milk products and a vitamin supplement can be used to meet this goal.

Other Factors that Influence Nutrient Needs in Older Adults

Medications and old age often go together. Medications can improve health and quality of life, but some of them also profoundly affect nutrient needs at all ages, including the later years (Table 16-4). Forty-five percent of the elderly population regularly take multiple prescription drugs; many drugs affect appetite or absorption of nutrients. Often, people must take several medications for long periods. They should make sure to work with their physician and pharmacist to coordinate all medications taken.[22] Pharmacists can advise when to take drugs—with or between meals—for greatest effectiveness.

Drug-related nutritional problems include (1) increased need for potassium when certain types of diuretics leach it out of the body and (2) changes in appetite caused by antidepressant agents or certain antibiotics. Blood loss from long-term use of aspirin or aspirin-like medications strains iron reserves and can lead to anemia. People who must take one or more medications for more than just a few weeks should closely watch their diets, eat nutrient-dense foods and possibly take nutrient supplements to counteract effects of certain medications. A physician should supervise this last practice, because some supplements can interfere with the function of certain medications. For example, vitamin K can reduce the activity of oral anticoagulants (see Chapter 8).

Nutrition

Insight

Alzheimer's Disease

Alzheimer's disease has become a dreaded reality for many people approaching old age. Many of us have had first-hand experience as loved ones have been "lost" to this form of progressive dementia. Although it seems a disease of our times, it has actually existed for quite a while.

In 1907 Dr. Alois Alzheimer documented several cases of what seemed to be early senility. Typical symptoms of the disease included personality changes, unreasonable fears, explosive outbursts, depression, wandering, and general forgetfulness. Today the disease Dr. Alzheimer first described affects about 4 million people in the United States, including about 45% of all people over the age of 85 and 50% of all people in nursing homes. Age at diagnosis is generally about 75 years. Wandering is a frequent reason people with Alzheimer's disease are put in nursing homes. Death in Alzheimer's disease is frequently attributable to bacterial infection or pneumonia associated with accidental food inhalation.

More reports of Alzheimer's disease surface every day. Is this a disease of modern society, or has it always been around but misdiagnosed? Old age is often accompanied by a general decline in mental function. What makes Alzheimer's disease different is that it can be diagnosed specifically by the presence of specific protein deposits and tangled masses of nerves in areas of the brain that are linked to memory and thinking. However, this type of diagnosis can be done only at autopsy, and so it is difficult to know precisely how many cases of dementia in old age are actually Alzheimer's. Clinical assessments can and should be made by an experienced physician. Because much is now known about the typical course of the disease, clinical methods have recently become more reliable in differentiating between Alzheimer's disease and other causes of dementia.

Causes and Physical Effects

In general terms, Alzheimer's disease is best described as a progressive brain disorder marked by an inability to remember, reason, or understand what is going on. Age is the primary risk factor. Scientists propose causes, including altered cell development, altered brain proteins, and unidentified blood-borne agents. Research over the last few years suggests that a specific blood protein, called *apolipoprotein E-4*, increases the risk of developing Alzheimer's disease.[15] It is thought that this compound interferes with the maintenance of nerve cells, whereas the E-2 or E-3 variant of this protein do not. If the E-4 gene is inherited from both parents, the risk of Alzheimer's disease is about nine times greater in the offspring than if neither gene is E-4. About 2% to 3% of Americans have two E-4 genes. Researchers note, however, that testing individuals for the presence of the E-4 variant is premature, because this provides no guarantee that the person will or will not develop the disease. The presence of the E-4 variant is merely a risk factor. Still, there is some interest in developing medications that may compensate for the presence of E-4. Other risk factors under investigation include less educational and occupational attainment, as well as loss of estrogen at menopause in women. Scientists are also studying the possibility that regular use of ibuprofen and related drugs may reduce the risk of Alzheimer's by reducing related brain inflammation.[20]

In people with Alzheimer's disease, aluminum is highly concentrated in abnormal protein accumulations in the brain, but this high amount of aluminum is more likely an effect than a cause of the disease. Evidence supporting this is that people mining aluminum develop cancer from aluminum toxicity but typically don't develop Alzheimer's disease. Accordingly, a role for aluminum in the neuropathology of Alzheimer's disease remains a subject of speculation. Whether there are other causes of Alzheimer's disease remains to be discovered, but this is likely.

Treatment

The environment of the person with Alzheimer's disease should be safe, with attention paid to risks such as wandering or forgetting about food cooking on a stove. Establishing routines is also helpful, along with regular physical activity. Today, medical treatment of Alzheimer's disease is usually limited to the use of antidepressants and other drugs that target related symptoms of the disease. A new medication currently in use is tacrine (Cognex), a drug that may slow the brain's breakdown of a major neurotransmitter used in sending nerve messages. Side effects currently limit its usefulness to a subset of patients, and it does not cure the disease.

Continued.

Nutrition Considerations

The main nutrition goal for people with this disease is a healthful diet that maintains body weight. Abnormal food behavior, such as gorging, is often seen early in the course of Alzheimer's disease. A craving for sweets may lead to a temporary weight gain that can be managed by offering lower-energy snacks and meals. At the other extreme, many people refuse to eat. Frequent, small meals and nutrient-dense snacks using favorite foods when possible may encourage more regular eating. People who are still leading reasonably independent lives may not be able to shop or to remember to eat meals. Congregate feeding programs and home-delivered meals may be helpful during the early stages of disease. Keep in mind that by the time the disease has been diagnosed, some people have already developed nutritional problems.

As the disease progresses, people with Alzheimer's disease grow increasingly confused and distracted. At this stage it is wise for others to oversee food planning and mealtimes. Caretakers should also try to control distractions—such as television, radio, children, pets, and the telephone—that can disrupt a meal for someone with Alzheimer's disease. Caretakers also should monitor food temperatures, because people with Alzheimer's disease may ignore discomfort and burn themselves. Tough or crunchy foods that may easily cause choking should be avoided.

As people with Alzheimer's disease become less able to manage eating by themselves, feeding them becomes more of a challenge. They may hold food in the mouth, forget how to eat or swallow, spit out food, and play with and then refuse food.

We all should pay attention to dietary recommendations to promote and maintain health. People with Alzheimer's disease may not be able to do this on their own. In later stages of this disease people may not be attuned to their needs. The responsibilty for providing good nutrition ultimately falls to family, health-care providers, and nursing home staff.

Finally, in addition to its physical implications, Alzheimer's disease takes an immense emotional toll on people with the disease and their family members.

Ten warning signs of Alzheimer's disease

1. Recent memory loss that affects job performance
2. Difficulty performing familiar tasks
3. Problems with language
4. Disorientation to time and place
5. Faulty or decreased judgment
6. Problems with abstract thinking
7. Misplacing things
8. Changes in mood or behavior
9. Changes in personality
10. Loss of initiative

To find out more about Alzheimer's disease, call the Alzheimer's Association at (800) 272-3900, or the National Institute on Aging's Alzheimer's Disease Education and Referral center at (800) 438-4380.

TABLE 16-4

Potential Drug-Nutrient Interactions for Some Commonly Used Drugs

Drug	Use	Nutrient affected	Potential side effect
Antacids (Maalox)	Reduce stomach acidity	Calcium, vitamin B-12, and iron	Decreased absorption due to altered gastrointestinal pH
Anticoagulants (Coumadin)	Prevent blood clots	Vitamin K	Poor utilization
Aspirin	Antiinflammatory; pain reduction	Iron	Anemia from blood loss
Cathartics (laxatives)	Induce bowel movement	Calcium and potassium	Poor absorption
Cholestyramine	Reduces blood cholesterol	Vitamin A, D, E, and K	Poor absorption
Cimetidine (Tagamet)	Treatment of ulcers	Vitamin B-12	Poor absorption
Colchicine	Treatment of gout	Vitamin B-12, carotenoids, and magnesium	Decreased absorption due to damaged intestinal mucosa
Corticosteroids (prednisone)	Antiinflammatory	Zinc Calcium	Poor absorption Poor utilization
Furosemide (Lasix)	Decreases blood pressure; potassium-wasting diuretic	Potassium and sodium	Increased loss
Hydrochlorothiazide	Decreases blood pressure; diuretic	Potassium and magnesium	Increased loss; decreased absorption
MAO inhibitors (Parnate)	Antidepressant	Tyramine (in aged foods)	High blood pressure caused by limited tyramine metabolism
Tricyclic antidepressants (Elavil)	Antidepressant	—	Weight gain from appetite stimulation

About 15% of older adults experience significant depression. That—combined with isolation and loneliness as family and friends die, move away, or become less mobile—frequently contributes to apathetic eating and weight loss. People living alone do not necessarily make poor food choices, but they often consume less energy, in part from skipping meals. Older men are especially prone to this habit. About one third of all older people not in nursing homes live alone. Depression can be a downward spiral in which poor appetite produces weakness that leads to even poorer appetite (Figure 16-4). In older adults the resulting poor nutritional state can produce further mental confusion and increased isolation and loneliness.[12]

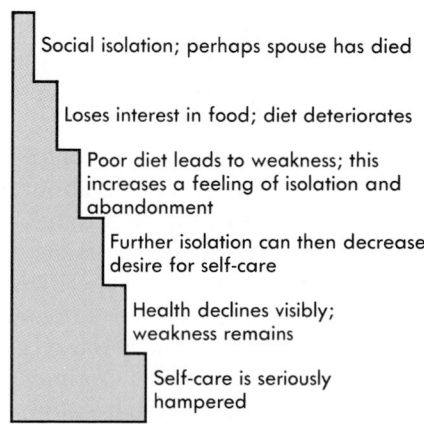

Figure 16-4 *The decline of health often seen in older adults. This decline needs to be prevented whenever possible.*

Social isolation; perhaps spouse has died

Loses interest in food; diet deteriorates

Poor diet leads to weakness; this increases a feeling of isolation and abandonment

Further isolation can then decrease desire for self-care

Health declines visibly; weakness remains

Self-care is seriously hampered

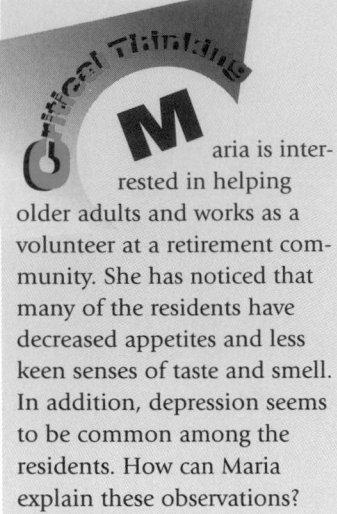

Maria is interested in helping older adults and works as a volunteer at a retirement community. She has noticed that many of the residents have decreased appetites and less keen senses of taste and smell. In addition, depression seems to be common among the residents. How can Maria explain these observations?

Nutrition contributes to the preservation of mental function in older people. Specific nutritional deficiencies of thiamin, niacin, vitamins B-6 and B-12, and folate, as well as excessive alcohol use, cause well-recognized central nervous system disorders. The subtle effects of eating minimal food energy, leading to semistarvation, are often overlooked. In addition, as mentioned earlier, an inadequate fluid intake may lead to dehydration and consequent confusion.[26]

Mental illness can lead to a poor nutritional state, but the extent to which subtle nutritional deficiencies can lead to a poor mental state is not as clear cut. It is important to prevent overt nutritional deficiencies, especially those mentioned previously. You should also note that a long and healthy life for almost everyone means that age, far from implying disengagement, should become a time to get even more involved. This, along with nutrient intake, supports mental function.

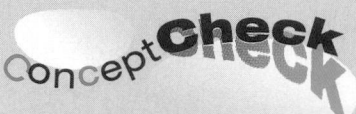

Specific nutrient requirements for older adults are only now being extensively studied. Diet plans should be modified for decreased physical abilities, presence of drug-nutrient interactions, possible depression, and economic constraints. Particular attention should be paid to the opportunity for sun exposure and intake of the vitamins D, B-6, folate, and B-12, as well as the minerals calcium and zinc, and dietary fiber. A nutrient-dense diet helps to meet these needs. In the United States, many nutrition services—such as congregate and home-delivered meals—are available to help our aging population obtain a healthful diet.

Meeting the Nutrient Needs of Older People

The RDAs for nutrients and energy include a category for both men and women who are 51 years of age and older. Because the lifestyle of an active 70-year-old person differs considerably from that of a 90-year-old nursing home resident, this wide age range in the RDAs is likely to be problematic.[4] The recommendations for energy intake assume an active lifestyle, a characteristic the RDA committee supports. Note also that the nutrient recommendations for older people have largely been projected from studies of young adults.

Do the RDAs Increase in Later Life?

Only during the last few years has much research focused on this question. Because the RDAs apply only to healthy people, many older people—for example, those who have ulcers or are heavy aspirin users—are not covered by RDAs. Indeed it is particularly tricky to develop RDAs that are valid for most older people because so many are ill and/or regularly take medication.

Researchers have suggested that the current RDAs for healthy older people are probably too high for vitamin A; a bit too low in protein (for active people); too low for vitamins D, B-6, and B-12; and about right for the other vitamins. For most minerals the RDAs are probably about right or a bit generous. The "about right" category reveals that we lack evidence to make a more definitive statement (Table 16-5). There is, however, concern that the RDA for calcium should be increased to help slow the acceleration of bone loss suffered by older women and men.[28] As just mentioned, 1500 milligrams per day was recently recommended for both genders by an NIH Consensus Conference on Optimal Calcium Needs.

Still, a well-planned diet that follows the Food Guide Pyramid can meet all nutrient needs for older people within about 1600 to 1800 kcal, except for probably

Older women need less iron because they no longer menstruate. However, chronic ulcers, hemorrhoids, and aspirin use may necessitate an increased iron intake.

TABLE 16-5

Comparing the Current RDAs for Older Adults to Projected Needs Based on Recent Research

Nutrient	Differing needs of Older people vs. RDA	Reason for differing needs
Protein	1.0-1.25 grams per kilogram vs. 0.8 gram per kilogram	• Help blunt loss in lean body mass • Possibly lower efficiency of dietary protein utilization
Vitamin A	Caution with supplement use is advised	• Increased absorption because of changes in lining of small intestine
Vitamin D	10-20 micrograms vs 5 micrograms (400-800 IU vs 200 IU)	• Limited exposure to direct sunlight • Reduced dermal synthesis • Reduced kidney conversion to active hormone
Vitamin B-6	No amount set	• Falling blood concentrations due to age • Blunted response to intake
Vitamin B-12*	3 micrograms vs 2 micrograms	• Reduced absorption caused by fall in gastric acid • Vitamin B-12 injections recommended if intrinsic factor synthesis inadequate.
Calcium	1500 milligrams vs 800 milligrams	• Reduced absorption, especially in women after menopause • Slows bone loss, such as in hip region

*Some scientists argue that the RDA is adequate and attention should instead be paid to screening older people for low vitamin B-12 concentration in the blood. They believe increasing the amount consumed by 1 microgram will not help, because the fall in vitamin B-12 status results from a profound decrease in absorption. Instead, regular intramuscular injections are needed to maintain vitamin B-12 status once the loss of gastric function is in advanced stages.

1500 milligrams of calcium (see Table 2-2). That would take at least four servings from the milk, yogurt, and cheese group—a recommendation that most older people would find difficult to meet. Calcium-fortified foods and calcium supplements can help when necessary (see Chapter 9 for details).

If a 1600 to 1800 kcal diet plan represents too much food energy, a special attempt should be made to regularly choose nutrient-rich foods such as 1% and nonfat milk, leafy vegetables, fish and lean meat, along with some nutrient-fortified foods, like ready-to-eat breakfast cereals and calcium-fortified orange juice. Nutrient supplements are another possibility, but these only complement—not substitute for—healthy food choices. Also, too much of some supplements can lead to toxicity. Between about 35% and 70% of older people regularly take supplements, some in potentially toxic amounts. If supplements are necessary, the older person should work closely with a physician or registered dietitian to determine which nutrients to include and the least amounts that are necessary. For example, the possibility of vitamin D deficiency is easily assessed by asking about the intake of vitamin D–fortified milk and the availability of regular sun exposure.

Planning a Diet for Older People

To supply energy needs for males age 51 and older, the current RDA suggestion is 2300 kcal; for females, the recommendation is 1900 kcal. (These values are based on a 170-pound, 68-inch tall man and a 143-pound, 63-inch tall woman.) Studies show that older men eat closer to 1800 to 2100 kcal, whereas women eat about 1300 to 1600 kcal. Thus diet plans for older adults should focus on nutrient density. A good practice is to decrease sugar and fat consumption to increase the diet's nutrient density and to make sure dietary fiber intake is adequate. In addition, some protein should come from lean meats to help meet vitamin B-6 and zinc needs, two nutrients of special concern.[24]

Fluid needs are about 8 cups (2 liters) per day. A high-fiber diet especially requires attention to fluid needs. Fiber intake should be slowly increased up to about 35 grams a day, with each serving of fiber accompanied by a glass of water (or other fluid).

Singles of all ages face logistical problems with food: purchasing, preparing, storing, and using food with minimal waste are challenging. Economy packages of meats and vegetables are normally too large to be useful for a single person. Many singles live in small dwellings, some without kitchens and freezers. Creating a diet to accommodate a limited budget and facilities and a single appetite requires special considerations.[12] Following are some practical suggestions for diet planning for singles:

- If you own a freezer, cook large amounts, divide into portions, and freeze.
- Buy only what you can use; small containers may be expensive, but letting food spoil is also costly.
- Ask the grocer to break open a family-sized package of wrapped meat or fresh vegetables and separate it into smaller units.
- Buy only several pieces of fruit—perhaps a ripe one, a medium-ripe one, and an unripe one—so that the fruit can be eaten over a period of several days.
- Keep a box of dry milk handy to add a nutritious punch to recipes for baked foods and other foods for which this addition is acceptable.

Nutritional deficiencies and protein-energy undernutrition have been identified among some aging populations, particularly those in nursing homes or long-term care facilities and those who are hospitalized.[29] These nutritional problems increase the risk for many diseases, including bed sores (pressure ulcers), and compromise recovery from illness and surgery. Feeding sick, infirm, and mentally confused people is time-consuming and demanding work that requires special training. Friends, relatives, and health personnel should look for poor nutrient intake in all older people, including those who live in nursing home settings. About 40% of adults now age 65 will spend some time in a nursing home. Family members have a unique opportunity to make sure nutrient needs are met by looking for weight maintenance based on regular, healthful meal patterns.[12] If problems arise in instituting a healthful diet, registered dietitians can offer professional and personalized advice.

Surveys show that the majority of older adults like most vegetables, despite misconceptions that they do not like broccoli (because it forms gas) or tomatoes (because they contain too much acid). By the time we reach adulthood, our eating habits reflect regional tastes, social class, ethnic group, and life experiences. There is no generic food list for older people.

Overall, good nutrition benefits older adults in many ways. It delays the onset of some diseases; improves management of some existing diseases; hastens recovery from many illnesses; can increase mental, physical, and social well-being; and often decreases the need for and length of hospitalization. Thus a good nutritional intake should be a vital part of the health maintenance program for older people.[12] A variety of strategies can promote healthful eating in later life (Table 16-6). These should focus on presenting nutritious, tasty foods in a pleasant environment.

Community Nutrition Services for Older People

Health-care advice and services for older people can come from clinics, private practitioners, hospitals, and health maintenance organizations. Home health-care agen-

TABLE 16-6

Guidelines for Healthful Eating in Later Years

- Eat regularly; small, frequent meals may be best. Use nutrient-dense foods as a basis for each menu.
- Find out which convenience foods and labor-saving devices can be of help.
- Try new foods, new seasonings, and new ways of preparing foods. Don't use just convenience foods and canned goods.
- Keep some easy-to-prepare foods on hand for times when you feel tired.
- Have a treat occasionally, perhaps an expensive cut of meat or a favorite fresh fruit.
- Eat in a well-lit or sunny area; serve meals attractively; use foods with different flavors, colors, shapes, textures, and smells.
- Arrange things so food preparation and clean-up are easier.
- Eat with friends, relatives, or at a senior center when possible.
- Share cooking responsibilities with a neighbor.
- Use community resources for help in shopping and other daily care needs.
- Stay physically active.
- If possible, take a walk before eating to stimulate appetite.
- When necessary, chop, grind, or blend hard-to-chew foods. Softer, protein-rich foods can be substituted for meat when poor dental function limits normal food intake. Prepare soups, stews, cooked whole-grain cereals, and casseroles.
- If your eating movements are limited, cut the food ahead of time, use utensils with deep sides or handles, and obtain more specialized utensils if needed.

cies, adult day-care programs, adult overnight-care programs, and **hospice** centers (for the terminally ill) can supply daily care. Professionals in the above-mentioned organizations can help identify older people whose health needs may require extra attention. Figure 16-5 shows a valuable screening tool, based on the acronym "DE-TERMINE."[7] When this tool suggests a problem, careful follow-up by a physician is indicated.[1]

Nutrition programs for those age 60 and over offer congregate meal programs, which provide lunch at a central location, and home-delivered meals (often known as Meals-on-Wheels if sponsored by the local private or public agencies) (Figure 16-6). Federal commodity distribution is available in some areas of the United States to low-income older people. Food stamps can benefit older people whose incomes are below the poverty level. Food cooperatives and a variety of clubs and social organizations provide additional aid.

- *Disease*
- *Eating poorly*
- *Tooth loss or mouth pain*
- *Economic hardship*
- *Reduced social contact and interaction*
- *Multiple medications*
- *Involuntary weight loss or gain*
- *Need for assistance with self care*
- *Elder at an advanced age*

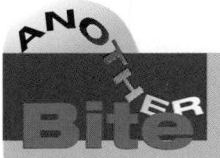

Studies have found that congregate meal programs can positively influence the nutritional status of otherwise homebound people. Still, congregate meal programs provide at most one meal a day and usually not every day of the week. If people come to depend on them exclusively, they eat too few meals. The problem with home-delivered meals is that the one or two meals delivered may never be eaten, and if not eaten on delivery and left at room temperature, they may become unsafe to eat later. Thus these programs can help older adults but probably don't meet all their nutritional needs.

Congregate meal programs and home-delivered meals are funded partially by the U.S. government under Title III of the Older Americans Act and through volunteer community efforts (Figure 16-7). The federal government sets specific standards for home-delivered meals and for those served in congregate feeding centers. The meals are designed to provide one third of the RDA. The social aspect often improves appetite and general outlook.

Many eligible older people are missing meals and are poorly nourished simply because they don't know of available programs. Irregular meal patterns and weight

To learn about meal programs for senior citizens in your area, call the Administration on Aging's Elder Care Locator, (800) 677-1116.

A Nutrition Test For Older Adults

Here's a nutrition check for anyone over age 65. Circle the number of points for each statement that applies. Then compute the total and check it against the nutritional score.

1. The person has a chronic illness or current condition that has changed the kind or amount of food eaten. (2 points)

2. The person eats fewer than two full meals per day. (3 points)

3. The person eats few fruits, vegetables, or milk products. (2 points)

4. The person drinks 3 or more servings of beer, liquor, or wine almost every day. (2 points)

5. The person has tooth or mouth problems that make eating difficult. (2 points)

6. The person does not have enough money for food. (4 points)

7. The person eats alone most of the time. (1 point)

8. The person takes three or more different prescription or over-the-counter drugs each day. (1 point)

9. The person has unintentionally lost or gained 10 pounds within the last 6 months. (2 points)

10. The person cannot always shop, cook, or feed himself or herself. (2 points)

Nutritional score:

0–2: Good. Recheck in 6 months.

3–5: Marginal. A local agency on aging has information about nutrition programs for the elderly. The National Association of Area Agencies on Aging can assist in finding help; call (800) 677-1116. Recheck in 6 months.

6 or more: High risk. A doctor should review this test and suggest how to improve nutritional health.

(Modified from the Nutrition Screening Initiative, 1010 Wisconsin Avenue, NW, Suite 800, Washington, DC 20002.)

Figure 16-5
A nutrition checklist for older people. Suspected problems should then be carefully evaluated in a more detailed physical examination.

loss, often caused by difficulties in preparing food, are warning signs that undernutrition may be developing. An effort should be made to identify and inform poorly nourished people of community services.[12]

The ideal is to remain healthy and live independently for as long as possible without becoming socially isolated. Personal living situations can greatly determine whether an older person is well-nourished. For some, just getting to the store or carrying groceries may be a major problem. Relatives and friends can be a real help. Special transportation arrangements may also be available through a local transit company or taxi service.

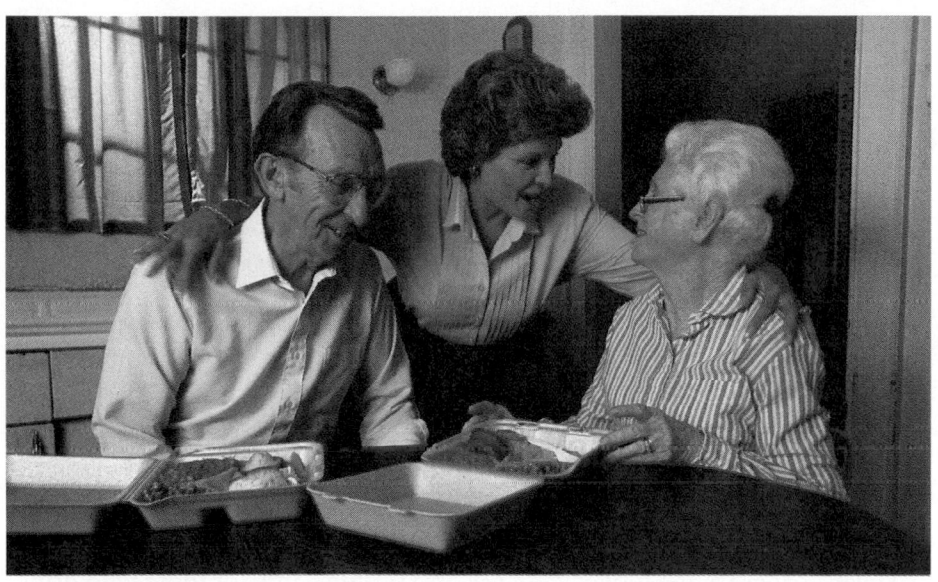

Figure 16-6
The home-delivered meals program is a gift of nutrition and caring from a community to its older citizens.

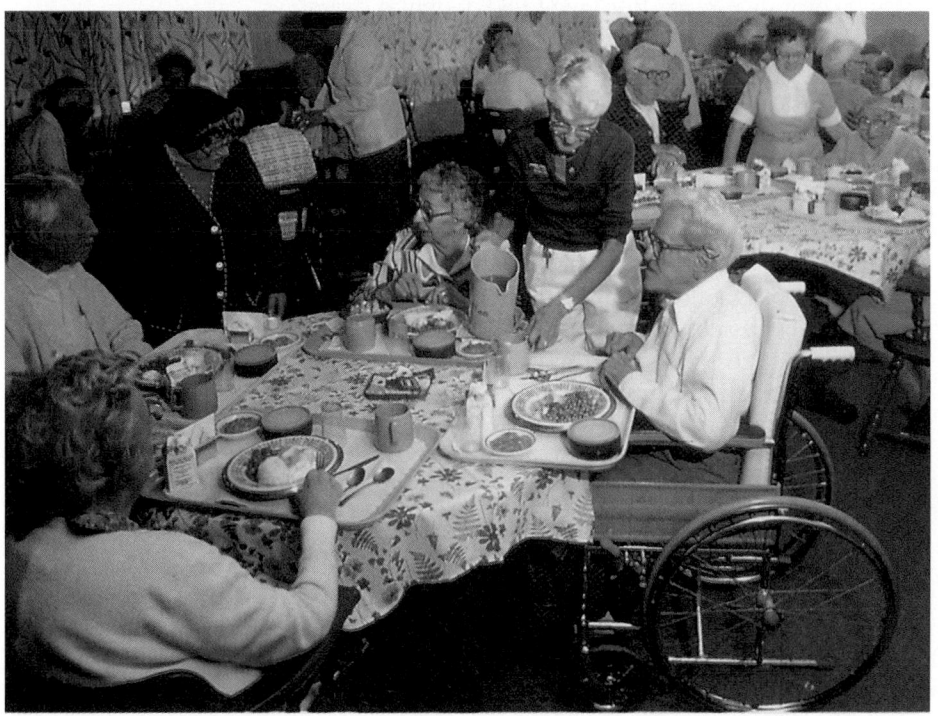

Figure 16-7
Congregate meals for older persons. Sites in many communities in the United States provide nutritious meals and an opportunity to socialize.

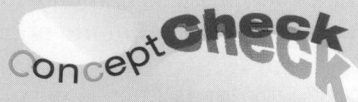

Nutritional problems common to aging adults relate to both the process of chronic diseases and the normal decrease in organ function that occurs with time. All these organ systems and functions can decrease as we age: appetite; sense of taste, smell, thirst, hearing, and sight; digestion and absorption; liver, gallbladder, pancreas, kidneys, lungs, heart; and the immune system. In addition, bone mass and muscle mass gradually decrease, the latter largely because of inactivity. Diet changes and regular physical activity can often help reduce the impact of these results of aging.

Summary

➤ A goal for all of us should be to delay symptoms of and disabilities from chronic diseases for as many years as possible. Good nutritional habits, especially those that follow the Food Guide Pyramid and Dietary Guidelines, play a role in this process.

➤ A basic plan for health promotion and disease prevention includes eating a proper diet that focuses on a variety of foods and moderation in fat intake, performing regular physical activity, consuming an adequate amount of fluids, abstaining from smoking, obtaining adequate sleep, and limiting alcohol intake.

➤ The Dietary Guidelines for Americans recommend that individuals eat a variety of foods; balance the food eaten with physical activity to maintain or improve weight; choose a diet with plenty of grain products, vegetables, and fruits; choose a diet low in fat, saturated fat, and cholesterol; choose a diet moderate in sugars; choose a diet moderate in salt and sodium; and, for those who drink alcoholic beverages, do so in moderation. In addition, specific recommendations to reduce cancer risk emphasize moderation in use of cured and smoked meats. Fluoride use can minimize risk of dental caries.

➤ Although maximum life span hasn't changed, life expectancy has increased dramatically over the past century. For many societies, this means that an increasing proportion of the population is over 65 years of age. As health care costs rise, the goal of delaying disease becomes even more important for all of us.

➤ Aging begins before birth. Cell aging probably results from automatic cellular changes and environmental influences, such as DNA damage. Add to this list damage caused by electron-seeking free-radical compounds, high blood glucose, hormonal changes, and alterations in the immune system as possible causes.

➤ Nutritional problems of older adults are related to the presence of chronic diseases and to the normal decreases in organ function that occur with time. These include loss of teeth, lessened sensitivity in the senses of taste and smell, changes in gastrointestinal tract function, and deterioration in heart and bone health. Although disease affects nutritional state, the reverse is also true. Undernutrition adversely affects immune function, allowing for infection.

➤ Alzheimer's disease is a progressive and irreversible brain disorder. Its causes are only beginnning to be understood. It differs from other types of senile dementia in that the brain tissue accumulates abnormal protein plaques and tangled nerves (observable by autopsy). Nutritional health for people in advanced stages of disease is often complicated by special feeding problems.

➤ Scientists are only now beginning extensive study of specific nutrient needs for older people. Diet plans should be based on a nutrient-dense approach and individualized for existing health problems, decreased physical abilities, presence of drug-nutrient interactions, possible depression, and economic constraints. Specific nutrients, such as protein, vitamin D, vitamin B-6, folate, vitamin B-12, zinc, and calcium, along with dietary fiber, often deserve special attention in diet planning.

Study Questions

1 Controversy surrounds the appropriateness of issuing recommendations for specific nutrient intakes, such as for sodium, to the general public. Describe the pros and cons of general dietary recommendations.

2 Define the term *reserve capacity* of organs, and describe how it tends to hide the early effects of aging.

3 Describe two hypotheses proposed to explain the causes of aging and note evidence for each in your daily life experiences.

4 List four organ systems that can decline in function in later years, along with a diet/lifestyle response to help cope with the decline.

5 Defend the recommendation for regular physical activity during late adulthood, including some resistance activity (weight training).

6 How might nutrition needs of older people differ from those of younger people? How are their needs similar? Be specific.

7 What three resources in a community are widely available to aid older adults in maintaining nutritional health?

8 Describe some early warning signs of Alzheimer's disease, and note some of the nutrition implications as this disease advances.

9 List four warning signs of undernutrition in older people that are part of the acronym "DETERMINE." Briefly justify the inclusion of each.

References

1 Barrocas A and others: Appropriate and effective use of NSI checklist and screens, *Journal of the American Dietetic Association* 95:467, 1995.

2 Cefalu WT and others: Contribution of visceral fat mass to the insulin resistance of aging, *Metabolism* 44:954, 1995.

3 Chandra R: Nutrition and immunity in the elderly: clinical significance, *Nutrition Reviews* 53(4):S80, 1995.

4 Chernoff R: Nutritional needs of elderly women. In Krummel DA, Kris-Etherton PM, editors: *Nutrition in women's health*, Gaithersburg, Md, 1995, Aspen Publishers.

5 Corder LS: Compression of disability: evidence from the national long-term care survey, *Nutrition Reviews* 54(1):S9, 1996.

6 Council on Scientific Affairs, American Medical Association: Alcoholism in the elderly, *Journal of the American Medical Association* 275:797, 1996.

7 Dwyer J: Strategies to detect and prevent malnutrition in the elderly: the nutrition screening initiative, *Nutrition Today* 29:14, 1994.

8 Evans WJ: Effects of aging and exercise on nutrition needs of the elderly, *Nutrition Reviews* 54(1):S35, 1996.

9 Fielding RA: The role of progressive resistance training and nutrition in the preservation of lean body mass in the elderly, *Journal of the American College of Nutrition* 14:587, 1995.

10 Hazzard WR: Weight control and exercise, *Journal of the American Medical Association* 274:1964, 1995.

11 Kritchevsky D: Caloric restriction and experimental tumorigenesis, *Nutrition Today*, p 25, Jan/Feb 1993.

12 Kurtzweil P: Growing older, eating better, *FDA Consumer*, p 12, March 1996.

13 Musto DF: Alcohol in American history, *Scientific American*, p 78, April 1996.

14 Pate RR and others: Physical activity and public health: a recommendation from the Centers for Disease Control and Prevention and the American College of Sports Medicine, *Journal of the American Medical Association* 273:402, 1995.

15 Reiman EM and others: Preclinical evidence of Alzheimer's disease in persons homozygous for the allele for apolipoprotein E, *New England Journal of Medicine* 334:752, 1996.

16 Rolls BJ and others: Age-related impairments in the regulation of food intake. *American Journal of Clinical Nutrition* 62:923, 1995.

17 Rosenberg IH: Keys to a longer, healthier, more vital life, *Nutrition Reviews* 52:S50, 1994.

18 Russell RM: Nutrition, *Journal of the American Medical Association* 273:1699, 1995.

19 Scrimshaw NS: Nutrition and health from womb to tomb, *Nutrition Today* 31:55, 1996.

20 Stephenson J: More evidence links NSAID, estrogen use with reduced Alzheimer's risk, *Journal of the American Medical Association* 275:1389, 1996.

21 Taylor A and others: Relations among aging, antioxidant status, and cataract, *American Journal of Clinical Nutrition* 62(suppl):1439S, 1995.

22 Thomas JA: Drug-nutrient interactions, *Nutrition Reviews* 53:271, 1995.

23 Troncale JA: The aging process, *Postgraduate Medicine* 99:111, 1996.

24 Tucker K: Micronutrient status and aging, *Nutrition Reviews* 53(9):S9, 1995.

25 Wallace JI and others: Involuntary weight loss in older outpatients: incidence and clinical significance, *Journal of the American Geriatric Society* 43:329, 1995.

26 Weinberg AD and others: Dehydration: evaluation and management in older adults, *Journal of the American Medical Association* 274:1552, 1995.

27 Weinruch R: Caloric restriction and aging, *Scientific American*, p 46, Jan 1996.

28 Wood RJ and others: Mineral requirements of elderly people, *American Journal of Clinical Nutrition* 62:493, 1995.

29 Zwanda ET: Malnutrition in the elderly, *Postgraduate Medicine* 100:207, 1996.

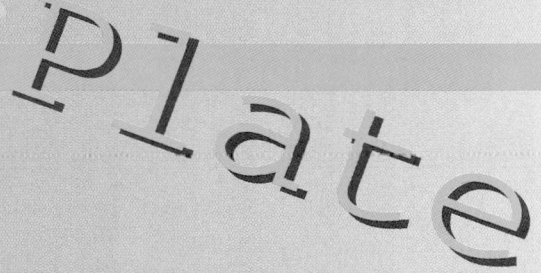
Helping Older Adults Eat Better

During their lifetimes, most people usually eat meals with families or loved ones. As elderly people reach even older ages, many of them are faced with living and eating alone. In a study of the diets of 4400 older Americans, one man in every five living alone and over age 55 ate poorly. One of four women between the ages of 55 and 64 years followed a low-quality diet. These poor diets can contribute to deteriorating mental and physical health. Consider the following example of the living situation of an older adult:

Neal, a 70-year-old man, lives alone in a house in a local suburban area. He lost his wife 1 year ago. He doesn't have many friends; his wife was his primary confidante. His neighbors across the street and next door are friendly, and Neal used to help them with yard projects in his spare time. Neal's health has been good, but he has had trouble with his teeth recently. His diet has been poor, and in the last 3 months his physical and mental vigor has deteriorated. He has been slowly lapsing into a depression and so keeps the shades drawn and rarely leaves his house. Neal keeps very little food in the house, because his wife did most of the cooking and shopping and he just isn't that interested in food.

If you were one of Neal's relatives and learned of Neal's situation, what six things could you do or suggest to help improve his nutritional status and mental outlook? Look back into the chapter to get some ideas.

1. _____

2. _____

3. _____

4. _____

5. _____

6. _____

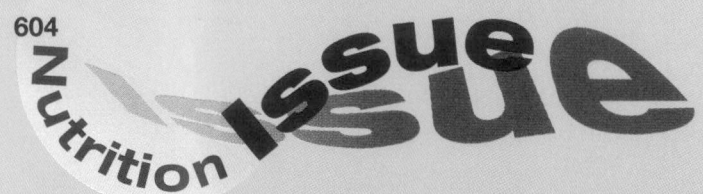

Alcohol—Metabolic, Nutritional, and Social Implications

Alcohol use is an issue requiring careful examination by all adults, including the aged.[6] Excessive consumption of alcohol is by far the most common drug abuse—wrecking families and friendships, spurring risky behaviors, spousal abuse, rape and other violence on college campuses, and filling jails. In 1990 its use cost American society an estimated 136 billion dollars and more than 65,000 lives, 22,000 of them from highway deaths. This accounts for as much as 20% of all health-care expenditures. About 15 million Americans currently have alcoholism; about 3 million are over age 60 years. From early adulthood through later years, excess alcohol intake has an enormous detrimental effect on nutritional and overall health.[13]

The American Medical Association defines alcoholism as an illness characterized by significant impairment directly related to persistent, excessive use of alcohol. Impairment can involve physiological, psychological, and social dysfunction. Causes of alcoholism include genetic, psychosocial, and environmental factors.

Some studies suggest that as much as 50% of a person's risk for alcoholism comes from genetic factors. Children of people with alcoholism have a fourfold increased risk of alcoholism, even when adopted by people with no history of alcoholism. This suggests that people with a family history of alcoholism need to be especially alert for evidence of the early signs of alcohol dependence.

Other studies question the importance of the genetic components. Children of people with alcoholism account for only a fraction of the alcohol abusers in the United States. Any one of us can become addicted if we drink long enough and hard enough.

After a person drinks an alcoholic beverage, the concentration of alcohol in the blood rises rapidly. Alcohol, technically known as *ethanol*, is readily absorbed into the blood from all parts of the gastrointestinal tract. You've probably been warned, with good reason, not to drink on an empty stomach. Alcohol absorption depends partly on the rate of stomach emptying. Food slows the stomach's emptying rate and stimulates secretions that dilute the alcohol and slow its absorption into the bloodstream.

METABOLISM

A social drinker who weighs 150 pounds and has normal liver function metabolizes about 7 to 14 grams (the equivalent of 1/2 to 1 12-ounce beer) of alcohol per hour (100 to 200 milligrams of alcohol per kilogram of body weight per hour). If a person drinks slightly less alcohol each hour than the amount that can be metabolized by the liver, the blood alcohol content remains low. In that case, a person can drink large amounts of alcohol over long periods without becoming noticeably intoxicated. When the rate of alcohol consumption exceeds the liver's metabolic capacity, the blood alcohol content rises and symptoms of intoxication appear (Table 16-7).

When a man and woman of similar size drink the same amount of alcohol, the woman retains more alcohol in her bloodstream; women cannot metabolize as much alcohol in their stomach cells. They have lower amounts of the key alcohol-metabolizing enzyme, alcohol dehydrogenase. Women are also much quicker to develop alcohol-related ailments, such as cirrhosis of the liver, than are men with the same drinking history.

Alcohol affects the brain more than any other organ. Acting as a sedative, alcohol tends to relieve the drinker's anxiety, cause slurred speech, reduce coordination in walking, impair judgment, and encourage uninhibited behavior. The mechanism for these effects is thought to be linked to changes in neurotransmitter synthesis and altered cell membrane fluidity in the brain. Because alcohol lowers inhibition, it appears to act as a stimulant, but in fact it is a powerful depressant. As William Shakespeare wrote, "It stirs up desire, but takes away the performance." Because it reduces secretion of the body's antidiuretic hormone, alcohol increases urination. It also causes the blood vessels to dilate, releasing body heat.

When a person drinks a lot of alcohol, the alcohol dehydrogenase in the liver cannot break it all down. For this and other reasons, another liver enzyme begins to metabolize alcohol. The liver usually uses the same system to metabolize medications and other "foreign" compounds to which the body is exposed. Once the extra system is activated, alcohol tolerance increases because the rate of alcohol metabolism increases.

> While the liver is metabolizing alcohol, it cannot rapidly metabolize medications, such as sedatives. Consequently, high amounts of alcohol mixed with some sedatives may cause a person to lapse into a coma and die.

ALCOHOL AND OVERALL HEALTH

About 32% of all Americans have three drinks or less each week, and about 22% have two drinks or less a day.

TABLE 16-7

Blood Alcohol Concentration and Symptoms

Concentration*	Sporadic drinker	Chronic drinker	Hours for alcohol to be metabolized
50 (party high)	Congenial euphoria; decreased tension	No observable effect	2-3
75	Gregarious	Often no effect	
100 (0.1%)	Uncoordinated; legally drunk (as in drunk driving) in most states; note that 0.08% is legal drunkenness in a growing number of areas in the United States	Minimal signs	4-6
125-150	Unrestrained behavior; episodic uncontrolled behavior; legally drunk at 0.15% in all states.	Pleasurable euphoria or beginning of uncoordination	6-10
200-250	Alertness lost; lethargic	Effort required to maintain emotional and motor control	10-24
300-350	Stupor to coma	Drowsy and slow	
> 500	Some will die	Coma	> 24

*Milligrams of alcohol per 100 milliliters of blood.
Modified from Wyngaarder JB, Smith LH: *Cecil textbook of medicine*, Philadelphia, 1988, WB Saunders.

Only about 11% have more than two drinks a day. Although the public health impact of alcohol abuse is still being calculated, misuse of alcohol, in and of itself, is one of the most preventable health problems in the United States. Excessive consumption of alcohol contributes significantly to 5 of the 10 leading causes of death in the United States—certain forms of cancer, cirrhosis of the liver, motor vehicle and other accidents, suicides, and homicides. Tobacco interacts with alcohol in a way that reinforces its effects in causing esophageal and oral cancer. In addition, excessive alcohol drinking increases the risk of some types of heart disease, high blood pressure (especially in African-Americans), nerve diseases, nutritional deficiencies (discussed later), damage to a pregnant woman's fetus, obesity, and many other disorders (Figure 16-8). A major cause of lasting mental retardation that begins in infancy stems from fetal exposure to alcohol[13] (see Chapter 14).

Social consequences of dependence on alcohol include family violence, divorce, unemployment, and poverty. An estimated 27 million American children are more likely to develop abnormally in psychosocial skills and relationships because their parents abuse alcohol.

All this must tell us—use alcohol cautiously and in moderation, if at all. Drinking even small amounts of alcohol can lead to dependence. Sometimes, there is only a fine line between social drinking and alcoholism.

People aged 20 to 40 drink the most alcohol. Excessive drinking often begins earlier; many high school seniors report having consumed alcohol in the past month; about 5% call themselves daily drinkers.

CIRRHOSIS

Long-term alcohol use causes fatty liver, alcoholic hepatitis, and cirrhosis. Cirrhosis is a chronic and usually relentlessly progressive disease characterized by fatty infiltration of the liver. Eventually the fat chokes off the blood supply, depriving the liver cells of oxygen and nutrients. Liver cells then die and are replaced by connective (scar) tissue. This scarring process is called *cirrhosis*. In America, most cases of cirrhosis are caused by alcohol consumption. Cirrhosis develops in about 12% to 31% of cases of alcoholism. In addition to the amount and duration of alcohol consumption, genetic factors and individual differences determine the body's response to alcohol. Once a person has cirrhosis, there is a 50% chance of death

Continued.

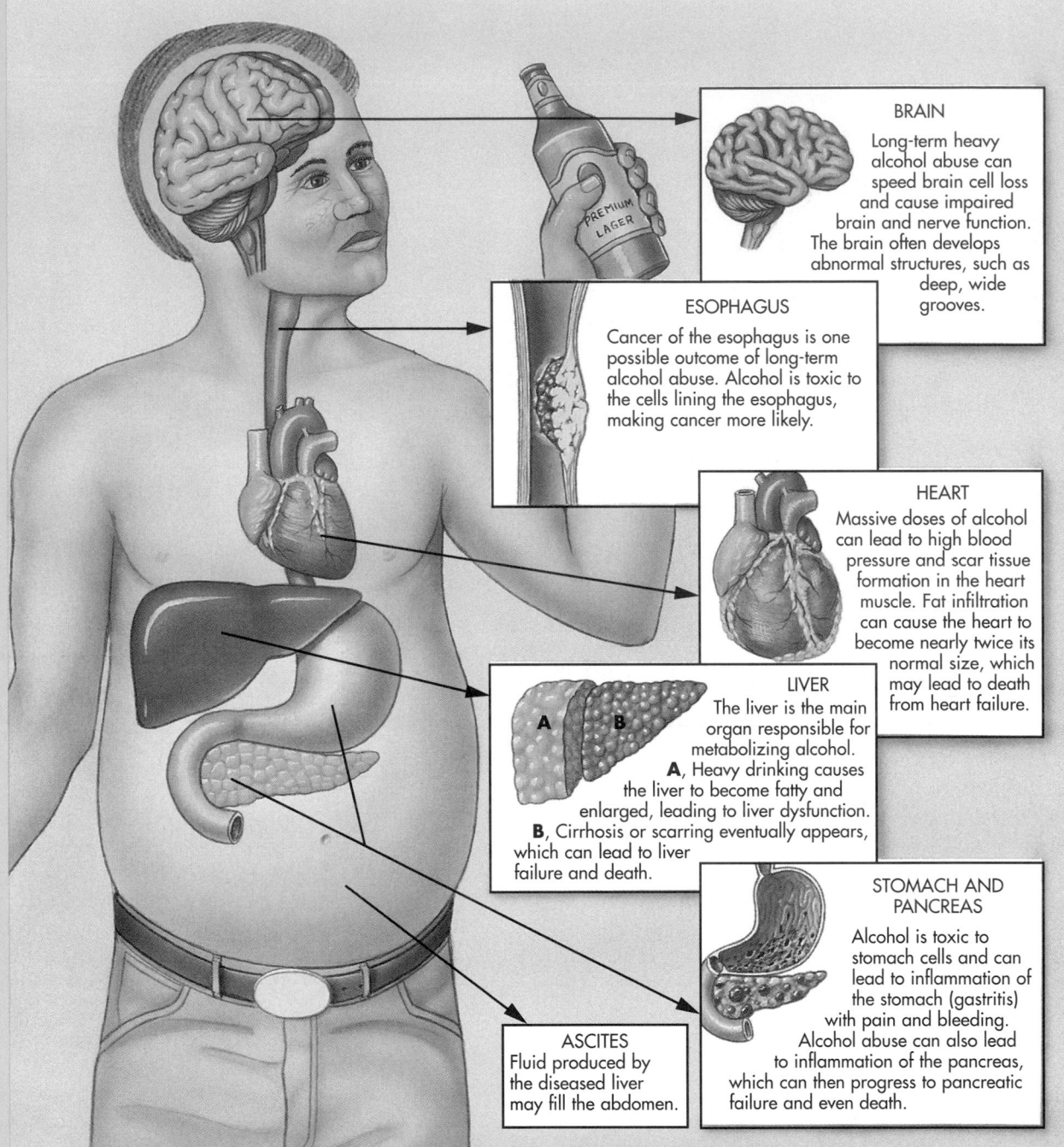

BRAIN

Long-term heavy alcohol abuse can speed brain cell loss and cause impaired brain and nerve function. The brain often develops abnormal structures, such as deep, wide grooves.

ESOPHAGUS

Cancer of the esophagus is one possible outcome of long-term alcohol abuse. Alcohol is toxic to the cells lining the esophagus, making cancer more likely.

HEART

Massive doses of alcohol can lead to high blood pressure and scar tissue formation in the heart muscle. Fat infiltration can cause the heart to become nearly twice its normal size, which may lead to death from heart failure.

LIVER

The liver is the main organ responsible for metabolizing alcohol. **A,** Heavy drinking causes the liver to become fatty and enlarged, leading to liver dysfunction. **B,** Cirrhosis or scarring eventually appears, which can lead to liver failure and death.

STOMACH AND PANCREAS

Alcohol is toxic to stomach cells and can lead to inflammation of the stomach (gastritis) with pain and bleeding. Alcohol abuse can also lead to inflammation of the pancreas, which can then progress to pancreatic failure and even death.

ASCITES

Fluid produced by the diseased liver may fill the abdomen.

Figure 16-8 *Effects of alcohol abuse on the body. The mind-altering effects of alcohol begin soon after it enters the bloodstream. Within minutes, alcohol numbs nerve cells in the brain. Heart muscle strains to cope with alcohol's depressive action. If drinking continues, rising blood alcohol causes impaired speech, vision, balance, and judgment. With an extremely high blood-alcohol contents, respiratory failure is possible. Over time, alcohol abuse increases the risk of liver and pancreas failure and certain forms of heart disease and cancer.*

within 4 years, which is a worse prognosis than in many forms of cancer. Most of the deaths from alcohol cirrhosis occur in people ages 40 to 54.

There are a number of possible mechanisms that underlie the liver damage from alcohol abuse, such as production of free radicals that damage liver cells. Other by-products of alcohol metabolism may also contribute to liver destruction.

No specific amount of alcohol consumption guarantees cirrhosis of the liver. Rather, some people are very susceptible to its effects, and others are not. One observable pattern is that cirrhosis commonly results from a 15-year consumption of approximately 80 grams of alcohol per day (Table 16-8). This is equivalent to seven beers per day. Some evidence suggests that the dose may be effective in causing cirrhosis when it's as low as 40 grams a day for men and 20 grams a day for women. Early stages of alcoholic liver injury are reversible, whereas advanced stages usually are not. The only known prevention for alcoholic cirrhosis is to limit consumption of alcohol.

A nutritious diet helps prevent some complications associated with alcoholism, but usually alcoholism wreaks serious destruction on the body in spite of an adequate diet. Laboratory animal studies show clearly that even when a nutritious diet is consumed, alcoholism can lead to cirrhosis. Still, deficient nutritional status compounds the problem of cirrhosis as it makes the liver more vulnerable to toxic substances by depleting supplies of antioxidants, such as vitamin E and vitamin C, which can reduce free radical damage to the liver if present in adequate amounts.

ALCOHOL AND NUTRITION

Nutritional problems in a person with alcoholism result from deficiencies of a variety of nutrients[6]:

- *Vitamin A deficiency,* which may be caused by a deficient diet and an inability of the liver to produce certain proteins. In addition, the chemical-detoxifying systems in the liver induced by chronic alcohol consumption may hasten the degradation of vitamin A in the liver.
- *Thiamin deficiency,* which can be caused by decreased thiamin absorption or decreased liver synthesis of the active thiamin coenzyme. People with alcoholism often exhibit nervous system problems similar to those seen in someone with a thiamin deficiency.
- *Niacin deficiency* and resulting pellagra caused by a deficient diet.
- *Vitamin B-6 deficiency,* probably stemming from a deficient dietary intake of the vitamin and increased breakdown of the vitamin B-6 coenzyme.
- *Folate deficiency,* which can be caused by a deficient diet and reduced nutrient absorption.
- *Vitamin D deficiency,* usually caused by the liver's decreased capacity to convert vitamin D into the final usable form. Alcohol may also encourage bone cell dysfunction, which diminishes bone formation and reduces bone mineralization. This can lead to osteoporosis.

TABLE 16-8

Energy, Carbohydrate, and Alcohol Content of Alcoholic Beverages*

Beverage	Amount (ounce)	Alcohol (grams)	Carbohydrates (grams)	Energy (kcal)
BEER				
Regular	12	13	13	146
Light	12	11	5	99
DISTILLED				
Gin, rum, vodka, whiskey, tequila	1.5	15	—	105
Brandy, cognac	1.0	9	—	64
WINE				
Red	3	8	2	64
White	3	8	1	60
Dessert, sweet	3	14	11	138
Rosé	3	8	1	63
MANHATTAN	3	26	3	191
MARTINI	3	27	—	189
BOURBON & SODA	3	11	—	78
WHISKEY SOUR	3	15	5	122

*There is little to no fat or protein contribution to energy content.
From Mosby's NutriTrac, Positive Input Corp.

Alcoholic beverages are high in food energy and low in or devoid of essential nutrients.

Continued.

- *Vitamin C deficiency,* resulting primarily from a decrease in dietary intake or from altered liver metabolism, or both.
- *Vitamin K deficiency,* probably occurring because less of the vitamin is synthesized by intestinal bacteria, less is consumed, and less is absorbed.

GENERAL GUIDELINES FOR ALCOHOL USE

Neither the Surgeon General's office, the National Academy of Science, nor the USDA/DHHS recommends drinking alcohol. All groups caution that if adults do consume alcohol, they should (1) drink alcohol only in moderation with meals (no more than two drinks a day for men and one for women); (2) avoid drinking any alcohol before or while driving, operating machinery, taking medications, or engaging in any other activity requiring sound judgment; and (3) avoid drinking alcohol while pregnant. Although this obviously isn't a plea for teetotalers to start drinking, people who have a drink or so a day and are not prone to abuse should know that there's nothing wrong with moderate drinking as long as they aren't putting themselves or others at risk. In fact, there are some benefits to moderate alcohol intake, such as a reduction in the risk of coronary heart disease. The effective dose of alcohol is between one half and three drinks a day. No further benefit can be seen for consumption beyond that amount. The reason for this reduction in coronary heart disease risk is still debatable but probably involves an increase in HDL concentration and a reduction in blood clotting and overall stress. Certain compounds in red wine may also act as antioxidants and thus may make this source of alcohol more potent in reducing coronary artery disease risk than others.

Unfortunately, however, when some of us allow ourselves to drink, we end up drinking too much. Furthermore, people who regularly take certain medications (such as aspirin and related substances or anticonvulsants) or who have diabetes or ulcers should consult a physician if they choose to drink.[6]

DO YOU HAVE A PROBLEM WITH ALCOHOL?

Asking a person about the quantity and frequency of alcohol consumption is an important means of detecting abuse and dependence. The following questionnaire (CAGE) is popular for use in routine health care.

CAGE QUESTIONNAIRE TO SCREEN FOR ALCOHOL ABUSE

C: Have you ever felt you ought to *Cut* down on drinking?

A: Have people *Annoyed* you by criticizing your drinking?

G: Have you ever felt bad or *Guilty* about your drinking?

E: Have you ever had a drink first thing in the morning to steady your nerves or get rid of a hangover *(Eye-opener)?*

More than one positive response to the CAGE questionnaire suggests an alcohol problem. Another key point to probe is tolerance. Does it take more to make you inebriated than it did in the past?

TREATMENT

Once a diagnosis of alcohol abuse or dependence is established, a physician should arrange appropriate treatment and counseling for the patient and family. An important goal of counseling is to identify ways to compensate for loss of pleasures from drinking. This helps the drinker confront the immediate problem of how to stop the drinking. Total abstinence must be the ultimate objective. For people with alcoholism, there is no such thing as "controlled drinking." A problem drinker cannot return safely to social drinking. The person should enter an Alcoholics Anonymous (AA) program or a reputable therapy program for people with alcoholism (one can check with a local mental health treatment center for programs available in the community or call 800-245-4656). The spouse should join the treatment program as well. Success is usually proportionate to participation in AA, other social agencies' programs, and religious counseling. About 2 years of treatment should be expected.

Current research does not support the generally negative public opinion about the prognosis for alcoholism. In most industrial alcoholism treatment programs, where workers are socially stable and—because of the risk to jobs and pensions—well motivated, recovery rates run at 60% or more. This remarkably high recovery rate is probably accounted for by early detection. Once a person moves from problem drinking to an advanced stage of alcoholism, success rates seldom exceed 40% to 50%. Early identification and intervention remain the most important steps in the treatment of alcoholism.

The medication disulfiram (Antabuse) can help the person with alcoholism to make the essential decision to stop drinking. An early step in alcohol metabolism is blocked by the action of this drug. As a result, a highly toxic alcohol by-product accumulates in the blood, producing nausea, vomiting, diffuse flushing, and a shocklike reaction. FDA recently approved naltrexone (Revia) as another agent to aid in the treatment of alcohol dependence. This agent reduces the craving for alcohol and blunts the associated inebriation ("high") from alcohol intake. However, neither medication substitutes for a comprehensive treatment plan, such as Alcoholics Anonymous.

NUTRITION
Beyond the Nutrients

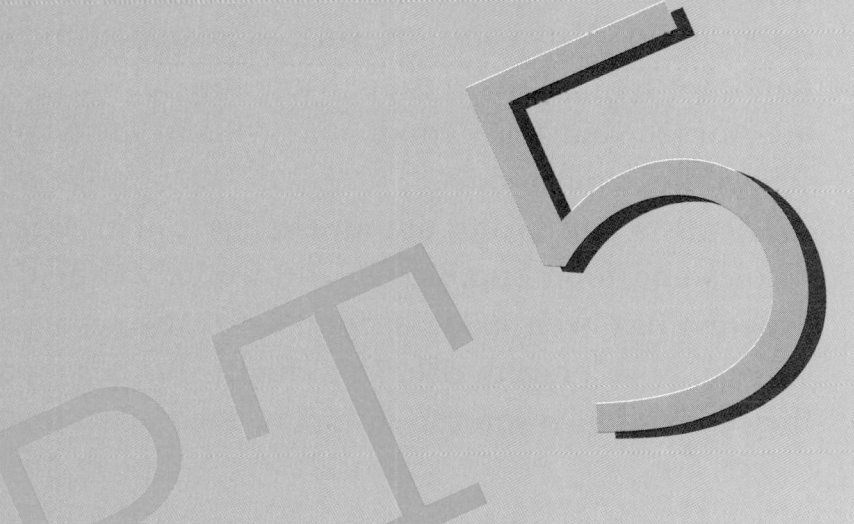

PART 5

Food Safety

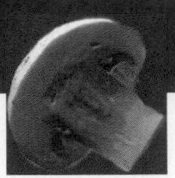

AT THE TURN OF THE CENTURY, conditions in Chicago's meat-packing industry were sickening. Moldy, spoiled meat was commonly doused with borax to cover up the smell, and glycerine was added to make it look fresh. By 1906 increasing public pressure forced the passage of the first Food and Drug Act in the United States. Federal inspection then safeguarded the public from worm-infested and diseased meat and generally improved food preparation standards.[28]

Today food safety warnings appear everywhere. Attention has turned to more contemporary food safety concerns, such as microbial and chemical contamination. On the one hand, we are told to eat more fruits, vegetables, fish, and poultry; on the other hand, we are warned that these foods may contain dangerous substances. So we still must ask, "How safe is our food?"

Scientists and health authorities agree that Americans enjoy one of the safest, most wholesome food supplies in the world.[11] Over the past 90 or so years, tremendous progress has been made in food safety. Nonetheless, microbes and chemicals in foods still can pose a health risk. This chapter focuses on these food-related hazards—how real they are and how you can minimize their effect on your life.

Test Your Food Safety Knowledge

Take this quiz to see how aware you are about the safety of some basic foods. Place a check in the appropriate column to indicate whether you think the item is safe or risky to eat.

		Safe	Risky
1.	Hot dogs that have been stored unopened in the refrigerator for over 7 days	✓	
2.	A bruised piece of fruit	✓	
3.	Frozen hamburger that was thawed on the counter	✓	✗
4.	An opened jar of mayonnaise that has been in the refrigerator for 3 months		✓
5.	A foil-covered baked potato left out on the counter since the night before	✓	✗
6.	Meat loaf that's pink in the middle after cooking		✓
7.	Raw ground beef that turns brown after 1 to 2 days of refrigeration	✓	
8.	An uncooked potato with a greenish cast, cooked and then eaten with the peel left on		✓
9.	Lettuce moistened by poultry drippings in a grocery bag	✓	✗
10.	Steak that was thawed in the refrigerator and then refrozen with some ice crystals still present	✓	
11.	Cooked shrimp that was never deveined	✓	
12.	Mustard or ketchup with a black, crusty ring around the rim of the jar	✓	
13.	Moldy or shriveled peanuts		✓

Now that you've completed this assessment, compare your responses with the answers below.

SAFE: 1, 2, 4, 7, 10, 11, 12.
RISKY: 3, 5, 6, 8, 9, 13.

Answering these questions may have been hard for you. Many people don't know much about preserving, handling, and cooking food to avoid significant illness. In this chapter you'll find explanations of the safety or risk of consuming these foods.

Key Chapter Concepts

- Bacteria and other microbes in food pose the greatest risk for food-borne illness. In the past, salt, sugar, smoke, fermentation, and drying were used to protect against food-borne illness. Today careful cooking, pasteurization, and temperature control (keeping hot foods hot and cold foods cold) provide additional insurance.

- Cross-contamination, the transfer of microbes from one food to another, commonly causes food-borne illness, especially when bacteria on raw animal products contact foods that can support their growth. Because of the risk of cross-contamination, no perishable food should be kept at room temperature for more than 1 to 2 hours (depending on the environmental temperature), especially if the food may have come in contact with raw animal products.

- Treatment for food-borne illness usually requires drinking lots of fluids, avoiding contact with food while diarrhea is present, washing hands thoroughly, and getting bed rest. Botulism and hepatitis are two types of food-borne illness that require prompt medical attention.

- Food additives are used primarily to extend shelf life by preventing microbial growth and destruction of food components by oxygen, metals, and other substances. In most cases the Delaney Clause allows FDA to ban manufacturers from adding to foods any substance that causes cancer.

- Certain food additives, such as antioxidants, prevent oxygen and enzyme destruction of food products. Other preservatives prevent bacterial growth. Sequestrants bind metals and thus prevent spoilage of food from metal contamination. Emulsifiers suspend fat in water, improving the uniformity, smoothness, and body of foods such as ice cream.

- Toxic substances occur naturally in a variety of foods, such as green potatoes, raw fish, and mushrooms. In many cases, cooking foods limits their toxic effects. Over the centuries, people have purposely avoided some of these foods, such as toxic mushroom species and the green parts of potatoes.

- A variety of environmental contaminants can be found in foods. Because most of them are fat soluble, exposure can be minimized by trimming fat from meats and discarding fat that is rendered during cooking of meats, fish, and poultry. In addition, it's helpful to wash fruits and vegetables thoroughly and discard the outer leaves of leafy vegetables.

Setting the Stage

Pasteurization

The process of heating food products to kill pathogenic microorganisms. One method heats milk at 161° F for at least 20 seconds.

Bacteria

A group of single-cell microorganisms, some of which produce poisonous substances called toxins that cause illness in humans. They contain only one chromosome and lack many organelles found in human cells. Bacteria produce enzymes that can digest substances around them. Some can live without oxygen and survive harsh conditions by means of spore formation.

During the early stages of urbanization in the United States, contaminated water and food—notably milk—were responsible for many large outbreaks of typhoid fever, septic sore throat, scarlet fever, diphtheria, and other devastating human diseases. These experiences led to the development of processes for purifying water, treating sewage, and **pasteurizing** milk. Since that time, safe water and milk have become universally available, with only rare problems from either. The greatest health risk from food is contamination from **bacteria** and, to a lesser extent, from various forms of **fungi** and **viruses**. These microbes can all cause **food-borne illness**. Even though microbial contamination is the cause of most incidents of food-borne illness, however, Americans seem more concerned about health risks from chemicals in foods.[19] Of consumers surveyed in a recent Gallup poll, about 75% said that pesticide contamination was a major concern to them. In the long run, this concern has some merit. On a day-to-day basis, however, only about 4% of all cases of food-borne illness in the United States are caused by food additives.

Microbial contamination of food is by far the more important issue for our day-to-day health and so will be discussed first. This chapter then covers the use and safety of food additives.

FOOD-BORNE ILLNESS

About one third to one half of all cases of diarrhea in the United States, upward of 33 million each year, are induced by food-borne organisms. According to recent estimates, diarrhea caused by these agents afflicts about 1 in 8 Americans each year, at a cost of up to $23 billion annually in medical expenses and lost productivity, and leads to about 9000 deaths. Clearly, microbes in food remain a considerable health risk.[17]

Most of us experience a brief but distressing episode of diarrhea from food-borne illness, such as so-called traveler's diarrhea. Food-borne illness generally presents no real long-term health risk for the average person, but for many it can be serious. Some people suffer greatly from food-borne illness, including the following:

- Infants and children
- The elderly
- Those with liver disease, diabetes, or HIV infection (and AIDS)
- Cancer patients
- Pregnant women
- People taking immunosuppresant agents

Some bouts of food-borne illness, coupled with the previous conditions, are lengthy and lead to food allergies, seizures, blood poisoning (from **toxins** or microbes in the bloodstream), or other illnesses.[27]

Because food-borne illness often results from unsafe handling of food at home, we each bear some responsibility for preventing food-borne illness (Table 17-1). Usually you can't tell by taste, smell, or sight that a particular food contains harmful microbes, so you might not even be aware that food caused your distress. In fact, however, your last case of diarrhea may have been caused by something you ate.

TABLE 17-1

The World Health Organization's Golden Rules for Safe Food Preparation

1. Choose foods processed for safety
2. Cook food thoroughly
3. Eat cooked foods immediately
4. Store cooked foods carefully
5. Reheat cooked foods thoroughly
6. Avoid contact between raw and cooked foods
7. Wash hands repeatedly
8. Keep all kitchen surfaces meticulously clean
9. Protect foods from insects, rodents, and other animals
10. Use pure water

Why Is Food-Borne Illness So Common?

The risk of contracting food-borne illness is high, because—in addition to problems from consumers' mishandling food—recent trends have added new causes. First, there is greater consumer interest in eating foods of animal origin raw or under-cooked.[16] In addition, more people receive medication that suppresses their ability to combat food-borne infectious agents. Another factor is the continuing increase of the elderly population.

Furthermore, the food industry tries where possible to increase the shelf life of products. A longer shelf life at room temperature allows more time for bacteria in foods to multiply. Some bacteria grow even at refrigeration temperatures. Partially

Food contamination presents a unique risk to the eldery for a variety of reasons. Poor eyesight and reduced senses of smell and taste may make it harder to spot spoiled food or dirty utensils. Their reduced appetite can lead to a weakened immune system. The elderly face further risks because their stomachs may be low in acid, which destroys harmful bacteria, and because of poor blood circulation, which can prevent antibodies from reaching sites of infection.

Fungi
Simple parasitic life forms including molds, mildews, yeasts, and mushrooms. They live on dead or decaying organic matter. Fungi can grow as single cells, like yeast, or as a multicellular colony as seen with molds.

Virus
The smallest known type of infectious agent. Many viruses cause disease in humans. They do not metabolize, grow, or move by themselves. They reproduce by the aid of a living cellular host. Viruses are essentially a piece of genetic material surrounded by a coat of protein.

Food-borne illness
Sickness caused by ingestion of food containing toxic substances produced by microorganisms.

Nutrition **Insight**

Protecting the U.S. Food Supply

A variety of federal, state, and local agencies in the United States monitor food safety. Some of the agencies involved are:

United States Department of Agriculture (USDA)

USDA enforces standards for wholesomeness and quality of grains, produce, meat, poultry, milk, and eggs produced in the United States through inspection and grading. As part of this effort, more than 7000 inspectors visually examine the carcasses of more than 120 million animals a year in an effort to keep obviously diseased meat from going to market. USDA also routinely monitors animal foods for antibiotics. Once the food product leaves the field and enters into food production and distribution, FDA takes over for all foods containing less than 2% meat or poultry. Foods containing more remain under USDA jurisdiction. USDA now requires companies to put a "Safe Handling Label" on meat and poultry products (see page 622). The labels explain how to properly handle, cook, and store these products.

Bureau of Alcohol, Tobacco, and Firearms (ATF)

ATF is responsible for enforcing laws that cover the production, distribution, and labeling of most alcoholic beverages. This agency and FDA sometimes share responsibility in cases of adulteration, or when an alcoholic beverage contains food or color additives, pesticides, or contaminants.

Environmental Protection Agency (EPA)

EPA regulates pesticides. EPA must approve all pesticides before they are sold in the United States. It determines the safety of new pesticide products and sets allowable limits for pesticide residue in foods. This limit is not necessarily the maximal safe amount of a pesticide in a food; EPA sets limits no higher than needed for a product's intended use. These amounts are then enforced by FDA. EPA also establishes water quality standards, including those for drinking water.[28]

Food and Drug Administration (FDA)

FDA is responsibile for ensuring the safety and wholesomeness of all foods sold in interstate commerce (except meat and poultry, which are primarily under USDA jurisdiction).[28] Follow their actions by reading *FDA Consumer*.

FDA is primarily responsible for the regulation of seafood and has been committing more resources to this task. FDA has about 350 inspectors to monitor seafood processing plants and imported seafood, oversee the National Shellfish Sanitation Program, sample and test seafood products, enforce labeling requirements, and provide education on seafood issues. FDA works with individual states to implement these regulatory programs.

FDA also sets standards for specific foods and enforces federal regulations for labeling food, color additives, food sanitation, and food safety. The agency inspects food plants, imported food products, and mills that make feeds containing medications or nutritional supplements for animals destined for human consumption. Over 90,000 businesses are inspected each year; about half are food-related businesses.

FDA acts primarily when the public health is endangered, for example, when proper medical care is being discouraged in favor of quackery. It regulates products, not people. FDA cannot control what people say, just what is on a product's label and how it is promoted. FDA gives low priority to products that are simply economically deceptive, such as weight-loss gimmicks.

To monitor foods for contaminants, FDA routinely samples items of dietary importance, such as produce. Foods suspected of containing illegal residues receive a more intensive evaluation. An important part of FDA's safety sampling is a "market basket" study of foods that typify the American diet. Four times a year, identical purchases of 234 foods, including processed foods, are analyzed for pesticide residues, radioactive elements, toxic metals, and other undesirable substances. Imported foods with illegal residues can be refused entry into the country.

Traditionally, FDA does not regularly inspect food-processing plants. It relies instead on its "Good Manufacturer's Procedures" plan that food processors and manufacturers are expected to follow. FDA inspectors may visit a specific food-processing establishment only infrequently. The agency relies on consumer complaints to alert it to potential dangers, then it researches these in greater detail. FDA simply doesn't have enough staff to conduct frequent, thorough inspections of every facility that is subject to federal regulation.

Centers for Disease Control and Prevention (CDC)

A branch of the Department of Health and Human Services, CDC becomes involved as a protector of food safety, including responding to emergencies when food-borne diseases are a factor. CDC surveys and studies environmental health problems. It directs and enforces quarantines, and it administers national programs for prevention and control of vector-borne diseases (diseases transmitted by a host organism) and other preventable conditions.

National Marine Fishery Service

This agency is part of the Department of Commerce. It is responsible for overseeing fisheries management and harvesting. It provides a voluntary program for inspection and grading of fish products. Its guidelines closely match regulations for which FDA has enforcement authority.

State and Local Government

States inspect restaurants, retail food establishments, dairies, grain processing plants, and other food-related establishments within their borders. States have the primary responsibility for milk safety. FDA provides guidelines to state and local governments for regulating dairy products and restaurants.[12]

Foreign Governments

Governments of at least 40 nations are now partners with the United States in ensuring food safety through agreements that cover 24 food products, including shellfish. International cooperation in food inspection and regulatory standards is expanding.

As noted earlier, the limited budgets of government enforcement agencies at all levels limit the number and thoroughness of inspections. More money is being devoted to this effort, but it still falls short of what is needed. This means individuals must assume some responsibility for their protection. We must remain alert in cases of apparent abuse and contact the appropriate government agency. Finally, we must promote safe food practices in our daily lives.

International label for noting prior irradiation of the food product.

of drying drives off free water. Bacteria need abundant stores of water to grow; yeasts and molds can grow with less water, but some is still necessary.

Decreasing the water content of some high-moisture foods, however, causes them to lose essential characteristics. To preserve such foods—cucumber pickles, sauerkraut, milk (yogurt), and wine—fermentation has been a traditional alternative. Selected bacteria are used to ferment or pickle foods. The fermenting bacteria make acids and alcohol, which minimize the growth of other microbes. The acid produced is especially helpful in preventing the growth of the deadly bacterium *Clostridium botulinum.*

Today we can add **pasteurization**, sterilization, refrigeration, freezing, **irradiation**, canning, and chemical preservatives to the list of food preservation techniques. A new method of food preservation—**aseptic processing**—simultaneously sterilizes the food and package separately before the food enters the package. Liquid foods, such as fruit juices, are especially easy to process in this manner. With aseptic packaging, boxes of sterile milk and juices can remain on supermarket shelves, free of microbial growth, for many years.

Food irradiation is also a fairly recent development. For over a decade FDA has permitted limited irradiation of certain food products. The radiation used does not make the food radioactive. However, the energy is strong enough to break chemical bonds, destroy cell walls and cell membranes, break down DNA, and link proteins together. Irradiation thereby controls growth of insects, microorganisms, and parasites in foods. This practice extends the shelf life and enhances the safety of spices, dry vegetable seasonings, pork and poultry products, and fresh fruits and vegetables.[1]

Irradiated food, except for dried seasonings, must be so labeled (see margin). Foods treated this way are safe in the opinion of FDA and many other health authorities. Japan, France, Italy, and Mexico all use food irradiation technology. To date, consumer acceptance of food irradiation in the United States is mixed. Certain consumer groups continually try to block its use. Continued attempts to employ this technology are likely, but whether the public will accept it as it does canning (which also originally met with skepticism) remains to be seen.

Food-Borne Illness: When Undesirable Microbes Alter Foods

In 1871 an Italian scientist named Selmi proposed that food-borne illness was caused by ptomaines, breakdown residues of proteins produced during bacterial spoilage of food. Although people still refer to ptomaine poisoning, scientists have long since rejected Selmi's theory because ptomaines are not as poisonous as was once assumed. Today scientists know that food-borne illness is caused by specific toxin-producing bacteria and other microbes. These organisms cause health problems either directly by invading the intestinal wall and producing an infection or indirectly by producing a toxin in the food that later harms us (called an *intoxication*).[23]

Many different types of bacteria cause food-borne illness, such as *Bacillus, Campylobacter, Clostridium, Escherichia, Listeria, Vibrio, Yersinia, Salmonella,* and *Staphylococcus.*[27] Because each teaspoon of soil contains about 2 billion bacteria, we are constantly at risk for food-borne illness. Luckily, only a small number of all bacteria actually pose a threat. Determining which microbe has caused an incident entails identifying the clinical features of the outbreak, the incubation period for symptoms, and the food source (see Table 17-2).

General Rules for Preventing Food-Borne Illness

You can greatly reduce the risk of food-borne illness by following some very important rules. It's a long list, because many risky habits need to be addressed.[17]

Purchasing Food

- When shopping, select frozen foods and perishable foods last, such as meat, poultry, or fish. Always have these products put in separate plastic bags so that drippings don't contaminate other foods in the shopping cart. Then, don't let groceries sit in a warm car; this allows bacteria to grow. Get the perishable foods home and promptly refrigerate or freeze.
- Don't buy or use food from flawed containers that leak, bulge, or are severely dented or buy or use food from jars that are cracked or have loose or bulging lids. Don't taste or use food that has a foul odor or spurts liquid when the can is opened; the deadly *Clostridium botulinum* toxin may be present.
- Purchase only pasteurized milk and cheese. This is especially important for pregnant women because highly toxic bacteria and viruses that can harm the fetus thrive in unpasteurized milk.

Preparing Food

- Thoroughly wash hands with hot, soapy water before and after handling food. This practice is especially important when handling raw meat, fish, poultry, or eggs.
- Make sure counters, cutting boards, dishes, and other equipment are thoroughly cleaned and rinsed before use. Be especially careful to use hot, soapy water to wash surfaces and equipment that have come in contact with raw meat, fish, poultry, and eggs as soon as possible to remove *Salmonella* bacteria that may be present.
- If possible, cut foods to be eaten raw on a clean cutting board reserved for that purpose. Then clean this cutting board using hot, soapy water. If the same board must be used for both meat and other foods, cut the raw items before cutting any potentially contaminated items, such as meat. After cutting the meat, wash the cutting board thoroughly.

  USDA recommends cutting boards with unmarred surfaces that are made of easy-to-clean, nonporous materials, such as plastic, marble, or glass. If you prefer a wooden board, reserve it for a specific purpose; for example, set it aside for cutting raw meat and poultry. Then keep a separate board for chopping produce or slicing bread to prevent these products from picking up bacteria from raw meat. Note that many foods are served raw, so any bacteria clinging to them are not destroyed.

  Furthermore, USDA recommends that all cutting boards, plastic or wood, be replaced when they become streaked with hard-to-clean grooves or cuts, which may harbor bacteria. In addition, both wood and plastic boards should be sanitized once a week in a solution of 2 teaspoons chlorine bleach per quart of water. Flood the board with the solution, let it sit a few minutes, and then rinse thoroughly.
- When thawing foods, do so in the refrigerator for 1 to 3 days, under cold running water or in a microwave oven. Never let frozen foods thaw unrefrigerated all day or night. Also, marinate food in the refrigerator.
- Avoid coughing or sneezing over foods, even when you're healthy. Cover cuts on hands with a sterile bandage. This helps stop *Staphylococcus* from entering food.
- Carefully wash fresh fruit and vegetables under running water to remove dirt and bacteria clinging to the surface. Use a vegetable brush for potatoes if the skin is to be eaten. People recently became ill from *Salmonella* that was introduced from melons used in making a fruit salad and from oranges used for fresh-squeezed orange juice. The bacteria were on the outside of the melons and oranges.
- Completely remove moldy portions of food or don't eat the food. **When in doubt, throw the food out.** Mold growth is prevented by properly storing food at cold temperatures and using the food within a reasonable length of time (Figure 17-1).

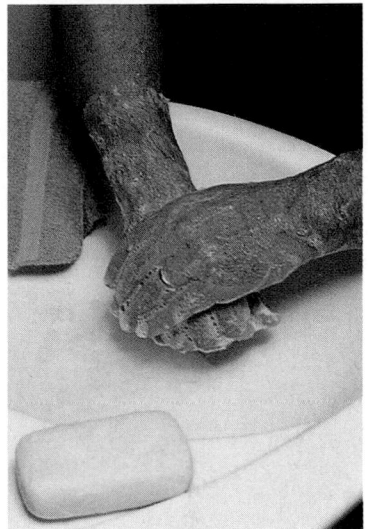

Washing hands thoroughly with hot water and soap should be the first step in food preparation.

Jon wants to buy a cutting board for his new kitchen. He's been looking at all the possibilities: Plexiglass, plastic, and wood. How would you advise him so that he can minimize the risk of any food-borne illness from his food preparation?

THE MIDDLETONS

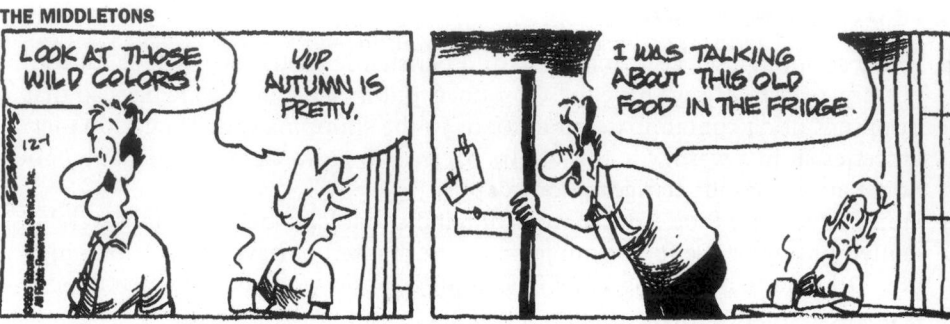

Figure 17-1 *The Middletons.*

- Use refrigerated ground meat and patties in 1 to 2 days and frozen meat and patties within 3 to 4 months.

Cooking Food

- Cook food thoroughly, especially beef, fish, and pork (160° F [71° C]), poultry (180° F [82° C]), and eggs (until the yolk and white are hard). Cooking destroys most food-borne bacteria, such as toxic strains of *Escherichia coli*, whereas freezing only halts growth. A good general precaution is to eat no raw animal products. Chickens are often contaminated by *Salmonella*, which is killed by thorough cooking (white flesh, not pink). Undercooked pork can allow infection by the parasite that causes trichinosis. USDA answers questions about safe use of animal products (800-535-4555, 10 AM to 4 PM weekdays, Eastern time).

  Seafood also poses a risk of food-borne illness. Properly cooked fish should flake easily and be opaque or dull and firm. If it's translucent or shiny, it's not done.

  Raw fish dishes, such as sushi, can be safe for most people to eat if they are made with very fresh fish that is commercially frozen and then thawed. The freezing is important to eliminate protential health risks from parasites. FDA recommends that the fish be frozen to an internal temperature of −10° F for 7 days. If you choose to eat uncooked fish, purchase the fish from reputable establishments that have high standards for quality and sanitation. People at high risk for food-borne illness would be wise to avoid raw fish products (Figure 17-2).

  Many people, especially those with liver disease, fall ill each year from eating raw shellfish. Clams and oysters may contain bacteria that can cause severe food-borne illness.[16,22]

- Cook stuffing separately from poultry (or wash poultry thoroughly, stuff immediately before cooking, and then transfer the stuffing to a clean bowl immediately after cooking). Make sure the stuffing reaches 165° F (74° C). Again, *Salmonella* is the major concern with poultry.

- Once a food is cooked, consume it right away, or cool it to 40° F (4° C) within 2 hours. If it is not to be eaten immediately, in hot weather (85° F and above) make sure this cooling is done within 1 hour. Do this by separating the food into as many shallow pans as needed to provide a large surface area. Be careful not to recontaminate cooked food by contact with raw meat or juices from hands, cutting boards, dirty utensils, or in other ways.

- Serve meat, poultry, and fish on a clean plate—never the same plate that was used to hold the raw product. For example, when grilling hamburgers, don't put cooked items on the same plate that was used to carry the raw product out to the grill.

- Cook food completely at the picnic site, with no partial cooking in advance.

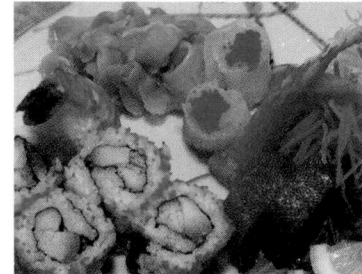

Figure 17-2
Sushi, like all raw fish or meat dishes, is a high-risk food. For maximum protection from food-borne illness, animal foods should be cooked thoroughly before eating. If you choose to eat uncooked fish, purchase fish from reputable establishments that have high standards for quality and sanitation. People at high risk for food-borne illness would be wise to avoid these products.

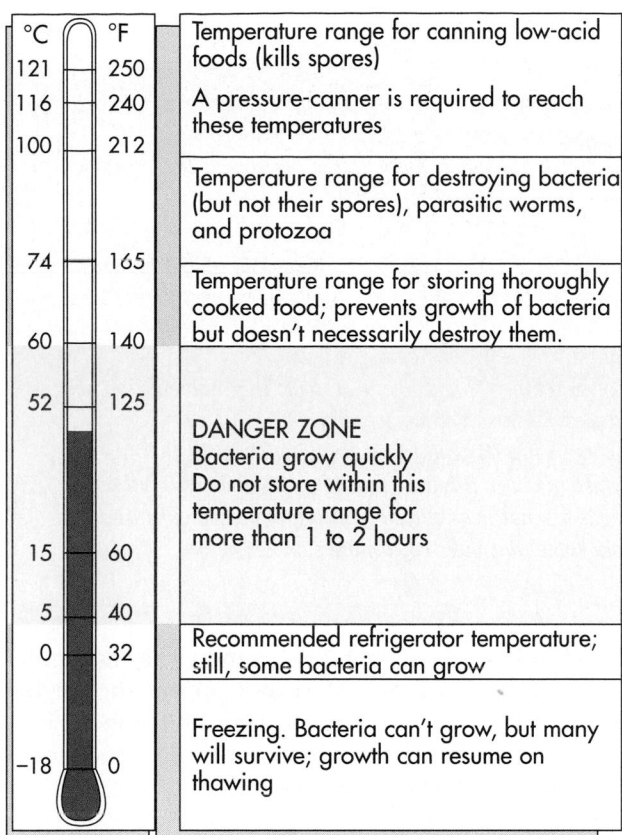

°C	°F	
121	250	Temperature range for canning low-acid foods (kills spores)
116	240	A pressure-canner is required to reach these temperatures
100	212	
		Temperature range for destroying bacteria (but not their spores), parasitic worms, and protozoa
74	165	
		Temperature range for storing thoroughly cooked food; prevents growth of bacteria but doesn't necessarily destroy them.
60	140	
52	125	DANGER ZONE Bacteria grow quickly Do not store within this temperature range for more than 1 to 2 hours
15	60	
5	40	
0	32	Recommended refrigerator temperature; still, some bacteria can grow
−18	0	Freezing. Bacteria can't grow, but many will survive; growth can resume on thawing

Figure 17-3 *Effects of temperature on microbes that cause food-borne illness. (Adapted from* Temperature guide to food safety: food and home notes, No. 25, *Washington, DC, June 20, 1977, USDA.)*

Storing and Reheating Cooked Food

- Keep hot foods hot and cold foods cold. Hold food below 40° F (4° C) or above 140° F (60° C) (Figure 17-3). Food-borne illness microbes thrive in more moderate temperatures (60° to 110° F [16° to 43° C]). Some microbes can even grow in the refrigerator. Again, don't leave cooked or refrigerated foods, such as meats and salads, at room temperature for more than 2 hours (or 1 hour in hot weather) because that gives microbes an opportunity to grow. Store dry food at 60° F to 70° F (16° C to 21° C).
- Reheat leftovers to 165° F (74° C); reheat gravy to a rolling boil to kill *Clostridium perfringens* bacteria that may be present. Merely reheating to a good eating temperature isn't enough to kill sufficient bacteria.
- Make sure the refrigerator stays below 40° F (4° C). Either use a refrigerator thermometer or keep it as cold as possible without freezing milk or lettuce.

Microbes that cause food-borne illness commonly enter food through cross-contamination—from one source to another—and grow in temperatures favorable to them. A recent example occurred at a large gathering where turkey franks were contaminated with bacteria. When the franks were later added to a salad, it too became contaminated, causing food-borne illness. It's important to avoid recontaminating prepared foods; potential sources are dirty kitchen towels and sponges.

It's essential to practice sanitary food-handling procedures when preparing any food (see Table 17-1). As one final precaution, watch for safe food-handling techniques when you eat out. Check that foods in a salad bar are iced; custard and pudding pies are chilled; hot foods served on a hot food bar are in fact hot; and vending

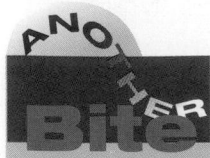

Several practices can reduce the risk of bacteria surviving during microwave cooking:

* *Cover food with glass or ceramic when possible. The trapped steam helps decrease evaporation and heats the surface.*
* *Stir and rotate food at least once or twice for even cooking. Then, allow microwaved food to stand, covered, after cooking is completed. The heat concentrated inside the food will radiate outward, helping cook the exterior and equalize the temperature throughout.*
* *Use the oven temperature probe or a meat thermometer to check that food is done. Insert it at several spots.*
* *Thaw meats in the refrigerator. If thawing them in the microwave, use the oven's defrost setting. Note that ice crystals in frozen foods are not heated well by the microwave oven and can create cold spots that later cook more slowly.*

- - - - - - - - - - - - - -

Safe Handling Instructions

This product was prepared from inspected and passed meat and/or poultry. Some food products may contain bacteria that could cause illness if the product is mishandled or cooked improperly. For your protection, follow these safe handling instructions.

Keep refrigerated or frozen.
Thaw in refrigerator or microwave.

Keep raw meat and poultry separate from other foods. Wash working surfaces (including cutting boards), utensils, and hands after touching raw meat or poultry.

Cook thoroughly.

Keep hot foods hot. Refrigerate leftovers immediately or discard.

Current safe handling instructions issued by USDA for meat and poultry products.

- - - - - - - - - - - - - -

machines are checked regularly, especially those containing sandwiches and milk. Send back any meat, poultry, seafood, or fish that does not appear thoroughly cooked. Keep track of how long cooked foods or salads have been sitting on the buffet table, and avoid anything that has been there for 2 hours or more. Food stored and served in dormitory cafeterias should also be properly handled.

Treatment of Food-Borne Illness

To offset the effects of diarrhea, drink a lot of fluids. To prevent further contamination, thoroughly wash hands before handling or eating food until the diarrhea disappears. Bed rest speeds recovery. A fever of 102° F (39° C) or greater, blood in the stool, and dehydration from frequent vomiting or diarrhea (a symptom of dehydration is dizziness when standing) deserve a physician's evaluation, especially if these symptoms persist for more than 2 or 3 days. In cases of suspected botulism, a physician should be consulted immediately because use of an antitoxin may speed recovery.

There are three particular situations in which it's vital for consumers to report incidents of food-borne illness to the local health department:

* If the food in question was eaten at a large gathering
* If the item came from a restaurant, delicatessen, sidewalk vendor, or kitchen that serves large numbers of people
* If the food was a commercial product, such as a canned or frozen item.

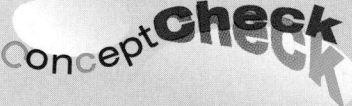

Bacteria and the toxins they produce pose the greatest risk for food-borne illness. In the past the addition to foods of sugar and salt, as well as smoking and drying, were used to prevent the growth of microorganisms. Today we know that ensuring cleanliness, keeping hot foods hot and cold foods cold, and cooking foods thoroughly offer additional protection from food-borne illness. Treat all raw animal products, cooked food, and raw fruits and vegetables as potential sources of food-borne illness. Symptoms of an attack are diarrhea, vomiting, and headache. Treatment generally requires only bed rest and extra fluids.

A Closer Look at Microbes that Cause Food-Borne Illness

As noted earlier, finding the agent that led to a food-borne illness requires some detective skills. Identifying the agent depends on knowing the food source, the incubation time for and types of symptoms, and the duration of illness associated with an outbreak. Let's look at the characteristics of the major "problem microbes" individually.

Staphylococcus aureus (S. aureus)

The organism *Staphylococcus aureus (S. aureus)* causes about 20% of food-borne illness cases each year. This microbe produces toxins in food. Once ingested, the toxin causes nausea, vomiting, diarrhea, headache, and abdominal cramps. Symptoms usually develop within 2 to 6 hours of eating the contaminated food. People seldom die from the toxin, but they don't develop immunity against future attacks. Bed rest and fluids are generally the only treatment needed. Recovery usually takes place within 2 to 3 days.

S. aureus bacteria live mainly in the nasal passages and in skin sores. These microbes enter food when people sneeze and cough over food or handle food while they have open skin sores. Once present in significant numbers in a food, *S. aureus* can make enough toxin to cause human illness in about 4 hours if the food temperature stays near 100° F (38° C). The toxin is undetectable by flavor, odor, and appearance and can even withstand prolonged cooking.[23]

Foods commonly associated with *S. aureus* intoxications are custard, ham, egg salad, cheese, seafood, cream-filled pastries, and milk. A frequent source is whipped cream left standing for hours at room temperature. Keeping these and other foods above 140° F (60° C) or below 40° F (4° C) prevents both the bacterium's growth and further toxin production. To limit the spread of this microbe, it's important to work with clean hands, working surfaces, and utensils; direct coughs and sneezes away from food; and cover skin cuts on hands and arms when handling food.

Salmonella

Many varieties of *Salmonella* bacteria cause food-borne illness. All 2000 types of *Salmonella* can be killed by normal cooking. Nonetheless, they are responsible for almost 55% of cases of food-borne illness. Commonly found in animal and human feces, these bacteria enter food via infected water, contaminated cutting boards, contaminated meat products, cracked eggs, and actual bits of feces in food. Ingesting the live bacteria causes the problem.[23] Feces from pet reptiles are also sources.

Symptoms of *Salmonella* infections are the same as those of *S. aureus* food intoxications but can take longer to develop, from 5 to 72 hours. Again, bed rest and fluids are the only effective treatment, and recovery usually occurs within 2 to 3 days. Deaths are rare. *Salmonella* attacks occur most frequently from consuming eggs, chicken, meat, meat products, custard made with infected eggs, raw milk, and inadequately refrigerated and reheated leftovers. Raw chicken is often contaminated, and undercooked food—including eggs—poses a particular risk. Again, thorough cooking kills *Salmonella* bacteria.

Most outbreaks of *Salmonella* infection can be traced to improper food handling.[17] Picnics pose a special challenge, because food is frequently held for hours at a dangerously high temperature (between 40° F and 140° F or 4° C and 60° C) (Figure 17-4). It takes only about 8 hours for *Salmonella* bacteria to multiply sufficiently to cause illness. Observing the temperature precautions for *S. aureus* organisms also prevents the growth of *Salmonella* bacteria.

Salmonella also poses a great risk for cross-contamination of foods. In 1986 five residents of a nursing home in Windsor, Connecticut, died and 25 others became ill from *Salmonella*. Health officials suspect that a blender used to purée food had previously been used to mix raw eggs and had not been properly cleaned.

Campylobacter jejuni receives more attention today as a cause of food-borne illness. This microbe likely causes about 24% of cases. Thoroughly cooking animal products and carefully storing leftovers are key preventive measures.

FDA warns us not to consume homemade ice cream, eggnog, and mayonnaise if made with unpasteurized, raw eggs because of the risk of *Salmonella* food-borne illness. Commercial forms of these products are safe because the egg products used have been pasteurized, which kills *Salmonella* bacteria. In addition, commercial mayonnaise contains enough acid to prevent bacterial growth.

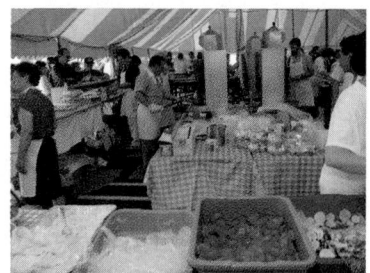

Figure 17-4
A picnic, especially in the warm days of summer, is a likely setting for food-borne illness. To minimize the risk, remember to keep hot foods hot and cold foods cold.

Clostridium perfringens (C. perfringens)

The bacterium *C. perfringens*, another potential cause of food-borne illness, lives throughout the environment, especially in soil, the intestines of farm animals and humans, and sewage. It is called the "cafeteria germ," because most food-borne outbreaks caused by this organism are associated with the food service industry or with events where large quantities of food are prepared and served. Symptoms of an infection resemble those of *Salmonella* cases, but the victim usually doesn't vomit. Symptoms occur within 8 to 24 hours of consuming enough live bacteria.[23] Again, bed rest and fluids are the only effective treatment, and recovery usually occurs within a day or so.

C. perfringens thrives in an oxygen-free environment. It forms heat-resistant **spores** that become bacteria at temperatures between 70° F and 120° F (21° C to 49° C). The bacteria then can quickly multiply to disease-causing amounts. Foods stored in deep serving dishes are especially fertile media for growth of these bacteria, because the centers are isolated from air and stay warm.

C. perfringens organisms are often found in cooked beef, turkey, gravy, dressing, stews, and casseroles. The best way to prevent their growth is to maintain proper holding temperatures and divide large leftover portions into smaller ones. The more surface exposed to air, the less oxygen-deprived the centers will be. Be especially careful to cook meats completely and cool them rapidly in small containers. Thoroughly reheat leftover meat to 165° F (74° C) before serving. Always bring leftover gravy to a rolling boil. Refrigerate cold cuts and sliced meats at 40° F or 4° C, and serve them cold.

Clostridium botulinum (C. botulinum)

The *C. botulinum* bacterium can cause botulism, a food-borne illness that can be fatal. This microbe comes from soil and may exist as a bacterium or spore in any food. As these bacteria multiply in food, they release a deadly toxin. The death rate for botulism receives much public attention; however, only a few cases are reported each year in the United States. At one time botulism was a serious problem in the canning industry, but now adequate heating and intact containers have virtually eliminated this danger from American manufactured canned foods.

Symptoms of botulism appear within 12 to 36 hours of ingesting contaminated food. The toxin blocks nerve function, causing vomiting, abdominal pain, double vision, dizziness, and acute respiratory failure. If the person survives, recovery occurs within 10 days.[23] Normally, bed rest is the only therapy. Sometimes treatment for botulism requires intensive care, including mechanical ventilation; the early administration of antitoxin is recommended. Still, ultimate recovery may be slow.

C. botulinum grows only in the absence of air, so it thrives primarily in canned food, especially improperly home-canned, low-acid foods such as string beans, corn, mushrooms, beets, and asparagus. Recently other foods with oxygen-deprived centers—such as potato salad, sautéed onions, stew, and chopped garlic—have caused botulism. FDA now requires that chopped garlic in oil be acidified to protect against *C. botulinum*. Cured meats also pose a risk for botulism; however, the nitrates and vitamin C used to preserve commercial products inhibit bacterial growth.

Critical Thinking

Diana had a party at her house for her son's birthday. After cleaning up after the kids went home, she realized she had forgotten to put away the potato salad and coleslaw, and decided to discard it. However, her husband Tim wanted her just to refrigerate it. "After all," he reasoned, "it was only left out for a couple of hours." Why was Diana right in wanting to throw away the leftover unrefrigerated food?

Toxin

A poisonous compound produced by an organism that can cause disease.

Spore

A dormant reproductive cell capable of forming into an adult organism without the help of another cell. Various fungi and bacteria form spores.

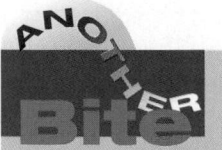

A man in Arkansas recently developed botulism after eating stew that was cooked and then kept at room temperature for 3 days. He spent 49 days in the hospital—42 of them on mechanical ventilation. Refrigeration to reduce growth of the bacteria is the key to preventing development of C. botulinum *in these foods.*

Home-canned foods are the most common sources of botulism. Although the canning process may kill all bacteria and the heat may drive out all oxygen, spores of *C. botulinum* can still survive if the heating is insufficient. When the can or jar cools, the spores germinate into bacteria that produce the toxin. Commercial canning factories are less likely to allow this to happen. Still, you should always check all cans carefully. Look for holes, rust on the seams, and swollen sides or tops. Make sure the can sucks in air when opened and the liquid inside is clear and not milky or foul-smelling. If you see any signs of spoilage, return the can to the store or take it to the nearest public health department. Whatever you do, *do not taste the food. One string bean can contain enough toxin to kill you.*

Other Problem Microbes

The bacteria discussed above are the key offenders. However, as noted earlier, the list of problem microbes—bacteria, fungi, molds, parasites, and viruses—is much longer. Molds growing on foods can produce toxins that have a wide range of effects when consumed. Aflatoxins are produced by a mold that often grows on peanuts, corn, wheat, and oil seeds, such as cottonseed. Although aflatoxins cause cancer, FDA allows them at acceptable concentrations because they are considered unavoidable contaminants.[11]

Parasites in foods pose additional problems. Most of us know the importance of cooking pork thoroughly. This kills a small parasitic worm, *Trichinella spiralis,* which can live in raw or undercooked pork and cause the disease trichinosis (Figure 17-5). Symptoms can take weeks or months to develop and include muscle weakness, fever, and fluid retention in the face.[25] Equally harmful is the parasitic worm *Anisakis,* found in its early growth stages in some raw fish. People who eat the popular Japanese dishes made of raw fish, sushi or sashimi, are particularly vulnerable to this type of food-borne illness. Symptoms usually occur within 12 hours of consumption and can include severe stomach pain if the young parasites penetrate the stomach lining. Thoroughly cooking fish or freezing it for at least 72 hours is a reliable method for eliminating the threat of *Anisakis* disease.

Viruses, such as hepatitis A, can also be transmitted in food. Symptoms include intestinal problems, weakness, fatigue, jaundice, and sometimes even development of serious liver disease requiring hospitalization. Because symptoms can take a month to show up, pinpointing the cause can be difficult. Raw seafood, such as oysters, and unsanitary food handling in restaurants are the usual culprits.

Botulism also may develop in vivo (inside the living body). Infants between 2 and 9 months of age are at the highest risk because of low stomach acid production. About 250 cases are reported each year. Fortunately the death rate is low: 1% to 2%. Adults with low stomach acid production are also at risk. Bacterial spores germinate in the stomach and produce the toxin. For this reason, honey and corn syrup should not be given to young infants because these products can contain the spores of this bacterium.

THE FAR SIDE　　By GARY LARSON

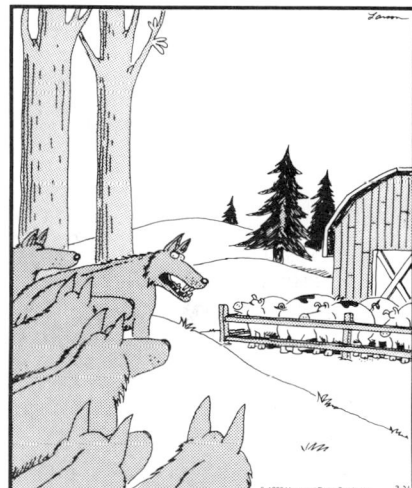

"I say we do it . . . and trichinosis be damned!"

Figure 17-5
The Far Side.

Concept Check

To prevent food-borne illness from *Staphylococcus aureus* organisms, cover cuts on hands and avoid sneezing on foods. To avoid *Salmonella* food-borne illness, work with clean hands and utensils and separate raw meats, especially poultry products, from other foods. Thoroughly cook meat and poultry products to destroy any *Salmonella* present. To avoid illness from *Clostridium perfringens,* rapidly cool leftover foods and thoroughly reheat them. To avoid botulism from *Clostridium botulinum,* carefully examine canned foods and don't allow cooked foods to stand for more than 1 to 2 hours at room temperature. To avoid other possible causes of food-borne illness, carefully handle raw animal products so that their juices don't contaminate other foods; thoroughly cook foods, especially fish and other seafood; consume only pasteurized dairy products; wash all fruits and vegetables; and thoroughly wash your hands with soap and water before and after preparing food, and after using the bathroom.

FOOD ADDITIVES

By the time you see a food on the market shelf, it usually contains substances added to make it more palatable or increase its nutrient content or shelf life. Manufacturers also add some substances to foods to make them easier to process.[9] Other substances may have accidentally found their way into the foods you buy. All these extraneous substances are known as *additives,* and although some may be beneficial, others may be harmful. All purposefully added substances must be evaluated by FDA. Appendix K provides a comprehensive list of food additives and their purposes.

Today, sugar, salt, corn syrup, and citric acid constitute 98% of all additives (by weight) used in food processing.

Why Are Food Additives Used?

Most additives are used to limit food spoilage. Food additives, such as potassium sorbate, are used to maintain the safety and acceptability of foods by retarding the growth of problem microbes implicated in food-borne illness.

Additives are also used to combat some enzymes that lead to undesirable changes in color and flavor in foods but don't cause anything so serious as food-borne illness. This second type of food spoilage occurs when enzymes in a food react to oxygen—for example, when apple and peach slices darken or turn rust color as they are exposed to air. Antioxidants are a type of preservative that retards the action of oxygen-requiring enzymes on food surfaces. These preservatives are not necessarily novel chemicals. They include vitamins E and C and a variety of sulfites.[9]

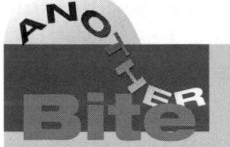

When buying food products, especially perishables, check the product date for safety. Four types of dates are commonly used. The pack date is the day the product was manufactured. The pull or sell date indicates the last date the product should be sold. It allows some time for storing food at home before eating. Check the expiration date of foods stored at home, because that is the last date the food can safely be consumed. Last, baked goods may have a freshness date, indicating that the product may safely be eaten for a short time after the date but may not taste the same.

Without the use of some food additives, it would be impossible to safely produce massive quantities of foods and distribute them nationwide or worldwide, as is now done. Despite consumer concerns about the safety of food additives, many have been extensively studied and proved safe when FDA guidelines for their use are followed.

Intentional food additives
Additives knowingly (directly) incorporated into food products by manufacturers.

Incidental food additives
Additives that appear in food products indirectly, from environmental contamination of food ingredients or during the manufacturing process.

Intentional Versus Incidental Food Additives

Food additives are classified into two types: those that are **intentionally** (directly) added to foods and those that have **incidentally** (indirectly) entered foods as contaminants. Both types of agents are regulated by FDA. Currently, more than 2800 different substances are intentionally added to foods. As many as 10,000 other substances enter foods as contaminants. This includes substances that may reasonably be expected to enter food through surface contact with processing equipment or packaging materials.

The GRAS List

In 1958, all food additives used in the United States and considered safe at that time were put on a **generally recognized as safe (GRAS)** list.[28] Congress established the GRAS list because it believed manufacturers did not need to prove the safety of substances that were already generally regarded as safe by knowledgeable scientists. Since that time, FDA has been responsible for proving that a substance does not belong on the GRAS list.

Since 1958, some substances on the list have been reviewed. A few, such as cyclamates, failed the review process and were removed from the list. Recently the additive red dye #3 was banned because it is linked to cancer. Many chemicals on the GRAS list have not yet been rigorously tested, primarily because of expense. These chemicals have received a low priority for testing, mostly because they have long histories of use without evidence of **toxicity** or because their chemical forms do not suggest they are potential health hazards.

Are Synthetic Chemicals Always Harmful?

Nothing about a natural product makes it inherently safer than a synthetic (man-made) product. Many synthetic products are simply laboratory copies of chemicals that also occur in nature (see the discussion in Chapter 18 on biotechnology for some examples). Moreover, although human endeavors contribute some toxins to foods, such as synthetic pesticides and industrial chemicals, nature's poisons are often even more potent and prevalent. Some cancer researchers suggest that we ingest at least 10,000 times more (by weight) natural toxins produced by plants than we do man-made pesticide residues. This comparison doesn't make man-made chemicals any less toxic, but it does lend perspective.

Consider the familiar food additive baking powder, which is used to make the batter rise in cakes, pancakes, and other quick breads. When manufacturers list potassium acid tartrate, sodium aluminum phosphate, or monocalcium phosphate on cake mix labels, they are referring to baking powder by its chemical names. Baking soda could be listed by its proper name, *sodium bicarbonate,* just as ordinary table salt could be called *sodium chloride.* The question should not be whether a food additive—such as salt—is a chemical but rather whether the chemical additive is safe to use.

Vitamin E is often added to food to prevent rancidity of fats. This chemical is safe when used within certain limits. However, high doses have been associated with health problems (see Chapter 8). Thus even well-known chemicals we are comfortable using can be toxic in some circumstances and at some concentrations.

Testing Food Additives for Safety

Food additives are tested under FDA scrutiny for safety on at least two animal species, usually rats and mice. Scientists determine the highest dose of the additive that produces **no observable effects** in the animals. High doses are needed to reduce the cost and length of the tests. Still, these doses are proportionately much higher than humans are ever exposed to. The maximum dosage is then divided by at least 100 to establish a margin of safety for human use.[28] The rationale for reducing the no-observable-effect level by a 100-fold margin is that we assume humans are at least 10 times more sensitive to food additives than are laboratory animals and that any one person might be 10 times more sensitive than another. This very broad margin essentially ensures that the food additive in question will cause no harmful health effects in humans. In fact, many synthetic chemicals are probably less dangerous at these low doses than the natural compounds in apples or celery.

Generally recognized as safe (GRAS)
A list of food additives that in 1958 were considered safe for consumption. Manufacturers were allowed to continue using these food additives, without special clearance, when needed in food products. FDA bears responsibility for proving they are not safe and can remove unsafe products from the list.

Toxicity
The capacity of a substance to produce injury or illness at some dosage.

No-observable-effects level (NOEL)
The highest dose of an additive that produces no deleterious health effects in animals.

Delaney Clause

This clause in the 1958 Food Additives Amendment of the federal Pure Food and Drug Act prevents the intentional (direct) addition to foods of a compound that has been shown to cause cancer in animals or humans.

Note that the margin of safety for some vitamins and trace minerals is much lower than for additives. In a few cases, consuming just 5 to 10 times more than our needs for a nutrient can be toxic. For this reason, the use of food additives is subjected to much stricter limits than are essential nutrients purchased in supplement form, such as copper and vitamin D.

One important exception applies to the schema for testing intentional food additives: if an additive is shown to cause cancer, even though only in very high doses, no margin of safety is allowed. The food additive cannot be used, because it would violate the **Delaney Clause** in the 1958 Food Additive Amendments. This clause prohibits intentionally adding to foods a compound that was introduced after 1958 and causes cancer. Evidence for cancer could come from either laboratory animal or human studies.[28]

Recently the value of animal cancer tests has been questioned. Research suggests that when rats are fed massive doses of chemicals, as they typically are in the tests, it may be the dose itself, rather than the chemical action, that causes cancer. The scientific community is currently debating which is the best method to test additives to evaluate cancer risk in humans. The question boils down to how to test chemicals efficiently and how to apply information obtained from laboratory animals to humans. Nevertheless, until a better method is established, we are left with our current ban on the intentional addition of chemicals that cause cancer.

Incidental food additives are another matter altogether. FDA cannot simply ban various industrial chemicals, pesticide residues, and mold toxins from foods, even though some of these contaminants can cause cancer. These products are not purposely added to foods—they are present whether we like it or not. FDA sets an acceptable level for these substances. Basically, it establishes a cancer safety margin of 1 million, which means that an incidental substance found in a food cannot contribute to more than one cancer case during the lifetimes of 1 million people. If a higher risk exists, the amount of the compound in a food must be reduced until the guideline is met. Previous laws applied the Delaney Clause to the presence of some pesticide residues, but recent legislation overrides that in favor of the previously cited cancer safety margin (one cancer case during the lifetimes of 1 million people).

Obtaining Approval for a New Food Additive

Today, before a new substance can be added to foods, FDA must approve its use. Besides rigorously testing an additive to establish its safety margins, manufacturers must give FDA information that (1) identifies the new additive, (2) gives its chemical composition, (3) states how it is manufactured, and (4) specifies laboratory methods used to measure its presence in the food supply at the amount of intended use.

Manufacturers must also offer proof that the additive will accomplish its intended purpose in a food, that it is safe, and that it is to be used in no higher amount than needed. Additives cannot be used to hide defective food ingredients, such as rancid oils; deceive customers; or replace good manufacturing practices. A manufacturer must establish that the ingredient is necessary for producing a specific food product.

Common Food Additives

A list of food additive categories appears in Appendix K. Some serve the general function of preservatives: acidic or alkaline agents, antioxidants, antimicrobial agents, curing and pickling agents, and **sequestrants.** Let's look at some of the specific categories of additives to understand exactly why these are used and to learn more about the specific substances employed.

Acidic or Alkaline Agents

Acids, such as calcium lactate, have many uses in foods. As flavor-enhancing agents, they impart a tart taste to soft drinks, sherbets, and cheese spreads, for example. As preservatives, they inhibit microbial growth. As antioxidants, they prevent discoloration and rancidity. They also adjust acid and base balance. Adding acids during food processing reduces the risk of botulism from eating naturally low-acid vegetables, such as beets.

Alkaline products, such as sodium hydroxide, can alter the texture and flavor of foods, including chocolate. In processing, alkaline products are sometimes used to produce a milder flavor by neutralizing the acids produced during fermentation.

Alternative Sweeteners

Currently saccharin and acesulfame (Sunette) are the only nonnutritive sweeteners used in foods. Because aspartame (Nutrasweet) yields energy, it is considered a nutritive sweetener (see Chapter 5). Saccharin is carcinogenic to rats when administered over two generations. The cancers are found primarily in the bladder. However, population studies of humans have not found an increased risk of developing bladder cancer from exposure to saccharin. As noted in Chapter 5, Congress has prevented FDA from banning saccharin by applying the Delaney Clause, and in 1991 FDA decided to make no further attempts to ban saccharin. Still, a cancer-warning label must appear on any product that contains saccharin.

Anticaking Agents

By absorbing moisture, compounds such as calcium silicate, ammonium citrate, magnesium stearate, and silicon dioxide keep table salt, baking powder, powdered sugar, and other powdered food products free flowing. These chemicals prevent the caking and lumping that would make powdered or crystalline products hard to use.

Antimicrobial Agents

Sodium benzoate, sorbic acid, and calcium propionate are common preservatives. Sorbic acid is a potent inhibitor of molds and fungal growth. Calcium propionate, a natural part of some cheeses, inhibits mold growth.

Antioxidants

This type of food preservative helps delay food discoloration from oxygen exposure, such as occurs when potatoes are diced. It also helps keep fats from turning rancid. Two widely used antioxidants are BHA (butylated hydroxyanisole) and BHT (butylated hydroxytoluene).[9] Vitamin E and related compounds also serve as antioxidants.

Sulfites, a group of sulfur-based chemicals, are widely used as antioxidants in foods. Some people are extremely sensitive to sulfites and may have difficulty breathing, wheeze, and vomit, as well as develop hives, diarrhea, abdominal pain, cramps, and dizziness.[18] As a result, FDA now limits the use of sulfites on raw fruits and vegetables—an action directed mainly at salad bars. FDA also requires manufacturers to declare the presence of sulfites on labels of packaged foods containing at least 10 parts per million of sulfites. Labels on wine bottles often list a sulfite warning.

Colors

Color additives don't improve nutritional qualities, but they can make foods more visually appealing. Food colorings cannot be used to deceive consumers—for example, by covering blemishes, concealing any inferiority, or misleading people in any way. Although colorings are arguably unnecessary additives, manufacturers have satisfied FDA that color is "necessary" for the production of certain foods.[13]

Controversy has surrounded the use of some food colors. Currently the safety of using tartrazine (FD&C yellow No. 5) is disputed. It has caused allergic symptoms—such as hives, itching, and nasal discharge—in sensitive individuals, especially in people allergic to aspirin. Although few Americans are sensitive to tartrazine, FDA requires manufacturers to list FD&C yellow No. 5 on labels of food products containing it. Some red dyes have also raised alarms, and some have been banned. Currently FDA requires manufacturers to list all forms of synthetic colors on the labels of foods that contain them. Pigments extracted from plant sources are exempted from specific description on food labels.

Curing and Pickling Agents

Nitrates and the related form, nitrites, are used as preservatives, especially to prevent growth of *Clostridium botulinum*. Sodium and potassium nitrates and nitrites are used to preserve meats such as bacon, ham, salami, and hot dogs (Figure 17-6). Nitrates and nitrites have been used for centuries, in conjunction with salt, to preserve meat. An added effect of nitrates is their reaction with pigments in meat to form a bright pink color. This gives ham, hot dogs, and other cured meats their characteristic appearance.

Nitrate consumption from both cured foods and natural vegetables has been associated with the synthesis of nitrosamines in the stomach. Some nitrosamines are cancer-causing agents, particularly for the stomach and esophagus. The actual risk appears to be low, however, except for people who secrete little stomach acid (some older people, for example).[6] A slightly increased risk for childhood leukemia and brain tumors is also suspected, but the data are preliminary.

FDA surmises that consumers take for granted a margin of microbial safety gained from nitrite use in cured meats. People often serve these meats cold or at least underheated. Consequently, government agencies have chosen not to ban nitrate or nitrite use in foods but rather to change manufacturing practices to lower amounts of preformed nitrosamines and suggest moderation in the use of these food products. Much progress has been made in this area during the last 25 years.[6]

The addition of vitamin C (sodium ascorbate) to cured meats, such as bacon, is one way to reduce the amount of nitrosamines formed in foods. This is a common manufacturing practice today. Other antioxidants, such as sodium erythrobate, also inhibit synthesis of nitrosamines.

Much nitrite and nitrate in the U.S. food supply occurs naturally in foods, primarily in vegetables and baked goods. About one third to two thirds of nitrites and one seventh of nitrates in our food supply are added in manufacturing.

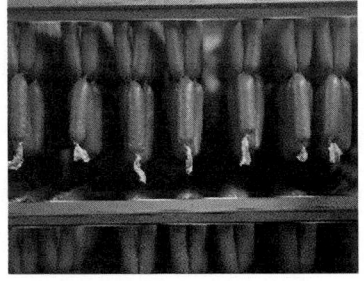

Figure 17-6
Cured meats derive their pink color from nitrates. The National Cancer Institute advises consuming these foods in moderation, as the nitrates/nitrites present some cancer risk.

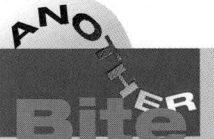

You might wonder why, if nitrates and nitrites form chemical substances that can cause cancer, they aren't banned by the Delaney Clause. In the United States, USDA regulates the use of chemicals in meats. The laws that govern USDA regulation of foods are separate from those that govern FDA regulation. Because of this, the Delaney Clause does not apply to USDA actions. Currently USDA sees no clear threat to public safety from the regulated use of nitrates and nitrites in meats, so no action has been taken.

Emulsifiers

By distributing and suspending fat in water, these products improve the uniformity, smoothness, and body of foods such as bakery goods, ice cream, and candies. In mayonnaise, for example, egg yolks act as emulsifiers in holding together the oil and the acids, such as vinegar or lemon juice. Lecithin, derived from soybeans, acts as an emulsifier in chocolate and margarine. Monoglycerides and diglycerides, found also as by-products of fat digestion, are used as emulsifiers in cake mixes.

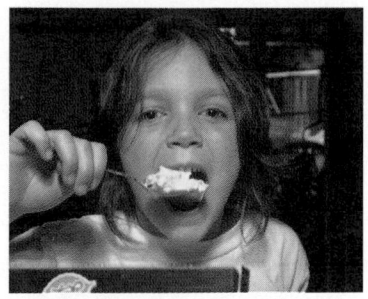

Emulsifiers improve the texture of foods such as ice cream, baked goods, and candies.

Fat Replacements

Fat replacements—such as Paselli SA2, Dur-Low, Oatrim, and Sta-Slim 143—are being produced for commercial use. These carbohydrate-based products are an addition to other players—Simplesse and Olean—discussed in Chapter 6.

Flavors and Flavoring Agents

Both naturally occurring and artificial agents can impart more flavor to foods. These agents include extracts from spices and herbs, as well as man-made agents. You've probably recognized flavors of some spices and of liquid derivatives of onion, garlic, cloves, and peppermint in foods. To meet the demand of industry, manufacturers have developed synthetic flavors that not only taste like natural flavors but also have the advantage of stability. Often artificial flavors, such as butter and banana flavors, have the same chemical composition as the natural flavor.

Some recent studies also suggest that certain flavor additives that share chemical similarities to aspirin might reduce the risk of heart attack. Chapter 6 discussed the usefulness of aspirin in reducing blood clotting and the related risk of heart attack in those at high risk. Scientists surmise that on average we consume the equivalent of about one third of a typical aspirin tablet per day from the various artificial flavors in our diets.[15]

Flavor Enhancers

Flavor enhancers are substances such as monosodium glutamate (MSG) that help bring out the natural flavors of foods. Note that the glutamate portion is simply a nonessential amino acid. A small percentage of people are sensitive to the glutamate in MSG and, after exposure, experience flushing, chest pain, facial pressure, dizziness, sweating, rapid heart rate, nausea, vomiting, and high blood pressure. MSG is often used in Chinese food. The onset of symptoms occurs about 10 to 20 minutes after ingestion and may last from 2 to 3 hours. People who find themselves sensitive to MSG should avoid it. It may be present alone (look for the word *glutamate*), as well as in any isolated protein source (caseinate, texturized vegetable protein, etc.), yeast extract, bouillon, soup stock, and seasonings. Tomatoes, mushrooms, and parmesan cheese are also sources of free glutamate. Fortunately, most of us find that moderate use of MSG or glutamate in foods poses no significant risk to our health.[21]

Humectants

These chemicals—such as glycerol, propylene glycol, and sorbitol—are added to foods to help retain proper moisture, fresh flavor, and texture. They are often used in candies, shredded coconut, and marshmallows.

Leavening Agents

Air and steam can be used to create a light texture in breads and cakes; however, carbon dioxide bubbles are much more reliable for this purpose. Common leavening agents that produce carbon dioxide gas include yeast, baking powder, and baking soda. Baking soda must react with acids to generate carbon dioxide. Baking powder can be used in either acid or alkaline conditions.

Maturing and Bleaching Agents

Such compounds as bromates, peroxides, and ammonium chloride hasten the natural aging and whitening processes of milled flour. This shortens the time needed for flour to become usable in baking products. Without these agents, freshly milled flour lacks the qualities necessary to make a stable, elastic dough and requires several months to be useful in baking.

Nutrient Supplements

Vitamin and mineral supplements are added to foods to improve their nutritional quality. Sometimes they replace nutrients lost in processing, as occurs when enriching flour. Vitamin A is added to margarine and some forms of milk. Vitamin D is added to some dairy products. Potassium iodide is added to salt, and calcium to some flours, fruit juices, and other products. Breakfast cereals often contain a variety of added nutrients.

Stabilizers and Thickeners

These additives impart a smooth texture and uniform color and flavor to candies, ice creams and other frozen desserts, chocolate milk, and artificially sweetened beverages. Commonly used substances are pectins, vegetable gums (such as guar gum and carrageenan), gelatins, and agars. They work by absorbing water. Without stabilizers and thickeners, ice crystals form in ice cream and other frozen desserts, and particles of chocolate separate from chocolate milk. Stabilizers are also used to prevent evaporation and deterioration of flavorings used in cakes, puddings, and gelatin mixes.

Sequestrants
Compounds that bind free metal ions. By so doing, they reduce the ability of ions to cause rancidity in foods containing fat.

Sequestrants

These compounds include EDTA and citric acid. They bind many free chemical ions, and by doing so help preserve food quality by reducing the ability of ions to cause rancidity in products containing fat.

Conclusion

In general, if you consume a variety of foods in moderation, the chances of food additives jeopardizing your health are minimal. Pay attention to your body. If you suspect an intolerance or sensitivity, consult your physician for further evaluation. Remember that, in the short run, you are more likely to suffer either from poor food-handling practices that allow bacteria to grow in food or from consuming raw animal foods than from eating additives. Excess energy, saturated fat, sodium, and other potential "problem" nutrients in our diets pose the greatest long-term risk.

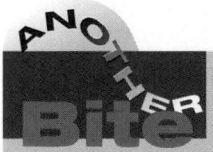

If you are bewildered or concerned about all the additives creeping into your diet, you can easily avoid most of them by emphasizing unprocessed whole foods (Figure 17-7). However, no evidence shows that this will necessarily make you healthier. It amounts to a personal decision. Do you have faith that FDA and food manufacturers are adequately protecting your health and welfare, or do you want to take more personal control by minimizing your intake of compounds not naturally found in foods?

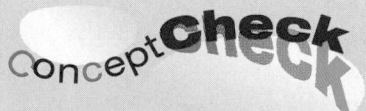

Food additives are used to reduce spoilage from microbial growth, oxygen, metals, and other compounds. Additives are also used to adjust pH, improve flavor and color, leaven, provide nutritional fortification, thicken, and emulsify food components. Additives are classified as intentional (direct), which are purposely added to foods, and incidental (indirect), which turn up in foods from environmental contamination or various manufacturing practices. The amount of an additive allowed in a food is limited to $\frac{1}{100}$ of the highest amount that has no observable effect when fed to animals. The Delaney Clause allows FDA to limit intentional addition of cancer-causing compounds to food under its jurisdiction. Also limited by law are the permissible amounts of carcinogens that incidentally enter foods.

A

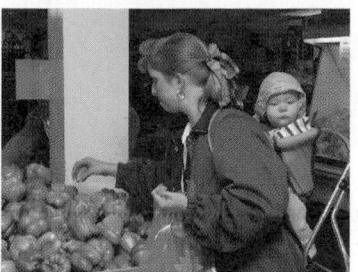

B

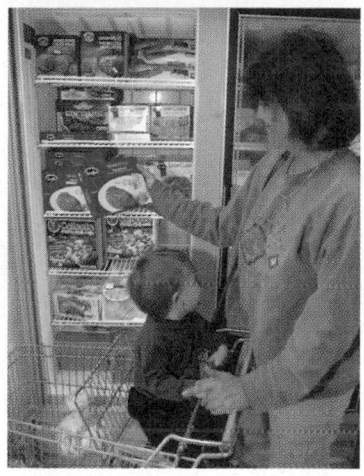

Figure 17-7
Depending on food choices, a diet can be either (**A**) *essentially devoid of or* (**B**) *high in food additives.*

SUBSTANCES THAT OCCUR NATURALLY IN FOODS AND CAN CAUSE ILLNESS

Foods contain a variety of naturally occurring substances that can cause illness. Here are some of the more important examples[11]:

Safrole—found in sassafras, mace, and nutmeg; causes cancer.

Solanine—found in potato shoots and green spots on potato skins; inhibits the action of neurotransmitters.

Mushroom toxins—found in some species of mushrooms; can cause stomach upset, dizziness, hallucinations, and other neurological symptoms. The more lethal varieties can cause liver and kidney failure, coma, and even death. FDA regulates commercially grown and harvested mushrooms. These are cultivated in concrete buildings or caves. However, there are no systematic controls on individual gatherers harvesting wild species, except in Michigan and Illinois.[24]

Avidin—found in raw egg whites; binds the vitamin biotin in a way that prevents its absorption.

Thiaminase—found in raw clams and mussels; destroys the vitamin thiamin.

Glycyrrhizic acid—found in pure licorice extracts; causes high blood pressure.

Tetrodotoxin—found in puffer fish; causes respiratory paralysis.

Protease inhibitor—found in raw soybeans; inhibits digestive enzymes.

Saponins—found in alfalfa sprouts; can destroy red blood cell membranes.

Oxalic acid—found in spinach; binds calcium and iron.

Herbal teas—containing senna or comfrey; can cause diarrhea and liver damage (see Chapter 3).

Browning products—found in toasted grains; can cause DNA mutations.

People have coexisted for centuries with these naturally occurring substances and have learned to avoid some of them and limit intake in other cases. Today they pose little health risk. Farmers know potatoes must be stored in the dark so that solanine won't be synthesized. Furthermore, we've developed cooking and food preparation methods to limit the potency of other substances. Nevertheless, it's important to understand that some potentially harmful chemicals in foods occur naturally.

Environmental Contaminants in Food

A variety of environmental contaminants may be found in foods. Aside from pesticide residue and products of fungal growth, other important contaminants deserve attention.[7]

Lead

Ingesting lead can cause anemia, kidney disease, and damage to the nervous system and can interfere with nerve impulse conduction. Because it has a high atomic weight, it is a "heavy" metal. Many heavy metals are toxic at low doses.

Lead toxicity is a particular problem for children because it is associated with IQ deficits, behavior disorders, slowed growth, impaired hearing, and possibly high blood pressure and kidney disease later in life. Exposed children who eat a high-fat diet low in calcium and low in iron absorb more lead than do those who eat a more healthful diet.[20]

Despite the reduction of lead exposure in children over the last 20 years associated with the decline in leaded gasoline and lead solder used in homes and in the canning industry, approximately 1.7 million children age 1 to 5 years still have elevated blood lead. Medical costs for a child with lead intoxication average $2,500 per treatment, and most children require two or more treatments.

Poor African-American children, who reside disproportionately in inner cities, are at increased risk for harmful lead exposure because of the lead-based paint present on the interiors and exteriors of older buildings. As this paint flakes off walls or is abraded from window trim as windows are opened and closed, lead paint chips enter the environment and may be ingested.

Other sources of lead include brass fittings on water pumps used in wells, imported wine from areas where leaded gasoline is still used (especially Eastern Europe), and lead caps on wine bottles in general. Wiping the neck of the bottle with a towel limits this type of exposure. An additional risk is posed by acidic products such as fruit juice, sauerkraut, or pickled vegetables stored in galvanized, tin, or other metal containers (except stainless steel). Acid can dissolve the metal, and lead leaches into the food product.

Lead can also leach from solder joints into copper pipes, so let tap water run a minute or so before drinking it or cooking with it, especially first thing in the morning or when the water has been off for a few hours. Use only cold water for drinking, cooking, and preparing infant formula. Lead in drinking water makes up about 20% of the average person's total lead exposure. Drinking water can be tested for lead content for about $20 to $50 by laboratories certified by the Environmental Protection Agency (EPA). Avoid softening drinking water, because soft water can leach lead from pipes.

Finally, lead can enter the food supply via leaded crystal and pottery glazes. Because of this hazard, lead is no longer used on commercially produced dishes in the United States. However, there is no way to ensure the safety of homemade or imported pottery items. Be sure not to use antiques or collectibles, including any made of leaded glass, for food or beverage storage.[17]

Dioxin

Dioxin is a chemical that contains chlorine and benzene. It can be created by incinerating chlorine-based material like plastics together with hydrocarbon-based material, such as paper. Dioxin causes cancer and other harmful effects in animals, even in small doses, and probably does so in humans as well.[7] Besides trash-burning incinerators, other sources of dioxin are bottom-feeding fish from the Great Lakes—an area with a great deal of industrial activity and chemical production.

Dioxin exposure from food is primarily a problem for people who frequently consume fish caught locally. People who eat commercial fish normally eat a variety, and even people who stick to one type of fish don't usualy have a problem because fish in interstate commerce generally come from different waters, only a few of which may contain dioxin.

Mercury

FDA first limited mercury, another heavy metal, in foods in 1969 after 120 people in Japan became ill from eating fish contaminated with high amounts. Birth defects in offspring of some of those people were also blamed on the mercury exposure. The fish most often contaminated was swordfish. Shark may also contain high amounts. Such large predatory fish that live for a long time can accumulate high amounts of mercury. These species are tested more frequently to ensure that the commercial supply is safe. FDA scientists responsible for seafood agree that these fish are safe, provided they are eaten infrequently (no more than once a week).[10] Pregnant women and women of childbearing age who may become pregnant, however, are advised by FDA to limit their consumption of shark and swordfish to no more than once a month. Note that other types of fish and seafood, especially smaller, younger varieties, generally contain little mercury.

Urethane in Alcoholic Beverages

Urethane forms during fermentation of alcoholic beverages. If the fermented product is heated, as in the production of sherry and bourbon, urethane concentration increases. Although urethane causes cancer in laboratory animals, it's unclear whether it causes cancer in humans. FDA research on urethane in food products is now a high priority. A prudent choice might be to limit consumption of products such as fruit brandies and sake because these show consistently high amounts of urethane.

Polychlorinated Biphenyls (PCBs)

PCBs were widely used for years in a variety of industrial products, but because they are linked to liver tumors and reproductive problems in animals, they are no longer produced. FDA has banned their use in machinery associated with food and animal feed and has established limits for PCBs in susceptible foods and in paper used for food-packaging material. The most significant food source of PCB residues is fish, primarily freshwater fish such as coho and chinook salmon from the Great Lakes and bottom-feeding freshwater species from waters in other industrial areas.[7] Again, a key guideline for fish consumption is variety and moderation when local sources have the potential for contamination.

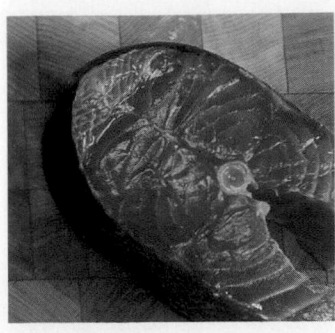

Fresh fish should be carefully refrigerated and used soon after purchase.

Protecting Yourself from Environmental Toxins in Foods

Environmental toxins that cause disease can be present in foods. To reduce exposure, find out which foods pose a risk. The Nutrition Insight reviewed some of them. In addition, emphasize variety and moderation in food selection. The presence of mercury in swordfish or shark may concern you, but it's normally not a health risk unless your diet is dominated by these fish. The small amount of mercury in most swordfish or shark isn't harmful if you're exposed to it infrequently. Here are some other practical tips for limiting the amount of pesticides and environmental contaminants in your diet: (1) thoroughly rinse and scrub fruits and vegetables, (2) remove outer leaves of leafy vegetables, (3) eat smaller, rather than larger, species of freshwater game fish (toxins accumulate more over the longer lifetime of the larger fish), (4) trim fat and skin from meat, poultry, and fish, and (5) discard any fat that is rendered from meat or fish during cooking. This practice helps, because many food contaminants dissolve in fat. Finally, pay attention to any warnings by local authorities about the high risk for contamination in specific waters or species of fish.

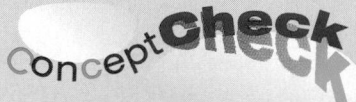

Concept **Check**

A general program to minimize exposure to environmental contaminants includes knowing which foods pose greater risks; consuming a wide variety of foods; thoroughly rinsing and scrubbing fruits and vegetables; removing outer leaves of leafy vegetables; trimming fat from meat and poultry, including the skin; and discarding any fat that is rendered from meat or fish during cooking.

Summary

➤ Bacteria and other microbes in food pose the greatest risk for food-borne illness. In the past, salt, sugar, smoke, fermentation, and drying were used to protect against food-borne illness. Today careful cooking, pasteurization, and keeping hot foods hot and cold foods cold provide additional insurance.

➤ The three major causes of food-borne illness today are the bacteria *Salmonella*, *Staphylococcus aureus*, and *Clostridium perfringens*. To protect against these bacteria, cover cuts on the hands, do not sneeze or cough on foods, avoid contact between raw meat or poultry products and other food products, and rapidly cool and thoroughly reheat leftovers. Thorough cooking of foods and the use of pasteurized dairy products protect against other bacteria and viruses that scientists are only now beginning to understand.

➤ Cross-contamination commonly causes food-borne illness. It occurs particularly when bacteria on raw animal products contact foods that can support bacterial growth. Because of the risk of cross-contamination, no perishable food should be kept at room temperature for more than 1 to 2 hours (depending on the environmental temperature), especially if it may have come in contact with raw animal products.

➤ Treatment for food-borne illness usually requires drinking lots of fluids, avoiding touching food while diarrhea is present, thorough handwashing, and bed rest. Botulism, hepatitis A infections, and trichinosis are types of food-borne illness that require prompt medical attention.

➤ Food additives are used primarily to extend shelf life by preventing microbial growth and destruction of food components by oxygen, metals, and other substances. Food additives are classified as those intentionally added to foods and those that incidentally end up in foods. An intentional additive is limited to no more than $1/100$ of the greatest amount that causes no observed symptoms in animals. The Delaney Clause allows FDA to ban use of any intentional food additive under its jurisdiction that causes cancer.

➤ Antioxidants, such as BHA, BHT, vitamins E and C, and sulfites, prevent oxygen and enzyme destruction of food products. Emulsifiers suspend fat in water, improving the uniformity, smoothness, and body of foods such as ice cream. Common preservatives include sodium benzoate and sorbic acid, which prevent bacterial growth. Sequestrants bind metals and thus prevent spoilage of food from metal contamination.

➤ Toxic substances occur naturally in a variety of foods, such as green potatoes, raw fish, mushrooms, raw soybeans, and raw egg whites. Cooking foods limits their toxic effects in some cases. Over the centuries, people have purposely avoided some of these foods, such as toxic mushroom species and the green parts of potatoes.

➤ A variety of environmental contaminants can be found in foods. Because most of them are fat soluble, trimming fat from meats and discarding fat that is rendered during cooking of meats, fish, and poultry are good steps to minimize exposure. In addition, it's helpful to know which foods pose a special risk, wash fruits and vegetables thoroughly, and discard the outer leaves of leafy vegetables.

Study Questions

1. Identify three major classes of microorganisms that are responsible for food borne illness.
2. Which kinds of foods are most likely to be involved in food-borne illness? Why are they targets for contamination?
3. What three trends in food purchasing and production have led to a greater number of cases of food-borne illness in recent years?
4. Why is thoroughly cooking food an important practice for reducing the risk of food-borne illness?
5. List four techniques other than thorough cooking that are important in preventing food-borne illness.
6. Define the term *food additive* and give examples of four intentional food additives. What are their specific functions in foods? What is their relationship to the GRAS list?
7. Describe the federal process that governs the use of food additives, including the Delaney Clause.
8. Put into perspective the benefits and risks of the use of additives in food. Point out any easy way to reduce consumption of food additives. Do you think this is worth the effort in terms of maintaining health? Why or why not?
9. Describe four recommendations for reducing the risk of toxicity from environmental contaminants.

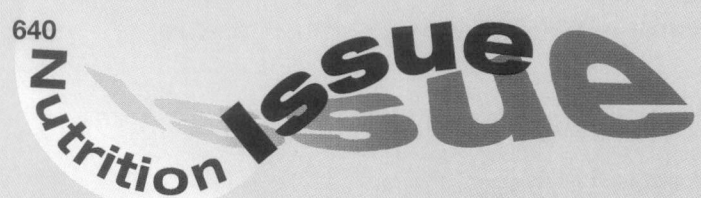

Pesticides in Food

Pesticides used in food production produce both beneficial and unwanted effects. Most health authorities believe the benefits greatly outweight the risks. Pesticides help ensure a safe and adequate food supply and help make foods available at reasonable cost. However, sentiment is growing nationwide that pesticides pose avoidable health risks. Consumers have come to assume that man-made is dangerous and "organic" is safe. Some researchers believe this sentiment is grounded in fear and fueled by unbalanced reports. Other researchers say concern about pesticides is valid and overdue.[2]

Some people are struggling to make sense of conflicting information on this topic. Most concern about pesticide residues in food appropriately focuses on chronic rather than acute toxicity because the amounts of residue present, if any, are extremely small. These low concentrations found in foods are not known to produce adverse effects in the short term, although harm has been caused by the high amounts that occasionally result from accidents or misuse. For humans, pesticides pose a danger mainly in their cumulative effects,[2] so their threats to health are difficult to determine. However, growing evidence, including the problems of contamination of underground water supplies and destruction of wildlife habitats, indicates that we would likely be better off as a nation if we could reduce use of pesticides. Both the federal government and many farmers are working toward that end.

WHAT IS A PESTICIDE?

Federal law defines a pesticide as any substance or mixture of substances intended to prevent, destroy, repel, or mitigate any pest.[26] The built-in toxic properties of pesticides lead to the possibility that other, nontarget organisms, including humans, might also be harmed. The term *pesticide* tends to be used as a generic reference to many types of products, including insecticides, herbicides, fungicides, and rodenticides. A pesticide product may be chemical or bacterial, natural or man-made. For agriculture, EPA allows about 10,000 pesticide uses, involving some 300 active ingredients.[26] Pesticide use in general substantially contributes to the chemical load applied intentionally to the earth's surface. About 1.2 billion pounds of pesticides are used each year in the United States, much of which is applied to agricultural crops (Figure 17-8).

Once a pesticide is applied, it can turn up in a number of unintended and unwanted places. It may be carried in the air and dust by wind currents, remain in soil attached to soil particles, be taken up by organisms in the soil, decompose to other compounds, be taken up by plant roots, enter ground water, or invade aquatic habitats. Each is a route to the food chain; some are more direct than others.

WHY USE PESTICIDES?

In the United States alone, pests destroy nearly $20 billion of food crops yearly, despite extensive pesticide use. The primary reason for using pesticides is economic—use of agricultural chemicals increases production and lowers the cost of food, at least in the short run. Many farmers believe they would have a tough time staying in business without pesticides. Quick and direct, pesticides help protect farmers from ruinous losses caused by a sudden pest outbreak.

Unless pesticides are applied, farming must depend much more on crop rotation to limit damage from pests. Federal government subsidies that encourage planting the same crops year after year discourage crop rotation, and so stimulate pesticide use. Further, pesticides also create new pests because they destroy the spiders, wasps, and predatory beetles that naturally keep most plant-feeding insect populations in check. The brown plant hopper that has recently plagued Indonesian rice fields was not a serious problem before heavy pesticide use began in the early 1970s. In the United States, such major pests as spider mites and the cotton bollworm were merely nuisances until pesticides decimated their predators.

Consumer demands also have changed over the years. At one time we wouldn't have thought twice about buying an apple with a worm hole; we simply took it home, cut out the wormy part, and ate the apple. Today consumers find worm holes less acceptable, so farmers rely more and more on pesticides to produce cosmetically attractive fruits and vegetables. On the practical side, pesticides can protect against rotting and decay of fresh fruits and vegetables. This is helpful because our food distribution system doesn't usually permit consumer purchase within hours of harvest. Also, food grown without pesticides can contain naturally occurring organisms that produce carcinogens at concentrations far above current standards for pesticide residues. For example, fungicides

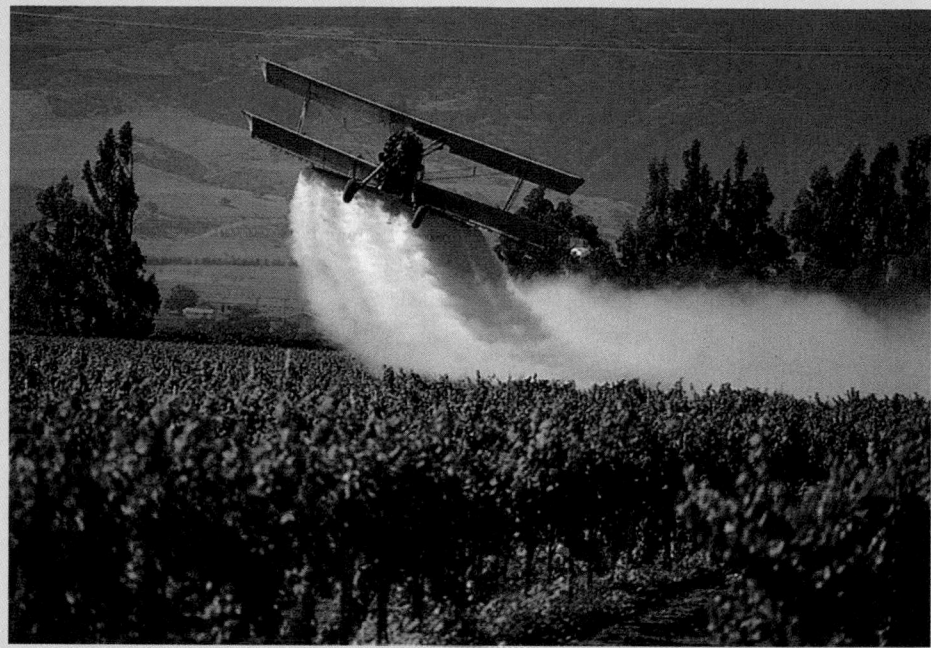

Figure 17-8 *Pesticide use poses a risk-versus-benefit question. Each side has points that deserve to be considered.*

help prevent the carcinogen aflatoxin (caused by growth of a fungus) from forming on some crops. So while some pesticides may improve the appearance of food products, others help keep some foods fresher and safer to eat.

REGULATING PESTICIDES

The responsibility for ensuring that residues of pesticides in foods are below amounts that pose a danger to health is shared by FDA, EPA, and the Food Safety and Inspection Service of USDA.[28] FDA is responsible for enforcing pesticide tolerances in all foods except meat, poultry, and certain egg products, which are monitored by USDA. A newly proposed pesticide is exhaustively tested, perhaps over 10 years or more, before it is approved for use. EPA must decide both that the pesticide causes no unreasonable adverse effects on people and the environment and that benefits of use outweigh the risks of using it. However, there is concern about older chemicals registered before 1970, when less stringent testing conditions were permitted.[2,26] EPA is now asking chemical companies to retest the old compounds using more rigorous tests. Unfortunately, inadequate funding at EPA has hampered the review of older pesticides. The slow pace of this retesting has angered the critics of pesticide use. When weighing whether to approve or cancel a pesticide, EPA considers how much more it would cost the farmer to use an alternative pesticide or process and whether cancellation would decrease productivity.[26] After determining the dollar cost to the farmer, EPA then looks at costs to processors and consumers.

Once a pesticide is approved for use, at least a 100-fold margin of safety is a standard requirement for contamination in food to minimize health effects other than cancer (such as kidney damage or birth defects). In other words, the tolerances (limits) used for foods set the safety standard at 100 times less than the highest dose at which the pesticide causes no ill effects in animals—or lower. If the pesticide causes cancer, its use must not cause more than one cancer case in 1 million people.

HOW SAFE ARE PESTICIDES?

Dangers from exposure to pesticides through food depend on how potent the chemical toxin is, how concentrated it is in the food, how much and how frequently it's eaten, and the consumer's resistance or susceptibility to the substance. Pesticide use is clearly associated with declining water quality. Accumulating information also links pesticide use to increased cancer rates in farm communities. For rural counties in the United States, the incidence of lymph, genital, brain, and digestive tract cancers increases with higher-than-average herbicide use.[2] Respiratory cancer cases increase with greater insecticide use. In tests using laboratory animals, scientists have found that some of the chemicals present in pesticide residues cause birth defects, sterility, tumors, organ damage, and injury to the central nervous system. Some pesticides persist in the environment for years.

Still, some researchers argue that the cancer risk from pesticide residues is hundreds of times less than the risk from eating such common foods as peanut butter, brown

Continued.

mustard, and basil. Plants manufacture their own toxic substances to defend themselves against insects, birds, and grazing animals (including humans). When plants are stressed or damaged, they produce even more of these toxins. Because of this, many foods contain naturally occurring chemicals considered toxic, even carcinogenic. Other scientists argue that if natural carcinogens are already in the food supply, then we should reduce the number of added carcinogens whenever possible. In other words, we should do what we can to decrease the problem.

The mere presence of a pesticide in food or water at any concentration frightens some people. But the concentrations of pesticide residues found in foods are almost always well below the tolerances that have been set to meet safety concerns. High and obviously hazardous concentrations are very rare and are usually the result of spills or improper uses. The major challenge for scientists and regulators goes beyond detecting and measuring pesticide residues; it is rather a question of what, if any, biological significance they have.[26]

THE RISKS OF PESTICIDES TO CHILDREN

Any discussions of pesticides and associated health risks must focus on children. They are not simply small adults in a biological sense. Children face a higher risk from pesticide exposure than do adults for several reasons.[4]

1. Their exposure is greater; children eat more food in proportion to their body weight than do adults.

2. Children consume more foods that are potential sources of pesticide residues than do adults. For example, they eat more fruit.

3. Exposure at an early age carries a greater risk than does exposure later in life; residues can accumulate to toxic amounts over a longer period. Also, cancer has more time to develop.

4. Physiological susceptibility to the effects of carcinogens and neurotoxins in pesticides may be greater; the cells in children are dividing rapidly, and the enzyme systems that detoxify chemicals are not fully developed.

Until recent years, EPA did not consider these factors in risk calculations. However, EPA now looks at age-related consumption data for approval of new pesticides. Although children are at greater risk from pesticides, the magnitude of that risk and how best to calculate it are open to debate. A recent report by the National Academy of Sciences advocates changes to the current pesticide regulatory system to ensure the safety of foods eaten by children. In addition, its authors stress the value of including fruits and vegetables in children's diets and caution parents not to change their children's diets to avoid certain foods.[4] Carefully washing fruits and vegetables and consuming a wide variety are sufficient recommendations. Peeling fruits and vegetables is another option. A final general precaution is to keep children away from lawns, gardens, and flower beds that have recently been treated with pesticides and herbicides.

TESTING AMOUNTS OF PESTICIDES IN FOODS

FDA tests thousands of raw products each year for pesticide residues. (A pesticide is considered illegal in this case it if is not approved for use on the crop in question or if the amount used exceeds the allowed tolerance.) A 1993 FDA study showed no residues in 64% of domestic samples and 69% of imported samples. Less than 1% of domestic and imported samples had residues that were over tolerance, and 1% of domestic and 3% of import samples had residues for which there was no tolerance.[8] The findings for 1994 continued to demonstrate that pesticide residues in foods are generally well below EPA tolerances, and they confirm the safety of the food supply relative to pesticide residues.

Residues sometimes appear on the wrong crops or in excessive amounts because of contamination from nearby farms via wind or water. When a problem is identified, FDA takes steps to make sure it's corrected and that the tainted food in question never reaches the consumer. However, of 600 pesticides available on international markets, many are not even detected by any of FDA's multiresidue tests.[2] This has raised concern by pesticide critics with regard to imported foods. Better tests that detect single residues are less frequently used because of cost.

PERSONAL ACTION

We often take risks in our own lives, but we prefer to have a choice in the matter after weighing the pros and cons. For instance, we can choose not to immunize a child, but we do so with the understanding that the child might get sick. We can also choose to risk cancer from smoking or to avoid that risk; or we can drive recklessly. These are personal risks that we choose to take. In regard to pesticides in food, however, someone else is deciding what is acceptable and what is not. Our only choice is whether to buy or avoid pesticide-containing foods. In reality it's almost impossible to avoid pesticides entirely, because even "organic" produce often contains traces of pesticides, probably as the result of cross-contamination from nearby farms.

Short-term studies of the effects of pesticides on laboratory animals cannot pinpoint long-term cancer risks precisely. It should be clearly understood, however, that the presence of minute traces of an environmental chemical in a food doesn't mean that any adverse effect will result from eating that food.

FDA and other scientific organizations believe that the hazards are comparatively low and in the short run are less than the hazards of food-borne illness created in our own kitchens. We can't avoid pesticide risks entirely, but we can limit exposure by following the advice given earlier in this chapter.

We can also encourage farmers to use fewer pesticides to reduce exposure to our foods and water supplies, but we'll have to settle for produce that isn't perfect in appearance. Are you concerned enough about pesticides on food to change your shopping habits or take more political action?

Undernutrition Throughout the World

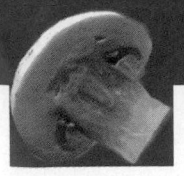

THE IMAGES ARE BOTH VIVID and heartrending. Emaciated children with enormous eyes and stomachs, too weak to cry, stare at us from news photos and television screens. Each year, more than 15 million children die of undernutrition and related preventable disease.

Today, nearly one in five people worldwide is chronically undernourished—too hungry to lead a productive, active life.[3] This is twice as many people as a decade ago. Throughout the world the problems of poverty and undernutrition are widespread and growing.[1]

The majority (two thirds) of undernourished people live in Asia. However, the largest increases in numbers of chronically hungry people currently occur in eastern Africa, particularly in Ethiopia, Sudan, Rwanda, Burundi, Kenya, Somalia, and Tanzania. Their eyes haunt us.[25]

This chapter examines the problem of undernutrition and the conditions that create it, as well as some possible solutions. If we are to eradicate undernutrition, we all have to understand the problem and assume responsibility for supplying some answers. It is important to recognize that many political leaders and citizens worldwide contribute directly and indirectly to the economic and social destruction that spawns hunger.[3]

CHAPTER 18

ASSESS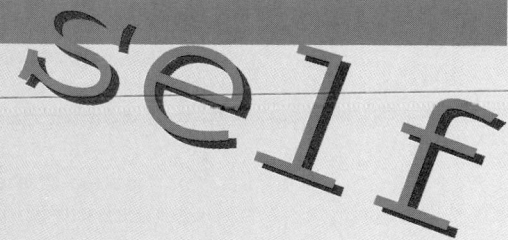

Broadening Your Vision

Many people in the United States don't realize the magnitude of undernutrition in the world and their own country. Reading this chapter will open your eyes to the nutritional state of the world's peoples. You'll discover what you can do to help correct the problem. First, though, think about the following questions and provide the best answers you can.

1. Who is most likely to experience undernutrition in the United States?

_____

_____

_____

2. What are the major causes of undernutrition in the United States?

_____

_____

_____

3. What are the major causes of undernutrition in the developing countries of the world?

_____

_____

_____

4. To what degree are you concerned about undernutrition in the United States and the world?

_____

_____

_____

These questions are designed to spur you to think about the issues addressed in this chapter. Other questions are also addressed.

Key Chapter Concepts

- Poverty is common wherever people suffer from undernutrition.
- The greatest risk of undernutrition occurs during critical periods of growth and development: gestation, infancy, and childhood. Low birth weight is a leading cause of infant deaths worldwide.
- Although famine has not existed in the United States since the 1930s, undernutrition is still a problem. In response, soup kitchens, the food stamp program, school lunch and breakfast programs, and the Supplemental Feeding Program for Women, Infants, and Children (WIC) have been created to help those in need.
- Reducing out-of-wedlock pregnancies and focusing more on the responsibilities of parents remain national priorities, because single parents and their children are likely to live in poverty.
- Multiple factors contribute to the problem of undernutrition in the developing world. Food resources may be inadequate. Farming methods often encourage erosion. Naturally occurring devastation from droughts, excessive rainfall, fire, crop infestation, and human causes—such as urbanization, war and civil unrest, debt, and poor sanitation—worsen the problem of undernutrition.
- Direct food aid is only a short-term solution to undernutrition in developing countries. A focus on sustainable subsistence-level farming and small scale industrial development are ways to gain the resources to feed one's family.
- The world has both the food and the technical expertise to end hunger. What is lacking is the political will to do so.

World Hunger: a Continuing Plague

In November 1974 the United Nations World Food Conference proclaimed its bold objective "that within a decade no child will go to bed hungry, that no family will fear for its next day's bread, and that no human being's future and capacities will be stunted by malnutrition." Obviously this promise remains unfulfilled: 22 years later hunger is a daily experience for one in five people in the developing world and one in eight people in the United States. Currently a third of Africa's population jeopardizes their physical and mental health by eating less than the minimum amount considered necessary for healthy life.[3]

The famines that occurred in Ethiopia in the 1980s called special attention to the problem of undernutrition in the developing world. The plight of millions of starving people elicited widespread public support for immediate aid to famine victims. Still, far from ending, hunger remains frequently in the news. Civil wars in Africa and Eastern Europe, coupled with drought in many parts of the world, have brought more than 30 million people to the brink of starvation, about two thirds of whom live in Africa.[3] Relief aid has been arriving but often with too little, too late. The deadly combination of war and poor weather has also recently led to increasing hunger in Bangladesh, Afghanistan, the Philippines, and Cambodia. As you might surmise, the problem of undernutrition in developing nations is ongoing, one that requires a long-range approach employing both political and technological solutions.[1]

Undernutrition and Poverty

Let's begin our look at these problems by first defining some key words.

Hunger is the physiological state that results when not enough food is eaten to meet energy needs. It also describes an uneasiness, discomfort, weakness, or pain caused by lack of food. If hunger is not relieved, the resulting medical and social costs from undernutrition are high—preterm births and mental retardation, inadequate growth and development in childhood, poor school performance, decreased work output in adulthood, and chronic disease[14] (Table 18-1). Symptoms of chronic hunger are found not only among people in the developing world but also among many people living at or below the poverty level in America. In the United States, about 4 million children younger than 12 years go hungry during at least part of the year. Almost 10 million more children in low-income families are at risk of hunger and its far-reaching health and psychosocial consequences.[5]

The primary cause of chronic hunger is poverty. Unemployment and underemployment, homelessness, drug addiction, functional illiteracy, single-parent families (often headed by a woman who has limited earning potential), wage discrimination, failing health, inadequate governmental programs, and war or civil strife all contribute to this poverty. In developing nations the problems of civil strife—frequently caused by ethnic and religious conflict leading to war—combine with a lack of resources and inadequate governmental programs to intensify hunger.[3]

TABLE 18-1

The Realities of Undernutrition

- Nearly one in five people in the developing world is chronically undernourished—too hungry to lead a productive, active life. This includes one third of the world's children.
- About 55,000 people die of hunger each day—two thirds of them children.
- 3 million newborns in the developing world die in the first week of life.
- Approximately half of all children who die each year in developing countries do so from causes that could be prevented at low cost.
- At least 250,000 children are permanently blinded each year simply through lack of vitamin A.
- Women in poor countries average up to four times more births than women in the United States.
- Every day the world produces about 2400 kcal for each person, generally meeting average energy needs.
- Poor women in developing countries face a 300-fold increased risk of death in pregnancy compared with women in the United States.
- In many developing countries, life expectancy of the population is one half to two thirds of that in the United States.
- Almost half of the world's people earn less than $200 a year—many use 80% to 90% of that income to obtain food. About $2000 to $3000 each year per person is needed for life expectancy to reach that seen in the United States.
- Of the nearly 5.8 billion people on earth, more than 1 billion drink contaminated water.
- About 2 billion people in the world are without proper sanitation facilities.
- Developing countries have two thirds of the 19 million AIDS cases world-wide.

Malnutrition is a condition of impaired development or function caused by either a long-term deficiency or an excess in energy and/or nutrient intake, the latter representing the state of overnutrition described in Chapter 1. The occurrence of specific diseases of malnutrition depends mostly on the food/population ratio.[16] When food supplies are low and the population is large, undernutrition is common, leading to nutritional deficiency diseases, such as goiter (from an iodide deficiency) and xerophthalmia (eye problems caused by a poor vitamin A intake).[8,23] However, when the food supply is ample or overabundant, incorrect food choices coupled with an excessive intake can lead to overnutrition-related chronic diseases, such as a certain form of diabetes. Note also, despite an ample supply of food, pockets of undernutrition among the poor may still be found in the United States.[3]

Malnutrition
Failing health that results from a long-standing dietary intake that either fails to meet or greatly exceeds nutritional needs.

TABLE 18-2

Effects of Nutrient-Deficiency Diseases that Commonly Accompany Undernutrition

Disease and key nutrient involved	Typical effects	Foods rich in deficient nutrient	Where the problem still exists
XEROPHTHALMIA			
Vitamin A	Blindness from chronic eye infections, poor growth, dryness and keratinization of epithelial tissues	Liver, fortified milk, sweet potatoes, spinach, greens, carrots, cantaloupe, apricots	Asia, Africa
RICKETS			
Vitamin D	Weakened bones, bowed legs, other bone deformities	Fortified milk, fish oils, sun exposure	Asia and Africa where religious practices encourage avoidance of sun exposure for women and children; elderly in developed nations
BERIBERI			
Thiamin	Nerve degeneration, altered muscle coordination, cardiovascular problems	Sunflower seeds, pork, whole and enriched grains, dried beans	Areas of famine in Africa
ARIBOFLAVINOSIS			
Riboflavin	Inflammation of face and oral cavity	Milk, mushrooms, spinach, liver, enriched grains	Areas of famine in Africa
PELLAGRA			
Niacin	Diarrhea, skin inflammation, dementia	Mushrooms, bran, tuna, chicken, beef, peanuts, whole and enriched grains	Areas of famine in Africa
SCURVY			
Vitamin C	Delayed wound healing, internal bleeding, abnormal formation of bones and teeth	Citrus fruits, strawberries, broccoli	Areas of famine in Africa
IRON-DEFICIENCY ANEMIA			
Iron	Reduced work output, reduced growth, increased health risk in pregnancy	Meats, spinach, seafood, broccoli, peas, bran, whole-grain and enriched breads	Worldwide
GOITER			
Iodide	Enlarged thyroid gland, poor growth in infancy and childhood, possible mental retardation, cretinism	Iodized salt, saltwater fish	South America, Eastern Europe, Africa

Often two or more nutrition-deficiency diseases are found in an undernourished person in the developing world. This separate discussion of nutrients just makes it easier to see the important role of each nutrient.

Genetic background contributes to both forms of malnutrition. Not every child in Thailand who eats mainly rice develops **protein-energy malnutrition (PEM)**; similarly, not every adult in New York City who consumes a high-fat, energy-rich diet suffers a heart attack. Genetic background influences the development of these diseases.[16]

Undernutrition is the malnutrition that results from an inadequate intake, absorption, or use of the nutrients or energy needed for optimal growth, development, and body function. The earliest response to undernutrition is to reduce physical activity. This allows the individual to preserve energy for growth and other vital functions.[24] With persistent undernutrition the second response is a reduced rate of weight gain or failure of weight maintenance. In addition, in children the rate of increase in height is reduced.[26]

Undernutrition is the most common form of malnutrition among the poor in both developing and developed countries. Currently about half of the 4 million African children under 5 years of age who die annually are undernourished. Undernutrition is also the primary cause of specific nutrient deficiencies that can result in muscle wasting, blindness (from xerophthalmia), scurvy, pellagra, beriberi, anemia, rickets, goiter, and a host of other problems[14] (Table 18-2). For example, more than 250,000 children develop blindness from xerophthalmia each year. This vitamin deficiency also raises the risk for other diseases, such as measles. The United Nations International Children's Fund reports that the lives of 1 to 3 million children could be saved annually in the developing world if vitamin A supplements were provided a few times a year. The annual cost per child would be about 6 cents. About 30% to 60% of all women in the developing world suffer from anemia caused by iron deficiency and malaria.

Of the 5.7 billion people in the world, at least 800 million exhibit some form of undernutrition.[3] Death and disease from infections, particularly those causing acute and prolonged diarrhea or acute lower respiratory disease, increase dramatically when the infections are superimposed on a state of chronic undernutrition.[16]

Protein-energy malnutrition (PEM) is a form of undernutrition caused by an extremely deficient intake of energy or protein generally accompanied by an illness. The typically dramatic results of protein-energy malnutrition—kwashiorkor and marasmus—were covered in Chapter 7. This chapter focuses on the more subtle effects of a chronic lack of food.

Famine is not the same thing as chronic hunger. Although both result from poverty and a lack of food, famine is the extreme form of chronic hunger. Periods of famine are characterized by large-scale loss of life, social disruption, and economic chaos that slows food production. As a result of these extreme events, the affected community experiences a downward spiral characterized by human distress; sales of land, livestock, and other important farm assets; migration; division and impoverishment of the poorest families; crime; and the weakening of customary moral codes, as seen recently in Sudan and Rwanda. Antisocial behavior—hoarding and crime, for example—increases. In the midst of all this, undernutrition rates soar, infectious diseases such as cholera spread, and people die in staggering numbers.[3] Halting this spiral requires more than just feeding those in need. Special efforts are needed to eradicate the fundamental causes of famine.

Causes of famine vary by region and decade, but the most common underlying cause is crop failure. The most obvious causes of crop failure are bad weather, war, and civil strife, or all three. War deserves a special focus: It contributes to food crisis by diverting labor from food production, disrupting the marketing of crops, destroying fields, creating refugees, and hindering relief efforts. In this situation, food relief can even be used as a weapon.[3] War has been linked to many famines in recent years. In fact, this type of man-made disaster has absorbed more than three quarters of the disaster assistance channeled through the World Food Program.

Protein-energy **malnutrition (PEM)**
A condition associated with body wasting and increased susceptibility to infections that results from prolonged consumption of insufficient amounts of food energy and protein.

Undernutrition
Failing health that results from a long-standing dietary intake that does not meet nutritional needs.

Famine
An extreme shortage of food that leads to massive starvation in a population; often associated with crop failures, war, and political strife.

More than 3 million people may have perished in the great famine of 1943 in Bengal, India. In 1974, another 1.5 million from that region starved in the new country of Bangladesh. China suffered an almost unbelievable famine from 1959 to 1961—estimates of mortality range from 16 million to 64 million.

Critical Life Stages When Undernutrition Is Particularly Devastating

Prolonged undernutrition is detrimental to health at all stages of life but particularly critical during some periods of growth and old age (Figure 18-1).

Pregnancy

The period when undernutrition poses the greatest health risk is during pregnancy. A pregnant woman needs extra nutrients to meet both her own needs and those of her developing fetus. Inadequate nutrient intake during pregnancy can seriously jeopardize her health. Nourishing the fetus may deplete stores of maternal nutrients. Maternal iron-deficiency anemia is one possible consequence. Pregnancy-induced hypertension (preeclampsia), a life-threatening condition involving rapid weight gain from fluid retention and a sharp increase in blood pressure, is also likely to be influenced by inadequate prenatal nutrition (see Chapter 14).

In Africa, women give birth, on average, to more than six live babies. Coupled with chronic undernutrition, these high birthrates create a 1 in 20 chance that a woman will die from pregnancy-related causes. In contrast, American women face a risk of 1 death in about 8000 births from pregnancy-related causes. No other social indicator, including literacy, life expectancy, and infant mortality, betrays a wider gap between the developing and industrialized world.[3]

Fetal and Infant Stages

Gestation
The time between conception and birth.

The fetus faces major health risks from undernutrition during **gestation.** To support growth and development of the brain and other body tissues, a growing fetus requires a rich supply of protein, vitamins, and minerals. When these needs are not met, the infant is often born before 37 weeks of gestation, well before the 40 weeks of gestation that is considered ideal.[26] Consequences of preterm birth include reduced lung function and a weakened immune system. These conditions not only compromise health but also increase the likelihood of death. Long-term problems in growth and development can result if the infant survives. In extreme cases, low–birth-weight babies (2500 grams [about 5.5 pounds] or less)—face 5 to 10 times the normal risk of dying before the age of 1 year, primarily because of reduced lung development. When low birth weight is accompanied by other physical abnormalities, medical intervention can cost $100,000 or more. When severe retardation occurs, the lifetime cost of care can exceed $2 million.

In the United States, low birth weight accounts for more than half of all infant deaths and for 75% of deaths of babies under 1 month of age. Currently about 7% of infants born in the United States have low birth weights. Worldwide, more than half of infant deaths result from low birth weight.[3]

Childhood

Critical Thinking

While studying early childhood development, Nakia was surprised to learn that some children in the United States are undernourished. What evidence might Nakia observe in children that would suggest undernourishment?

Early childhood, when growth is rapid, is another period when undernutrition is extremely risky. The brain and central nervous system are particularly vulnerable because of their rapid growth from conception through early childhood. After the preschool years, brain growth and development slow dramatically until maturity, when they cease. Nutritional deprivation, especially in early infancy, can lead to permanent brain impairment.[5,24] After early childhood, environmental factors may affect learning, but the basic size and structure of the brain are set.

In general, poor children experience more nutritional deprivation and overall illness and are more severely affected than other children. For example, iron-

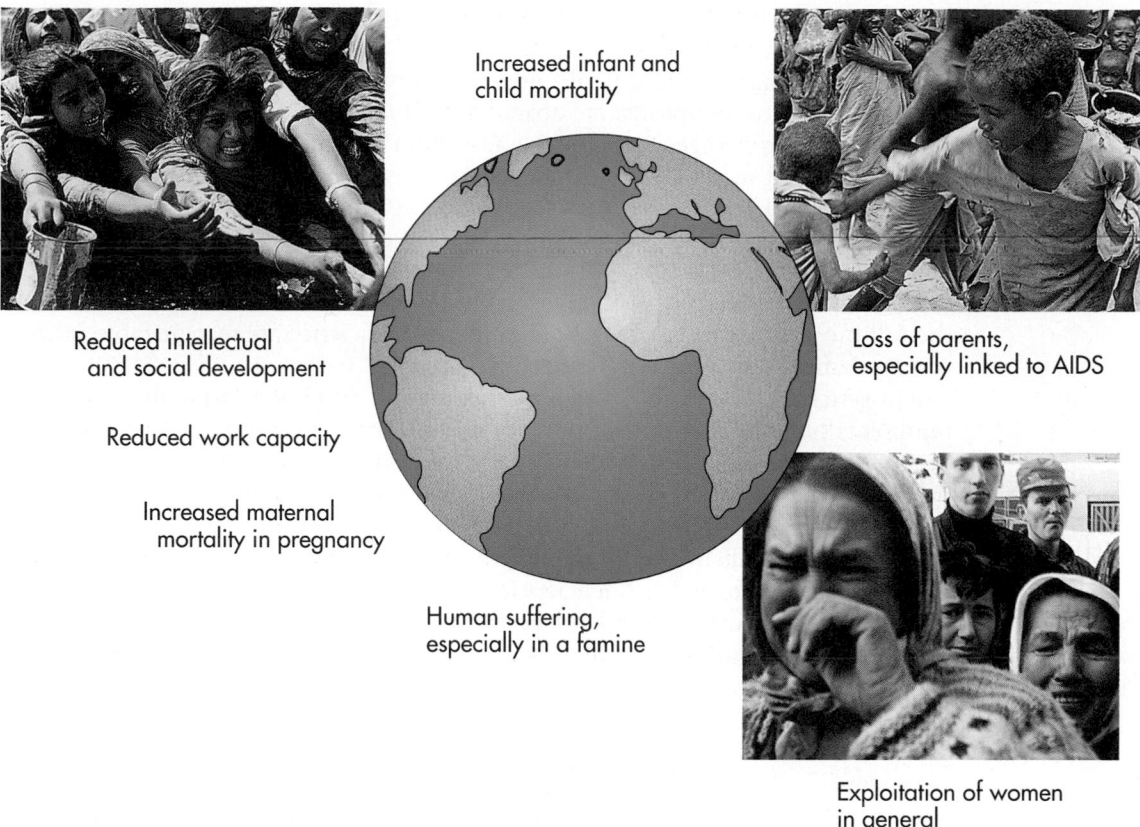

Increased infant and child mortality

Reduced intellectual and social development

Reduced work capacity

Increased maternal mortality in pregnancy

Human suffering, especially in a famine

Loss of parents, especially linked to AIDS

Exploitation of women in general

Figure 18-1 *Undernutrition affects many aspects of human health and humanity in general.*

deficiency anemia is much more common among poor children than children from less deprived families. This deficiency can lead to fatigue, reduced stamina, stunted growth, and learning problems. Undernutrition in childhood can also weaken resistance to infection, because immune function decreases when such nutrients as protein, vitamin A, and zinc are very low in a diet.[14,19] Poorly nourished youngsters are then at risk for more frequent colds, ear infections, and other infectious diseases, which may lead to frequent absences from school. Clearly, undernutrition and illness have a cyclical relationship: Not only does undernutrition cause illness, but illness worsens undernutrition, particularly diarrhea and infectious diseases.[3] Overall, chronic poor health depletes children of nutrients and leaves them with poor appetites.

When adequate nutrients are restored to children's diets, improvements in health can be obvious. For example, in recent years the average height of several groups of growth-retarded children in the United States, including Hispanic children in Colorado, has been shown to increase after zinc supplementation.

According to a recent survey of 76 developing countries, stunting was seen in more than one third of children from the ages of 2 to 5 years.

Later Years

Older people are also at risk for undernutrition.[3] They often require nutrient-dense foods, in amounts depending on their state of health and degree of physical activity. Because many of them have fixed incomes and incur significant medical costs, food often becomes a low-priority item. In addition, older people are often unable to take care of all their own needs, are sometimes isolated, and are more apt to be depressed—all important factors that can influence food intake (see Chapter 16).

General Effects of Semistarvation

In the initial stages the results of undernutrition from semistarvation are often so mild that physical symptoms are absent and blood tests do not usually detect the slight metabolic changes. Even in the absence of clinical symptoms, however, undernourishment may affect reproductive capacity, resistance to and recovery from disease, physical activity and work output, and attitudes and behavior.[14] Recall from Chapter 1 that as tissues continue to be depleted of nutrients, blood tests eventually detect biochemical changes, such as a drop in blood hemoglobin concentration. Physical symptoms, such as body weakness, appear with further depletion. Finally, the full-blown symptoms of the predominating deficiency are recognizable, such as when **edema** accompanies a protein deficiency.[16]

In general, when a few people in a population develop a severe deficiency, this represents only the tip of the iceberg. Typically a much greater number have milder degrees of undernutrition. As previously noted, mild nutrient deficiencies may not be life threatening, but they can in certain critical combinations still cause serious practical difficulties in health, as well as in life in general. These deficiencies should not, therefore, be dismissed as trivial, especially in the developing world.[12] It is becoming clear that combined deficiencies of specific vitamins and the minerals iron and zinc can seriously reduce work performance, even when they don't cause obvious physical symptoms. **Marginal** deficiencies of iodide, iron, and zinc affect hundreds of millions of people worldwide.[14] A leading group of international nutrition scientists has set a goal to reverse this pattern.[12]

In the 1940s a group of scientists, led by Dr. Ansel Keys, performed detailed experiments on the effects of chronic undernutrition. The researchers maintained 32 previously healthy men on a diet averaging about 1600 kcal daily for 6 months. During this time the men lost an average of 24% of their body weight. After about 3 months the subjects complained of fatigue, muscle soreness, irritability, and hunger pains. They exhibited a lack of ambition and self-discipline and poor concentration. They were often moody and depressed. They became less able to laugh heartily, sneeze, and tolerate heat. Heart rate and muscle tone also decreased.

These cumulative stresses of undernutrition eventually caused emotional instability and general apathy. Persistent hunger made it difficult for the subjects to pursue cultural interests, perform manual activities, and study. When the subjects were permitted to eat normally again, the desire for more food and a feeling of fatigue continued, even after 12 weeks of rehabilitation. By 20 weeks they had largely, but not fully, recovered—full recovery required about 33 weeks.

The effects of undernutrition in poor countries are probably even greater than Dr. Keys and his colleagues reported, because their subjects had adequate vitamin and mineral intakes. In addition, the inhabitants of poorer countries must contend with recurrent infections, poor sanitary conditions, extreme weather conditions, and regular exposure to extremely infectious diseases.[3] They require greater amounts of certain nutrients—especially iron—to combat rampant parasite and other infections, which compounds the problem. As mentioned before, deficiencies in both iron and zinc can lead to reduced immune function and thereby increase the risk of disease caused by infections such as diarrhea, pneumonia, and dysentery. This state of ill health in turn diminishes the ability of individuals, communities, and even whole countries to perform at peak levels of physical and mental capacity, creating a dearth in human resources.[3]

As described earlier, a common consequence of undernutrition in the United States and worldwide is an increased rate of infant mortality. The U.S. infant mortality rate is currently higher than that of 23 other industrialized countries. Contributing to infant mortality here are teenage pregnancy and inadequate food intake. Young mothers frequently don't meet their nutrient needs, which increases their risk of delivering a low–birth-weight infant.[15] These babies are much more likely to con-

Edema
The buildup of excess fluid in extracellular spaces.

Marginal
Noticeable but not severe.

tract life-threatening infections. Worldwide a lack of food, whether caused by poverty or poor food choices, compromises the health of many young children.[26]

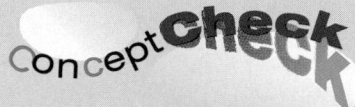

Hunger is the uneasiness and pain that result when insufficient food is eaten to meet energy needs. Chronic hunger leads to undernutrition, which can cause growth failure in children and weakness in adults. Risk of infection increases, and nutrient-deficiency diseases result. The primary cause of undernutrition is poverty. The critical periods for undernutrition occur during pregnancy, infancy, childhood, and old age. The adverse effects in pregnancy and infancy are quite dramatic, as evidenced by mortality rates much higher than those of healthy populations.

Undernutrition in the United States

About 38 million Americans live at or near the poverty level, currently estimated at about $15,141 annually for a family of four (Table 18-3). This represents 19% of families with children, up from 11% in 1973. More than two thirds of these people live in metropolitan areas. These poor include about 20% of all children; children, in fact, comprise 48% of the poor.[3] Overall, African-Americans have the highest poverty rate of any racial group, currently 32%. The poverty rate for Hispanics is 28%; Asians and Pacific Islanders, 12%; and Caucasians, 11%. About two thirds of these Americans experience chronic hunger.

Poor Americans often face difficult choices: whether to buy groceries for the family or pay this month's rent; whether to have dental work done or pay the current utility bill; or whether to replace clothes the children have outgrown or pay for transportation to apply for a job. Food is one of the few flexible items in a poor person's budget. Rents are fixed, utility costs aren't negotiable, the price of medical care and prescription drugs can't be bargained down, and bus drivers won't accept less than the going rate to transport riders. A person can always eat less, however. The short-term consequences may be less dramatic than having the utilities shut off. The long-term cumulative effects, however, are disturbing.[5]

In sheer numbers, undernutrition in the United States is a troubling problem. Its existence is all the more disturbing because, although the threat of undernutrition for most Americans was virtually eliminated in the 1970s, it reemerged and spread rapidly in the 1980s. The fact that undernutrition and hunger remain in the 1990s indicates that their roots are mainly political and socioeconomic, rather than technical.[4] Clearly, American society is productive enough to generate the resources

The official measures of poverty don't include the effects of either noncash benefits or tax breaks, such as the Earned Income Tax Credit. Adjusted to include these, the poverty rate is 11.5%, or 30.1 million persons. This shows the importance of targeted support for the poor and portends the dangers of reducing such benefits (see discussion later in this chapter).

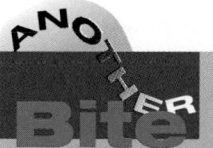

Because Americans experiencing chronic hunger eat enough to prevent overt starvation, undernutrition in the United States is quite different from that in the developing world. Kwashiorkor and marasmus, evident in the pictures of Rwandan children in the mid-1990s, rarely occur. Instead, undernutrition is represented by the young child whose weight is several pounds below the low end of the normal range on a growth chart. The untrained eye may not recognize the condition or may simply see the child as skinny. The trained professional will recognize that the child's size reflects growth failure.[4]

TABLE 18-3

The Realities of Poverty and Undernutrition in the United States

- About 7% of infants born in the United States are low–birth-weight. This accounts for more than half of all infant deaths and for 75% of deaths of babies under 1 month of age.

- The infant mortality rate in the United States is higher than that of 21 other industrialized countries. Teenage pregnancy contributes to infant mortality because young mothers frequently don't meet their nutrient needs.

- Single-parent families constitute about 25% of all families with children. The poverty rate (60%) for the approximately 19 million children in such families is four times higher than that for children in two-parent families.

- About 38 million Americans live at or near the poverty level. These poor include about 20% of all children; children, in fact, comprise 40% of the poor. Hunger frequently accompanies poverty.

- A poor family of four in the United States has an average income of $10,923. Contrast that to the average earnings of an affluent family: $65,536.

- In the United States an estimated 12 million people, or 6.5 percent of all adults, have experienced homelessness sometime during their lives. An episode of homelessness nearly always lasts for at least 1 week and often for a month or more.

- The Food Stamp program for low-income people provides each household with $170 per month. About 1 American in 10 participates in this program.

- Second Harvest, the largest U.S. food bank, estimates that 26 million people, or more than 1 American in 10, rely on food depositories and soup kitchens to feed themselves and their families. Most of these people, the organization reports, are skilled workers who have lost their jobs.

required to feed all its citizens. In the developing world, far more factors complicate this problem, a subject that will be discussed later in the chapter.

Helping Hungry Americans: a Historical Perspective

Until the twentieth century, individuals and a wide variety of charitable, often church-related organizations provided most of the help to poor, undernourished people in the United States. Local governments sponsored only limited programs. Few of these early efforts distributed direct cash payments to poor people because these were thought to reduce recipients' motivation to improve their circumstances or change behavior, such as excessive drinking, that contributed to their poverty. Beginning in the early 1900s the involvement of local, county, and state governments in providing assistance to the poor has steadily increased.[15]

Depression Era to the Mid-1970s

The Great Depression of the 1930s marked a decisive change, as the federal government assumed for the first time a major role in various programs aimed at reducing undernutrition and poverty. Studies at the time documented both undernutrition and the existence of widespread pellagra (niacin deficiency) and rickets (vitamin D deficiency). In response, the federal government sponsored soup kitchens and other programs that distributed food commodities throughout the country. During World War II a large percentage of the men rejected for physical reasons by the draft were found to have been undernourished 10 to 12 years earlier, during the Depression era. This practical demonstration of the long-term detrimental effects of

TABLE 18-4

Some Current Federally Subsidized Programs that Supply Food for Americans

Program	Eligibility	Description
Food Stamps	Low income	Coupons are given to purchase food at grocery stores, the amount based on size of household and income
Emergency Food System	Low income	Food stamps issued on 24-hour notice for 1 month while eligibility for further use of the program can be investigated
Commodity Supplemental Food Program	Certain low-income populations, such as pregnant women and young children	USDA surplus foods are distributed by county agencies
Special Supplemental Feeding Program for Women, Infants, and Children (WIC)	Low-income pregnant/lactating women, infants, and children less than 5 years old at nutritional risk	Coupons are given to purchase milk, cheese, fruit juice, cereal, infant formula, and other specific food items at grocery stores
School Lunch	Low income	Free or reduced-price lunch distributed by the school; meal follows USDA pattern based on the Food Guide Pyramid; cost for the child depends on family income. In schools without a lunch program, special milk programs may be available.
School Breakfast	Low income	Free or reduced-price breakfast distributed by the school; meal follows USDA pattern; cost for the child depends on family income.
Child Care Food Program	Child enrolled in organized child care program; income guidelines are the same as School Lunch Program	Reimbursement given for meals supplied to children at the site; meals must follow USDA guidelines based on the Food Guide Pyramid.
Congregate Meals for the Elderly	Age 60 or over (no income guidelines)	Free noon meal is furnished at a site; meal follows specific pattern based on $1/3$ of the RDA.
Home-delivered Meals	Age 60 or over, homebound	Noon meal is delivered at no cost or for a fee, depending on income, at least 5 days a week. Sometimes other meals for later consumption are delivered at the same time; private organizations that sponsor these programs often refer to them as "Meals on Wheels."

childhood undernutrition led Congress to enact legislation setting up the school lunch program in 1946.[15]

In the 1950s, it was assumed that all Americans had enough to eat. Nevertheless, occasional reports of undernutrition surfaced, mostly among the chronic poor: migrant workers, Native Americans, African-Americans in the South, unemployed minorities in general, and some older people.

After observing extensive hunger and poverty during his presidential campaign in the 1960s, John F. Kennedy revitalized the food stamp program, which actually began two decades earlier, and expanded commodity distribution programs.[15] The Food Stamp program for low-income people allows recipients to use food stamps to purchase food and seeds—but not tobacco, cleaning items, alcoholic beverages, and nonedible products—at stores authorized to accept them. Each household currently receives about $170 per month, on average. About 1 in 10 Americans participates in this program[21] (Table 18-4).

Congress established the school breakfast program in 1965 as politicians began to notice the number of children coming to school hungry. School lunch and breakfast programs still enable low-income students to receive meals free or at reduced cost if certain income guidelines are met (under $26,500 annual income for

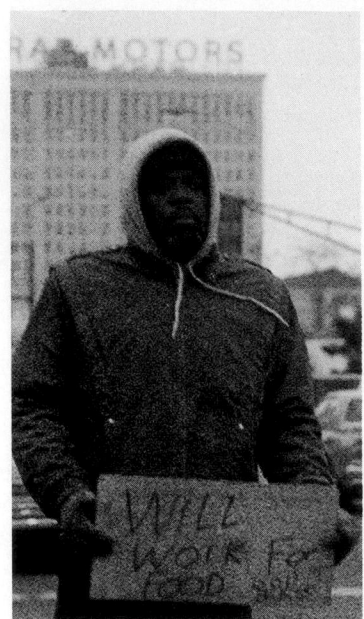

Major job layoffs in blue-collar industries have contributed to the twin problems of hunger and homelessness in the United States.

a family of four). In the same year, Congress funded group noontime (called *congregate*) meals and home-delivered meals for all citizens over 60 years of age, regardless of income.[15] Both remain active programs, serving about 1 million meals each day, but they still do not reach all who need help.[21]

Political and social awareness of hunger and undernutrition in the late 1960s was spurred on by the book *Hunger USA* and a resulting television documentary, *Hunger in America*, shown in May 1968. The film graphically demonstrated that hunger existed in all areas and ethnic groups in the United States. The response was dramatic. Between 1969 and 1971, some already large federal food programs were expanded and others were created. For example, the Food Stamp program served only 2 million people in 1968, but by 1971 it was serving 11 million. The School Lunch program, which served only 2 million poor children before 1970, was serving 8 million children by 1971. Soon after, the School Breakfast program, a pilot program for children living in impoverished areas, became nationally available. In addition, in 1972 the Special Supplemental Feeding Program for Women, Infants, and Children (WIC) was authorized. This program provides food vouchers and nutrition education to low-income pregnant and lactating women and their young children.[15] Today it serves about 7 million people.

WIC has been repeatedly shown to be cost effective, especially in reducing the numbers of preterm, low–birth-weight babies. WIC is also credited for the widespread drop in iron-deficiency anemia among children in the last decade.[15] However, the federal budget shortfalls over the last few years have threatened not only the scope but the existence of this program. Every year the program struggles for support. "Of all the dumb ways of saving money, not feeding pregnant women and kids is the dumbest," said the late Dr. Jean Mayer, one of the world's pioneers in nutrition research and policy.[15]

A Reevaluation: 1975 to Now

In 1977, a team of physicians resurveyed areas of undernutrition studied 10 years earlier. They found that the degree of poverty in certain regions, such as Appalachia and the slums of big cities, had not changed. If anything, poverty was often worse than in 1967. Yet undernutrition had essentially disappeared as a social phenomenon. As a population, Americans had more food resources available to them. The large federal food programs—Food Stamps, the School Lunch and School Breakfast programs, and WIC—contributed to this difference. Politicians had responded to the demands of the American people by directing federal resources toward a massive human problem, and the effort succeeded. Certainly, some Americans still fell through the cracks, but a "safety net" was catching many whose nutritional needs had not been met before.[4]

The first official recognition that widespread hunger had reappeared in the United States came from a conference of mayors in 1982, although the news media had been reporting the appearance of soup kitchens and bread lines in the nation's cities since the beginning of the decade.[4] Why was there a sudden increase in hungry people in the United States? First, unemployment in the United States rose in early 1980. Second, the eligibility and funding for federal food assistance programs such as the Food Stamp program and the School Lunch and Breakfast programs were tightened and reduced. During that time, funding for meal programs for older people also lagged far behind increases in food prices, operating costs, and the number of people in this age group. Finally, working poor families suffered from a decrease in benefits from Aid to Families with Dependent Children (AFDC).

Currently, federal funds still fall short of the amount needed to end hunger in the United States. For instance, the need for WIC services greatly outstrips resources allocated to the program. This forces children out of the program, because pregnant women and infants are given the highest priority.

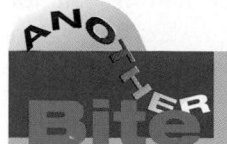

Privately funded programs augment state and federal efforts to combat hunger in the United States. There are currently more than 180 food banks, 23,000 food pantries, and 3300 soup kitchens helping to cope with this problem.[15] A recent survey found that slightly more than two of every three people requesting such emergency food assistance were members of families—children and their parents. Second Harvest, the largest U.S. food bank, estimates that 26 million people, or more than one in 10 of all Americans, rely on food depositories and soup kitchens to feed themselves and their families. Most of these people are skilled workers who have lost their jobs.

Socioeconomic Factors Related to Undernutrition

In the United States today, persistent hunger and undernutrition are largely associated with two interrelated conditions: poverty and homelessness. Thus economic, social, and political changes that lead to an increase in the number of poor or homeless people also tend to intensify the problem of undernutrition.

Poverty

Although highly trained people are quite competitive in the increasingly global economy of the 1990s, there is a glut of unskilled manual labor available throughout the world. As noted earlier, in 1995 more than 38 million Americans were living at or below the poverty threshold. Many families have suffered economic hardship caused by massive layoffs in U.S. manufacturing industries that began in the late 1980s and continue in the 1990s as the economy becomes more global. Furthermore, many jobs created in the 1980s were in the service sector, such as quick-service restaurants.[15] When one or both parents have one of these low-paying jobs—even full-time—their family may still be at or below the poverty level. Note that parents in most poor families do work; nearly two in three contain at least one worker. In sum, working poor people in the United States have not only had to subsist with less federal assistance, but they have also been forced to cope with a dwindling amount of purchasing power.

A poor family of four in the United States currently has an average income of $10,923. Contrast that with the average earnings of an affluent family: $65,536. Needless to say, the poor family's limited budget must affect food purchases.

Another primary factor contributing to poverty has been the dramatic increase in the number of single-parent families in the United States, the result of high rates of divorce and out-of-wedlock births. Currently, single-parent families constitute about 25% of all families with children. The poverty rate (60%) for the approximately

19 million children in single-parent families is four times higher than the rate for those in two-parent families.[3]

About one third of children are now born out of wedlock, 30% to teenagers. The number of children born to unwed teenagers rose from about 250,000 in 1980 to about 367,000 a decade later. When unmarried teenagers have babies, mothers and children alike often face a lifetime of poverty. The reasons for the large increase in out-of-wedlock births are complex: increased sexual promiscuity by unmarried individuals, especially teenagers; diminishing economic prospects for young people, especially inner-city men; cultural devaluation of marriage as an institution; and a popular culture that celebrates instant gratification without emphasizing future consequences. Indeed, some experts suggest that child poverty would largely disappear in the United States if out-of-wedlock births dropped to zero.

Some observers believe that many publicly funded assistance programs have actually provided an incentive for poor single women to have more children: the more children they have, the more welfare and other assistance benefits they receive. Although only limited evidence supports this belief, many people are recommending policies that shift emphasis from direct assistance to other options. A recent overhaul of the nation's welfare program reflects this thinking by imposing limits on direct assistance to 5 years or so, in part to decrease welfare dependence and encourage a return to work.

Many politicians and political writers point out we need greater wisdom in our approach to illegitimacy and single parenthood. They consider this issue a crisis with the potential for disaster and stress the need for solutions we haven't yet found or fully implemented. Some suggestions have been to improve child care, teach parenting skills, and expand job opportunities.[3]

Homelessness

The availability of cooking facilities affects nutrient intake among the poor. Without cooking facilities, people may buy expensive foods that require no preparation. These are typically processed snack foods, which provide energy but are often lacking in nutrients.

The economics of poverty and undernutrition have recently changed in one additional important way. Homelessness is much more evident now than in 1980. Families with children currently account for about 43 percent of the homeless. An estimated 12 million people, or 6.5 percent of all adults, in the United States have experienced homelessness sometime during their lives. Episodes of homelessness nearly always last for at least 1 week and often for a month or more. The estimated lifetime homelessness rate rises to about 15 percent of the adult population in the United States when it includes people who have moved into someone else's residence during periods when they had nowhere else to live.

Homelessness exists partly because the cost of housing has substantially increased and partly because federal support for subsidized housing was cut dramatically (by 75%) during the 1980s. The government considers housing costs, which include rent and utilities, to be affordable if they consume no more than 30% of a family's income. Today many poor people who rent pay a much larger percentage of their income in rent and utilities.[15] These families, although not homeless, are likely to suffer from undernutrition without direct food assistance. Moreover, even a small change in the economic circumstances of such poor families may force them into actual homelessness, at least temporarily. In this situation, homelessness is essentially a consequence of poverty. This scenario often involves single-parent families; as noted earlier, these families are most likely to suffer poverty and homelessness.

Other important causes of homelessness include the widespread release of mentally ill patients from mental institutions in the 1980s, unemployment, substance abuse, and personal crises. The abuse of alcohol and crack cocaine is another notable cause. Nationally, up to 85% of all homeless people in large cities abuse alcohol or drugs or have a mental illness. Most people with such problems are unable to find and hold employment; without support from family or friends, they and their dependents will probably become homeless.[9]

The stereotypical image of a homeless person is someone who is out of step with society and who might refuse to work. Each year, however, more and more typical Americans find themselves among the homeless.

Food and Shelter as a Basic Human Right

Numerous factors in the United States contribute to poverty and homelessness—and the undernutrition that usually results. Providing better housing, education, and training is an important first step in solving the problem. Although many people in these situations may bear at least part of the responsibility, blaming the victims does not deliver food or shelter to those in need. Opponents of federal nutrition programs raise the issue of cost, often citing the federal deficit as a reason for limiting spending and arguing that much of the money is wasted by bureaucrats and drug-addicted recipients. In your opinion, do these factors outweigh the need to meet the nutritional and housing needs of American citizens?

Consider that when money is needed for crisis situations, such as sending military aid to end strife in war-torn countries in the 1990s, it is there. Also consider that there is no easy way to penalize the parent, if that is the intent, without hurting the innocent child. According to a recent survey conducted by the National League of Cities, officials in 47 large cities expressed little optimism that current attempts by Congress to reform welfare would help revitalize impoverished neighborhoods. Instead, about 3 in 4 officials concluded that the legislation would worsen homelessness and increase child abuse and poverty in their cities.

Undernutrition especially is a condition that need not exist. If used fully and effectively, nutrition programs and community intervention could go a long way toward meeting the nutritional needs of those at highest risk.[13] An increase in training and employment opportunities could help stabilize these improvements.[13] The near elimination of large-scale undernutrition in the United States in the 1970s demonstrates that this national problem can be solved.[4] Until all citizens can support themselves, the government will continue to be an important safety net for the undernourished.

Private emergency-food network systems are also important, as noted earlier, but are not sufficient to meet all food needs in the United States. Private donations often taper off during economic hardship in a given geographical area.[3] Furthermore, most of the donated items are limited in nutritional value. By necessity, processed and canned grocery items predominate, rather than protein-rich foods and perishable items, such as fresh produce and milk.

Still, a long-term solution to the problem of hunger in the United States can't be achieved by the government or private agencies alone. Education, training, housing, and food assistance provide only part of the answer. Change also requires a cultural shift emphasizing the responsibility of all citizens to provide as best they can for themselves, their families, and the less fortunate around them. Many Americans consider an increase in individual responsibility as a critical goal for our society at this time. Government programs can't easily fix poverty and resulting hunger that stem from irresponsible individual behavior. Government programs can, however, help reduce or prevent poverty that results largely from lack of opportunity.[9] We have seen a recent cultural shift against smoking and drunk driving. Could illegitimacy and abandonment of family be similarly discouraged?

Clearly the victims of poverty don't deserve all the blame. Poorer Americans confront substantial difficulties: substandard education and training, poor communication skills, lack of reliable and safe child care, inability to relocate, little employment experience, and no economic reserves to fall back on during crises.[4] Even with a strong desire for a better life, people may get discouraged and apathetic in the face of apparently insurmountable obstacles. Moreover, many poor Americans are unable to meet the demands of a modern, dynamic society—in particular, elderly,

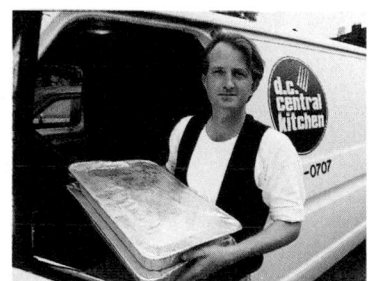

This Washington, D.C., operation collects leftover food from hotels, restaurants, and catering firms for delivery to homeless shelters, soup kitchens, and churches.

sick, and disabled people and young single mothers and their children. Regardless of how repugnant government assistance appears to some people, it will probably always be necessary to some extent. The columnist George Will notes, "Conservatives say, well, nothing could be worse than the current system. They are underestimating their ingenuity." In abolishing a so-called failed welfare system, are we not obligated to put something workable in its place?

Because long-term undernutrition—especially among children—has both individual and societal consequences, all Americans are affected by this problem, either directly or indirectly. The next few years are likely to bring further changes in both government and private assistance programs, demanding new initiatives from all Americans. Your contribution to this process as an informed voter and, ideally, an active participant is an important part of the process.

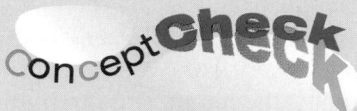

Federal programs designed to reduce hunger and undernutrition began in the 1930s, during the Great Depression. In response to reports of widespread poverty and hunger during the early 1960s, Congress established several new federal food assistance programs and substantially increased funding for already existing programs. Largely as a result of these federal programs, undernutrition decreased substantially by the mid-1970s. The improvement was short-lived, and the number of Americans experiencing poverty, homelessness, and undernutrition grew during the 1980s and 1990s. The presence of these three interrelated problems is influenced by economic, cultural, and individual factors, as well as government policies. The serious questions about the long-term effectiveness of many government assistance programs are causing major changes in their future administration, funding mechanisms, and program design. All citizens can help to reduce the problem of undernutrition.

Undernutrition in the Developing World: Underlying Causes

Undernutrition in the developing world is also tied to poverty, and any true solution must address this problem. However, these countries have a multitude of problems so complex and interrelated that they cannot be treated separately. Programs that have proved immensely helpful in the United States are only a starting point in this context. The following major obstacles challenge those seeking a solution[3]:

- Extreme imbalances in the food/population ratio in different regions of a country
- War and political/civil unrest
- The rapid depletion of natural resources
- Cultural attitudes toward certain foods
- Poor **infrastructure,** especially poor housing, sanitation and storage facilities, education, communications, and transportation systems
- High external debt

Each problem deserves individual consideration. In this context, Figure 18-2 depicts key factors relating to a household's food intake.

The Food/Population Ratio

Whether the earth can yield enough food for all people has been a long-standing question. As early as 1798, the English clergyman and political economist Thomas

Infrastructure
The basic framework of a system of organization. For a society, this includes roads, bridges, telephones, and other basic technologies.

Malthus proposed a rather pessimistic view of our prospects. He said that given the passion between the sexes (which he felt should be discouraged), the population would always increase faster than the food supply. Malthus felt that the growing population would therefore be subject to recurring checks imposed by widespread starvation, war, or natural catastrophe brought on by disease.

Malthus's proposals became the object of intense controversy in England and elsewhere, often meeting vigorous opposition. Eminent British scientists pointed out that scientific advances in agriculture would greatly increase food production. In fact, that has proved true. Nevertheless, the aptly named population explosion has undermined this progress. Population growth has not slowed significantly through natural checks, disease, or recent human interventions, such as birth control[2] (Figure 18-3).

No one knows how many people the earth can support; it depends on an unknown potential for changes in technology and on the ability of economies to substitute new resources for ones that are running out. Some experts argue that the real threat is not a finite amount of land, topsoil, and water but rather the failure of nations to pursue the economic, trade, and research policies necessary to increase the production of food, limit environmental damage, and ensure resources reach the people who need them. In a free society, people are an asset, not a liability. Significant poverty and undernutrition persist mainly in areas where governments dominate and suffocate economic progress, such as in North Korea. Still, ingenuity of this

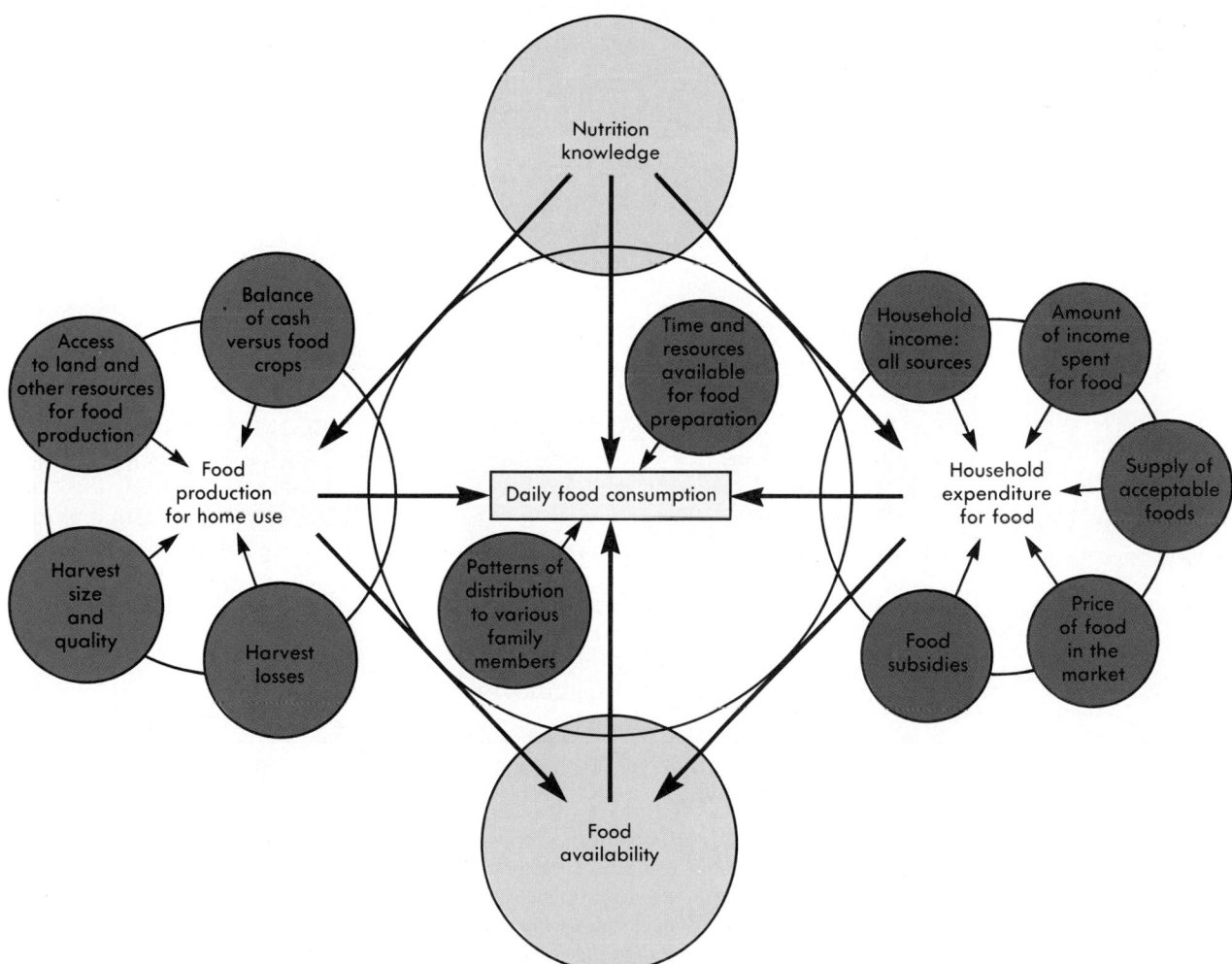

Figure 18-2 *The many factors affecting household food consumption.*

sort does not materialize automatically. Furthermore, even if new solutions can be devised, some countries lack the means to take timely advantage of them.[3]

Currently, population growth exceeds economic growth in much of the world, and poverty is increasing.[2] Because efforts to speed up economic development have failed, the only remaining way to improve the situation may be slowing down the growth of population, as Malthus recommended. If we want to ensure a decent life for a widening segment of humanity, the growth in the earth's population should

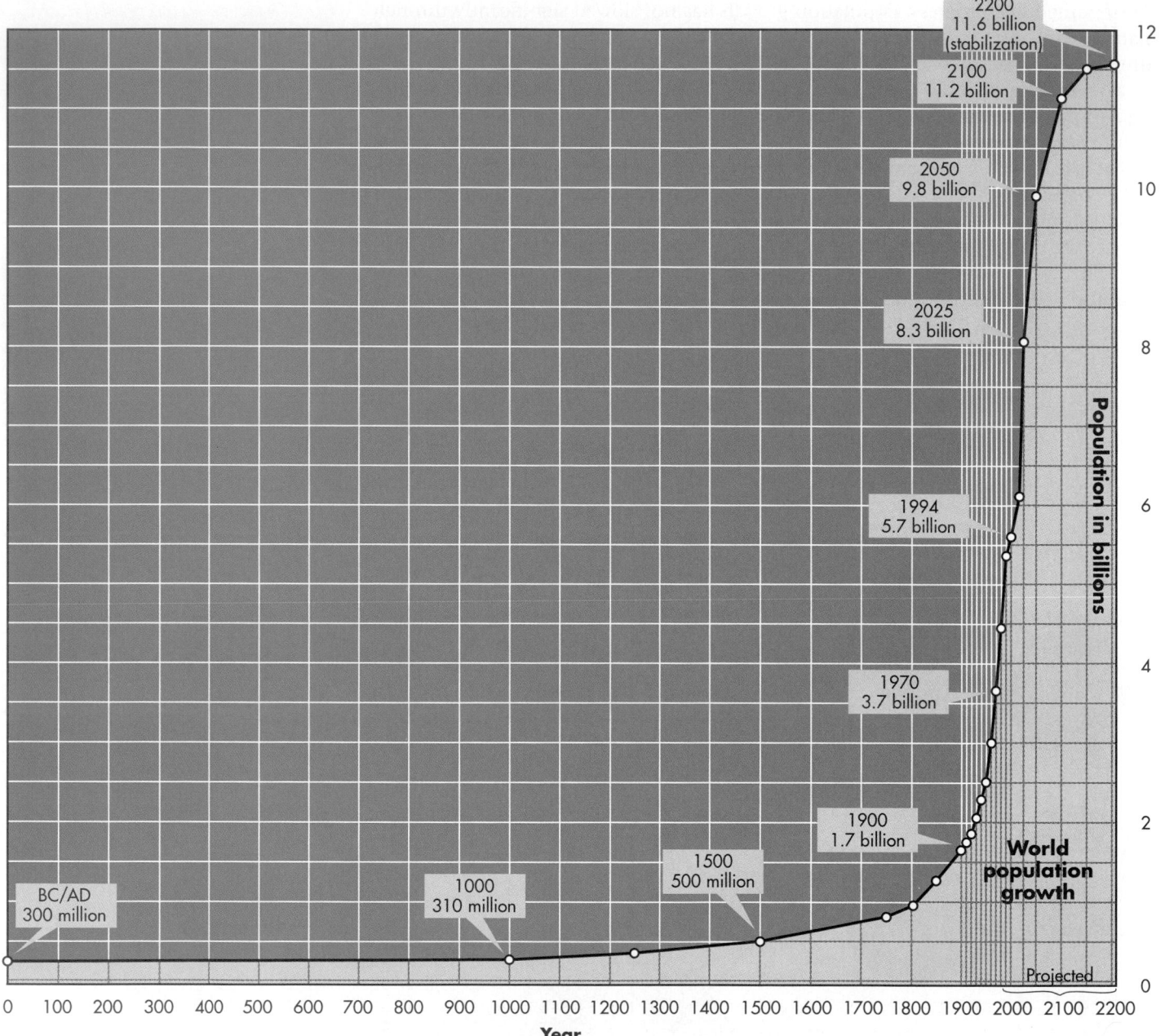

Figure 18-3 *World population trends. Population growth is stabilizing in the industrialized countries of the world but continues to skyrocket in the developing countries. The current world population is 5.8 billion. These long-range projections of expected population values assume a continued decline in fertility. Without this decline, population growth could be much more rapid in the first half of the next century than shown here. (Data modified from Overseas Development Council, United Nations Population Fund.)*

slow. According to the World Bank, the world's population increases by 1 billion people every 12 years, mostly in cities and in seacoast and river-basin areas, where the environment is most under stress. By 2030 the world will have nearly 3 billion more people than today—2 billion of them in countries where the average person earns less than $2 a day. Unless a catastrophe occurs, more than 9 of 10 infants in the next generation will be born in the poorest parts of the world.[3]

As one brake on population expansion, birth control programs have been effective in developed countries but relatively ineffective in developing countries that could really profit from them. Whereas women in the United States average 2.1 live births each, women in some East African countries average 8.5 live births each and women worldwide average 4.0 live births. At this time, there are about 5.8 billion people in the world. More than three quarters live in countries in the developing world, and more than half live in Asia. Many experts believe that the global supply of food would provide adequate nutrition for all 5.8 billion of us, about 2400 kcal each per day.[3] However, food supplies are not distributed equally among consumers. Gross disparities exist between developed and developing countries, among the rich and poor within countries, and even within families. In some instances, women and children get less to eat than men, and sometimes female children get less than their male counterparts.[16]

Food supply and population trends within the developing world also vary greatly. Latin America and Russia both have had declining population growth rates since 1970, and their share of the world population will have risen only marginally between 1950 and 2025. On the other hand, the population in Africa will have more than doubled, constituting 19% of the world population over the same 75-year period. The population will probably rise from 650 million in 1992 to 900 million by the year 2000.[3]

Economists estimate that world food production will in fact continue to increase more rapidly than the world population in the near future, allowing the food/population ratio to increase through the year 2020. In the short run then, the primary problem appears to be not food production, but distribution and use, especially in poverty-stricken areas of the developing nations.

Eventually, though, food production will probably begin to lag behind population growth.[2] We are currently drifting in that direction. Most good farmland in the world is already in use, and because of poor farming practices or competing land-use demands, the number of farmable acres worldwide decreases annually. For many reasons, sustainable world food output—an amount that doesn't deplete the earth's resources—is now running well behind food consumption.[18] This discrepancy suggests that food production in less-developed countries will barely keep up with population growth and will soon lag behind. That in turn will reduce the reserves needed to combat and prevent undernutrition, particularly widespread starvation, in developing countries.

A renewed focus on population control. Although efforts on the supply side of the food/population ratio are essential, many researchers still emphasize the need to reduce the demand side.[2] They argue that the survival of our civilization depends on limiting reproduction.

For millions of years, maximizing reproduction has been a measure of biological success. Because disease and difficult living conditions often claimed young lives, couples produced many offspring in an attempt to ensure the longevity of the family. These conditions still exist in countries in the developing world, where children also provide the primary means of support to their parents in old age. More children also means more helpers to farm, hunt, and prepare food. In India a rigid class structure that leaves many people destitute encourages large families. Traditionally, poorer people bear more children, contrary to what you might predict.

Now, in an evolutionary blink of the eye—mere decades—poor people in developing nations are being asked to reverse their attitude toward having children. It is a difficult undertaking. In 1888, 1.5 billion people inhabited the earth. Now the population exceeds 5.8 billion and is growing fast.[3] Currently the population increases by three people every second, or about a quarter of a million people every day. In essence the world must accommodate a new population roughly equivalent to that of the United States and Canada every 3 years!

Even though the overall rate of growth has begun to decline, population experts believe population size will still pass 8.3 billion by the year 2025. The poorest countries are increasing the most and will contain 7 billion of us, further straining their ability to cope. The world's population is likely to exceed 9.8 billion in 2050 and 11 billion in 2100 before it is finally stabilized at 11.6 billion between 2150 and 2200. If population growth continues as these predictions indicate, governments will be forced to confront economic problems that would have been difficult even in less crowded times. Generally speaking, an increasing population stresses existing resources in developing countries; many people's needs are not met, social unrest is intensified, and significant environmental destruction is more likely.[3]

Keys to successful family planning programs. Attempts to implement family-planning programs in developing nations have been only partially successful. Some small countries—such as Singapore, Taiwan, Thailand, Colombia, Costa Rica, and several Caribbean countries—have reduced their birthrates substantially. Larger countries, including India and Mexico, are struggling.

With its nearly 1.2 billion people, China is seriously overpopulated—22% of the world's population is living on 7% of the world's arable land. Recognizing the gravity of the situation, the Chinese government has imposed the world's most stringent family-planning program, which allows only one child per urban couple—two in rural areas if the first child is a girl. The birthrate now averages 1.8 children in a woman's lifetime. Penalties for having extra children include restricted housing and employment opportunities. Abortion is very common and is sometimes forced on unwilling women, as is sterilization. These policies have lowered China's population growth rate from 27.6 per thousand in 1964 to 11.5 per thousand in 1993. Despite its statistical success, China's program is controversial, and its coercive aspects have been criticized as human rights abuses.

In general, experience with family-planning programs in developing countries and historical changes in birthrates in many industrialized countries suggests an important conclusion: Only when people have enough to eat and are financially secure do they feel safe having fewer children.[2] If poor people have adequate access to food, shelter, health care, and sufficient resources to support themselves in old age, experts believe more couples will choose to have fewer children. Increasing per capita income and improving education, especially for women in developing nations, are currently considered to be the most likely long-term solutions to excessive population growth.[3]

The history of South Korea illustrates this approach. In 1960, families in South Korea averaged six children each. Economic policies, coupled with a strong family-planning program, transformed South Korea from a struggling country to an economic success. Today, Korean families average slightly fewer than two children each, and the population will soon stabilize. However, nations do not have to wait to become industrialized before launching population-control programs. Indonesia, South Korea, and Thailand made great economic strides and at the same time controlled population growth. Currently, however, population stabilization—as in Western countries—has mainly been accompanied by relative wealth and security. In fact, in some parts of Germany the government has proposed paying couples to have children, because the birthrate has fallen since reunification of the country. Apparently, people there realize the difficulties of maintaining an acceptable standard of living as the number of children in a household increases.

In addition to economics, other obstacles to family-planning programs are ancient cultural, religious, and traditional beliefs. In subSaharan Africa, childlessness signifies the end of a line of descent, and women who don't have children are often perceived as evil. The Yoruba believe, for example, that a childless woman made a pact with evil spirits before her own birth to kill her children and, devoid of descendants, will return to join these evil spirits in some otherworldly sphere. These women fear being rendered functionally infertile by the death of all their children almost as much as they fear bearing none. Thus female sterilization and even contraception have not been successful. Even women with four or five children fear, not unreasonably, that all their children may suddenly die. Also, Moslem religious practices typically promote a large, abundant family as a sign of prosperity and health.

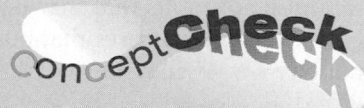

Breastfeeding is important to family health. It also aids in family planning because it helps space births farther apart. If no supplemental nourishment is given, breastfeeding an infant decreases ovulation—and therefore, the likelihood of fertilization—for an average of about 6 months, although breastfeeding is not a completely reliable form of birth control. When childbirths are more widely spaced, mother and infant are healthier and fewer total births occur. Women who do not breastfeed generally begin to ovulate within a month or so after giving birth.

Only by taking on the twin challenges of economic insecurity and population growth can the developed world hope to escape the expensive trap of humanitarian intervention and crisis management for peoples in need.[3] Today it is likely that Malthus' gloomy prediction may soon become a fact. If we cannot find ways of humanely controlling population growth, nature may solve the problem by killing off large portions of humanity in the ways Malthus predicted.[2] Only the future will tell.

Concept Check

Currently, world food production is sufficient to meet the energy needs of the world's population. Despite adequate food resources, undernutrition exists because of poverty, politics, and unequal distribution. In addition, projected population growth may soon overwhelm food production. Most scientists and world leaders recommend limiting population growth, especially in developing countries where birth rates are high.

War and Political/Civil Unrest

The president of Mali recently stated,

"Only by translating our sense of common destiny into action will we be able to resolve the paradox of currently spending $1000 billion each year in the production of lethal weapons, while only a fraction of that sum would make our planet a land of prosperity for millions of people who today suffer from illness, hunger, thirst, and ignorance."

Worldwide military spending has doubled over the past 20 years. In 1994, global military expenditures were estimated at $767 billion—more than the total income of the poorest 45% of the world's population. Although Africa has been ravaged by economic decay and famines for years, military spending in Africa more than doubled in the 1970s and held firm through the early 1990s. Presently, less than one half of 1% of the world's yearly production of goods and services is devoted to economic development assistance, whereas approximately 6% goes to military expenditures.[3]

In the worst cases, civil disruptions and war contribute to massive undernutrition. War-related famine affects at least 20 million people in southern and northeastern Africa. Currently, Sudan, Rwanda, and Somalia are examples of once productive economies now struggling with mass starvation. Ethnic and politically motivated fighting has led to bloody civil wars, upending these countries' infrastructures and creating millions of refugees. Most of these people are left without shelter, clothing, food, and any means of obtaining them.[3]

Such civil strife is not limited to Africa. Following the breakup of the former Yugoslavia, warring ethnic and religious groups caused Europe's worst war since 1945. The destruction and disruption of daily life brought manufacturing, commerce, and food production to a near standstill throughout Bosnia and areas of Croatia and Serbia. Globally, civil strife currently puts 100 million people at risk of hunger.[3]

Even when food is available, political divisions may impede distribution to the point that undernutrition will plague many people for years to come. Especially during emergencies, programs designed to help the poor have been undermined by poor administration, corruption, and political influence. During the 1960s and 1970s the problem of undernutrition in less developed countries was perceived as a technical one: how to produce enough food for the growing world population. As previously explained, impressive gains in agricultural productivity and world food production have occurred in the past three decades. The problem is now seen as largely political: how to achieve cooperation among and within nations so that gains in food production and infrastructure are not wiped out by war.[3] For example, when U.S. troops ended their mission in Somalia in the early 1990s, they left knowing that although they helped end a famine in the short run, they could not pacify a hostile country. Today in much of Africa, war is destroying what the last 30 years of aid helped to build.

Only a combination of approaches—finding technical solutions that may help with problems of chronic hunger and poverty and solving political crises that push disadvantaged nations into a state of acute hunger and chaos—will help.

The Rapid Depletion of Natural Resources

As we quickly deplete the earth's resources, population control grows increasingly critical. The productive capacity of agriculture is approaching its limits in many areas worldwide. Environmentally unsustainable farming methods undermine food production, especially in parts of the developing world.[18]

The term *green revolution* describes a phenomenon that began in the 1960s when crop yields rose dramatically in some countries, such as the Philippines, India, and Mexico. The increased use of fertilizers and the development of superior crops through careful plant breeding made this rise possible.[6] Many of the technologies associated with the green revolution have now achieved most of their potential. For example, rice yield has not increased significantly since the release of superior varieties in 1966. Wheat is another example: India more than tripled its wheat harvest between 1965 and 1983, a period when high-yielding crop strains were introduced. Since then, its grain output has not increased.

Future gains in productivity may be much harder to accomplish because of the need to farm less productive soils. Until the introduction of another superior wheat

Green revolution

Increases in crop yields accompanying the introduction of new agricultural technologies in less developed countries, beginning in the 1960s. The key technologies were high-yielding, disease-resistant strains of rice, wheat, and corn; greater use of fertilizer; and improved cultivation practices.

or rice strain, developing countries will not benefit greatly from recent, more modest breakthroughs in biotechnology (see the Nutrition Issue at the end of this chapter). Actually, the green revolution was never intended to solve the world's food problems, according to Dr. Norman Borlaug, its chief architect. It was just a stopgap measure until world leaders could control population growth.

Areas of the world that remain uncultivated or ungrazed are mostly unsuited to farming: rocky, steep, infertile, too dry, too wet, or inaccessible. Much of this land is nonetheless invaluable for the crucial **ecosystem** benefits it provides. This is particularly true for humid tropical areas, such as the Amazon basin rain forests, which significantly influence the earth's climate, most notably through oxygen production. Some nations, such as Brazil, can still expand onto arable land, but such countries are in the minority. Even then, this expansion in Brazil causes further rain forest devastation. The general trend over the last few decades has been overextension of agriculture onto erodible land, followed by predictable degradation, erosion, and abandonment.[18]

In Africa an area of land twice the size of New Jersey is turned into unproductive desert each year because of soil erosion (Figure 18-4). The erosion results from overgrazing by livestock, destructive farming techniques, and destruction of mature rain forests. Also, cultivation of many **cash crops** in African countries damages the land, draining the soil of vital nutrients. Then, when the land has been used up,

Ecosystem
A community in nature that includes plants, animals, and their environment.

Cash crop
A crop grown specifically for export so that goods from other countries can be purchased. Cultivation of cash crops diverts agricultural resources necessary to feed a country's own citizens. Examples of cash crops are coffee, tea, cocoa, and bananas.

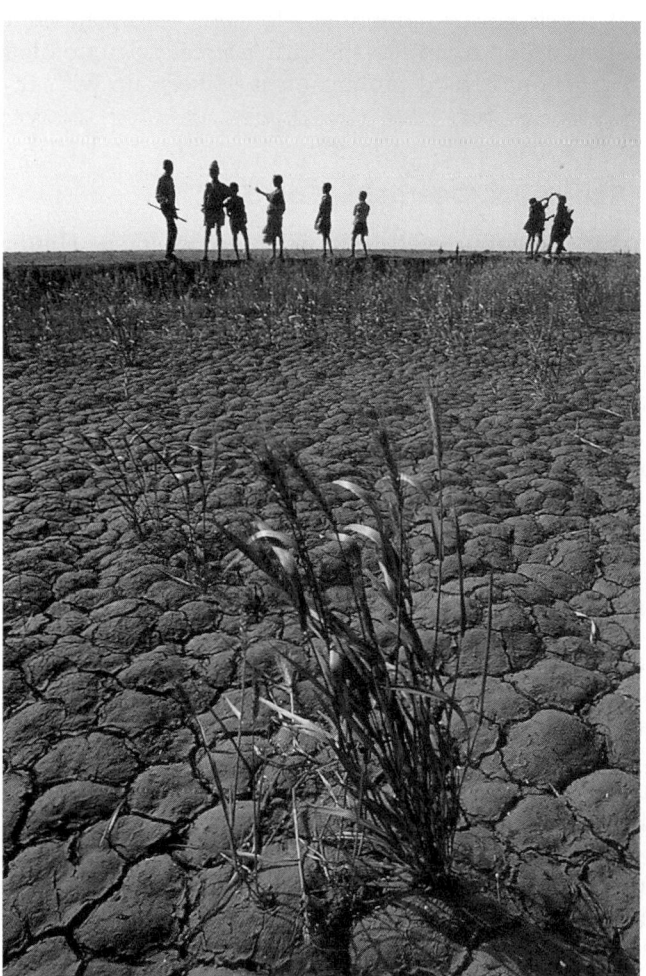

Figure 18-4 *The need for sustainable agriculture exists worldwide. Literally losing ground in their effort to grow food, farmers survey erosion of fields. Some 1.5 to 1.7 million acres of agricultural land in developing countries are lost each year to soil erosion.*

farmers move on to other areas, leaving behind desolate land vulnerable to soil erosion. In the short run, farmers can overplow and overpump with impressive results, but in doing so they use up natural resources on which long-term productivity depends.[3] Soil erosion is also a problem in the United States. Farmland equivalent in size to Ireland is currently lost in the United States to erosion every year. New farming techniques, such as "no till" planting, are helping to reverse this trend.

Nearly all irrigation water available worldwide is currently being used, and groundwater supplies are becoming depleted at rapid rates in many regions. China, which has more than 20% of the world's irrigated land, is plagued with a growing scarcity of fresh water.[6] In developing countries, poultry, swine, and milk production is often overconcentrated around metropolitan areas, in turn polluting and overdrawing groundwater.

The prospects of obtaining substantially more food from the oceans are also poor. In recent years the amount of fish caught worldwide has leveled off at about 80 million metric tons a year.[3]

Clearly, we can exploit the earth's resources only so far—world population probably can't continue to expand as it does today without the potential for serious famine and death. The Food and Agriculture Organization (FAO) of the United Nations works on this principle: "The fight to ensure that all people have enough nutritious food to eat is worthy of our greatest efforts, but it must be fought with the full recognition that it cannot be won unless agricultural, fishery, and forestry production returns to the earth as much as—or more than—it takes." This statement highlights the need for immediate action to protect the earth's already deteriorated environment from further destruction, if food production is to keep up with expanding population.[18]

Cultural Attitudes Toward Certain Foods

Culture affects food use just as it does family size. In India, for example, the Hindu reverence for cattle has worsened some already significant nutrition problems. These sacred cows consume food rather than provide it; the wandering cows also damage vegetation that could otherwise feed humans. Although the cows provide milk, no attempt is made to improve milk production through selective breading practices. In certain areas of India a child may not be fed milk curds, because of a superstitious belief that they inhibit growth, or bananas, because they supposedly cause convulsions. These are obstacles, but not barriers, to good nutrition. Given adequate food resources, a healthful diet allowing for individual food taboos and prejudices is possible.

In the United States, many people shun potential foods such as horse meat, insects, and algae.

Inadequate Shelter and Sanitation

When people die from undernutrition in developing countries, other influences, such as inadequate shelter and sanitation, almost always contribute. Poor sanitation raises the risk of infection, as does undernutrition. Together these represent a lethal combination (Figure 18-5). For example, the 1994 plague that killed almost 5000 people and sparked the panicked exodus of another half a million in Surat, in northwest India, was linked mainly to unsanitary housing conditions.

Inadequate and deteriorating shelters threaten the lives of more than 500 million people today. The future looks even worse.[3] By the year 2000, Mexico City will house more than 26 million people, with Sao Paulo, Calcutta, and Bombay not far behind. Many of the 15 million annual deaths of children—half of them under 5 years old—in developing countries could be prevented by improved standards of environmental hygiene.

Urban populations of some developing countries are currently growing at an annual rate of 5% to 7%. Such a skewed population distribution will result in more poverty. The current urban explosion is the result of both high birthrates and continuing migration of people to the cities from the countryside. People come to the cities to find employment and resources the countryside can no longer provide. Worldwide, 38 percent of people lived in urban areas in 1975. The figure is expected to reach 48 percent by the year 2000 and climb to 61 percent by 2025. Nine of the 10 largest cities 20 years from now will be in poor countries. Los Angeles, which is

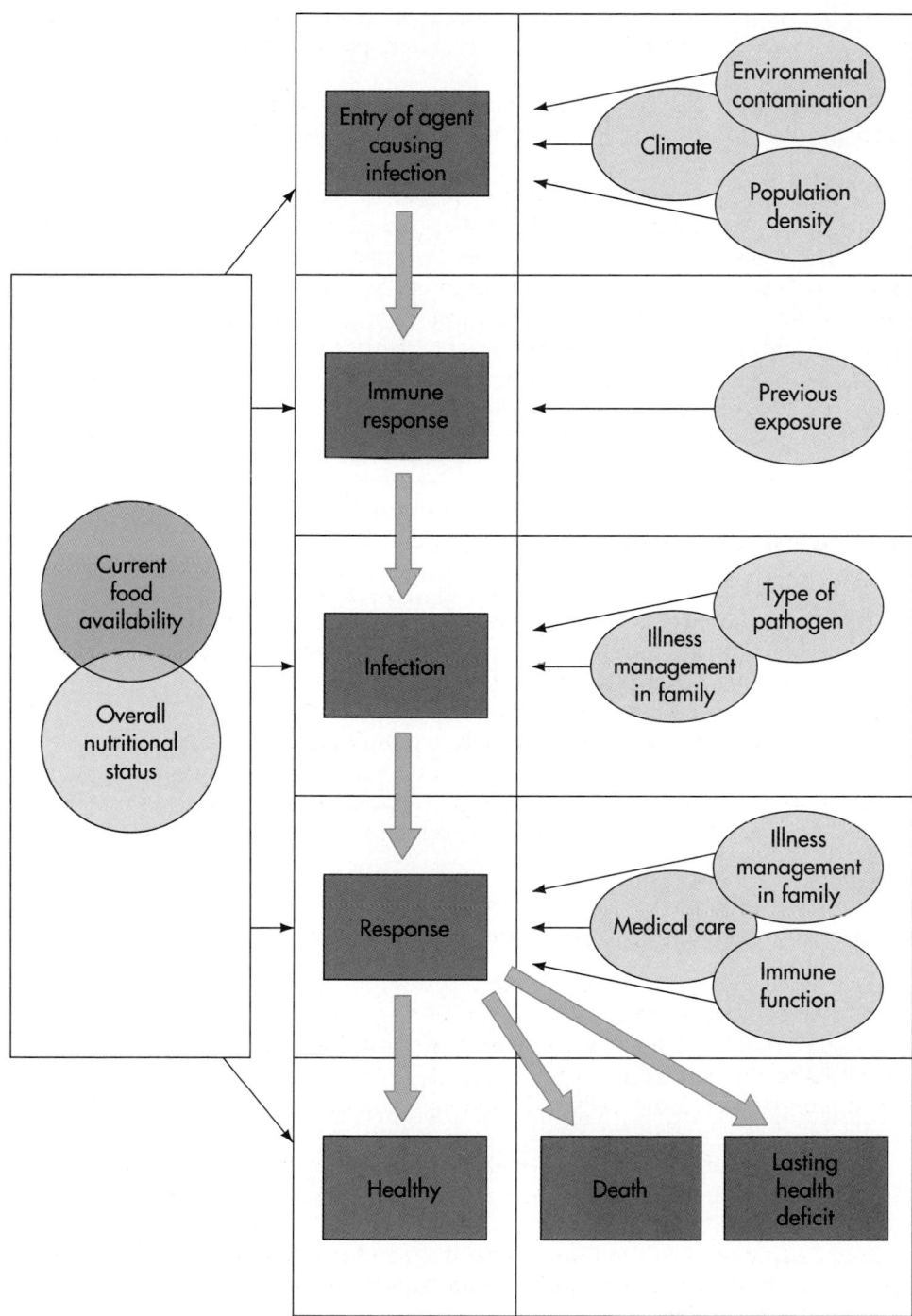

Figure 18-5 *Nutritional status and overall food supply combine with a variety of environmental factors to influence the risk of infection and ultimate outcome.*

The Impact of AIDS Worldwide

The Black Plague left its grim mark on civilization by claiming the lives of approximately 25 million people in the fourteenth century. By the year 2000 an estimated 30 to 120 million people around the world will be infected with the human immunodeficiency virus (HIV), and possibly 25 million people will have acquired immunodeficiency syndrome (AIDS). **About 1 million Americans are currently infected with HIV; of these people, 140,000 have AIDS.** About 40,000 new HIV infections are detected each year in this country, totaling 500,000 to date. African-American and Hispanic people account for more cases than whites based on their percentage of the population (101, 51, and 17 per 100,000, respectively). Stopping the spread of this disease is imperative for all the nation's citizens, especially in minority communities.[10]

In the United States AIDS is now the leading cause of death among men ages 25 to 44 and the fourth-leading cause of death among women in this age range. Because no cure currently exists, the majority of people infected with HIV—the twentieth century plague—face certain death from it. Current medication regimens can only slow progress of the disease and are expensive. About 240,000 Americans have already died from AIDS.[10]

The devastating effects of AIDS on our civilization have been very rapid when measured by Earth's scale of time, and the true costs to societies—other than the cost of human lives—have yet to emerge. Though AIDS has not replaced heart disease and stroke as the primary cause of death in America, the very nature of the disease is likely to wreak significant human devastation here and worldwide, partly because its primary route of transmission is a basic human behavior—sexual activity.

The Route of Infection

The vectors, or vehicles of transmission, for HIV are blood and body fluids, including sexual secretions. Most cases have been transmitted through homosexual and heterosexual contact and intravenous drug use, when a needle infected with the virus is shared. Safer sex and use of clean drug needles are known to reduce the spread of the disease and are keys to conquering AIDS. It is unlikely that vaccines alone will be able to eradicate HIV. A behavioral change offers the only hope. After initial contact with HIV, a person may notice no symptoms for as long as 5 to 10 years and may be an unsuspecting carrier. When the immune system can no longer fight off related subsequent infections, such as tuberculosis and pneumonia, the condition of AIDS is well on its way.[10]

Who Is Affected?

The belief that AIDS is a novel disease affecting a limited population of homosexual males on the east and west coasts in the United States is dangerously inaccurate. Though homosexual people currently account for more than half the cases here, the number of AIDS cases in heterosexual people—especially women and the children that HIV-infected women bear—is rapidly increasing.[10] In fact, recent studies show that about 20% of people in some south Florida towns have HIV infections, with heterosexual contact being the main method of contracting the virus.

AIDS needs no passport. Heterosexually transmitted HIV flows freely in Thai sex parlors, along the truck routes of India, around Dominican Republic sugar-cane plantations, and in the copper mines of Zambia. It is likely that one fourth of all adults in Zambia are infected with HIV. Heterosexual contact accounts for the majority of cases. A recent study warns us that 57 countries risk major HIV outbreaks. Reported HIV cases are increasing rapidly in Africa, Asia, and Russia, with 2 million men, women, and children becoming infected yearly worldwide.[3] The World Health Organization estimates that 70% of the world's 19 million people infected with the HIV virus are in Africa, with civil war refugees and migration contributing to its spread. The AIDS epicenter, however, is now shifting to Asia, especially India. By the year 2000, experts predict, 1 million people will have AIDS in India and 5 million will be HIV-positive.

What Are the Costs of AIDS?

Though human life can't be tagged with a price, the cost of AIDS research and medical care for AIDS patients, the loss of labor force for industry, and the economic hardship experienced by families of victims can be quantified. By 2000 the AIDS plague could siphon off an estimated $81 to $107 billion from the U.S. economy and may drain $356 to $514 billion from the global economy. This is money that could be spent on goods and services to help maintain stable economies around the world.

The impact of AIDS will hit poor countries worst, because their economies are already small and their living standards low.[14] Brazil, for example, would need to spend $600 million to adequately help its AIDS victims today. Such an economic burden would certainly mean rising budget deficits and expanding levels of debt, especially for a country that is still struggling with a foreign debt load of more than $100 billion. Other developing nations may well face a similar dilemma.

Hidden Costs

Behind the mind-boggling statistics on AIDS are less obvious costs to businesses, families, and society in general. In India and Thailand, for example, a significant number of the adult male populations will be forfeited to AIDS. Worker productivity will plummet because AIDS victims produce less and demand more, especially as they waste away in the latter stages of the disease. Business productivity drops even further when relatives take time away from work and school to care for family members afflicted with AIDS. Furthermore, AIDS demands a considerable amount of family income. Hard-pressed families that have to devote much of their income to doctors and medicines have little left for living expenses. Other fam-

ily members must struggle to keep up with daily duties because they must care for orphans left behind in the disease's wake. The number of youngsters orphaned by AIDS could more than double in the next 3 years to reach 3.7 million worldwide.

Individual and Government Response—Has It Been Adequate?

Governments worldwide have come under fire for their slow response in fighting AIDS. At present, neither governments nor the medical profession in developing countries has taken the lead in finding a solution. In India, for example, Bombay's first AIDS clinic, funded by a private interest group, didn't open until January 1993. Governments of developing nations frequently can't afford to supply AIDS counseling or treatment. Even worse, some continue to act as if their countries remain immune to the scourge. The weak response of government leaders and the resignation of citizens will undoubtedly lead to a greater degree of poverty and illness worldwide.

We all must act in concert to stop the spread of HIV. To do any less is to worsen the problem of undernutrition throughout the world.[3] The medical ramifications of caring for those already infected with HIV will be troubling enough, especially in the developing world. If the AIDS epidemic continues to spread at the current rate, however, the resulting social and economic burdens could very well spark crises that spread beyond national borders.

On a more individual scale, can eating a balanced diet prevent HIV or stave off AIDS? The answer is no. Again, there is no known cure for HIV and AIDS. Preventive measures include abstinence or safer sexual practices (especially use of condoms) and avoidance of contact with infected blood products and body fluids. Eating a balanced diet helps lessen the impact of infections but does not cure the disease or make it less deadly. A poor nutritional status contributes to quicker onset of such symptoms as body wasting and ultimately leads to a quicker demise.

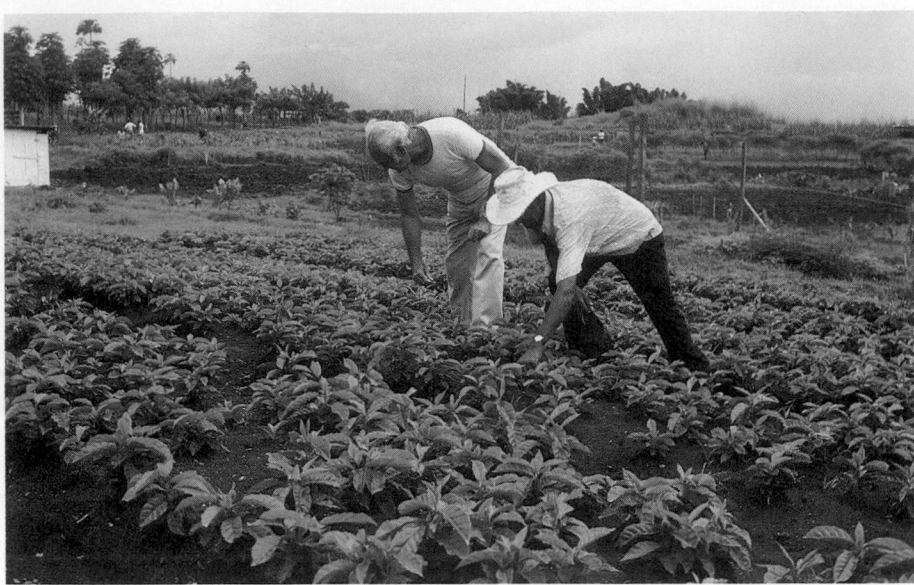

Poor people in less developed countries benefit from access to the land, which provides an important source for food. This advantage is lost when people move to cities.

now the seventh-largest city in the world, and New York, which is third, will drop far down the list.

In developing countries the poor make up most of the urban population, and their needs for housing and community services often outstrip available governmental resources.[3] Most of these urban poor live in overcrowded, self-made shelters that lack a safe and adequate water supply and are only partially served by public utilities. The shantytowns and ghettos of the developing world are often worse than the rural areas the people left behind. Because the urban poor need cash to purchase food, they often subsist on diets that are even more meager than the homegrown rural fare. Making matters worse, haphazard shelters often lack facilities to protect food from spoilage or the ravages of insects and rodents. In some developing countries, food losses can amount to as much as 30% to 40% of the perishable foods.

The shift from rural to urban life takes its greatest toll on infants and children.[26] Infants are often weaned early from the breast, partly because the mother must find employment and partly because she may be influenced by the images of sophisticated, formula-using women promoted in advertisements. Unfortunately, because infant formulas are relatively expensive, poor parents may overdilute the mixture or use too little to meet the baby's needs. Because the water supply may not be safe, the prepared formula is also likely to be grossly contaminated with bacteria.

In many nations, bottle-fed infants contract far more illnesses and are as much as 25 times more likely to die in childhood than those who are exclusively breast-fed for the first 6 months of life.[22] Human milk, in contrast, is generally much more hygienic, readily available, and nutritious and also provides infants with immunity to some ailments. In spite of these grim statistics, major corporations continue to aggressively market infant formulas in these regions.

Overall, the single most effective health advantage for people, wherever they live, is a safe and convenient water supply. Inadequate sanitation and consumption of contaminated water cause 75 percent of all diseases and over one third of all deaths in developing countries. The World Health Organization (WHO) estimates that 1.2 billion people, about one fifth of all people, have an unsafe and inadequate water supply.

Poor sanitation, another example of inadequate infrastructure in the developing world, creates another critical public health problem. Human feces, rotting garbage, and associated insect and rodent infestations are commonly seen in urban

In Brazil, migrants displaced by multinational land developers have flooded from the North and Northeast into Rio de Janeiro and São Paulo, attracted by the prospect of jobs. There they have built shantytowns next to apartment towers and affluent suburbs, but the jobs do not materialize, and urban poverty simply replaces rural impoverishment.

areas of the developing world. Potent sources of disease organisms, human urine and feces are two of the most dangerous substances people encounter in routine daily living.[20] The inability to dispose of the massive numbers of dead people resulting from recent civil wars causes additional sanitation problems. In some developing countries, diarrheal diseases account for as many as one third of all deaths in children under 5 years of age.[3] WHO estimates that even with improvements in housing, 1.8 billion people in the world still lack proper sanitation.

To this already unbalanced equation, add the threat of sickness from acquired immunodeficiency syndrome (AIDS), an incurable disease. Developing countries currently contain the bulk of the world's 19 million cases of human immunodeficiency virus (HIV) infections, and numbers are increasing rapidly. As more people contract AIDS, the economic and social impact will be enormous. In an already undernourished population the long-term effects may rival those of a prolonged war.

High External Debt

People sometimes take out high-interest loans from the neighborhood finance company to pay for necessary items of daily living. If they can't keep up with payments, they may be able to get another loan to pay off the first. Eventually, however, unless their income increases, they will be forced to sell off assets or perhaps declare bankruptcy.

During the 1970s and 1980s, many developing countries became trapped in the same cycle, borrowing repeatedly from foreign countries.[17] Servicing these external debts, which now total about $2 trillion, has brought several countries to the verge of economic collapse. Even the United States is not immune to such national financial problems. As the result of large annual federal deficits, our national debt is now so large that the yearly interest payments account for about 15% of all federal spending. This debt limits our country's ability to help less developed countries.

The external debt of Latin America represents 45% of the region's gross regional output of goods and services. Nearly 40% of total export earnings are spent in paying off this debt. One option is for Latin American nations to form a comprehensive plan aimed at renegotiating the external debt on more realistic terms.

Many African nations also carry large debt burdens. Recent drops in prices for raw commodities they export, higher prices for imported oil, and embezzlement of funds by high political officials are at the root of this problem. Still, countries need to import—and pay for—machinery, concrete, trucks, and consumer goods. To make up the difference between export income and import expenses, countries have been forced to borrow billions of dollars from international banks.

Although the African debts are much smaller in absolute terms than those of Brazil, Argentina, and Mexico, for example, the actual burden is greater when national incomes and export earnings are considered. Nearly half the money African nations earn from exports goes to paying off the continent's multibillion dollar debt. As a result, African nations have had to impose cuts in domestic programs, which can cause widespread undernutrition in many of these poor nations.[3]

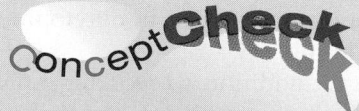

ConceptCheck

War and civil strife, along with a decline in the world's natural resources, contribute to the difficulty of ending undernutrition in many developing countries. In addition, inadequate housing conditions, impure water, and inadequate sanitation worldwide increase the risk for infection and disease. Infection then combines with undernutrition to further compromise the health of impoverished people. Finally, many developing countries are burdened by extremely high external debts, which severely limit their ability to implement programs to reduce undernutrition.

Reducing Undernutrition in the Developing World

As you have probably guessed, greatly reducing undernutrition in the developing world will be complicated and will take considerable time to accomplish. In the 1980s, it was a common practice for the more affluent nations to supply famished areas with direct food aid. However highly publicized and praised at the time, direct food aid is not a long-term solution. Although it reduces the number of deaths from famine, it can also reduce incentives for local production by driving down local prices. In addition, the affected countries may have little or no means of transporting the food to those who need it most. Furthermore, the donated foods may receive little cultural acceptance.

In the short run, there is no choice—aid must be given because people are starving. Still, improving the infrastructure for poor people, especially rural people, needs to be the long-term focus. This long-term approach is necessary because the most significant factor affecting undernutrition of people in impoverished areas of the world is their reliance on outside sources for basic needs. Their dependence makes them constantly vulnerable.

One American program that has helped improve the infrastructure of developing nations is the Peace Corps, which provides education, distributes food and medical supplies, and builds structures for local use. The aim of the Peace Corps is to improve the infrastructure and education of developing countries and thereby help create independent, self-sustaining economies around the world.

Tailoring Development to Local Conditions

Recall that in the last 30 years, world food supplies have grown faster than the population. Thus the increase in undernutrition during this period is caused by an increase in the number of people cut off from their fair share of this supply. Millions of farmers are losing access to resources they need to be self-reliant. The number of households with insufficient means to support themselves is growing. In response, careful, small-scale regional development is one option. There is a growing realization that rural people who own no land will flock to the overcrowded cities unless economic opportunities can be created as part of a plan for sustainable development.[20]

Small-scale rural enterprises and off-farm activities would ensure that poor people in rural areas who have no access to land or other assets can acquire food. Such enterprises can be run by the people who stand to benefit, either as individuals or members of small groups, using very limited capital. Access to credit, appropriate technologies, a market, and the ability to transport the product to that market are prerequisites. Landowning families could be helped in different ways to increase their ability to feed themselves.

For the most part, the solution lies in helping people to meet their own needs and directing them to resources and employment opportunities, rather than simply giving them resources. Experience has shown that credit—along with training, food storage facilities, and marketing—allows rural people to participate in development to their benefit and that of their families and communities.[3]

Impoverished women are a special concern. In addition to working longer hours than men, they grow most of the food for family consumption and make up three fourths of the labor force in the informal sector and an increasing proportion in the formal economy. Economic opportunities for women must be augmented. Of the 1.3 billion people living in poverty worldwide, 70% are women. Moreover, among the developing world's 900 million illiterate people, women outnumber men 2 to 1. Thus an important means of propelling nations out of poverty is to end the cycle of female neglect. If there is one critical message from the recent United

Nations Conference on Women in Beijing, it may be that providing women with education, entrepreneurship, and political power could pay off in numerous ways, ranging from slower population growth and higher incomes to healthier families.

Suitable technologies for processing, preserving, marketing, and distributing nutritious local staples also need to be encouraged so small farmers can flourish. Education on how to use these foods to create healthful diets, such as for preparing vitamin A–rich vegetables, adds further benefit. Supplementing indigenous foods with nutrients that are in short supply, such as iron and iodide, also deserves consideration.[23] One current program involves adding iron to sugar in various parts of the world.[27]

Promoting extensive landownership is a key part of the solution. Increasing the availability of food is one of the many advantages. If food resources are concentrated among a minority of people, as often happens with unequal landownership, food won't be equally distributed unless efficient transportation systems are in place. Inequitable distribution then proves a very difficult problem to resolve.

Raising the economic status of impoverished people by employing them is as important as expanding the food supply. If an increase in food supply is achieved without an accompanying rise in employment, there may be no long-term change in the number of undernourished people. Although food prices may fall with increased mechanization, use of fertilizers, and other modern technologies, these same advances can also displace people from jobs. When this happens, the food that is produced will still be unaffordable for those who need it most.

A shipment of high-technology tractors, for example, might put local laborers out of work. Rice might be planted more efficiently using farm machinery, but using human power eventually leaves more humans with the resources to buy food. The successful reduction of undernutrition in the developing world can occur only when more poor people are employed more productively on available land or when they have other jobs. From this perspective, it is of little consequence that these jobs are technologically primitive by Western standards. As mentioned before, increasing both per capita income and education is necessary. That effort must include employment.[3]

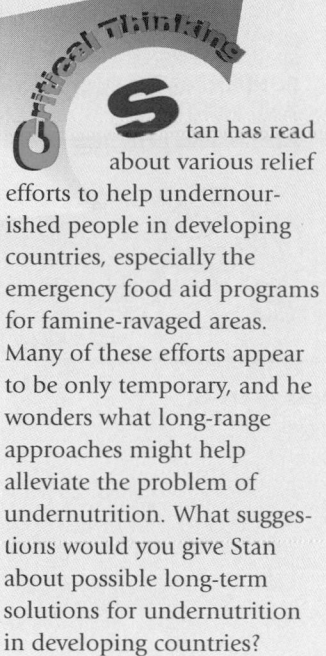

Critical Thinking

Stan has read about various relief efforts to help undernourished people in developing countries, especially the emergency food aid programs for famine-ravaged areas. Many of these efforts appear to be only temporary, and he wonders what long-range approaches might help alleviate the problem of undernutrition. What suggestions would you give Stan about possible long-term solutions for undernutrition in developing countries?

Some Concluding Thoughts

Clearly the developing world will have to rely largely on its own resources to finance development, especially in light of the current budget deficit in the United States. For decades, countries in Africa could count on the Cold War as an economic resource. The United States and the former Soviet Union opposed each other through African proxies, pouring in money to prop up proWestern or proCommunist governments. Now the big powers' priorities have turned inward. Making full use of the human resources available in the developing world itself is more essential than ever. The right choice for production depends on the relative need to employ people and the number of people available to do the work.

Overemphasizing cash crops, such as coffee, tea, rubber, and cocoa—as some developing countries have done, especially in Latin America—is not likely to solve the nutritional problems of poor people. Cash crops are usually grown at the expense of food crops on the assumption that money earned from the cash crops will be used to purchase food for the families of the workers. However, this is not always the case. Food can be bought, but it may not be enough and it is more expensive. In such a situation, poorer families are at greater risk than others, because the money earned from cash crops is often not enough to meet other basic family needs, let alone their food needs.[3] As with poor families in the United States, buying quality foods often takes a secondary position, resulting in nutritional deprivation.

Also detrimental is the economics of drug crops, such as cocaine, marijuana, and opium. Perceiving drugs as valuable cash crops, workers often believe that the large sums of money netted from these crops—which are often more easily

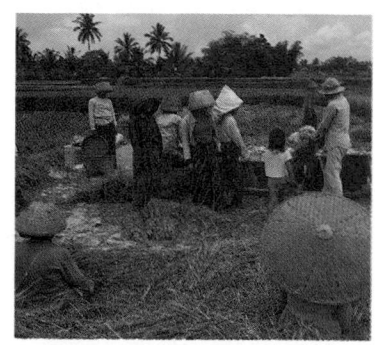

Labor-intensive agriculture, which is necessary in these rice fields, may be the best choice for some less developed countries.

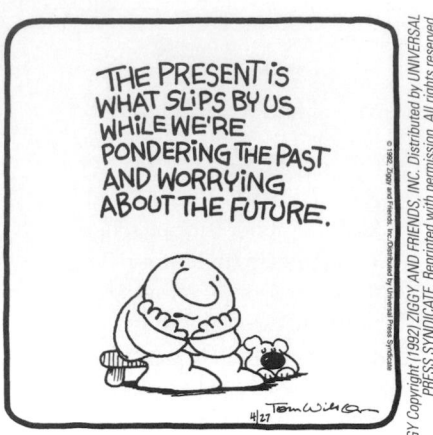

Figure 18-6
Ziggy.

grown than food crops—can meet family needs and increase the standard of living. An unfortunate reality is that many workers see little or no cash earnings and become victims of their trade. Cash from drug crops often lines the pockets of criminals and corrupt government officials and results in little incentive to initiate subsistence-level food crops that could provide employment and nourishment for many.

Today the economic loss from undernutrition is staggering, and the amount of human pain and suffering is incalculable.[3] With all the international relief efforts and assistance from governments and private organizations combined, we are still in the Dark Ages when it comes to our battle against undernutrition (Figure 18-6).

Currently, world leaders are concerned about the "marginalization" of problems in the developing world, fearing rich nations might dismiss war, disease, and famine as a way of life for poorer nations. In a recent survey, Americans identified world famine as less of a concern than violence, drugs, and inflation. Note that U.S. food aid, which averaged $1.9 billion annually in the early 1990s, fell to $1.25 billion in 1995 as the political support for such aid dwindles. Ultimately, however, depletion of world resources, the massive debt incurred by poorer countries, the threat of danger to more prosperous countries nearby, and the toll taken in human lives does affect our world economy and well-being.

Leaders of rich and poor nations alike need to come to an agreement on the best possible means to serve all of the world's citizens. Perhaps if we rid ourselves of negative government actions worldwide, the task could become easier. Life is not necessarily fair, but the aim of civilization should be to make it fairer.[3] The world has both the food and the technical expertise to end hunger. What is lacking is the political will to do so.[25]

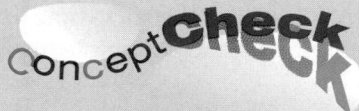

Overall, one important solution to reducing undernutrition in the developing world lies in providing sufficient employment so that people can purchase the food their families need or provide access to land and other food production resources. Development programs must be sensitive to regional conditions to ensure that the new technologies introduced don't intensify existing problems for the poorest people. Simple approaches are appropriate if people acquire the resources they need to feed their families.

Summary

➤ Poverty is a common thread wherever people suffer from undernutrition. Malnutrition can occur when the food supply is either scarce or abundant. The resulting deficiency conditions and degenerative diseases are influenced by genetic makeup.

➤ Undernutrition is the most common form of malnutrition in developing countries. It results from inadequate intake, absorption, or use of nutrients or food energy. Many deficiency conditions consequently appear, and infectious diseases thrive because the immune system cannot function properly.

➤ The greatest risk of undernutrition occurs during critical periods of growth and development: gestation, infancy, and childhood. Low birth weight is a leading cause of infant deaths worldwide. Many developmental problems are caused by nutritional deprivation during critical periods of brain growth.

➤ Undernutrition diminishes both physical and mental capabilities. In poor countries, this is worsened by recurrent infections, unsanitary conditions, extreme weather, inadequate shelter, and exposure to diseases.

➤ In the United States, famine has been nonexistent since the 1930s, but undernutrition remains. Soup kitchens, food stamps, school lunch and breakfast programs, and the Supplemental Feeding Program for Women, Infants, and Children (WIC) have focused on improving the nutritional health of poor and at-risk people. When adequately funded, these programs have proved effective in reducing undernutrition. The need to reduce out-of-wedlock pregnancies remains a national priority, because single parents and their children are likely to live in poverty.

➤ Multiple factors contribute to the problem of undernutrition in the developing world. In densely populated countries, food resources, as well as the means for distributing food, may be inadequate. Farming methods often encourage erosion, which deprives the soil of valuable nutrients and thereby hampers future efforts to grow food. Limited water availability limits food production. Naturally occurring devastation from droughts, excessive rainfall, fire, crop infestation, and human causes—such as urbanization, war and civil unrest, debt, and poor sanitation—all contribute to the major problem of undernutrition.

➤ Proposed solutions to world undernutrition must include consideration of the interaction of multiple factors, many of which are thoroughly embedded in cultural traditions. Family planning efforts, for example, may not succeed until life expectancy increases. Through education, efforts should be made to upgrade farming methods, encourage breastfeeding, and improve sanitation and hygiene. Direct food aid is only a short-term solution. In what may appear to be a step backward, many experts recommend sustainable subsistence-level farming, away from the specialization of cash crops, to increase the economic status of poor people. Small-scale industrial development is another way to create meaningful employment and purchasing power for vast numbers of the rural poor.

Study Questions

1 Describe in a short paragraph any evidence of undernutrition that you saw while you were growing up. What are/were the roots of these problems?

2 What do you believe are the major factors contributing to undernutrition in wealthy nations, such as the United States? What are some solutions to this problem?

3 What three points would you make to a group of seventh-grade girls concerning the economic perils of teenage pregnancy and parenting?

4 Personal responsibility is a common theme in political circles these days. How does this relate to the problem of undernutrition in the United States? Does it apply to all causes of the problem?

5 A person you recently met asks you where to find food and shelter. Where in your community would you first direct this person? If you are unsure, try to find out.

6 Choose one problem that contributes to the complex issue of famine. In two paragraphs, describe the problem and discuss possible solutions.

7 Outline how war and civil unrest in developing countries have worsened problems of chronic hunger over the last few years.

8 How important is population control in addressing the problem of world hunger? Support your answer with three main points.

References

1 American Dietetic Association Reports: Position of the American Dietetic Association: World hunger, *Journal of the American Dietetic Association* 95:1160, 1995.

2 Bongaarts J: Population policy options in the developing world, *Science* 263:771, 1994.

3 Bread for the World Institute: *Hunger 1995: causes of hunger,* Silver Spring, Md, 1994, Bread for the World Institute.

4 Brown JL, Allen D: Hunger in America, *Annual Review of Public Health* 9:503, 1988.

5 Brown JL, Pollitt E: Malnutrition, poverty, and intellectual development, *Scientific American,* p 38, Feb 1996.

6 Clausi AS: The power of food, *Food Technology,* p 129, May 1995.

7 Comai L: Impact of plant genetic engineering on foods and nutrition, *Annual Review of Nutrition* 13:191, 1993.

8 Fawzi WW and others: Vitamin A supplementation and child mortality, *Journal of the American Medical Association* 269:898, 1993.

9 Gelgerg L and others: Determinants of undernutrition among homeless adults, *Public Health Reports* 110:448, 1995.

10 Greeley A: Concern about AIDS in minority communities, *FDA Consumer,* p 11, Dec 1995.

11 Henkel J: Genetic engineering: fast forwarding to future foods, *FDA Consumer,* p 6, April 1995.

12 IUNS Declaration: Nutritional goals for the nineties: a call for advocacy and action, *Nutrition Today* 29:5, 1994.

13 Joy AB and others: Hunger in California: what interventions are needed? *Journal of the American Dietetic Association* 94:749, 1994.

14 Maberly GF and others: Programs against micronutrient malnutrition: ending hidden hunger, *Annual Review of Public Health* 15:277, 1994.

15 Mayer J: Nutritional problems in the United States: then and now two decades later, *Nutrition Today,* p 15, Jan/Feb 1990.

16 Olson RE: World food production and problems in human nutrition, *Nutrition Today,* p 18, Jan/Feb 1989.

17 Pearce D and others: Debt and the environment, *Scientific American,* p 51, June 1995.

18 Plunknett DL, Winkelmann DL: Technology for sustainable agriculture, *Scientific American,* p 182, Sept 1995.

19 Sazawal S and others: Zinc supplementation in young children with acute diarrhea in India, *The New England Journal of Medicine* 333:839, 1995.

20 Solomons NW, Gross R: Urban nutrition in developing countries, *Nutrition Reviews* 53:90, 1995.

21 Splett, PL: Federal food assistance programs, *Nutrition Today,* p 6, March/April 1994.

22 Taren D, Chen J: A positive association between extended breast-feeding and nutritional status in rural Hubei Province, People's Republic of China, *American Journal of Clinical Nutrition* 58:862, 1993.

23 Tebeb HN: Goiter problems in Ethiopia, *American Journal of Clinical Nutrition* 57:315S, 1993.

24 Trowbridge FL and others: Coordinated strategies for controlling micronutrient malnutrition: a technical workshop, *Journal of Nutrition* 123:775, 1993.

25 Uvin P: The state of world hunger, *Nutrition Reviews* 52:151, 1994.

26 Waterlow JC: Childhood malnutrition in developing nations: looking back and looking forward, *Annual Review of Nutrition* 14:1, 1994.

27 Yip R: The challenge of controlling iron deficiency: sweet news from Guatemala, *American Journal of Clinical Nutrition* 61:1164, 1995.

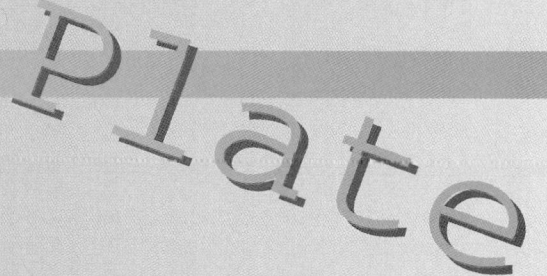

RATE Your Plate

Fighting World Undernutrition On a Personal Level

If you want to do something about world and domestic undernutrition, the following activities are suggested. It is a noble act to try to make a difference, even if you make just one small step. As with any change in behavior, don't try to do too many things at once. Try one or two activities that represent your commitment to solving this gigantic problem.

1. Volunteer at a local soup kitchen or homeless shelter for a time-limited period (1 month for example). What insights did you gain?

2. Donate some money to a voluntary agency that does antihunger work, such as those listed below:

Bread for the World
802 Rhode Island Ave., NE
Washington, DC 20018

Oxfam America
115 Broadway
Boston, MA 02116

Save the Children Federation
P.O. Box 970
Westport, CT 06881

Catholic Relief Services
209 W Fayette St.
Baltimore, MD 21201

CARE
660 First Ave.
New York, NY 10016

Second Harvest
116 Michigan Ave.
Suite #4
Chicago, IL 60603

3. Write a letter to a senator or member of Congress asking what he or she is doing about ending domestic and world undernutrition.

4. Contribute to World Food Day activities each October 16th to stay informed about the issues. In addition, Internet users can find information on hunger at several sites, including the following:

- HungerWeb, at Brown University, which offers information on hunger research, programs, education, and advocacy and an overview of the Alan Shawn Feinstein World Hunger Program at Brown. HungerWeb is a World Wide Web home page that links to Internet sites run by the UN, US AID, and the World Bank.
  http://www.netspace.org/hungerweb
- The UN Food and Agriculture Organization, which provides an extensive list of publications related to agriculture and global foods security.
  http://www.fao.org/ or gopher.fao.org
- The World Food Programme, which provides information about food aid and other issues. gopher.unep.org; or on the World Wide Web: gopher://unep.unep.no:70/11/un/wfp
- The Congressional Hunger Center, which tracks domestic and global hunger issues.
  http://www.fh.org/chc/index.html

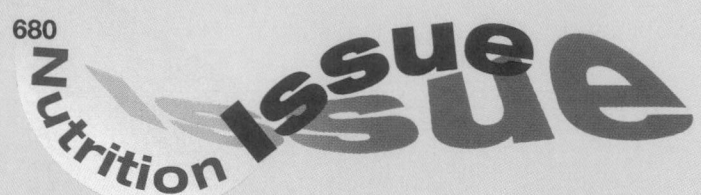

Biotechnology: an Answer to Food Shortages?

The ability of humans to manipulate nature has enabled us to improve the production and yield of many important foods. Traditional **biotechnology** is almost as old as agriculture. The first farmer to improve his stock by selectively breeding the best bull with the best cows was implementing biotechnology in a simple sense. The first baker to use yeast to make bread rise took similar advantage of biotechnology.

By the 1930s, biotechnology made possible the selective breeding of better plant hybrids; as a result, corn production in the United States quickly doubled. Through similar methods, agricultural wheat was crossed with wild grasses to confer more desirable properties, such as greater yield, increased resistance to mildew and bacterial diseases, and tolerance to salt or adverse climatic conditions.

Another type of biotechnology uses hormones rather than breeding. In the last decade, Canadian salmon have been treated with a hormone that allows them to mature three times faster than normal—without changing the fish in any other way. In general terms, biotechnology can be understood as the use of living things—plants, animals, bacteria—to manufacture products.

THE NEW BIOTECHNOLOGY

The new biotechnology used in agriculture includes a number of methods that directly modify products. It differs from traditional methods because it directly changes some of the genetic material (DNA) of organisms to improve characteristics. Cross-breeding plants or animals is no longer the only tool. Development of the new process, called *genetic engineering*, began in the 1970s.[7] The field now features a wide range of cell and subcell techniques for the synthesis and placement of genetic material in organisms (Figure 18-7). This allows access to a wider gene pool, and it permits faster and more accurate production of new and more useful microbial, plant, and animal species. Traditional breeding has had inconsistent results, but biotechnology is precise. Scientists select the traits they want and genetically engineer or introduce the gene that produces the desired trait into animals. It is important to note, however, that genetic engineering doesn't replace conventional breeding practices; both work together.

Already, genetic engineering at the agricultural level has allowed us to make use of new types of seeds, growth hormones, and microbial inoculants to stop pests and frost damage. Biotechnology is also used to develop drought-tolerant crops, as well as to detect *Listeria* and other microbes that cause food-borne illness. Scientists are engineering plants that grow without chemical pesticides and new forms of potatoes that can last without preservatives.[11] There is even interest in putting certain animal genes into plants to improve various plant characteristics. Because cautious use is the order of the day, these early benefits of the new biotechnology will strike us as only subtly different. The ultimate benefits, however, could be substantial.

Questions surround the use of the new biotechnology. Take, for instance, the new Flavr Savr tomato, which was genetically engineered to stay firm longer. Is it still a tomato? It looks the same, feels the same, tastes the same, and even has the same nutritional value. The only change researchers made is to counteract the action of a single gene in the DNA that makes tomatoes rot rapidly. Reversing just one gene out of 10,000 makes the biotech tomato significantly different from the standard garden variety.

Still, the question remains: how many and which properties can be changed in a plant, animal, or bacterium before it becomes something else? A tomato altered in only one specific way still seems to be a tomato, but does it remain one if it is improved in 10 or 20 ways? When traditional methods crossed a tangerine with a grapefruit, the new genetic structure was clearly something else, now commonly known as a *tangelo*.

Controversy surrounding the new biotechnology

Public response to use of the new biotechnology has been mixed. Although the use of genetically modified organisms may reduce the need for environmentally harmful activities, such as spraying crops with chemical pesticides, critics point out past mistakes with the release of foreign agents, such as insects and plants, into areas with no natural predators. While the risks may appear to be momentarily negligible, they may be cumulative and therefore dangerous in the long run. In addition, will allergens, such as those found in peanuts, eggs, milk, wheat, and shellfish, be added to genetically engineered foods that previously did not contain them? Evidence that this can happen has been seen in soybeans. Note, however, that FDA carefully examines all products developed using this technology and will enforce labeling of potential allergens that may be newly present in a biotech food.[11]

The public has long been opposed to processes perceived as harmful to the environment, such as producing unnatural products. Because food reserves are high in the United States, Canada, and Europe, some question the need to increase food production. Skepticism surrounds unnatural products, as exemplified by western Europe's ban of a growth hormone previously used in beef production. Citizens believed the increase in meat supply was not worth the perceived risks associated with the product. In the United States, FDA recently approved the first genetically engineered food product for humans, a substitute for the enzyme renin, called *chymosin*. Renin is traditionally used in making cheese. Will a protest arise over the current use of chymosin? Both scientists and concerned consumer groups are currently studying other potentially beneficial applications of the new biotechnology. Bovine somatotropin (BST), a hormone produced by cattle, has been known since the 1930s to increase milk production when injected into dairy cattle. Today an identical BST (Posilac) produced through genetic engineering can be used to greatly increase milk yield. Because it is a protein, any BST in the milk produced would be digested and therefore inactivated. People even produce their own form of somatotropin, but its structure differs considerably from

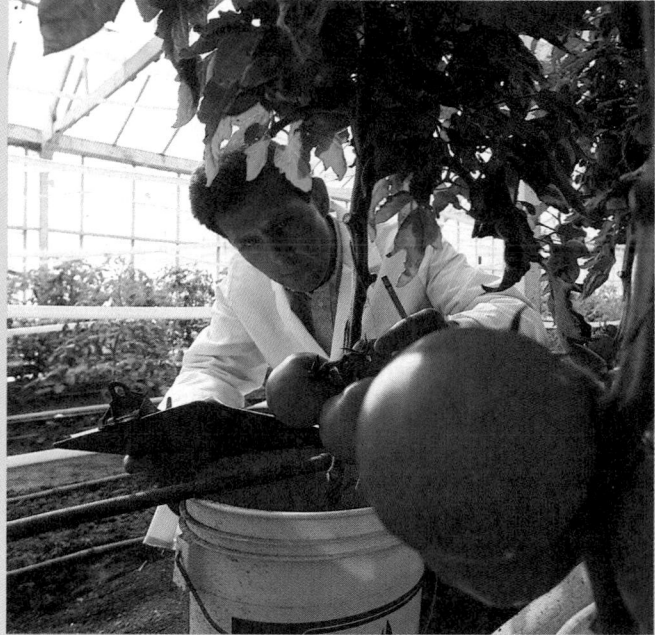

Figure 18-7 *Traditional biotechnology has helped create the tomato we enjoy today.*

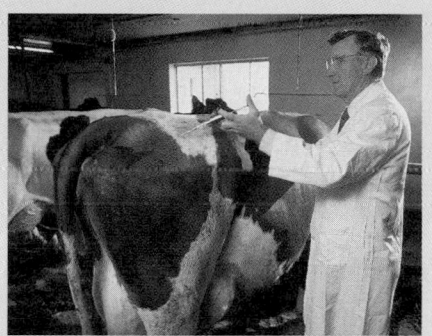

Milk yields can be increased using genetically engineered bovine somatotropin.

that of BST. Because cows produce BST naturally, it has always been present in their milk. Treating the animals with the proposed higher levels of BST won't increase the concentration of hormone occurring naturally in the milk, nor will it alter the milk's nutrient composition.

While FDA is still evaluating the safety of BST with respect to animals and the environment, the agency has determined that milk from treated animals is safe for human consumption.[11] Currently about 1 in 10 dairy farms uses the product. Some critics question whether the increased milk production will stress the health of the cows, leading farmers to use more antibiotics, which can show up in milk. The public already appears to oppose BST, and the European Economic Community has banned its use. Again, with a surplus of milk in the United States and Europe, garnering public support will be difficult. Furthermore, dairy farmers in Wisconsin and other dairy-producing regions generally oppose the introduction of the hormone, because they fear negative consumer reaction will lower milk consumption. The industry is also concerned that a sharp increase in milk

output will adversely affect prices and thereby harm thousands of small dairy farms facing an already precarious economic situation.

Role of the new biotechnology in the developing world

Whether genetically engineered applications will help to significantly reduce undernutrition in the developing world remains to be seen. Unless price cuts accompany the increased production, only landowners and suppliers of biotechnology will enjoy the benefits of biotechnology. This point deserves emphasis: the person who couldn't afford a tangelo yesterday probably won't be able to afford one tomorrow. The same can be said for improved tomatoes. As with most innovations, the more successful farmers, often those with larger farms, will adopt the new biotechnology first. Because of this, the present trend of fewer and larger farms will continue in the developing world, a trend that undermines the most pressing undernutrition issues there. Furthermore, biotechnology does not promise dramatic increases in the production of most grains, the primary food resource in the world.

For the developing world the focus needs to be on providing people with resources to produce and purchase their own food, not on simply growing more food. Biotechnology is a useful tool against the complex scourge of world undernutrition but it's no panacea. Improved crops produced by this technology will contribute to the battle, together with political and other efforts.[3]

Food Composition Table

THIS FOOD COMPOSITION table, developed by Positive Input Corp., lists the foods in Mosby's NutriTrac software, which is available as a supplement to this text.

The quickest way to find a food is to use the "Search For" feature in Mosby's NutriTrac software. However, if you do not have access to a computer or your computer time is limited, you can easily find a food using this food composition table. The foods in the table are arranged alphabetically. Note, however, that in some cases foods are arranged alphabetically within groups, such as Babyfood, Beef, and Bread, rather than by name alone.

Food from restaurants, including fast food (quick service), is cataloged separately, starting on p. A-68. These foods are listed alphabetically by restaurant name. If the fast-food/quick-service restaurant you are looking for is not listed, use the generic "Fast Food" category within the "Restaurant" section.

The code number in the left-hand column corresponds to the food data bank in Mosby's NutriTrac software. When you enter your intake into the software program, you may choose to use code numbers. Alternatively, you may choose to enter your intake into Mosby's NutriTrac by typing a food's name or partial name and selecting the "Search For" option.

Code	Name	Amount	Unit	Grams	Energy (kcal)	Carbohydrates (g)	Protein (g)	Fat (g)	Saturated fat (g)	Monounsaturated fat (g)
11001	Alfalfa Seeds, Sprouted, Fresh	1/2	Cup	16.5	5	1	1	0	0	0
19065	Almond Joy Candy Bar	1	Bar	50.0	232	29	2	14	8	3
12067	Almonds, Toasted, Unblanched	1/2	Cup	71.0	418	16	14	36	3	23
19066	Alpine White Bar w/ Almonds	1	Bar	35.0	197	18	4	13	7	5
15002	Anchovy, European, Cnd In Oil	3	Ounce	85.1	179	0	25	8	2	3
55188	Angel Hair Pasta, Lean Cuisine-Stouffer's	1	Each	283.5	240	38	10	5	1	-
18150	Animal Crackers	1	Each	2.5	11	2	0	0	0	0
19294	Apple Butter	1	Tbsp.	18.0	33	9	0	0	-	-
19186	Apple Crisp	1	Cup	282.0	460	91	5	10	2	4
9400	Apple Juice, Unsweetened	3/4	Cup	185.8	87	22	0	0	0	0
18302	Apple Pie	1	Slice	155.0	411	58	4	19	5	8
9007	Apples, Cnd, Sweetened	1/2	Cup	102.0	68	17	0	0	0	0
9009	Apples, Dehydrated, Sulfured	1/4	Cup	15.0	52	14	0	0	0	0
9003	Apples, Fresh, w/ Skin	1	Medium	138.0	81	21	0	0	0	0
9004	Apples, Fresh, w/o Skin	1	Medium	128.0	73	19	0	0	0	0
9020	Applesauce, Sweetened	1/2	Cup	127.5	97	25	0	0	0	0
9019	Applesauce, Unsweetened	1/2	Cup	122.0	52	14	0	0	0	0
9403	Apricot Nectar, Cnd, w/ Added Vit C	3/4	Cup	188.2	105	27	1	0	0	0
9036	Apricot Nectar, Cnd, w/o Added Vit C	3/4	Cup	188.2	105	27	1	0	0	0
9028	Apricots, Cnd, Heavy Syrup Pack	1/2	Cup	129.0	107	28	1	0	0	0
9024	Apricots, Cnd, Juice Pack	1/2	Cup	124.0	60	15	1	0	0	0
9026	Apricots, Cnd, Light Syrup Pack	1/2	Cup	126.5	80	21	1	0	0	0
9022	Apricots, Cnd, Water Pack	1/2	Cup	121.5	33	8	1	0	0	0
9030	Apricots, Dehydrated, Sulfured	1/4	Cup	29.8	95	25	1	0	0	0
9032	Apricots, Dried, Sulfured	1/4	Cup	32.5	77	20	1	0	0	0
9021	Apricots, Fresh	3	Medium	106.0	51	12	1	0	0	0
9035	Apricots, Frozen, Sweetened	1/2	Cup	121.0	119	30	1	0	0	0
11705	Asparagus, Ckd	1/2	Cup	90.0	23	4	2	0	0	0
11015	Asparagus, Cnd	1/2	Cup	121.0	23	3	3	1	0	0
11011	Asparagus, Fresh	1/2	Cup	67.0	15	3	2	0	0	0
11019	Asparagus, Frz, Ckd	1/2	Cup	100.0	28	5	3	0	0	0
9037	Avocados, Fresh	1	Medium	201.0	324	15	4	31	5	19
3117	Babyfood, Applesauce	3	Ounce	85.1	31	9	0	0	-	-
3280	Babyfood, Bananas w/ Tapioca	3	Ounce	85.1	57	15	0	0	-	-
3681	Babyfood, Barley, Ppd w/ Whole Milk	3	Ounce	85.1	94	14	4	3	-	-
3003	Babyfood, Beef	3	Ounce	85.1	90	0	12	4	2	2
3043	Babyfood, Beef Lasagna	3	Ounce	85.1	65	9	4	2	-	-
3287	Babyfood, Beef Noodle	3	Ounce	85.1	48	6	2	2	-	-
3052	Babyfood, Beef Stew	3	Ounce	85.1	43	5	4	1	0	0
3049	Babyfood, Beef and Rice	3	Ounce	85.1	70	7	4	2	-	-
3098	Babyfood, Beets	3	Ounce	85.1	29	7	1	0	-	-
3100	Babyfood, Carrots	3	Ounce	85.1	27	6	1	0	-	-
3013	Babyfood, Chicken	3	Ounce	85.1	127	0	13	8	2	4
3069	Babyfood, Chicken Noodle	3	Ounce	85.1	43	6	2	1	-	-
3070	Babyfood, Chicken Soup	3	Ounce	85.1	43	6	1	1	-	-
3014	Babyfood, Chicken Sticks	3	Stick	30.0	56	0	4	4	-	-
3214	Babyfood, Cookies, Arrowroot	3	Ounce	85.1	376	61	6	12	3	8
3120	Babyfood, Corn, Creamed	3	Ounce	85.1	55	14	1	0	-	-
3028	Babyfood, Cottage Cheese w/ Fruit	3	Ounce	85.1	66	14	3	1	-	-
3018	Babyfood, Egg Yolks	3	Ounce	85.1	173	1	9	15	4	6
3201	Babyfood, Egg Yolks and Bacon	3	Ounce	85.1	67	5	2	4	-	-
3236	Babyfood, Fruit Dessert	3	Ounce	85.1	54	15	0	0	-	-
3092	Babyfood, Green Beans	3	Ounce	85.1	21	5	1	0	-	-
3009	Babyfood, Ham	3	Ounce	85.1	106	0	13	6	2	3
3166	Babyfood, Juice, Apple	3/4	Cup	185.8	87	22	0	0	-	-
3179	Babyfood, Juice, Mixed Fruit	3/4	Cup	185.8	87	22	0	0	-	-

Polyunsaturated fat (g)	Dietary Fiber (g)	Cholesterol (mg)	Folate (µg)	Vitamin A (RE)	Vitamin B-6 (mg)	Vitamin B-12 (µg)	Vitamin C (mg)	Vitamin E (mg)	Riboflavin (mg)	Thiamin (mg)	Calcium (mg)	Iron (mg)	Magnesium (mg)	Niacin (mg)	Phosphorus (mg)	Potassium (mg)	Sodium (mg)	Zinc (mg)
0	0	0	6	3	0	0	1	0	0	0	5	.2	4	.1	12	13	1	.2
1	-	1	4	2	0	.1	0	-	.1	0	40	.6	33	.2	70	186	67	.4
8	8	0	45	0	.1	0	0	11.4	.4	.1	201	3.5	216	2	390	549	8	3.5
1	2	4	5	9	0	.3	0	-	.1	0	81	.2	13	0	82	146	26	.4
2	0	72	11	18	.2	.7	0	4.3	.3	.1	197	3.9	59	16.9	214	463	3120	2.1
1	-	10	-	250	-	-	6	-	.3	.3	80	1.5	-	2.9	-	500	410	-
0	-	0	0	0	0	0	0	-	0	0	1	.1	0	.1	3	3	10	0
-	0	0	0	0	0	0	0	0	0	0	1	0	1	0	1	16	0	0
3	-	0	14	87	.1	-	6	-	.2	.2	79	2.1	20	2.2	71	274	513	.5
0	-	0	0	0	.1	0	77	0	0	0	13	.7	6	-	13	221	6	.1
5	-	0	6	19	0	0	3	-	.2	.2	11	1.7	11	1.9	43	122	327	.3
0	2	0	0	5	0	0	0	.1	0	0	4	.2	2	.1	5	69	3	0
0	2	0	0	1	0	0	0	.5	0	0	3	.3	3	.1	8	96	19	0
0	4	0	4	7	.1	0	8	.8	0	0	10	.2	7	.1	10	159	0	.1
0	2	0	1	5	.1	0	5	.3	0	0	5	.1	4	.1	9	145	0	.1
0	2	0	1	1	0	0	2	.1	0	0	5	.4	4	.2	9	78	4	.1
0	1	0	1	4	0	0	1	.1	0	0	4	.1	4	.2	9	92	2	0
0	-	0	2	248	0	0	102	-	0	0	13	.7	9	.5	17	215	6	.2
0	1	0	2	248	0	0	1	.2	0	0	13	.7	9	.5	17	215	6	.2
0	-	0	2	160	0	0	4	-	0	0	12	.6	10	.5	17	173	14	.1
0	2	0	2	210	.1	0	6	1.1	0	0	15	.4	12	.4	25	205	5	.1
0	2	0	2	167	.1	0	3	1.1	0	0	14	.5	10	.4	16	175	5	.1
0	2	0	2	157	.1	0	4	1.1	0	0	10	.4	9	.5	16	233	4	.1
0	-	0	1	377	.2	0	3	-	0	0	18	1.9	19	1.1	47	550	4	.3
0	3	0	3	235	.1	0	1	0	0	0	15	1.5	15	1	38	448	3	.2
0	3	0	9	277	.1	0	11	.9	0	0	15	.6	8	.6	20	314	1	.3
0	2	0	2	203	.1	0	11	1.1	0	0	12	1.1	11	1	23	277	5	.1
0	-	0	88	75	.1	0	24	-	.1	.1	22	.6	17	.9	55	279	216	.4
0	2	0	116	64	.1	0	22	-	.1	.1	19	2.2	12	1.2	52	208	472	.5
0	1	0	86	39	.1	0	9	1.3	.1	.1	14	.6	12	.8	38	183	1	.3
0	-	0	135	82	0	0	24	-	.1	.1	23	.6	13	1	55	218	4	.6
4	12	0	124	123	.6	0	16	2.7	.2	.2	22	2.1	78	3.9	82	1204	20	.8
-	1	-	1	1	0	0	32	.5	0	0	4	.2	3	.1	5	65	2	0
-	1	-	5	3	.1	0	22	.5	0	0	7	.3	10	.2	8	92	8	.1
-	-	-	8	-	.1	.3	-	-	.5	.4	196	10.5	26	5.1	128	163	42	.7
0	0	-	5	26	.1	1.3	2	.3	.1	0	7	1.4	8	2.8	61	162	56	1.7
-	-	-	5	133	.1	.4	2	-	.1	.1	15	.7	9	1.2	34	104	386	.6
-	1	-	5	75	0	.1	1	.3	0	0	7	.4	6	.5	26	39	14	.3
0	1	11	5	196	.1	.4	3	.2	.1	0	8	.6	9	1.1	37	121	293	.7
-	-	-	5	67	.1	.4	3	-	.1	0	9	.6	7	1.1	30	102	304	.8
-	2	-	26	3	0	0	2	.4	0	0	12	.3	12	.1	12	155	71	.1
-	1	-	15	1004	.1	0	5	.4	0	0	20	.3	9	.4	17	172	42	.1
2	0	-	9	48	.2	.3	1	.3	.1	0	47	.8	9	2.9	77	104	43	.9
-	1	-	5	91	0	.1	1	.2	0	0	14	.3	8	.4	20	30	14	.3
-	1	-	4	188	0	.1	1	.2	0	0	31	.2	4	.2	20	56	14	.2
-	0	-	3	286	0	.1	1	.1	.1	0	22	.5	4	.6	36	32	144	.3
1	0	1	9	-	0	.1	5	.4	.4	.4	27	2.6	19	4.9	99	133	315	.5
-	2	-	11	7	0	0	2	.4	0	0	15	.2	7	.4	28	69	44	.2
-	0	-	4	2	0	.1	20	.5	0	0	26	.1	3	0	33	36	43	.1
2	0	625	78	320	.1	1.3	1	.7	.2	.1	65	2.3	6	0	244	65	33	1.6
-	1	-	3	24	0	.1	1	.2	.1	0	24	.4	4	.2	43	30	41	.2
-	1	-	3	20	0	0	3	.2	0	0	8	.2	4	.1	7	81	11	0
-	2	-	28	37	0	0	7	.4	.1	0	55	.9	19	.3	16	109	2	.2
1	0	-	2	9	.2	.1	2	.3	.2	.1	4	.9	9	2.4	76	179	57	1.4
-	0	-	0	4	.1	0	108	1.1	0	0	7	1.1	6	.2	9	169	6	.1
-	0	-	12	7	.1	0	118	.4	0	0	16	.6	0	.2	0	100	7	.1

Code	Name	Amount	Unit	Grams	Energy (kcal)	Carbohydrates (g)	Protein (g)	Fat (g)	Saturated fat (g)	Monounsaturated fat (g)
3172	Babyfood, Juice, Orange	3/4	Cup	185.8	82	19	1	1	-	-
3090	Babyfood, Macaroni and Cheese	3	Ounce	85.1	52	7	2	2	-	-
3045	Babyfood, Macaroni and Tomato and Beef	3	Ounce	85.1	50	8	2	1	-	-
3021	Babyfood, Meat Sticks	3	Stick	30.0	55	0	4	4	2	2
3279	Babyfood, Mixed Vegetable	3	Ounce	85.1	28	7	1	0	-	-
3076	Babyfood, Noodles and Chicken	3	Ounce	85.1	54	8	1	2	-	-
3228	Babyfood, Peach Cobbler	3	Ounce	85.1	57	16	0	0	-	-
3230	Babyfood, Peach Melba	3	Ounce	85.1	51	14	0	0	-	-
3131	Babyfood, Peaches w/ Sugar	3	Ounce	85.1	60	16	0	0	-	-
3133	Babyfood, Pears	3	Ounce	85.1	37	10	0	0	-	-
3124	Babyfood, Peas, Buttered	3	Ounce	85.1	51	10	3	1	-	-
3135	Babyfood, Plums w/ Tapioca	3	Ounce	85.1	63	17	0	0	-	-
3694	Babyfood, Rice, Ppd w/ Whole Milk	3	Ounce	85.1	98	14	3	3	-	-
3210	Babyfood, Rice, w/ Mixed Fruit	3	Ounce	85.1	71	16	1	0	-	-
3050	Babyfood, Spaghetti and Tomato and Meat	3	Ounce	85.1	54	9	2	1	-	-
3103	Babyfood, Spinach, Creamed	3	Ounce	85.1	36	5	3	1	-	-
3058	Babyfood, Split Pea and Ham	3	Ounce	85.1	60	10	3	1	-	-
3105	Babyfood, Squash	3	Ounce	85.1	20	5	1	0	-	-
3109	Babyfood, Sweetpotatoes	3	Ounce	85.1	51	12	1	0	-	-
3216	Babyfood, Teething Biscuits	3	Biscuit	33.0	129	25	4	1	-	-
3238	Babyfood, Tropical Fruit	3	Ounce	85.1	51	14	0	0	-	-
3016	Babyfood, Turkey	3	Ounce	85.1	110	0	13	6	2	2
3017	Babyfood, Turkey Sticks	3	Stick	30.0	55	0	4	4	-	-
3083	Babyfood, Turkey and Rice	3	Ounce	85.1	42	6	2	1	0	0
10124	Bacon	1	Slice	6.0	35	0	2	3	1	1
10131	Bacon, Canadian-style Bacon, Grilled	1	Slice	21.0	39	0	5	2	1	1
62528	Bacon, Turkey	1	Slice	14.0	25	0	3	2	1	-
62631	Bagel Chips	1	Ounce	28.4	150	20	4	6	1	3
18005	Bagels, Cinnamon-raisin	1	3-1/2 In.	71.0	195	39	7	1	0	0
18006	Bagels, Cinnamon-raisin, Toasted	1	3-1/2 In.	66.0	194	39	7	1	0	0
18003	Bagels, Egg	1	3-1/2 In.	71.0	197	38	8	1	0	0
18004	Bagels, Egg, Toasted	1	3-1/2 In.	66.0	197	38	8	1	0	0
18007	Bagels, Oat Bran	1	3-1/2 In.	71.0	181	38	8	1	0	0
18008	Bagels, Oat Bran, Toasted	1	3-1/2 In.	66.0	181	38	8	1	0	0
18001	Bagels, Plain	1	3-1/2 In.	71.0	195	38	7	1	0	0
18409	Bagels, Plain, Toasted	1	3-1/2 In.	66.0	195	38	7	1	0	0
55189	Baked Cheese Ravioli, Lean Cuisine-Stouffer's	1	Each	241.0	240	30	13	8	3	-
41297	Baked Cheese Ravioli-Healthy Choice	1	Each	255.1	250	44	14	2	1	-
55190	Baked Potato w/ Sour Cream, Lean Cuisine-Stouffer's	1	Each	294.1	230	38	9	5	2	-
11028	Bamboo Shoots, Cnd	1/2	Cup	65.5	12	2	1	0	0	0
11026	Bamboo Shoots, Fresh	1/2	Cup	75.5	20	4	2	0	0	0
19400	Banana Chips	1	Ounce	28.4	147	17	1	10	8	1
18304	Banana Cream Pie	1	Slice	148.0	398	49	7	20	6	8
41240	Banana Nut Muffin-Healthy Choice	1	Each	70.9	180	32	3	6	-	-
19311	Banana Pudding	1	Cup	298.1	379	63	7	11	2	5
9040	Bananas, Fresh	1	Medium	114.0	105	27	1	1	0	0
7001	Barbecue Loaf, Lunch Meat	1	Slice	23.0	40	1	4	2	1	1
6150	Barbecue Sauce	1/2	Cup	125.0	94	16	2	2	0	1
20004	Barley	1	Cup	184.0	651	135	23	4	1	1
15187	Bass, Freshwater, Ckd, Dry Heat	3	Ounce	85.1	124	0	21	4	1	2
15188	Bass, Striped, Ckd, Dry Heat	3	Ounce	85.1	105	0	19	3	1	1
62678	Bean Dip	2	Tbsp.	30.0	20	4	1	0	0	0
11924	Bean Sprouts	1/2	Cup	66.7	83	6	9	5	-	-
41276	Bean and Ham Soup-Healthy Choice	1	Each	212.6	220	35	12	4	1	-
16006	Beans, Baked, Cnd, Vegetarian	1/2	Cup	127.0	118	26	6	1	0	0
16007	Beans, Baked, Cnd, w/ Beef	1/2	Cup	133.0	161	22	8	5	2	2

Polyunsaturated fat (g)	Dietary Fiber (g)	Cholesterol (mg)	Folate (µg)	Vitamin A (RE)	Vitamin B-6 (mg)	Vitamin B-12 (µg)	Vitamin C (mg)	Vitamin E (mg)	Riboflavin (mg)	Thiamin (mg)	Calcium (mg)	Iron (mg)	Magnesium (mg)	Niacin (mg)	Phosphorus (mg)	Potassium (mg)	Sodium (mg)	Zinc (mg)
-	0	-	49	11	.1	0	116	1.1	.1	.1	22	.3	17	.4	20	342	2	.1
-	0	-	1	3	0	0	1	.2	.1	0	43	.3	6	.5	50	37	65	.3
-	1	-	6	93	0	.2	1	.2	0	0	12	.3	6	.6	37	61	14	.3
0	0	-	3	6	0	.1	1	.1	.1	0	10	.4	3	.4	31	34	164	.6
-	-	-	6	208	.1	0	3	-	0	0	14	.3	9	.4	19	95	8	.2
-	1	-	3	111	0	.1	1	.2	0	0	22	.4	9	.6	28	50	22	.3
-	1	-	1	12	0	0	17	.2	0	0	3	.1	2	.2	5	48	8	0
-	-	-	2	17	0	0	22	-	0	0	9	.3	2	.2	4	79	8	.2
-	1	-	3	15	0	0	16	.5	0	0	4	.2	4	.6	9	132	4	0
-	3	-	3	3	0	0	19	.5	0	0	7	.2	8	.2	10	98	2	.1
-	-	-	31	35	-	-	11	-	.1	.1	38	.9	-	1.2	-	100	4	-
-	1	-	1	8	0	0	1	.5	0	0	5	.2	3	.2	5	71	7	.1
-	-	-	7	-	.1	.3	-	-	.4	.4	203	10.4	38	4.4	149	162	39	.5
-	1	-	2	2	.2	0	17	.3	.5	.2	17	4	4	2.3	20	28	9	.2
-	1	-	6	113	.1	0	2	.2	.1	.1	15	.5	7	.9	31	92	17	.4
-	2	-	59	313	0	.1	3	.4	.1	0	96	1.2	54	.2	42	188	47	.3
-	1	-	11	68	0	0	2	.2	0	0	20	.4	-	.4	42	116	12	.5
-	2	-	13	171	.1	0	7	.4	.1	0	20	.3	10	.3	14	157	1	.1
-	1	-	9	565	.1	0	8	.4	0	0	14	.3	10	.3	20	207	19	.1
-	0	-	7	4	0	0	3	.1	.2	.1	87	1.2	12	1.4	54	107	119	.3
-	-	-	3	2	0	0	16	-	0	0	9	.2	4	.1	7	49	6	0
1	0	-	10	145	.1	.9	2	.3	.2	0	24	1.1	10	3	81	153	61	1.5
-	0	-	3	20	0	.3	0	.1	0	0	22	.4	5	.5	31	27	145	.5
0	1	-	3	126	0	.1	1	.2	0	0	20	.2	7	.2	14	29	13	.2
0	0	5	0	0	0	.1	2	0	0	0	1	.1	1	.4	20	29	96	.2
0	0	12	1	0	.1	.2	5	.1	0	.2	2	.2	4	1.5	62	82	325	.4
-	-	10	-	0	-	-	0	-	-	-	0	0	-	-	-	-	170	-
2	1	0	-	0	-	-	0	-	-	-	0	.4	-	-	-	-	190	-
0	-	0	15	6	0	0	0	-	.2	.3	13	2.7	15	2.2	55	108	229	.5
0	-	0	11	5	0	0	0	-	.2	.2	13	2.7	15	2	55	108	228	.5
0	-	17	16	23	.1	.1	0	-	.2	.4	9	2.8	18	2.4	60	48	359	.5
0	-	17	11	21	.1	.1	0	-	.1	.3	9	2.8	18	2.2	59	48	358	.5
0	-	0	33	0	.1	0	0	-	.2	.2	9	2.2	40	2.1	117	145	360	1.5
0	-	0	23	0	.1	0	0	-	.2	.2	9	2.2	41	1.9	117	145	360	1.5
0	1	0	16	0	0	0	0	-	.2	.4	53	2.5	21	3.2	68	72	379	.6
0	-	0	11	0	0	0	0	-	.2	.3	13	2.5	20	2.9	68	72	379	.6
-	-	55	-	60	-	-	36	-	.3	.1	160	.8	-	1.1	-	380	590	-
-	-	20	-	500	-	-	5	-	.3	.3	200	1.5	-	1.9	240	590	420	-
-	-	15	-	350	-	-	30	-	.3	.2	160	.6	-	1.1	-	900	570	-
0	2	0	2	1	.1	0	1	.2	0	0	5	.2	3	.1	16	52	3	.4
0	2	0	5	2	.2	0	3	.8	.1	.1	10	.4	2	.5	45	402	3	.8
0	2	0	4	2	.1	0	2	1.5	0	0	5	.4	22	.2	16	152	2	.2
5	-	75	16	104	.2	.4	2	-	.3	.2	111	1.5	24	1.6	136	244	355	.7
3	-	0	-	-	-	-	-	-	.1	.2	80	1	-	.8	160	250	80	-
4	-	0	6	89	.1	.5	1	-	.4	.1	253	.4	24	.5	206	328	584	.8
0	3	0	22	9	.7	0	10	.3	.1	.1	7	.4	33	.6	23	451	1	.2
0	0	9	2	2	.1	.4	4	-	.1	.1	13	.3	4	.5	30	76	307	.6
1	1	0	5	109	.1	0	9	1.4	0	0	24	1.1	22	1.1	25	217	1019	.2
2	32	0	35	4	.6	0	0	1	.5	1.2	61	6.6	245	8.5	486	832	22	5.1
1	0	74	14	30	.1	2	2	-	.1	.1	88	1.6	32	1.3	218	388	77	.7
1	0	88	9	26	.3	3.8	0	-	0	.1	16	.9	43	2.2	216	279	75	.4
0	1	0	0	0	0	0	0	-	0	0	0	.2	0	0	0	-	150	0
-	-	0	85	1	.1	0	8	-	.1	.3	55	.3	64	.7	144	378	167	1.4
1	-	5	-	60	-	-	2	-	.2	.2	48	1	-	1.1	220	630	480	-
0	6	0	30	22	.2	0	4	-	.1	.2	64	.4	41	.5	132	376	504	1.8
0	-	29	58	28	.1	0	2	-	.1	.1	60	2.1	30	1.0	100	420	932	1.6

Code	Name	Amount	Unit	Grams	Energy (kcal)	Carbohydrates (g)	Protein (g)	Fat (g)	Saturated fat (g)	Monounsaturated fat (g)
16008	Beans, Baked, Cnd, w/ Franks	1/2	Cup	128.5	182	20	9	8	3	4
16009	Beans, Baked, Cnd, w/ Pork	1/2	Cup	126.5	134	25	7	2	1	1
16005	Beans, Baked, Home Prepared	1/2	Cup	126.5	191	27	7	7	2	3
16315	Beans, Black, Ckd	1/2	Cup	86.0	114	20	8	0	0	0
11056	Beans, Green, Cnd	1/2	Cup	68.0	14	3	1	0	0	0
11052	Beans, Green, Fresh	1/2	Cup	55.0	17	4	1	0	0	0
11061	Beans, Green, Fzn	1/2	Cup	67.5	18	4	1	0	0	0
16029	Beans, Kidney, Cnd	1/2	Cup	128.0	104	19	7	0	0	0
16073	Beans, Lima, Cnd	1/2	Cup	120.5	95	18	6	0	0	0
11040	Beans, Lima, Fzn	1/2	Cup	90.0	95	18	6	0	0	0
16039	Beans, Navy, Cnd	1/2	Cup	131.0	148	27	10	1	0	0
16044	Beans, Pinto, Cnd	1/2	Cup	120.0	94	17	5	0	0	0
16103	Beans, Refried, Cnd	1/2	Cup	126.5	135	23	8	1	1	1
11932	Beans, Yellow, Cnd	1/2	Cup	68.0	14	3	1	0	0	0
11722	Beans, Yellow, Fresh	1/2	Cup	55.0	17	4	1	0	0	0
14114	Beef Broth and Tomato Juice, Cnd	3/4	Cup	183.0	68	16	1	0	0	0
55192	Beef Cannelloni w/ Sauce, Lean Cuisine-Stouffer's	1	Each	272.9	200	28	14	3	1	-
62692	Beef Chow Mein	1	Cup	247.0	110	15	10	2	1	-
41249	Beef Enchilada-Healthy Choice	1	Each	379.2	370	66	15	5	2	-
19002	Beef Jerky, Chopped and Formed	3	Ounce	85.1	287	12	34	11	5	5
55149	Beef Pie-Stouffer's	1	Each	283.5	460	37	18	27	-	-
57806	Beef Pot Pie-Swanson	1	Pie	198.5	370	36	12	19	-	-
43405	Beef Ravioli, Micro Cup-Hormel	1	Each	212.6	270	34	9	11	4	5
41251	Beef Sirloin Tips-Healthy Choice	1	Each	318.9	270	29	22	7	3	-
43413	Beef Stew, Micro Cup-Hormel	1	Each	212.6	230	11	13	15	5	4
55158	Beef Stroganoff w/ Parsley Noodles-Stouffer's	1	Each	276.4	390	28	24	20	-	-
41335	Beef and Bean Burritos (medium)-Healthy Choice	1	Each	148.8	270	42	12	7	3	0
41334	Beef and Bean Burritos (mild)-Healthy Choice	1	Each	148.8	250	45	11	5	1	-
55191	Beef and Bean Enchiladas, Lean Cuisine-Stouffer's	1	Each	262.2	240	32	15	6	3	-
41270	Beef and Potato Soup-Healthy Choice	1	Each	212.6	110	17	9	1	-	-
13347	Beef, Corned, Brisket, Ckd	3	Ounce	85.1	213	0	15	16	5	8
13353	Beef, Cured, Lunch Meat, Jellied	3	Ounce	85.1	94	0	16	3	1	1
13355	Beef, Cured, Pastrami	3	Ounce	85.1	297	3	15	25	9	12
13357	Beef, Cured, Sausage, Smoked	3	Ounce	85.1	265	2	12	23	10	11
13358	Beef, Cured, Smoked, Chopped Beef	3	Ounce	85.1	105	2	17	4	2	2
13360	Beef, Cured, Thin-sliced Beef	3	Ounce	85.1	151	5	24	3	1	1
13298	Beef, Ground, Extra Lean, Broiled	3	Ounce	85.1	218	0	22	14	5	6
13300	Beef, Ground, Extra Lean, Pan-fried	3	Ounce	85.1	217	0	21	14	5	6
13305	Beef, Ground, Lean, Broiled	3	Ounce	85.1	231	0	21	16	6	7
13307	Beef, Ground, Lean, Pan-fried	3	Ounce	85.1	234	0	21	16	6	7
13312	Beef, Ground, Regular, Broiled	3	Ounce	85.1	246	0	20	18	7	8
13314	Beef, Ground, Regular, Pan-fried	3	Ounce	85.1	260	0	20	19	8	8
13326	Beef, Liver, Ckd, Braised	3	Ounce	85.1	137	3	21	4	2	1
13327	Beef, Liver, Ckd, Pan-fried	3	Ounce	85.1	185	7	23	7	2	1
7042	Beef, Loaved, Lunch Meat	1	Slice	28.4	87	1	4	7	3	3
13504	Beef, Steaks and Roasts, Ckd, 1/2 in. Fat	3	Ounce	85.1	297	0	21	23	9	10
13361	Beef, Steaks and Roasts, Ckd, Fat Trimmed	3	Ounce	85.1	232	0	23	15	6	6
13004	Beef, Steaks and Roasts, Ckd., 1/4 in. Fat	3	Ounce	85.1	259	0	22	18	7	8
7043	Beef, Thin Sliced	1	Slice	4.2	7	0	1	0	0	0
14006	Beer, Light	12	Fl Oz	354.0	99	5	1	0	0	0
14003	Beer, Regular	12	Fl Oz	356.4	146	13	1	0	0	0
11081	Beets, Ckd	1/2	Cup	85.0	37	8	1	0	0	0
18009	Biscuits, Plain or Buttermilk	1	Each	35.0	127	17	2	6	1	2
14008	Bloody Mary	1	Fl Oz	29.7	23	1	0	0	0	0
9052	Blueberries, Cnd, Heavy Syrup	1/2	Cup	128.0	113	28	1	0	-	-
9050	Blueberries, Fresh	1/2	Cup	72.5	41	10	0	0	-	-

Polyunsaturated fat (g)	Dietary Fiber (g)	Cholesterol (mg)	Folate (µg)	Vitamin A (RE)	Vitamin B-6 (mg)	Vitamin B-12 (µg)	Vitamin C (mg)	Vitamin E (mg)	Riboflavin (mg)	Thiamin (mg)	Calcium (mg)	Iron (mg)	Magnesium (mg)	Niacin (mg)	Phosphorus (mg)	Potassium (mg)	Sodium (mg)	Zinc (mg)
1	9	8	39	19	.1	0	3	.6	.1	.1	62	2.2	36	1.2	134	302	553	2.4
0	7	9	46	23	.1	0	3	.7	0	.1	67	2.2	43	.6	137	391	524	1.8
1	7	6	61	0	.1	0	1	.3	.1	.2	77	2.5	54	.5	138	453	534	.9
0	-	0	128	1	.1	0	0	-	.1	.2	23	1.8	60	.4	120	305	204	1
0	1	0	22	24	0	0	3	.1	0	0	18	.6	9	.1	13	74	171	.2
0	2	0	20	37	0	0	9	.2	.1	0	20	.6	14	.4	21	115	3	.1
0	2	0	6	36	0	0	6	.1	0	0	30	.6	14	.3	16	76	9	.4
0	-	0	63	0	.1	0	2	-	.1	.1	35	1.6	40	.6	134	329	444	.7
0	6	0	61	0	.1	0	0	.9	0	.1	25	2.2	47	.3	89	265	405	.8
0	-	0	14	15	.1	0	5	-	0	.1	25	1.8	50	.7	101	370	26	.5
0	7	0	82	0	.1	0	1	.5	.1	.2	62	2.4	62	.6	176	377	587	1
0	4	0	72	0	.1	0	1	-	.1	.1	44	1.9	32	.4	110	361	499	.8
0	7	0	106	0	.1	0	8	0	.1	.1	58	2.2	49	.6	106	497	536	1.7
0	1	0	22	7	0	0	3	.2	0	0	18	.6	9	.1	13	74	171	.2
0	1	0	20	6	0	0	9	0	.1	0	20	.6	14	.4	21	115	3	.1
0	-	0	8	24	0	.1	2	-	.1	0	20	1.1	5	.3	24	176	240	0
-	-	25	-	350	-	-	6	-	.2	.1	120	1.5	-	2.9	-	800	490	-
-	4	10	0	40	0	0	12	-	0	0	24	.4	0	0	0	-	760	0
2	-	30	-	250	-	-	24	-	.3	.3	120	1	-	1.9	260	600	450	-
0	0	96	14	0	.4	3.4	0	.1	.8	.1	9	4.7	43	7.8	323	508	2445	6.9
-	-	-	-	700	-	-	2	-	.4	.3	32	1.5	-	3.8	-	300	1130	-
-	-	-	-	250	-	-	-	-	.2	.2	16	1.5	-	2.9	-	-	730	-
1	-	20	-	100	-	-	11	.5	.3	.2	48	.9	28	2.5	-	359	920	1.1
2	-	65	-	700	-	-	42	-	.2	.2	16	1	-	2.9	190	520	360	-
-	-	45	-	320	-	-	2	.3	.1	0	16	.9	21	2.3	-	487	1140	2.4
-	-	-	-	40	-	-	1	-	.3	.1	48	1.5	-	2.9	-	300	1090	-
3	-	15	-	20	-	-	4	-	.2	.4	48	1.5	-	1.9	180	270	520	-
2	-	10	-	20	-	-	1	-	.2	.4	32	2	-	2.9	130	330	450	-
1	-	45	-	80	-	-	6	-	.3	.2	80	1	-	1.9	-	470	480	-
-	-	20	-	-	-	-	2	-	-	0	-	.2	-	.4	-	100	550	-
1	0	83	5	0	.2	1.4	14	.1	.1	0	7	1.6	10	2.6	106	123	964	3.9
0	0	29	6	0	.2	4.4	15	-	.2	.1	9	2.9	15	4.1	118	342	1124	3
1	0	79	6	0	.2	1.5	3	.2	.1	.1	8	1.6	15	4.3	128	194	1044	3.6
1	0	57	3	0	.1	1.6	10	-	.1	0	6	1.5	11	2.7	89	150	962	2.4
0	0	39	7	0	.3	1.5	18	.1	.1	.1	7	2.4	18	3.9	154	321	1070	3.3
0	0	35	9	0	.3	2.2	12	.1	.2	.1	9	2.3	16	4.5	143	365	1224	3.4
1	0	71	8	0	.2	1.8	0	.2	.2	.1	6	2	18	4.2	137	266	60	4.6
1	0	69	8	0	.2	1.7	0	.2	.2	.1	6	2	18	4	136	265	60	4.6
1	0	74	8	0	.2	2	0	.2	.2	0	9	1.8	18	4.4	134	256	65	4.6
1	0	71	8	0	.2	1.9	0	.2	.2	0	9	1.9	17	4.1	135	254	65	4.4
1	0	77	8	0	.2	2.5	0	.2	.2	0	9	2.1	17	4.9	145	248	71	4.4
1	0	76	8	0	.2	2.3	0	.2	.2	0	9	2.1	17	5	145	255	71	4.3
1	0	331	185	9017	.8	60.4	20	-	3.5	.2	6	5.8	17	9.1	344	200	60	5.2
1	0	410	187	9125	1.2	95.1	20	.5	3.5	.2	9	5.3	20	12.3	392	310	90	4.6
0	0	18	1	0	.1	1.1	4	.1	.1	0	3	.7	4	1	34	59	377	.7
1	0	77	6	0	.3	2	0	-	.2	.1	9	2.2	18	2.9	164	244	50	4.7
1	0	74	6	0	.3	2.1	0	.2	.2	.1	8	2.3	20	3.1	179	275	53	5.2
1	0	75	6	0	.3	2.1	0	.2	.2	.1	9	2.2	19	3.1	173	266	53	5
0	0	2	0	0	0	.1	1	0	0	0	0	.1	1	.2	7	18	60	.2
0	0	0	15	0	.1	0	0	0	.1	0	18	.1	18	1.4	42	64	11	.1
0	1	0	21	0	.2	.1	0	0	.1	0	18	.1	21	1.6	43	89	18	.1
0	1	0	68	3	.1	0	3	.3	0	0	14	.7	20	.3	32	259	65	.3
2	-	0	2	0	0	0	0	-	.1	.1	17	1.2	6	1.2	151	78	368	.2
0	-	0	4	10	0	0	4	-	0	0	2	.1	2	.1	4	43	67	0
-	2	0	2	8	0	0	1	1.3	.1	0	6	.4	5	.1	13	51	4	.1
-	2	0	5	7	0	0	0	.7	0	0	4	.1	4	.3	7	65	4	.1

Code	Name	Amount	Unit	Grams	Energy (kcal)	Carbohydrates (g)	Protein (g)	Fat (g)	Saturated fat (g)	Monounsaturated fat (g)
9055	Blueberries, Frozen, Sweetened	1/2	Cup	115.0	93	25	0	0	–	–
9054	Blueberries, Frozen, Unsweetened	1/2	Cup	77.5	40	9	0	0	–	–
41241	Blueberry Muffin-Healthy Choice	1	Each	70.9	190	39	3	4	–	–
18305	Blueberry Pie	1	Slice	125.0	290	44	2	13	2	7
15189	Bluefish, Ckd, Dry Heat	3	Ounce	85.1	135	0	22	5	1	2
10126	Bologna	1	Slice	23.0	57	0	4	5	2	2
7007	Bologna, Beef	1	Slice	28.4	88	0	3	8	3	4
41286	Boneless Beef Ribs w/ Barbecue Sauce-Healthy Choice	1	Each	311.8	330	40	28	6	2	–
14413	Bourbon and Soda	1	Fl Oz	29.0	26	0	0	0	0	0
12078	Brazilnuts, Dried, Unblanched	1/2	Cup	70.0	459	9	10	46	11	16
19167	Bread Pudding	1	Cup	252.0	423	62	13	15	6	5
18080	Bread Sticks, Plain	1	Stick	10.0	41	7	1	1	0	0
18083	Bread Stuffing, Plain	1	Cup	232.0	390	52	9	17	3	7
18020	Bread, Banana	1	Slice	60.0	203	33	3	7	2	3
18024	Bread, Cornbread	1	Piece	65.0	173	28	4	5	1	1
18025	Bread, Cracked-wheat	1	Slice	25.0	65	12	2	1	0	0
18026	Bread, Cracked-wheat, Toasted	1	Slice	23.0	65	12	2	1	0	0
18344	Bread, Dinner Roll, Egg	1	Each	35.0	107	18	3	2	1	1
18349	Bread, Dinner Roll, French	1	Each	38.0	105	19	3	2	0	1
18345	Bread, Dinner Roll, Oat Bran	1	Each	33.0	78	13	3	2	0	0
18342	Bread, Dinner Roll, Plain	1	Each	35.0	105	18	3	3	1	1
18346	Bread, Dinner Roll, Rye	1	Each	35.0	100	19	4	1	0	0
18347	Bread, Dinner Roll, Wheat	1	Each	33.0	90	15	3	2	1	1
18348	Bread, Dinner Roll, Whole-wheat	1	Each	33.0	88	17	3	2	0	0
18027	Bread, Egg	1	Slice	40.0	115	19	4	2	1	1
18028	Bread, Egg, Toasted	1	Slice	37.0	117	19	4	2	1	1
18029	Bread, French or Vienna	1	Slice	25.0	69	13	2	1	0	0
18030	Bread, French or Vienna, Toasted	1	Slice	23.0	69	13	2	1	0	0
18033	Bread, Italian	1	Slice	30.0	81	15	3	1	0	0
18034	Bread, Italian, Toasted	1	Slice	27.0	80	15	3	1	0	0
18049	Bread, Lo Cal, Oat Bran	1	Slice	23.0	46	9	2	1	0	0
18050	Bread, Lo Cal, Oat Bran, Toasted	1	Slice	19.0	45	9	2	1	0	0
18051	Bread, Lo Cal, Oatmeal	1	Slice	23.0	48	10	2	1	0	0
18052	Bread, Lo Cal, Oatmeal, Toasted	1	Slice	19.0	48	10	2	1	0	0
18053	Bread, Lo Cal, Rye	1	Slice	23.0	47	9	2	1	0	0
18054	Bread, Lo Cal, Rye, Toasted	1	Slice	19.0	46	9	2	1	0	0
18055	Bread, Lo Cal, Wheat	1	Slice	23.0	46	10	2	1	0	0
18056	Bread, Lo Cal, Wheat, Toasted	1	Slice	19.0	45	10	2	1	0	0
18057	Bread, Lo Cal, White	1	Slice	23.0	48	10	2	1	0	0
18058	Bread, Lo Cal, White, Toasted	1	Slice	19.0	47	10	2	1	0	0
18035	Bread, Mixed-grain	1	Slice	26.0	65	12	3	1	0	0
18036	Bread, Mixed-grain, Toasted	1	Slice	24.0	65	12	3	1	0	0
18037	Bread, Oat Bran	1	Slice	30.0	71	12	3	1	0	0
18038	Bread, Oat Bran, Toasted	1	Slice	27.0	70	12	3	1	0	0
18039	Bread, Oatmeal	1	Slice	27.0	73	13	2	1	0	0
18040	Bread, Oatmeal, Toasted	1	Slice	25.0	73	13	2	1	0	0
18041	Bread, Pita, White, Enriched	1	Pita	60.0	165	33	5	1	0	0
18042	Bread, Pita, Whole-wheat	1	Pita	64.0	170	35	6	2	0	0
18044	Bread, Pumpernickel	1	Slice	32.0	80	15	3	1	0	0
18045	Bread, Pumpernickel, Toasted	1	Slice	29.0	80	15	3	1	0	0
18046	Bread, Pumpkin	1	Slice	60.0	199	31	2	8	1	2
18047	Bread, Raisin	1	Slice	26.0	71	14	2	1	0	1
18048	Bread, Raisin, Toasted	1	Slice	24.0	71	14	2	1	0	1
18059	Bread, Rice Bran	1	Slice	27.0	66	12	2	1	0	0
18384	Bread, Rice Bran, Toasted	1	Slice	25.0	66	12	2	1	0	0
18353	Bread, Rolls, Hard (includes Kaiser)	1	Each	57.0	167	30	6	2	0	1

Polyunsaturated fat (g)	Dietary Fiber (g)	Cholesterol (mg)	Folate (µg)	Vitamin A (RE)	Vitamin B-6 (mg)	Vitamin B-12 (µg)	Vitamin C (mg)	Vitamin E (mg)	Riboflavin (mg)	Thiamin (mg)	Calcium (mg)	Iron (mg)	Magnesium (mg)	Niacin (mg)	Phosphorus (mg)	Potassium (mg)	Sodium (mg)	Zinc (mg)
-	2	0	8	5	.1	0	1	.8	.1	0	7	.4	2	.3	8	69	1	.1
-	2	0	5	6	0	0	2	.8	0	0	6	.1	4	.4	9	42	1	.1
2	-	0	-	-	-	-	4	-	.2	.2	80	.8	-	.8	160	200	110	-
2	-	0	5	43	0	0	3	-	0	0	10	.4	6	.4	26	63	406	.2
1	0	65	2	117	.4	5.3	0	-	.1	.1	8	.5	36	6.2	247	406	65	.9
0	0	14	1	0	.1	.2	8	.1	0	.1	3	.2	3	.9	32	65	272	.5
0	0	16	1	0	0	.4	6	.1	0	0	3	.5	3	.7	25	45	278	.6
2	-	70	-	60	-	-	5	-	.3	.2	48	1	-	2.9	220	670	530	-
-	-	0	0	0	0	0	0	-	0	0	1	0	0	0	1	1	4	0
17	4	0	3	0	.2	0	0	5.3	.1	.7	123	2.4	158	1.1	420	420	1	3.2
2	-	166	33	164	.2	-	2	-	.6	.2	287	2.8	48	1.6	275	564	582	1.3
0	-	0	3	0	0	0	0	-	.1	.1	2	.4	3	.5	12	12	66	.1
5	-	0	39	160	.1	0	4	-	.3	.4	148	3.8	35	3.7	114	304	1070	.7
2	-	26	7	14	.1	.1	1	-	.1	.1	11	.8	8	.9	34	79	119	.2
2	-	26	12	35	.1	.1	0	-	.2	.2	162	1.6	16	1.5	110	96	428	.4
0	1	0	10	0	.1	0	0	-	.1	.1	11	.7	13	.9	38	44	135	.3
0	-	0	7	0	.1	0	0	-	.1	.1	11	.7	13	.8	38	44	135	.3
0	1	18	19	8	0	.1	0	-	.2	.2	21	1.2	9	1.2	35	37	191	.3
0	-	0	13	0	0	0	0	-	.1	.2	35	1	8	1.7	32	43	231	.3
1	1	0	10	0	0	0	0	-	.1	.1	28	1.4	10	1.6	34	36	136	.3
0	1	0	11	0	0	0	0	-	.1	.2	42	1.1	8	1.4	41	47	182	.3
0	-	0	8	0	0	0	0	-	.1	.1	11	.9	19	1.4	56	63	312	.4
0	-	0	5	0	0	0	0	-	.1	.1	58	1.2	14	1.3	39	44	112	.3
1	-	0	10	0	.1	0	0	-	.1	.1	35	.8	28	1.2	74	90	158	.7
0	-	20	28	9	0	0	0	-	.2	.2	37	1.2	8	1.9	42	46	197	.3
0	-	21	20	9	0	0	0	-	.2	.2	38	1.2	8	1.8	43	47	200	.3
0	1	0	8	0	0	0	0	-	.1	.1	19	.6	7	1.2	26	28	152	.2
0	-	0	6	0	0	0	0	-	.1	.1	19	.6	7	1.1	26	28	152	.2
0	1	0	9	0	0	0	0	-	.1	.1	23	.9	8	1.3	31	33	175	.3
0	-	0	6	0	0	0	0	-	.1	.1	23	.9	8	1.2	31	33	173	.3
0	-	0	8	0	0	0	0	-	0	.1	13	.7	11	.9	28	23	81	.2
0	-	0	5	0	0	0	0	-	0	.1	13	.7	10	.8	27	23	79	.2
0	-	0	8	0	0	-	0	-	.1	.1	26	.5	7	.7	27	35	89	.2
0	-	0	5	0	0	0	0	-	.1	.1	26	.5	6	.6	27	35	88	.2
0	-	0	5	0	0	0	0	-	.1	.1	17	.7	4	.6	19	23	93	.2
0	-	0	4	0	0	0	0	-	0	.1	17	.7	4	.5	19	22	92	.2
0	3	0	6	-	0	0	0	-	.1	.1	18	.7	6	.9	-	29	118	.2
0	-	0	4	0	0	0	0	-	.1	.1	18	.7	6	.8	21	28	116	.2
0	2	0	8	-	0	.1	0	-	.1	.1	22	.7	6	.8	31	17	104	.3
0	-	0	6	0	0	.1	0	-	.1	.1	21	.7	6	.7	30	17	102	.3
0	2	0	12	0	.1	0	0	-	.1	.1	24	.9	14	1.1	46	53	127	.3
0	-	0	9	0	.1	0	0	-	.1	.1	24	.9	14	1	46	53	127	.3
1	1	0	8	0	0	0	0	-	.1	.2	20	.9	9	1.4	32	34	122	.3
1	-	0	5	-	0	0	0	-	.1	.1	19	.9	9	1.3	31	33	121	.3
0	1	0	7	1	0	-	0	-	.1	.1	18	.7	10	.8	34	38	162	.3
0	-	0	5	1	0	0	0	-	.1	.1	18	.7	10	.8	34	39	163	.3
0	1	0	14	0	0	0	0	-	.2	.4	52	1.6	16	2.8	58	72	322	.5
1	5	0	22	0	.1	0	0	-	.1	.2	10	1.8	44	1.8	115	109	340	1
0	2	0	11	0	0	0	0	-	.1	.1	22	.9	17	1	57	67	215	.5
0	-	0	8	0	0	0	0	-	.1	.1	21	.9	17	.9	57	66	214	.5
4	-	26	7	334	0	0	1	-	.1	.1	11	1	8	.8	32	55	188	.2
0	1	0	9	0	0	0	0	-	.1	.1	17	.8	7	.9	28	59	101	.2
0	-	0	6	0	0	0	0	-	.1	.1	17	.8	7	.8	28	59	102	.2
0	-	0	8	-	.1	0	0	-	.1	.2	19	1	19	1.8	43	53	119	.3
0	-	0	6	0	.1	0	0	-	.1	.1	19	1	19	1.7	44	53	120	.3
1	-	0	9	0	0	0	0	-	.2	.3	54	1.9	15	2.4	57	62	310	.5

Code	Name	Amount	Unit	Grams	Energy (kcal)	Carbohydrates (g)	Protein (g)	Fat (g)	Saturated fat (g)	Monounsaturated fat (g)
18060	Bread, Rye	1	Slice	32.0	83	15	3	1	0	0
18061	Bread, Rye, Toasted	1	Slice	29.0	82	15	3	1	0	0
18064	Bread, Wheat (includes Wheat Berry)	1	Slice	25.0	65	12	2	1	0	0
18066	Bread, Wheat Bran	1	Slice	36.0	89	17	3	1	0	1
18067	Bread, Wheat Bran, Toasted	1	Slice	33.0	90	17	3	1	0	1
18065	Bread, Wheat, Toasted	1	Slice	23.0	65	12	2	1	0	0
18069	Bread, White	1	Slice	25.0	67	12	2	1	0	0
18070	Bread, White, Toasted	1	Slice	23.0	67	13	2	1	0	0
18075	Bread, Whole Wheat	1	Slice	25.0	62	12	2	1	0	0
18078	Bread, Whole Wheat, Toasted	1	Slice	25.0	76	14	2	1	0	0
41348	Breaded Fish-Healthy Choice	1	Stick	9.8	15	2	1	1	-	-
43400	Breast of Chicken w/ Spanish Rice, Top Shelf-Hormel	1	Each	283.5	400	38	27	15	7	4
41252	Breast of Turkey-Healthy Choice	1	Each	297.7	290	39	21	5	2	-
62616	Broccoli and Cheese Baked Potato-Weight Watchers	1	Each	283.5	230	34	12	7	2	-
11091	Broccoli, Ckd	1/2	Cup	78.0	22	4	2	0	0	0
11740	Broccoli, Flower Clusters, Fresh	1/2	Cup	44.0	12	2	1	0	0	0
11093	Broccoli, Frz, Chopped, Ckd	1/2	Cup	92.0	26	5	3	0	0	0
18151	Brownies	1	Each	56.0	227	36	3	9	2	5
11099	Brussels Sprouts, Ckd	1/2	Cup	78.0	30	7	2	0	0	0
62601	Buffalo (Chicken) Wings	4	Each	91.0	190	2	18	12	3	-
18351	Buns, Hamburger or Hot Dog, Mixed-grain	1	Each	43.0	113	19	4	3	1	1
18350	Buns, Hamburger or Hot Dog, Plain	1	Each	43.0	123	22	4	2	1	1
18155	Butter Cookies	1	Each	5.0	23	3	0	1	1	0
1002	Butter, Whipped	1	Tbsp.	11.0	79	0	0	9	6	3
4136	Butter, w/ Salt	1	Pat	5.0	36	0	0	4	3	1
1145	Butter, w/o Salt	1	Pat	5.0	36	0	0	4	3	1
19069	Butterfinger Bar	1	Bar	61.0	267	41	5	11	5	4
19070	Butterscotch Candy	1	Piece	6.0	24	6	0	0	0	0
18307	Butterscotch Pudding Pie	1	Slice	127.0	354	42	6	18	5	8
11110	Cabbage, Ckd	1/2	Cup	75.0	17	3	1	0	0	0
11749	Cabbage, Fresh	1	Cup	70.0	17	4	1	0	0	0
18086	Cake, Angelfood	1	Slice	28.4	73	16	2	0	0	0
18090	Cake, Boston Cream Pie	1	Slice	92.0	232	39	2	8	2	4
18094	Cake, Carrot, w/ Cream Cheese Frosting	1	Slice	111.0	484	52	5	29	5	7
18096	Cake, Chocolate w/ Chocolate Frosting	1	Slice	64.0	235	35	3	10	3	6
18110	Cake, Fruitcake	1	Piece	43.0	139	26	1	4	0	2
18113	Cake, German Chocolate, w/ Frosting	1	Slice	111.0	404	55	4	21	5	9
18115	Cake, Gingerbread	1	Slice	67.0	207	34	3	7	2	4
18119	Cake, Pineapple Upside-down	1	Slice	115.0	367	58	4	14	3	6
18120	Cake, Pound	1	Slice	28.4	110	14	2	6	3	2
18133	Cake, Sponge	1	Slice	38.0	110	23	2	1	0	0
18102	Cake, White, w/ Coconut Frosting	1	Slice	112.0	399	71	5	12	4	4
18139	Cake, White, w/o Frosting	1	Slice	74.0	264	42	4	9	2	4
18140	Cake, Yellow, w/ Chocolate Frosting	1	Slice	64.0	243	35	2	11	3	6
18141	Cake, Yellow, w/ Vanilla Frosting	1	Slice	64.0	239	38	2	9	2	4
55177	Canadian Style Bacon, French Bread Pizzas-Stouffer's	1	Each	163.0	370	40	18	15	-	-
62633	Candy, Candy Corn	26	Each	39.0	140	36	-	-	-	-
19074	Caramels	1	Piece	8.0	31	6	0	1	1	0
11655	Carrot Juice, Cnd	3/4	Cup	184.5	74	17	2	0	0	0
11960	Carrots, Baby, Fresh	1	Medium	10.0	4	1	0	0	0	0
11125	Carrots, Ckd	1/2	Cup	78.0	35	8	1	0	0	0
11128	Carrots, Cnd, Reg Pk	1/2	Cup	73.0	17	4	0	0	0	0
11124	Carrots, Fresh	1	Medium	60.0	26	6	1	0	0	0
11131	Carrots, Frz, Ckd	1/2	Cup	73.0	26	6	1	0	0	0
12586	Cashew Oil Roasted	1/2	Cup	65.0	374	19	10	31	6	18
12585	Cashews, Dry Roasted	1/2	Cup	68.5	393	22	10	32	6	19

Polyunsaturated fat (g)	Dietary Fiber (g)	Cholesterol (mg)	Folate (μg)	Vitamin A (RE)	Vitamin B-6 (mg)	Vitamin B-12 (μg)	Vitamin C (mg)	Vitamin E (mg)	Riboflavin (mg)	Thiamin (mg)	Calcium (mg)	Iron (mg)	Magnesium (mg)	Niacin (mg)	Phosphorus (mg)	Potassium (mg)	Sodium (mg)	Zinc (mg)
0	2	0	16	0	0	0	-	-	.1	.1	23	.9	13	1.2	40	53	211	.4
0	-	0	11	-	0	0	0	-	.1	.1	23	.9	12	1.1	40	53	210	.4
0	1	0	10	0	0	0	0	-	.1	.1	26	.8	12	1	38	50	133	.3
0	3	0	9	0	.1	0	0	-	.1	.1	27	1.1	29	1.6	67	82	175	.5
0	-	0	7	0	.1	0	0	-	.1	.1	27	1.1	29	1.4	67	82	176	.5
0	-	0	7	0	0	0	0	-	.1	.1	26	.8	12	.9	37	50	132	.3
0	1	0	9	0	0	-	0	-	.1	.1	27	.8	6	1	24	30	135	.2
0	-	0	6	0	0	0	0	-	.1	.1	27	.8	6	.9	24	30	136	.2
0	2	0	13	0	0	0	0	-	.1	.1	18	.8	22	1	57	63	132	.5
1	-	0	9	0	0	0	0	-	.1	.1	9	.9	22	1	51	86	95	.4
0	-	3	-	-	-	-	-	-	0	0	-	.1	-	.1	-	20	31	-
3	-	75	-	100	-	-	4	.1	.3	.1	80	.4	35	7.6	-	584	810	1.7
-	-	45	-	40	-	-	48	-	.3	.5	32	1	-	5.7	270	540	420	-
-	6	10	-	200	-	-	9	-	-	-	300	.8	-	-	-	830	510	-
0	2	0	39	108	.1	0	58	.4	.1	0	36	.7	19	.4	46	228	20	.3
0	-	0	31	132	.1	0	41	-	.1	0	21	.4	11	.3	29	143	12	.2
0	3	0	52	174	.1	0	37	.4	.1	.1	47	.6	18	.4	51	166	22	.3
1	1	10	7	11	0	.1	0	-	.1	.1	16	1.3	17	1	57	83	175	.4
0	3	0	47	56	.1	0	48	.7	.1	.1	28	.9	16	.5	44	247	16	.3
-	-	100	-	60	-	-	1	-	-	-	24	.4	-	-	-	-	900	-
0	2	0	12	0	0	0	0	-	.1	.2	41	1.7	21	1.9	52	65	197	.5
0	-	0	12	0	0	0	0	-	.1	.2	60	1.4	9	1.7	38	61	241	.3
0	0	4	0	8	0	0	0	-	0	0	1	.1	1	.2	5	6	18	0
0	0	24	0	83	0	0	0	.2	0	0	3	0	0	0	3	3	91	0
0	0	11	0	38	0	0	0	.1	0	0	1	0	0	0	1	1	41	0
0	0	11	0	38	0	0	0	.1	0	0	1	0	0	0	1	1	1	0
2	2	1	19	12	0	.1	2	.8	0	.1	15	.6	27	2	58	129	83	.4
0	0	1	0	2	0	0	0	0	0	0	0	0	0	0	0	0	3	0
4	-	77	14	107	.1	.4	1	-	.3	.2	128	1.6	22	1.3	135	221	335	.7
0	2	0	15	10	.1	0	15	.1	0	0	23	.1	6	.2	11	73	6	.1
0	-	0	40	9	.1	0	36	-	0	0	33	.4	11	.2	16	172	13	.1
0	0	0	1	0	0	-	0	-	.1	0	40	.1	3	.3	66	26	212	0
1	1	34	7	21	0	.1	0	-	.2	.4	21	.3	6	.2	45	36	132	.1
15	-	60	13	426	.1	.1	1	-	.2	.2	28	1.4	20	1.1	79	124	273	.5
1	2	29	5	18	-	.1	0	-	.1	0	28	1.4	22	.4	78	128	214	.4
1	2	2	1	8	0	0	0	-	0	0	14	.9	7	.3	22	66	116	.1
5	-	53	4	23	0	.1	0	-	.1	.1	53	1.2	19	1.1	173	151	369	.5
1	2	23	7	11	0	0	0	-	.1	.1	46	2.2	11	1	113	161	307	.3
4	-	25	8	75	0	.1	1	-	.2	.2	138	1.7	15	1.4	94	129	367	.4
0	-	63	3	44	0	.1	0	-	.1	0	10	.4	3	.4	39	34	113	.1
0	-	39	5	17	0	.1	0	-	.1	.1	27	1	4	.7	52	38	93	.2
2	-	1	6	12	0	.1	0	-	.2	.1	101	1.3	13	1.2	78	111	318	.4
2	1	1	5	12	0	.1	0	-	.2	.1	96	1.1	9	1.1	69	70	242	.2
1	1	35	5	17	0	.1	0	-	.1	.1	24	1.3	19	.8	103	114	216	.4
3	-	36	6	12	0	.1	0	-	0	.1	40	.7	4	.3	92	34	220	.2
-	-	-	-	80	-	-	6	-	.4	.6	160	1	-	3.8	-	300	1070	-
-	-	-	-	0	-	-	0	-	-	-	0	0	-	-	-	-	80	-
0	0	1	0	1	0	0	0	0	0	0	11	0	1	0	9	17	20	0
0	1	0	7	4751	.4	0	16	0	.1	.2	44	.8	26	.7	77	539	54	.3
0	-	0	3	20	0	0	1	-	0	0	2	.1	1	.1	4	28	4	0
0	3	0	11	1915	.2	0	2	.3	0	0	24	.5	10	.4	23	177	51	.2
0	1	0	7	1005	.1	0	2	-	0	0	18	.5	6	.4	18	131	176	.2
0	2	0	8	1688	.1	0	6	.3	0	.1	16	.3	9	.6	26	194	21	.1
0	3	0	8	1292	.1	0	2	.3	0	0	20	.3	7	.3	19	115	43	.2
5	2	0	44	0	.2	0	0	1	.1	.3	27	2.7	166	1.2	277	345	407	3.1
5	2	0	47	0	.2	0	0	4	1	1	31	1.1	178	1	336	807	400	3.8

Code	Name	Amount	Unit	Grams	Energy (kcal)	Carbohydrates (g)	Protein (g)	Fat (g)	Saturated fat (g)	Monounsaturated fat (g)
15235	Catfish, Channel, Farmed, Ckd, Dry Heat	3	Ounce	85.1	129	0	16	7	2	4
15233	Catfish, Channel, Wild, Ckd, Dry Heat	3	Ounce	85.1	89	0	16	2	1	1
15011	Catfish, Fried	3	Ounce	85.1	195	7	15	11	3	5
11935	Catsup	1	Tbsp.	15.0	16	4	0	0	0	0
11949	Catsup, Low Sodium	1	Tbsp.	15.0	16	4	0	0	0	0
11136	Cauliflower, Ckd, Boiled	1/2	Cup	62.0	14	3	1	0	0	0
11135	Cauliflower, Fresh	1/2	Cup	50.0	13	3	1	0	0	0
11138	Cauliflower, Frz, Ckd	1/2	Cup	90.0	17	3	1	0	0	0
15012	Caviar, Black and Red, Granular	1	Tbsp.	16.0	40	1	4	3	1	1
11144	Celery, Ckd	1/2	Cup	75.0	14	3	1	0	0	0
11143	Celery, Fresh	1/2	Cup	60.0	10	2	0	0	0	0
8053	Cereals, 100% Bran	1	Cup	66.0	178	48	8	3	1	1
8054	Cereals, 100% Natural Cereal, Plain	1	Cup	104.0	489	65	12	22	15	4
8055	Cereals, 100% Natural Cereal, w/ Apple and Cinn.	1	Cup	104.0	477	70	11	20	15	2
8056	Cereals, 100% Natural Cereal, w/ Raisins and Dates	1	Cup	110.0	496	72	11	20	14	4
8028	Cereals, 40% Bran Flakes, Kellogg's	1	Cup	39.0	127	31	5	1	-	-
8029	Cereals, 40% Bran Flakes, Post	1	Cup	47.0	152	37	5	1	-	-
8153	Cereals, 40% Bran Flakes, Ralston Purina	1	Cup	49.0	159	39	6	1	-	-
8001	Cereals, All-bran	1	Cup	85.2	212	63	12	2	-	-
8006	Cereals, Bran Chex	1	Cup	49.0	156	39	5	1	-	-
8008	Cereals, C.W. Post, Plain	1	Cup	97.0	432	69	9	15	11	2
8009	Cereals, C.W. Post, w/ Raisins	1	Cup	103.0	446	74	9	15	11	2
8010	Cereals, Cap'n Crunch	1	Cup	37.0	156	30	2	3	2	0
8011	Cereals, Cap'n Crunch's Crunchberries	1	Cup	35.0	146	29	2	3	2	0
8012	Cereals, Cap'n Crunch's Peanut Butter	1	Cup	35.0	154	26	3	5	2	1
8013	Cereals, Cheerios	1	Cup	22.7	89	16	3	1	0	1
8014	Cereals, Cocoa Krispies	1	Cup	36.0	139	32	2	1	-	-
8017	Cereals, Cookie-crisp, Choc Chip and Van.	1	Cup	30.0	120	26	2	1	-	-
8018	Cereals, Corn Bran	1	Cup	36.0	125	30	2	1	-	-
8019	Cereals, Corn Chex	1	Cup	28.4	111	25	2	0	-	-
8020	Cereals, Corn Flakes, Kellogg's	1	Cup	22.7	88	20	2	0	-	-
8022	Cereals, Corn Flakes, Low Sodium	1	Cup	25.0	100	22	2	0	-	-
8021	Cereals, Corn Flakes, Ralston Purina	1	Cup	25.0	98	22	2	0	-	-
8023	Cereals, Cracklin' Bran	1	Cup	60.0	229	41	6	9	-	-
8168	Cereals, Cream Of Rice, Ckd	1	Cup	244.0	127	28	2	0	-	-
8171	Cereals, Cream Of Wheat, Instant	1	Cup	241.0	154	32	4	0	-	-
8170	Cereals, Cream Of Wheat, Quick	1	Cup	239.0	129	27	4	0	-	-
8169	Cereals, Cream Of Wheat, Regular	1	Cup	251.0	133	28	4	0	-	-
8024	Cereals, Crisp Rice, Low Sodium	1	Cup	26.0	105	24	1	0	-	-
62634	Cereals, Crispex	1	Cup	30.0	110	26	2	0	0	-
8025	Cereals, Crispy Rice	1	Cup	28.0	111	25	2	0	-	-
8026	Cereals, Crispy Wheats 'n Raisins	1	Cup	43.0	150	35	3	1	-	-
8027	Cereals, Fortified Oat Flakes	1	Cup	48.0	177	35	9	1	-	-
62637	Cereals, Frosted Mini-Wheats	1	Cup	52.0	190	45	-	1	0	-
8030	Cereals, Fruit Loops	1	Cup	28.4	111	25	2	1	-	-
8035	Cereals, Golden Grahams	1	Cup	39.0	150	33	2	1	1	0
8036	Cereals, Graham Crackos	1	Cup	30.0	108	26	2	0	-	-
8037	Cereals, Granola, Homemade	1	Cup	122.0	594	67	15	33	6	9
8038	Cereals, Grape-nuts	1	Cup	113.6	406	93	13	0	-	-
8039	Cereals, Grape-nuts Flakes	1	Cup	32.5	116	27	3	0	-	-
62639	Cereals, Great Grains	1	Cup	79.5	330	57	7	9	1	-
8040	Cereals, Heartland Natural Cereal, Plain	1	Cup	115.0	499	79	12	18	-	-
8041	Cereals, Heartland Natural Cereal, w/ Cocnt	1	Cup	105.0	463	71	11	17	-	-
8042	Cereals, Heartland Natural Cereal, w/ Raisins	1	Cup	110.0	468	76	11	16	-	-
8045	Cereals, Honey Nut Cheerios	1	Cup	33.0	125	26	4	1	0	0
8043	Cereals, Honey and Nut Corn Flakes	1	Cup	37.9	151	31	2	2	-	-

Polyunsaturated fat (g)	Dietary Fiber (g)	Cholesterol (mg)	Folate (μg)	Vitamin A (RE)	Vitamin B-6 (mg)	Vitamin B-12 (μg)	Vitamin C (mg)	Vitamin E (mg)	Riboflavin (mg)	Thiamin (mg)	Calcium (mg)	Iron (mg)	Magnesium (mg)	Niacin (mg)	Phosphorus (mg)	Potassium (mg)	Sodium (mg)	Zinc (mg)
1	0	54	6	13	.1	2.4	1	-	.1	.4	8	.7	22	2.1	208	273	68	.9
1	0	61	9	13	.1	2.5	1	-	.1	.2	9	.3	24	2	259	356	43	.5
3	-	69	14	7	.2	1.6	0	-	.1	.1	37	1.2	23	1.9	184	289	238	.7
0	0	0	2	15	0	0	2	.2	0	0	3	.1	3	.2	6	72	178	0
0	0	0	2	15	0	0	2	.2	0	0	3	.1	3	.2	6	72	3	0
0	2	0	27	1	.1	0	27	0	0	0	10	.2	6	.3	20	88	9	.1
0	1	0	29	1	.1	0	23	0	0	0	11	.2	8	.3	22	152	15	.1
0	2	0	37	2	.1	0	28	0	0	0	15	.4	8	.3	22	125	16	.1
1	0	94	8	90	.1	3.2	0	1.1	.1	0	44	1.9	48	0	57	29	240	.2
0	1	0	17	10	.1	0	5	.3	0	0	32	.3	9	.2	19	213	68	.1
0	1	0	17	8	.1	0	4	.2	0	0	24	.2	7	.2	15	172	52	.1
2	20	0	47	0	2.1	6.3	63	1.5	1.8	1.6	46	8.1	312	20.9	801	824	457	5.7
2	9	1	31	-	.2	.1	0	.7	.6	.3	181	3.1	125	2.4	383	514	45	2.4
1	7	1	17	-	.1	.3	1	.7	.6	.3	157	2.9	72	1.9	350	514	52	2
2	7	1	45	-	.2	.1	0	.8	.6	.3	160	3.1	124	2.1	348	538	47	2.1
-	5	0	138	516	.7	2.1	0	.4	.6	.5	19	24.8	71	6.9	192	248	303	5.1
-	9	0	166	622	.8	2.5	0	.5	.7	.6	21	7.5	102	8.3	296	251	431	2.5
-	7	0	173	649	.9	2.6	26	.6	.7	.6	23	7.8	118	8.6	273	286	456	2
-	30	0	301	1128	1.5	0	45	2	1.3	1.1	69	13.5	318	15	794	1051	961	11.2
-	8	0	173	11	.9	2.6	26	.6	.3	.6	29	7.8	126	8.6	327	394	455	2.1
1	7	0	342	1284	1.7	5.1	0	.7	1.5	1.3	47	15.4	67	17.1	224	198	167	1.6
1	14	0	364	1364	1.9	5.5	0	.7	1.5	1.3	50	16.4	74	18.1	232	261	161	1.6
1	1	0	238	5	1	2.3	0	.1	.7	.7	6	9.8	15	8.6	47	48	278	4
0	1	0	128	5	.9	2.5	0	.1	.7	.6	11	9	14	8.1	47	49	244	3.6
1	0	0	244	6	1	2.3	0	.1	.7	.6	7	9.1	19	9	49	57	268	3.8
1	2	0	5	301	.4	1.2	12	.2	.3	.3	39	3.6	31	4	107	81	246	.6
-	0	0	127	477	.6	0	19	0	.5	.5	6	2.3	12	6.3	47	53	275	1.9
-	0	0	3	397	.5	1.6	16	.1	.4	.4	6	4.8	8	5.3	24	29	207	.3
-	7	0	232	8	.9	1.4	0	.8	.7	.4	41	12.2	18	10.9	52	70	310	4
-	1	0	100	14	.5	1.5	15	.1	.1	.4	3	1.8	4	5	11	23	272	.1
-	1	0	80	301	.4	0	12	.1	.3	.3	1	1.4	3	4	14	21	232	.1
-	0	0	2	10	0	0	0	0	0	0	11	.6	3	.1	12	18	3	.1
-	0	0	2	10	0	0	0	.1	0	.1	2	.6	3	1.1	10	22	239	.1
-	10	0	212	794	1.1	0	32	.7	.9	.8	40	3.8	116	10.6	241	355	487	3.2
-	-	0	7	0	.1	0	0	-	0	0	7	.5	7	1	41	49	422	.4
-	-	0	10	0	0	0	0	-	0	.2	60	12.1	14	1.7	43	48	364	.4
-	-	0	10	0	0	0	0	-	0	.2	50	10.3	12	1.4	100	45	464	.3
-	-	0	10	0	0	0	0	-	0	.3	50	10.3	10	1.5	43	43	336	.3
-	-	0	3	0	0	0	0	-	0	0	17	.8	10	.4	27	20	3	.4
-	1	0	50	150	.5	.5	15	-	.4	.4	0	1	0	4.8	16	-	230	1.5
-	0	0	3	0	0	.1	1	0	0	.1	5	.7	12	2	31	27	206	.5
-	3	0	15	569	.8	2.3	0	11.4	.6	.6	71	6.8	34	7.6	117	174	204	.5
-	1	0	169	636	.9	2.5	0	.3	.7	.6	68	13.7	58	8.4	176	343	429	1.5
-	5	0	50	0	.5	.5	0	-	.4	.4	24	1	35	4.8	120	180	10	1.5
-	1	0	100	376	.5	0	15	.1	.4	.4	3	4.5	7	5	24	26	145	3.7
0	1	0	6	516	.7	2.1	21	.1	.6	.5	24	6.2	16	6.9	56	86	385	.3
-	2	0	106	397	.5	0	16	0	.4	.4	14	1.9	25	5.3	66	108	196	1.6
17	13	0	99	-	.4	0	1	5.7	.3	.7	76	4.8	142	2.1	494	612	12	4.5
-	11	0	401	1504	2	6	0	.3	1.7	1.5	11	4.9	76	20	285	379	790	2.5
-	3	0	115	430	.6	1.7	0	.1	.5	.4	13	9.3	36	5.7	97	113	183	.6
-	6	0	75	375	.7	.7	0	-	.6	.6	36	2.2	52	7.1	180	180	225	1.8
-	7	0	64	-	.2	0	1	.8	.2	.4	75	4.3	147	1.6	416	385	293	3
-	7	0	57	-	.2	0	1	.7	.1	.3	66	5.4	138	1.8	380	384	213	2.7
	6	0	44	-	.2	0	1	.8	.1	.3	66	4	141	1.5	376	415	226	2.8
0	1	0	21	437	.6	1.7	17	.2	.5	.4	23	5.2	39	5.8	122	115	299	.9
-	0	0	134	501	.7	0	20	.1	.6	.5	5	2.4	8	6.7	17	48	301	.1

Code	Name	Amount	Unit	Grams	Energy (kcal)	Carbohydrates (g)	Protein (g)	Fat (g)	Saturated fat (g)	Monounsaturated fat (g)
8044	Cereals, Honeybran	1	Cup	35.0	119	29	3	1	–	–
8046	Cereals, Honeycomb	1	Cup	22.0	86	20	1	0	–	–
62641	Cereals, Just Right	1	Cup	55.0	200	46	4	2	0	–
62642	Cereals, Kellogg's Low-Fat Granola	1	Cup	82.5	315	64	7	4	1	–
8048	Cereals, Kix	1	Cup	18.9	74	16	2	0	0	0
8049	Cereals, Life, Plain and Cinn Products	1	Cup	44.0	162	32	8	1	–	–
8050	Cereals, Lucky Charms	1	Cup	32.0	125	26	3	1	0	0
8178	Cereals, Malt-o-meal, Plain and Choc	1	Cup	240.0	122	26	4	0	–	–
8179	Cereals, Maypo, Ckd w/ water, w/ Salt	1	Cup	240.0	170	32	6	2	–	–
8119	Cereals, Maypo, Ckd w/ water, w/o Salt	1	Cup	240.0	170	32	6	2	–	–
8052	Cereals, Nature Valley Granola	1	Cup	113.0	503	75	12	20	13	3
8149	Cereals, Nutri-grain, Barley	1	Cup	41.0	153	34	4	0	–	–
8150	Cereals, Nutri-grain, Corn	1	Cup	42.0	160	35	3	1	–	–
8151	Cereals, Nutri-grain, Rye	1	Cup	40.0	144	34	3	0	–	–
8152	Cereals, Nutri-grain, Wheat	1	Cup	44.0	158	37	4	0	–	–
8123	Cereals, Oats, Instant, Plain	1	Pkt.	177.0	104	18	4	2	–	–
8125	Cereals, Oats, Instant, w/ Apples and cinn	1	Pkt.	149.0	136	26	4	2	–	–
8127	Cereals, Oats, Instant, w/ bran&rsns	1	Pkt.	195.0	158	30	5	2	–	–
8129	Cereals, Oats, Instant, w/ cinn and spice	1	Pkt.	161.0	177	35	5	2	–	–
8131	Cereals, Oats, Instant, w/ mapl&brn sug flav	1	Pkt.	155.0	163	32	5	2	–	–
8133	Cereals, Oats, Instant, w/ raisins and spice	1	Pkt	158.0	161	32	4	2	–	–
8180	Cereals, Oats, Reg and Quick and Instant	1	Cup	234.0	145	25	6	2	0	1
8058	Cereals, Product 19	1	Cup	33.0	126	27	3	0	–	–
8059	Cereals, Quisp	1	Cup	30.0	124	25	2	2	1	0
8060	Cereals, Raisin Bran, Kellogg's	1	Cup	49.2	154	37	5	1	–	–
8061	Cereals, Raisin Bran, Post	1	Cup	56.8	174	43	5	1	–	–
8062	Cereals, Raisin Bran, Ralston Purina	1	Cup	56.0	178	46	4	0	–	–
8063	Cereals, Raisins, Rice and Rye	1	Cup	46.0	155	39	3	0	–	–
8064	Cereals, Rice Chex	1	Cup	25.2	100	23	1	0	–	–
8065	Cereals, Rice Krispies	1	Cup	28.4	112	25	2	0	–	–
8156	Cereals, Rice, Puffed	1	Cup	14.0	56	13	1	0	–	–
8067	Cereals, Special K	1	Cup	21.3	83	16	4	0	–	–
8068	Cereals, Sugar Corn Pops	1	Cup	28.4	108	26	1	0	–	–
8069	Cereals, Sugar Frosted Flakes	1	Cup	35.0	133	32	2	0	–	–
8074	Cereals, Tasteeos	1	Cup	24.0	94	19	3	1	–	–
8075	Cereals, Team	1	Cup	42.0	164	36	3	1	–	–
8077	Cereals, Total	1	Cup	33.0	116	26	3	1	0	0
8078	Cereals, Trix	1	Cup	28.0	108	25	2	0	–	–
8080	Cereals, Wheat 'n Raisin Chex	1	Cup	54.0	185	43	5	0	–	–
8082	Cereals, Wheat Chex	1	Cup	46.0	169	38	5	1	–	–
8147	Cereals, Wheat, Shredded, Large Biscuit	1	Biscuit	23.6	83	19	3	0	–	–
8148	Cereals, Wheat, Shredded, Small Biscuit	1	Cup	33.1	119	26	4	1	–	–
8143	Cereals, Wheatena, Ckd w/ water	1	Cup	243.0	136	29	5	1	–	–
8182	Cereals, Wheatena, Ckd w/ water, w/ Salt	1	Cup	243.0	136	29	5	1	–	–
8089	Cereals, Wheaties	1	Cup	29.0	101	23	3	0	0	0
8183	Cereals, Whole Wheat Hot Natural Cereal	1	Cup	242.0	150	33	5	1	–	–
55832	Cheddar Cheese Sauce-Stouffer's	1	Cup	283.9	731	22	26	60	–	–
55764	Cheddar Cheese Soup-Stouffer's	1	Cup	283.9	441	18	21	31	–	–
55772	Cheddar Cheese, Heat'n Serve Soup -Stouffer's	1	Cup	307.6	488	22	22	36	–	–
62670	Cheddar Cheese, Non-Fat	1-1/2	Ounce	42.5	68	3	12	0	0	0
62668	Cheerios, Apple Cinnamon	1	Cup	40.0	160	87	3	3	0	0
55196	Cheese Cannelloni, Lean Cuisine-Stouffer's	1	Each	258.7	270	27	23	8	4	–
55108	Cheese Enchiladas-Stouffer's	1	Each	276.4	490	33	23	29	–	–
41331	Cheese French Bread Pizza-Healthy Choice	1	Each	159.5	290	46	19	4	2	–
41300	Cheese Manicotti-Healthy Choice	1	Each	262.2	220	34	15	3	2	–
55796	Cheese Manicotti-Stouffer's	1	Ounce	28.4	29	3	2	1	–	–

Polyunsaturated fat (g)	Dietary Fiber (g)	Cholesterol (mg)	Folate (μg)	Vitamin A (RE)	Vitamin B-6 (mg)	Vitamin B-12 (μg)	Vitamin C (mg)	Vitamin E (mg)	Riboflavin (mg)	Thiamin (mg)	Calcium (mg)	Iron (mg)	Magnesium (mg)	Niacin (mg)	Phosphorus (mg)	Potassium (mg)	Sodium (mg)	Zinc (mg)
-	4	0	23	463	.6	1.9	19	.8	.5	.5	16	5.6	46	6.2	132	151	202	.9
-	1	0	78	291	.4	1.2	0	.1	.3	.3	4	2.1	7	3.9	22	70	124	1.2
-	3	0	50	250	.5	.5	0	-	.4	.4	0	9	28	4.8	80	-	250	.6
-	4	0	75	225	.7	.7	0	-	.6	.6	36	1.5	52	7.1	180	255	202	5.6
0	0	0	67	251	.3	1	10	0	.3	.2	24	5.4	8	3.3	26	30	194	.2
-	3	0	37	-	.1	0	-	.3	1	1	154	11.6	14	11.6	238	197	229	1.5
0	1	0	6	424	.6	1.7	17	.2	.5	.4	36	5.1	27	5.6	89	66	227	.6
-	-	0	5	0	0	0	0	-	.2	.5	5	9.6	5	5.8	24	31	324	.2
-	-	0	10	703	1	2.9	29	-	.7	.7	125	8.4	50	9.4	247	211	259	1.5
-	6	0	10	703	1	2.9	29	1.7	.7	.7	125	8.4	50	9.4	247	211	10	1.5
3	6	0	85	-	.1	0	0	3.4	.2	.4	71	3.8	115	.8	354	389	233	2.2
-	2	0	145	543	.7	2.2	22	10.8	.6	.5	11	1.4	32	7.2	126	108	277	5.4
-	3	0	148	556	.8	2.2	22	11.1	.6	.5	1	.9	27	7.4	121	98	276	5.5
-	3	0	141	530	.7	2.1	21	10.6	.6	.5	8	1.1	30	7	104	72	272	5.3
-	3	0	155	583	.8	2.3	23	11.6	.7	.6	12	1.2	34	7.7	165	120	299	5.8
-	3	0	150	453	.7	0	0	.2	.3	.5	163	6.3	42	5.5	133	99	285	.9
-	-	0	137	435	.7	0	0	-	.3	.5	158	6.1	34	5.1	118	107	222	.7
-	-	0	156	480	.8	0	0	-	.6	.6	174	7.6	57	8.1	207	236	248	1.3
-	3	0	153	473	.8	0	0	.4	.3	.6	172	6.6	52	5.7	145	105	280	1
-	-	0	146	451	.7	0	0	-	.3	.5	161	6.4	42	5.3	143	102	279	.9
-	2	0	150	441	.7	0	0	.2	.4	.5	166	6.6	36	5.5	133	150	226	.7
1	-	0	9	-	0	0	0	-	0	.3	19	1.6	56	.3	178	131	374	1.1
-	1	0	466	1748	2.3	7	70	34.9	2	1.7	4	21	12	23.3	47	51	378	.5
0	1	0	8	5	.9	2.6	0	.1	.8	.5	9	6.3	12	5.8	25	45	241	.2
-	5	0	133	500	.7	2	0	1.1	.6	.5	17	22.3	63	6.7	183	256	273	5
-	8	0	201	752	1	3	0	1.3	.9	.7	27	9	97	10	238	350	370	3
-	8	0	148	556	.7	2.2	2	1.3	.6	.6	27	27.3	85	7.4	248	287	486	1.7
-	3	0	125	468	.6	1.9	0	.3	.6	.5	10	5.6	20	6.3	50	144	350	4.7
-	0	0	89	2	.5	1.3	13	0	0	.3	4	1.6	6	4.4	25	29	211	.3
-	0	0	100	376	.5	0	15	0	.4	.4	4	1.8	10	5	34	30	341	.5
-	-	0	3	0	0	0	0	-	.3	.4	1	4.4	4	4.9	14	16	0	.1
-	1	0	75	282	.4	0	11	.1	.3	.3	6	3.4	12	3.7	41	37	199	2.8
-	0	0	100	376	.5	0	15	.1	.4	.4	1	1.8	2	5	28	17	104	1.5
-	1	0	124	463	.6	0	19	.1	.5	.5	1	2.2	3	6.2	26	22	284	0
-	3	0	9	318	.4	1.3	13	.2	.4	.3	11	3.8	26	4.2	96	71	183	.7
-	1	0	7	556	.8	2.2	22	.1	.6	.5	6	2.6	18	7.4	65	71	260	.6
0	4	0	466	1748	2.3	7	70	34.9	2	1.7	282	21	37	23.3	137	123	326	.8
-	0	0	3	371	.5	1.5	15	.1	.4	.4	6	4.5	6	4.9	19	26	179	.1
-	4	0	143	0	.7	2.2	2	.3	.6	.5	24	7.7	53	7.1	163	227	306	1.2
-	4	0	162	0	.8	2.4	24	.2	.2	.6	18	7.3	58	8.1	182	173	308	1.2
-	2	0	12	0	.1	0	0	.1	.1	.1	10	.7	40	1.1	86	77	0	.6
-	3	0	17	0	.1	0	0	.2	.1	.1	13	1.4	44	1.7	117	120	3	1.1
-	7	0	17	0	0	0	0	.9	0	0	10	1.4	49	1.3	146	187	5	1.7
-	-	0	17	0	0	0	0	-	0	0	10	1.4	49	1.3	146	187	578	1.7
0	3	0	102	384	.5	1.5	15	.1	.4	.4	44	4.6	32	5.1	100	108	276	.6
-	-	0	27	0	.2	0	0	-	.1	.2	17	1.5	53	2.2	167	172	564	1.2
-	-	130	-	-	-	-	0	-	0	0	6	.1	-	0	-	341	1392	-
-	-	70	-	-	-	-	0	-	0	0	5	0	-	.2	-	511	681	-
-	-	98	-	-	-	-	0	-	0	0	5	.1	-	.2	-	553	770	-
0	0	6	0	91	0	0	0	-	0	0	365	0	0	0	0	-	425	0
0	1	0	67	200	.7	0	20	-	.6	.5	32	3.3	19	6.3	64	87	213	5
-	-	25	-	60	-	-	21	-	.3	.1	240	.4	-	1.5	-	400	590	-
-	-	-	-	150	-	-	6	-	.3	.1	480	.8	-	1.5	-	400	550	-
1	-	15	-	20	-	-	0	-	.3	.5	240	2	-	2.9	240	310	390	-
-	-	30	-	250	-	-	6	-	.3	.3	120	1.5	-	1.9	210	590	310	-
-	-	4	-	-	-	-	2	-	0	0	296	0	-	0	-	45	108	-

Code	Name	Amount	Unit	Grams	Energy (kcal)	Carbohydrates (g)	Protein (g)	Fat (g)	Saturated fat (g)	Monounsaturated fat (g)
55822	Cheese Ravioli-Stouffer's	1	Ounce	28.4	54	6	3	2	-	-
1150	Cheese Spread, Past. Processed, American	2	Ounce	56.7	165	5	9	12	8	4
62671	Cheese Stick, Mozzarella	1	Each	28.0	80	0	8	5	3	0
55808	Cheese Stuffed Shells-Stouffer's	1	Ounce	28.4	28	3	2	1	-	-
55819	Cheese Tortellini w/ Egg Pasta-Stouffer's	1	Each	145.3	212	22	11	8	-	-
55821	Cheese Tortellini w/ Spinach Pasta-Stouffer's	1	Ounce	28.4	56	6	3	2	-	-
1147	Cheese, American, Pasteurized Processed	2	Ounce	56.7	213	1	13	18	11	5
1004	Cheese, Blue	1-1/2	Ounce	42.5	150	1	9	12	8	3
1005	Cheese, Brick	1-1/2	Ounce	42.5	158	1	10	13	8	4
1006	Cheese, Brie	1-1/2	Ounce	42.5	142	0	9	12	7	3
1008	Cheese, Caraway	1-1/2	Ounce	42.5	160	1	11	12	8	4
1009	Cheese, Cheddar	1-1/2	Ounce	42.5	171	1	11	14	9	4
62577	Cheese, Cheddar, Reduced Fat	1-1/2	Ounce	42.5	120	2	12	8	5	-
1011	Cheese, Colby	1-1/2	Ounce	42.5	167	1	10	14	9	4
1012	Cheese, Cottage, Creamed	1-1/2	Ounce	42.5	44	1	5	2	1	1
1013	Cheese, Cottage, Creamed, w/ Fruit	1-1/2	Ounce	42.5	53	6	4	1	1	0
62690	Cheese, Cottage, Fat Free	1/2	Cup	113.0	70	0	13	0	0	0
1016	Cheese, Cottage, Lowfat, 1% Fat	1-1/2	Ounce	42.5	31	1	5	0	0	0
1015	Cheese, Cottage, Lowfat, 2% Fat	1-1/2	Ounce	42.5	38	2	6	1	1	0
1014	Cheese, Cottage, Uncreamed, Dry	1-1/2	Ounce	42.5	36	1	7	0	0	0
1017	Cheese, Cream	1-1/2	Ounce	42.5	148	1	3	15	9	4
62554	Cheese, Cream, Fat Free	2	Tbsp.	35.0	35	2	5	0	0	-
62553	Cheese, Cream, Light	2	Tbsp.	32.0	70	2	3	5	4	-
1018	Cheese, Edam	1-1/2	Ounce	42.5	152	1	11	12	7	3
62579	Cheese, Fat Free Slices, White	1	Slice	21.3	30	2	5	0	0	-
62578	Cheese, Fat Free Slices, Yellow	1	Slice	21.3	30	2	5	0	0	-
1019	Cheese, Feta	1-1/2	Ounce	42.5	112	2	6	9	6	2
1020	Cheese, Fontina	1-1/2	Ounce	42.5	165	1	11	13	8	4
1156	Cheese, Goat, Hard Type	1-1/2	Ounce	42.5	192	1	13	15	10	3
1157	Cheese, Goat, Semisoft Type	1-1/2	Ounce	42.5	155	1	9	13	9	3
1159	Cheese, Goat, Soft Type	1-1/2	Ounce	42.5	114	0	8	9	6	2
1022	Cheese, Gouda	1-1/2	Ounce	42.5	152	1	11	12	7	3
1023	Cheese, Gruyere	1-1/2	Ounce	42.5	176	0	13	14	8	4
1024	Cheese, Limburger	1-1/2	Ounce	42.5	139	0	9	12	7	4
1025	Cheese, Monterey	1-1/2	Ounce	42.5	159	0	10	13	8	4
62576	Cheese, Monterey, Reduced Fat	1-1/2	Ounce	42.5	120	2	12	8	5	-
1028	Cheese, Mozzarella, Part Skim Milk	1-1/2	Ounce	42.5	108	1	10	7	4	2
1029	Cheese, Mozzarella, Part Skim Milk, Low Moisture	1-1/2	Ounce	42.5	119	1	12	7	5	2
1161	Cheese, Mozzarella, Substitute	1-1/2	Ounce	42.5	105	10	5	5	2	3
1026	Cheese, Mozzarella, Whole Milk	1-1/2	Ounce	42.5	120	1	8	9	6	3
1027	Cheese, Mozzarella, Whole Milk, Low Moisture	1-1/2	Ounce	42.5	135	1	9	10	7	3
1030	Cheese, Muenster	1-1/2	Ounce	42.5	157	0	10	13	8	4
1032	Cheese, Parmesan, Grated	1	Tbsp.	5.0	23	0	2	2	1	0
62608	Cheese, Parmesan, Grated, Fat Free	1	Tbsp.	5.0	5	1	1	0	0	0
1033	Cheese, Parmesan, Piece	1-1/2	Ounce	42.5	167	1	15	11	7	3
1146	Cheese, Parmesan, Shredded	1-1/2	Ounce	42.5	176	1	16	12	7	4
1035	Cheese, Provolone	1-1/2	Ounce	42.5	149	1	11	11	7	3
1037	Cheese, Ricotta, Part Skim Milk	1-1/2	Ounce	42.5	59	2	5	3	2	1
1036	Cheese, Ricotta, Whole Milk	1-1/2	Ounce	42.5	74	1	5	6	4	2
1038	Cheese, Romano	1-1/2	Ounce	42.5	164	2	14	11	7	3
1039	Cheese, Roquefort	1-1/2	Ounce	42.5	157	1	9	13	8	4
1040	Cheese, Swiss, Domestic	1-1/2	Ounce	42.5	160	1	12	12	8	3
1044	Cheese, Swiss, Pasteurized Processed	2	Ounce	56.7	189	1	14	14	9	4
18147	Cheesecake, Commercially Prepared	1	Slice	85.0	273	22	5	19	10	7
18149	Cheesecake, Homemade	1	Slice	85.0	303	21	6	22	12	7
18148	Cheesecake, No-bake Type	1	Slice	80.0	219	28	4	10	6	3

Polyunsaturated fat (g)	Dietary Fiber (g)	Cholesterol (mg)	Folate (µg)	Vitamin A (RE)	Vitamin B-6 (mg)	Vitamin B-12 (µg)	Vitamin C (mg)	Vitamin E (mg)	Riboflavin (mg)	Thiamin (mg)	Calcium (mg)	Iron (mg)	Magnesium (mg)	Niacin (mg)	Phosphorus (mg)	Potassium (mg)	Sodium (mg)	Zinc (mg)
-	-	14	-	-	-	-	0	-	0	0	336	0	-	0	-	16	52	-
0	0	31	4	107	.1	.2	0	-	.2	0	319	.2	16	.1	496	137	921	1.5
0	0	15	0	40	0	0	0	-	0	0	240	0	0	0	0	-	170	0
-	-	3	-	-	-	-	1	-	0	0	248	0	-	.1	-	53	59	-
-	-	63	-	-	-	-	0	-	0	0	2	.1	-	.2	-	71	272	-
-	-	19	-	-	-	-	0	-	0	0	0	0	-	.1	-	26	79	-
1	0	54	4	164	0	.4	0	-	.2	0	349	.2	13	0	252	92	369	1.7
0	0	32	15	97	.1	.5	0	.3	.2	0	224	.1	10	.4	165	109	593	1.1
0	0	40	9	128	0	.5	0	.2	.1	0	286	.2	10	.1	192	58	238	1.1
0	0	43	28	77	.1	.7	0	.3	.2	0	78	.2	9	.2	80	65	268	1
0	0	40	8	123	0	.1	0	-	.2	0	286	.3	9	.1	208	40	293	1.3
0	0	45	8	129	0	.4	0	.2	.2	0	307	.3	12	0	218	42	264	1.3
	0	23	-	90	-	-	0	-	-	-	360	0	-	-	-	35	270	-
0	0	40	8	117	0	.4	0	.1	.2	0	291	.3	11	0	194	54	257	1.3
0	0	6	5	20	0	.3	0	.1	.1	0	26	.1	2	.1	56	36	172	.2
0	0	5	4	15	0	.2	0	0	.1	0	20	0	2	0	44	28	172	.1
0	0	10	0	0	0	0	0	-	0	0	120	0	0	0	0	-	420	0
0	0	2	5	5	0	.3	0	0	.1	0	26	.1	2	.1	57	36	173	.2
0	0	4	6	9	0	.3	0	0	.1	0	29	.1	3	.1	64	41	173	.2
0	0	3	6	3	0	.4	0	0	.1	0	13	.1	2	.1	44	14	5	.2
1	0	47	6	186	0	.2	0	.4	.1	0	34	.5	3	0	44	51	126	.2
-	-	5	-	100	-	-	0	-	-	-	120	0	-	-	-	-	180	-
-	-	15	-	80	-	-	0	-	-	-	48	0	-	-	-	-	150	-
0	0	38	7	108	0	.7	0	.3	.2	0	311	.2	13	0	228	80	410	1.6
-	0	0	-	40	-	-	0	-	-	-	120	0	-	-	-	18	310	-
-	0	0	-	40	-	-	0	-	-	-	120	0	-	-	-	18	310	-
0	0	38	14	54	.2	.7	0	0	.4	.1	209	.3	8	.4	143	26	475	1.2
1	0	49	3	123	0	.7	0	.1	.1	0	234	.1	6	.1	147	27	340	1.5
0	-	45	2	663	0	.1	0	-	.5	.1	381	.8	23	1	310	20	147	.7
0	0	34	1	702	0	.1	0	-	.3	0	127	.7	12	.5	159	67	219	.3
0	0	20	5	578	.1	.1	0	-	.2	0	60	.8	7	.2	109	11	156	.4
0	0	48	9	74	0	.7	0	.1	.1	0	298	.1	12	0	232	51	348	1.7
1	0	47	4	128	0	.7	0	.1	.1	0	430	.1	15	0	257	34	143	1.7
0	0	38	24	134	0	.4	0	.3	.2	0	211	.1	9	.1	167	54	340	.9
0	0	38	8	108	0	.4	0	.1	.2	0	317	.3	11	0	189	34	228	1.3
-	0	23	-	90	-	-	0	-	-	-	360	0	-	-	-	27	270	-
0	0	25	4	75	0	.3	0	.2	.1	0	275	.1	10	0	197	36	198	1.2
0	0	23	4	81	0	.4	0	.2	.1	0	311	.1	11	.1	223	40	224	1.3
1	0	0	5	186	0	.3	0	-	.2	0	259	.2	17	.1	248	193	291	.8
0	0	33	3	102	0	.3	0	.1	.1	0	220	.1	8	0	158	29	159	.9
0	0	38	3	117	0	.3	0	.3	.1	0	244	.1	9	0	175	32	176	1
0	0	41	5	134	0	.6	0	.2	.1	0	305	.2	12	0	199	57	267	1.2
0	0	4	0	9	0	.1	0	0	0	0	69	0	3	0	40	5	93	.2
0	0	2	-	0	-	-	0	-	-	-	16	0	-	-	-	10	15	-
0	0	29	3	63	0	.5	0	.3	.1	0	503	.3	19	.1	295	39	681	1.2
0	0	31	3	74	0	.6	0	-	.1	0	533	.4	22	.1	313	41	721	1.4
0	0	29	4	112	0	.6	0	.1	.1	0	321	.2	12	.1	211	59	372	1.4
0	0	13	6	48	0	.1	0	.1	.1	0	116	.2	6	0	78	53	53	.6
0	0	22	5	57	0	.1	0	.1	.1	0	88	.2	5	0	67	44	36	.5
0	0	44	3	60	0	.5	0	.3	.2	0	452	.3	17	0	323	37	510	1.1
1	0	38	21	127	.1	.3	0	-	.2	0	281	.2	13	.3	167	39	769	.9
0	0	39	3	108	0	.7	0	.2	.2	0	409	.1	15	0	257	47	111	1.7
0	0	48	3	130	0	.7	0	.4	.2	0	438	.3	17	0	432	122	777	2
1	2	47	13	137	0	.1	1	-	.2	0	43	.5	9	.2	79	77	176	.4
2	-	103	10	273	0	.2	0	-	.2	0	49	1.1	7	.3	82	87	241	.5
1	2	34	14	79	0	.2	0	-	.2	.1	138	.4	15	.4	187	160	004	.4

Code	Name	Amount	Unit	Grams	Energy (kcal)	Carbohydrates (g)	Protein (g)	Fat (g)	Saturated fat (g)	Monounsaturated fat (g)
18382	Cheesecake, Plain, w/ Cherry Topping	1	Slice	90.0	258	24	5	17	9	5
9066	Cherries, Sour, Red, Cnd, Heavy Syrup Pack	1/2	Cup	128.0	116	30	1	0	0	0
9065	Cherries, Sour, Red, Cnd, Light Syrup Pack	1/2	Cup	126.0	95	24	1	0	0	0
9064	Cherries, Sour, Red, Cnd, Water Pack	1/2	Cup	122.0	44	11	1	0	0	0
9067	Cherries, Sour, Red, Cnd, X-heavy Syrup Pack	1/2	Cup	130.5	149	38	1	0	0	0
9063	Cherries, Sour, Red, Fresh	1/2	Cup	51.5	26	6	1	0	0	0
9074	Cherries, Sweet, Cnd, Heavy Syrup Pack	1/2	Cup	128.5	107	27	1	0	0	0
9072	Cherries, Sweet, Cnd, Juice Pack	1/2	Cup	125.0	67	17	1	0	0	0
9073	Cherries, Sweet, Cnd, Light Syrup Pack	1/2	Cup	126.0	84	22	1	0	0	0
9071	Cherries, Sweet, Cnd, Water Pack	1/2	Cup	124.0	57	15	1	0	0	0
9075	Cherries, Sweet, Cnd, X-heavy Syrup Pack	1/2	Cup	130.5	133	34	1	0	0	0
9070	Cherries, Sweet, Fresh	1/2	Cup	72.5	52	12	1	1	0	0
9076	Cherries, Sweet, Frozen, Sweetened	1/2	Cup	129.5	115	29	1	0	0	0
18308	Cherry Pie	1	Slice	125.0	325	50	3	14	3	7
18444	Cherry Pie, Fried	1	Pie	128.0	404	55	4	21	3	10
19163	Chewing Gum	1	Stick	3.0	10	3	0	0	–	–
62672	Chewing Gum, Sugar-Free	1	Stick	1.7	5	1	–	–	–	–
19033	Chex Mix	1	Cup	42.5	181	28	5	7	–	–
55199	Chicken Cacciatore, Lean Cuisine-Stouffer's	1	Each	308.3	280	31	22	7	2	–
43398	Chicken Cacciatore, Top Shelf-Hormel	1	Each	283.5	210	25	21	3	–	–
55200	Chicken Chow Mein w/ Rice, Lean Cuisine-Stouffer's	1	Each	255.1	240	34	14	5	1	–
55110	Chicken Chow Mein w/ Rice-Stouffer's	1	Each	304.8	250	39	13	5		
41303	Chicken Chow Mein-Healthy Choice	1	Each	241.0	220	31	18	3	1	–
62611	Chicken Chow Mein-Weight Watchers	1	Each	255.2	200	34	12	2	1	–
55807	Chicken Classica -Stouffer's	1	Ounce	28.4	22	2	2	1	–	–
41336	Chicken Con Queso Burritos (mild)-Healthy Choice	1	Each	148.8	280	40	15	8	2	–
41254	Chicken Dijon-Healthy Choice	1	Each	311.8	250	40	21	3	1	–
55111	Chicken Divan-Stouffer's	1	Each	226.8	220	11	24	10	–	–
62618	Chicken Enchiladas Suiza-Weight Watchers	1	Each	255.2	250	28	15	8	3	–
55201	Chicken Enchiladas, Lean Cuisine-Stouffer's	1	Each	280.0	290	34	17	9	3	–
41304	Chicken Enchiladas-Healthy Choice	1	Each	269.3	310	44	14	9	3	–
55112	Chicken Enchiladas-Stouffer's	1	Each	283.5	490	31	21	31	–	–
41305	Chicken Fajitas-Healthy Choice	1	Each	198.5	200	25	17	3	1	–
55203	Chicken Fettucini, Lean Cuisine-Stouffer's	1	Each	255.1	280	33	23	6	3	–
41306	Chicken Fettucini-Healthy Choice	1	Each	241.0	240	29	22	4	2	–
62620	Chicken Fettucini-Weight Watchers	1	Each	233.9	280	25	22	9	3	–
55763	Chicken Gumbo Soup-Stouffer's	1	Cup	283.9	110	9	7	5	–	–
55204	Chicken Italiano, Lean Cuisine-Stouffer's	1	Each	255.1	270	33	22	6	1	–
55789	Chicken Italienne-Stouffer's	1	Ounce	28.4	22	1	2	1	–	–
55755	Chicken Noodle Soup-Stouffer's	1	Cup	283.9	130	10	7	7	–	–
55768	Chicken Noodle, Heat'n Serve Soup-Stouffer's	1	Cup	283.9	320	28	13	17	–	–
55205	Chicken Oriental, Lean Cuisine-Stouffer's	1	Each	255.1	280	31	22	7	2	–
41256	Chicken Oriental-Healthy Choice	1	Each	318.9	200	32	19	1	–	–
41257	Chicken Parmigiana-Healthy Choice	1	Each	326.0	280	45	22	4	2	–
41271	Chicken Pasta Soup-Healthy Choice	1	Each	212.6	100	13	7	2	–	–
55113	Chicken Pie-Stouffer's	1	Each	283.5	440	32	16	27	–	–
57807	Chicken Pot Pie-Swanson	1	Each	198.5	380	35	11	22	–	–
55790	Chicken Primavera-Stouffer's	1	Ounce	28.4	17	1	2	1	–	–
5280	Chicken Roll, Light Meat	3	Ounce	85.1	135	2	17	6	2	3
5283	Chicken Salad Sandwich Spread	3	Ounce	85.1	170	6	10	11	3	3
5281	Chicken Spread, Cnd	3	Ounce	85.1	163	5	13	10	3	4
41295	Chicken Stir Fry w/ Broccoli-Healthy Choice	1	Each	340.2	280	35	21	6	3	–
55206	Chicken Tenderloins, Lean Cuisine-Stouffer's	1	Each	269.3	240	19	29	5	2	–
55820	Chicken Tortellini w/ Egg Pasta-Stouffer's	1	Ounce	28.4	51	6	3	2	–	–
55109	Chicken a la King w/ Rice-Stouffer's	1	Each	269.3	270	38	18	5	–	–
43397	Chicken a la King, Top Shelf-Hormel	1	Each	283.5	360	49	18	10	4	4

Polyunsaturated fat (g)	Dietary Fiber (g)	Cholesterol (mg)	Folate (µg)	Vitamin A (RE)	Vitamin B-6 (mg)	Vitamin B-12 (µg)	Vitamin C (mg)	Vitamin E (mg)	Riboflavin (mg)	Thiamin (mg)	Calcium (mg)	Iron (mg)	Magnesium (mg)	Niacin (mg)	Phosphorus (mg)	Potassium (mg)	Sodium (mg)	Zinc (mg)
1	-	77	9	217	0	.2	1	-	.1	0	39	1.1	6	.3	64	84	183	.4
0	1	0	10	91	.1	0	3	.2	0	0	13	1.7	8	.2	13	119	9	.1
0	-	0	10	92	.1	0	3	-	0	0	13	1.7	8	.2	13	120	9	.1
0	1	0	10	92	.1	0	3	.2	.1	0	13	1.7	7	.2	12	120	9	.1
0	-	0	10	91	.1	0	2	-	0	0	13	1.6	7	.2	12	119	9	.1
0	1	0	4	66	0	0	5	.1	0	0	8	.2	5	.2	8	89	2	.1
0	1	0	5	19	0	0	5	.1	.1	0	12	.4	12	.5	23	186	4	.1
0	1	0	5	16	0	0	3	.1	0	0	17	.7	15	.5	27	164	4	.1
0	1	0	5	20	0	0	5	.2	.1	0	11	.5	11	.5	23	186	4	.1
0	1	0	5	20	0	0	3	.2	.1	0	14	.4	11	.5	19	162	1	.1
0	-	0	5	20	0	0	5	-	.1	0	12	.5	10	.5	22	185	4	.1
0	2	0	3	15	0	0	5	.1	0	0	11	.3	8	.3	14	162	0	0
0	1	0	5	25	0	0	1	.2	.1	0	16	.5	13	.2	21	258	1	.1
3	1	0	10	-	.1	0	1	-	0	0	15	.6	10	.3	36	101	308	.2
7	-	-	4	22	0	.1	2	-	.1	.2	28	1.6	13	1.8	55	83	479	.3
-	0	0	0	0	0	0	0	0	0	0	0	0	0	0	0	0	0	0
-	-	-	-	-	-	-	-	-	-	-	-	-	-	-	-	-	-	-
-	-	0	0	6	.7	5.3	20	-	.2	.7	15	10.5	27	7.2	80	114	432	.9
1	-	45	-	100	-	-	9	-	.2	.2	32	8	-	5.7	-	560	570	-
-	-	50	-	100	-	-	2	.5	.3	.2	80	1	-	6.7	-	-	810	-
1	-	30	-	60	-	-	6	-	.2	.2	32	.6	-	4.8	-	350	530	-
-	-	-	-	80	-	-	12	-	.2	0	16	.4	-	1.9	-	340	720	-
1	-	45	-	80	-	-	4	-	.1	.2	16	.8	-	3.8	290	290	440	-
-	3	25	-	300	-	-	36	-	-	-	48	.4	-	-	-	360	430	-
-	-	5	-	-	-	-	1	-	0	0	112	0	-	.1	-	50	83	-
3	-	20	-	20	-	-	6	-	.3	.5	80	1.5	-	2.9	170	260	500	-
-	-	40	-	100	-	-	9	-	.1	.2	16	1	-	9.5	300	350	470	-
-	-	-	-	60	-	-	4	-	.2	.5	200	2	-	3.8	32	490	610	-
-	4	25	-	40	-	-	1	-	-	-	360	.8	-	-	-	470	570	-
2	-	55	-	250	-	-	6	-	.3	.2	120	1.5	-	2.9	-	450	500	-
1	-	35	-	80	-	-	21	-	.2	.2	80	.8	-	4.8	160	380	480	-
-	-	-	-	60	-	-	2	-	.3	.1	240	.6	-	2.9	-	420	860	-
1	-	35	-	150	-	-	9	-	.2	.2	64	1.5	-	3.8	210	360	310	-
-	-	35	-	-	-	-	-	-	.4	.3	120	.8	-	5.7	-	420	500	-
2	-	45	-	-	-	-	-	-	.2	.2	64	1	-	2.9	210	190	370	-
-	2	40	-	40	-	-	0	-	-	-	240	1	-	-	-	730	590	-
-	-	20	-	-	-	-	0	-	0	0	160	.1	-	.2	-	180	1422	-
2	-	40	-	100	-	-	24	-	.3	.3	80	.8	-	5.7	-	600	590	-
-	-	7	-	-	-	-	1	-	0	0	48	0	-	.1	-	57	128	-
-	-	20	-	-	-	-	0	-	0	0	80	.1	-	.2	-	140	1282	-
-	-	60	-	-	-	-	6	-	0	0	240	.2	-	.6	-	310	1793	-
2	-	35	-	40	-	-	6	-	.2	.2	32	1	-	6.7	-	470	480	-
-	-	35	-	250	-	-	36	-	.1	.2	32	.8	-	7.6	200	400	440	-
-	-	45	-	900	-	-	12	-	.2	.2	80	1	-	9.5	260	500	370	-
-	-	15	-	60	-	-	-	-	-	0	-	-	-	.4	-	70	560	-
-	-	-	-	500	-	-	1	-	.4	.3	80	1	-	4.8	-	320	750	-
-	-	-	-	400	-	-	-	-	.2	.2	16	1	-	2.9	-	-	760	-
-	-	5	-	-	-	-	1	-	0	0	48	0	-	.1	-	40	119	-
1	0	43	2	20	.2	.1	0	.2	.1	.1	37	.8	16	4.5	134	194	497	.6
5	0	26	4	36	.1	.3	1	-	.1	0	9	.5	9	1.4	28	156	321	.9
2	0	44	3	21	.1	.1	0	-	.1	0	106	2	10	2.3	76	90	328	1
-	-	55	-	20	-	-	-	-	.3	.2	48	1.5	-	2.9	260	630	500	-
1	-	60	-	200	-	-	5	-	.3	.2	120	.4	-	7.6	-	750	490	-
-	-	20	-	-	-	-	0	-	0	0	72	0	-	.1	-	31	57	-
-	-	-	-	20	-	-	1	-	.2	.1	160	.8	-	2.9	32	260	800	-
2	-	37	-	250	-	-	1	.2	.2	.1	48	.2	28	8.6	-	476	890	1.2

Code	Name	Amount	Unit	Grams	Energy (kcal)	Carbohydrates (g)	Protein (g)	Fat (g)	Saturated fat (g)	Monounsaturated fat (g)
57799	Chicken a la King-Swanson	1	Each	250.0	319	15	17	20	-	-
55197	Chicken a la Orange, Lean Cuisine-Stouffer's	1	Each	226.8	280	33	27	4	1	-
41301	Chicken a la Orange-Healthy Choice	1	Each	255.1	240	36	20	2	2	-
55792	Chicken and Dumplings-Stouffer's	1	Each	220.0	303	24	15	16	-	-
57801	Chicken and Dumplings-Swanson	1	Each	200.0	207	18	10	10	-	-
41253	Chicken and Pasta Divan-Healthy Choice	1	Each	340.2	300	41	25	4	2	-
55794	Chicken and Veg. Oriental-Stouffer's	1	Each	220.0	186	14	12	9	-	-
55198	Chicken and Veg. w/ Vermicelli, Lean Cuisine-Stouffer's	1	Each	333.1	240	30	18	5	1	-
41302	Chicken and Vegetables-Healthy Choice	1	Each	326.0	210	31	20	1	-	-
55202	Chicken in BBQ Sauce, Lean Cuisine-Stouffer's	1	Each	248.1	260	32	20	6	1	-
41248	Chicken w/ Barbecue Sauce-Healthy Choice	1	Each	361.5	410	65	24	6	2	-
41277	Chicken w/ Rice Soup-Healthy Choice	1	Each	212.6	90	14	5	1	-	-
5054	Chicken, Back, Meat Only, Ckd, Fried	3	Ounce	85.1	245	5	26	13	4	5
5055	Chicken, Back, Meat Only, Ckd, Roasted	3	Ounce	85.1	203	0	24	11	3	4
5056	Chicken, Back, Meat Only, Ckd, Stewed	3	Ounce	85.1	178	0	22	10	3	3
5049	Chicken, Back, Meat&skin, Ckd, Fried, Batter	3	Ounce	85.1	282	9	19	19	5	8
5050	Chicken, Back, Meat&skin, Ckd, Fried, Flr	3	Ounce	85.1	282	6	24	18	5	7
5051	Chicken, Back, Meat&skin, Ckd, Roasted	3	Ounce	85.1	255	0	22	18	5	7
5052	Chicken, Back, Meat&skin, Ckd, Stewed	3	Ounce	85.1	219	0	19	15	4	6
5063	Chicken, Breast, Meat Only, Ckd, Fried	3	Ounce	85.1	159	0	28	4	1	1
5064	Chicken, Breast, Meat Only, Ckd, Roasted	3	Ounce	85.1	140	0	26	3	1	1
5065	Chicken, Breast, Meat Only, Ckd, Stewed	3	Ounce	85.1	128	0	25	3	1	1
5058	Chicken, Breast, Meat&skin, Ckd, Fried, Batter	3	Ounce	85.1	221	8	21	11	3	5
5059	Chicken, Breast, Meat&skin, Ckd, Fried, Flr	3	Ounce	85.1	189	1	27	8	2	3
5060	Chicken, Breast, Meat&skin, Ckd, Roasted	3	Ounce	85.1	168	0	25	7	2	3
5061	Chicken, Breast, Meat&skin, Ckd, Stewed	3	Ounce	85.1	156	0	23	6	2	2
5277	Chicken, Cnd.	3	Ounce	85.1	140	0	19	7	2	3
5044	Chicken, Dark Meat, Meat Only, Ckd, Fried	3	Ounce	85.1	203	2	25	10	3	4
5045	Chicken, Dark Meat, Meat Only, Ckd, Roasted	3	Ounce	85.1	174	0	23	8	2	3
5046	Chicken, Dark Meat, Meat Only, Ckd, Stewed	3	Ounce	85.1	163	0	22	8	2	3
5035	Chicken, Dark Meat, Meat&skin, Ckd, Fried, Batter	3	Ounce	85.1	253	8	19	16	4	6
5036	Chicken, Dark Meat, Meat&skin, Ckd, Fried, Flr	3	Ounce	85.1	242	3	23	14	4	6
5037	Chicken, Dark Meat, Meat&skin, Ckd, Roasted	3	Ounce	85.1	215	0	22	13	4	5
5038	Chicken, Dark Meat, Meat&skin, Ckd, Stewed	3	Ounce	85.1	198	0	20	12	3	5
5072	Chicken, Drumstick, Meat Only, Ckd, Fried	3	Ounce	85.1	166	0	24	7	2	3
5073	Chicken, Drumstick, Meat Only, Ckd, Roasted	3	Ounce	85.1	146	0	24	5	1	2
5074	Chicken, Drumstick, Meat Only, Ckd, Stewed	3	Ounce	85.1	144	0	23	5	1	2
5067	Chicken, Drumstick, Meat&skin, Ckd, Fried, Batter	3	Ounce	85.1	228	7	19	13	4	5
5068	Chicken, Drumstick, Meat&skin, Ckd, Fried, Flr	3	Ounce	85.1	208	1	23	12	3	5
5069	Chicken, Drumstick, Meat&skin, Ckd, Roasted	3	Ounce	85.1	184	0	23	9	3	4
5070	Chicken, Drumstick, Meat&skin, Ckd, Stewed	3	Ounce	85.1	174	0	22	9	2	3
5021	Chicken, Giblets, Ckd, Fried	3	Ounce	85.1	236	4	28	11	3	4
5022	Chicken, Giblets, Ckd, Simmered	3	Ounce	85.1	134	1	22	4	1	1
5026	Chicken, Heart, Ckd, Simmered	3	Ounce	85.1	157	0	22	7	2	2
5081	Chicken, Leg, Meat Only, Ckd, Fried	3	Ounce	85.1	177	1	24	8	2	3
5082	Chicken, Leg, Meat Only, Ckd, Roasted	3	Ounce	85.1	162	0	23	7	2	3
5083	Chicken, Leg, Meat Only, Ckd, Stewed	3	Ounce	85.1	157	0	22	7	2	2
5076	Chicken, Leg, Meat&skin, Ckd, Fried, Batter	3	Ounce	85.1	232	7	19	14	4	6
5077	Chicken, Leg, Meat&skin, Ckd, Fried, Flour	3	Ounce	85.1	216	2	23	12	3	5
5078	Chicken, Leg, Meat&skin, Ckd, Roasted	3	Ounce	85.1	197	0	22	11	3	4
5079	Chicken, Leg, Meat&skin, Ckd, Stewed	3	Ounce	85.1	187	0	21	11	3	4
5028	Chicken, Liver, Ckd, Simmered	3	Ounce	85.1	134	1	21	5	2	1
5012	Chicken, Meat Only, Ckd, Fried	3	Ounce	85.1	186	1	26	8	2	3
5013	Chicken, Meat Only, Roasted	3	Ounce	85.1	162	0	25	6	2	2
5014	Chicken, Meat Only, Stewed	3	Ounce	85.1	151	0	23	6	2	2
5097	Chicken, Thigh, Meat Only, Ckd, Fried	3	Ounce	85.1	185	1	24	9	2	3

Polyunsaturated fat (g)	Dietary Fiber (g)	Cholesterol (mg)	Folate (μg)	Vitamin A (RE)	Vitamin B-6 (mg)	Vitamin B-12 (μg)	Vitamin C (mg)	Vitamin E (mg)	Riboflavin (mg)	Thiamin (mg)	Calcium (mg)	Iron (mg)	Magnesium (mg)	Niacin (mg)	Phosphorus (mg)	Potassium (mg)	Sodium (mg)	Zinc (mg)
-	-	-	-	-	-	-	-	-	.2	.1	54	.3	-	3.2	-	-	1159	-
-	-	55	-	80	-	-	12	-	.2	.2	32	.4	-	9.5	-	490	290	-
-	-	45	-	150	-	-	27	-	.1	.2	16	.8	-	5.7	230	430	220	-
-	-	70	-	-	-	-	0	-	0	0	1	.2	-	.4	-	248	660	-
-	-	-	-	75	-	-	-	-	.1	0	15	.4	-	1.8	-	-	922	-
1	-	50	-	800	-	-	72	-	.3	.4	120	1	-	4.8	270	500	520	-
-	-	31	-	-	-	-	5	-	0	0	372	.1	-	.6	-	349	1079	-
1	-	30	-	150	-	-	6	-	.3	.3	64	1	-	5.7	-	500	500	-
-	-	35	-	150	-	-	9	-	.2	.3	32	1.5	-	3.8	190	390	490	-
2	-	50	-	250	-	-	18	-	.2	.2	48	.8	-	5.7	-	650	500	-
2	-	55	-	100	-	-	12	-	.1	.1	48	1.5	-	8.6	250	670	550	-
-	-	10	-	80	-	-	6	-	.1	0	16	.2	-	1.9	70	140	510	-
3	0	79	8	25	.3	.3	0	-	.2	.1	22	1.4	21	6.5	150	213	84	2.4
3	0	77	6	24	.3	.3	0	.2	.2	.1	20	1.2	19	6	140	202	82	2.3
2	0	72	6	23	.2	.2	0	.2	.1	0	18	1.1	14	3.9	111	134	57	2
4	-	75	8	31	.2	.2	0	-	.2	.1	22	1.3	16	5	117	153	270	1.7
4	-	76	7	31	.3	.2	0	-	.2	.1	20	1.4	20	6.2	141	192	77	2.1
4	0	75	5	84	.2	.2	0	.2	.2	.1	18	1.2	17	5.7	131	179	74	1.9
3	0	66	4	75	.1	.2	0	.2	.1	0	15	1	14	3.7	102	123	54	1.6
1	0	77	3	6	.5	.3	0	.4	.1	.1	14	1	26	12.6	209	235	67	.9
1	0	72	3	5	.5	.3	0	.2	.1	.1	13	.9	25	11.7	194	218	63	.9
1	0	65	3	5	.3	.2	0	.2	.1	0	11	.7	20	7.2	140	159	54	.8
3	0	72	5	17	.4	.3	0	.9	.1	.1	17	1.1	20	8.9	157	171	234	.8
2	-	76	3	13	.5	.3	0	-	.1	.1	14	1	26	11.7	198	220	65	.9
1	0	71	3	23	.5	.3	0	.2	.1	.1	12	.9	23	10.8	182	208	60	.9
1	0	64	3	20	.2	.2	0	.2	.1	0	11	.8	19	6.6	133	151	53	.8
1	0	53	3	29	.3	.2	2	.2	.1	0	12	1.3	10	5.4	94	117	428	1.2
2	0	82	8	20	.3	.3	0	-	.2	.1	15	1.3	21	6	159	215	82	2.5
2	0	79	7	19	.3	.3	0	.2	.2	.1	13	1.1	20	5.6	152	204	79	2.4
2	0	75	6	18	.2	.2	0	.2	.2	0	12	1.2	17	4	122	154	63	2.3
4	-	76	8	26	.2	.2	0	-	.2	.1	18	1.2	17	4.8	123	157	251	1.8
3	-	78	7	26	.3	.3	0	-	.2	.1	14	1.3	20	5.8	150	196	76	2.2
3	0	77	6	49	.3	.2	0	-	.2	.1	13	1.2	19	5.4	143	187	74	2.1
3	0	70	5	46	.1	.2	0	-	.2	0	12	1.1	15	3.8	113	141	60	1.9
2	0	80	8	15	.3	.3	0	-	.2	.1	10	1.1	20	5.2	158	212	82	2.7
1	0	79	8	15	.3	.3	0	.2	.2	.1	10	1.1	20	5.2	156	209	81	2.7
	0	75	7	14	.2	.2	0	.2	.2	0	9	1.2	18	3.7	128	169	68	2.6
3	-	73	8	22	.2	.2	0	-	.2	.1	14	1.1	17	4.3	125	158	229	2
3	-	77	7	21	.3	.3	0	-	.2	.1	10	1.1	20	5.1	150	195	76	2.5
2	0	77	7	26	.3	.3	0	.2	.2	.1	10	1.1	20	5.1	149	195	77	2.4
2	0	71	6	23	.2	.2	0	.2	.2	0	9	1.1	17	3.6	120	156	65	2.3
3	0	379	322	3044	.5	11.3	7	-	1.3	.1	15	8.8	21	9.3	243	281	96	5.3
1	0	334	320	1896	.3	8.6	7	1.1	.8	.1	10	5.5	17	3.5	195	134	49	3.9
2	0	206	68	8	.3	6.2	2	-	.6	.1	16	7.7	17	2.4	169	112	41	6.2
2	0	84	8	17	.3	.3	0	-	.2	.1	11	1.2	21	5.7	164	216	82	2.5
2	0	80	7	16	.3	.3	0	.2	.2	.1	10	1.1	20	5.4	156	206	77	2.4
2	0	76	7	15	.2	.2	0	.2	.2	.1	9	1.2	18	4.1	127	162	66	2.4
3	-	77	8	23	.2	.2	0	-	.2	.1	15	1.2	17	4.6	129	161	237	1.8
3	-	80	7	24	.3	.3	0	-	.2	.1	11	1.2	20	5.6	155	198	75	2.3
3	0	78	6	33	.3	.3	0	.2	.2	.1	10	1.1	20	5.3	148	191	74	2.2
2	0	71	5	31	.2	.2	0	.2	.2	0	9	1.1	17	3.9	118	150	62	2.1
1	0	537	655	4179	.5	16.5	13	1.2	1.5	.1	12	7.2	18	3.8	265	119	43	3.7
2	0	80	6	15	.4	.3	0	.4	.2	.1	14	1.1	23	8.2	174	219	77	1.9
1	0	76	5	14	.4	.3	0	.2	.2	.1	13	1	21	7.8	166	207	73	1.8
1	0	71	5	13	.2	.2	0	.2	.1	0	12	1	18	5.2	128	153	60	1.7
2	0	87	8	18	.0	.0	0	-	.2	.1	11	1.2	22	6.1	169	220	81	2.4

Code	Name	Amount	Unit	Grams	Energy (kcal)	Carbohydrates (g)	Protein (g)	Fat (g)	Saturated fat (g)	Monounsaturated fat (g)
5098	Chicken, Thigh, Meat Only, Ckd, Roasted	3	Ounce	85.1	178	0	22	9	3	4
5099	Chicken, Thigh, Meat Only, Ckd, Stewed	3	Ounce	85.1	166	0	21	8	2	3
5092	Chicken, Thigh, Meat&skin, Ckd, Fried, Batter	3	Ounce	85.1	236	8	18	14	4	6
5093	Chicken, Thigh, Meat&skin, Ckd, Fried, Flr	3	Ounce	85.1	223	3	23	13	3	5
5094	Chicken, Thigh, Meat&skin, Ckd, Roasted	3	Ounce	85.1	210	0	21	13	4	5
5095	Chicken, Thigh, Meat&skin, Ckd, Stewed	3	Ounce	85.1	197	0	20	13	3	5
5106	Chicken, Wing, Meat Only, Ckd, Fried	3	Ounce	85.1	179	0	26	8	2	3
5107	Chicken, Wing, Meat Only, Ckd, Roasted	3	Ounce	85.1	173	0	26	7	2	2
5108	Chicken, Wing, Meat Only, Ckd, Stewed	3	Ounce	85.1	154	0	23	6	2	2
5101	Chicken, Wing, Meat&skin, Ckd, Fried, Batter	3	Ounce	85.1	276	9	17	19	5	8
5102	Chicken, Wing, Meat&skin, Ckd, Fried, Flr	3	Ounce	85.1	273	2	22	19	5	8
5103	Chicken, Wing, Meat&skin, Ckd, Roasted	3	Ounce	85.1	247	0	23	17	5	6
5104	Chicken, Wing, Meat&skin, Ckd, Stewed	3	Ounce	85.1	212	0	19	14	4	6
41272	Chili Beef Soup-Healthy Choice	1	Each	212.6	150	22	11	1	-	-
55114	Chili Con Carne w/ Beans-Stouffer's	1	Each	248.1	280	28	20	10	-	-
43411	Chili Mac, Micro Cup-Hormel	1	Each	212.6	192	18	10	9	4	4
43408	Chili no Beans, Micro Cup-Hormel	1	Each	209.1	290	15	18	17	8	8
55767	Chili w/ Beans Soup-Stouffer's	1	Cup	283.9	240	25	14	9	-	-
16059	Chili w/ Beans, Cnd	1/2	Cup	127.5	143	15	7	7	3	3
43409	Chili w/ Beans, Micro Cup-Hormel	1	Each	209.1	250	23	15	11	4	4
43369	Chili w/ Beans-Hormel	1	Cup	253.2	357	32	18	18	6	7
43368	Chili w/o Beans-Hormel	1	Cup	253.2	429	17	19	32	13	15
62691	Chili, Fat Free	1/2	Cup	120.0	80	15	7	0	0	0
18198	Chocolate Chip Cookies, Dietary	1	Each	7.0	32	5	0	1	1	0
18159	Chocolate Chip Cookies, Higher Fat, Enr	1	Each	10.0	48	7	1	2	1	1
18158	Chocolate Chip Cookies, Lower Fat	1	Each	10.0	45	7	1	2	0	1
18160	Chocolate Chip Cookies, Soft-type	1	Each	15.0	69	9	1	4	1	2
18310	Chocolate Creme Pie	1	Slice	113.0	344	38	3	22	6	12
18312	Chocolate Mousse Pie	1	Slice	95.0	247	28	3	15	8	5
19183	Chocolate Pudding	1	Cup	298.1	396	68	8	12	2	5
18157	Chocolate Wafers	1	Each	6.0	26	4	0	1	0	0
19119	Chunky Bar	1	Bar	35.0	173	20	3	10	8	0
43370	Chunky Chili w/ Beans-Hormel	1	Cup	253.2	345	30	18	17	-	-
14187	Clam and Tomato Juice, Cnd	3/4	Cup	181.1	83	20	1	0	0	0
15158	Clam, Ckd, Breaded and Fried	3	Ounce	85.1	172	9	12	9	2	4
15159	Clam, Ckd, Moist Heat	3	Ounce	85.1	126	4	22	2	0	0
15160	Clam, Cnd, Drained Solids	3	Ounce	85.1	126	4	22	2	0	0
14121	Club Soda	12	Fl Oz	355.2	0	0	0	0	0	0
19219	Coconut Cream Pudding	1	Cup	280.0	291	50	9	7	5	1
18313	Coconut Creme Pie	1	Slice	64.0	191	24	1	11	5	4
18316	Coconut Custard Pie	1	Slice	104.0	270	31	6	14	6	6
15016	Cod, Atlantic, Ckd, Dry Heat	3	Ounce	85.1	89	0	19	1	0	0
15017	Cod, Atlantic, Cnd	3	Ounce	85.1	89	0	19	1	0	0
14209	Coffee, Brewed	6	Fl Oz	177.6	4	1	0	0	0	0
62685	Coffee, Brewed, Decaf.	6	Fl Oz	177.6	4	1	0	0	0	0
14418	Coffee, Instant, Cappuccino Flavor	6	Fl Oz	175.8	56	10	0	2	2	0
14219	Coffee, Instant, Decaffeinated	6	Fl Oz	179.2	4	1	0	0	0	0
14420	Coffee, Instant, Mocha Flavor	6	Fl Oz	175.8	47	8	1	2	2	0
14215	Coffee, Instant, Regular	6	Fl Oz	179.2	4	1	0	0	0	0
18104	Coffeecake	1	Slice	63.0	263	29	4	15	4	8
18103	Coffeecake, Cheese	1	Slice	76.0	258	34	5	12	4	6
18106	Coffeecake, Fruit	1	Slice	50.0	156	26	3	5	1	3
14400	Cola	12	Fl Oz	369.6	152	38	0	0	0	-
62530	Cola, Diet	12	Fl Oz	355.2	0	0	0	0	-	-
11159	Coleslaw	1/2	Cup	64.0	44	8	1	2	0	0
11162	Collards, Ckd	1/2	Cup	64.0	17	4	1	0	-	-

Polyunsaturated fat (g)	Dietary Fiber (g)	Cholesterol (mg)	Folate (µg)	Vitamin A (RE)	Vitamin B-6 (mg)	Vitamin B-12 (µg)	Vitamin C (mg)	Vitamin E (mg)	Riboflavin (mg)	Thiamin (mg)	Calcium (mg)	Iron (mg)	Magnesium (mg)	Niacin (mg)	Phosphorus (mg)	Potassium (mg)	Sodium (mg)	Zinc (mg)
2	0	81	7	17	.3	.3	0	.2	.2	.1	10	1.1	20	5.5	156	202	75	2.2
2	0	77	6	16	.2	.2	0	.2	.2	.1	9	1.2	18	4.4	127	156	64	2.2
3	-	79	8	25	.2	.2	0	-	.2	.1	15	1.2	18	4.9	132	163	245	1.7
3	-	82	7	25	.3	.3	0	-	.2	.1	12	1.3	21	5.9	159	202	75	2.1
3	0	79	6	41	.3	.2	0	.2	.2	.1	10	1.1	19	5.4	148	189	71	2
3	0	71	5	37	.1	.2	0	.2	.2	0	9	1.2	16	4.2	118	145	60	1.9
2	0	71	3	15	.5	.3	0	-	.1	0	13	1	18	6.2	139	177	77	1.8
2	0	72	3	15	.5	.3	0	.2	.1	0	14	1	18	6.2	141	179	78	1.8
1	0	63	3	14	.3	.2	0	.2	.1	0	11	1	15	4.4	114	130	62	1.7
4	-	67	5	29	.3	.2	0	-	.1	.1	17	1.1	14	4.5	103	117	272	1.2
4	-	69	3	32	.3	.2	0	-	.1	0	13	1.1	16	5.7	128	151	65	1.5
4	0	71	3	40	.4	.2	0	.2	.1	0	13	1.1	16	5.7	128	156	70	1.5
3	0	60	3	34	.2	.2	0	.2	.1	0	10	1	14	3.9	103	118	57	1.4
-	-	15	-	20	-	-	6	-	0	.1	16	.6	-	.4	-	290	560	-
-	-	-	-	200	-	-	15	-	.3	.2	64	2	-	2.9	-	700	910	-
-	-	22	-	210	-	-	-	.2	.2	.1	-	1.5	35	2.1	-	443	977	2.1
1	-	60	-	400	-	-	-	0	.2	.1	48	1.6	35	2.5	-	507	830	3.9
-	-	30	-	-	-	-	0	-	0	0	0	.3	-	.6	-	711	991	-
0	6	22	29	43	.2	0	2	.9	.1	.1	60	4.4	57	.5	196	465	666	2.6
-	-	49	-	190	-	-	-	18.9	.2	.1	48	1.9	46	1.7	-	677	977	2.7
1	-	65	-	250	-	-	-	0	.2	.1	57	1.9	58	2	-	913	1226	2.5
1	-	71	-	786	-	-	-	.6	.3	.1	48	1.7	42	2.9	-	592	1024	3.2
0	7	0	0	1000	0	0	12	-	0	0	24	1	0	0	0	-	160	0
0	-	0	0	0	0	0	0	0	0	0	2	.2	2	.2	6	14	1	0
0	0	0	1	0	0	0	0	-	0	0	3	.3	3	.3	11	14	32	.1
0	-	0	1	0	0	0	0	-	0	0	2	.3	3	.3	8	12	38	.1
0	0	0	1	0	0	0	0	-	0	0	2	.4	5	.2	8	14	49	.1
3	2	6	8	-	0	0	0	-	.1	0	41	1.2	24	.8	77	144	154	.3
1	-	21	3	96	0	.2	0	-	.1	0	73	1	30	.6	219	271	437	.6
4	3	9	9	33	.1	0	5	.4	.5	.1	268	1.5	63	1	238	537	385	1.3
0	-	0	1	0	0	0	0	-	0	0	2	.2	3	.2	8	13	35	.1
2	2	4	8	4	0	.1	0	-	.1	0	50	.4	26	.7	73	187	19	.6
-	-	60	-	-	-	-	-	-	-	-	-	-	-	-	-	-	929	-
0	-	0	29	40	.2	55.4	7	-	.1	.1	22	1.1	40	.3	141	163	724	2
2	-	52	15	77	.1	34.2	9	-	.2	.1	54	11.8	12	1.8	160	277	310	1.2
0	0	57	24	145	.1	84.1	19	-	.4	.1	78	23.8	15	2.9	287	534	95	2.3
0	0	57	24	145	.1	84.1	19	.9	.4	.1	78	23.8	15	2.9	287	534	95	2.3
0	0	0	0	0	0	0	0	0	0	0	18	0	4	0	0	7	75	.4
0	-	20	11	140	.4	.7	2	-	.4	.1	316	.6	45	.3	249	445	456	1
1	-	0	3	13	0	-	0	-	.1	0	19	.5	13	.1	54	42	163	.4
1	2	36	4	28	0	.1	0	-	.2	.1	84	.8	19	.4	127	182	348	.7
0	0	47	7	12	.2	.9	1	.3	.1	.1	12	.4	36	2.1	117	208	66	.5
0	0	47	7	12	.2	.9	1	.2	.1	.1	18	.4	35	2.1	221	449	185	.5
0	0	0	0	0	0	0	0	0	0	0	4	.1	9	.4	2	96	4	0
0	0	0	0	0	0	0	0	-	0	0	4	.1	9	.4	2	96	4	0
0	-	0	0	0	0	0	0	-	0	0	7	.1	9	.3	25	109	95	.1
0	-	0	0	0	0	0	0	-	0	0	5	.1	7	.5	5	63	5	.1
0	-	0	0	0	0	0	0	-	0	0	7	.2	9	.2	26	111	33	.1
0	-	0	0	0	0	0	0	-	0	0	5	.1	7	.5	5	64	5	.1
2	2	20	20	18	0	.1	0	-	.1	.1	34	1.2	14	1.1	68	77	221	.5
1	1	26	44	54	0	.1	0	-	.1	.1	45	.5	11	.5	75	220	258	.4
1	1	11	10	10	0	0	0	-	.1	0	23	1.2	9	1.3	59	45	193	.3
-	0	0	0	0	0	0	0	0	0	0	11	.1	4	0	44	4	15	0
-	0	-	-	-	-	-	-	-	-	-	-	-	-	-	-	-	30	-
1	-	5	17	52	1	0	21	-	0	0	29	.4	6	.2	20	116	15	.1
-	1	0	4	175	0	0	8	.6	0	0	15	.1	4	.2	5	84	10	.1

Code	Name	Amount	Unit	Grams	Energy (kcal)	Carbohydrates (g)	Protein (g)	Fat (g)	Saturated fat (g)	Monounsaturated fat (g)
11161	Collards, Fresh	1	Cup	36.0	11	3	1	0	–	–
11164	Collards, Frz, Chopped, Ckd	1/2	Cup	85.0	31	6	3	0	–	–
19049	Combos Snacks Cheddar Pretzel	1	Ounce	28.4	136	18	3	6	–	–
55799	Confetti Rice-Stouffer's	1	Ounce	28.4	24	5	1	0	–	–
62656	Corn Chips	13	Chips	29.0	160	15	2	11	2	–
55824	Corn Pudding-Stouffer's	1	Ounce	28.4	38	5	1	2	–	–
55168	Corn Souffle-Stouffer's	1	Each	170.1	240	27	7	11	–	–
20092	Corn, Ckd	1/2	Cup	70.0	88	20	2	1	0	0
11901	Corn, Sweet, White, Ckd	1/2	Cup	82.0	89	21	3	1	0	0
11905	Corn, Sweet, White, Cnd	1/2	Cup	82.0	66	15	2	1	0	0
11906	Corn, Sweet, White, Cnd, Cream Style	1/2	Cup	128.0	92	23	2	1	0	0
11900	Corn, Sweet, White, Fresh	1/2	Cup	77.0	66	15	2	1	0	0
11168	Corn, Sweet, Yellow, Ckd	1/2	Cup	82.0	89	21	3	1	0	0
11172	Corn, Sweet, Yellow, Cnd, Brine Pk	1/2	Cup	82.0	66	15	2	1	0	0
11174	Corn, Sweet, Yellow, Cnd, Cream Style	1/2	Cup	128.0	92	23	2	1	0	0
11167	Corn, Sweet, Yellow, Fresh	1/2	Cup	77.0	66	15	2	1	0	0
43366	Corned Beef Hash-Hormel	1	Cup	253.2	420	18	27	27	9	18
7020	Corned Beef Loaf, Jellied	1	Slice	28.4	43	0	6	2	1	1
19401	Cornnuts, Barbecue-flavor	1	Ounce	28.4	124	20	3	4	1	2
19402	Cornnuts, Nacho-flavor	1	Ounce	28.4	124	20	3	4	1	2
19009	Cornnuts, Plain	1	Ounce	28.4	124	21	2	4	1	2
41278	Country Vegetable Soup-Healthy Choice	1	Each	212.6	120	23	3	1	–	–
15137	Crab, Alaska King, Ckd, Moist Heat	3	Ounce	85.1	82	0	16	1	0	0
15138	Crab, Alaska King, Imitation	3	Ounce	85.1	87	9	10	1	0	0
15140	Crab, Blue, Ckd, Moist Heat	3	Ounce	85.1	87	0	17	2	0	0
15141	Crab, Blue, Cnd	3	Ounce	85.1	84	0	17	1	0	0
15142	Crab, Blue, Crab Cakes	3	Ounce	85.1	132	0	17	6	1	2
15226	Crab, Dungeness, Ckd, Moist Heat	3	Ounce	85.1	94	1	19	1	0	0
15227	Crab, Queen, Ckd, Moist Heat	3	Ounce	85.1	98	0	20	1	0	0
9077	Crabapples, Fresh	1/2	Cup	55.0	42	11	0	0	0	0
18214	Crackers, Cheese, Regular	1	Each	1.0	5	1	0	0	0	0
18215	Crackers, Cheese, w/ Peanut Butter Filling	1	Each	7.0	34	4	1	2	0	1
18216	Crackers, Crispbread, Rye	1	Each	10.0	37	8	1	0	0	0
18218	Crackers, Matzo, Egg	1	Each	28.4	111	22	3	1	0	0
18400	Crackers, Matzo, Egg and Onion	1	Each	28.4	111	22	3	1	0	0
18217	Crackers, Matzo, Plain	1	Each	28.4	112	24	3	0	0	0
18219	Crackers, Matzo, Whole-wheat	1	Each	28.4	100	22	4	0	0	0
18220	Crackers, Melba Toast, Plain	1	Each	5.0	20	4	1	0	0	0
18424	Crackers, Melba Toast, Plain, w/o Salt	1	Each	5.0	20	4	1	0	0	0
18221	Crackers, Melba Toast, Rye	1	Each	5.0	19	4	1	0	0	0
18222	Crackers, Melba Toast, Wheat	1	Each	5.0	19	4	1	0	0	0
18229	Crackers, Ritz	1	Each	3.0	15	2	0	1	0	0
18427	Crackers, Ritz, Low Sodium	1	Each	3.0	15	2	0	1	0	0
18226	Crackers, Rye, Wafers, Plain	1	Each	25.0	84	20	2	0	0	0
18227	Crackers, Rye, Wafers, Seasoned	1	Each	22.0	84	16	2	2	0	1
18225	Crackers, Rye, w/ Cheese Filling	1	Each	7.0	34	4	1	2	0	1
18228	Crackers, Saltines	1	Each	3.0	13	2	0	0	0	0
62688	Crackers, Saltines, Fat Free	1	Each	3.0	12	2	0	0	0	0
18425	Crackers, Saltines, Low Salt	1	Each	3.0	13	2	0	0	0	0
18230	Crackers, Snack-type, w/ Cheese Filling	1	Each	7.0	33	4	1	1	0	1
18231	Crackers, Snack-type, w/ Peanut Butter Filling	1	Each	7.0	34	4	1	2	0	1
18428	Crackers, Wheat, Low Salt	1	Each	2.0	9	1	0	0	0	0
18232	Crackers, Wheat, Regular	1	Each	2.0	9	1	0	0	0	0
18233	Crackers, Wheat, w/ Cheese Filling	1	Each	7.0	35	4	1	2	0	1
18234	Crackers, Wheat, w/ Peanut Butter Filling	1	Each	7.0	35	4	1	2	0	1
18235	Crackers, Whole-wheat	1	Each	4.0	18	3	0	1	0	0

Polyunsaturated fat (g)	Dietary Fiber (g)	Cholesterol (mg)	Folate (µg)	Vitamin A (RE)	Vitamin B-6 (mg)	Vitamin B-12 (µg)	Vitamin C (mg)	Vitamin E (mg)	Riboflavin (mg)	Thiamin (mg)	Calcium (mg)	Iron (mg)	Magnesium (mg)	Niacin (mg)	Phosphorus (mg)	Potassium (mg)	Sodium (mg)	Zinc (mg)
-	1	0	4	120	0	0	8	.8	0	0	10	.1	3	.1	4	61	7	0
-	-	0	65	508	.1	0	22	-	.1	0	179	1	26	.5	23	213	43	.2
-	-	3	2	2	0	0	0	-	.2	0	54	.9	6	.9	41	37	317	.2
-	-	1	-	-	-	-	0	-	0	0	24	0	-	0	-	14	136	-
-	1	0	0	0	0	0	0	-	0	0	72	.2	0	0	0	-	200	0
-	-	15	-	-	-	-	1	-	0	0	88	0	-	.1	-	51	125	-
-	-	-	-	60	-	-	-	-	.3	.2	48	.4	-	1.1	-	200	760	-
0	3	0	4	4	0	0	0	.2	0	0	1	.2	25	.4	53	22	0	.4
0	5	0	38	0	0	0	5	.1	.1	.2	2	.5	26	1.3	84	204	14	.4
0	1	0	40	0	0	0	7	.1	.1	0	4	.7	16	1	53	160	265	.3
0	2	0	57	0	.1	0	6	.1	.1	0	4	.5	22	1.2	65	172	365	.7
0	2	0	35	0	0	0	5	.2	0	.2	2	.4	28	1.3	69	208	12	.3
0	2	0	38	18	0	0	5	.1	.1	.2	2	.5	26	1.3	84	204	14	.4
0	2	0	40	13	0	0	7	.1	.1	0	4	.7	16	1	53	160	265	.3
0	2	0	57	13	.1	0	6	.1	.1	0	4	.5	22	1.2	65	172	365	.7
0	2	0	35	22	0	0	5	.1	0	.2	2	.4	28	1.3	69	208	12	.3
-	-	80	-	-	-	-	-	.4	.2	-	71	1.8	31	3.4	-	625	991	4
0	0	13	2	0	0	.4	2	.1	0	0	3	.6	3	.5	21	29	270	1.2
1	2	0	0	10	.1	0	0	-	0	.1	5	.5	31	.4	80	81	277	.5
1	2	1	4	1	.1	0	4	-	0	.1	10	.5	31	.3	88	88	180	.5
1	2	0	0	0	.1	0	0	.3	0	0	3	.5	32	.5	78	79	156	.5
-	-	0	-	200	-	-	6	-	.1	.1	32	.4	-	1.5	100	380	540	-
0	0	45	43	8	.2	9.8	6	-	0	0	50	.6	54	1.1	238	223	912	6.5
1	0	17	1	17	0	1.4	0	-	0	0	11	.3	37	.2	240	77	715	.3
1	0	85	43	2	.2	6.2	3	.9	0	.1	88	.8	28	2.8	175	276	237	3.6
0	0	76	36	2	.1	.4	2	.9	.1	.1	86	.7	33	1.2	221	318	283	3.4
2	0	128	35	69	.1	5	2	-	.1	.1	89	.9	28	2.5	181	276	281	3.5
0	0	65	36	26	.1	8.8	3	-	.2	0	50	.4	49	3.1	149	347	321	4.7
0	0	60	36	44	.1	8.8	6	-	.2	.1	28	2.4	54	2.5	109	170	588	3.1
0	-	0	-	2	-	0	4	-	0	0	10	.2	4	.1	8	107	1	-
0	0	0	0	0	0	0	0	-	0	0	2	0	0	0	2	1	10	0
0	0	0	2	-	.1	0	0	-	0	0	6	.2	4	.5	23	17	69	.1
0	2	0	2	0	0	0	0	-	0	0	3	.2	8	.1	27	32	26	.2
0	-	25	8	4	0	.1	0	-	.2	.2	11	.8	7	1.4	45	43	6	.2
0	1	15	3	5	0	.1	0	-	.1	.2	10	1.2	9	1.4	25	24	81	.2
0	1	0	4	0	0	0	0	-	.1	.1	4	.9	7	1.1	25	32	1	.2
0	3	0	10	0	0	0	0	-	.1	.1	7	1.3	38	1.5	86	90	1	.7
0	0	0	1	0	0	0	0	-	0	0	5	.2	3	.2	10	10	41	.1
0	-	0	1	0	0	0	0	-	0	0	5	.2	3	.2	10	10	1	.1
0	0	0	1	-	0	0	0	-	0	0	4	.2	2	.2	9	10	45	.1
0	0	0	1	0	0	0	0	-	0	0	2	.2	3	.3	8	7	42	.1
0	0	0	0	0	0	0	0	-	0	0	4	.1	1	.1	7	4	25	0
0	-	0	0	0	0	0	0	-	0	0	4	.1	1	.1	7	11	11	0
0	-	0	11	1	.1	0	0	-	.1	.1	10	1.5	30	.4	84	124	199	.7
0	-	0	11	-	0	0	0	-	0	.1	10	.7	23	.5	68	100	195	.6
0	-	1	1	0	0	0	0	-	0	0	16	.2	3	.2	24	24	73	0
0	0	0	1	0	0	0	0	-	0	0	4	.2	1	.2	3	4	39	0
0	0	0	0	0	0	0	0	-	0	0	0	.1	0	0	0	26	36	0
0	-	0	1	0	0	0	0	-	0	0	4	.2	1	.2	3	22	19	0
0	-	0	1	0	0	0	0	-	0	0	18	.2	3	.3	28	30	98	0
0	-	0	2	0	0	0	0	-	0	0	7	.2	4	.4	17	16	66	.1
0	-	0	0	0	0	0	0	-	0	0	1	.1	1	.1	4	4	6	0
0	0	0	0	0	0	0	0	-	0	0	1	.1	1	.1	4	4	16	0
0	-	0	1	1	0	0	0	-	0	0	14	.2	4	.2	27	21	64	.1
0	-	0	3	0	0	0	0	-	0	0	12	.2	3	.4	24	21	56	.1
0	0	0	1	0	0	0	0	-	0	0	2	.1	4	.2	12	12	26	.1

Code	Name	Amount	Unit	Grams	Energy (kcal)	Carbohydrates (g)	Protein (g)	Fat (g)	Saturated fat (g)	Monounsaturated fat (g)
18429	Crackers, Whole-wheat, Low Salt	1	Each	4.0	18	3	0	1	0	0
9078	Cranberries, Fresh	1/2	Cup	47.5	23	6	0	0	–	–
9080	Cranberry Juice Bottled	3/4	Cup	189.4	108	27	0	0	–	–
9081	Cranberry Sauce, Cnd, Sweetened	1/2	Cup	138.5	209	54	0	0	–	–
14238	Cranberry-apple Juice Drink, Bottled	3/4	Cup	183.4	123	31	0	0	0	–
14240	Cranberry-apricot Juice Drink, Bottled	3/4	Cup	183.4	117	30	0	0	0	–
14241	Cranberry-grape Juice Drink, Bottled	3/4	Cup	183.4	103	26	0	0	0	–
9082	Cranberry-orange Relish, Cnd	1/2	Cup	137.5	245	64	0	0	–	–
15243	Crayfish, Farmed, Ckd, Moist Heat	3	Ounce	85.1	74	0	15	1	0	0
15146	Crayfish, Wild, Ckd, Moist Heat	3	Ounce	85.1	75	0	14	1	0	0
18238	Cream Puffs, Shell, w/ Custard Filling	1	Each	130.0	335	30	9	20	5	8
14130	Cream Soda	12	Fl Oz	370.8	189	49	0	0	0	0
1067	Cream Substitute, Nondairy, Liquid	1	Tbsp.	15.0	20	2	0	1	0	1
1069	Cream Substitute, Nondairy, Powdered	1	Tsp.	2.0	11	1	0	1	1	0
55762	Cream of Broccoli Soup-Stouffer's	1	Cup	283.9	300	16	12	21	–	–
55765	Cream of Potato Soup-Stouffer's	1	Cup	283.9	300	34	11	13	–	–
1049	Cream, Half and Half, Cream and Milk	1	Tbsp.	15.0	20	1	0	2	1	0
1053	Cream, Heavy Whipping	1	Tbsp.	15.0	52	0	0	6	3	2
1052	Cream, Light Whipping	1	Tbsp.	15.0	44	0	0	5	3	1
1050	Cream, Light, Coffee or Table	1	Tbsp.	15.0	29	1	0	3	2	1
1051	Cream, Medium, 25% Fat	1	Tbsp.	15.0	37	1	0	4	2	1
1054	Cream, Whipped, Pressurized	1	Tbsp.	3.0	8	0	0	1	0	0
55788	Creamed Chicken-Stouffer's	1	Ounce	28.4	48	1	3	4	–	–
55777	Creamed Chipped Beef-Stouffer's	1	Ounce	28.4	45	2	2	3	–	–
55169	Creamed Spinach-Stouffer's	1	Each	127.6	190	8	4	16	–	–
55756	Creamy Chicken Soup-Stouffer's	1	Cup	283.9	240	25	17	8	–	–
14034	Creme De Menthe, 72 Proof	1	Fl Oz	33.6	125	14	0	0	0	0
18240	Croissant, Apple	1	Medium	57.0	145	21	4	5	3	1
18239	Croissant, Butter	1	Medium	57.0	231	26	5	12	7	3
18241	Croissant, Cheese	1	Medium	57.0	236	27	5	12	5	4
18242	Croutons, Plain	1/2	Cup	15.0	61	11	2	1	0	1
18243	Croutons, Seasoned	1/2	Cup	20.0	93	13	2	4	1	2
62635	Crystal Lite	8	Fl Oz	236.6	5	–	–	–	–	–
11205	Cucumber, Fresh	1/2	Cup	52.0	7	1	0	0	0	0
14010	Daiquiri	1	Fl Oz	30.2	56	2	0	0	0	0
14009	Daiquiri, Bottled	1	Fl Oz	30.5	38	5	0	0	0	–
18245	Danish Pastry, Cheese	1	Each	71.0	266	26	6	16	5	8
18244	Danish Pastry, Cinnamon	1	Each	65.0	262	29	5	15	4	8
18246	Danish Pastry, Fruit,	1	Each	71.0	263	34	4	13	3	7
18433	Danish Pastry, Lemon	1	Each	71.0	263	34	4	13	3	7
18247	Danish Pastry, Nut	1	Each	65.0	280	30	5	16	4	8
18435	Danish Pastry, Raspberry	1	Each	71.0	263	34	4	13	3	7
9087	Dates, Domestic, Natural and Dry	1/2	Cup	89.0	245	65	2	0	–	–
1073	Dessert Topping, Nondairy	1	Tbsp.	4.0	13	1	0	1	1	0
43375	Dinty Moore Beef Stew-Hormel	1	Cup	253.2	246	18	12	15	7	6
43376	Dinty Moore Chicken Stew-Hormel	1	Cup	253.2	310	18	13	21	5	7
43377	Dinty Moore Meatball Stew-Hormel	1	Cup	253.2	268	16	12	18	8	8
43378	Dinty Moore Vegetable Stew-Hormel	1	Cup	253.2	173	22	6	7	2	1
19032	Doo Dads Snack Mix, Original Flavor	1	Cup	56.7	259	36	6	10	–	–
62686	Dough Holes	1	Each	15.0	64	8	1	3	1	2
18251	Doughnuts, Chocolate, Sugared or Glazed	1	Each	42.0	175	24	2	8	2	5
18253	Doughnuts, French Crullers, Glazed	1	Each	41.0	169	24	1	8	2	4
18255	Doughnuts, Glazed	1	Each	60.0	242	27	4	14	3	8
18248	Doughnuts, Plain	1	Each	47.0	198	23	2	11	2	5
18249	Doughnuts, Plain, Chocolate-coated or Frosted	1	Each	43.0	204	21	2	13	4	7
18250	Doughnuts, Plain, Sugared or Glazed	1	Each	45.0	192	23	2	10	2	5

Polyunsaturated fat (g)	Dietary Fiber (g)	Cholesterol (mg)	Folate (μg)	Vitamin A (RE)	Vitamin B-6 (mg)	Vitamin B-12 (μg)	Vitamin C (mg)	Vitamin E (mg)	Riboflavin (mg)	Thiamin (mg)	Calcium (mg)	Iron (mg)	Magnesium (mg)	Niacin (mg)	Phosphorus (mg)	Potassium (mg)	Sodium (mg)	Zinc (mg)
0	-	0	1	0	0	0	0	-	0	0	2	.1	4	.2	12	12	10	.1
-	2	0	1	2	0	0	6	0	0	0	3	.1	2	0	4	34	0	.1
-	-	0	0	0	0	0	67	-	0	0	6	.3	4	.1	4	34	4	.1
-	1	0	-	3	0	0	3	.1	0	0	6	.3	4	.1	8	36	40	.1
-	0	0	0	0	0	0	59	0	0	0	13	.1	4	.1	6	50	4	.1
-	0	0	1	84	0	0	0	0	0	0	17	.3	6	.2	9	112	4	.1
-	0	0	1	0	.1	0	59	0	0	0	15	0	6	.2	7	44	6	.1
-	-	0	-	10	-	0	25	-	0	0	15	.3	5	.1	11	52	44	-
0	0	117	9	13	.1	2.6	0	-	.1	0	43	.9	28	1.4	205	202	82	1.3
0	0	113	37	13	.1	1.8	1	1.3	.1	0	51	.7	28	1.9	230	252	80	1.5
5	-	174	20	259	.1	.5	0	-	.4	.2	86	1.5	16	1.1	142	150	443	.8
0	0	0	0	0	0	0	0	0	0	0	19	.2	4	0	0	4	44	.3
0	0	0	0	1	0	0	0	.2	0	0	1	0	0	0	10	29	12	0
0	0	0	0	0	0	0	0	0	0	0	0	0	0	0	8	16	4	0
-	-	60	-	-	-	-	0	-	0	0	2	0	-	0	-	431	791	-
-	-	30	-	-	-	-	0	-	0	0	2	.1	-	.2	-	791	1422	-
0	0	6	0	16	0	0	0	0	0	0	16	0	2	0	14	19	6	.1
0	0	21	1	63	0	0	0	.1	0	0	10	0	1	0	9	11	6	0
0	0	17	1	44	0	0	0	.1	0	0	10	0	1	0	9	15	5	0
0	0	10	0	27	0	0	0	0	0	0	14	0	1	0	12	18	6	0
0	0	13	0	35	0	0	0	.1	0	0	14	0	1	0	11	17	6	0
0	0	2	0	6	0	0	0	0	0	0	3	0	0	0	3	4	4	0
-	-	14	-	-	-	-	0	-	0	0	352	0	-	.1	-	37	119	-
-	-	13	-	-	-	-	0	-	0	0	184	0	-	.2	-	57	176	-
-	-	-	-	400	-	-	6	-	.2	0	80	.4	-	-	-	400	400	-
-	-	20	-	-	-	-	0	-	0	0	2	0	-	.2	-	511	1282	-
0	0	0	0	0	0	0	0	0	0	0	0	0	0	0	0	0	2	0
0	1	29	7	42	0	.1	0	-	.1	.1	17	.6	7	.9	33	51	156	.6
1	2	43	16	78	0	.2	0	-	.1	.2	21	1.2	9	1.2	60	67	424	.4
2	2	36	19	89	0	.2	0	-	.2	.3	30	1.2	14	1.2	74	75	316	.5
0	1	0	3	0	0	0	0	-	0	.1	11	.6	5	.8	17	19	105	.1
0	1	1	8	1	0	0	0	-	.1	.1	19	.6	8	.9	28	36	248	.2
-	-	-	0	0	0	0	6	-	0	0	0	0	0	0	0	-	-	0
0	0	0	7	11	0	0	3	0	0	0	7	.1	6	.1	10	75	1	.1
0	0	0	1	0	0	0	0	0	0	0	1	0	1	0	2	6	2	0
-	0	0	0	0	0	0	0	0	0	0	0	0	0	0	1	3	12	0
2	-	32	18	44	0	.2	0	-	.2	.1	25	1.1	11	1.4	77	70	320	.6
2	1	20	21	7	0	.1	0	-	.2	.2	46	1.3	12	1.9	70	81	241	.5
2	1	15	11	11	-	.1	3	-	.2	.2	33	1.3	11	1.4	63	59	251	.4
2	-	-	11	38	-	-	3	-	.1	0	33	.5	11	.5	63	59	251	.4
4	1	30	18	9	.1	.1	1	-	.2	.1	61	1.2	21	1.5	72	62	236	.6
2	-	-	11	43	-	-	3	-	.1	0	33	.5	11	.5	63	59	251	.4
-	7	0	11	4	.2	0	0	.1	.1	.1	28	1	31	2	36	580	3	.3
0	0	0	0	3	0	0	0	0	0	0	0	0	0	0	0	1	1	0
1	-	33	-	815	-	-	3	-	.1	0	27	1	23	2.5	-	588	971	2.8
8	-	95	-	476	-	-	2	-	.3	.1	38	.7	25	3.6	-	610	1012	1.3
1	-	33	-	279	-	-	1	2.6	.2	.1	27	1.2	27	3.2	-	586	1094	2.7
2	-	16	-	714	-	-	2	.6	.1	.1	36	.7	31	1.7	-	509	949	.8
-	4	1	23	24	.1	0	0	-	.1	.2	42	1.4	34	3	168	157	721	1.3
0	-	5	2	0	0	0	0	-	0	0	9	.2	3	.2	18	15	60	.1
1	1	24	7	11	0	.1	0	-	0	0	89	1	14	.2	68	50	143	.2
1	-	5	3	-	0	0	0	-	.1	.1	11	.6	5	.6	50	32	141	.1
2	1	4	13	-	0	.1	0	-	.1	.2	26	1.2	13	1.7	56	65	205	.5
4	1	17	4	8	0	.1	0	-	.1	.1	21	.9	9	.9	126	60	257	.3
2	1	25	7	13	0	.2	0	-	0	.1	15	1.1	17	.6	87	49	184	.3
1	-	14	5	1	0	.1	0	-	.1	.1	27	.5	8	.7	53	46	181	.2

Code	Name	Amount	Unit	Grams	Energy (kcal)	Carbohydrates (g)	Protein (g)	Fat (g)	Saturated fat (g)	Monounsaturated fat (g)
18252	Doughnuts, Whole Wheat, Sugared or Glazed	1	Each	45.0	162	19	3	9	1	4
18254	Doughnuts, w/ Creme Filling	1	Each	85.0	307	26	5	21	6	11
18256	Doughnuts, w/ Jelly Filling	1	Each	85.0	289	33	5	16	4	9
14153	Dr. Pepper	12	Fl Oz	368.4	151	38	0	0	0	-
5142	Duck, Domesticated, Meat Only, Roasted	3	Ounce	85.1	171	0	20	10	4	3
5140	Duck, Domesticated, Meat&skin, Roasted	3	Ounce	85.1	287	0	16	24	8	11
7021	Dutch Brand Loaf, Lunch Meat	1	Slice	28.4	68	2	4	5	2	2
18257	Eclairs, Custard-filled w/ Chocolate Glaze	1	Each	62.0	162	15	4	10	3	4
18317	Egg Custard Pie	1	Slice	105.0	221	22	6	12	3	6
19168	Egg Custards	1	Cup	282.0	296	30	14	13	7	4
62636	Egg Roll	1	Each	85.0	160	21	7	5	1	-
1142	Egg Substitute, Frozen	1	Cup	240.0	384	8	27	27	5	6
1143	Egg Substitute, Liquid	1	Cup	251.0	211	2	30	8	2	2
1124	Egg, White Only, w/o Yolk	2	Large	66.8	33	1	7	0	-	-
1057	Eggnog	1	Cup	254.0	342	34	10	19	11	6
62680	Eggnog, Reduced-Fat	1	Cup	246.0	320	48	12	8	5	0
11210	Eggplant, Ckd	1/2	Cup	48.0	13	3	0	0	0	0
11209	Eggplant, Fresh	1/2	Cup	41.0	11	2	0	0	0	0
1128	Eggs, Chicken, Whole, Ckd, Fried	1	Large	46.0	92	1	6	7	2	3
1129	Eggs, Chicken, Whole, Ckd, Hard-boiled	1	Large	50.0	78	1	6	5	2	2
1130	Eggs, Chicken, Whole, Ckd, Omelet	1	Large	59.0	90	1	6	7	2	3
1131	Eggs, Chicken, Whole, Ckd, Poached	1	Large	50.0	75	1	6	5	2	2
1132	Eggs, Chicken, Whole, Ckd, Scrambled	1/2	Cup	110.0	183	2	12	13	4	5
1123	Eggs, Chicken, Whole, Fresh, and Frozen	1	Large	50.0	75	1	6	5	2	2
41242	English Muffin Sandwich-Healthy Choice	1	Each	120.5	200	30	16	3	1	-
18260	English Muffins, Mixed-grain (includes Granola)	1	Each	66.0	155	31	6	1	0	1
18261	English Muffins, Mixed-grain, Toasted	1	Each	61.0	156	31	6	1	0	1
18258	English Muffins, Plain	1	Each	57.0	134	26	4	1	0	0
18259	English Muffins, Plain, Toasted	1	Each	52.0	133	26	4	1	0	0
18262	English Muffins, Raisin-cinnamon	1	Each	57.0	139	28	4	2	0	0
18263	English Muffins, Raisin-cinnamon, Toasted	1	Each	52.0	137	28	4	2	0	0
18264	English Muffins, Wheat	1	Each	57.0	127	26	5	1	0	0
18265	English Muffins, Wheat, Toasted	1	Each	52.0	126	25	5	1	0	0
18266	English Muffins, Whole-wheat	1	Each	66.0	134	27	6	1	0	0
18267	English Muffins, Whole-wheat, Toasted	1	Each	61.0	135	27	6	1	0	0
55170	Escalloped Apples-Stouffer's	1	Each	170.1	200	41	0	4	-	-
55117	Escalloped Chicken and Noodles-Stouffer's	1	Each	283.5	420	30	21	24	-	-
62592	Fat Free Cinnamon Graham Snacks-SnackWell	20	Each	13.4	49	12	1	0	0	0
62606	Fat Free Cracked Pepper Crackers-SnackWell	7	Each	15.0	60	13	2	0	0	0
62589	Fat Free Devils Food Cookie Cakes-SnackWell	1	Each	16.0	50	13	1	0	0	0
62591	Fat Free Double Fudge Cookie Cakes-SnackWell	1	Each	16.0	50	12	1	0	0	0
62590	Fat Free Wheat Crackers-SnackWell	5	Each	15.0	60	12	2	0	0	0
62621	Fettucini Alfredo with Broccoli-Weight Watchers	1	Each	241.0	220	24	15	6	3	-
55208	Fettucini Alfredo, Lean Cuisine-Stouffer's	1	Each	255.1	280	41	14	7	3	-
55171	Fettucini Alfredo-Stouffer's	1	Each	141.8	245	22	8	14	-	-
55209	Fettucini Primavera, Lean Cuisine-Stouffer's	1	Each	283.5	260	32	14	8	3	-
55831	Fettucini Sauce (Alfredo Style)-Stouffer's	1	Cup	283.9	701	11	14	67	-	-
41288	Fettucini w/ Turkey and Vegetables-Healthy Choice	1	Each	354.4	350	45	29	6	3	-
62612	Fiesta Chicken-Weight Watchers	1	Each	241.0	220	38	12	2	1	-
55773	Fiesta Mexicali Heat'n Serve Soup -Stouffer's	1	Cup	283.9	110	18	3	3	-	-
19098	Fifth Avenue Bar	1	Bar	60.0	280	41	5	13	-	-
18170	Fig Bars	1	Each	16.0	56	11	1	1	0	1
55210	Filet of Fish Divan, Lean Cuisine-Stouffer's	1	Each	294.1	210	13	27	5	2	-
55211	Filet of Fish Florentine, Lean Cuisine-Stouffer's	1	Each	272.9	220	13	26	7	3	-
15027	Fish Fillets and Sticks, Fried	3	Ounce	85.1	231	20	13	10	3	4
15029	Flounder, Ckd, Dry Heat	3	Ounce	85.1	100	0	21	1	0	0

Polyunsaturated fat (g)	Dietary Fiber (g)	Cholesterol (mg)	Folate (µg)	Vitamin A (RE)	Vitamin B-6 (mg)	Vitamin B-12 (µg)	Vitamin C (mg)	Vitamin E (mg)	Riboflavin (mg)	Thiamin (mg)	Calcium (mg)	Iron (mg)	Magnesium (mg)	Niacin (mg)	Phosphorus (mg)	Potassium (mg)	Sodium (mg)	Zinc (mg)
3	-	9	7	9	0	.1	0	-	.1	.1	22	.5	10	.8	47	67	160	.3
3	-	20	12	7	0	.1	0	-	.1	.3	21	1.6	17	1.9	65	68	263	.7
2	-	22	14	7	0	.1	1	-	.1	.3	21	1.5	17	1.8	72	67	249	.6
-	0	0	0	0	0	0	0	0	0	0	11	.1	0	0	41	4	37	.1
1	0	76	9	20	.2	.3	0	.6	.4	.2	10	2.3	17	4.3	173	214	55	2.2
3	0	71	5	54	.2	.3	0	.6	.2	.1	9	2.3	14	4.1	133	174	50	1.6
1	0	13	1	0	.1	.4	5	.1	.1	.1	24	.4	6	.7	46	107	354	.5
2	-	79	9	118	0	.2	0	-	.2	.1	39	.7	9	.5	66	73	209	.4
2	1	35	21	53	.1	.5	0	-	.2	0	84	.6	12	.3	118	111	252	.5
1	-	245	28	169	.1	.9	1	-	.6	.1	316	.8	39	.2	319	431	217	1.5
-	2	10	0	100	0	0	1	-	0	0	24	.2	0	0	0	-	350	0
15	0	5	39	324	.3	.8	1	5.1	.9	.3	175	4.8	36	.3	172	512	479	2.4
4	0	3	37	542	0	.7	0	1.2	.8	.3	133	5.3	22	.3	304	828	444	3.3
-	0	-	2	0	0	.1	0	0	.3	0	4	0	7	.1	9	96	110	0
1	0	149	2	203	.1	1.1	4	.6	.5	.1	330	.5	47	.3	278	420	138	1.2
0	0	90	0	160	0	0	2	-	0	0	480	.4	0	0	0	-	280	0
0	1	0	7	3	0	0	1	0	0	0	3	.2	6	.3	11	119	1	.1
0	1	0	8	3	0	0	1	0	0	0	3	.1	6	.2	9	89	1	.1
1	0	211	17	114	.1	.4	0	1.6	.2	0	25	.7	5	0	89	61	162	.5
1	0	212	22	84	.1	.6	0	1	.3	0	25	.6	5	0	86	63	62	.5
1	0	207	17	110	.1	.4	0	1.5	.2	0	25	.7	5	0	87	60	159	.5
1	0	212	18	95	.1	.4	0	.5	.2	0	25	.7	5	0	89	60	140	.6
2	0	387	33	215	.1	.8	0	.9	.5	.1	78	1.3	13	.1	187	152	308	1.1
1	0	213	24	96	.1	.5	0	1	.3	0	25	.7	5	0	89	61	63	.6
1	-	20	-	60	-	-	4	-	.4	.5	120	2	-	2.9	220	200	510	-
0	-	0	23	1	.1	0	0	-	.2	.3	129	2	29	2.4	98	103	275	.6
0	-	0	16	1	.1	0	0	-	.2	.2	130	2	29	2.1	99	103	276	.6
1	-	0	21	0	0	0	0	-	.2	.3	99	1.4	12	2.2	76	75	264	.4
1	-	0	15	0	0	0	0	-	.1	.2	98	1.4	11	2	75	74	262	.4
1	-	0	18	0	0	0	0	-	.2	.2	84	1.4	9	2	44	119	255	.6
1	-	0	13	0	0	0	0	-	.1	.2	83	1.4	9	1.8	44	118	253	.6
0	-	0	22	0	.1	0	0	-	.2	.2	101	1.6	22	1.9	66	106	218	.6
0	-	0	16	0	0	0	0	-	.1	.2	100	1.6	22	1.7	64	105	216	.6
1	4	0	32	0	.1	0	0	-	.1	.2	175	1.6	47	2.3	186	139	420	1.1
1	-	0	23	0	.1	0	0	-	.1	.2	176	1.6	47	2	187	139	422	1.1
-	-	-	-	-	-	-	30	-	-	0	-	-	-	-	-	90	15	-
-	-	-	-	20	-	-	-	-	.3	.2	80	.8	-	3.8	-	300	840	-
0	0	0	-	0	-	-	0	-	-	-	0	.3	-	-	-	-	40	-
0	0	0	-	0	-	-	0	-	-	-	24	.4	-	-	-	-	150	-
0	1	0	-	0	-	-	0	-	-	-	0	0	-	-	-	-	25	-
0	1	0	-	0	-	-	0	-	-	-	0	.2	-	-	-	-	70	-
0	1	0	-	0	-	-	0	-	-	-	24	.4	-	-	-	45	170	-
-	6	15	-	60	-	-	1	-	-	-	300	1.5	-	-	-	510	540	-
-	-	15	-	-	-	-	-	-	.4	.3	200	.8	-	1.5	-	270	570	-
-	-	-	-	-	-	-	-	-	.3	.2	120	.4	-	1	-	100	400	-
-	-	45	-	400	-	-	18	-	.4	.3	240	.8	-	1.5	-	400	510	-
-	-	180	-	-	-	-	0	-	0	0	3	0	-	0	-	341	1813	-
2	-	60	-	150	-	-	-	-	.5	.5	120	1.5	-	3.8	310	450	480	-
-	5	25	-	450	-	-	42	-	-	-	72	1.5	-	-	-	490	480	-
-	-	10	-	-	-	-	6	-	0	0	2	1	-	.2	-	431	711	-
-	-	2	33	5	.1	.1	0	-	.1	0	42	.6	38	2	90	197	112	.6
0	1	0	2	1	0	0	0	-	0	0	10	.5	4	.3	10	33	56	.1
1	-	65	-	20	-	-	27	-	.3	.2	120	.4	-	1.9	-	800	490	-
2	-	65	-	500	-	-	1	-	.3	.2	120	.4	-	1.9	-	780	590	-
3	0	95	15	26	.1	1.5	0	-	.2	.1	17	.6	21	1.8	154	222	495	.6
0	0	58	8	9	.2	2.1	0	-	.1	.1	15	.9	49	1.9	246	293	89	.5

Code	Name	Amount	Unit	Grams	Energy (kcal)	Carbohydrates (g)	Protein (g)	Fat (g)	Saturated fat (g)	Monounsaturated fat (g)
20081	Flour, White	1	Cup	125.0	455	95	13	1	0	0
20080	Flour, Whole Grain	1	Cup	120.0	407	87	16	2	0	0
55178	French Bread Pizza, Cheese-Stouffer's	1	Each	145.3	350	40	16	14	–	–
41332	French Bread Pizza, Deluxe-Healthy Choice	1	Each	180.7	330	41	23	7	3	–
55181	French Bread Pizza, Deluxe-Stouffer's	1	Each	173.6	420	40	21	19	–	–
55180	French Bread Pizza, Double Cheese-Stouffer's	1	Each	166.6	420	43	22	18	–	–
55182	French Bread Pizza, Hamburger-Stouffer's	1	Each	173.6	410	39	23	18	–	–
55183	French Bread Pizza, Pepperoni-Stouffer's	1	Each	159.5	400	39	19	19	–	–
55185	French Bread Pizza, Sausage-Stouffer's	1	Each	170.1	430	40	20	21	–	–
55187	French Bread Pizza, Vegetable Deluxe-Stouffer's	1	Each	180.7	420	41	18	20	–	–
62677	French Onion Dip	2	Tbsp.	30.0	60	2	1	5	3	0
55761	French Onion Soup-Stouffer's	1	Cup	283.9	100	10	4	4	–	–
18268	French Toast, Frozen, Ready-to-heat	1	Slice	59.0	126	19	4	4	1	1
18269	French Toast, Made w/ Lowfat (2%) Milk	1	Slice	65.0	149	16	5	7	2	3
18381	French Toast, Made w/ Whole Milk	1	Slice	65.0	151	16	5	7	2	3
62638	Frosted Pop Tart, Fruit	1	Each	52.0	200	38	2	5	2	–
19226	Frostings, Chocolate, Creamy	1	Ounce	28.4	113	18	0	5	2	3
19713	Frostings, Cream Cheese-flavor	1	Ounce	28.4	117	19	0	5	1	3
19229	Frostings, Sour Cream-flavor	1	Ounce	28.4	117	19	0	5	1	3
19230	Frostings, Vanilla, Creamy	1	Ounce	28.4	119	20	0	5	1	2
41319	Frozen Dessert, Bordeaux Cherry-Healthy Choice	1	Cup	133.0	240	46	6	4	0	–
41320	Frozen Dessert, Butter Pecan Crunch-Healthy Choice	1	Cup	133.0	280	52	6	4	–	–
41321	Frozen Dessert, Chocolate Chip-Healthy Choice	1	Cup	133.0	260	48	6	4	0	–
41322	Frozen Dessert, Coffee Toffee-Healthy Choice	1	Cup	133.0	260	50	6	4	–	–
41323	Frozen Dessert, Cookies 'n Cream-Healthy Choice	1	Cup	133.0	260	48	8	4	0	–
41324	Frozen Dessert, Double Fudge Swirl-Healthy Choice	1	Cup	133.0	260	48	6	4	–	–
41325	Frozen Dessert, Fudge Brownie-Healthy Choice	1	Cup	133.0	280	54	6	4	0	–
41326	Frozen Dessert, Mint Chocolate Chip-Healthy Choice	1	Cup	133.0	280	50	6	4	0	–
41327	Frozen Dessert, Neapolitan-Healthy Choice	1	Cup	133.0	240	44	6	4	0	–
41328	Frozen Dessert, Praline and Caramel-Healthy Choice	1	Cup	133.0	260	52	6	4	0	–
41329	Frozen Dessert, Rocky Road-Healthy Choice	1	Cup	133.0	320	64	6	4	0	–
41330	Frozen Dessert, Vanilla-Healthy Choice	1	Cup	133.0	240	42	8	4	0	–
9100	Fruit cocktail, Hvy Syrup	1/2	Cup	127.5	93	24	0	0	0	0
9097	Fruit cocktail, Juice Pack	1/2	Cup	124.0	57	15	1	0	0	0
9099	Fruit cocktail, Lt Syrup	1/2	Cup	126.0	72	19	1	0	0	0
18319	Fruit Pie, Fried	1	Pie	128.0	404	55	4	21	3	10
14267	Fruit Punch Drink, Cnd	3/4	Cup	185.8	87	22	0	0	0	0
9105	Fruit Salad, Hvy Syrup	1/2	Cup	127.5	93	24	0	0	0	0
9103	Fruit Salad, Juice Pack	1/2	Cup	124.5	62	16	1	0	0	0
9104	Fruit Salad, Lt Syrup	1/2	Cup	126.0	73	19	0	0	0	0
9102	Fruit Salad, Water Pack	1/2	Cup	122.5	37	10	0	0	0	0
9096	Fruit Water Pack	1/2	Cup	122.5	39	10	1	0	0	0
19263	Fruit and Juice Bars	1	Bar	77.0	63	16	1	0	–	–
9188	Fruit, Mixed, Dried	1/4	Cup	37.5	91	24	1	0	0	0
9189	Fruit, Mixed, Frzn, Swtnd, Thawd	1/2	Cup	125.0	123	30	2	0	0	0
9187	Fruit, Mixed, Hvy Syrup	1/2	Cup	127.5	92	24	0	0	0	0
19381	Fudge, Brown Sugar w/ Nuts	1	Piece	14.0	55	11	0	1	0	0
19100	Fudge, Chocolate	1	Piece	17.0	65	14	0	1	1	0
19101	Fudge, Chocolate w/ Nuts	1	Piece	19.0	81	14	1	3	1	1
19102	Fudge, Peanut Butter	1	Piece	16.0	59	13	1	1	0	0
19103	Fudge, Vanilla	1	Piece	16.0	59	13	0	1	1	0
19104	Fudge, Vanilla w/ Nuts	1	Piece	15.0	62	11	0	2	1	0
16058	Garbanzo Beans, Cnd	1/2	Cup	120.0	143	27	6	1	0	0
41337	Garden Potato Casserole-Healthy Choice	1	Each	262.2	180	23	12	4	2	–
55774	Garden Tomato Heat'n Serve Soup-Stouffer's	1	Cup	283.9	110	16	4	3	–	–
41273	Garden Vegetable Soup-Healthy Choice	1	Each	212.6	100	18	3	1	–	–

Polyunsaturated fat (g)	Dietary Fiber (g)	Cholesterol (mg)	Folate (µg)	Vitamin A (RE)	Vitamin B-6 (mg)	Vitamin B-12 (µg)	Vitamin C (mg)	Vitamin E (mg)	Riboflavin (mg)	Thiamin (mg)	Calcium (mg)	Iron (mg)	Magnesium (mg)	Niacin (mg)	Phosphorus (mg)	Potassium (mg)	Sodium (mg)	Zinc (mg)
1	4	0	33	0	.1	0	0	.5	.6	1	19	5.8	28	7.4	135	134	3	.9
1	15	0	53	0	.4	0	0	1.5	.3	.5	41	4.7	166	7.6	415	486	6	3.5
-	-	-	-	60	-	-	4	-	.3	.5	200	1.5	-	2.9	-	300	630	-
1	-	35	-	80	-	-	-	-	.3	.5	200	2.5	-	3.8	280	350	500	-
-	-	-	-	100	-	-	6	-	.4	.5	160	1.5	-	3.8	-	350	950	-
-	-	-	-	40	-	-	6	-	.5	.5	360	1.5	-	3.8	-	320	850	-
-	-	-	-	60	-	-	6	-	.3	.4	160	1.5	-	3.8	-	340	650	-
-	-	-	-	100	-	-	6	-	.4	.5	160	1.5	-	3.8	-	300	880	-
-	-	-	-	80	-	-	6	-	.4	.6	160	1.5	-	3.8	-	340	840	-
-	-	-	-	250	-	-	4	-	.4	.5	280	1.5	-	3.8	-	230	830	-
0	0	15	0	40	0	0	1	-	0	0	24	0	0	0	0	-	105	0
-	-	0	-	-	-	-	0	-	0	0	240	0	-	0	-	170	2073	-
1	2	48	14	32	.3	1	0	-	.2	.2	63	1.3	10	1.6	82	79	292	.5
2	-	75	15	86	0	.2	0	-	.2	.1	65	1.1	11	1.1	76	87	311	.4
2	-	76	15	81	0	.2	0	-	.2	.1	64	1.1	11	1.1	76	86	311	.4
-	1	0	20	100	.2	0	0	-	.2	.2	0	1	0	1.9	16	-	170	0
1	-	0	0	56	0	0	0	-	0	0	2	.4	6	0	22	56	52	.1
1	-	0	0	0	0	0	0	-	0	0	1	0	1	0	1	10	11	0
1	-	0	0	35	0	0	0	-	0	0	1	0	1	.2	1	55	58	0
1	-	0	0	64	0	0	0	-	0	0	1	0	0	0	11	10	26	0
2	-	10	-	-	-	-	-	-	.3	.1	160	-	-	-	200	300	100	-
2	-	10	-	-	-	-	2	-	.3	.1	160	-	-	-	160	300	160	-
2	-	10	-	-	-	-	2	-	.3	.1	160	.4	-	-	160	320	140	-
2	-	10	-	-	-	-	2	-	.3	.1	160	-	-	-	160	320	160	-
2	-	10	-	-	-	-	-	-	.3	.1	240	-	-	-	200	360	160	-
2	-	10	-	-	-	-	-	-	.3	.1	160	.8	-	-	200	420	140	-
2	-	10	-	-	-	-	-	-	.3	.1	160	.4	-	-	160	380	140	-
4	-	10	-	-	-	-	-	-	.3	.1	160	.4	-	-	-	340	160	-
2	-	10	-	-	-	-	-	-	.3	.1	160	-	-	-	200	320	120	-
2	-	10	-	-	-	-	-	-	.3	.1	160	-	-	-	200	320	140	-
2	-	10	-	-	-	-	-	-	.3	.1	160	-	-	-	200	380	140	-
2	-	10	-	-	-	-	-	-	.5	.1	240	-	-	-	200	360	120	-
0	1	0	3	26	.1	0	2	.4	0	0	8	.4	6	.5	14	112	8	.1
0	1	0	3	38	.1	0	3	.2	0	0	10	.3	9	.5	17	118	5	.1
0	1	0	3	26	.1	0	2	.4	0	0	8	.4	6	.5	14	112	8	.1
7	3	0	4	4	0	.1	2	-	.1	.2	28	1.6	13	1.8	55	83	479	.3
0	0	0	2	2	0	0	55	0	0	0	15	.4	4	0	2	46	41	.2
0	1	0	3	64	0	0	3	.6	0	0	8	.4	6	.4	11	102	8	.1
0	-	0	3	75	0	0	4	-	0	0	14	.3	10	.4	17	144	6	.2
0	-	0	3	54	0	0	3	-	0	0	9	.4	6	.5	11	103	8	.1
0	-	0	3	54	0	0	2	-	0	0	9	.4	6	.5	11	96	4	.1
0	1	0	3	31	.1	0	3	.4	0	0	6	.3	9	.4	13	115	5	.1
-	-	0	5	2	0	0	7	-	0	0	4	.1	3	.1	5	41	3	0
-	-	0	1	92	.1	0	1	-	.1	0	14	1	15	.7	29	299	7	.2
0	2	0	9	40	0	0	94	.6	0	0	9	.3	7	.5	15	164	4	.1
0	-	0	4	24	0	0	88	-	.1	0	1	.5	6	.8	13	107	5	.1
1	-	1	2	2	0	0	0	-	0	0	16	.3	7	0	12	52	14	.1
0	0	2	0	8	0	0	0	0	0	0	7	.1	4	0	10	18	11	.1
1	0	3	2	9	0	0	0	.1	0	0	10	.1	9	0	18	30	11	.1
0	-	1	2	2	0	0	0	-	0	0	7	0	4	.2	10	21	12	.1
0	0	3	0	8	0	0	0	0	0	0	6	0	1	0	5	8	11	0
1	0	2	2	7	0	0	0	.1	0	0	7	.1	4	0	11	17	9	.1
1	5	0	80	2	.6	0	5	-	0	0	38	1.6	35	.2	108	206	359	1.3
-	-	20	-	-	-	-	-	-	-	-	-	-	-	-	-	600	360	-
-	-	10	-	-	-	-	0	-	0	0	240	.3	-	.2	-	431	1052	-
-	-	0	-	350	-	-	9	-	.1	.1	10	.4	-	.0	-	200	560	

Code	Name	Amount	Unit	Grams	Energy (kcal)	Carbohydrates (g)	Protein (g)	Fat (g)	Saturated fat (g)	Monounsaturated fat (g)
62687	Gardenburger	1	Each	90.0	140	8	18	4	2	–
19215	Gelatin Pops	1	Each	44.0	31	7	1	0	–	–
14011	Gin and Tonic	1	Fl Oz	30.0	23	2	0	0	0	0
14136	Ginger Ale	12	Fl Oz	366.0	124	32	0	0	0	–
62532	Ginger Ale, Diet	12	Fl Oz	355.2	0	0	0	0	–	–
18172	Gingersnaps	1	Each	7.0	29	5	0	1	0	0
43399	Glazed Breast of Chicken, Top Shelf-Hormel	1	Each	283.5	170	19	19	2	1	1
55212	Glazed Chicken w/ Veg. Lean Cuisine-Stouffer's	1	Each	241.0	250	24	21	7	2	–
41307	Glazed Chicken-Healthy Choice	1	Each	241.0	220	27	21	3	1	–
55784	Glazed Chicken-Stouffer's	1	Ounce	28.4	26	1	3	1	–	–
19105	Goobers	1	Piece	1.0	5	0	0	0	0	0
18173	Graham Crackers, Plain or Honey	1	Each	7.0	30	5	0	1	0	0
62684	Granola Bar, Low-Fat	1	Each	28.0	110	21	2	2	0	0
19016	Granola Bars, Hard, Almond	1	Each	28.4	140	18	2	7	4	2
19017	Granola Bars, Hard, Chocolate Chip	1	Each	28.4	124	20	2	5	3	1
19019	Granola Bars, Hard, Peanut	1	Each	28.4	136	18	3	6	1	2
19420	Granola Bars, Hard, Peanut Butter	1	Each	28.4	137	18	3	7	1	2
19015	Granola Bars, Hard, Plain	1	Each	28.4	134	18	3	6	1	1
19404	Granola Bars, Soft, Chocolate Chip	1	Each	28.4	119	20	2	5	3	1
19406	Granola Bars, Soft, Nut and Raisin	1	Each	28.4	129	18	2	6	3	1
19021	Granola Bars, Soft, Peanut Butter	1	Each	28.4	121	18	3	4	1	2
19027	Granola Bars, Soft, Peanut Butter and Choc Chip	1	Each	28.4	122	18	3	6	2	2
19020	Granola Bars, Soft, Plain	1	Each	28.4	126	19	2	5	2	1
19022	Granola Bars, Soft, Raisin	1	Each	28.4	127	19	2	5	3	1
14277	Grape Drink, Cnd	3/4	Cup	187.6	84	22	0	0	0	0
14282	Grape Juice Drink, Cnd	3/4	Cup	187.6	94	24	0	0	0	0
9135	Grape Juice, Cnd or Bottled, Unsweetened	3/4	Cup	189.4	116	28	1	0	0	0
14142	Grape Soda	12	Fl Oz	372.0	160	42	0	0	0	0
9124	Grapefruit Juice, Cnd, Sweetened	3/4	Cup	187.0	86	21	1	0	0	0
9123	Grapefruit Juice, Cnd, Unsweetened	3/4	Cup	185.2	70	17	1	0	0	0
9404	Grapefruit Juice, Pink, Fresh	3/4	Cup	185.3	72	17	1	0	0	0
9128	Grapefruit Juice, White, Fresh	3/4	Cup	185.3	72	17	1	0	0	0
9112	Grapefruit, Fresh, Pink&red	1	Medium	146.0	44	11	1	0	0	0
9116	Grapefruit, Fresh, White	1	Medium	136.0	45	11	1	0	0	0
9120	Grapefruit, Sections, Cnd, Juice Pack	1/2	Cup	124.5	46	11	1	0	0	0
9121	Grapefruit, Sections, Cnd, Light Syrup Pack	1/2	Cup	127.0	76	20	1	0	0	0
9119	Grapefruit, Sections, Cnd, Water Pack	1/2	Cup	122.0	44	11	1	0	0	0
9131	Grapes, Fresh	1/2	Cup	46.0	29	8	0	0	0	0
6114	Gravy, Au Jus, Cnd	1/4	Cup	59.6	10	1	1	0	0	0
6116	Gravy, Beef, Cnd	1/4	Cup	58.3	31	3	2	1	1	1
6119	Gravy, Chicken, Cnd	1/4	Cup	59.6	47	3	1	3	1	2
6121	Gravy, Mushroom, Cnd	1/4	Cup	59.6	30	3	1	2	0	1
6125	Gravy, Turkey, Cnd	1/4	Cup	59.6	30	3	2	1	0	1
6527	Gravy, Unspecified Type	1/4	Cup	65.4	22	4	1	0	0	0
55172	Green Bean Mushroom Casserole-Stouffer's	1	Each	134.7	160	13	5	10	–	–
55118	Green Pepper Steak w/ Rice-Stouffer's	1	Each	297.7	310	35	20	10	–	–
55780	Green Pepper Steak-Stouffer's	1	Ounce	28.4	28	1	3	1	–	–
62617	Grilled Salisbury Steak-Weight Watchers	1	Each	241.0	250	24	19	9	3	–
20030	Grits	1/2	Cup	80.0	58	11	1	1	0	0
15032	Grouper, Ckd, Dry Heat	3	Ounce	85.1	100	0	21	1	0	0
62534	Guava Juice	3/4	Cup	179.9	66	16	–	0	–	–
19106	Gumdrops	1	Each	3.5	14	3	0	0	–	–
15034	Haddock, Ckd, Dry Heat	3	Ounce	85.1	95	0	21	1	0	0
15035	Haddock, Smoked	3	Ounce	85.1	99	0	21	1	0	0
15037	Halibut, Ckd, Dry Heat	3	Ounce	85.1	119	0	23	3	0	1
15196	Halibut, Greenland, Ckd, Dry Heat	3	Ounce	85.1	203	0	16	15	3	9

Polyunsaturated fat (g)	Dietary Fiber (g)	Cholesterol (mg)	Folate (μg)	Vitamin A (RE)	Vitamin B-6 (mg)	Vitamin B-12 (μg)	Vitamin C (mg)	Vitamin E (mg)	Riboflavin (mg)	Thiamin (mg)	Calcium (mg)	Iron (mg)	Magnesium (mg)	Niacin (mg)	Phosphorus (mg)	Potassium (mg)	Sodium (mg)	Zinc (mg)
1	5	0	-	0	-	-	0	-	-	.3	96	1.5	-	4	-	-	380	7.5
-	0	0	0	0	0	0	0	0	0	0	1	0	0	0	0	1	20	0
0	-	0	0	0	0	0	0	-	0	0	1	0	0	0	0	2	1	0
-	0	0	0	0	0	0	0	0	0	0	11	.7	4	0	0	4	26	.2
-	0	-	-	-			-	-	-	-	-	-	-	-	-	-	30	-
0	0	0	0	0	0	0	0	-	0	0	5	.4	3	.2	6	24	46	0
1	-	35	-	400	-	-	4	.8	.2	.1	32	.4	35	7.6	-	804	780	1.1
4	-	50	-	20	-	-	4	-	.2	.2	16	.2	-	7.6	-	580	590	-
1	-	45	-	-	-	-	1	-	.1	.2	-	.6	-	6.7	240	370	510	-
-	-	9	-	-	-	-	0	-	0	0	24	0	-	.2	-	45	105	-
0	-	0	0	0	0	0	0	-	0	0	1	0	1	.1	3	5	0	0
0	0	0	1	0	0	0	0	-	0	0	2	.3	2	.3	7	9	42	.1
0	1	0	0	0	0	0	0	-	0	0	0	.2	0	0	0	-	70	0
1	-	0	3	1	0	0	0	-	0	.1	9	.7	23	.2	65	77	73	.4
0	1	0	4	1	0	0	0	-	0	.1	22	.9	20	.2	58	71	98	.5
3	-	0	7	1	0	0	0	-	0	.1	11	.7	31	.4	85	86	79	.6
3	-	0	5	1	0	0	0	-	0	.1	12	.7	16	.6	39	82	80	.4
3	2	0	7	4	0	0	0	-	0	.1	17	.8	27	.4	79	95	83	.6
1	1	0	6	1	0	0	0	-	0	.1	26	.7	22	.3	65	96	77	.4
2	2	0	9	1	0	.1	0	-	.1	.1	24	.6	26	.7	68	111	72	.5
1	1	0	9	1	0	.1	0	-	0	.1	26	.6	24	.9	71	82	116	.5
1	1	0	9	1	0	.1	0	-	0	0	23	.5	25	.9	74	107	93	.5
2	1	0	7	0	0	.1	0	-	0	.1	30	.7	21	.1	65	92	79	.4
1	1	0	6	0	0	.1	0	-	0	.1	29	.7	20	.3	62	103	80	.4
0	0	0	1	0	0	0	64	0	0	0	6	.3	4	0	2	9	11	.2
0	0	0	2	0	0	0	30	0	0	0	6	.2	8	.2	8	66	2	.1
0	0	0	5	2	.1	0	0	0	.1	0	17	.5	19	.5	21	250	6	.1
0	0	0	0	0	0	0	0	0	0	0	11	.3	4	0	0	4	56	.3
0	0	0	19	0	0	0	50	.1	0	.1	15	.7	19	.6	21	303	4	.1
0	0	0	19	2	0	0	54	.1	0	.1	13	.4	19	.4	20	283	2	.2
0	-	0	19	82	.1	0	70	-	0	.1	17	.4	22	.4	28	300	2	.1
0	0	0	19	2	.1	0	70	.1	0	.1	17	.4	22	.4	28	300	2	.1
0	-	0	18	38	.1	0	56	-	0	0	16	.2	12	.3	13	188	0	.1
0	1	0	14	1	.1	0	45	.3	0	.1	16	.1	12	.4	11	201	0	.1
0	0	0	11	0	0	0	42	.3	0	0	19	.3	14	.3	15	210	9	.1
0	1	0	11	0	0	0	27	.3	0	0	18	.5	13	.3	13	164	3	.1
0	0	0	11	0	0	0	27	.3	0	0	18	.5	12	.3	12	161	2	.1
0	1	0	2	5	.1	0	2	.2	0	0	6	.1	2	.1	5	88	1	0
0	-	0	1	0	0	.1	1	-	0	0	2	.4	1	.5	18	48	30	.6
0	0	2	1	0	0	.1	0	0	0	0	3	.4	1	.4	17	47	326	.6
1	0	1	1	66	0	.1	0	.1	0	0	12	.3	1	.3	17	65	344	.5
1	0	0	7	0	0	0	0	0	0	0	4	.4	1	.4	9	63	340	.4
0	0	1	1	0	0	.1	0	0	0	0	2	.4	1	.8	17	65	344	.5
0	-	0	1	0	0	0	0	-	0	0	9	.1	3	.2	12	16	356	.1
-	-	-	-	40	-	-	2	-	.2	.1	64	.2	-	.4	-	200	550	-
-	-	-	-	40	-	-	6	-	.2	.2	16	1	-	3.8	-	410	700	-
-	-	7	-	-	-	-	4	-	0	0	48	0	-	.1	-	51	164	-
-	4	30	-	60	-	-	0	-	-	-	120	1.5	-	-	-	450	590	-
0	2	0	1	0	0	0	0	-	0	0	8	.5	13	0	28	7	168	.8
0	0	40	9	43	.3	.6	0	-	0	.1	18	1	31	.3	122	404	45	.4
-	-	0	-	0	-	-	30	-	0	-	0	0	-	-	-	-	18	-
-	0	0	0	0	0	0	0	0	0	0	0	0	0	0	0	0	2	0
0	0	63	11	16	.3	1.2	0	-	0	0	36	1.1	43	3.9	205	339	74	.4
0	0	65	13	19	.3	1.4	0	.3	0	0	42	1.2	46	4.3	213	353	649	.4
1	0	35	12	46	.3	1.2	0	-	.1	.1	51	.9	91	6.1	242	490	59	.5
1	0	50	1	15	.4	.8	0	-	.1	.1	3	.7	28	1.6	179	293	88	.4

Code	Name	Amount	Unit	Grams	Energy (kcal)	Carbohydrates (g)	Protein (g)	Fat (g)	Saturated fat (g)	Monounsaturated fat (g)
7031	Ham Salad Spread	1	Tbsp.	15.0	32	2	1	2	1	1
55159	Ham and Asparagus Bake-Stouffer's	1	Each	269.3	520	32	18	35	-	-
7032	Ham and Cheese Loaf(or Roll), Lunch Meat	1	Slice	28.4	73	0	5	6	2	3
7033	Ham and Cheese Spread, Lunch Meat	1	Tbsp.	15.0	37	0	2	3	1	1
7029	Ham, Approx 11% Fat, Sliced	1	Slice	28.4	52	1	5	3	1	1
7027	Ham, Chopped, Not Cnd	3	Ounce	85.1	195	0	15	15	5	7
7026	Ham, Chopped, Spiced, Cnd	3	Ounce	85.1	203	0	14	16	5	8
7028	Ham, Extra Lean, Appx 5% Fat	1	Slice	28.4	37	0	5	1	0	1
7030	Ham, Minced	3	Ounce	85.1	224	2	14	18	6	8
62683	Hamburger Helper, Beef Noodle	1	Cup	220.0	260	23	4	11	4	0
62682	Hamburger Helper, Cheesy Italian	1	Cup	220.0	330	30	5	21	2	0
62681	Hamburger Helper, Chili Mac	1	Cup	220.0	290	30	3	16	4	0
62626	Hamburger Patty, Meatless	1	Each	90.0	140	8	18	4	2	-
55809	Heartland Medley-Stouffer's	1	Ounce	28.4	17	2	1	0	-	-
41279	Hearty Beef Soup-Healthy Choice	1	Each	212.6	120	17	9	1	-	-
41280	Hearty Chicken Soup-Healthy Choice	1	Each	212.6	110	17	7	2	-	-
41258	Herb Roasted Chicken-Healthy Choice	1	Each	347.3	300	50	22	5	2	-
15040	Herring, Ckd, Dry Heat	3	Ounce	85.1	173	0	20	10	2	4
15042	Herring, Kippered	3	Ounce	85.1	185	0	21	11	2	4
15197	Herring, Pacific, Ckd, Dry Heat	3	Ounce	85.1	213	0	18	15	4	7
15041	Herring, Pickled	3	Ounce	85.1	223	8	12	15	2	10
41311	Homestyle Turkey w/ Vegetables-Healthy Choice	1	Each	269.3	260	34	26	2	-	-
20330	Hominy, Cnd, Yellow	1/2	Cup	80.0	58	11	1	1	0	0
19296	Honey	1	Tbsp.	21.0	64	17	0	0	-	-
7035	Honey Loaf, Lunch Meat	1	Slice	28.4	36	2	4	1	0	1
55214	Honey Mustard Chicken, Lean Cuisine-Stouffer's	1	Each	212.6	230	30	18	4	1	-
41312	Honey Mustard Chicken-Healthy Choice	1	Each	269.3	310	41	26	4	1	-
43371	Hot Chili no Beans-Hormel	1	Each	212.6	360	14	16	27	11	13
43410	Hot Chili w/ Beans, Micro Cup-Hormel	1	Each	209.1	250	24	15	11	4	4
43372	Hot Chili w/ Beans-Hormel	1	Each	212.6	300	27	15	15	5	6
7022	Hot Dog, Beef	1	Each	57.0	180	1	7	16	7	8
7024	Hot Dog, Chicken	1	Each	45.0	116	3	6	9	2	4
62605	Hot Dog, Fat Free	1	Each	50.0	40	2	7	0	0	0
7025	Hot Dog, Turkey	1	Each	45.0	102	1	6	8	3	3
16137	Hummus, Fresh	1/2	Cup	123.0	210	25	6	10	2	4
18270	Hush Puppies	1	Each	22.0	74	10	2	3	0	1
18271	Ice Cream Cones, Cake or Wafer-type	1-1/2	Each	6.0	25	5	0	0	0	0
18272	Ice Cream Cones, Sugar, Rolled-type	1-1/2	Each	15.0	60	13	1	1	0	0
62640	Ice Cream Sandwich	1	Each	63.0	170	27	3	6	3	-
19270	Ice Cream, Chocolate	1-1/2	Cup	198.0	428	56	8	22	13	6
19090	Ice Cream, French Vanilla, Soft-serve	1-1/2	Cup	199.5	429	44	8	26	15	7
19271	Ice Cream, Strawberry	1-1/2	Cup	198.0	380	55	6	17	-	-
19095	Ice Cream, Vanilla	1-1/2	Cup	198.0	398	47	7	22	13	6
19089	Ice Cream, Vanilla, Rich	1-1/2	Cup	199.5	481	45	7	32	20	9
19088	Ice Milk, Vanilla	1/2	Cup	66.5	92	15	3	3	2	1
19096	Ice Milk, Vanilla, Soft Serve	1/2	Cup	66.5	84	14	3	2	1	1
19283	Ice Pops	1	Bar	52.0	37	10	0	0	-	-
19717	Ice Pops, w/ Added Ascorbic Acid	1	Bar	52.0	37	10	0	0	-	-
62547	Iced Tea, Bottled, All Flavors	1	Cup	236.6	118	29	0	0	0	-
62548	Iced Tea, Bottled, All Flavors, Diet	1	Cup	236.6	0	1	0	0	0	-
62622	Italian Cheese Lasagna-Weight Watchers	1	Each	311.9	300	28	29	8	3	-
43395	Italian Lasagna, Top Shelf-Hormel	1	Each	283.5	350	30	23	16	8	5
55798	Italian Style Vegetables-Stouffer's	1	Ounce	28.4	10	2	0	0	-	-
19297	Jams and Preserves	1	Tbsp.	20.0	48	13	0	0	0	0
19300	Jellies	1	Tbsp.	19.0	51	13	0	0	-	-
19173	Jello	1/2	Cup	135.0	80	19	2	0	-	-

Polyunsaturated fat (g)	Dietary Fiber (g)	Cholesterol (mg)	Folate (µg)	Vitamin A (RE)	Vitamin B-6 (mg)	Vitamin B-12 (µg)	Vitamin C (mg)	Vitamin E (mg)	Riboflavin (mg)	Thiamin (mg)	Calcium (mg)	Iron (mg)	Magnesium (mg)	Niacin (mg)	Phosphorus (mg)	Potassium (mg)	Sodium (mg)	Zinc (mg)
0	0	6	0	0	0	.1	1	.3	0	.1	1	.1	2	.3	18	22	137	.2
-	-	-	-	60	-	-	36	-	.5	.5	160	.8	-	2.9	-	360	1100	-
1	0	16	1	7	.1	.2	7	.1	.1	.2	16	.3	5	1	72	83	381	.6
0	0	9	0	14	0	.1	1	-	0	0	33	.1	3	.3	74	24	180	.3
0	0	16	1	0	.1	.2	8	.1	.1	.2	2	.3	5	1.5	70	94	373	.6
2	0	43	1	0	.3	.8	17	-	.2	.5	6	.7	14	3.3	132	271	1166	1.6
2	0	42	1	0	.3	.6	2	.2	.1	.5	6	.8	11	2.7	118	242	1161	1.6
0	0	13	1	0	.1	.2	7	.1	.1	.3	2	.2	5	1.4	62	99	405	.5
2	0	60	1	0	.2	.8	26	-	.2	.6	9	.7	14	3.5	134	265	1059	1.6
0	1	5	0	60	0	0	0	-	.2	.2	24	1	0	3.8	0	240	900	0
0	1	5	0	60	0	0	0	-	.3	.3	120	1.5	0	3.8	0	400	900	0
0	1	4	0	200	0	0	0	-	.3	.3	24	1.5	0	4.8	0	-	900	0
1	5	0	-	0	-	-	0	-	-	.3	96	1.5	-	4	-	-	380	7.5
-	-	3	-	-	-	-	1	-	0	0	40	0	-	.1	-	60	85	-
-	-	20	-	150	-	-	9	-	.1	.1	32	.4	-	1.9	90	280	540	-
-	-	25	-	200	-	-	2	-	.2	.1	32	.4	-	1.9	90	190	520	-
1	-	40	-	250	-	-	24	-	.1	.2	32	.8	-	7.6	280	370	560	-
2	0	65	10	26	.3	11.2	1	1.1	.3	.1	63	1.2	35	3.5	258	356	98	1.1
2	0	70	12	33	.4	15.9	1	.9	.3	.1	71	1.3	39	3.7	276	380	781	1.2
3	0	84	5	30	.4	8.2	0	-	.2	.1	90	1.2	35	2.4	248	461	81	.6
1	0	11	2	219	.1	3.6	0	.9	.1	0	65	1	7	2.8	76	59	740	.5
-	-	30	-	100	-	-	5	-	.1	0	32	-	-	-	-	100	550	-
0	-	0	1	9	0	0	0	-	0	0	8	.5	13	0	28	7	168	.8
-	0	0	0	0	0	0	0	0	0	0	1	.1	0	0	1	11	1	0
0	0	10	2	0	.1	.3	6	.1	.1	.1	5	.4	5	.9	41	97	374	.7
1	-	40	-	200	-	-	2	-	.2	.2	16	.4	-	3.8	-	340	540	-
-	-	45	-	100	-	-	4	-	0	.2	16	.8	-	1.5	-	110	520	-
1	-	60	-	330	-	-	-	10.6	.2	0	40	1.4	35	2.5	-	497	860	2.7
-	-	49	-	190	-	-	-	2	.2	.1	48	1.9	46	1.7	-	677	977	2.7
1	-	55	-	210	-	-	-	0	.2	.1	48	1.8	49	1.7	-	777	1030	2.3
1	0	35	2	0	.1	.9	14	.1	.1	0	11	.8	2	1.4	50	95	585	1.2
2	0	45	2	17	.1	.1	0	.1	.1	0	43	.9	5	1.4	48	38	617	.5
0	0	15	-	0	-	-	0	-	-	-	0	.2	-	-	-	-	460	-
2	0	48	4	0	.1	.1	0	.3	.1	0	48	.8	6	1.9	60	81	642	1.4
4	6	0	73	2	.5	0	10	1.2	.1	.1	61	1.9	36	.5	138	214	300	1.4
2	1	10	4	9	0	0	0	-	.1	.1	61	.7	5	.6	42	32	147	.1
0	0	0	0	0	0	0	0	-	0	0	2	.2	2	.3	6	7	9	0
0	1	0	1	0	0	0	0	-	.1	.1	7	.7	5	.8	15	22	48	.1
-	1	10	0	20	0	0	0	-	0	0	48	.4	0	0	0	-	140	0
1	-	67	32	236	.1	.6	1	-	.4	.1	216	1.8	57	.4	212	493	150	1.1
1	-	182	18	307	.1	1	2	-	.4	.1	261	.4	24	.2	231	353	122	1
-	-	57	24	154	.1	.6	15	-	.5	.1	238	.4	28	.3	198	372	119	.7
1	0	87	10	232	.1	.8	1	0	.5	.1	253	.2	28	.2	208	394	158	1.4
1	0	122	10	367	.1	.7	1	0	.3	.1	233	.1	22	.2	189	317	112	.8
0	0	9	4	31	0	.4	1	0	.2	0	92	.1	10	.1	72	140	57	.3
0	0	8	4	19	0	.3	1	0	.1	0	104	0	9	.1	80	147	47	.4
-	0	0	0	0	0	0	0	0	0	0	0	0	1	0	0	2	6	0
-	-	0	0	0	0	0	6	-	0	0	0	0	1	0	0	2	6	0
-	0	0	-	0	-	-	0	-	-	-	0	0	-	-	-	-	10	-
-	0	0	-	0	-	-	0	-	-	-	0	0	-	-	-	-	0	-
-	7	25	-	350	-	-	15	-	-	-	780	1.5	-	-	-	720	560	-
1	-	60	-	100	-	-	2	.7	.5	.3	240	1.5	49	3.8	-	728	840	3.2
-	-	0	-	-	-	-	2	-	0	0	72	0	-	0	-	62	147	-
0	0	0	7	0	0	0	2	0	0	0	4	.1	1	0	2	15	8	0
-	0	0	0	0	0	0	0	0	0	0	2	0	1	0	1	12	7	0
-	0	0	0	0	0	0	0	0	0	0	3	0	1	0	30	1	57	0

Code	Name	Amount	Unit	Grams	Energy (kcal)	Carbohydrates (g)	Protein (g)	Fat (g)	Saturated fat (g)	Monounsaturated fat (g)
19108	Jellybeans	1	Each	1.1	4	1	0	0	–	–
19109	Kit Kat Wafer Bar	1	Bar	46.0	235	28	3	13	8	4
9148	Kiwifruit, Fresh	1	Medium	76.0	46	11	1	0	–	–
62643	Kool-Aid	8	Fl Oz	236.6	60	16	–	–	–	–
19110	Krackel Chocolate Bar	1	Bar	47.0	236	29	3	13	6	3
17225	Lamb, Ground, Ckd, Broiled	3	Ounce	85.1	241	0	21	17	7	7
17018	Lamb, Leg, Shank, Meat Only, Ckd, Rstd	3	Ounce	85.1	153	0	24	6	2	2
17016	Lamb, Leg, Shank, Meat and Fat, Ckd, Rstd	3	Ounce	85.1	191	0	22	11	4	4
17022	Lamb, Leg, Sirloin, Meat Only, Ckd, Rstd	3	Ounce	85.1	174	0	24	8	3	3
17020	Lamb, Leg, Sirloin, Meat and Fat, Ckd, Rstd	3	Ounce	85.1	248	0	21	18	7	7
17014	Lamb, Leg, Whole, Meat Only, Ckd, Rstd	3	Ounce	85.1	162	0	24	7	2	3
17012	Lamb, Leg, Whole, Meat and Fat, Ckd, Rstd	3	Ounce	85.1	219	0	22	14	6	6
17027	Lamb, Loin, Meat Only, Ckd, Broiled	3	Ounce	85.1	184	0	26	8	3	4
17028	Lamb, Loin, Meat Only, Ckd, Roasted	3	Ounce	85.1	172	0	23	8	3	3
17024	Lamb, Loin, Meat and Fat, Ckd, Broiled	3	Ounce	85.1	269	0	21	20	8	8
17025	Lamb, Loin, Meat and Fat, Ckd, Roasted	3	Ounce	85.1	263	0	19	20	9	8
17004	Lamb, Meat Only, Ckd	3	Ounce	85.1	175	0	24	8	3	4
17002	Lamb, Meat and Fat, Ckd	3	Ounce	85.1	250	0	21	18	8	8
17033	Lamb, Rib, Meat Only, Ckd, Broiled	3	Ounce	85.1	200	0	24	11	4	4
17034	Lamb, Rib, Meat Only, Ckd, Roasted	3	Ounce	85.1	197	0	22	11	4	5
17030	Lamb, Rib, Meat and Fat, Ckd, Broiled	3	Ounce	85.1	307	0	19	25	11	10
17031	Lamb, Rib, Meat and Fat, Ckd, Roasted	3	Ounce	85.1	305	0	18	25	11	11
4002	Lard	1/4	Cup	51.3	462	0	0	51	20	23
62613	Lasagna Florentine-Weight Watchers	1	Each	283.5	210	37	13	2	1	–
55215	Lasagna w/ Meat Sauce, Lean Cuisine-Stouffer's	1	Each	290.6	280	36	20	6	3	–
41308	Lasagna w/ Meat Sauce-Healthy Choice	1	Each	283.5	260	37	18	5	2	–
62623	Lasagna with Meat Sauce-Weight Watchers	1	Each	290.6	290	34	24	7	3	–
43403	Lasagna, Micro Cup-Hormel	1	Each	212.6	250	25	8	13	6	4
55134	Lasagna-Stouffer's	1	Each	283.5	340	40	18	12	–	–
11247	Leeks, Ckd	1/2	Cup	52.0	16	4	0	0	0	0
11246	Leeks, Fresh	1/2	Cup	52.0	32	7	1	0	0	0
18320	Lemon Meringue Pie	1	Slice	113.0	303	53	2	10	2	4
41259	Lemon Pepper Fish-Healthy Choice	1	Each	304.8	300	52	13	5	1	–
18445	Lemon Pie, Fried	1	Pie	128.0	404	55	4	21	3	10
19380	Lemon Pudding	1	Cup	298.1	373	75	0	9	1	4
14145	Lemon-lime Soda	12	Fl Oz	368.4	147	38	0	0	0	0
62529	Lemon-lime Soda, Diet	12	Fl Oz	355.2	0	0	0	0	–	–
14297	Lemonade Flavor Drink	1	Cup	266.0	112	29	0	0	0	0
14543	Lemonade, Pink	1	Cup	247.8	99	26	0	0	0	0
14290	Lemonade, Low Calorie	1	Cup	243.7	5	1	0	0	0	–
14293	Lemonade, White	1	Cup	247.8	99	26	0	0	0	0
9150	Lemons, Fresh, w/o Peel	1	Medium	58.0	17	5	1	0	0	0
41274	Lentil Soup-Healthy Choice	1	Each	212.6	140	23	8	1	–	–
11250	Lettuce, Butterhead, Fresh	1	Cup	56.0	7	1	1	0	0	0
11252	Lettuce, Iceberg, Fresh	1	Cup	56.0	7	1	1	0	0	0
11253	Lettuce, Looseleaf, Fresh	1	Cup	56.0	10	2	1	0	0	0
11251	Lettuce, Romaine, Fresh	1	Cup	56.0	9	1	1	0	0	0
55216	Linguini w/ Clam Sauce, Lean Cuisine-Stouffer's	1	Each	272.9	280	36	17	8	2	–
14415	Liqueur, Coffee w/ Cream, 34 Proof	1	Fl Oz	31.1	102	6	1	5	3	1
14414	Liqueur, Coffee, 53 Proof	1	Fl Oz	34.8	117	16	0	0	0	0
14534	Liqueur, Coffee, 63 Proof	1	Fl Oz	34.8	107	11	0	0	0	0
14533	Liquor, Distilled, All 100 Proof	1	Fl Oz	27.8	82	0	0	0	0	0
14037	Liquor, Distilled, All 80 Proof	1	Fl Oz	27.8	64	0	0	0	0	0
14550	Liquor, Distilled, All 86 Proof	1	Fl Oz	27.8	70	0	0	0	0	0
14551	Liquor, Distilled, All 90 Proof	1	Fl Oz	27.8	73	0	0	0	0	0
14532	Liquor, Distilled, All 94 Proof	1	Fl Oz	27.8	76	0	0	0	0	0

Polyunsaturated fat (g)	Dietary Fiber (g)	Cholesterol (mg)	Folate (µg)	Vitamin A (RE)	Vitamin B-6 (mg)	Vitamin B-12 (µg)	Vitamin C (mg)	Vitamin E (mg)	Riboflavin (mg)	Thiamin (mg)	Calcium (mg)	Iron (mg)	Magnesium (mg)	Niacin (mg)	Phosphorus (mg)	Potassium (mg)	Sodium (mg)	Zinc (mg)
-	0	0	0	0	0	0	0	0	0	0	0	0	0	0	0	0	0	0
0	0	12	0	14	0	.3	1	.4	.1	0	83	.4	20	.2	80	142	46	.5
-	3	0	-	14	-	0	74	.9	0	0	20	.3	23	.4	30	252	4	-
-	-	-	0	0	0	0	6	-	0	0	0	0	0	0	0	-	-	0
3	-	9	4	6	0	.3	0	-	.1	0	84	.4	26	.2	104	161	64	.6
1	0	82	16	0	.1	2.2	-	.2	.2	.1	19	1.5	20	5.7	171	288	69	4
0	0	74	20	0	.1	2.3	0	.2	.2	.1	7	1.8	22	5.4	177	291	56	4.3
1	0	77	19	0	.1	2.3	0	.1	.2	.1	9	1.7	21	5.6	168	277	55	4
1	0	78	18	0	.1	2.2	0	.1	.3	.1	7	1.9	21	5.3	173	283	60	4.1
1	0	82	14	0	.1	2.2	0	.1	.2	.1	9	1.7	19	5.6	156	256	58	3.5
0	0	76	20	0	.1	2.2	0	.2	.2	.1	7	1.8	22	5.4	175	287	58	4.2
1	0	79	17	0	.1	2.2	0	.1	.2	.1	9	1.7	20	5.6	162	266	56	3.7
1	0	81	20	0	.1	2.1	0	.1	.2	.1	16	1.7	24	5.8	192	320	71	3.5
1	0	74	21	0	.1	1.8	0	.1	.2	.1	14	2.1	23	5.8	175	227	56	3.5
1	0	85	15	0	.1	2.1	0	.1	.2	.1	17	1.5	20	6	167	278	65	3
2	0	81	16	0	.1	1.9	0	.1	.2	.1	15	1.8	20	6	153	209	54	2.9
1	0	78	20	0	.1	2.2	0	.2	.2	.1	13	1.7	22	5.4	179	293	65	4.5
1	0	82	15	0	.1	2.2	0	-	.2	.1	14	1.6	20	5.7	160	264	61	3.8
1	0	77	18	0	.1	2.2	0	.2	.2	.1	14	1.9	25	5.6	181	266	72	4.5
1	0	75	19	0	.1	1.8	0	.1	.2	.1	18	1.5	20	5.2	166	268	69	3.8
2	0	84	12	0	.1	2.2	0	.1	.2	.1	16	1.6	20	6	151	230	65	3.4
2	0	82	13	0	.1	1.9	0	.1	.2	.1	19	1.4	17	5.7	141	230	62	3
6	0	49	0	0	0	0	0	.6	0	0	0	0	0	0	0	0	0	.1
-	5	10	-	300	-	-	15	-	-	-	300	1.5	-	-	-	440	420	-
-	-	25	-	100	-	-	6	-	.3	.2	120	1	-	2.9	-	700	560	-
1	-	20	-	150	-	-	2	-	.3	.3	80	1.5	-	1.9	210	500	420	-
-	7	15	-	250	-	-	12	-	-	-	480	1.5	-	-	-	720	580	-
2	-	23	-	100	-	-	2	-	.2	.1	40	.8	25	1.9	-	331	949	1.1
-	-	-	-	150	-	-	6	-	.3	.2	200	1	-	6.7	-	570	840	-
0	-	0	13	3	.1	0	2	-	0	0	16	.6	7	.1	9	45	5	0
0	1	0	33	5	.1	0	6	.5	0	0	31	1.1	15	.2	18	94	10	.1
3	1	51	9	59	0	.2	4	-	.2	.1	63	.7	17	.7	119	101	165	.6
2	-	40	-	80	-	-	48	-	.1	.2	32	.6	-	1.1	180	410	370	-
-	-	-	4	4	0	.1	0	-	.1	.2	28	1.6	13	1.8	55	83	479	.3
3	-	0	0	0	0	0	0	-	0	0	6	.2	3	0	15	3	417	.1
0	0	0	0	0	0	0	0	0	0	0	7	.3	4	.1	0	4	41	.2
-	0	-	-	-	-	-	-	-	-	-	-	-	-	-	-	-	30	-
0	-	0	0	0	0	0	34	-	0	0	29	.1	3	0	3	3	19	.1
0	-	0	5	0	0	0	10	-	.1	0	7	.4	5	0	5	37	7	.1
-	0	0	0	0	0	0	6	0	0	0	5	.1	2	0	24	0	7	.1
0	-	0	5	5	0	0	10	-	.1	0	7	.4	5	0	5	37	7	.1
0	2	0	6	2	0	0	31	.1	0	0	15	.3	5	.1	9	80	1	0
-	-	0	-	60	-	-	2	-	0	.1	-	.6	-	.4	-	160	480	-
0	1	0	41	54	0	0	4	.2	0	0	18	.2	7	.2	13	144	3	.1
0	1	0	31	18	0	0	2	.1	0	0	11	.3	5	.1	11	88	5	.1
0	1	0	28	106	0	0	10	.2	0	0	38	.8	6	.2	14	148	5	.2
0	1	0	76	146	0	0	13	.2	.1	.1	20	.6	3	.3	25	162	4	.1
2	-	30	-	-	-	-	-	-	.2	.3	32	1.5	-	1.9	-	90	560	-
0	0	5	0	13	0	0	0	0	0	0	5	0	1	0	16	10	29	0
0	0	0	0	0	0	0	0	0	0	0	0	0	1	.1	2	10	3	0
0	-	0	0	0	0	0	0	-	0	0	0	0	1	.1	2	10	3	0
0	-	0	0	0	0	0	0	-	0	0	0	0	0	0	1	1	0	0
0	0	0	0	0	0	0	0	0	0	0	0	0	0	0	1	1	0	0
0	0	0	0	0	0	0	0	0	0	0	0	0	0	0	1	1	0	0
0	0	0	0	0	0	0	0	0	0	0	0	0	0	0	1	1	0	0
0	-	0	0	0	0	0	0	-	0	0	0	0	0	0	1	1	0	0

Code	Name	Amount	Unit	Grams	Energy (kcal)	Carbohydrates (g)	Protein (g)	Fat (g)	Saturated fat (g)	Monounsaturated fat (g)
15148	Lobster, Northern, Ckd, Moist Heat	3	Ounce	85.1	83	1	17	1	0	0
15228	Lobster, Spiny, Ckd, Moist Heat	3	Ounce	85.1	122	3	22	2	0	0
19107	Lollipop	1	Each	6.0	22	6	0	0	–	–
19140	M&M's Peanut	1	Pkg	49.0	243	29	5	13	–	–
19141	M&M's Plain	1	Pkg	48.0	228	33	3	11	–	–
62667	M&M's, Almond	1	Pkg	42.0	230	25	4	13	4	0
12131	Macadamias, Dried	1/2	Cup	67.0	470	9	6	49	7	39
12633	Macadamias, Oil Roasted	1/2	Cup	67.0	481	9	5	51	8	40
55217	Macaroni and Beef in Sauce, Lean Cuisine-Stouffer's	1	Each	283.5	250	35	14	6	1	–
55137	Macaroni and Beef w/ Tomatoes-Stouffer's	1	Each	326.0	340	38	21	12	–	–
41338	Macaroni and Beef-Healthy Choice	1	Each	241.0	200	32	12	3	1	–
62533	Macaroni and Cheese	1	Cup	111.9	360	44	1	13	8	–
57808	Macaroni and Cheese Pot Pie-Swanson	1	Each	198.5	200	24	7	8	–	–
55218	Macaroni and Cheese, Lean Cuisine-Stouffer's	1	Each	255.1	290	37	15	9	4	–
43406	Macaroni and Cheese, Micro Cup-Hormel	1	Each	212.6	260	28	12	11	6	3
41339	Macaroni and Cheese-Healthy Choice	1	Each	255.1	280	45	12	6	3	–
55155	Macaroni and Cheese-Stouffer's	1	Each	170.1	250	23	11	13	–	–
62624	Macaroni and Cheese-Weight Watchers	1	Each	255.2	260	43	15	6	2	–
20100	Macaroni, Ckd, Enriched	1	Cup	140.0	197	40	7	1	0	0
20400	Macaroni, Ckd, Unenriched	1	Cup	140.0	197	40	7	1	0	0
20106	Macaroni, Vegetable, Ckd, Enriched	1	Cup	134.0	172	36	6	0	0	0
20108	Macaroni, Whole-wheat, Ckd	1	Cup	140.0	174	37	7	1	0	0
41309	Mandarin Chicken-Healthy Choice	1	Each	311.8	260	39	23	2	–	–
62535	Mango Juice	3/4	Cup	179.9	66	16	–	0	–	–
9176	Mangos, Fresh	1/2	Cup	82.5	54	14	0	0	0	0
14012	Manhattan	1	Fl Oz	28.5	64	1	0	0	0	0
4067	Margarine, Hard, Corn&sybn	1	Tsp.	4.7	34	0	0	4	1	2
4071	Margarine, Hard, Corn(hydr)	1	Tsp.	4.7	34	0	0	4	1	2
4128	Margarine, Imitation (appx 40% Fat)	1	Tsp.	4.8	17	0	0	2	0	1
4132	Margarine, Regular, w/ Salt Added	1	Tsp.	4.7	34	0	0	4	1	2
4131	Margarine, Regular, w/o Added Salt	1	Tsp.	4.7	34	0	0	4	1	2
4130	Margarine, Soft, w/ Salt Added	1	Tsp.	4.7	34	0	0	4	1	1
4129	Margarine, Soft, w/o Added Salt	1	Tsp.	4.7	34	0	0	4	1	2
62645	Margarita Mix, Liquid	1	Fl Oz	29.6	29	5	0	0	–	–
11256	Marinara Sauce	1/2	Cup	125.0	85	13	2	4	1	2
55830	Marinara Sauce-Stouffer's	1	Cup	283.9	180	18	3	11	–	–
19303	Marmalade, Orange	1	Tbsp.	20.0	49	13	0	0	–	–
19116	Marshmallows	1	Cup	46.0	146	37	1	0	–	–
14014	Martini	1	Fl Oz	28.2	63	0	0	0	0	0
4018	Mayonnaise	1	Tbsp.	14.7	57	4	0	5	1	1
62610	Mayonnaise, Fat Free	1	Tbsp.	15.0	10	3	0	0	0	–
62609	Mayonnaise, Light	1	Tbsp.	15.0	25	1	0	2	0	–
55219	Meatloaf w/ Mac. and Cheese, Lean Cuisine-Stouffer's	1	Each	265.8	280	26	26	8	3	–
41260	Meatloaf-Healthy Choice	1	Each	340.2	340	48	17	8	3	–
55779	Meatloaf-Stouffer's	1	Ounce	28.4	57	2	4	3	–	–
9185	Melon Balls, Frozen, Unthawed	1/2	Cup	86.5	29	7	1	0	–	–
9181	Melons, Cantaloupe, Fresh	1	Wedge	80.0	28	7	1	0	–	–
9183	Melons, Casaba, Fresh	1	Wedge	164.0	43	10	1	0	–	–
9184	Melons, Honeydew, Fresh	1	Wedge	129.0	45	12	1	0	–	–
55812	Mexicali Chicken-Stouffer's	1	Ounce	28.4	20	2	1	1	–	–
19120	Milk Chocolate	1	Bar	44.0	226	26	3	13	8	4
19126	Milk Chocolate Coated Peanuts	1	Ounce	28.4	147	14	4	9	4	4
19127	Milk Chocolate Coated Raisins	1	Ounce	28.4	111	19	1	4	2	1
19132	Milk Chocolate w/ Almonds	1	Bar	41.0	216	22	4	14	7	6
1110	Milk Shakes, Thick Chocolate	1-1/2	Cup	518.2	615	110	16	14	9	4
1111	Milk Shakes, Thick Vanilla	1-1/2	Cup	518.2	579	92	20	16	10	5

Polyunsaturated fat (g)	Dietary Fiber (g)	Cholesterol (mg)	Folate (µg)	Vitamin A (RE)	Vitamin B-6 (mg)	Vitamin B-12 (µg)	Vitamin C (mg)	Vitamin E (mg)	Riboflavin (mg)	Thiamin (mg)	Calcium (mg)	Iron (mg)	Magnesium (mg)	Niacin (mg)	Phosphorus (mg)	Potassium (mg)	Sodium (mg)	Zinc (mg)
0	0	61	9	22	.1	2.6	0	.9	.1	0	52	.3	30	.9	157	299	323	2.5
1	0	77	1	5	.1	3.4	2	-	0	0	54	1.2	43	4.2	195	177	193	6.2
-	0	0	0	0	0	0	0	0	0	0	0	0	0	0	0	0	2	0
-	2	6	27	4	.1	.2	0	2.7	.1	0	65	.7	40	1.6	134	191	46	.7
-	1	7	4	12	0	.2	0	.6	.1	0	81	.7	32	.3	94	188	49	.6
0	2	5	0	0	0	0	0	-	0	0	72	.4	0	0	0	-	20	0
1	6	0	11	0	.1	0	0	.3	.1	.2	47	1.6	78	1.4	91	247	3	1.1
1	6	0	11	1	.1	0	0	.3	.1	.1	30	1.2	78	1.4	134	220	174	.7
1	-	25	-	100	-	-	4	-	.2	.2	48	1.5	-	2.9	-	450	540	-
-	-	-	-	60	-	-	6	-	.1	.1	32	.8	-	1.9	-	300	1440	-
-	-	15	-	200	-	-	15	-	.3	.3	32	1	-	0	-	530	420	-
-	16	40	-	100	-	-	0	-	-	-	240	1.5	-	-	-	-	1029	-
-	-	-	-	80	-	-	-	-	.2	.1	120	.6	-	.8	-	-	740	-
-	-	30	-	-	-	-	-	-	.4	.3	200	.8	-	1.5	-	160	550	-
1	-	45	-	80	-	-	6	0	.3	.1	80	.6	25	1.1	-	209	650	1.1
1	-	20	-	-	-	-	-	-	.3	.3	120	1	-	1.1	230	220	520	-
-	-	-	-	20	-	-	-	-	.3	.2	160	.4	-	.4	-	140	640	-
-	7	20	-	100	-	-	0	-	-	-	300	1	-	-	-	410	550	-
0	2	0	10	0	0	0	0	0	.1	.3	10	2	25	2.3	76	43	1	.7
0	2	0	10	-	0	0	0	0	0	0	10	.7	25	.6	76	43	1	.7
0	6	0	8	7	0	0	0	.1	.1	.2	15	.7	25	1.4	67	42	8	.6
0	6	0	7	0	.1	0	0	.1	.1	.2	21	1.5	42	1	125	62	4	1.1
-	-	50	-	250	-	-	9	-	.2	.2	16	1	-	4.8	200	400	400	-
-	-	0	-	0	-	-	30	-	-	-	0	0	-	-	-	-	18	-
0	1	0	-	321	.1	0	23	.9	0	0	8	.1	7	.5	9	129	2	0
0	-	0	0	0	0	0	0	-	0	0	1	0	1	0	2	7	1	0
1	0	0	0	47	0	0	0	.5	0	0	1	0	0	0	1	2	44	0
1	0	0	0	47	0	0	0	.5	0	0	1	0	0	0	1	2	44	-
1	0	0	0	48	0	0	0	.1	0	0	1	0	0	0	1	1	46	0
1	0	0	0	47	0	0	0	.6	0	0	1	0	0	0	1	2	44	0
1	0	0	0	47	0	0	0	.6	0	0	1	0	0	0	1	1	0	0
2	0	0	0	47	0	0	0	.6	0	0	1	0	0	0	1	2	51	0
1	0	0	0	47	0	0	0	.4	0	0	1	0	0	0	1	2	1	0
-	0	-	0	0	0	0	0	-	0	0	0	0	0	0	0	-	12	0
1	-	0	17	120	.3	0	16	-	.1	.1	22	1	30	2	44	530	786	.3
-	-	0	-	-	-	-	66	-	0	0	0	.2	-	.4	-	681	1222	-
-	0	0	7	1	0	0	1	0	0	0	8	0	0	0	1	7	11	0
-	0	0	0	0	0	0	0	0	0	0	1	.1	1	0	4	2	22	0
0	-	0	0	0	0	0	0	-	0	0	1	0	1	0	1	5	1	0
3	0	4	1	12	0	0	0	.6	0	0	0	0	0	0	4	1	104	0
-	0	0	-	0	-	-	0	-	-	-	0	0	-	-	-	10	105	-
-	-	5	-	0	-	-	0	-	-	-	0	0	-	-	-	5	130	-
1	-	55	-	60	-	-	9	-	.4	.2	120	2	-	3.8	-	550	540	-
1	-	40	-	-	-	-	-	-	-	-	-	-	-	-	240	690	560	-
-	-	15	-	-	-	-	0	-	0	0	48	.1	-	.1	-	4	193	-
-	1	0	22	153	.1	0	5	.1	0	.1	9	.3	12	.6	10	242	27	.1
-	1	0	14	258	.1	0	34	.1	0	0	9	.2	9	.5	14	247	7	.1
-	1	0	-	5	-	0	26	.2	0	.1	8	.7	13	.7	11	344	20	-
-	1	0	-	5	.1	0	32	.2	0	.1	8	.1	9	.8	13	350	13	-
-	-	5	-	-	-	-	4	-	0	0	88	0	-	.1	-	68	48	-
0	2	10	3	21	0	.2	0	.5	.1	0	84	.6	26	.1	95	169	36	.6
1	1	3	2	0	.1	.1	0	.7	0	0	29	.4	26	1.2	60	142	12	.5
0	1	1	1	2	0	.1	0	.3	0	0	24	.5	13	.1	41	146	10	.2
1	3	8	5	6	0	.2	0	5.2	.2	0	92	.7	37	.3	108	182	30	.5
1	2	54	25	109	.1	1.6	0	.5	1.2	.2	684	1.6	83	.6	653	1161	575	2.5
1	0	61	34	145	.2	2.7	0	.5	1	.2	767	.6	61	.8	507	947	494	2

Code	Name	Amount	Unit	Grams	Energy (kcal)	Carbohydrates (g)	Protein (g)	Fat (g)	Saturated fat (g)	Monounsaturated fat (g)
1075	Milk Substitutes, Fluid w/ hydr Vegetable Oils	1	Cup	244.0	150	15	4	8	2	5
1076	Milk Substitutes, Fluid, w/ lauric Acid Oil	1	Cup	244.0	150	15	4	8	7	0
1088	Milk, Buttermilk	1	Cup	245.0	99	12	8	2	1	1
1104	Milk, Chocolate Drink, Lowfat, 1% Fat	1	Cup	250.0	158	26	8	2	2	1
1103	Milk, Chocolate Drink, Lowfat, 2% Fat	1	Cup	250.0	179	26	8	5	3	1
1102	Milk, Chocolate Drink, Whole	1	Cup	250.0	208	26	8	8	5	2
1105	Milk, Chocolate Homemade Hot Cocoa	1	Cup	250.0	218	26	9	9	6	3
1095	Milk, Cnd, Condensed, Sweetened	1/4	Cup	76.3	245	42	6	7	4	2
1153	Milk, Cnd, Evaporated	1/4	Cup	63.0	85	6	4	5	3	1
1097	Milk, Cnd, Evaporated, Skim	1/4	Cup	63.8	50	7	5	0	0	0
1082	Milk, Lowfat, 1% Fat	1	Cup	244.0	102	12	8	3	2	1
1079	Milk, Lowfat, 2% Fat	1	Cup	244.0	121	12	8	5	3	1
1099	Milk, Malted, Beverage	1	Cup	265.0	236	27	10	10	6	3
1101	Milk, Malted, Chocolate Flavor, Beverage	1	Cup	265.0	228	30	9	9	6	3
1085	Milk, Skim	1	Cup	245.0	86	12	8	0	0	0
1077	Milk, Whole, 3.3% Fat	1	Cup	244.0	150	11	8	8	5	2
1078	Milk, Whole, 3.7% Fat	1	Cup	244.0	157	11	8	9	6	3
19135	Milky Way Bar	1	Bar	60.0	251	44	3	9	5	3
18322	Mince Meat Pie	1	Slice	165.0	477	79	4	18	4	8
55770	Minestrone Heat'n Serve Soup-Stouffer's	1	Cup	283.9	130	18	5	4	–	–
41281	Minestrone Soup-Healthy Choice	1	Each	212.6	160	30	6	1	–	–
55760	Minestrone Soup-Stouffer's	1	Cup	283.9	140	20	6	3	–	–
12635	Mixed w/ Peanuts, Dry Roasted	1/2	Cup	68.5	407	17	12	35	5	22
12637	Mixed w/ Peanuts, Oil Roasted	1/2	Cup	71.0	438	15	12	40	6	23
12638	Mixed w/o Peanuts, Oil Roasted	1/2	Cup	72.0	443	16	11	40	7	24
18177	Molasses Cookies	1	Each	15.0	65	11	1	2	0	1
19142	Mounds Candy Bar	1	Bar	20.0	72	12	1	4	2	1
62659	Mountain Dew	12	Fl Oz	355.2	165	47	–	–	–	–
19143	Mr. Goodbar Chocolate Bar	1	Bar	50.0	257	26	6	16	9	6
18274	Muffins, Blueberry	1	Large	65.0	180	31	4	4	1	2
18279	Muffins, Corn	1	Large	65.0	198	33	4	5	1	2
18283	Muffins, Oat Bran	1	Large	65.0	176	31	5	5	1	1
18273	Muffins, Plain	1	Large	65.0	192	27	4	7	1	2
18287	Muffins, Wheat Bran	1	Large	65.0	184	27	5	8	1	2
15056	Mullet, Striped, Ckd, Dry Heat	3	Ounce	85.1	128	0	21	4	1	1
41313	Mushroom Gravy over Beef Sirloin Tips-Healthy Choice	1	Each	269.3	310	43	22	5	2	–
11261	Mushrooms, Ckd	1/2	Cup	78.0	21	4	2	0	0	0
11264	Mushrooms, Cnd, Drained Solids	1/2	Cup	78.0	19	4	1	0	0	0
11950	Mushrooms, Enoki, Fresh	1	Medium	3.0	1	0	0	0	0	0
11260	Mushrooms, Fresh	1/2	Cup	35.0	9	2	1	0	0	0
11269	Mushrooms, Shiitake, Ckd	1/2	Cup	72.5	40	10	1	0	0	0
11268	Mushrooms, Shiitake, Dried	1	Medium	3.6	11	3	0	0	0	0
15165	Mussel, Blue, Ckd, Moist Heat	3	Ounce	85.1	146	6	20	4	1	1
62646	Mustard	1	Tbsp.	5.0	0	0	0	0	–	–
62679	Nacho Cheese Dip	2	Tbsp.	33.0	40	4	0	3	1	0
62619	Nacho Grande Chicken Enchiladas-Weight Watchers	1	Each	255.2	290	42	15	8	3	–
41340	Nacho Macaroni and Cheese-Healthy Choice	1	Each	255.1	280	44	13	5	3	–
55754	Navy Bean w/ Ham Soup-Stouffer's	1	Cup	283.9	240	31	11	8	–	–
19145	Nestle Crunch	1	Bar	40.0	198	26	2	10	6	4
55757	New England Clam Chowder Soup-Stouffer's	1	Cup	283.9	341	21	14	23	–	–
55829	Newburg Sauce Supreme-Stouffer's	1	Cup	283.9	481	20	7	41	–	–
55804	Noodles Romanoff-Stouffer's	1	Cup	283.9	441	36	17	25	–	–
43407	Noodles and Chicken, Micro Cup-Hormel	1	Each	212.6	174	19	7	7	2	3
20113	Noodles, Chinese, Chow Mein	1/2	Cup	22.5	119	13	2	7	1	2
20310	Noodles, Egg, Ckd, Enriched	1/2	Cup	80.0	106	20	4	1	0	0
20510	Noodles, Egg, Ckd, Unenriched	1/2	Cup	80.0	106	20	4	1	0	0

Polyunsaturated fat (g)	Dietary Fiber (g)	Cholesterol (mg)	Folate (µg)	Vitamin A (RE)	Vitamin B-6 (mg)	Vitamin B-12 (µg)	Vitamin C (mg)	Vitamin E (mg)	Riboflavin (mg)	Thiamin (mg)	Calcium (mg)	Iron (mg)	Magnesium (mg)	Niacin (mg)	Phosphorus (mg)	Potassium (mg)	Sodium (mg)	Zinc (mg)
1	0	0	0	0	0	0	0	2.6	.2	0	79	1	16	0	181	279	191	2.9
0	0	0	0	0	0	0	0	-	.2	0	79	1	16	0	181	279	191	2.9
0	0	9	12	20	.1	.5	2	.1	.4	.1	285	.1	27	.1	219	371	257	1
0	0	7	12	147	.1	.9	2	-	.4	.1	287	.6	33	.3	256	425	152	1
0	4	17	12	142	.1	.8	2	.1	.4	.1	284	.6	33	.3	254	422	150	1
0	4	30	12	72	.1	.8	2	.2	.4	.1	280	.6	33	.3	251	417	149	1
0	4	33	12	85	.1	.9	2	.3	.4	.1	298	.8	55	.4	270	480	123	1.2
0	0	26	9	62	0	.3	2	.2	.3	.1	216	.1	20	.2	193	284	97	.7
0	0	19	5	34	0	.1	1	-	.2	0	164	.1	15	.1	127	191	67	.5
0	0	2	5	75	0	.2	1	0	.2	0	185	.2	17	.1	124	211	73	.6
0	0	10	12	144	.1	.9	2	.1	.4	.1	300	.1	34	.2	235	381	123	1
0	0	18	12	139	.1	.9	2	.2	.4	.1	297	.1	33	.2	232	377	122	1
1	0	37	22	95	.2	1	3	-	.6	.2	355	.3	53	1.3	302	530	223	1.1
0	0	34	16	80	.1	.9	3	-	.4	.6	305	.6	48	.6	265	498	172	1.1
0	0	4	13	149	.1	.9	2	.1	.3	.1	302	.1	28	.2	247	406	126	1
0	0	33	12	76	.1	.9	2	.2	.4	.1	291	.1	33	.2	228	370	120	.9
0	0	35	12	83	.1	.9	4	-	.4	.1	290	.1	33	.2	227	368	119	.9
0	1	12	5	28	0	.3	1	.4	.1	0	78	.5	20	.2	98	145	144	.4
5	-	0	8	3	.1	0	10	-	.2	.2	36	2.5	23	2	69	335	419	.4
-	-	0	-	-	-	-	0	-	0	0	0	.2	0	-	-	310	1192	-
-	-	0	-	60	-	-	15	-	.1	.1	32	.6	-	1.5	130	440	520	-
-	-	10	-	-	-	-	0	-	0	0	0	.2	-	.2	-	371	1282	-
7	6	0	35	1	.2	0	0	4.1	.1	.1	48	2.5	154	3.2	298	409	458	2.6
9	6	0	59	1	.2	0	0	4.3	.2	.4	77	2.3	167	3.6	329	413	463	3.6
8	4	0	41	1	.1	0	0	4.3	.3	.4	76	1.9	181	1.4	323	392	504	3.4
0	-	0	1	0	0	0	0	-	0	.1	11	1	8	.5	14	52	69	.1
0	1	0	1	0	0	0	0	.4	0	0	5	.8	14	0	24	42	25	.2
-	-	-	-	-	-	-	-	-	-	-	-	-	-	-	-	-	75	-
1	2	10	36	5	.1	.2	0	.6	.1	0	56	.6	48	2.4	140	225	17	.9
1	2	20	10	-	0	.4	1	-	.1	.1	37	1	10	.7	128	80	291	.3
2	-	33	22	23	.1	.1	0	-	.2	.2	48	1.8	24	1.3	185	45	339	.5
3	5	0	12	-	.1	0	0	-	.1	.2	41	2.7	102	.3	244	330	255	1.2
4	2	25	8	26	0	.1	0	-	.2	.2	130	1.6	11	1.5	99	79	304	.4
4	-	21	34	163	.2	.1	5	-	.3	.2	122	2.7	51	2.6	185	207	382	1.8
1	0	54	8	36	.4	.2	1	-	.1	.1	26	1.2	28	5.4	208	390	60	.7
-	-	35	-	60	-	-	2	-	0	-	-	.2	-	.4	-	80	500	-
0	2	0	14	0	.1	0	3	.1	.2	.1	5	1.4	9	3.5	68	278	2	.7
0	2	0	10	0	0	0	0	.1	0	.1	9	.6	12	1.2	51	101	332	.6
0	-	0	1	0	0	0	0	-	0	0	0	0	0	.1	3	11	0	0
0	0	0	7	0	0	0	1	0	.2	0	2	.4	4	1.4	36	130	1	.3
0	2	0	15	0	.1	0	0	.1	.1	0	2	.3	10	1.1	21	85	3	1
0	0	0	6	0	0	0	0	0	0	0	0	.1	5	.5	11	55	0	.3
1	0	48	64	77	.1	20.4	12	.7	.4	.3	28	5.7	31	2.6	242	228	314	2.3
-	-	-	0	0	0	0	0	-	0	0	0	0	0	0	0	-	75	0
0	0	0	0	0	0	0	0	-	0	0	24	0	0	0	0	-	200	0
-	4	20	-	300	-	-	12	-	-	-	360	.6	-	-	-	600	560	-
-	-	20	-	0	-	-	0	-	.5	.6	160	.8	-	0	-	420	560	-
-	-	20	-	-	-	-	0	-	0	0	70	3	-	.2	-	571	1252	-
0	1	8	4	6	0	.2	0	-	.1	0	68	.3	18	.2	71	138	59	.4
-	-	40	-	-	-	-	0	-	0	0	2	.1	-	.2	-	571	961	-
-	-	120	-	-	-	-	0	-	0	0	2	0	-	0	-	371	1052	-
-	-	40	-	-	-	-	0	-	0	0	2	.2	-	.2	-	260	1993	-
2	-	29	-	270	-	-	8	-	.1	.1	32	.7	21	1.7	-	254	1009	.8
4	1	0	5	2	0	0	0	0	.1	.1	5	1.1	12	1.3	36	27	99	.3
0	-	26	6	5	0	.1	0	-	.1	.1	10	1.3	15	1.2	55	22	132	.5
0	-	26	6	5	0	.1	0	-	0	0	10	.5	15	.3	55	22	132	.5

Code	Name	Amount	Unit	Grams	Energy (kcal)	Carbohydrates (g)	Protein (g)	Fat (g)	Saturated fat (g)	Monounsaturated fat (g)
20112	Noodles, Egg, Spinach, Ckd, Enriched	1/2	Cup	80.0	106	19	4	1	0	0
20115	Noodles, Japanese, Soba, Ckd	1/2	Cup	57.0	56	12	3	0	0	0
62647	Noodles, Ramen	1	Each	86.0	380	52	10	16	8	-
18200	Oatmeal Cookies, Dietary	1	Each	7.0	31	5	0	1	1	1
18178	Oatmeal Cookies, Regular	1	Each	18.0	81	12	1	3	1	2
18179	Oatmeal Cookies, Soft-type	1	Each	15.0	61	10	1	2	0	1
3189	Oatmeal, Dry	1	Cup	38.4	153	27	5	3	-	-
3689	Oatmeal, Prepared w/ Milk	1/2	Cup	180.0	209	28	9	7	-	-
15058	Ocean Perch, Atlantic, Ckd, Dry Heat	3	Ounce	85.1	103	0	20	2	0	1
4053	Oil, Olive	1	Tbsp.	13.5	119	0	0	14	2	10
4042	Oil, Peanut	1	Tbsp.	13.5	119	0	0	14	2	6
4058	Oil, Sesame	1	Tbsp.	13.6	121	0	0	14	2	5
4044	Oil, Soybean	1	Tbsp.	13.6	121	0	0	14	2	3
4034	Oil, Soybean, (hydr)	1	Tbsp.	13.6	121	0	0	14	2	6
4543	Oil, Soybean, (hydr)&cttnsd	1	Tbsp.	13.6	121	0	0	14	2	4
4518	Oil, Vegetable Corn	1	Tbsp.	13.6	121	0	0	14	2	3
4582	Oil, Vegetable, Canola	1	Tbsp.	13.6	121	0	0	14	1	8
4501	Oil, Vegetable, Cocoa Butter	1	Tbsp.	13.6	121	0	0	14	8	4
4502	Oil, Vegetable, Cottonseed	1	Tbsp.	13.6	121	0	0	14	4	2
4055	Oil, Vegetable, Palm	1	Tbsp.	13.6	121	0	0	14	7	5
4513	Oil, Vegetable, Palm Kernel	1	Tbsp.	13.6	118	0	0	14	11	2
4510	Oil, Vegetable, Safflower, Linoleic	1	Tbsp.	13.6	121	0	0	14	1	2
4511	Oil, Vegetable, Safflower, Oleic	1	Tbsp.	13.6	121	0	0	14	1	10
4584	Oil, Vegetable, Sunflower	1	Tbsp.	13.6	121	0	0	14	1	11
11279	Okra, Ckd	1/2	Cup	80.0	26	6	1	0	0	0
11278	Okra, Fresh	1/2	Cup	50.0	19	4	1	0	0	0
11281	Okra, Frz, Ckd	1/2	Cup	92.0	34	8	2	0	0	0
11280	Okra, Frz, Unprepared	1/2	Cup	71.3	21	5	1	0	0	0
41282	Old Fashioned Chicken Noodle Soup-Healthy Choice	1	Each	212.6	90	11	5	2	-	-
55806	Old-Fashion Stuff'n-Stouffer's	1/2	Cup	142.0	310	31	6	19	-	-
10161	Olive Loaf, Lunch Meat	1	Slice	28.4	67	3	3	5	2	2
7051	Olive Loaf, Pork, Lunch Meat	1	Slice	28.4	67	3	3	5	2	2
62648	Olives, Green	5	Each	15.0	25	0	0	3	-	-
9194	Olives, Ripe, Canned (jumbo-super colossal)	1	Jumbo	8.3	7	0	0	1	0	0
9193	Olives, Ripe, Canned (small-extra large)	1	Small	3.2	4	0	0	0	0	0
11283	Onions, Ckd	1/2	Cup	119.9	53	12	2	0	0	0
11285	Onions, Cnd, Sol&liq	1/2	Cup	112.0	21	4	1	0	0	0
11282	Onions, Fresh	1/2	Cup	79.9	30	7	1	0	0	0
14323	Orange Drink, Cnd	3/4	Cup	185.8	95	24	0	0	0	0
9206	Orange Juice, Fresh	3/4	Cup	186.0	84	19	1	0	0	0
9215	Orange Juice, From Concentrate	3/4	Cup	186.4	84	20	1	0	0	0
62558	Orange Juice, w/ Added Calcium	3/4	Cup	186.4	84	20	1	0	0	0
14327	Orange and Apricot Juice Drink, Cnd	3/4	Cup	187.0	95	24	1	0	0	0
9200	Oranges, Fresh	1	Medium	131.0	62	15	1	0	0	0
18199	Oreos, Dietary	1	Each	10.0	46	7	0	2	1	1
18166	Oreos, Regular	1	Each	10.0	47	7	0	2	0	1
18168	Oreos, w/ Extra Creme Filling	1	Each	13.0	65	9	0	3	1	2
55220	Oriental Beef w/ Veg., Lean Cuisine-Stouffer's	1	Each	244.5	290	31	20	9	2	-
41314	Oriental Chicken w/ Spicy Peanut Sauce-Healthy Choice	1	Each	269.3	340	40	33	5	1	-
19031	Oriental Mix, Rice-based	1	Ounce	28.4	155	9	6	12	5	3
55221	Oven Baked Chicken, Lean Cuisine-Stouffer's	1	Each	226.8	200	21	17	5	2	-
15168	Oyster, Eastern, Breaded and Fried	3	Ounce	85.1	168	10	7	11	3	4
15170	Oyster, Eastern, Cnd	3	Ounce	85.1	59	3	6	2	1	0
15245	Oysters, Raw	3	Ounce	85.1	50	5	4	1	0	0
18288	Pancakes Plain, Frozen	1	4 In.	9.0	21	4	0	0	0	0
18294	Pancakes, Blueberry	1	4 In.	9.5	21	3	1	1	0	0

Polyunsaturated fat (g)	Dietary Fiber (g)	Cholesterol (mg)	Folate (µg)	Vitamin A (RE)	Vitamin B-6 (mg)	Vitamin B-12 (µg)	Vitamin C (mg)	Vitamin E (mg)	Riboflavin (mg)	Thiamin (mg)	Calcium (mg)	Iron (mg)	Magnesium (mg)	Niacin (mg)	Phosphorus (mg)	Potassium (mg)	Sodium (mg)	Zinc (mg)
0	2	26	17	11	.1	.1	0	0	.1	.2	15	.9	19	1.2	46	30	10	.5
0	-	0	4	0	0	0	0	-	0	.1	2	.3	5	.3	14	20	34	.1
-	2	0	0	0	0	0	0	-	0	0	0	1.6	0	0	0	-	1560	0
0	-	0	1	0	0	0	0	-	0	0	3	.2	2	.1	10	12	1	0
0	1	0	1	0	0	0	0	-	0	0	7	.5	6	.4	25	26	69	.1
0	0	1	1	1	0	0	0	-	0	0	14	.4	5	.3	31	20	52	.1
-	3	-	14	-	.1	0	1	.1	1	1.1	281	28.2	56	13.8	191	180	13	1.4
-	-	-	18	-	.1	.5	-	-	1	.9	396	21.9	63	10.8	288	367	83	1.7
0	0	46	9	12	.2	1	1	-	.1	.1	117	1	33	2.1	236	298	82	.5
1	0	0	0	0	0	0	0	1.6	0	0	0	.1	0	0	0	0	0	0
4	0	0	0	0	0	0	0	1.7	0	0	0	0	0	0	0	0	0	0
6	0	0	0	0	0	0	0	.6	0	0	0	0	0	0	0	0	0	0
8	0	0	0	0	0	0	0	.8	0	0	0	0	0	0	0	0	0	0
5	0	0	0	0	0	0	0	2.2	0	0	0	0	0	0	0	0	0	0
7	0	0	0	0	0	0	0	.6	0	0	0	0	0	0	0	0	0	0
8	0	0	0	0	0	0	0	2.9	0	0	0	0	0	0	0	0	0	0
4	0	-	0	0	0	0	0	-	0	0	0	0	0	0	0	0	0	0
0	0	0	0	0	0	0	0	.2	0	0	0	0	0	0	0	0	0	0
7	0	0	0	0	0	0	0	5.2	-	0	0	0	0	0	0	0	0	0
1	0	0	0	0	0	0	0	3	0	0	0	0	0	0	0	0	0	-
0	0	0	0	0	0	0	0	.5	0	0	0	0	0	0	0	0	0	0
10	0	0	0	0	0	0	0	4.7	0	0	0	0	0	0	0	0	0	0
2	0	0	0	0	0	0	0	4.7	0	0	0	0	0	0	0	0	0	0
1	0	-	0	0	0	0	0	-	0	0	0	0	0	0	0	0	0	0
0	2	0	37	46	.1	0	13	.6	0	.1	50	.4	46	.7	45	258	4	.4
0	1	0	44	33	.1	0	11	.3	0	.1	41	.4	29	.5	32	152	4	.3
0	3	0	134	47	0	0	11	.6	.1	.1	88	.6	47	.7	42	215	3	.6
0	2	0	105	33	0	0	9	.5	.1	.1	58	.4	31	.5	30	150	2	.4
-	-	20	-	80	-	-	12	-	.1	0	16	.2	-	1.9	60	130	540	-
-	-	5	-	-	-	-	0	-	0	0	0	.2	-	.4	-	100	561	-
1	0	11	1	6	.1	.4	2	-	.1	.1	31	.2	5	.5	36	84	421	.4
1	0	11	1	0	.1	.4	3	.1	.1	.1	31	.2	5	.5	36	84	421	.4
-	-	-	0	0	0	0	0	-	0	0	0	0	0	0	0	-	65	0
0	-	0	0	3	0	0	0	-	0	0	8	.3	0	0	0	1	75	0
0	-	0	0	1	0	0	0	-	0	0	3	.1	0	0	0	0	28	0
0	2	0	18	0	.2	0	6	.2	0	.1	26	.3	13	.2	42	199	4	.3
0	1	0	11	0	.2	0	5	.2	0	0	50	.1	7	.1	31	124	416	.3
0	1	0	15	0	.1	0	5	.1	0	0	16	.2	8	.1	26	125	2	.2
0	0	0	4	4	0	0	63	0	0	0	11	.5	4	.1	2	33	30	.2
0	0	0	56	37	.1	0	93	.2	.1	.2	20	.4	20	.7	32	372	2	.1
0	0	0	82	15	.1	0	73	.4	0	.1	17	.2	19	.4	30	354	2	.1
0	0	0	82	15	.1	0	73	-	0	.1	224	.2	19	.4	30	354	2	.1
0	0	0	11	108	.1	0	37	0	0	0	9	.2	7	.4	15	150	4	.1
0	3	0	40	28	.1	0	70	.3	.1	.1	52	.1	13	.4	18	237	0	.1
0	-	0	1	0	0	0	0	-	0	0	6	.5	7	.3	18	30	24	.1
0	0	0	1	0	0	0	0	-	0	0	3	.4	5	.2	10	18	60	.1
0	-	0	1	0	0	0	0	-	0	0	3	.4	4	.2	12	16	64	.1
-	-	40	-	150	-	-	1	-	.2	.1	16	1	-	2.9	-	400	590	-
1	-	45	-	-	-	-	2	-	-	-	-	.2	-	.4	-	50	470	-
3	4	0	25	1	.1	0	0	-	0	.1	22	.8	40	3	112	147	235	1.3
-	-	35	-	350	-	-	6	-	.2	.2	16	.8	-	7.6	-	550	480	-
3	-	69	12	77	.1	13.3	3	-	.2	.1	53	5.9	49	1.4	135	208	355	74.1
1	0	47	8	77	.1	16.3	4	.7	.1	.1	38	5.7	46	1.1	118	195	95	77.4
1	0	21	15	7	.1	13.8	4	-	.1	.1	-	4.9	28	1.1	79	105	151	32.3
0	-	1	1	3	0	0	0	-	0	0	6	.3	1	.4	33	7	46	.1
0	-	5	1	5	0	0	0	-	0	0	20	.2	2	.1	14	13	39	.1

Code	Name	Amount	Unit	Grams	Energy (kcal)	Carbohydrates (g)	Protein (g)	Fat (g)	Saturated fat (g)	Monounsaturated fat (g)
18390	Pancakes, Buttermilk	1	4 In.	9.5	22	3	1	1	0	0
18298	Pancakes, Dietary	1	3 In.	22.0	44	9	1	0	0	0
18293	Pancakes, Plain	1	4 In.	9.5	22	3	1	1	0	0
18300	Pancakes, Whole-wheat	1	4 In.	44.0	92	13	4	3	1	1
9229	Papaya Nectar, Cnd	3/4	Cup	187.0	107	27	0	0	0	0
9226	Papayas, Fresh	1	Medium	304.0	119	30	2	0	0	0
11808	Parsnips, Ckd, w/ Salt	1/2	Cup	78.0	63	15	1	0	0	0
11299	Parsnips, Ckd, w/o Salt	1/2	Cup	78.0	63	15	1	0	0	0
11298	Parsnips, Fresh	1/2	Cup	66.5	50	12	1	0	0	0
9232	Passion-fruit Juice, Purple, Fresh	3/4	Cup	185.2	94	25	1	0	-	-
9233	Passion-fruit Juice, Yellow, Fresh	3/4	Cup	185.2	111	27	1	0	-	-
55800	Pasta Florentine-Stouffer's	1/2	Cup	142.0	190	16	8	11	-	-
41294	Pasta Italiano-Healthy Choice	1	Each	340.2	350	59	16	5	2	-
55810	Pasta Roma-Stouffer's	1/2	Cup	142.0	130	16	8	4	-	-
41292	Pasta Shells w/ Tomato Sauce-Healthy Choice	1	Each	340.2	330	53	24	3	2	-
55142	Pasta Shells, Cheese w/ Sauce-Stouffer's	1	Each	262.2	300	28	17	13	-	-
41287	Pasta w/ Cacciatore Chicken-Healthy Choice	1	Each	354.4	310	47	26	3	-	-
41293	Pasta w/ Teriyaki Chicken-Healthy Choice	1	Each	357.9	350	58	24	3	1	-
20321	Pasta, Ckd, Enriched, w/ Added Salt	1/2	Cup	70.0	99	20	3	0	0	0
20121	Pasta, Ckd, Enriched, w/o Added Salt	1/2	Cup	70.0	99	20	3	0	0	0
20094	Pasta, Fresh-refrigerated, Plain, Ckd	1/2	Cup	73.0	96	18	4	1	0	0
20096	Pasta, Fresh-refrigerated, Spinach, Ckd	1/2	Cup	73.0	95	18	4	1	0	0
20097	Pasta, Homemade, Made w/ Egg, Ckd	1/2	Cup	73.6	96	17	4	1	0	0
20098	Pasta, Homemade, Made w/o Egg, Ckd	1/2	Cup	73.6	91	18	3	1	0	0
20127	Pasta, Spinach, Ckd	1/2	Cup	70.0	91	18	3	0	0	0
20125	Pasta, Whole-wheat, Ckd	1/2	Cup	70.0	87	19	4	0	0	0
9251	Peach Nectar, Cnd, w/o Added Vit C	3/4	Cup	186.4	101	26	1	0	0	0
9241	Peaches, Cnd, Heavy Syrup Pack	1/2	Cup	128.0	95	26	1	0	0	0
9238	Peaches, Cnd, Juice Pack	1/2	Cup	124.0	55	14	1	0	0	0
9240	Peaches, Cnd, Light Syrup Pack	1/2	Cup	125.5	68	18	1	0	0	0
9237	Peaches, Cnd, Water Pack	1/2	Cup	122.0	29	7	1	0	0	0
9242	Peaches, Cnd, X-heavy Syrup Pack	1/2	Cup	131.0	126	34	1	0	0	0
9239	Peaches, Cnd, X-light Syrup	1/2	Cup	123.5	52	14	0	0	0	0
9244	Peaches, Dehydrated, Sulfured	1/4	Cup	29.0	94	24	1	0	0	0
9246	Peaches, Dried, Sulfured	1/4	Cup	40.0	96	25	1	0	0	0
9236	Peaches, Fresh	1	Medium	87.0	37	10	1	0	0	0
9250	Peaches, Frozen, Sliced, Sweetened	1/2	Cup	125.0	118	30	1	0	0	0
19147	Peanut Bar	1	Bar	40.0	209	19	6	13	2	7
19148	Peanut Brittle	1	Ounce	28.4	128	20	2	5	1	2
18185	Peanut Butter Cookies, Regular	1	Each	15.0	72	9	1	4	1	1
18186	Peanut Butter Cookies, Soft-type	1	Each	15.0	69	9	1	4	1	2
18201	Peanut Butter Sandwich Cookies, Dietary	1	Each	10.0	54	5	1	3	1	2
18190	Peanut Butter Sandwich Cookies, Regular	1	Each	14.0	67	9	1	3	1	2
16097	Peanut Butter, Chunk Style, w/ Salt	2	Tbsp.	32.3	190	7	8	16	3	8
16397	Peanut Butter, Chunk Style, w/o Salt	2	Tbsp.	32.3	190	7	8	16	3	8
62689	Peanut Butter, Reduced Fat	2	Tbsp.	36.0	190	15	8	12	3	-
16098	Peanut Butter, Smooth Style, w/ Salt	2	Tbsp.	32.3	190	7	8	16	3	8
16398	Peanut Butter, Smooth Style, w/o Salt	2	Tbsp.	32.3	190	7	8	16	3	8
12681	Peanut Kernels, Oil Roasted	1/2	Cup	72.0	418	14	19	35	5	18
16088	Peanuts, All Types, Ckd, Boiled, w/ Salt	1/2	Cup	31.5	100	7	4	7	1	3
16090	Peanuts, All Types, Dry-roasted, w/ Salt	1/2	Cup	73.0	427	16	17	36	5	18
16390	Peanuts, All Types, Dry-roasted, w/o Salt	1/2	Cup	73.0	427	16	17	36	5	18
16087	Peanuts, All Types, Fresh	1/2	Cup	73.0	414	12	19	36	5	18
16089	Peanuts, All Types, Oil-roasted, w/ Salt	1/2	Cup	72.0	418	14	19	35	5	18
16389	Peanuts, All Types, Oil-roasted, w/o Salt	1/2	Cup	72.0	418	14	19	35	5	18
16091	Peanuts, Spanish, Fresh	1/2	Cup	73.0	416	12	19	36	6	16

Polyunsaturated fat (g)	Dietary Fiber (g)	Cholesterol (mg)	Folate (µg)	Vitamin A (RE)	Vitamin B-6 (mg)	Vitamin B-12 (µg)	Vitamin C (mg)	Vitamin E (mg)	Riboflavin (mg)	Thiamin (mg)	Calcium (mg)	Iron (mg)	Magnesium (mg)	Niacin (mg)	Phosphorus (mg)	Potassium (mg)	Sodium (mg)	Zinc (mg)
0	-	6	1	3	0	0	0	-	0	0	15	.2	1	.1	13	14	50	.1
0	-	0	1	2	0	0	0	-	0	0	13	.4	6	.4	75	85	58	.2
0	-	6	1	5	0	0	0	-	0	0	21	.2	2	.1	15	13	42	.1
1	-	27	9	28	0	.1	0	-	.2	.1	110	1.4	20	1	164	123	252	.5
0	1	0	4	21	0	0	6	0	0	0	19	.6	6	.3	0	58	9	.3
0	5	0	116	85	.1	0	188	3.4	.1	.1	73	.3	30	1	15	781	9	.2
0	-	0	45	0	.1	0	10	-	0	.1	29	.5	23	.6	54	286	192	.2
0	3	0	45	0	.1	0	10	.8	0	.1	29	.5	23	.6	54	286	8	.2
0	3	0	44	0	.1	0	11	.7	0	.1	24	.4	19	.5	47	249	7	.4
-	0	0	-	133	-	0	55	.1	.2	0	7	.4	31	2.7	24	515	11	-
	0	0	-	446	-	0	34	.1	.2	0	7	.7	31	4.1	46	515	11	-
-	-	25	-	-	-	-	0	-	0	0	2	.1	-	.1	-	200	446	-
3	-	30	-	60	-	-	-	-	.5	.5	48	2	-	2.9	180	540	530	-
-	-	15	-	-	-	-	3	-	0	.1	1	.2	-	.5	-	300	391	-
-	-	35	-	100	-	-	21	-	.4	.5	320	1.5	-	2.9	240	640	470	-
-	-	-	-	150	-	-	9	-	.3	.1	280	1	-	1.9	-	480	820	-
1	-	35	-	100	-	-	6	-	.4	.5	32	1.5	-	6.7	250	660	430	-
2	-	45	-	100	-	-	6	-	.3	.3	48	1.5	-	3.8	200	390	370	-
0	-	0	5	-	0	0	0	-	.1	.1	5	1	13	1.2	38	22	70	.4
0	1	0	5	-	0	0	0	0	.1	.1	5	1	13	1.2	38	22	1	.4
0	-	24	5	4	0	.1	0	-	.1	.2	4	.8	13	.7	46	18	4	.4
0	-	24	13	10	.1	.1	0	-	.1	.1	13	.8	18	.7	42	27	4	.5
0	-	30	14	13	0	0	0	-	.1	.1	7	.9	10	.9	38	15	61	.3
0	-	0	13	0	0	0	0	-	.1	.1	4	.8	10	1	29	14	54	.3
0	-	0	8	11	.1	0	0	-	.1	.1	21	.7	43	1.1	76	41	10	.8
0	3	0	4	0	.1	0	0	0	0	.1	11	.7	21	.5	62	31	2	.6
0	1	0	3	48	0	0	10	0	0	0	9	.4	7	.5	11	75	13	.1
0	1	0	4	42	0	0	4	1.1	0	0	4	.3	6	.8	14	118	8	.1
0	1	0	4	47	0	0	4	1.9	0	0	7	.3	9	.7	21	159	5	.1
0	1	0	4	44	0	0	3	1.1	0	0	4	.5	6	.7	14	122	6	.1
0	1	0	4	65	0	0	4	1.1	0	0	2	.4	6	.6	12	121	4	.1
0	-	0	4	17	0	0	2	-	0	0	4	.4	7	.7	14	109	10	.1
0	-	0	4	33	0	0	4	-	0	0	6	.4	6	1	14	91	6	.1
0	-	0	2	41	0	0	3	-	0	0	11	1.6	17	1.4	47	392	3	.2
0	3	0	0	86	0	0	2	0	.1	0	11	1.6	17	1.8	48	398	3	.2
0	2	0	3	47	0	0	6	.6	0	0	4	.1	6	.9	10	171	0	.1
0	2	0	4	35	0	0	118	1.1	0	0	4	.5	6	.8	14	162	7	.1
4	1	3	24	20	0	0	0	.4	.1	0	31	.4	30	3.2	61	163	96	.5
1	1	4	20	13	0	0	0	.5	0	.1	9	.4	14	1	31	59	128	.3
1	-	0	5	1	0	0	0	-	0	0	5	.4	7	.6	13	25	62	.1
1	0	0	1	0	0	0	0	-	0	0	2	.1	5	.3	13	16	50	.1
1	-	0	3	0	0	0	0	-	0	0	5	.2	5	.5	19	29	41	.2
1	-	0	2	0	0	0	0	-	0	0	7	.4	7	.5	26	27	52	.1
5	2	0	30	0	.1	0	0	3.2	0	0	13	.6	51	4.4	102	241	157	.9
5	2	0	30	0	.1	0	0	3.2	0	0	13	.6	51	4.4	102	241	5	.9
-	2	-	12	0	.1	0	0	-	0	0	0	.4	53	4.8	0	721	250	.9
5	2	0	25	0	.1	0	0	3.2	0	0	11	.5	51	4.2	104	233	154	.8
5	-	0	25	0	.1	0	0	-	0	0	11	.5	51	4.2	104	233	5	.8
11	6	0	91	0	.2	0	0	5.3	.1	.2	63	1.3	133	10.3	372	491	312	4.8
2	3	0	23	0	0	0	0	1	0	.1	17	.3	32	1.7	62	57	237	.6
11	6	0	106	0	.2	0	0	5.4	.1	.3	39	1.6	128	9.9	261	480	593	2.4
11	6	0	106	0	.2	0	0	5.7	.1	.3	39	1.6	128	9.9	261	480	4	2.4
11	6	0	175	0	.3	0	0	6.7	.1	.5	67	3.3	123	8.8	274	515	13	2.4
11	7	0	91	0	.2	0	0	5.3	.1	.2	63	1.3	133	10.3	372	491	312	4.8
11	7	0	91	0	.2	0	0	5.3	.1	.2	63	1.3	133	10.3	372	491	4	4.8
13	7	0	175	0	.3	0	0	-	.1	.5	77	2.9	137	11.0	283	543	16	1.5

Code	Name	Amount	Unit	Grams	Energy (kcal)	Carbohydrates (g)	Protein (g)	Fat (g)	Saturated fat (g)	Monounsaturated fat (g)
16092	Peanuts, Spanish, Oil-roasted, w/ Salt	1/2	Cup	73.5	426	13	21	36	6	16
16392	Peanuts, Spanish, Oil-roasted, w/o Salt	1/2	Cup	73.5	426	13	21	36	6	16
16093	Peanuts, Valencia, Fresh	1/2	Cup	73.0	416	15	18	35	5	16
16094	Peanuts, Valencia, Oil-roasted, w/ Salt	1/2	Cup	72.0	424	12	19	37	6	17
16394	Peanuts, Valencia, Oil-roasted, w/o Salt	1/2	Cup	72.0	424	12	19	37	6	17
16095	Peanuts, Virginia, Fresh	1/2	Cup	73.0	411	12	18	36	5	18
16096	Peanuts, Virginia, Oil-roasted, w/ Salt	1/2	Cup	71.5	413	14	18	35	5	18
16396	Peanuts, Virginia, Oil-roasted, w/o Salt	1/2	Cup	71.5	413	14	18	35	5	18
9340	Pears, Asian, Fresh	1	Medium	122.0	51	13	1	0	0	0
9257	Pears, Cnd, Heavy Syrup Pack	1/2	Cup	127.5	94	24	0	0	0	0
9254	Pears, Cnd, Juice Pack	1/2	Cup	124.0	62	16	0	0	0	0
9256	Pears, Cnd, Light Syrup Pack	1/2	Cup	125.5	72	19	0	0	0	0
9253	Pears, Cnd, Water Pack	1/2	Cup	122.0	35	10	0	0	0	0
9258	Pears, Cnd, X-heavy Syrup Pack	1/2	Cup	130.5	127	33	0	0	0	0
9255	Pears, Cnd, X-light Syrup Pack	1/2	Cup	123.5	58	15	0	0	0	0
9252	Pears, Fresh	1	Medium	166.0	98	25	1	1	0	0
11318	Peas and Carrots, Cnd	1/2	Cup	76.0	29	6	2	0	0	0
11323	Peas and Carrots, Frz, Ckd	1/2	Cup	80.0	38	8	2	0	0	0
11324	Peas and Onions, Cnd	1/2	Cup	60.0	31	5	2	0	0	0
11327	Peas and Onions, Frz, Ckd	1/2	Cup	90.0	41	8	2	0	0	0
11300	Peas, Edible-podded, Fresh	1/2	Cup	72.5	30	5	2	0	0	0
11305	Peas, Green, Ckd	1/2	Cup	80.0	67	13	4	0	0	0
11308	Peas, Green, Cnd	1/2	Cup	85.0	59	11	4	0	0	0
11310	Peas, Green, Cnd, Seasoned	1/2	Cup	85.0	43	8	3	0	0	0
11304	Peas, Green, Fresh	1/2	Cup	72.5	59	10	4	0	0	0
11313	Peas, Green, Frz, Ckd	1/2	Cup	80.0	62	11	4	0	0	0
18324	Pecan Pie	1	Slice	113.0	452	65	5	21	4	12
12142	Pecans, Dried	1/2	Cup	54.0	360	10	4	37	3	23
41333	Pepperoni French Bread Pizza-Healthy Choice	1	Each	170.1	310	38	20	7	3	-
62625	Pepperoni Pizza-Weight Watchers	1	Each	157.6	390	46	23	12	4	-
11329	Peppers, Hot Chili, Green, Cnd	1	Each	73.0	18	4	1	0	0	0
11670	Peppers, Hot Chili, Green, Fresh	1	Each	45.0	18	4	1	0	0	0
11820	Peppers, Hot Chili, Red, Cnd	1	Each	73.0	18	4	1	0	0	0
11819	Peppers, Hot Chili, Red, Fresh	1	Each	45.0	18	4	1	0	0	0
11632	Peppers, Jalapeno, Cnd	1/4	Cup	34.0	8	2	0	0	0	0
11333	Peppers, Sweet, Green, Fresh	1	Medium	74.0	20	5	1	0	0	0
11821	Peppers, Sweet, Red, Fresh	1	Medium	74.0	20	5	1	0	0	0
11951	Peppers, Sweet, Yellow, Fresh	1	Medium	74.0	20	5	1	0	-	-
15061	Perch, Ckd, Dry Heat	3	Ounce	85.1	100	0	21	1	0	0
55827	Pesto Sauce-Stouffer's	1/4	Cup	71.0	193	5	9	15	-	-
11958	Pickle Relish, Hamburger	1	Tbsp.	15.0	19	5	0	0	0	0
11944	Pickle Relish, Hot Dog	1	Tbsp.	15.0	14	4	0	0	0	0
11945	Pickle Relish, Sweet	1	Tbsp.	15.0	19	5	0	0	0	0
10162	Pickle and Pimento Loaf, Lunch Meat	1	Slice	28.4	74	2	3	6	2	3
7058	Pickle and Pimiento Loaf, Pork, Lunch Meat	1	Slice	28.4	74	2	3	6	2	3
11941	Pickle, Cucumber ,Sour	1	Slice	7.0	1	0	0	0	0	0
11937	Pickle, Cucumber, Dill	1	Slice	6.0	1	0	0	0	0	0
11947	Pickle, Cucumber, Dill, Low Sodium	1	Slice	6.0	1	0	0	0	0	0
11946	Pickle, Cucumber, Sour, Low Sodium	1	Slice	7.0	1	0	0	0	0	0
11940	Pickle, Cucumber, Sweet	1	Slice	6.0	7	2	0	0	0	0
11948	Pickle, Cucumber, Sweet, Low Sodium	1	Slice	6.0	7	2	0	0	0	0
7062	Picnic Loaf, Lunch Meat	1	Slice	28.4	66	1	4	5	2	2
15063	Pike, Northern, Ckd, Dry Heat	3	Ounce	85.1	96	0	21	1	0	0
15204	Pike, Walleye, Ckd, Dry Heat	3	Ounce	85.1	101	0	21	1	0	0
14017	Pina Colada	1	Fl Oz	31.4	58	9	0	1	0	0
12147	Pine Nuts	1	Tbsp.	10.0	52	1	2	5	1	2

Polyunsaturated fat (g)	Dietary Fiber (g)	Cholesterol (mg)	Folate (μg)	Vitamin A (RE)	Vitamin B-6 (mg)	Vitamin B-12 (μg)	Vitamin C (mg)	Vitamin E (mg)	Riboflavin (mg)	Thiamin (mg)	Calcium (mg)	Iron (mg)	Magnesium (mg)	Niacin (mg)	Phosphorus (mg)	Potassium (mg)	Sodium (mg)	Zinc (mg)
13	-	0	93	0	.2	0	0	-	.1	.2	74	1.7	123	11	284	570	318	1.5
13	-	0	93	0	.2	0	0	-	.1	.2	74	1.7	123	11	284	570	4	1.5
12	-	0	179	0	.2	0	0	-	.2	.5	45	1.5	134	9.4	245	242	1	2.4
13	-	0	90	0	.2	0	0	-	.1	.1	39	1.2	115	10.3	230	441	556	2.2
13	-	0	90	0	.2	0	0	-	.1	.1	39	1.2	115	10.3	230	441	4	2.2
11	-	0	174	0	.3	0	0	-	.1	.5	65	1.9	125	9	277	504	7	3.2
10	-	0	90	0	.2	0	0	-	.1	.2	61	1.2	134	10.5	362	466	310	4.7
10	-	0	90	0	.2	0	0	-	.1	.2	61	1.2	134	10.5	362	466	4	4.7
0	4	0	10	0	0	0	5	.6	0	0	5	0	10	.3	13	148	0	0
0	3	0	2	0	0	0	1	.6	0	0	6	.3	5	.3	9	83	6	.1
0	2	0	1	1	0	0	2	.6	0	0	11	.4	9	.2	15	119	5	.1
0	3	0	2	0	0	0	1	.6	0	0	6	.4	5	.2	9	83	6	.1
0	2	0	1	0	0	0	1	.6	0	0	5	.3	5	.1	9	65	2	.1
0	-	0	2	0	0	0	1	-	0	0	7	.3	5	.3	9	84	7	.1
0	-	0	1	0	0	0	2	-	0	0	9	.2	6	.5	9	56	2	.1
0	4	0	12	3	0	0	7	.8	.1	0	18	.4	10	.2	18	208	0	.2
0	3	0	14	438	.1	0	5	.3	0	.1	17	.6	11	.4	35	76	197	.4
0	3	0	21	621	.1	0	6	.3	.1	.2	18	.8	13	.9	39	126	54	.4
0	-	0	16	10	.1	0	2	-	0	.1	10	.5	10	.8	31	58	265	.3
0	3	0	18	32	.1	0	6	.1	.1	.1	13	.8	12	.9	31	105	33	.3
0	2	0	30	10	.1	0	44	.3	.1	.1	31	1.5	17	.4	38	145	3	.2
0	4	0	51	48	.2	0	11	.3	.1	.2	22	1.2	31	1.6	94	217	2	1
0	3	0	38	65	.1	0	8	.3	.1	.1	17	.8	14	.6	57	147	186	.6
0	-	0	24	37	.1	0	10	-	.1	.1	13	1	13	.6	46	104	216	.6
0	4	0	47	46	.1	0	29	.3	.1	.2	18	1.1	24	1.5	78	177	4	.9
0	4	0	47	54	.1	0	8	.1	.1	.2	19	1.3	23	1.2	72	134	70	.8
3	4	36	7	53	0	.1	1	-	.1	.1	19	1.2	20	.3	87	84	479	.6
9	4	0	21	7	.1	0	1	1.7	.1	.5	19	1.2	69	.5	157	212	1	3
1	-	30	-	150	-	-	-	-	.3	.5	160	2.5	-	3.8	240	350	470	-
-	4	45	-	80	-	-	5	-	-	-	540	1	-	-	-	320	650	-
0	1	0	7	45	.1	0	50	.5	0	0	5	.4	10	.6	12	137	856	.1
0	1	0	11	35	.1	0	109	.3	0	0	8	.5	11	.4	21	153	3	.1
0	1	0	7	868	.1	0	50	.3	0	0	5	.4	10	.6	12	137	856	.1
0	1	0	11	484	.1	0	109	.3	0	0	8	.5	11	.4	21	153	3	.1
0	-	0	5	58	.1	0	4	-	0	0	9	1	4	.2	6	46	497	.1
0	1	0	16	47	.2	0	66	.5	0	0	7	.3	7	.4	14	131	1	.1
0	2	0	16	422	.2	0	141	.5	0	0	7	.3	7	.4	14	131	1	.1
-	-	0	19	18	.1	0	136	-	0	0	8	.3	9	.7	18	157	1	.1
0	0	98	5	9	.1	1.9	1	-	.1	.1	87	1	32	1.6	219	293	67	1.2
-	-	18	-	-	-	-	3	-	0	0	1	.1	-	.1	-	155	341	-
0	0	0	0	4	0	0	0	-	0	0	1	.2	1	.1	3	11	164	0
0	0	0	0	3	0	0	0	-	0	0	1	.2	3	.1	6	12	164	0
0	-	0	0	2	0	0	0	-	0	0	0	.1	1	0	2	4	122	0
1	0	10	1	2	.1	.3	4	-	.1	.1	27	.3	5	.6	40	96	394	.4
1	0	10	1	8505	.1	.3	4	.1	.1	.1	27	.3	5	.6	40	96	394	.4
0	0	0	0	1	0	0	0	0	0	0	0	0	0	0	1	2	85	0
0	0	0	0	2	0	0	0	0	0	0	1	0	1	0	1	7	77	0
0	-	0	0	2	0	0	0	-	0	0	1	0	1	0	1	7	1	0
0	0	0	-	1	-	0	0	0	0	0	0	0	0	0	1	2	1	0
0	0	0	0	1	0	0	0	0	0	0	0	0	0	0	1	2	56	0
0	0	0	0	1	0	0	0	0	0	0	0	0	0	0	1	2	1	0
1	0	11	1	0	.1	.4	5	-	.1	.1	13	.3	4	.7	35	76	330	.6
0	0	43	15	20	.1	2	3	-	.1	.1	62	.6	34	2.4	240	282	42	.7
0	0	94	14	20	.1	2	0	-	.2	.3	120	1.4	32	2.4	229	424	55	.7
0	-	0	3	0	0	0	1	-	0	0	3	.1	3	0	2	22	2	0
2	0	0	6	0	0	0	0	.4	0	.1	3	.9	23	.4	51	60	0	.4

Code	Name	Amount	Unit	Grams	Energy (kcal)	Carbohydrates (g)	Protein (g)	Fat (g)	Saturated fat (g)	Monounsaturated fat (g)
9273	Pineapple Juice, Cnd	3/4	Cup	187.6	105	26	1	0	0	0
14334	Pineapple and Grapefruit Juice Drink, Cnd	3/4	Cup	187.6	88	22	0	0	0	0
14341	Pineapple and Orange Juice Drink, Cnd	3/4	Cup	187.6	94	22	2	0	0	0
9270	Pineapple, Cnd, Heavy Syrup Pack	1/2	Cup	127.5	99	26	0	0	0	0
9268	Pineapple, Cnd, Juice Pack	1/2	Cup	125.0	75	20	1	0	0	0
9269	Pineapple, Cnd, Light Syrup Pack	1/2	Cup	126.0	66	17	0	0	0	0
9267	Pineapple, Cnd, Water Pack	1/2	Cup	123.0	39	10	1	0	0	0
9271	Pineapple, Cnd, X-heavy Syrup Pack	1/2	Cup	130.0	108	28	0	0	0	0
9266	Pineapple, Fresh	1	Slice	84.0	41	10	0	0	0	0
12151	Pistachios, Dried	1/2	Cup	64.0	369	16	13	31	4	21
12652	Pistachios, Dry Roasted	1/2	Cup	64.0	388	18	10	34	4	23
9284	Plums, Cnd, Purple, Heavy Syrup Pack	1/2	Cup	129.0	115	30	0	0	0	0
9282	Plums, Cnd, Purple, Juice Pack	1/2	Cup	126.0	73	19	1	0	0	0
9283	Plums, Cnd, Purple, Light Syrup Pack	1/2	Cup	126.0	79	21	0	0	0	0
9281	Plums, Cnd, Purple, Water Pack	1/2	Cup	124.5	51	14	0	0	0	0
9285	Plums, Cnd, Purple, X-heavy Syrup Pack	1/2	Cup	130.5	132	34	0	0	0	0
9279	Plums, Fresh	1	Medium	66.0	36	9	1	0	0	0
15205	Pollock, Atlantic, Ckd, Dry Heat	3	Ounce	85.1	100	0	21	1	0	0
15069	Pompano, Florida, Ckd, Dry Heat	3	Ounce	85.1	179	0	20	10	4	3
19034	Popcorn, Air-popped	1	Cup	8.0	31	6	1	0	0	0
19806	Popcorn, Air-popped, White Popcorn	1	Cup	8.0	31	6	1	0	0	0
19036	Popcorn, Cakes	1	Cake	10.0	38	8	1	0	0	0
19038	Popcorn, Caramel-coated, w/ Peanuts	1	Cup	35.2	141	28	2	3	0	1
19039	Popcorn, Caramel-coated, w/o Peanuts	1	Cup	35.2	152	28	1	5	1	1
19040	Popcorn, Cheese-flavor	1	Cup	11.0	58	6	1	4	1	1
62649	Popcorn, Microwave	4	Cup	56.0	170	17	3	12	3	-
62650	Popcorn, Microwave, Low-Fat	4	Cup	56.0	93	15	3	4	1	-
19035	Popcorn, Oil-popped	1	Cup	11.0	55	6	1	3	1	1
19807	Popcorn, Oil-popped, White Popcorn	1	Cup	11.0	55	6	1	3	1	1
62602	Popsicles	1	Each	56.0	40	11	0	0	0	0
19408	Pork Skins, Barbecue-flavor	1	Ounce	28.4	153	0	16	9	3	4
9041	Pork Skins, Plain	1	Ounce	28.4	155	0	17	9	3	4
10193	Pork, Backribs	3	Ounce	85.1	315	0	21	25	9	11
10127	Pork, Braunschweiger	3	Ounce	85.1	305	3	11	27	9	13
7045	Pork, Cnd, Lunch Meat	1	Slice	21.0	70	0	3	6	2	3
10220	Pork, Ground, Ckd	3	Ounce	85.1	253	0	22	18	7	8
10147	Pork, Ham Patties, Grilled	3	Ounce	85.1	291	1	11	26	9	12
10148	Pork, Ham Salad Spread	3	Ounce	85.1	184	9	7	13	4	6
10154	Pork, Ham and Cheese Loaf or Roll	3	Ounce	85.1	220	1	14	17	6	8
10143	Pork, Ham, Chopped, Cnd	3	Ounce	85.1	203	0	14	16	5	8
10138	Pork, Ham, Cnd, Extra Lean (appx 4% Fat), Roasted	3	Ounce	85.1	116	0	18	4	1	2
10185	Pork, Ham, Cnd, Extra Lean and Reg, Roasted	3	Ounce	85.1	142	0	18	7	2	3
10184	Pork, Ham, Cnd, Extra Lean and Reg, Unheated	3	Ounce	85.1	122	0	15	6	2	3
10140	Pork, Ham, Cnd, Regular (approx 13% Fat), Roasted	3	Ounce	85.1	192	0	17	13	4	6
10134	Pork, Ham, Extra Lean (5% Fat), Roasted	3	Ounce	85.1	123	1	18	5	2	2
10133	Pork, Ham, Extra Lean (5% Fat), Unheated	3	Ounce	85.1	111	1	16	4	1	2
10183	Pork, Ham, Extra Lean and Reg, Roasted	3	Ounce	85.1	140	0	19	7	2	3
10182	Pork, Ham, Extra Lean and Reg, Unheated	3	Ounce	85.1	138	2	16	7	2	3
10153	Pork, Ham, Meat Only, Roasted	3	Ounce	85.1	134	0	21	5	2	2
10151	Pork, Ham, Meat and Fat, Roasted	3	Ounce	85.1	207	0	18	14	5	7
10136	Pork, Ham, Regular (11% Fat), Roasted	3	Ounce	85.1	151	0	19	8	3	4
10135	Pork, Ham, Regular (11% Fat), Unheated	3	Ounce	85.1	155	3	15	9	3	4
10172	Pork, Smoked Link Sausage, Grilled	3	Ounce	85.1	331	2	19	27	10	12
10089	Pork, Spareribs, Meat and Fat, Ckd, Braised	3	Ounce	85.1	338	0	25	26	9	11
10223	Pork, Tenderloin, Meat Only, Ckd, Broiled	3	Ounce	85.1	159	0	26	5	2	2
10221	Pork, Tenderloin, Meat and Fat, Ckd, Broiled	3	Ounce	85.1	171	0	25	7	2	3

Polyunsaturated fat (g)	Dietary Fiber (g)	Cholesterol (mg)	Folate (µg)	Vitamin A (RE)	Vitamin B-6 (mg)	Vitamin B-12 (µg)	Vitamin C (mg)	Vitamin E (mg)	Riboflavin (mg)	Thiamin (mg)	Calcium (mg)	Iron (mg)	Magnesium (mg)	Niacin (mg)	Phosphorus (mg)	Potassium (mg)	Sodium (mg)	Zinc (mg)
0	0	0	43	0	.2	0	20	0	0	.1	32	.5	24	.5	15	251	2	.2
0	0	0	20	8	.1	0	86	0	0	.1	13	.6	11	.5	11	114	26	.1
0	0	0	20	99	.1	0	42	0	0	.1	9	.5	11	.4	8	86	6	.1
0	1	0	6	1	.1	0	9	.1	0	.1	18	.5	20	.4	9	133	1	.2
0	1	0	6	5	.1	0	12	.1	0	.1	17	.3	17	.4	7	152	1	.1
0	1	0	6	1	.1	0	9	.1	0	.1	18	.5	20	.4	9	132	1	.2
0	1	0	6	2	.1	0	9	.1	0	.1	18	.5	22	.4	5	156	1	.1
0	-	0	6	1	.1	0	9	-	0	.1	18	.5	20	.4	9	133	1	.1
0	1	0	9	2	.1	0	13	.1	0	.1	6	.3	12	.4	6	95	1	.1
5	7	0	37	15	.2	0	5	3.3	.1	.5	86	4.3	101	.7	322	700	4	.9
5	7	0	38	15	.2	0	5	4.1	.2	.3	45	2	83	.9	305	621	499	.9
0	1	0	3	34	0	0	1	.9	0	0	12	1.1	6	.4	17	117	25	.1
0	1	0	3	127	0	0	4	.9	.1	0	13	.4	10	.6	19	194	1	.1
0	1	0	3	33	0	0	1	.9	0	0	11	1.1	6	.4	16	117	25	.1
0	1	0	3	113	0	0	3	.9	.1	0	9	.2	6	.5	16	157	1	.1
0	-	0	3	33	0	0	1	-	0	0	12	1.1	7	.4	16	116	25	.1
0	1	0	1	21	.1	0	6	.4	.1	0	3	.1	5	.3	7	114	0	.1
1	0	77	3	10	.3	3.1	0	-	.2	0	65	.5	73	3.4	241	388	94	.5
1	0	54	15	31	.2	1	0	-	.1	.6	37	.6	26	3.2	290	541	65	.6
0	1	0	2	2	0	0	0	0	0	0	1	.2	10	.2	24	24	0	.3
0	-	0	2	0	0	0	0	-	0	0	1	.2	10	.2	24	24	0	.3
0	0	0	2	1	0	0	0	0	0	0	1	.2	16	.6	28	33	29	.4
1	1	0	6	2	.1	0	0	.5	0	0	23	1.4	28	.7	45	125	104	.4
2	2	2	1	4	0	0	0	.4	0	0	15	.6	12	.8	29	38	73	.2
2	1	1	1	5	0	.1	0	0	0	0	12	.2	10	.2	40	29	98	.2
-	3	0	0	0	0	0	0	-	0	0	0	.2	0	0	0	-	290	0
-	2	0	0	0	0	0	0	-	0	0	0	.3	0	0	0	-	220	0
1	1	0	2	2	0	0	0	0	0	0	1	.3	12	.2	27	25	97	.3
1	-	0	2	0	0	0	0	-	0	0	1	.3	12	.2	27	25	97	.3
0	0	0	-	0	-	-	1	-	-	-	0	0	-	-	-	-	10	-
1	-	33	9	52	0	0	0	-	.1	0	12	.3	0	1	62	51	756	.2
1	-	27	0	11	0	.2	0	-	.1	0	9	.2	3	.4	24	36	521	.2
2	-	100	3	3	.3	.5	0	-	.2	.4	38	1.2	18	3	166	268	86	2.9
3	0	133	37	3589	.3	17.1	8	-	1.3	.2	8	8	9	7.1	143	169	972	2.4
1	0	13	1	0	0	.2	0	-	0	.1	1	.2	2	.7	17	45	271	.3
2	0	80	5	2	.3	.5	1	-	.2	.6	19	1.1	20	3.6	192	308	62	2.7
3	0	61	3	0	.1	.6	0	.2	.2	.3	8	1.4	9	2.8	86	208	904	1.6
2	0	31	1	0	.1	.6	5	-	.1	.4	7	.5	9	1.8	102	128	776	.9
2	0	48	3	20	.2	.7	21	-	.2	.5	49	.8	14	2.9	215	250	1142	1.7
2	0	42	1	0	.3	.6	2	-	.1	.5	6	.8	11	2.7	118	242	1161	1.6
0	0	26	4	0	.4	.6	23	.2	.2	.9	5	.8	18	4.2	178	296	965	1.9
1	0	35	4	0	.3	.7	19	.2	.2	.8	6	.9	17	4.3	188	299	908	2
1	0	32	5	0	.4	.7	21	.2	.2	.7	5	.8	14	3.9	176	284	1085	1.6
2	0	53	4	0	.3	.9	12	-	.2	.7	7	1.2	14	4.5	207	304	800	2.1
0	0	45	3	0	.3	.6	18	.2	.2	.6	7	1.3	12	3.4	167	244	1023	2.4
0	0	40	3	0	.4	.6	22	.2	.2	.8	6	.6	14	4.1	185	298	1215	1.6
1	0	48	3	0	.3	.6	19	.2	.2	.6	7	1.2	16	4.5	211	308	1178	2.2
1	0	45	3	0	.3	.7	23	.2	.2	.8	6	.8	15	4.3	201	253	1087	1.7
1	0	47	3	0	.4	.6	-	.2	.2	.6	6	.8	19	4.3	193	269	1129	2.2
2	0	53	3	0	.3	.5	-	.2	.2	.5	6	.7	16	3.8	182	243	1010	2
1	0	50	3	0	.3	.6	19	.2	.3	.6	7	1.1	19	5.2	239	348	1276	2.1
1	0	48	3	0	.3	.7	24	.2	.2	.7	6	.8	16	4.5	210	282	1120	1.8
3	0	58	4	0	.3	1.4	2	.3	.2	.6	26	1	16	3.9	138	286	1276	2.4
2	0	103	3	3	.3	.9	-	.2	.3	.3	40	1.6	20	4.7	222	272	79	3.9
0	-	80	5	2	.4	.9	1	-	.3	.8	4	1.2	31	4.4	251	384	55	2.5
1	-	80	5	2	.4	.8	1		.0	.0	4	1.2	30	4.3	247	378	54	2.5

Code	Name	Amount	Unit	Grams	Energy (kcal)	Carbohydrates (g)	Protein (g)	Fat (g)	Saturated fat (g)	Monounsaturated fat (g)
19042	Potato Chips, Barbecue-flavor	1	Ounce	28.4	139	15	2	9	2	2
19421	Potato Chips, Cheese-flavor	1	Ounce	28.4	141	16	2	8	2	2
19422	Potato Chips, Light	1	Ounce	28.4	134	19	2	6	1	1
19411	Potato Chips, Plain, Salted	1	Ounce	28.4	152	15	2	10	3	3
19811	Potato Chips, Plain, Unsalted	1	Ounce	28.4	152	15	2	10	3	3
19412	Potato Chips, Pringles, Cheese-flavor	1	Ounce	28.4	156	14	2	10	3	2
19045	Potato Chips, Pringles, Light	1	Ounce	28.4	142	18	2	7	1	2
19410	Potato Chips, Pringles, Plain	1	Ounce	28.4	158	14	2	11	3	2
19046	Potato Chips, Pringles, Sour-cream&onion-flavor	1	Ounce	28.4	155	15	2	10	3	2
19043	Potato Chips, Sour-cream-and-onion-flavor	1	Ounce	28.4	151	15	2	10	3	2
11920	Potato Chips, w/o Salt Added	1	Ounce	28.4	148	15	2	10	3	2
11672	Potato Pancakes, Home-prepared	1	Ounce	28.4	77	8	2	4	1	1
11399	Potato Puffs, Frz, Prepared	1	Each	7.0	16	2	0	1	0	0
11414	Potato Salad	1/2	Cup	125.0	179	14	3	10	2	3
19415	Potato Sticks	1	Ounce	28.4	148	15	2	10	3	2
55174	Potatoes Au Gratin-Stouffer's	1	Each	163.0	170	17	5	9	-	-
11843	Potatoes, Au Gratin, Home-prepared	1/2	Cup	122.5	162	14	6	9	4	3
11363	Potatoes, Baked w/o Skin	1	Medium	202.0	188	44	4	0	0	0
11364	Potatoes, Baked, Skin only	1	Each	58.0	115	27	2	0	0	0
11674	Potatoes, Baked, w/ Skin	1	Medium	202.0	220	51	5	0	0	0
11365	Potatoes, Boiled, Ckd In Skin w/o Skin	1	Medium	202.0	176	41	4	0	0	0
11367	Potatoes, Boiled, Ckd w/o Skin	1	Medium	202.0	174	40	3	0	0	0
11366	Potatoes, Boiled, Skin only	1	Each	34.0	27	6	1	0	0	0
11376	Potatoes, Cnd, Drained Solids	1/2	Cup	90.0	54	12	1	0	0	0
11374	Potatoes, Cnd, Solids and Liquids	1/2	Cup	150.0	60	13	2	0	0	0
11370	Potatoes, Hashed Brown	1/2	Cup	78.0	119	6	2	11	4	5
11657	Potatoes, Mashed, Home-prepared	1/2	Cup	105.0	81	18	2	1	0	0
11930	Potatoes, Mashed, Prepared From Flakes	1/2	Cup	105.0	119	16	2	6	2	2
11368	Potatoes, Microwaved w/o Skin	1/2	Cup	78.0	78	18	2	0	0	0
11369	Potatoes, Microwaved, Skin only	1	Each	58.0	77	17	3	0	0	0
11675	Potatoes, Microwaved, w/ Skin	1	Medium	202.0	212	49	5	0	0	0
11671	Potatoes, O'brien, Home-prepared	1/2	Cup	97.0	79	15	2	1	1	0
11844	Potatoes, Scalloped	1/2	Cup	122.5	105	13	4	5	2	2
62693	Power Bar	1	Each	65.0	230	45	10	3	1	2
19216	Praline	1	Piece	39.0	177	24	1	9	1	6
19047	Pretzels, Hard, Plain, Salted	1	Ounce	28.4	108	22	3	1	0	0
19814	Pretzels, Hard, Plain, Unsalted	1	Ounce	28.4	108	22	3	1	0	0
19050	Pretzels, Hard, Whole-wheat	1	Ounce	28.4	103	23	3	1	0	0
9294	Prune Juice, Cnd	3/4	Cup	191.8	136	33	1	0	0	0
9289	Prunes, Dehydrated	1/4	Cup	33.0	112	29	1	0	0	0
9293	Prunes, Dried, Stewed, w/ Added Sugar	1/4	Cup	59.5	74	20	1	0	0	0
9292	Prunes, Dried, Stewed, w/o Added Sugar	1/4	Cup	53.0	57	15	1	0	0	0
9291	Prunes, Dried, Uncooked	1/4	Cup	40.3	96	25	1	0	0	0
19072	Pudding Pops, Chocolate	1	Each	47.0	72	12	2	2	-	-
19073	Pudding Pops, Vanilla	1	Each	47.0	75	13	2	2	-	-
18326	Pumpkin Pie	1	Slice	109.0	229	30	4	10	2	5
11423	Pumpkin, Ckd	1/2	Cup	122.5	24	6	1	0	0	0
11424	Pumpkin, Cnd, w/o Salt	1/2	Cup	122.5	42	10	1	0	0	0
11429	Radishes, Fresh	1/2	Cup	58.0	10	2	0	0	0	0
11431	Radishes, Oriental, Ckd	1/2	Cup	73.5	12	3	0	0	0	0
11432	Radishes, Oriental, Dried	1/2	Cup	58.0	157	37	5	0	0	0
11430	Radishes, Oriental, Fresh	1/2	Cup	44.0	8	2	0	0	0	0
11637	Radishes, White Icicle, Fresh	1/2	Cup	50.0	7	1	1	0	0	0
18191	Raisin Cookies, Soft-type	1	Each	15.0	60	10	1	2	1	1
19149	Raisinets	10	Piece	10.0	41	7	0	2	1	1
9297	Raisins, Golden Seedless	1/2	Cup	72.5	219	58	2	0	0	0

Polyunsaturated fat (g)	Dietary Fiber (g)	Cholesterol (mg)	Folate (μg)	Vitamin A (RE)	Vitamin B-6 (mg)	Vitamin B-12 (μg)	Vitamin C (mg)	Vitamin E (mg)	Riboflavin (mg)	Thiamin (mg)	Calcium (mg)	Iron (mg)	Magnesium (mg)	Niacin (mg)	Phosphorus (mg)	Potassium (mg)	Sodium (mg)	Zinc (mg)
5	1	0	24	6	.2	0	10	1.4	.1	.1	14	.5	21	1.3	53	357	213	.3
3	-	1	0	2	.1	0	15	-	0	0	20	.5	21	1.4	85	433	225	.3
3	-	0	8	0	.2	0	7	-	.1	.1	6	.4	25	2	55	494	139	0
3	1	0	13	0	.2	0	9	1.4	.1	0	7	.5	19	1.1	47	361	168	.3
3	-	0	13	0	.2	0	9	-	.1	0	7	.5	19	1.1	47	361	2	.3
5	-	1	5	0	.1	0	2	-	0	.1	31	.5	15	.7	46	108	214	.2
4	1	0	7	0	.2	0	3	1.4	0	.1	10	.4	18	1.2	44	285	121	.2
6	1	0	2	0	0	0	2	1.4	0	.1	7	.4	16	.9	45	286	186	.2
5	-	1	7	28	.1	0	3	-	0	.1	18	.4	16	.7	48	141	204	.2
5	1	2	18	6	.2	.3	11	-	.1	.1	20	.5	21	1.1	50	377	177	.3
5	1	0	13	0	.1	0	12	2.2	0	0	7	.3	17	1.2	43	368	2	.3
2	1	27	7	4	.1	.1	6	0	0	0	7	.4	9	.6	31	223	144	.2
0	0	0	1	0	0	0	0	0	0	0	2	.1	1	.2	3	27	52	0
5	-	85	8	41	.2	0	12	-	.1	.1	24	.8	19	1.1	65	317	661	.4
5	1	0	11	0	.1	0	13	1.4	0	0	5	.6	18	1.4	49	351	71	.3
-	-	-	-	20	-	-	4	-	.1	-	48	.8	-	.8	-	260	670	-
1	-	18	10	47	.2	0	12	-	.1	.1	146	.8	24	1.2	138	485	530	.8
0	3	0	18	0	.6	0	26	.1	0	.2	10	.7	51	2.8	101	790	10	.6
0	2	0	13	0	.4	0	8	0	.1	.1	20	4.1	25	1.8	59	332	12	.3
0	5	0	22	0	.7	0	26	.1	.1	.2	20	2.7	55	3.3	115	844	16	.6
0	4	0	20	0	.6	0	26	.1	0	.2	10	.6	44	2.9	89	766	8	.6
0	4	0	18	0	.5	0	15	.1	0	.2	16	.6	40	2.7	81	663	10	.5
0	-	0	3	0	.1	0	2	-	0	0	15	2.1	10	.4	18	138	5	.1
0	-	0	6	0	.2	0	5	-	0	0	4	1.1	13	.8	25	206	234	.3
0	2	0	7	0	.2	0	19	.1	0	.1	45	1.5	21	1.3	33	364	451	.6
1	2	-	6	0	.2	0	4	.1	0	.1	6	.6	16	1.6	33	250	19	.2
0	2	2	9	20	.2	0	7	.1	0	.1	27	.3	19	1.2	50	314	318	.3
2	-	4	8	22	0	0	10	-	.1	.1	51	.2	19	.7	59	245	349	.2
0	-	0	10	0	.2	0	12	-	0	.1	4	.3	20	1.3	85	321	5	.3
0	-	0	10	0	.3	0	9	-	0	0	27	3.4	21	1.3	48	377	9	.3
0	-	0	24	0	.7	0	31	-	.1	.2	22	2.5	55	3.5	212	903	16	.7
0	-	4	8	55	.2	0	16	-	.1	.1	35	.5	17	1	49	258	210	.3
1	-	7	11	23	.2	0	13	-	.1	.1	70	.7	23	1.3	77	463	410	.5
1	3	0	200	0	2	2	0	-	1.7	1.5	360	3.5	123	19	280	-	90	5.3
2	-	0	5	2	0	0	0	-	0	.1	12	.5	20	.1	43	82	24	.8
0	1	0	24	0	0	0	0	.1	.2	.1	10	1.2	10	1.5	32	41	486	.2
0	1	0	24	0	0	0	0	.1	.2	.1	10	1.2	10	1.5	32	41	82	.2
0	-	0	15	0	.1	0	0	-	.1	.1	8	.8	9	1.9	35	122	58	.2
0	2	0	1	0	.4	0	8	0	.1	0	23	2.3	27	1.5	48	529	8	.4
0	-	0	1	58	.2	0	0	-	.1	0	24	1.2	21	1	37	349	2	.2
0	2	0	0	17	.1	0	2	0	.1	0	12	.6	11	.4	20	186	1	.1
0	3	0	0	16	.1	0	2	0	.1	0	12	.6	11	.4	19	177	1	.1
0	3	0	1	80	.1	0	1	.6	.1	0	21	1	18	.8	32	300	2	.2
-	0	1	1	16	0	.3	0	0	.1	0	66	.2	10	.1	53	105	78	.2
-	0	1	2	24	0	.2	0	0	.1	0	61	0	5	0	47	65	50	.2
2	3	22	16	523	.1	.4	2	-	.2	.1	65	.9	16	.2	77	168	307	.5
0	-	0	10	132	.1	0	6	-	.1	0	18	.7	11	.5	37	282	1	.3
0	3	0	15	2702	.1	0	5	1.3	.1	0	32	1.7	28	.4	43	252	6	.2
0	1	0	16	1	0	0	13	0	0	0	12	.2	5	.2	10	135	14	.2
0	1	0	13	0	0	0	11	0	0	0	12	.1	7	.1	18	209	10	.1
0	-	0	171	0	.4	0	0	-	.4	.2	365	3.9	99	2	118	2027	161	1.2
0	1	0	12	0	0	0	10	0	0	0	12	.2	7	.1	10	100	9	.1
0	-	0	7	0	0	0	15	-	0	0	14	.4	5	.2	14	140	8	.1
0	-	0	1	2	0	0	0	-	0	0	7	.3	3	.3	12	21	51	0
0	-	0	1	1	0	0	0	-	0	0	11	.1	5	0	14	51	4	.1
0	3	0	2	3	.2	0	2	.5	.1	0	38	1.3	25	.8	83	541	9	.2

Code	Name	Amount	Unit	Grams	Energy (kcal)	Carbohydrates (g)	Protein (g)	Fat (g)	Saturated fat (g)	Monounsaturated fat (g)
9299	Raisins, Seeded	1/2	Cup	72.5	215	57	2	0	0	0
9298	Raisins, Seedless	1/2	Cup	72.5	218	57	2	0	0	0
9304	Raspberries, Cnd, Red, Heavy Syrup Pack	1/2	Cup	128.0	116	30	1	0	0	0
9302	Raspberries, Fresh	1/2	Cup	61.5	30	7	1	0	0	0
9306	Raspberries, Frozen, Red, Sweetened	1/2	Cup	125.0	129	33	1	0	0	0
62536	Ravioli, Beef	1	Cup	243.9	230	36	9	5	2	-
62537	Ravioli, Cheese	1	Cup	243.9	220	38	9	3	1	-
62557	Red Beans and Rice	2	Ounce	56.7	189	40	8	1	0	-
62607	Reduced Fat Chocolate Chip Cookies	13	Each	5.8	26	4	0	1	0	0
62595	Reduced Fat Chocolate Sandwich Cookies-SnackWell	2	Each	25.0	100	-	1	3	1	1
62593	Reduced Fat Classic Golden Crackers-SnackWell	6	Each	14.0	60	11	1	1	0	0
62594	Reduced Fat Creme Sandwich Cookies-SnackWell	2	Each	26.0	110	21	1	3	1	1
62597	Reduced Fat French Onion Snack Crackers-SnackWell	32	Each	30.0	120	23	2	2	0	1
62598	Reduced Fat Oatmeal Raisin Cookies-SnackWell	2	Each	27.0	110	20	2	3	0	1
62525	Reduced Fat Zesty Cheese Snack Crackers-SnackWell	32	Each	30.0	120	23	3	2	1	1
19150	Reese's Peanut Butter Cups	1	Each	7.0	34	3	1	2	2	0
19151	Reese's Pieces Candy	1	Pkg	55.0	258	34	7	11	-	-
62632	Refried Beans, Fat Free	1/2	Cup	134.0	120	21	8	0	0	-
19052	Rice Cakes, Brown Rice, Buckwheat	1	Cake	9.0	34	7	1	0	0	0
19817	Rice Cakes, Brown Rice, Buckwheat, Unsalted	1	Cake	9.0	34	7	1	0	0	0
19413	Rice Cakes, Brown Rice, Corn	1	Cake	9.0	35	7	1	0	0	0
19414	Rice Cakes, Brown Rice, Multigrain	1	Cake	9.0	35	7	1	0	0	0
19818	Rice Cakes, Brown Rice, Multigrain, Unsalted	1	Cake	9.0	35	7	1	0	0	0
19051	Rice Cakes, Brown Rice, Plain	1	Cake	9.0	35	7	1	0	0	0
19816	Rice Cakes, Brown Rice, Plain, Unsalted	1	Cake	9.0	35	7	1	0	0	0
19416	Rice Cakes, Brown Rice, Rye	1	Cake	9.0	35	7	1	0	0	0
62669	Rice Krispie Treats	1	Cup	40.0	160	33	1	2	0	1
19193	Rice Pudding	1	Cup	298.1	486	66	6	22	3	10
20037	Rice, Brown, Long-grain, Ckd	1/2	Cup	97.5	108	22	3	1	0	0
20041	Rice, Brown, Medium-grain, Ckd	1/2	Cup	97.5	109	23	2	1	0	0
20045	Rice, White, Long-grain, Ckd	1/2	Cup	79.0	103	22	2	0	0	0
20049	Rice, White, Long-grain, Instant, Enriched	1/2	Cup	82.5	81	18	2	0	0	0
20051	Rice, White, Medium-grain, Ckd	1/2	Cup	93.0	121	27	2	0	0	0
20053	Rice, White, Short-grain, Ckd	1/2	Cup	93.0	121	27	2	0	0	0
20057	Rice, White, w/ Pasta, Ckd	1/2	Cup	101.0	123	22	3	3	1	1
62662	Rice-a-Roni Wild Rice	1	Cup	56.0	240	43	5	1	0	0
55222	Rigatoni Bake, Lean Cuisine-Stouffer's	1	Each	276.4	250	27	18	8	3	-
41341	Rigatoni in Meat Sauce-Healthy Choice	1	Each	269.3	260	34	16	6	2	-
55782	Rigatoni w/ Meat Sauce-Stouffer's	1/2	Cup	142.0	145	16	8	6	-	-
62614	Roast Turkey Medallions-Weight Watchers	1	Each	241.0	190	34	10	2	1	-
41310	Roasted Turkey and Mushrooms in Gravy-Healthy Choice	1	Each	241.0	200	26	18	3	1	-
15071	Rockfish, Pacific, Ckd, Dry Heat	3	Ounce	85.1	103	0	20	2	0	0
14157	Root Beer	12	Fl Oz	369.6	152	39	0	0	0	0
62531	Root Beer, Diet	12	Fl Oz	355.2	0	0	0	0	-	-
15232	Roughy, Orange, Ckd, Dry Heat	3	Ounce	85.1	76	0	16	1	0	1
62541	Salad Dressing, Blue Cheese	2	Tbsp.	32.0	90	5	1	7	4	-
62542	Salad Dressing, Blue Cheese, Fat Free	2	Tbsp.	35.0	50	12	1	0	0	-
4120	Salad Dressing, French	2	Tbsp.	31.3	134	5	0	13	3	3
62545	Salad Dressing, French, Fat Free	2	Tbsp.	35.0	50	12	0	0	0	-
4020	Salad Dressing, French, Lo Fat	2	Tbsp.	32.5	44	7	0	2	0	0
4114	Salad Dressing, Italian	2	Tbsp.	29.4	137	3	0	14	2	3
62543	Salad Dressing, Italian, Fat Free	2	Tbsp.	31.0	10	2	0	0	0	-
4021	Salad Dressing, Italian, Lo Cal	2	Tbsp.	30.0	32	1	0	3	0	1
62539	Salad Dressing, Ranch	2	Tbsp.	29.0	170	2	0	18	3	-
62540	Salad Dressing, Ranch, Fat Free	2	Tbsp.	35.0	50	11	0	0	0	-
4015	Salad Dressing, Russian	2	Tbsp.	30.7	151	3	0	16	2	4

Polyunsaturated fat (g)	Dietary Fiber (g)	Cholesterol (mg)	Folate (µg)	Vitamin A (RE)	Vitamin B-6 (mg)	Vitamin B-12 (µg)	Vitamin C (mg)	Vitamin E (mg)	Riboflavin (mg)	Thiamin (mg)	Calcium (mg)	Iron (mg)	Magnesium (mg)	Niacin (mg)	Phosphorus (mg)	Potassium (mg)	Sodium (mg)	Zinc (mg)
0	5	0	2	0	.1	0	4	.5	.1	.1	20	1.9	22	.8	54	598	20	.1
0	3	0	2	1	.2	0	2	.5	.1	.1	36	1.5	24	.6	70	544	9	.2
0	4	0	13	4	.1	0	11	.6	0	0	14	.5	15	.6	12	120	4	.2
0	4	0	16	8	0	0	15	.3	.1	0	14	.4	11	.6	7	93	0	.3
0	5	0	32	7	0	0	21	.6	.1	0	19	.8	16	.3	21	142	1	.2
-	4	20	-	150	-	-	2	-	-	-	0	1.5	-	-	-	-	1150	-
-	4	15	-	60	-	-	1	-	-	-	24	1.5	-	-	-	-	1280	-
-	7	0	-	99	-	-	6	-	-	.2	48	1.5	-	2.8	-	-	786	-
0	0	0	-	0	-	-	0	-	-	-	0	.1	-	-	-	-	34	-
0	1	0	-	0	-	-	0	-	-	-	0	.4	-	-	-	-	190	-
0	0	0	-	0	-	-	0	-	-	-	24	.4	-	-	-	-	140	-
0	1	0	-	0	-	-	0	-	-	-	24	.2	-	-	-	-	95	-
-	1	23	-	0	-	-	0	-	-	-	48	.6	-	-	-	-	290	-
1	1	0	-	0	-	-	0	-	-	-	24	.4	-	-	-	-	135	-
0	1	5	0	0	0	0	0	0	0	0	48	.6	0	0	0	0	350	0
0	0	1	2	1	0	0	0	.1	0	0	5	.1	6	.3	17	28	20	.1
-	2	2	31	2	.1	.2	0	.7	.1	0	73	.8	45	3.1	127	242	83	.6
-	7	0	-	0	-	-	0	-	-	-	0	1	-	-	-	-	480	-
0	0	0	2	0	0	0	0	-	0	0	1	.1	14	.7	34	27	10	.2
0	-	0	2	0	0	0	0	-	0	0	1	.1	14	.7	34	27	0	.2
0	0	0	2	0	0	0	0	-	0	0	1	.1	10	.6	29	25	26	.2
0	0	0	2	0	0	0	0	-	0	0	2	.2	12	.6	33	26	23	.2
0	-	0	2	0	0	0	0	-	0	0	2	.2	12	.6	33	26	0	.2
0	0	0	2	0	0	0	0	.1	0	0	1	.1	12	.7	32	26	29	.3
0	0	0	2	0	0	0	0	0	0	0	1	.1	12	.7	32	26	2	.3
0	0	0	0	0	0	0	0	-	0	0	2	.2	13	.6	34	28	10	.3
0	0	0	0	200	.7	.7	20	-	.6	.5	0	1.3	0	6.3	21	27	227	0
8	-	3	9	104	.1	.6	1	-	.2	.1	155	.9	24	.5	203	179	253	1.5
0	2	0	4	0	.1	0	0	.7	0	.1	10	.4	42	1.5	81	42	5	.6
0	-	0	4	0	.1	0	0	-	0	.1	10	.5	43	1.3	75	77	1	.6
0	0	0	2	0	.1	0	0	0	0	.1	8	.9	9	1.2	34	28	1	.4
0	0	0	3	0	0	0	0	0	0	.1	7	.5	4	.7	12	3	2	.2
0	0	0	2	0	0	0	0	-	0	.2	3	1.4	12	1.7	34	27	0	.4
0	-	0	2	0	.1	0	0	-	0	.2	1	1.4	7	1.4	31	24	0	.4
1	4	1	7	0	.1	.1	0	-	.1	.1	8	.9	12	1.8	37	42	574	.3
0	1	0	0	80	0	0	6	-	.1	.2	48	.8	0	1.5	0	-	1110	0
1	-	25	-	200	-	-	6	-	.3	.2	160	1.5	-	3.8	-	620	430	-
-	-	30	-	200	-	-	2	-	.3	.3	120	1.5	-	2.9	200	700	540	-
-	-	15	-	-	-	-	24	-	0	0	1	.2	-	.4	-	310	426	-
-	4	20	-	100	-	-	5	-	-	-	24	1	-	-	-	220	530	-
1	-	40	-	200	-	-	-	-	.1	.1	16	.8	-	2.9	150	260	380	-
1	0	37	9	56	.2	1	0	-	.1	0	10	.5	29	3.3	194	442	65	.5
0	0	0	0	0	0	0	0	0	0	0	18	.2	4	0	0	4	48	.3
-	0	-	-	-	-	-	-	-	-	-	-	-	-	-	-	-	30	-
0	0	22	7	20	.3	2	0	-	.2	.1	32	.2	32	3.1	218	327	69	.8
-	0	10	-	0	-	-	0	-	-	-	24	0	-	-	-	-	470	-
-	0	0	-	0	-	-	0	.4	-	-	0	0	-	-	-	-	340	-
7	0	18	1	6	0	0	0	2.6	0	0	3	.1	0	0	4	25	428	0
-	0	0	-	100	-	-	0	-	-	-	0	0	-	-	-	-	300	-
1	0	2	0	0	0	0	0	.5	0	0	4	.1	0	0	5	26	256	.1
8	0	0	1	7	0	0	0	3	0	0	3	.1	0	0	1	4	231	0
-	0	0	-	0	-	-	0	-	-	-	0	0	-	-	-	-	290	-
2	0	2	0	0	0	0	0	.5	0	0	1	.1	0	0	2	5	236	0
-	0	5	-	0	-	-	0	-	-	-	0	0	-	-	-	-	270	-
-	0	0	-	0	-	-	0	.6	-	-	0	0	-	-	-	-	310	-
0	0	0	0	03	0	.1	2	3.1	0	0	6	.2	0	.2	11	48	266	.1

Code	Name	Amount	Unit	Grams	Energy (kcal)	Carbohydrates (g)	Protein (g)	Fat (g)	Saturated fat (g)	Monounsaturated fat (g)
4022	Salad Dressing, Russian, Low Cal	2	Tbsp.	32.5	46	9	0	1	0	0
4016	Salad Dressing, Sesame Seed	2	Tbsp.	30.7	136	3	1	14	2	4
4017	Salad Dressing, Thousand Island	2	Tbsp.	31.3	118	5	0	11	2	3
62544	Salad Dressing, Thousand Island, Fat Free	2	Tbsp.	35.0	45	11	0	0	0	-
4023	Salad Dressing, Thousand Island, Lo Cal	2	Tbsp.	30.7	49	5	0	3	0	1
4135	Salad Dressing, Vinegar and Oil	2	Tbsp.	31.3	140	1	0	16	3	5
41290	Salisbury Steak w/ Mushroom Gravy-Healthy Choice	1	Each	311.8	280	35	21	6	3	-
43402	Salisbury Steak, Top Shelf-Hormel	1	Each	283.5	320	22	25	15	7	8
15209	Salmon, Atlantic, Wild, Ckd, Dry Heat	3	Ounce	85.1	155	0	22	7	1	2
15210	Salmon, Chinook, Ckd, Dry Heat	3	Ounce	85.1	196	0	22	11	3	5
15211	Salmon, Chum, Ckd, Dry Heat	3	Ounce	85.1	131	0	22	4	1	2
15087	Salmon, Cnd.	3	Ounce	85.1	130	0	17	6	1	2
15239	Salmon, Coho, Farmed, Ckd, Dry Heat	3	Ounce	85.1	151	0	21	7	2	3
15247	Salmon, Coho, Wild, Ckd, Dry Heat	3	Ounce	85.1	118	0	20	4	1	1
15082	Salmon, Coho, Wild, Ckd, Moist Heat	3	Ounce	85.1	156	0	23	6	1	2
15212	Salmon, Pink, Ckd, Dry Heat	3	Ounce	85.1	127	0	22	4	1	1
62546	Salsa	2	Tbsp.	33.0	20	5	0	0	0	-
41262	Salsa Chicken-Healthy Choice	1	Each	318.9	240	36	20	2	1	-
62651	Salt Substitute	1/4	Tsp.	1.2	0	-	-	0	-	-
2047	Salt, Table	1	Tsp.	6.0	0	0	0	0	0	0
15088	Sardine, Atlantic, Cnd In Oil	3	Ounce	85.1	177	0	21	10	1	3
6313	Sauce, White	1/2	Cup	131.9	120	11	5	7	3	2
11439	Sauerkraut, Cnd, Sol&liq	1/2	Cup	118.0	22	5	1	0	0	0
7003	Sausage, Beerwurst, Pork	1	Slice	23.0	55	0	3	4	1	2
7006	Sausage, Bockwurst	1	Link	65.0	200	0	9	18	7	8
7013	Sausage, Bratwurst	1	Link	85.0	256	2	12	22	8	10
7089	Sausage, Italian, Ckd	1	Link	83.0	268	1	17	21	8	10
7037	Sausage, Kielbasa, Kolbassy	1	Link	85.0	264	2	11	23	8	11
7038	Sausage, Knockwurst	1	Link	68.0	209	1	8	19	7	9
7075	Sausage, Link, Pork and Beef	1	Link	68.0	228	1	9	21	7	10
16107	Sausage, Meatless	1	Link	25.0	64	2	5	5	1	1
7057	Sausage, Pepperoni	1	Slice	5.5	27	0	1	2	1	1
7059	Sausage, Polish-style	1	Each	227.0	740	4	32	65	23	31
7064	Sausage, Pork, Links or Bulk, Ckd	1	Link	13.0	48	0	3	4	1	2
7072	Sausage, Salami, Beef and Pork, Dry	1	Slice	10.0	42	0	2	3	1	2
7068	Sausage, Salami, Beef, Ckd	1	Slice	23.0	60	1	3	5	2	2
7074	Sausage, Smoked Link, Pork	1	Link	68.0	265	1	15	22	8	10
62661	Sausage, Turkey	3	Ounce	85.1	135	5	12	8	4	0
15173	Scallop, Breaded and Fried	3	Ounce	85.1	183	9	15	9	2	4
15174	Scallop, Imitation	3	Ounce	85.1	84	9	11	0	0	0
43412	Scalloped Potatoes and Ham, Micro Cup-Hormel	1	Each	212.6	260	21	8	16	6	8
55175	Scalloped Potatoes-Stouffer's	1	Each	163.0	130	16	4	6	-	-
62652	Scallops, Sauteed	3	Ounce	85.1	150	2	29	1	0	-
14018	Screwdriver	1	Fl Oz	30.4	25	3	0	0	0	0
15092	Sea Bass, Ckd, Dry Heat	3	Ounce	85.1	105	0	20	2	1	0
12036	Seeds, Sunflower, Dried	1/2	Cup	72.0	410	14	16	36	4	7
12537	Seeds, Sunflower, Dry Roasted, w/ Salt added	1/2	Cup	64.0	372	15	12	32	3	6
12037	Seeds, Sunflower, Dry Roasted, w/o Salt	1/2	Cup	64.0	372	15	12	32	3	6
12538	Seeds, Sunflower, Oil Roasted, w/ Salt added	1/2	Cup	67.5	415	10	14	39	4	7
12038	Seeds, Sunflower, Oil Roasted, w/o Salt	1/2	Cup	67.5	415	10	14	39	4	7
12539	Seeds, Sunflower, Toasted, w/ Salt added	1/2	Cup	67.0	415	14	12	38	4	7
12039	Seeds, Sunflower, Toasted, w/o Salt	1/2	Cup	67.0	415	14	12	38	4	7
19418	Sesame Sticks, Wheat-based, Salted	1	Ounce	28.4	153	13	3	10	2	3
19820	Sesame Sticks, Wheat-based, Unsalted	1	Ounce	28.4	153	13	3	10	2	3
14346	Shake, Chocolate	1-1/2	Cup	339.6	431	70	12	13	8	4
14428	Shake, Strawberry	1-1/2	Cup	339.6	384	64	12	10	6	-

Polyunsaturated fat (g)	Dietary Fiber (g)	Cholesterol (mg)	Folate (µg)	Vitamin A (RE)	Vitamin B-6 (mg)	Vitamin B-12 (µg)	Vitamin C (mg)	Vitamin E (mg)	Riboflavin (mg)	Thiamin (mg)	Calcium (mg)	Iron (mg)	Magnesium (mg)	Niacin (mg)	Phosphorus (mg)	Potassium (mg)	Sodium (mg)	Zinc (mg)
1	0	2	1	5	0	0	2	.2	0	0	6	.2	0	0	12	51	282	0
8	-	0	0	63	0	0	0	1.5	0	0	6	.2	0	0	11	48	307	0
6	1	8	2	30	0	.1	0	.4	0	0	3	.2	1	0	5	35	219	0
-	0	0	-	0	-	-	0	-	-	-	0	0	-	-	-	-	300	-
2	0	5	2	29	0	.1	0	2.3	0	0	3	.2	0	0	5	35	307	0
8	0	0	0	0	0	0	0	2.8	0	0	0	0	0	0	0	2	0	0
-	-	55	-	-	-	-	-	-	-	-	-	-	-	-	260	630	500	-
1	-	70	-	0	-	-	4	0	.3	0	16	1.5	35	4.8	-	801	910	5.7
3	0	60	25	11	.8	2.6	0	-	.4	.2	13	.9	31	8.6	218	534	48	.7
2	0	72	30	127	.4	2.4	3	-	.1	0	24	.8	104	8.5	316	430	51	.5
1	0	81	4	29	.4	2.9	0	-	.2	.1	12	.6	24	7.3	309	468	54	.5
2	0	37	8	45	.3	.3	0	1.4	.2	0	203	.9	25	4.7	277	321	458	.9
2	0	54	12	50	.5	2.7	1	-	.1	.1	10	.3	29	6.3	282	391	44	.4
1	0	47	11	33	.5	4.3	1	-	.1	.1	-	.5	28	6.8	274	369	49	.5
2	0	48	8	27	.5	3.8	1	-	.1	.1	39	.6	30	6.6	253	387	45	.4
1	0	57	4	35	.2	2.9	0	-	.1	.2	14	.8	28	7.3	251	352	73	.6
-	0	0	-	80	-	-	4	-	-	-	0	0	-	-	-	-	240	-
-	-	50	-	200	-	-	66	-	.2	.2	64	.6	-	3.8	200	540	450	-
-	-	-	0	0	0	0	0	-	0	0	0	0	0	0	0	610	0	0
0	0	0	0	0	0	0	0	-	0	0	3	0	0	0	0	0	2325	0
4	0	121	10	57	.1	7.6	0	.3	.2	.1	325	2.5	33	4.5	417	338	430	1.1
1	-	17	8	46	0	.5	1	-	.2	0	212	.1	132	.3	128	222	398	.3
0	3	0	28	2	.2	0	17	.1	0	0	35	1.7	15	.2	24	201	780	.2
1	0	14	1	0	.1	.2	7	.1	0	.1	2	.2	3	.7	24	58	285	.4
2	0	38	4	4	.1	.5	0	.1	.1	.3	10	.4	12	2.7	95	176	718	1
2	0	51	2	0	.2	.8	1	.2	.2	.4	37	1.1	13	2.7	127	180	473	2
3	0	65	4	0	.3	1.1	2	.2	.2	.5	20	1.2	15	3.5	141	252	765	2
3	0	57	4	0	.2	1.4	18	.2	.2	.2	37	1.2	14	2.4	126	230	915	1.7
2	0	39	1	0	.1	.8	18	.4	.1	.2	7	.6	7	1.9	67	135	687	1.1
2	0	48	1	0	.1	1	13	.1	.1	.2	7	1	8	2.2	73	129	643	1.4
2	1	0	7	16	.2	0	0	.5	.1	.6	16	.9	9	2.8	56	58	222	.4
0	0	4	0	0	0	.1	0	0	0	0	1	.1	1	.3	7	19	112	.1
7	0	159	5	0	.4	2.2	2	-	.3	1.1	27	3.3	32	7.8	309	538	1989	4.4
0	0	11	0	0	0	.2	0	0	0	.1	4	.2	2	.6	24	47	168	.3
0	0	8	0	0	.1	.2	3	0	0	.1	1	.2	2	.5	14	38	186	.3
0	0	15	0	0	0	.7	4	0	0	0	2	.5	3	.7	26	52	270	.5
3	0	46	3	0	.2	1.1	1	.2	.2	.5	20	.8	13	3.1	110	228	1020	1.9
0	0	45	0	30	0	0	18	-	0	0	36	5.3	0	0	0	-	900	0
2	-	52	15	19	.1	1.1	2	-	.1	0	36	.7	50	1.3	201	283	395	.9
0	0	19	1	17	0	1.4	0	-	0	0	7	.3	37	.3	240	88	676	.3
2	-	33	-	-	-	-	11	.4	.1	.1	32	.4	21	2.1	-	425	768	.9
-	-	-	-	-	-	-	2	-	.1	0	80	.2	-	.8	-	375	610	-
-	-	60	0	0	0	0	2	-	0	0	24	0	0	0	0	-	275	0
0	-	0	11	2	0	0	9	-	0	0	2	0	2	0	4	47	0	0
1	0	45	5	54	.4	.3	0	-	.1	.1	11	.3	45	1.6	211	279	74	.4
24	8	0	164	4	.6	0	1	36.2	.2	1.6	84	4.9	255	3.2	508	496	2	3.6
21	4	0	152	0	.5	0	1	32.2	.2	.1	45	2.4	83	4.5	739	544	499	3.4
21	6	0	152	0	.5	0	1	32.2	.2	.1	45	2.4	83	4.5	739	544	2	3.4
26	5	0	158	3	.5	0	1	27	.2	.2	38	4.5	86	2.8	769	326	407	3.5
26	5	0	158	3	.5	0	1	33.9	.2	.2	38	4.5	86	2.8	769	326	2	3.5
25	-	0	159	0	.5	0	1	-	.2	.2	38	4.6	86	2.8	776	329	411	3.6
25	-	0	159	0	.5	0	1	-	.2	.2	38	4.6	86	2.8	776	329	2	3.6
5	1	0	6	3	0	0	0	1.1	0	0	48	.2	13	.4	39	50	422	.3
5	-	0	6	3	0	0	0	-	0	0	48	.2	13	.4	39	50	8	.3
0	-	44	12	78	.2	1.2	1	-	.8	.2	384	1.1	58	.5	346	679	329	1.4
-	-	37	10	08	.1	1.1	0	-	.7	.2	384	.4	44	.6	340	618	282	1.2

Code	Name	Amount	Unit	Grams	Energy (kcal)	Carbohydrates (g)	Protein (g)	Fat (g)	Saturated fat (g)	Monounsaturated fat (g)
14347	Shake, Vanilla	1-1/2	Cup	339.6	377	61	12	10	6	3
11640	Shallots, Freeze-dried	1/2	Cup	7.2	25	6	1	0	0	0
11677	Shallots, Fresh	1/2	Cup	79.9	58	13	2	0	0	0
15096	Shark, Ckd, Batter-dipped and Fried	3	Ounce	85.1	194	5	16	12	3	5
19097	Sherbet, All Flavors	1	Cup	192.0	265	58	2	4	2	1
18193	Shortbread Cookies, Pecan	1	Each	14.0	76	8	1	5	1	3
18192	Shortbread Cookies, Plain	1	Each	8.0	40	5	0	2	0	1
41263	Shrimp Marinara-Healthy Choice	1	Each	297.7	260	51	10	1	-	-
62615	Shrimp Marinara-Weight Watchers	1	Each	255.2	190	35	9	2	1	-
15150	Shrimp, Ckd, Breaded and Fried	3	Ounce	85.1	206	10	18	10	2	3
15151	Shrimp, Ckd, Moist Heat	3	Ounce	85.1	84	0	18	1	0	0
15152	Shrimp, Cnd	3	Ounce	85.1	102	1	20	2	0	0
15149	Shrimp, Fresh	3	Ounce	85.1	90	1	17	1	0	0
15153	Shrimp, Imitation	3	Ounce	85.1	86	8	11	1	0	0
55143	Single Serving Stuffed Pepper-Stouffer's	1	Each	283.5	220	28	10	8	-	-
41264	Sirloin Beef w/ Barbecue Sauce-Healthy Choice	1	Each	311.8	280	44	17	4	2	-
19370	Skittles Bite Size Candies	1	Pkg	65.0	255	62	0	2	-	-
41291	Sliced Turkey Breast w/ Gravy and Dressing-Healthy Choice	1	Each	283.5	270	30	27	4	2	-
41296	Sliced Turkey Breast w/ Gravy-Healthy Choice	1	Each	340.2	290	46	19	3	1	-
55225	Sliced Turkey w/ Dressing, Lean Cuisine-Stouffer's	1	Each	223.3	200	23	16	5	1	-
19407	Slim Jims, Smoked	1	Ounce	28.4	156	2	6	14	6	6
15100	Smelt, Rainbow, Ckd, Dry Heat	3	Ounce	85.1	105	0	19	3	0	1
15102	Snapper, Ckd, Dry Heat	3	Ounce	85.1	109	0	22	1	0	0
19155	Snickers Bar	1	Bar	61.0	278	37	6	14	7	4
62599	Sorbet, All Flavors	1/2	Cup	90.0	100	25	0	0	0	-
6474	Soup, Bean w/ Bacon	1	Cup	264.9	106	16	5	2	1	1
6007	Soup, Bean w/ Ham	1	Cup	243.0	231	27	13	9	3	4
6406	Soup, Bean w/ Hot Dogs	1	Cup	250.0	187	22	10	7	2	3
6404	Soup, Bean w/ Pork	1	Cup	253.0	172	23	8	6	2	2
6008	Soup, Beef Broth or Bouillon	1	Cup	240.0	17	0	3	1	0	0
6547	Soup, Beef Mushroom	1	Cup	244.0	73	6	6	3	1	1
6409	Soup, Beef Noodle	1	Cup	244.0	83	9	5	3	1	1
6070	Soup, Beef, Chunky	1	Cup	240.0	170	20	12	5	3	2
6402	Soup, Black Bean	1	Cup	247.0	116	20	6	2	0	1
6478	Soup, Cauliflower	1	Cup	256.1	69	11	3	2	0	1
6411	Soup, Cheese	1	Cup	247.0	156	11	5	10	7	3
6480	Soup, Chicken Broth or Bouillon	1	Cup	244.0	22	1	1	1	0	0
6417	Soup, Chicken Gumbo	1	Cup	244.0	56	8	3	1	0	1
6549	Soup, Chicken Mushroom	1	Cup	244.0	132	9	4	9	2	4
6419	Soup, Chicken Noodle	1	Cup	241.0	75	9	4	2	1	1
6018	Soup, Chicken Noodle, Chunky	1	Cup	240.0	175	17	13	6	1	3
6485	Soup, Chicken Rice	1	Cup	252.8	61	9	2	1	0	1
6022	Soup, Chicken Rice, Chunky	1	Cup	240.0	127	13	12	3	1	1
6425	Soup, Chicken Vegetable	1	Cup	241.0	75	9	4	3	1	1
6024	Soup, Chicken Vegetable, Chunky	1	Cup	240.0	166	19	12	5	1	2
6412	Soup, Chicken w/ Dumplings	1	Cup	241.0	96	6	6	6	1	3
6423	Soup, Chicken w/ Rice	1	Cup	241.0	60	7	4	2	0	1
6015	Soup, Chicken, Chunky	1	Cup	251.0	178	17	13	7	2	3
6426	Soup, Chili Beef	1	Cup	250.0	170	21	7	7	3	3
6027	Soup, Clam Chowder, Manhattan Style	1	Cup	240.0	134	19	7	3	2	1
6230	Soup, Clam Chowder, New England	1	Cup	248.0	164	17	9	7	3	2
6034	Soup, Crab	1	Cup	244.0	76	10	5	2	0	1
6201	Soup, Cream Of Asparagus	1	Cup	248.0	161	16	6	8	3	2
6210	Soup, Cream Of Celery	1	Cup	248.0	164	15	6	10	4	2
6216	Soup, Cream Of Chicken	1	Cup	248.0	191	15	7	11	5	4
6243	Soup, Cream Of Mushroom	1	Cup	248.0	203	15	6	14	5	3

Polyunsaturated fat (g)	Dietary Fiber (g)	Cholesterol (mg)	Folate (µg)	Vitamin A (RE)	Vitamin B-6 (mg)	Vitamin B-12 (µg)	Vitamin C (mg)	Vitamin E (mg)	Riboflavin (mg)	Thiamin (mg)	Calcium (mg)	Iron (mg)	Magnesium (mg)	Niacin (mg)	Phosphorus (mg)	Potassium (mg)	Sodium (mg)	Zinc (mg)
0	-	37	11	109	.2	1.2	3	-	.6	.2	414	.3	41	.6	346	591	278	1.2
0	-	0	8	404	.1	0	3	-	0	0	13	.4	7	.1	21	119	4	.1
0	-	0	27	998	.3	0	6	-	0	0	30	1	17	.2	48	267	10	.3
3	0	50	4	46	.3	1	0	-	.1	.1	43	.9	37	2.4	165	132	104	.4
0	-	10	8	27	.1	.2	8	-	.1	0	104	.3	15	.2	77	184	88	.9
1	0	5	1	0	0	0	0	-	0	0	4	.3	3	.3	12	10	39	.1
0	-	2	1	1	0	0	0	-	0	0	3	.2	1	.3	9	8	36	0
-	-	60	-	100	-	-	114	-	.1	.2	48	1.5	-	1.1	130	390	320	-
-	4	40	-	150	-	-	6	-	-	-	120	1	-	-	-	440	400	-
4	-	151	7	48	.1	1.6	1	-	.1	.1	57	1.1	34	2.6	185	191	293	1.2
0	0	166	3	56	.1	1.3	2	3.1	0	0	33	2.6	29	2.2	117	155	191	1.3
1	0	147	2	15	.1	1	2	2.1	0	0	50	2.3	35	2.3	198	179	144	1.1
1	0	129	3	46	.1	1	2	2.4	0	0	44	2	31	2.2	174	157	126	.9
1	0	31	1	17	0	1.4	0	-	0	0	16	.5	37	.1	240	76	600	.3
-	-	-	-	20	-	-	6	-	.2	.2	32	1	-	2.9	-	400	1010	-
1	-	25	-	-	-	-	-	-	-	-	-	-	-	-	190	630	240	-
-	0	0	0	0	0	0	0	0	0	0	2	.1	1	0	2	15	30	0
1	-	50	-	150	-	-	-	-	.3	.3	48	1	-	7.6	310	590	530	-
1	-	20	-	150	-	-	27	-	.1	.2	16	.6	-	1.5	-	360	520	-
2	-	25	-	500	-	-	6	-	.3	.2	32	.8	-	4.8	-	400	590	-
1	-	38	0	48	.1	.3	2	-	.1	0	19	1	6	1.3	51	73	420	.7
1	0	77	4	14	.1	3.4	0	-	.1	0	65	1	32	1.5	251	316	65	1.8
1	0	40	5	30	.4	3	1	-	0	0	34	.2	31	.3	171	444	48	.4
1	2	7	24	19	.1	.3	0	3.4	.1	0	70	.5	37	1.8	129	199	163	.7
-	1	0	-	0	-	-	12	-	-	-	0	0	-	-	-	-	10	-
0	9	3	8	5	0	0	1	.3	.3	.1	56	1.3	29	.4	90	326	927	.7
1	11	22	29	396	.1	.1	4	.1	.1	.1	78	3.2	46	1.7	143	425	972	1.1
2	-	12	30	87	.1	.1	1	-	.1	.1	87	2.3	47	1	165	477	1092	1.2
2	9	3	32	89	0	.1	2	.1	0	.1	81	2	46	.6	132	402	951	1
0	0	0	5	0	0	.2	0	0	.1	0	14	.4	5	1.9	31	130	782	0
0	-	7	10	0	0	.2	5	-	.1	0	5	.9	10	1	34	154	942	1.5
0	1	5	4	63	0	.2	0	0	.1	.1	15	1.1	5	1.1	46	100	952	1.5
0	1	14	13	262	.1	.6	7	.2	.2	.1	31	2.3	5	2.7	120	336	866	2.6
0	4	0	25	49	.1	0	1	.1	.1	.1	44	2.1	42	.5	106	274	1198	1.4
1	-	0	3	0	0	.2	3	-	.1	.1	10	.5	3	.5	51	105	843	.3
0	-	30	5	109	0	0	0	-	.1	0	141	.7	5	.4	136	153	958	.6
0	0	0	2	12	0	0	0	0	0	0	15	.1	5	.2	12	24	1484	0
0	2	5	5	15	.1	0	5	0	0	0	24	.9	5	.7	24	76	954	.4
2	-	10	0	112	0	0	0	-	.1	0	29	.9	10	1.6	27	154	942	1
1	1	7	2	72	0	.1	0	.1	.1	.1	17	.8	5	1.4	36	55	1106	.4
2	4	19	5	122	0	.3	0	.8	.2	.1	24	1.4	10	4.3	72	108	850	1
0	1	3	1	0	0	.1	0	0	0	0	8	0	0	.4	10	10	981	.1
1	1	12	4	586	0	.3	4	.1	.1	0	34	1.9	10	4.1	72	108	888	1
1	1	10	5	265	0	.1	1	.1	.1	0	17	.9	7	1.2	41	154	945	.4
1	-	17	12	600	.1	.2	6	-	.2	0	26	1.5	10	3.3	106	367	1068	2.2
1	1	34	2	53	0	.2	0	.1	.1	0	14	.6	5	1.8	60	116	860	.4
0	1	7	1	65	0	.1	0	.1	0	0	17	.7	0	1.1	22	101	815	.3
1	2	30	5	131	.1	.3	1	.2	.2	.1	25	1.7	8	4.4	113	176	889	1
0	9	12	17	150	.2	.3	4	.2	.1	.1	42	2.1	30	1.1	147	525	1035	1.4
0	3	14	9	329	.3	7.9	12	.1	.1	.1	67	2.6	19	1.8	84	384	1001	1.7
1	1	22	10	40	.1	10.2	3	.1	.2	.1	186	1.5	22	1	156	300	992	.8
0	1	10	15	51	.1	.2	0	.1	.1	.2	66	1.2	15	1.3	88	327	1235	1.5
2	1	22	30	84	.1	.5	4	.8	.3	.1	174	.9	20	.9	154	360	1042	.9
3	1	32	8	67	.1	.5	1	1	.2	.1	186	.7	22	.4	151	310	1009	.2
2	0	27	8	94	.1	.5	1	.2	.3	.1	181	.7	17	.9	151	273	1047	.7
5	0	20	10	37	.1	.5	2	1.3	.3	.1	179	.6	20	.9	156	270	1076	.6

Code	Name	Amount	Unit	Grams	Energy (kcal)	Carbohydrates (g)	Protein (g)	Fat (g)	Saturated fat (g)	Monounsaturated fat (g)
6246	Soup, Cream Of Onion	1	Cup	248.0	186	18	7	9	4	3
6253	Soup, Cream Of Potato	1	Cup	248.0	149	17	6	6	4	2
6256	Soup, Cream Of Shrimp	1	Cup	248.0	164	14	7	9	6	3
6501	Soup, Cream Of Vegetable	1	Cup	260.1	107	12	2	6	1	3
6036	Soup, Gazpacho	1	Cup	244.0	56	1	9	2	0	1
6037	Soup, Lentil w/ ham	1	Cup	248.0	139	20	9	3	1	1
6440	Soup, Minestrone	1	Cup	241.0	82	11	4	3	1	1
6039	Soup, Minestrone, Chunky	1	Cup	240.0	127	21	5	3	1	1
6493	Soup, Mushroom	1	Cup	253.0	96	11	2	5	1	2
6445	Soup, Onion	1	Cup	241.0	58	8	4	2	0	1
6249	Soup, Pea, Green	1	Cup	254.0	239	32	13	7	4	2
6451	Soup, Pea, Split w/ Ham	1	Cup	253.0	190	28	10	4	2	2
6050	Soup, Pea, Split w/ Ham, Chunky	1	Cup	240.0	185	27	11	4	2	2
6359	Soup, Tomato	1	Cup	248.0	161	22	6	6	3	2
6461	Soup, Tomato Beef w/ noodle	1	Cup	244.0	139	21	4	4	2	2
6463	Soup, Tomato Rice	1	Cup	247.0	119	22	2	3	1	1
6499	Soup, Tomato Vegetable	1	Cup	253.0	56	10	2	1	0	0
6465	Soup, Turkey Noodle	1	Cup	244.0	68	9	4	2	1	1
6466	Soup, Turkey Vegetable	1	Cup	241.0	72	9	3	3	1	1
6064	Soup, Turkey, Chunky	1	Cup	236.0	135	14	10	4	1	2
6500	Soup, Vegetable Beef	1	Cup	253.1	53	8	3	1	1	0
6067	Soup, Vegetable, Chunky	1	Cup	240.0	122	19	4	4	1	2
6468	Soup, Vegetarian Vegetable	1	Cup	241.0	72	12	2	2	0	1
1056	Sour Cream	1	Tbsp.	12.0	26	1	0	3	2	1
62556	Sour Cream, Fat Free	1	Tbsp.	16.0	13	3	1	0	0	-
1074	Sour Cream, Imitation, Nondairy, Cultured	1	Tbsp.	14.4	30	1	0	3	3	0
62555	Sour Cream, Light	1	Tbsp.	16.0	16	1	1	1	1	-
62660	Sour Cream, Non-Fat	2	Tbsp.	32.0	25	5	1	0	0	0
41265	Southwestern Style Chicken-Healthy Choice	1	Each	354.4	340	51	25	5	2	-
6134	Soy Sauce	1	Tbsp.	18.0	10	2	1	0	0	0
16109	Soybeans, Boiled	1/2	Cup	86.0	149	9	14	8	1	2
16111	Soybeans, Dry Roasted	1/2	Cup	86.0	387	28	34	19	3	4
11455	Spaghetti Sauce	1/2	Cup	124.5	136	20	2	6	1	3
62666	Spaghetti Sauce, Healthy Choice	1	Cup	146.0	59	13	2	1	0	0
62665	Spaghetti Sauce, Prego	1	Cup	146.0	154	26	4	4	1	0
62664	Spaghetti Sauce, Ragu	1	Cup	146.0	131	20	4	5	2	0
43404	Spaghetti and Meatballs, Micro Cup-Hormel	1	Each	212.6	210	27	10	7	3	3
55226	Spaghetti w/ Meat Sauce, Lean Cuisine-Stouffer's	1	Each	326.0	290	45	15	6	2	-
43396	Spaghetti w/ Meat Sauce, Top Shelf-Hormel	1	Each	283.5	260	37	14	6	2	2
41342	Spaghetti w/ Meat Sauce-Healthy Choice	1	Each	283.5	280	42	14	6	2	-
55247	Spaghetti w/ Meat Sauce-Stouffer's	1	Each	365.0	320	38	16	12	-	-
55150	Spaghetti w/ Meatballs, -Stouffer's	1	Each	276.4	290	37	14	9	-	-
19164	Special Dark Sweet Chocolate Bar	1	Bar	79.0	376	49	4	24	-	-
55176	Spinach Souffle-Stouffer's	1	Each	170.1	220	11	9	15	-	-
11458	Spinach, Ckd	1/2	Cup	90.0	21	3	3	0	0	0
11461	Spinach, Cnd, Drained Solids	1/2	Cup	107.0	25	4	3	1	0	0
11459	Spinach, Cnd, Reg Pk, Sol&liq	1/2	Cup	117.0	22	3	2	0	0	0
11457	Spinach, Fresh	1	Cup	56.0	12	2	2	0	0	0
11464	Spinach, Frz, Ckd	1/2	Cup	95.0	27	5	3	0	0	0
11463	Spinach, Frz, Unprepared	1/2	Cup	78.0	19	3	2	0	0	0
55766	Split Pea Soup w/ Ham-Stouffer's	1	Cup	283.9	220	35	15	3	-	-
41283	Split Pea and Ham Soup-Healthy Choice	1	Each	212.6	170	25	10	3	1	-
11483	Squash, Acorn, Ckd. w/o Salt	1/2	Cup	102.5	57	15	1	0	0	0
11486	Squash, Butternut, Ckd. w/o Salt	1/2	Cup	102.5	41	11	1	0	0	0
11493	Squash, Spaghetti, Ckd. w/o Salt	1/2	Cup	77.5	22	5	1	0	0	0
11642	Squash, Summer, Ckd	1/2	Cup	90.0	18	4	1	0	0	0

Polyunsaturated fat (g)	Dietary Fiber (g)	Cholesterol (mg)	Folate (µg)	Vitamin A (RE)	Vitamin B-6 (mg)	Vitamin B-12 (µg)	Vitamin C (mg)	Vitamin E (mg)	Riboflavin (mg)	Thiamin (mg)	Calcium (mg)	Iron (mg)	Magnesium (mg)	Niacin (mg)	Phosphorus (mg)	Potassium (mg)	Sodium (mg)	Zinc (mg)
2	1	32	12	67	.1	.5	2	.1	.3	.1	179	.7	22	.6	154	310	1004	.6
1	0	22	9	67	.1	.5	1	.1	.2	.1	166	.5	17	.6	161	322	1061	.7
0	0	35	10	55	.4	1	1	.9	.2	.1	164	.6	22	.5	146	248	1037	.8
1	1	0	8	3	0	.1	4	1.2	.1	1.2	31	.5	10	.5	55	96	1170	.3
1	4	0	10	20	.1	0	3	.5	0	0	24	1	7	.9	37	224	1183	.2
0	-	7	50	35	.2	.3	4	-	.1	.2	42	2.7	22	1.4	184	357	1319	.7
1	1	2	16	234	.1	0	1	.1	0	.1	34	.9	7	.9	55	313	911	.7
0	2	5	31	434	.2	0	5	.7	.1	.1	60	1.8	14	1.2	110	612	864	1.4
2	1	0	5	0	0	.3	1	.6	.1	.3	66	.5	5	.5	76	200	1020	.1
1	1	0	15	0	0	0	1	.3	0	0	27	.7	2	.6	12	67	1053	.6
1	3	18	8	58	.1	.4	3	.2	.3	.2	173	2	56	1.3	239	376	1046	1.8
1	-	8	3	46	.1	.3	2	-	.1	.1	23	2.3	48	1.5	213	400	1007	1.3
1	4	7	5	487	.2	.2	7	.1	.1	.1	34	2.1	38	2.5	178	305	965	3.1
1	0	17	21	109	.2	.4	68	2.6	.2	.1	159	1.8	22	1.5	149	449	932	.3
1	1	5	7	54	.1	.2	0	.8	.1	.1	17	1.1	7	1.9	56	220	917	.8
1	1	2	14	77	.1	0	15	.8	0	.1	22	.8	5	1.1	35	331	815	.5
0	1	0	10	20	.1	0	6	.8	0	.1	8	.6	20	.8	30	104	1146	.2
0	1	5	2	29	0	.1	0	.1	.1	.1	12	1	5	1.4	49	76	815	.6
1	0	2	5	243	0	.2	0	.1	0	0	17	.8	5	1	41	176	906	.6
1	-	9	11	715	.3	2.1	6	-	.1	0	50	1.9	24	3.6	104	361	923	2.1
0	1	0	8	23	.1	.3	1	0	0	0	13	.9	23	.5	35	76	1002	.3
1	1	0	17	588	.2	0	6	.6	.1	.1	55	1.6	7	1.2	72	396	1010	3.1
1	0	0	11	301	.1	0	1	.8	0	.1	22	1.1	7	.9	34	210	822	.5
0	0	5	1	23	0	0	0	.1	0	0	14	0	1	0	10	17	6	0
-	-	3	-	30	-	-	0	-	-	-	36	0	-	-	-	-	18	-
0	0	0	0	0	0	0	0	0	0	0	0	.1	1	0	6	23	15	.2
-	-	5	-	18	-	-	0	-	-	-	22	0	-	-	-	27	9	-
0	0	5	0	60	0	0	0	-	0	0	72	0	0	0	0	-	35	0
2	-	60	-	-	-	-	-	-	-	-	-	-	-	-	260	560	550	-
0	0	0	3	0	0	0	0	0	0	0	3	.4	6	.6	20	32	1029	.1
4	5	0	46	1	.2	0	1	1.7	.2	.1	88	4.4	74	.3	211	443	1	1
10	7	0	176	2	.2	0	4	1.7	.6	.4	232	3.4	196	.9	558	1173	2	4.1
2	4	0	27	153	.4	0	14	3.1	.1	.1	35	.8	30	1.9	45	478	618	.3
0	2	0	0	119	0	0	6	-	0	0	57	.7	0	0	0	-	463	0
0	4	0	0	356	0	0	21	-	0	0	85	.7	0	0	0	-	724	0
0	4	0	0	178	0	0	1	-	0	0	57	.7	0	0	0	-	653	0
1	-	20	-	140	-	-	4	0	.3	.1	32	1.1	25	2.3	-	341	930	1.1
2	-	20	-	100	-	-	6	-	.3	.3	48	2	-	3.8	-	500	500	-
1	-	20	-	100	-	-	2	.1	.3	.2	48	1.5	46	3.8	-	879	980	2.4
2	-	20	-	250	-	-	5	-	.3	.4	48	2	-	1.9	160	540	480	-
12	-	-	-	150	-	-	6	-	.2	.2	80	1.5	-	3.8	-	800	560	-
-	-	-	-	100	-	-	6	-	.3	.3	64	1.5	-	3.8	-	550	790	-
-	4	0	3	2	0	0	0	.8	.2	0	15	1.7	91	.5	126	269	8	1.2
-	-	-	-	200	-	-	6	-	.3	.1	120	.4	-	.4	-	345	820	-
0	2	0	131	737	.2	0	9	.9	.2	.1	122	3.2	78	.4	50	419	63	.7
0	-	0	105	939	.1	0	15	-	.1	0	136	2.5	81	.4	47	370	29	.5
0	3	0	68	752	.1	0	16	1.1	.1	0	97	1.8	66	.3	37	269	373	.5
0	2	0	109	376	.1	0	16	1.1	.1	0	55	1.5	44	.4	27	312	44	.3
0	3	0	102	739	.1	0	12	.9	.2	.1	139	1.4	66	.4	46	283	82	.7
0	2	0	93	605	.1	0	19	.7	.1	.1	87	1.6	45	.3	32	252	58	.3
-	-	10	-	-	-	-	0	-	0	0	240	.2	-	.4	-	571	1192	-
-	-	10	-	100	-	-	6	-	.1	.2	16	.6	-	1.9	190	450	460	-
0	-	0	19	44	.2	0	11	-	0	.2	45	1	44	.9	46	448	4	.2
0	-	0	20	718	.1	0	15	-	0	.1	42	.6	30	1	28	291	4	.1
0	1	0	6	9	.1	0	3	.1	0	0	16	.3	9	.6	11	91	14	.2
0	1	0	18	26	.1	0	5	.1	0	0	24	.3	22	.5	35	173	1	.4

Code	Name	Amount	Unit	Grams	Energy (kcal)	Carbohydrates (g)	Protein (g)	Fat (g)	Saturated fat (g)	Monounsaturated fat (g)
11641	Squash, Summer, Fresh	1/2	Cup	65.0	13	3	1	0	0	0
11644	Squash, Winter, Baked	1/2	Cup	102.5	40	9	1	1	0	0
11643	Squash, Winter, Fresh	1/2	Cup	58.0	21	5	1	0	0	0
11953	Squash, Zucchini, Baby, Fresh	1	Medium	11.0	2	0	0	0	0	0
15176	Squid, Fried	3	Ounce	85.1	149	7	15	6	2	2
9316	Strawberries, Fresh	1/2	Cup	74.5	22	5	0	0	0	0
9320	Strawberries, Frozen, Sweetened	1/2	Cup	127.5	122	33	1	0	0	0
9318	Strawberries, Frozen, Unsweetened	1/2	Cup	74.5	26	7	0	0	0	0
14351	Strawberry Flavor Beverage	1	Cup	266.0	234	33	8	8	5	2
18354	Strudel, Apple	1	Each	71.0	195	29	2	8	2	4
55781	Stuffed Cabbage no Sauce-Stouffer's	1	Ounce	28.4	39	3	2	2	-	-
55228	Stuffed Cabbage w/ Meat, Lean Cuisine-Stouffer's	1	Each	269.3	210	26	13	6	2	-
55778	Stuffed Cabbage-Stouffer's	1	Ounce	28.4	29	3	1	1	-	-
55157	Stuffed Green Peppers-Stouffer's	1	Each	219.7	200	22	9	8	-	-
18203	Sugar Cookies, Dietary	1	Each	7.0	30	5	1	1	0	1
18204	Sugar Cookies, Regular (includes Vanilla)	1	Each	15.0	72	10	1	3	1	2
19334	Sugar, Brown	1	Tsp.	5.0	19	5	0	0	-	-
19335	Sugar, Granulated	1	Tsp.	4.0	15	4	0	0	-	-
19336	Sugar, Powdered	1	Tbsp.	8.0	31	8	0	0	-	-
15218	Sunfish, Ckd, Dry Heat	3	Ounce	85.1	97	0	21	1	0	0
55229	Swedish Meatballs w/ Pasta, Lean Cuisine-Stouffer's	1	Each	258.7	290	31	23	8	3	-
55148	Swedish Meatballs w/ Pasta-Stouffer's	1	Each	262.2	420	32	24	21	-	-
18359	Sweet Rolls w/ Raisins and Nuts	1	Each	57.0	196	30	4	7	1	3
18355	Sweet Rolls, Cheese	1	Each	66.0	238	29	5	12	4	6
18356	Sweet Rolls, Cinnamon w/ Raisins	1	Each	60.0	223	31	4	10	3	5
41266	Sweet and Sour Chicken-Healthy Choice	1	Each	326.0	280	52	20	2	-	-
11508	Sweetpotatoes, Baked In Skin	1/2	Cup	100.0	103	24	2	0	0	0
11510	Sweetpotatoes, Boiled, w/o Skin	1/2	Cup	164.0	172	40	3	0	0	0
11659	Sweetpotatoes, Candied	1/2	Cup	113.4	155	32	1	4	2	1
11514	Sweetpotatoes, Mashed	1/2	Cup	127.5	129	30	3	0	0	0
11647	Sweetpotatoes, Syrup Pack, Drained Solids	1/2	Cup	98.0	106	25	1	0	0	0
15111	Swordfish, Ckd, Dry Heat	3	Ounce	85.1	132	0	22	4	1	2
19093	Symphony Milk Chocolate Bar	1	Bar	68.0	355	39	5	22	-	-
19348	Syrup, Chocolate, Fudge-type	1	Tbsp.	21.0	73	12	1	3	1	1
19349	Syrup, Corn, Dark	1	Tbsp.	20.0	56	15	0	0	-	-
19351	Syrup, Corn, High-fructose	1	Tbsp.	19.0	53	14	0	0	-	-
19350	Syrup, Corn, Light	1	Tbsp.	20.0	56	15	0	0	-	-
19352	Syrup, Malt	1	Tbsp.	24.0	76	17	1	0	-	-
19353	Syrup, Maple	1	Tbsp.	20.0	52	13	0	0	-	-
19128	Syrup, Pancake, Lo Cal	1	Tbsp.	20.0	33	9	0	0	-	-
19360	Syrup, Pancake, w/ 2% Maple	1	Tbsp.	20.0	53	14	0	0	-	-
19113	Syrup, Pancake, w/ Butter	1	Tbsp.	20.0	59	15	0	0	0	0
62653	Tabouli	1	Ounce	28.4	30	2	1	2	0	-
18360	Taco Shells, Baked	1	Medium	13.0	61	8	1	3	0	1
18448	Taco Shells, Baked, w/o Added Salt	1	Medium	13.0	61	8	1	3	0	1
43438	Taco Shells, Chi-Chi's-Hormel	1	Each	20.0	99	12	1	5	-	-
19382	Taffy	1	Piece	15.0	56	14	0	0	0	0
9223	Tangerine Juice, Cnd, Sweetened	3/4	Cup	186.4	93	22	1	0	0	0
9221	Tangerine Juice, Fresh	3/4	Cup	185.2	80	19	1	0	0	0
9219	Tangerines, Cnd, Juice Pack	1/2	Cup	124.5	46	12	1	0	0	0
9220	Tangerines, Cnd, Light Syrup Pack	1/2	Cup	126.0	77	20	1	0	0	0
9218	Tangerines, Fresh	1	Medium	84.0	37	9	1	0	0	0
19218	Tapioca Pudding	1	Cup	298.1	355	58	6	11	2	5
19524	Taro Chips	1	Ounce	28.4	141	19	1	7	2	1
62654	Tator Tots	10	Each	28.4	140	20	3	5	1	-
14355	Tea, Brewed	8	Fl Oz	236.8	2	1	0	0	0	0

Polyunsaturated fat (g)	Dietary Fiber (g)	Cholesterol (mg)	Folate (µg)	Vitamin A (RE)	Vitamin B-6 (mg)	Vitamin B-12 (µg)	Vitamin C (mg)	Vitamin E (mg)	Riboflavin (mg)	Thiamin (mg)	Calcium (mg)	Iron (mg)	Magnesium (mg)	Niacin (mg)	Phosphorus (mg)	Potassium (mg)	Sodium (mg)	Zinc (mg)
0	1	0	17	13	.1	0	10	.1	0	0	13	.3	15	.4	23	127	1	.2
0	3	0	29	365	.1	0	10	.1	0	.1	14	.3	8	.7	21	448	1	.3
0	1	0	13	235	0	0	7	.1	0	.1	18	.3	12	.5	19	203	2	.1
0	-	0	2	5	0	0	4	-	0	0	2	.1	4	.1	10	50	0	.1
2	0	221	5	9	0	1	4	-	.4	0	33	.9	32	2.2	213	237	260	1.5
0	2	0	13	2	0	0	42	.1	0	0	10	.3	7	.2	14	124	1	.1
0	2	0	19	3	0	0	53	.2	.1	0	14	.8	9	.5	17	125	4	.1
0	2	0	13	3	0	0	31	.2	0	0	12	.6	8	.3	10	110	1	.1
0	-	32	12	74	.1	.9	2	-	.4	.1	293	.2	32	.2	229	370	128	.9
1	2	20	4	6	0	.1	1	-	0	0	11	.3	6	.2	23	69	191	.1
-	-	5	-	-	-	-	1	-	0	0	72	0	-	.1	-	48	150	-
1	-	30	-	80	-	-	6	-	.2	.1	64	1.5	-	3.8	-	600	560	-
-	-	4	-	-	-	-	3	-	0	0	48	0	-	.1	-	51	145	-
-	-	-	-	60	-	-	6	-	.1	.1	32	.8	-	2.9	-	380	650	-
0	-	0	0	0	0	0	0	-	0	0	2	.3	1	.2	6	7	0	0
0	-	8	2	4	0	0	0	-	0	0	3	.3	2	.4	12	9	54	.1
-	0	0	0	0	0	0	0	0	0	0	4	.1	1	0	1	17	2	0
-	0	0	0	0	0	0	0	0	0	0	0	0	0	0	0	0	0	0
-	0	0	0	0	0	0	0	0	0	0	0	0	0	0	0	0	0	0
0	0	73	14	14	.1	2	1	-	.1	.1	88	1.3	32	1.2	196	382	88	1.7
1	-	55	-	20	-	-	-	-	.3	.2	48	1.5	-	3.8	-	450	550	-
-	-	-	-	20	-	-	1	-	.3	.2	48	1.5	-	2.9	-	350	740	-
3	-	13	18	60	.1	.1	0	-	.2	.2	36	1.5	16	1.3	63	123	185	.4
1	-	37	20	41	0	.1	0	-	.1	.1	78	.5	13	.5	65	87	236	.4
1	1	40	14	38	.1	.1	1	-	.2	.2	43	1	10	1.4	46	67	230	.4
-	-	35	-	250	-	-	30	-	.2	.2	32	1	-	8.6	220	480	320	-
0	3	0	23	2182	.2	0	25	4.6	.1	.1	28	.4	20	.6	55	348	10	.3
0	4	0	18	2796	.4	0	28	7.5	.2	.1	34	.9	16	1	44	302	21	.4
0	-	9	13	475	0	0	8	-	0	0	29	1.3	12	.4	29	214	79	.2
0	-	0	14	1929	.3	0	7	-	.1	0	38	1.7	31	1.2	66	268	96	.3
0	-	0	8	702	.1	0	11	-	0	0	17	.9	12	.3	25	189	38	.2
1	0	43	2	35	.3	1.7	1	-	.1	0	5	.9	29	10	287	314	98	1.3
-	-	19	5	9	0	.3	0	-	.3	.1	160	.7	37	.2	170	262	58	.8
1	0	3	1	5	0	.1	0	0	0	0	21	.3	10	0	36	45	27	.2
-	0	0	0	0	0	0	0	0	0	0	4	.1	2	0	2	9	31	0
-	0	0	0	0	0	0	0	0	0	0	0	0	0	0	0	0	0	0
-	-	0	0	0	0	0	0	-	0	0	1	0	0	0	0	1	24	0
-	-	0	3	0	.1	0	0	-	.1	0	15	.2	17	1.9	57	77	8	0
-	0	0	0	0	0	0	0	0	0	0	13	.2	3	0	0	41	2	.8
-	0	0	0	0	0	0	0	0	0	0	0	0	0	0	9	1	40	0
-	0	0	0	0	0	0	0	0	0	0	1	0	0	0	2	1	12	0
0	-	1	0	3	0	0	0	-	0	0	0	0	0	0	2	1	20	0
-	1	0	0	100	0	0	12	-	0	0	0	.4	0	0	0	-	75	0
1	1	0	1	5	0	0	0	-	0	0	21	.3	14	.2	32	23	48	.2
1	-	0	1	-	-	0	0	-	0	0	21	.3	14	.2	32	23	2	.2
-	-	0	-	-	-	-	-	.1	.1	.1	-	.1	-	.5	-	-	4	-
0	-	1	0	5	0	0	0	-	0	0	0	0	0	0	0	1	13	0
0	0	0	9	78	.1	0	41	.2	0	.1	34	.4	15	.2	26	332	2	.1
0	0	0	9	78	.1	0	57	.2	0	.1	33	.4	15	.2	26	330	2	.1
0	1	0	6	106	.1	0	43	.6	0	.1	14	.3	14	.6	12	166	6	.6
0	1	0	6	106	.1	0	25	.4	.1	.1	9	.5	10	.6	13	98	8	.3
0	2	0	17	77	.1	0	26	.2	0	.1	12	.1	10	.1	8	132	1	.2
4	0	3	12	0	.3	.3	2	.3	.3	.1	250	.7	24	.9	236	310	352	.8
4	2	0	6	0	.1	0	1	1.4	0	0	17	.3	24	.1	37	214	97	.1
-	3	0	0	0	0	0	0	-	0	0	0	0	0	0	0	240	240	0
0	0	0	12	0	0	0	0	0	0	0	0	0	7	0	2	88	7	0

Code	Name	Amount	Unit	Grams	Energy (kcal)	Carbohydrates (g)	Protein (g)	Fat (g)	Saturated fat (g)	Monounsaturated fat (g)
14381	Tea, Herb, Brewed	8	Fl Oz	236.8	2	0	0	0	0	0
14371	Tea, Instant, Sweetened	8	Fl Oz	259.0	88	22	0	0	0	0
14367	Tea, Instant, Unsweetened	8	Fl Oz	236.8	2	0	0	0	0	0
43401	Tender Beef Roast, Top Shelf-Hormel	1	Each	283.5	240	19	28	6	2	2
14020	Tequila Sunrise	1	Fl Oz	31.2	34	3	0	0	0	0
41267	Teriyaki Chicken-Healthy Choice	1	Each	347.3	290	39	24	4	1	-
6112	Teriyaki Sauce	1	Tbsp.	18.0	15	3	1	0	0	0
14382	Theist Quencher Drink, Bottled	12	Fl Oz	361.2	90	23	0	0	0	0
55811	Three Bean Chili-Stouffer's	1	Cup	283.9	210	32	10	5	-	-
19159	Three Musketeers Bar	1	Bar	60.0	250	46	2	8	4	3
18361	Toaster Pastries, Brown-sugar-cinn.	1	Each	52.0	214	35	3	7	2	4
18362	Toaster Pastries, Fruit	1	Each	52.0	204	37	2	5	1	2
19383	Toffee	1	Piece	12.0	65	8	0	4	2	1
16126	Tofu, Fresh, Firm	1	Ounce	28.4	41	1	4	2	0	1
16127	Tofu, Fresh, Regular	1	Ounce	28.4	22	1	2	1	0	0
16129	Tofu, Fried	1	Ounce	28.4	77	3	5	6	1	1
16429	Tofu, Fried, Prepared w/ Calcium Sulfate	1	Ounce	28.4	77	3	5	6	1	1
16130	Tofu, Okara	1	Ounce	28.4	22	4	1	0	0	0
16132	Tofu, Salted and Fermented (fuyu)	1	Ounce	28.4	33	1	2	2	0	1
14023	Tom Collins	1	Fl Oz	29.6	16	0	0	0	0	0
11954	Tomatillos, Fresh	1	Medium	34.0	11	2	0	0	-	-
41284	Tomato Garden Soup-Healthy Choice	1	Each	212.6	130	22	4	3	1	-
11540	Tomato Juice, Cnd, w/ Salt	3/4	Cup	183.0	31	8	1	0	0	0
11886	Tomato Juice, Cnd, w/o Salt	3/4	Cup	183.0	31	8	1	0	0	0
11883	Tomatoes, Cherry	1	Each	10.0	2	0	0	0	0	0
11530	Tomatoes, Ckd, Boiled	1/2	Cup	120.0	32	7	1	0	0	0
11660	Tomatoes, Ckd, Stewed	1/2	Cup	50.5	40	7	1	1	0	1
11533	Tomatoes, Cnd, Stewed	1/2	Cup	127.5	33	8	1	0	0	0
11535	Tomatoes, Cnd, Wedges In Tomato Juice	1/2	Cup	130.5	34	8	1	0	0	0
11531	Tomatoes, Cnd, Whole, Reg Pk	1/2	Cup	120.0	24	5	1	0	0	0
11537	Tomatoes, Cnd, w/ Green Chilies	1/2	Cup	120.5	18	4	1	0	0	0
11529	Tomatoes, Fresh	1	Medium	123.0	26	6	1	0	0	0
11527	Tomatoes, Green, Fresh	1	Medium	123.0	30	6	1	0	0	0
11955	Tomatoes, Sun-dried	1/4	Cup	13.5	35	8	2	0	0	0
11956	Tomatoes, Sun-dried, Packed In Oil	1/4	Cup	27.5	59	6	1	4	1	2
14155	Tonic Water	12	Fl Oz	366.0	124	32	0	0	0	0
19364	Toppings, Butterscotch or Caramel	1	Tbsp.	20.5	52	14	0	0	0	0
62550	Toppings, Caramel	1	Tbsp.	16.7	52	13	0	-	-	-
62549	Toppings, Hot Fudge	1	Tbsp.	19.0	70	11	1	2	1	-
19365	Toppings, Marshmallow Cream	1	Tbsp.	20.5	64	16	0	0	-	-
19367	Toppings, Nuts in Syrup	1	Tbsp.	20.5	84	11	1	5	0	1
19366	Toppings, Pineapple	1	Tbsp.	21.3	54	14	0	0	-	-
19137	Toppings, Strawberry	1	Tbsp.	21.3	54	14	0	0	-	-
62538	Tortellini, Beef	1	Cup	257.9	230	46	5	1	0	-
55160	Tortellini-Cheese in Alfredo Sauce-Stouffer's	1	Each	251.6	580	35	26	37	-	-
55161	Tortellini-Cheese w/ Tomato Sauce-Stouffer's	1	Each	262.2	360	39	18	15	-	-
62655	Tortilla Chips, Low-Fat, Baked	13	Chips	28.4	110	24	3	1	-	-
19057	Tortilla Chips, Nacho-flavor	1	Ounce	28.4	141	18	2	7	1	4
19424	Tortilla Chips, Nacho-flavor, Light	1	Ounce	28.4	126	20	2	4	1	3
19056	Tortilla Chips, Plain	1	Ounce	28.4	142	18	2	7	1	4
19058	Tortilla Chips, Ranch-flavor	1	Ounce	28.4	139	18	2	7	1	4
19063	Tortilla Chips, Taco-flavor	1	Ounce	28.4	136	18	2	7	1	4
18363	Tortillas, Corn	1	Medium	25.0	56	12	1	1	0	0
18449	Tortillas, Corn, w/o Added Salt	1	Medium	25.0	56	12	1	1	0	0
18364	Tortillas, Flour	1	Medium	35.0	114	19	3	2	0	1
18450	Tortillas, Flour, w/o Added Salt	1	Medium	35.0	114	19	3	2	0	1

Polyunsaturated fat (g)	Dietary Fiber (g)	Cholesterol (mg)	Folate (µg)	Vitamin A (RE)	Vitamin B-6 (mg)	Vitamin B-12 (µg)	Vitamin C (mg)	Vitamin E (mg)	Riboflavin (mg)	Thiamin (mg)	Calcium (mg)	Iron (mg)	Magnesium (mg)	Niacin (mg)	Phosphorus (mg)	Potassium (mg)	Sodium (mg)	Zinc (mg)
0	0	0	1	0	0	0	0	0	0	0	5	.2	2	0	0	21	2	.1
0	-	0	10	0	0	0	0	-	0	0	5	.1	5	.1	3	49	8	.1
0	0	0	1	0	0	0	0	0	0	0	5	0	5	.1	2	47	7	.1
1	-	60	-	400	-	-	2	0	.4	.8	16	1.5	42	5.7	-	933	880	4.5
0	-	0	3	3	0	0	6	-	0	0	2	.1	2	.1	3	32	1	0
2	-	55	-	20	-	-	6	-	.1	.1	32	.8	-	7.6	250	520	560	-
0	0	0	4	0	0	0	0	0	0	0	5	.3	11	.2	28	41	690	0
0	0	0	0	0	0	-	0	0	0	0	0	.2	4	0	33	40	144	.1
-	-	20	-	-	-	-	6	-	0	0	1	.4	-	.6	-	891	861	-
0	1	7	0	16	0	.1	0	.3	.1	0	50	.4	17	.1	55	80	116	.3
1	-	0	42	116	.2	.1	0	-	.3	.2	18	2.1	12	2.4	69	59	220	.3
2	-	0	42	55	.2	0	0	-	.2	.2	14	1.8	9	2	58	58	218	.3
0	-	13	0	38	0	0	0	-	0	0	4	0	0	0	4	6	22	0
1	1	0	8	5	0	0	0	-	0	0	58	3	27	.1	54	67	4	.4
1	0	0	4	3	0	0	0	0	0	0	30	1.5	29	.1	27	34	2	.2
3	1	0	8	0	0	0	0	0	0	0	105	1.4	17	0	81	41	5	.6
3	-	0	8	0	0	0	0	-	0	0	272	1.4	27	0	81	41	5	.6
0	-	0	7	0	0	0	0	-	0	0	23	.4	7	0	17	60	3	.2
1	-	0	8	5	0	0	0	-	0	0	13	.6	15	.1	21	21	814	.4
0	-	0	0	0	0	0	1	-	0	0	1	0	0	0	0	2	5	0
-	1	0	2	4	0	0	4	.1	0	0	2	.2	7	.6	13	91	0	.1
-	-	5	-	100	-	-	6	-	.1	.1	32	.4	-	1.1	70	440	510	-
0	1	0	36	102	.2	0	33	1.7	.1	.1	16	1.1	20	1.2	35	403	661	.3
0	1	0	36	102	.2	0	33	1.7	.1	.1	16	1.1	20	1.2	35	403	18	.3
0	-	0	2	6	0	0	3	0	0	0	1	0	1	.1	2	22	1	0
0	1	0	16	89	.1	0	27	.5	.1	.1	7	.7	17	.9	37	335	13	.1
1		0	6	34	0	0	9	.6	0	.1	13	.5	8	.6	19	125	230	.1
0	-	0	7	70	0	0	17	-	0	.1	42	.9	15	.9	26	305	324	.2
0	-	0	13	76	.2	0	19	-	0	.1	34	.6	14	.9	30	328	283	.2
0	1	0	9	72	.1	0	18	.4	0	.1	31	.7	14	.9	23	265	196	.2
0	-	0	11	47	.1	0	7	-	0	0	24	.3	13	.8	17	129	483	.2
0	1	0	18	76	.1	0	23	.5	.1	.1	6	.6	14	.8	30	273	11	.1
0	2	0	11	79	.1	0	29	.5	0	.1	16	.6	12	.6	34	251	16	.1
0	2	0	9	12	0	0	5	0	.1	.1	15	1.2	26	1.2	48	463	283	.3
1	-	0	6	35	.1	0	28	-	.1	.1	13	.7	22	1	38	430	73	.2
0	0	0	0	0	0	0	0	0	0	0	4	0	0	0	0	0	15	.4
0	-	0	0	6	0	0	0	-	0	0	11	0	1	0	10	17	72	0
-	-	-	-	-	-	-	0	-	0	0	2	-	-	-	5	6	11	0
-	-	0	0	-	-	-	0	-	-	-	36	.2	-	-	-	-	35	-
-	-	0	0	0	0	0	0	-	0	0	1	0	0	0	2	1	9	0
3	0	0	4	1	0	0	0	.2	0	0	8	.2	13	.1	23	43	9	.2
-	0	0	1	0	0	0	12	0	0	0	5	.1	0	0	2	67	13	.1
-	0	0	0	0	0	0	5	0	0	0	5	.2	1	.1	3	16	4	.1
-	9	15	-	150	-	-	4	-	-	-	96	1.5	-	-	-	-	770	-
-	-	-	-	40	-	-	4	-	.5	.3	320	.8	-	1.9	-	270	830	-
-	-	-	-	150	-	-	6	-	.3	.2	240	1	-	1.9	-	420	720	-
-	2	0	0	0	0	0	0	-	0	0	48	0	0	0	0	-	140	0
1	2	1	4	12	.1	0	1	-	.1	0	42	.4	23	.4	69	61	201	.3
1	-	1	7	12	.1	0	0	-	.1	.1	45	.5	27	.1	90	77	284	-
1	2	0	3	6	.1	0	0	.4	.1	0	44	.4	25	.4	58	56	150	.4
1	-	0	5	8	.1	0	0	-	.1	0	40	.4	25	.4	68	69	174	.4
1	-	1	6	26	.1	0	0	-	.1	.1	44	.6	25	.6	68	62	223	.4
0	1	0	4	6	.1	0	0	-	0	0	44	.4	16	.4	79	39	40	.2
0	-	0	4	-	.1	0	0	-	0	0	44	.4	16	.4	79	39	3	.2
1	1	0	4	0	0	0	0	-	.1	.2	44	1.2	9	1.3	43	46	167	.2
1	-	0	1	0	0	0	0	-	.1	.2	14	1.2	9	1.3	43	46	167	.2

Code	Name	Amount	Unit	Grams	Energy (kcal)	Carbohydrates (g)	Protein (g)	Fat (g)	Saturated fat (g)	Monounsaturated fat (g)
19059	Trail Mix, Regular	1	Cup	150.0	693	67	21	44	8	19
19821	Trail Mix, Regular, Unsalted	1	Cup	150.0	693	67	21	44	8	19
19062	Trail Mix, Regular, w/ Chocolate Chips	1	Cup	146.0	707	66	21	47	9	20
19061	Trail Mix, Tropical	1	Cup	140.0	570	92	9	24	12	3
62673	Triscuits	7	Each	31.0	140	21	3	5	1	1
62674	Triscuits, Low-Fat	8	Each	32.0	130	24	3	3	1	0
14269	Tropical Fruit Juice, Blend	3/4	Cup	185.2	85	22	0	0	0	0
15219	Trout, Ckd, Dry Heat	3	Ounce	85.1	162	0	23	7	1	4
15241	Trout, Rainbow, Farmed, Ckd, Dry Heat	3	Ounce	85.1	144	0	21	6	2	2
15116	Trout, Rainbow, Wild, Ckd, Dry Heat	3	Ounce	85.1	128	0	19	5	1	1
19138	Truffles	1	Piece	12.0	59	5	1	4	3	1
55162	Tuna Noodle Casserole-Stouffer's	1	Each	283.5	280	33	17	15	-	-
15128	Tuna Salad	3	Ounce	85.1	159	8	14	8	1	2
15183	Tuna, Light Meat, Cnd In Oil	3	Ounce	85.1	168	0	25	7	1	3
15184	Tuna, Light Meat, Cnd In Water	3	Ounce	85.1	111	0	25	0	0	0
15121	Tuna, Light, Cnd In Water	3	Ounce	85.1	99	0	22	1	0	0
15220	Tuna, Skipjack, Ckd, Dry Heat	3	Ounce	85.1	112	0	24	1	0	0
15185	Tuna, White Meat, Cnd In Oil	3	Ounce	85.1	158	0	23	7	1	2
15186	Tuna, White Meat, Cnd In Water	3	Ounce	85.1	116	0	23	2	1	1
15221	Tuna, Yellowfin, Ckd, Dry Heat	3	Ounce	85.1	118	0	25	1	0	0
5297	Turkey Bologna	1	Slice	21.0	42	0	3	3	1	1
7079	Turkey Breast Meat	1	Slice	21.0	23	0	5	0	0	0
55232	Turkey Dijon, Lean Cuisine-Stouffer's	1	Each	269.3	210	20	20	6	2	-
55791	Turkey Dijonnaise-Stouffer's	1	Each	260.0	113	7	8	5	-	-
5287	Turkey Lunch Meat	1	Slice	28.4	36	0	5	1	0	0
5289	Turkey Pastrami	1	Slice	28.4	40	0	5	2	1	1
5292	Turkey Patties, Breaded, Battered, Fried	3	Ounce	85.1	241	13	12	15	4	6
55163	Turkey Pie-Stouffer's	1	Each	283.5	410	33	16	24	-	-
57809	Turkey Pot Pie-Swanson	1	Each	198.0	191	18	6	11	-	-
5296	Turkey Roast, Roasted	3	Ounce	85.1	132	3	18	5	2	1
5290	Turkey Roll, Light Meat	3	Ounce	85.1	125	0	16	6	2	2
5291	Turkey Roll, Light and Dark Meat	3	Ounce	85.1	127	2	15	6	2	2
5299	Turkey Salami	1	Slice	28.4	56	0	5	4	1	1
41243	Turkey Sausage Omelet on English Muffin-Healthy Choice	1	Each	134.7	210	30	16	4	2	-
5300	Turkey Sticks, Breaded, Battered, Fried	3	Ounce	85.1	237	14	12	14	4	6
41268	Turkey Tetrazzini-Healthy Choice	1	Each	357.9	340	49	23	6	3	-
55164	Turkey Tetrazzini-Stouffer's	1	Each	283.5	400	26	22	23	-	-
5294	Turkey Thigh, Prebasted, Meat&skin, Ckd, Roasted	3	Ounce	85.1	134	0	16	7	2	2
41275	Turkey Vegetable Soup-Healthy Choice	1	Each	212.6	110	17	4	3	1	-
55814	Turkey and Gravy-Stouffer's	1	Each	255.0	78	2	12	2	-	-
5190	Turkey, Back, Meat&skin, Ckd, Roasted	3	Ounce	85.1	207	0	23	12	4	4
5192	Turkey, Breast, Meat&skin, Ckd, Roasted	3	Ounce	85.1	161	0	24	6	2	2
5164	Turkey, Ckd, Roasted, Meat&skin&giblets&neck	3	Ounce	85.1	174	0	24	8	2	3
5188	Turkey, Dark Meat, Ckd, Roasted	3	Ounce	85.1	159	0	24	6	2	1
5184	Turkey, Dark Meat, Meat&skin, Ckd, Roasted	3	Ounce	85.1	188	0	23	10	3	3
5172	Turkey, Giblets, Ckd, Simmered, Some Giblet Fat	3	Ounce	85.1	142	2	23	4	1	1
5306	Turkey, Ground, Ckd	3	Ounce	85.1	200	0	23	11	3	4
5194	Turkey, Leg, Meat&skin, Ckd, Roasted	3	Ounce	85.1	177	0	24	8	3	2
5186	Turkey, Light Meat, Ckd, Roasted	3	Ounce	85.1	134	0	25	3	1	0
5182	Turkey, Light Meat, Meat&skin, Ckd, Roasted	3	Ounce	85.1	168	0	24	7	2	2
5168	Turkey, Meat Only, Ckd, Roasted	3	Ounce	85.1	145	0	25	4	1	1
5166	Turkey, Meat&skin, Ckd, Roasted	3	Ounce	85.1	177	0	24	8	2	3
5288	Turkey, Thin Sliced	3	Ounce	85.1	94	0	19	1	0	0
5196	Turkey, Wing, Meat&skin, Ckd, Roasted	3	Ounce	85.1	195	0	23	11	3	4
11565	Turnips, Ckd	1/2	Cup	78.0	14	4	1	0	0	0
11564	Turnips, Fresh	1/2	Cup	65.0	18	4	1	0	0	0

Polyunsaturated fat (g)	Dietary Fiber (g)	Cholesterol (mg)	Folate (µg)	Vitamin A (RE)	Vitamin B-6 (mg)	Vitamin B-12 (µg)	Vitamin C (mg)	Vitamin E (mg)	Riboflavin (mg)	Thiamin (mg)	Calcium (mg)	Iron (mg)	Magnesium (mg)	Niacin (mg)	Phosphorus (mg)	Potassium (mg)	Sodium (mg)	Zinc (mg)
14	-	0	107	3	.4	0	2	-	.3	.7	117	4.6	237	7.1	518	1028	344	4.8
14	-	0	107	3	.4	0	2	-	.3	.7	117	4.6	237	7.1	518	1028	15	4.8
16	-	6	95	7	.4	0	2	-	.3	.6	159	4.9	235	6.4	565	946	177	4.6
7	-	0	59	7	.5	0	11	-	.2	.6	80	3.7	134	2.1	260	993	14	1.6
2	4	0	0	0	0	0	0	-	0	0	0	.8	0	0	80	-	170	0
1	4	0	0	0	0	0	0	-	0	0	0	1	0	0	120	-	180	0
0	-	0	2	2	0	0	81	-	0	0	7	.2	4	0	2	24	7	.1
2	0	63	13	16	.2	6.4	0	-	.4	.4	47	1.6	24	4.9	267	394	57	.7
2	0	58	20	73	.3	4.2	3	-	.1	.2	-	.3	27	7.5	226	375	36	.4
2	0	59	16	13	.3	5.4	2	-	.1	.1	-	.3	26	4.9	229	381	48	.4
0	-	6	0	17	0	0	0	-	0	0	19	.1	6	0	21	37	9	.1
-	-	-	-	20	-	-	-	-	.3	.2	120	.6	-	3.8	-	380	1090	-
4	0	11	6	23	.1	1	2	-	.1	0	14	.9	16	5.7	151	151	342	.5
2	0	15	5	20	.1	1.9	0	1	.1	0	11	1.2	26	10.5	265	176	43	.8
0	0	15	4	20	.3	1.9	0	.5	.1	0	10	2.7	25	10.5	158	267	43	.4
0	0	26	3	14	.3	2.5	0	.5	.1	0	9	1.3	23	11.3	139	202	287	.7
0	0	51	9	15	.8	1.9	1	-	.1	0	31	1.4	37	16	242	444	40	.9
3	0	26	4	20	.4	1.9	0	-	.1	0	3	.6	29	9.9	227	283	43	.4
1	0	36	3	20	.4	1.9	0	-	0	0	3	.5	29	4.9	227	241	43	.4
0	0	49	2	17	.9	.5	1	-	0	.4	18	.8	54	10.2	208	484	40	.6
1	0	21	1	0	0	.1	0	-	0	0	18	.3	3	.7	28	42	184	.4
0	0	9	1	0	.1	.4	0	-	0	0	1	.1	4	1.7	48	58	301	.2
-	-	45	-	400	-	-	2	-	.3	.2	120	.4	-	4.8	-	640	590	-
-	-	28	-	-	-	-	1	-	0	0	0	.1	-	.3	-	176	356	-
0	0	16	2	0	.1	.1	0	.2	.1	0	3	.8	5	1	54	92	282	.8
0	0	15	1	0	.1	.1	0	.1	.1	0	3	.5	4	1	57	74	296	.6
4	0	53	7	9	.2	.2	0	2	.2	.1	12	1.9	13	2	230	234	680	1.2
-	-	-	-	250	-	-	-	-	.4	.3	80	1	-	3.8	-	290	750	-
-	-	-	-	176	-	-	-	-	.1	.1	8	.5	-	1.4	-	-	363	-
1	0	45	4	0	.2	1.3	-	.3	.1	0	4	1.4	19	5.3	208	253	578	2.2
1	0	37	3	0	.3	.2	0	-	.2	.1	34	1.1	14	6	156	213	416	1.3
2	0	47	4	0	.2	.2	0	.3	.2	.1	27	1.1	15	4.1	143	230	498	1.7
1	0	23	1	0	.1	.1	0	-	0	0	6	.5	4	1	30	69	285	.5
1	-	20	-	60	-	-	-	-	.5	.4	160	2	-	2.9	250	590	470	-
4	-	54	8	10	.2	.2	0	-	.2	.1	12	1.9	13	1.8	199	221	713	1.2
2	-	40	-	-	-	-	72	-	.3	.2	80	1	-	3.8	250	510	490	-
-	-	-	-	20	-	-	-	-	.4	.2	80	.8	-	2.9	-	300	960	-
2	0	53	5	0	.2	.2	0	-	.2	.1	7	1.3	14	2	145	205	372	3.5
1	-	15	-	150	-	-	5	-	0	0	16	.2	-	.4	-	140	540	-
-	-	23	-	-	-	-	0	-	0	0	85	0	-	.9	-	406	296	-
3	0	77	7	0	.3	.3	0	.5	.2	0	28	1.9	19	2.9	161	221	62	3.3
2	0	63	5	0	.4	.3	0	-	.1	0	18	1.2	23	5.4	179	245	54	1.7
2	0	81	17	58	.3	1.1	0	-	.2	0	22	1.7	20	4.2	170	231	57	2.7
2	0	72	8	0	.3	.3	0	.5	.2	.1	27	2	20	3.1	174	247	67	3.8
3	0	76	8	0	.3	.3	0	.5	.2	0	28	1.9	20	3	167	233	65	3.5
1	0	356	293	1527	.3	20.4	1	1.2	.8	0	11	5.7	14	3.8	174	170	50	3.1
3	0	87	6	0	.3	.3	0	.3	.1	0	21	1.6	20	4.1	167	230	91	2.4
2	0	72	8	0	.3	.3	0	.5	.2	0	27	2	20	3.6	169	238	65	3.6
1	0	59	5	0	.5	.3	0	.1	.1	.1	16	1.1	24	5.8	186	259	54	1.7
2	0	65	5	0	.4	.3	0	.1	.1	0	18	1.2	22	5.3	177	242	54	1.7
1	0	65	6	0	.4	.3	0	.3	.2	.1	21	1.5	22	4.6	181	253	60	2.6
2	0	70	6	0	.3	.3	0	.3	.2	0	22	1.5	21	4.3	173	238	58	2.5
0	0	35	3	0	.3	1.7	0	.1	.1	0	6	.3	17	7.1	195	236	1217	1
3	0	69	5	0	.4	.3	0	.1	.1	0	20	1.2	21	4.9	168	226	52	1.8
0	2	0	7	0	.1	0	9	0	0	0	17	.2	6	.2	15	105	39	.2
0	1	0	0	0	.1	0	14	0	0	0	20	.2	7	.3	18	124	44	.2

Code	Name	Amount	Unit	Grams	Energy (kcal)	Carbohydrates (g)	Protein (g)	Fat (g)	Saturated fat (g)	Monounsaturated fat (g)
19160	Twix	1	Each	57.0	272	37	3	13	-	-
19112	Twizzlers Strawberry Candy	1	Pkg	71.0	263	66	2	1	-	-
62663	Uncle Ben's Wild Rice	1	Cup	56.0	190	41	6	1	0	0
62644	V8, Low Salt	8	Fl Oz	240.0	60	11	2	0	0	-
18328	Vanilla Cream Pie	1	Slice	126.0	350	41	6	18	5	8
19201	Vanilla Pudding	1	Cup	298.1	388	65	7	11	2	5
18210	Vanilla Sandwich Cookies w/ Creme Filling	1	Each	10.0	48	7	0	2	0	1
18213	Vanilla Wafers, Higher Fat	1	Each	6.0	28	4	0	1	0	1
18212	Vanilla Wafers, Lower Fat	1	Each	4.0	18	3	0	1	0	0
17091	Veal, Meat Only, Ckd	3	Ounce	85.1	167	0	27	6	2	2
17089	Veal, Meat and Fat, Ckd	3	Ounce	85.1	196	0	26	10	4	4
41285	Vegetable Beef Soup-Healthy Choice	1	Each	212.6	130	21	8	1	-	-
55759	Vegetable Beef w/ Barley Soup-Stouffer's	1	Cup	283.9	190	15	4	13	-	-
55797	Vegetable Chow Mein-Stouffer's	1	Ounce	28.4	14	2	0	1	-	-
11578	Vegetable Juice Cnd	3/4	Cup	181.5	34	8	1	0	0	0
55166	Vegetable Lasagna-Stouffer's	1	Each	274.0	400	33	23	20	-	-
41343	Vegetable Pasta Italiano-Healthy Choice	1	Each	283.5	220	46	7	1	-	-
11581	Vegetables, Mixed, Cnd	1/2	Cup	81.5	38	8	2	0	0	0
11584	Vegetables, Mixed, Frz	1/2	Cup	91.0	54	12	3	0	0	0
55758	Vegetarian Vegetable Soup-Stouffer's	1	Cup	283.9	120	20	6	2	-	-
55828	Veloute Sauce Supreme-Stouffer's	1	Cup	307.6	564	21	9	50	-	-
17165	Venison, Ckd, Roasted	3	Ounce	85.1	134	0	26	3	1	1
62629	Vitamin Supplement, Centrum	1	Each	1.0	-	-	-	-	-	-
62628	Vitamin Supplement, One-A-Day	1	Each	1.0	-	-	-	-	-	-
62630	Vitamin Supplement, StressTab	1	Each	1.0	-	-	-	-	-	-
18392	Waffles, Buttermilk	1	Each	75.0	217	25	6	10	2	3
18367	Waffles, Plain	1	Each	75.0	218	25	6	11	2	3
18403	Waffles, Plain, Frozen, Toasted	1	Each	33.0	87	13	2	3	0	1
12154	Walnuts, Black, Dried	1/2	Cup	62.5	379	8	15	35	2	8
12155	Walnuts, English, Dried	1/2	Cup	60.0	385	11	9	37	3	9
9326	Watermelon	1/2	Cup	80.0	26	6	0	0	-	-
55167	Welsh Rarebit-Stouffer's	1	Each	141.8	270	9	13	20	-	-
41244	Western Style Omelet on English Muffin-Healthy Choice	1	Each	134.7	200	29	16	3	2	-
62675	Wheat Thins	16	Each	29.0	140	19	2	6	1	1
62676	Wheat Thins, Low-Fat	18	Each	29.0	120	21	2	4	0	0
55826	Whipped Sweet Potatoes-Stouffer's	1/2	Cup	142.0	205	30	2	9	-	-
14032	Whiskey Sour	1	Fl Oz	29.9	41	2	0	0	0	0
15223	Whitefish, Ckd, Dry Heat	3	Ounce	85.1	146	0	21	6	1	2
15131	Whitefish, Smoked	3	Ounce	85.1	92	0	20	1	0	0
20089	Wild Rice, Ckd	1/2	Cup	82.0	83	17	3	0	0	0
14536	Wine, Dessert, Dry	3	Fl Oz	90.0	113	4	0	0	0	0
14057	Wine, Dessert, Sweet	3	Fl Oz	90.0	138	11	0	0	0	0
14084	Wine, Table, All	3	Fl Oz	88.5	62	1	0	0	0	0
14096	Wine, Table, Red	3	Fl Oz	88.5	64	2	0	0	0	0
14104	Wine, Table, Rose	3	Fl Oz	88.5	63	1	0	0	0	0
14106	Wine, Table, White	3	Fl Oz	88.5	60	1	0	0	0	0
11602	Yam, Baked	1/2	Cup	68.0	79	19	1	0	0	0
41269	Yankee Pot Roast-Healthy Choice	1	Each	311.8	260	36	19	4	2	-
15225	Yellowtail, Ckd, Dry Heat	3	Ounce	85.1	159	0	25	6	-	-
15135	Yellowtail, Fresh	3	Ounce	85.1	124	0	20	4	1	2
62657	Yogurt, Frozen	1/2	Cup	74.0	160	24	3	6	2	-
62552	Yogurt, Frozen, Fat Free	1/2	Cup	67.0	100	22	4	0	0	-
62658	Yogurt, Frozen, Low-Fat	1/2	Cup	74.0	140	24	3	3	2	-
62604	Yogurt, Fruit, Fat Free	1	Cup	248.0	233	48	10	0	0	0
62627	Yogurt, Fruit, Fat Free, Light	1	Cup	248.0	110	19	10	0	0	0
1121	Yogurt, Fruit, Lowfat, 10 Gm Protein Per 8 Oz	1	Cup	227.0	231	43	10	2	2	1

Polyunsaturated fat (g)	Dietary Fiber (g)	Cholesterol (mg)	Folate (µg)	Vitamin A (RE)	Vitamin B-6 (mg)	Vitamin B-12 (µg)	Vitamin C (mg)	Vitamin E (mg)	Riboflavin (mg)	Thiamin (mg)	Calcium (mg)	Iron (mg)	Magnesium (mg)	Niacin (mg)	Phosphorus (mg)	Potassium (mg)	Sodium (mg)	Zinc (mg)
-	1	5	4	18	0	.2	0	.4	.1	0	67	.4	17	.2	76	117	115	.4
-	-	0	0	0	0	0	0	-	0	0	25	.4	4	.1	220	45	197	.1
0	1	0	0	0	0	0	2	-	0	0	24	1	0	0	0	-	620	0
-	2	0	0	500	0	0	60	-	0	0	48	.6	0	0	0	740	140	0
4	-	78	14	107	.1	.4	1	-	.3	.2	113	1.3	16	1.2	131	159	328	.7
4	0	21	0	18	0	.3	0	.4	.4	.1	262	.4	24	.8	203	337	402	.7
0	0	0	0	0	-	0	0	-	0	0	3	.2	1	.3	8	9	35	0
0	-	0	0	-	0	0	0	-	0	0	2	.1	1	.2	4	6	18	0
0	-	2	0	1	0	0	0	-	0	0	2	.1	1	.1	4	4	12	0
1	0	100	14	0	.3	1.4	0	.4	.3	.1	20	1	24	7.2	213	287	76	4.3
1	0	97	13	0	.3	1.3	0	.3	.3	.1	19	1	22	6.8	203	276	74	4
-	-	15	-	150	-	-	15	-	.1	.1	32	.4	-	1.9	120	360	530	-
-	-	10	-	-	-	-	0	-	0	0	240	.1	-	.2	-	341	1252	-
-	-	0	-	-	-	-	1	-	0	0	24	0	-	0	-	26	156	-
0	1	0	38	212	.3	0	50	.6	.1	.1	20	.8	20	1.3	31	350	662	.4
-	-	-	-	250	-	-	-	-	.4	.1	160	.6	-	.8	-	350	760	-
0	-	0	-	250	-	-	0	-	.3	.5	32	2.5	-	1.5	-	380	330	-
0	-	0	19	949	.1	0	4	-	0	0	22	.9	13	.5	34	237	121	.3
0	5	0	17	389	.1	0	3	.3	.1	.1	23	.7	20	.8	46	154	32	.4
-	-	0	-	-	-	-	0	-	0	0	0	.1	-	.2	-	401	911	-
-	-	98	-	-	-	-	0	-	0	0	2	0	-	0	-	369	1410	-
1	0	95	-	0	-	-	0	-	.5	.2	6	3.8	20	5.7	192	285	46	2.3
-	-	-	400	1000	2	6	60	10	1.7	1.5	162	18	100	20	109	40	-	15
-	-	-	400	1000	2	6	60	10	1.7	1.5	-	-	-	20	-	-	-	15
-	-	-	400	-	5	12	500	10	-	10	-	18	-	100	-	-	-	-
5	-	50	11	26	0	.2	0	-	.3	.2	137	1.6	14	1.5	124	128	451	.6
5	-	52	11	49	0	.2	0	-	.3	.2	191	1.7	14	1.6	143	119	383	.5
1	-	8	12	120	.3	.8	0	-	.2	.1	77	1.5	7	1.5	139	42	260	.2
23	3	0	41	19	.3	0	2	1.6	.1	.1	36	1.9	126	.4	290	328	1	2.1
23	3	0	40	7	.3	0	2	1.6	.1	.2	56	1.5	101	.6	190	301	6	1.6
-	0	0	2	30	.1	0	8	.1	0	.1	6	.1	9	.2	7	93	2	.1
-	-	-	-	40	-	-	-	-	.3	0	280	.2	-	-	-	140	460	-
-	-	15	-	100	-	-	4	-	.5	.5	160	2	-	1.9	240	220	480	-
3	2	0	0	0	0	0	0	-	0	0	24	.4	0	0	0	-	170	0
2	2	0	0	0	0	0	0	-	0	0	24	.4	0	0	80	-	220	0
-	-	30	-	-	-	-	0	-	0	0	0	.1	-	.1	-	200	556	-
0	-	0	2	0	0	0	4	-	0	.1	2	0	1	0	2	16	3	0
2	0	65	14	33	.3	.8	0	-	.1	.1	28	.4	36	3.3	294	345	55	1.1
0	0	28	6	48	.3	2.8	0	.2	.1	0	15	.4	20	2	112	360	867	.4
0	1	0	21	0	.1	0	0	-	.1	0	2	.5	26	1.1	67	83	2	1.1
0	0	0	0	0	0	0	0	0	0	0	7	.2	8	.2	8	83	8	.1
0	0	0	0	0	0	0	0	0	0	0	7	.2	8	.2	8	83	8	.1
0	0	0	1	0	0	0	0	0	0	0	7	.4	9	.1	12	79	7	.1
0	-	0	2	0	0	0	0	-	0	0	7	.4	12	.1	12	99	4	.1
0	-	0	1	0	0	0	0	-	0	0	7	.3	9	.1	13	88	4	.1
0	-	0	0	0	0	0	0	-	0	0	8	.3	9	.1	12	71	4	.1
0	3	0	11	0	.2	0	8	3.1	0	.1	10	.4	12	.4	33	456	5	.1
-	-	55	-	100	-	-	9	-	.2	.2	32	1	-	1.5	150	350	400	-
-	0	60	3	26	.2	1.1	2	-	0	.1	25	.5	32	7.4	171	458	43	.6
1	0	47	3	25	.1	1.1	2	-	0	.1	20	.4	26	5.8	134	357	33	.4
-	-	10	0	20	0	0	0	-	0	0	96	0	0	0	0	-	50	0
-	-	0	-	20	-	-	0	-	-	-	96	0	-	-	-	-	70	-
-	-	10	0	20	0	0	0	-	0	0	96	0	0	0	0	-	50	0
0	0	7	-	0	-	-	0	-	-	-	438	0	-	-	-	423	153	-
0	0	5	-	0	-	-	15	-	-	-	420	.2	-	-	-	510	160	-
0	0	10	21	25	.1	1.1	1	.1	.4	.1	345	.2	33	.2	271	442	133	1.7

Code	Name	Amount	Unit	Grams	Energy (kcal)	Carbohydrates (g)	Protein (g)	Fat (g)	Saturated fat (g)	Monounsaturated fat (g)
1122	Yogurt, Fruit, Lowfat, 11 Gm Protein Per 8 Oz	1	Cup	227.0	239	42	11	3	2	1
1120	Yogurt, Fruit, Lowfat, 9 Gm Protein Per 8 Oz	1	Cup	227.0	225	42	9	3	2	1
62603	Yogurt, Plain, Fat Free	1	Cup	248.0	120	17	13	0	0	0
1117	Yogurt, Plain, Lowfat, 12 Gm Protein Per 8 Oz	1	Cup	227.0	144	16	12	4	2	1
1118	Yogurt, Plain, Skim Milk, 13 Gm Protein Per 8 Oz	1	Cup	227.0	127	17	13	0	0	0
1116	Yogurt, Plain, Whole Milk, 8 Gm Protein Per 8 Oz	1	Cup	227.0	139	11	8	7	5	2
19393	Yogurt, Soft-serve, Chocolate	1	Cup	144.1	231	36	6	9	5	3
19293	Yogurt, Soft-serve, Vanilla	1	Cup	144.1	229	35	6	8	5	2
1119	Yogurt, Vanilla, Lowfat, 11 Gm Protein Per 8 Oz	1	Cup	227.0	194	31	11	3	2	1
19091	York Peppermint Pattie	1	Sm Patty	11.0	38	9	0	1	-	-
55233	Zucchini Lasagna, Lean Cuisine-Stouffer's	1	Each	311.8	260	34	17	6	2	-
41344	Zucchini Lasagna-Healthy Choice	1	Each	326.0	250	41	14	3	2	-

Restaurants, Including Fast Food (Quick Service)

Code	Name	Amount	Unit	Grams	Energy (kcal)	Carbohydrates (g)	Protein (g)	Fat (g)	Saturated fat (g)	Monounsaturated fat (g)
32391	Arby's-Beef'N Cheddar Sandwich	1	Each	194.0	443	30	35	20	10	4
32433	Arby's-Boston Clam Chowder	1	Each	226.8	207	18	10	11	4	5
32400	Arby's-Chicken Breast Fillet Sandwich	1	Each	204.0	547	53	26	28	6	11
32434	Arby's-Cream of Broccoli Soup	1	Each	226.8	180	19	9	8	5	2
32413	Arby's-Curly Fries	1	Each	99.2	337	43	4	18	7	8
32405	Arby's-Fish Fillet Sandwich	1	Each	221.0	526	50	23	27	7	9
32411	Arby's-French Fries	1	Each	70.9	246	30	2	13	3	6
32406	Arby's-Ham'N Cheese Sandwich	1	Each	170.1	411	38	24	19	7	8
32390	Arby's-Regular Roast Beef	1	Each	155.9	388	38	25	16	4	8
32393	Arby's-Super Roast Beef	1	Each	241.0	516	51	26	23	9	8
32410	Arby's-Turkey Sub	1	Each	277.0	599	54	33	28	6	7
32438	Arby's-Wisconsin Cheese Soup	1	Each	226.8	287	19	9	19	8	8
34858	Burger King-Bacon Double Cheeseburger	1	Each	202.0	613	29	34	40	17	15
34856	Burger King-Cheeseburger	1	Each	134.7	360	35	18	16	-	-
34857	Burger King-Double Cheeseburger	1	Each	191.4	537	32	33	30	14	12
34855	Burger King-Hamburger	1	Each	122.9	310	35	16	12	-	-
34843	Burger King-Salad w/ 1000 Island	1	Each	176.0	145	9	2	12	-	-
34842	Burger King-Salad w/ Bleu Cheese	1	Each	176.0	184	7	3	16	-	-
34844	Burger King-Salad w/ French	1	Each	176.0	152	13	2	11	-	-
34845	Burger King-Salad w/ Golden Italian	1	Each	176.0	162	7	2	14	-	-
34841	Burger King-Salad w/ House Dressing	1	Each	176.0	159	8	3	13	-	-
34846	Burger King-Salad w/ Reduced-Calorie Italian	1	Each	176.0	42	7	2	1	-	-
34859	Burger King-Whopper	1	Each	283.5	684	54	28	39	18	15
37167	Dunkin' Donuts-Almond Croissant	1	Each	105.0	420	38	8	27	-	-

Polyunsaturated fat (g)	Dietary Fiber (g)	Cholesterol (mg)	Folate (µg)	Vitamin A (RE)	Vitamin B-6 (mg)	Vitamin B-12 (µg)	Vitamin C (mg)	Vitamin E (mg)	Riboflavin (mg)	Thiamin (mg)	Calcium (mg)	Iron (mg)	Magnesium (mg)	Niacin (mg)	Phosphorus (mg)	Potassium (mg)	Sodium (mg)	Zinc (mg)
0	0	12	24	34	.1	1.2	2	-	.4	.1	383	.2	37	.2	301	491	147	1.9
0	0	10	19	27	.1	1	1	.1	.4	.1	314	.1	30	.2	247	402	121	1.5
0	0	5	-	0	-	-	4	-	.2	-	480	0	-	-	0	600	170	-
0	0	14	25	36	.1	1.3	2	.1	.5	.1	415	.2	40	.3	326	531	159	2
0	0	4	28	5	.1	1.4	2	0	.5	.1	452	.2	43	.3	355	579	174	2.2
0	0	29	17	68	.1	.8	1	.2	.3	.1	274	.1	26	.2	215	351	105	1.3
0	-	7	16	62	.1	.4	0	-	.3	.1	212	1.8	39	.4	200	376	141	.7
0	0	3	9	82	.1	.4	1	.1	.3	.1	206	.4	20	.4	186	304	125	.6
0	0	11	24	30	.1	1.2	2	.1	.5	.1	389	.2	37	.2	306	498	149	1.9
-	-	0	0	0	0	0	0	-	0	0	2	.2	7	.1	10	13	4	.1
-	-	20	-	150	-	-	6	-	.3	.2	200	.8	-	1.9	-	650	520	-
-	-	15	-	350	-	-	6	-	.3	.4	200	1.5	-	1.9	250	830	400	-

Polyunsaturated fat (g)	Dietary Fiber (g)	Cholesterol (mg)	Folate (µg)	Vitamin A (RE)	Vitamin B-6 (mg)	Vitamin B-12 (µg)	Vitamin C (mg)	Vitamin E (mg)	Riboflavin (mg)	Thiamin (mg)	Calcium (mg)	Iron (mg)	Magnesium (mg)	Niacin (mg)	Phosphorus (mg)	Potassium (mg)	Sodium (mg)	Zinc (mg)
4	1	85	45	64	.4	2.3	1	.4	.5	.4	202	5.6	44	6.5	442	380	1801	6
2	1	28	9	100	.1	9.4	4	.1	.2	.1	170	1.4	20	.9	143	319	1157	.7
11	2	101	35	17	.7	.4	0	2.9	.4	.5	123	3.9	51	16.4	322	366	1130	1.9
1	2	3	46	50	.2	.6	9	1.4	.4	.1	237	.8	55	.8	193	455	1113	.7
2	-	0	-	-	-	-	-	-	.1	.1	16	.8	-	1.9	-	724	167	-
11	-	44	-	-	-	-	1	-	.3	.3	72	2.1	-	5.3	-	450	872	-
5	-	0	-	-	-	-	4	-	-	.1	-	.6	-	1.9	-	240	114	-
2	1	68	83	112	.2	.6	3	1.3	.6	.4	151	3.8	19	3.1	177	338	899	1.6
2	1	58	45	71	.3	1.4	2	.2	.3	.4	61	4.7	35	6.6	268	354	888	3.8
6	2	41	42	0	.5	4.4	0	.4	.6	.6	118	6.6	60	9.7	414	518	822	11
8	-	82	-	-	-	-	-	-	.4	.5	94	3.2	-	9.4	-	-	1432	-
3	2	31	7	90	.1	0	2	.4	.2	0	252	1.3	7	.7	241	441	1129	1.1
6	1	115	32	74	.4	3.4	8	1.6	.4	.3	162	4.1	39	8.4	386	480	833	6.6
-	-	-	-	-	-	-	-	-	-	-	-	-	-	-	-	-	705	-
2	2	111	34	111	.3	2	7	2	.3	.2	210	3.3	34	5.5	339	383	947	4.5
-	-	-	-	-	-	-	-	-	-	-	-	-	-	-	-	-	560	-
-	-	17	-	-	-	-	26	-	0	0	336	.1	98	.2	528	405	251	.1
-	-	22	-	-	-	-	25	-	0	0	528	.1	102	.2	664	382	333	.1
-	-	0	-	-	-	-	26	-	0	0	320	.1	98	.2	480	410	330	.1
-	-	0	-	-	-	-	25	-	0	0	320	.1	98	.2	480	389	292	.1
-	-	11	-	-	-	-	25	-	0	0	352	.1	95	.2	592	402	293	.1
-	-	0	-	-	-	-	25	-	0	0	320	.1	105	.2	472	390	430	.1
2	3	113	34	209	.3	3.1	14	4.2	0	0	113	6.5	54	5.6	339	565	1075	5.8
-	3	0	-	-	-	-	-	-	-	-	-	-	-	-	-	-	280	-

Code	Name	Amount	Unit	Grams	Energy (kcal)	Carbohydrates (g)	Protein (g)	Fat (g)	Saturated fat (g)	Monounsaturated fat (g)
37160	Dunkin' Donuts-Apple 'n Spice Muffin	1	Each	100.0	300	52	6	8	–	–
37146	Dunkin' Donuts-Apple Filled w/ Cinnamon Sugar	1	Each	79.0	250	33	5	11	–	–
37159	Dunkin' Donuts-Banana Nut Muffin	1	Each	103.0	310	49	7	10	–	–
37147	Dunkin' Donuts-Bavarian Fillled /w Chocolate	1	Each	79.0	240	32	5	11	–	–
37149	Dunkin' Donuts-Blueberry Filled	1	Each	67.0	210	29	4	8	–	–
37156	Dunkin' Donuts-Blueberry Muffin	1	Each	101.0	280	46	6	8	–	–
37157	Dunkin' Donuts-Bran Muffin w/ Raisins	1	Each	104.0	310	51	6	9	–	–
37151	Dunkin' Donuts-Cake Ring, Plain	1	Each	62.0	270	25	4	17	–	–
37163	Dunkin' Donuts-Chocolate Chunk Cookie	1	Each	43.0	200	25	3	10	–	–
37164	Dunkin' Donuts-Chocolate Chunk Cookie w/ Nuts	1	Each	43.0	210	23	3	11	–	–
37168	Dunkin' Donuts-Chocolate Crossant	1	Each	94.0	440	38	7	29	–	–
37145	Dunkin' Donuts-Chocolate Frosted Yeast Ring	1	Each	55.0	200	25	4	10	–	–
37158	Dunkin' Donuts-Corn Muffin	1	Each	96.0	340	51	7	12	–	–
37161	Dunkin' Donuts-Cranberry Nut Muffin	1	Each	98.0	290	44	6	9	–	–
37166	Dunkin' Donuts-Croissant, Plain	1	Each	72.0	310	27	7	19	–	–
37153	Dunkin' Donuts-Glazed Buttermilk Ring	1	Each	74.0	290	37	4	14	–	–
37152	Dunkin' Donuts-Glazed Chocolate Rings	1	Each	71.0	324	34	4	21	–	–
37144	Dunkin' Donuts-Glazed Coffee Roll	1	Each	81.0	280	37	5	12	–	–
37155	Dunkin' Donuts-Glazed French Cruller	1	Each	38.0	140	16	2	8	–	–
37143	Dunkin' Donuts-Glazed Yeast Ring	1	Each	55.0	200	26	4	9	–	–
37150	Dunkin' Donuts-Jelly Filled	1	Each	67.0	220	31	4	9	–	–
37148	Dunkin' Donuts-Lemon Filled	1	Each	79.0	260	33	4	12	–	–
37162	Dunkin' Donuts-Oat Bran Muffin	1	Each	100.0	330	50	7	11	–	–
37165	Dunkin' Donuts-Oatmeal Pecan Raisin Cookie	1	Each	46.0	200	28	3	9	–	–
21002	Fast Food-Biscuit w/ Egg	1	Each	136.0	316	24	11	20	6	8
21003	Fast Food-Biscuit w/ Egg and Bacon	1	Each	150.0	458	29	17	31	10	13
21004	Fast Food-Biscuit w/ Egg and Ham	1	Each	192.0	442	30	20	27	8	11
21005	Fast Food-Biscuit w/ Egg and Sausage	1	Each	180.0	581	41	19	39	15	16
21007	Fast Food-Biscuit w/ Egg, Cheese, and Bacon	1	Each	144.0	477	33	16	31	11	14
21008	Fast Food-Biscuit w/ Ham	1	Each	113.0	386	44	13	18	11	5
21009	Fast Food-Biscuit w/ Sausage	1	Each	124.0	485	40	12	32	14	13
21010	Fast Food-Biscuit w/ Steak	1	Each	141.0	455	44	13	26	7	11
21001	Fast Food-Biscuit, Plain	1	Each	74.0	276	34	4	13	9	3
21027	Fast Food-Brownie	1	Each	60.0	243	39	3	10	3	4
21060	Fast Food-Burrito w/ Beans	1	Each	108.5	224	36	7	7	3	2
21061	Fast Food-Burrito w/ Beans and Cheese	1	Each	93.0	189	27	8	6	3	1
21062	Fast Food-Burrito w/ Beans and Chili Peppers	1	Each	102.0	206	29	8	7	4	3
21063	Fast Food-Burrito w/ Beans and Meat	1	Each	115.5	254	33	11	9	4	4
21064	Fast Food-Burrito w/ Beans, Cheese, and Beef	1	Each	101.5	165	20	7	7	4	2
21065	Fast Food-Burrito w/ Beans, Cheese, and Chili Peppers	1	Each	167.0	329	42	17	11	6	4
21066	Fast Food-Burrito w/ Beef	1	Each	110.0	262	29	13	10	5	4
21067	Fast Food-Burrito w/ Beef and Chili Peppers	1	Each	100.5	213	25	11	8	4	3
21068	Fast Food-Burrito w/ Beef, Cheese, and Chili Peppers	1	Each	152.0	316	32	20	12	5	5
21069	Fast Food-Burrito w/ Fruit (Apple or Cherry)	1	Each	74.0	231	35	3	10	5	3
21100	Fast Food-Cheeseburger, Large, Double Patty	1	Each	258.0	704	40	38	44	18	17
21098	Fast Food-Cheeseburger, Large, Single Patty	1	Each	219.0	563	38	28	33	15	13
21097	Fast Food-Cheeseburger, Large, Single Patty w/ Bcn&cond	1	Each	195.0	608	37	32	37	16	14
21096	Fast Food-Cheeseburger, Large, Single Patty, Plain	1	Each	185.0	609	47	30	33	15	13
21095	Fast Food-Cheeseburger, Regular, Double Patty	1	Each	228.0	650	53	30	35	13	13
21091	Fast Food-Cheeseburger, Regular, Single Patty	1	Each	154.0	359	28	18	20	9	7
21089	Fast Food-Cheeseburger, Regular, Single Patty, Plain	1	Each	102.0	319	32	15	15	6	6
21101	Fast Food-Cheeseburger, Triple Patty, Plain	1	Each	304.0	796	27	56	51	22	22
21103	Fast Food-Chicken Fillet Sandwich w/ Cheese	1	Each	228.0	632	42	29	39	12	14
21102	Fast Food-Chicken Fillet Sandwich, Plain	1	Each	182.0	515	39	24	29	9	10
21037	Fast Food-Chicken Nuggets, Plain	1	Each	17.0	48	3	3	3	1	1
21038	Fast Food-Chicken Nuggets, w/ Barb. Sauce	1	Each	17.0	43	3	2	2	1	1

Polyunsaturated fat (g)	Dietary Fiber (g)	Cholesterol (mg)	Folate (µg)	Vitamin A (RE)	Vitamin B-6 (mg)	Vitamin B-12 (µg)	Vitamin C (mg)	Vitamin E (mg)	Riboflavin (mg)	Thiamin (mg)	Calcium (mg)	Iron (mg)	Magnesium (mg)	Niacin (mg)	Phosphorus (mg)	Potassium (mg)	Sodium (mg)	Zinc (mg)
-	2	25	-	-	-	-	-	-	-	-	-	-	-	-	-	-	360	-
-	1	0	-	-	-	-	-	-	-	-	-	-	-	-	-	-	280	-
-	3	30	-	-	-	-	-	-	-	-	-	-	-	-	-	-	410	-
-	2	0	-	-	-	-	-	-	-	-	-	-	-	-	-	-	260	-
-	2	0	-	-	-	-	-	-	-	-	-	-	-	-	-	-	240	-
-	2	30	-	-	-	-	-	-	-	-	-	-	-	-	-	-	340	-
-	4	15	-	-	-	-	-	-	-	-	-	-	-	-	-	-	560	-
-	1	0	-	-	-	-	-	-	-	-	-	-	-	-	-	-	330	-
-	1	30	-	-	-	-	-	-	-	-	-	-	-	-	-	-	110	-
-	2	30	-	-	-	-	-	-	-	-	-	-	-	-	-	-	100	-
-	3	0	-	-	-	-	-	-	-	-	-	-	-	-	-	-	220	-
-	1	0	-	-	-	-	-	-	-	-	-	-	-	-	-	-	190	-
-	1	40	-	-	-	-	-	-	-	-	-	-	-	-	-	-	560	-
-	2	25	-	-	-	-	-	-	-	-	-	-	-	-	-	-	360	-
-	2	0	-	-	-	-	-	-	-	-	-	-	-	-	-	-	240	-
-	1	10	-	-	-	-	-	-	-	-	-	-	-	-	-	-	370	
-	2	0	-	-	-	-	-	-	-	-	-	-	-	-	-	-	383	-
-	2	0	-	-	-	-	-	-	-	-	-	-	-	-	-	-	310	-
-	0	30	-	-	-	-	-	-	-	-	-	-	-	-	-	-	130	-
-	1	0	-	-	-	-	-	-	-	-	-	-	-	-	-	-	230	-
-	1	0	-	-	-	-	-	-	-	-	-	-	-	-	-	-	230	-
-	1	0	-	-	-	-	-	-	-	-	-	-	-	-	-	-	280	-
-	3	0	-	-	-	-	-	-	-	-	-	-	-	-	-	-	450	-
-	1	25	-	-	-	-	-	-	-	-	-	-	-	-	-	-	100	-
4	-	233	30	178	.1	.7	0	-	.3	.3	154	3.1	20	.7	185	160	654	1.1
6	-	353	30	53	.1	1	3	-	.2	.1	189	3.7	24	2.4	239	251	999	1.6
5	-	300	33	240	.3	1.2	0	-	.6	.7	221	4.6	31	2	317	319	1382	2.2
4	-	302	40	164	.2	1.4	0	-	.5	.5	155	4	25	3.6	490	320	1141	2.2
3	-	261	37	166	.1	1.1	2	-	.4	.3	164	2.5	20	2.3	459	230	1260	1.5
1	-	25	8	34	.1	0	0	-	.3	.5	160	2.7	23	3.5	554	197	1433	1.6
3	1	35	9	14	.1	.5	0	-	.3	.4	128	2.6	20	3.3	446	198	1071	1.6
6	-	25	11	16	.2	.9	0	-	.4	.4	116	4.3	27	4.2	204	234	795	2.7
1	-	5	6	24	0	.1	0	-	.2	.3	90	1.6	9	1.6	260	87	584	.3
3	-	10	4	2	0	.2	3	-	.1	.1	25	1.3	16	.6	88	83	153	.6
1	-	2	59	16	.2	.5	1	-	.3	.3	56	2.3	43	2	49	327	493	.8
1	-	14	41	119	.1	.4	1	-	.4	.1	107	1.1	40	1.8	90	248	583	.8
0	-	16	59	10	.1	.6	1	-	.4	.2	50	2.3	36	2.2	57	290	522	1.7
1	-	24	37	32	.2	.9	1	-	.4	.3	53	2.4	42	2.7	70	328	668	1.9
1	-	62	30	75	.1	.5	3	-	.4	.2	65	1.9	25	1.9	70	205	495	1.2
1	-	78	72	190	.2	1	3	-	.6	.3	144	3.8	48	3.8	142	402	1024	3
0	-	32	20	14	.2	1	1	-	.5	.1	42	3	41	3.2	87	370	746	2.4
0	-	27	18	23	.2	.6	1	-	.4	.2	43	2.2	30	2.5	70	249	558	2.2
1	-	85	29	56	.2	1	2	-	.6	.3	111	3.9	35	4.2	158	333	1046	4
1	-	4	4	37	.1	.5	1	-	.2	.2	16	1.1	7	1.9	15	104	212	.4
5	-	142	49	54	.4	3.4	1	-	.5	.4	240	5.9	52	7.2	395	596	1148	6.7
2	-	88	28	129	.3	2.6	8	1.2	.5	.4	206	4.7	44	7.4	311	445	1108	4.6
3	-	111	33	80	.3	2.3	2	-	.4	.3	162	4.7	45	6.6	400	332	1043	6.8
2	-	96	39	148	.3	2.5	0	-	.6	.5	91	5.5	39	11.2	422	644	1589	5.6
6	-	93	34	84	.3	2.1	3	2	.4	.6	169	4.7	36	8.3	349	390	921	4.1
1	-	52	22	71	.2	1.2	2	-	.2	.3	182	2.6	26	6.4	216	229	976	2.6
2	-	50	27	37	.1	1	0	-	.4	.4	141	2.4	21	3.7	196	164	500	2.4
3	-	161	52	85	.6	5.9	3	-	.6	.6	283	8.3	61	11.5	541	821	1213	10.9
10	-	78	46	128	.4	.5	3	-	.5	.4	258	3.6	43	9.1	406	333	1238	2.9
8	-	60	29	31	.2	.4	9	-	.2	.3	60	4.7	35	6.8	233	353	957	1.9
0	0	10	2	5	.1	.1	0	-	0	0	3	.2	3	1.1	34	42	90	.2
0	-	8	4	6	0	0	0	-	0	0	0	.2	3	.9	28	42	108	.1

Code	Name	Amount	Unit	Grams	Energy (kcal)	Carbohydrates (g)	Protein (g)	Fat (g)	Saturated fat (g)	Monounsaturated fat (g)
21039	Fast Food-Chicken Nuggets, w/ Honey	1	Each	17.0	49	4	2	3	1	1
21040	Fast Food-Chicken Nuggets, w/ Must. Sauce	1	Each	17.0	42	3	2	2	1	1
21041	Fast Food-Chicken Nuggets, w/ Sweet and Sour	1	Each	17.0	45	4	2	2	1	1
21042	Fast Food-Chili Con Carne	1	Cup	253.0	256	22	25	8	3	3
21070	Fast Food-Chimichanga, w/ Beef	1	Each	174.0	425	43	20	20	9	8
21071	Fast Food-Chimichanga, w/ Beef and Cheese	1	Each	183.0	443	39	20	23	11	9
21030	Fast Food-Chocolate Chip Cookies	1	Box	55.0	233	36	3	12	5	5
21043	Fast Food-Clams, Breaded and Fried	3	Ounce	85.1	333	29	9	20	5	8
21128	Fast Food-Corn On The Cob w/ Butter	1	Each	146.0	155	32	4	3	2	1
21045	Fast Food-Crab, Soft-shell, Fried	1	Each	125.0	334	31	11	18	4	8
21011	Fast Food-Croissant w/ Egg and Cheese	1	Each	127.0	368	24	13	25	14	8
21012	Fast Food-Croissant w/ Egg, Cheese, and Bacon	1	Each	129.0	413	24	16	28	15	9
21013	Fast Food-Croissant w/ Egg, Cheese, and Ham	1	Each	152.0	474	24	19	34	17	11
21014	Fast Food-Croissant w/ Egg, Cheese, and Sausage	1	Each	160.0	523	25	20	38	18	14
21015	Fast Food-Danish Pastry, Cheese	1	Each	91.0	353	29	6	25	5	16
21016	Fast Food-Danish Pastry, Cinnamon	1	Each	88.0	349	47	5	17	3	11
21017	Fast Food-Danish Pastry, Fruit	1	Each	94.0	335	45	5	16	3	10
21104	Fast Food-Egg and Cheese Sandwich	1	Each	146.0	340	26	16	19	7	8
21018	Fast Food-Egg, Scrambled	2	Eggs	94.0	199	2	13	15	6	6
21074	Fast Food-Enchilada w/ Cheese	1	Each	163.0	319	29	10	19	11	6
21075	Fast Food-Enchilada w/ Cheese and Beef	1	Each	192.0	323	30	12	18	9	6
21076	Fast Food-Enchirito w/ Cheese, Beef, and Beans	1	Each	193.0	344	34	18	16	8	7
21019	Fast Food-Eng. Muffin w/ Butter	1	Each	63.0	189	30	5	6	2	2
21020	Fast Food-Eng. Muffin w/ Cheese and Sausage	1	Each	115.0	393	29	15	24	10	10
21021	Fast Food-Eng. Muffin w/ Egg, Cheese, and Can. Bacon	1	Each	146.0	383	31	20	20	9	7
21022	Fast Food-Eng. Muffin w/ Egg, Cheese, and Sausage	1	Each	165.0	487	31	22	31	12	13
21047	Fast Food-Fish Fillet, Battered and Fried	1	Each	91.0	211	15	13	11	3	2
21105	Fast Food-Fish Sandwich w/ Tartar Sauce	1	Each	158.0	431	41	17	23	5	8
21106	Fast Food-Fish Sandwich w/ Tartar Sauce and Cheese	1	Each	183.0	523	48	21	29	8	9
21023	Fast Food-French Toast w/ Butter	1	Slice	67.5	178	18	5	9	-	-
21031	Fast Food-Fried Pie, Fruit (Apple, Cherry, or Lemon)	1	Each	85.0	266	33	2	14	7	6
21077	Fast Food-Frijoles w/ Cheese	3	Ounce	85.1	115	15	6	4	2	1
21116	Fast Food-Ham and Cheese Sandwich	1	Each	146.0	352	33	21	15	6	7
21117	Fast Food-Ham, Egg, and Cheese Sandwich	1	Each	143.0	347	31	19	16	7	6
21114	Fast Food-Hamburger, Double Patty w/ Cond and Veg	1	Each	226.0	540	40	34	27	11	10
21111	Fast Food-Hamburger, Double Patty w/ Condiments	1	Each	215.0	576	39	32	32	12	14
21110	Fast Food-Hamburger, Double Patty, Plain	1	Each	176.0	544	43	30	28	10	12
21113	Fast Food-Hamburger, Large, Single Patty w/ Cond&veg	1	Each	218.0	512	40	26	27	10	11
21112	Fast Food-Hamburger, Large, Single Patty, Plain	1	Each	137.0	426	32	23	23	8	10
21108	Fast Food-Hamburger, Single Patty w/ Condiments	1	Each	107.0	275	33	14	10	4	4
21107	Fast Food-Hamburger, Single Patty, Plain	1	Each	90.0	275	31	12	12	4	5
21115	Fast Food-Hamburger, Triple Patty w/ Condiments	1	Each	259.0	692	29	50	41	16	18
21119	Fast Food-Hot Dog w/ Chili	1	Each	114.0	296	31	14	13	5	7
21120	Fast Food-Hot Dog w/ Corn Flour Coating (corndog)	1	Each	175.0	460	56	17	19	5	9
21118	Fast Food-Hot Dog, Plain	1	Each	98.0	242	18	10	15	5	7
21028	Fast Food-Ice Milk, Vanilla, Soft-serve w/ Cone	1	Each	103.0	164	24	4	6	4	2
21078	Fast Food-Nachos w/ Cheese	3	Ounce	85.1	260	27	7	14	6	6
21079	Fast Food-Nachos w/ Cheese and Jalapeno Peppers	3	Ounce	85.1	253	25	7	14	6	6
21080	Fast Food-Nachos w/ Cheese, Beans, Ground Beef	3	Ounce	85.1	190	19	7	10	4	4
21081	Fast Food-Nachos w/ Cinnamon and Sugar	3	Ounce	85.1	462	49	6	28	14	9
21130	Fast Food-Onion Rings, Breaded and Fried	1	Each	10.0	33	4	0	2	1	1
21048	Fast Food-Oysters, Battered or Breaded, and Fried	3	Ounce	85.1	225	24	8	11	3	4
21025	Fast Food-Pancakes w/ Butter and Syrup	1	Each	74.0	166	29	3	4	2	2
21049	Fast Food-Pizza w/ Cheese	1	Slice	63.0	140	21	8	3	2	1
21050	Fast Food-Pizza w/ Cheese, Sausage, and Vegetables	1	Slice	79.0	184	21	13	5	2	3
21051	Fast Food-Pizza w/ Pepperoni	1	Slice	71.0	181	20	10	7	2	3

Polyunsaturated fat (g)	Dietary Fiber (g)	Cholesterol (mg)	Folate (µg)	Vitamin A (RE)	Vitamin B-6 (mg)	Vitamin B-12 (µg)	Vitamin C (mg)	Vitamin E (mg)	Riboflavin (mg)	Thiamin (mg)	Calcium (mg)	Iron (mg)	Magnesium (mg)	Niacin (mg)	Phosphorus (mg)	Potassium (mg)	Sodium (mg)	Zinc (mg)
0	-	9	2	4	0	0	0	-	0	0	3	.2	3	1	30	38	79	.2
0	-	8	2	4	0	0	0	-	0	0	3	.2	3	.9	29	37	103	.1
0	-	8	2	10	0	0	0	-	0	0	3	.2	3	.9	28	36	89	.1
1	-	134	30	167	.3	1.1	2	-	1.1	.1	68	5.2	46	2.5	197	691	1007	3.6
1	-	9	31	16	.3	1.5	5	-	.6	.5	63	4.5	63	5.8	124	586	910	5
1	-	51	33	126	.2	1.3	3	-	.9	.4	238	3.8	60	4.7	187	203	957	3.4
1	-	12	16	15	0	.1	1	.4	.2	.1	20	1.5	17	1.4	52	82	188	.3
5	-	65	7	27	0	.8	0	-	.2	.2	15	2.3	23	2.1	176	196	617	1.2
1	-	6	44	96	.3	0	7	-	.1	.2	4	.9	41	2.2	108	359	29	.9
5	-	45	20	4	.2	4.5	1	-	.1	.1	55	1.8	25	1.8	131	163	1118	1.1
1	-	216	37	255	.1	.8	0	-	.4	.2	244	2.2	22	1.5	348	174	551	1.8
2	-	215	35	120	.1	.9	2	-	.3	.3	151	2.2	23	2.2	276	201	889	1.9
2	-	213	36	117	.2	1	11	-	.3	.5	144	2.1	26	3.2	336	272	1081	2.2
3	-	216	38	109	.1	.9	0	-	.3	1	144	3	24	4	290	283	1115	2.1
2	-	20	15	43	.1	.2	3	-	.2	.3	70	1.8	15	2.5	80	116	319	.6
2	-	27	14	5	.1	.2	3	-	.2	.3	37	1.8	14	2.2	74	96	326	.5
2	-	19	15	24	.1	.2	2	-	.2	.3	22	1.4	14	1.8	69	110	333	.5
3	-	291	37	181	.1	1.1	1	-	.6	.3	225	3	22	2.1	302	188	804	1.6
2	0	400	53	252	.2	.9	3	.9	.5	.1	54	2.4	13	.2	227	138	211	1.6
1	-	44	34	186	.4	.7	1	-	.4	.1	324	1.3	51	1.9	134	240	784	2.5
1	-	40	192	142	.3	1	1	-	.4	.1	228	3.1	83	2.5	167	574	1319	2.7
0	-	50	253	133	.2	1.6	5	-	.7	.2	218	2.4	71	3	224	560	1251	2.8
1	-	13	17	33	0	0	1	.1	.3	.3	103	1.6	13	2.6	85	69	386	.4
3	-	59	18	86	.1	.7	1	-	.3	.7	168	2.3	24	4.1	186	215	1036	1.7
2	-	234	44	158	.2	.8	1	.6	.5	.5	207	3.3	34	3.9	320	213	784	1.8
3	-	274	54	172	.2	1.4	1	-	.5	.8	196	3.5	30	4.5	287	294	1135	2.4
6	-	31	51	11	.1	1	0	-	.1	.1	16	1.9	22	1.9	156	291	484	.4
8	-	55	44	30	.1	1.1	3	.9	.2	.3	84	2.6	33	3.4	212	340	615	1
9	-	68	31	97	.1	1.1	3	1.8	.4	.5	185	3.5	37	4.2	311	353	939	1.2
-	-	58	15	73	0	.2	0	-	.2	.3	36	.9	8	2	73	88	257	.3
1	-	13	4	33	0	.1	1	.4	.1	.1	13	.9	8	1	37	51	325	.2
0	-	19	57	36	.1	.3	1	-	.2	.1	96	1.1	43	.8	89	308	449	.9
1	-	58	72	76	.2	.5	3	.3	.5	.3	130	3.2	16	2.7	152	291	771	1.4
2	-	246	43	149	.2	1.2	3	-	.6	.4	212	3.1	26	4.2	346	210	1005	2
3	-	122	27	11	.5	4.1	1	-	.4	.4	102	5.9	50	7.6	314	570	791	5.7
3	-	103	45	4	.4	3.3	1	-	.4	.3	92	5.5	45	6.7	284	527	742	5.8
2	-	99	37	0	.3	2.9	0	1.3	.4	.3	86	4.6	37	8.3	234	363	554	5.7
2	-	87	37	33	.3	2.4	3	-	.4	.4	96	4.9	44	7.3	233	480	824	4.9
2	-	71	32	0	.2	2.1	0	-	.3	.3	74	3.6	27	6.2	175	267	474	4.1
2	-	43	17	13	.1	.8	3	.4	.3	.3	51	2.5	22	4.7	110	215	564	2.1
1	-	35	25	0	.1	.9	0	.5	.3	.3	63	2.4	19	3.7	103	145	387	2
3	-	142	31	16	.6	4.9	1	-	.5	.3	65	8.3	54	11	394	785	712	10.7
-	-	51	50	6	0	.3	3	-	.4	.2	19	3.3	10	3.7	192	166	480	.8
3	-	79	60	37	.1	.4	0	-	.7	.3	102	6.2	18	4.2	166	263	973	1.3
2	-	44	29	0	0	.5	0	-	.3	.2	24	2.3	13	3.6	97	143	670	2
0	-	28	5	52	.1	.2	1	.4	.3	.1	153	.2	15	.3	139	169	92	.6
2	-	14	8	69	.2	.6	1	-	.3	.1	205	1	42	1.2	208	129	614	1.3
2	-	35	8	196	.2	.4	0	-	.2	.1	259	1	45	1.2	164	122	724	1.2
2	-	7	13	156	.1	.3	2	-	.2	.1	128	.9	32	1.1	129	151	600	1.2
3	-	31	6	9	.1	1.3	6	-	.3	.1	66	2.3	15	3.1	26	61	343	.5
0	-	2	1	0	0	0	0	0	0	0	9	.1	2	.1	10	16	52	0
3	-	66	8	66	0	.6	3	-	.2	.2	17	2.7	14	2.7	120	111	414	9.6
1	-	19	11	22	0	.1	1	.4	.2	.1	41	.8	16	1.1	152	80	352	.3
0	-	9	59	74	0	.3	1	-	.2	.2	117	.6	16	2.5	113	110	336	.8
1	-	21	27	101	.1	.4	2	-	.2	.2	101	1.5	18	2	131	179	382	1.1
1	-	14	53	55	.1	.2	2	-	.2	.1	65	.9	9	3	75	150	207	.5

Code	Name	Amount	Unit	Grams	Energy (kcal)	Carbohydrates (g)	Protein (g)	Fat (g)	Saturated fat (g)	Monounsaturated fat (g)
21131	Fast Food-Potato, Baked w/ Cheese Sauce	1	Each	296.0	474	47	15	29	11	11
21132	Fast Food-Potato, Baked w/ Cheese Sauce and Bacon	1	Each	299.0	451	44	18	26	10	10
21133	Fast Food-Potato, Baked w/ Cheese Sauce and Broccoli	1	Each	339.0	403	47	14	21	9	8
21134	Fast Food-Potato, Baked w/ Cheese Sauce and Chili	1	Each	395.0	482	56	23	22	13	7
21135	Fast Food-Potato, Baked w/ Sour Cream and Chives	1	Each	302.0	393	50	7	22	10	8
21136	Fast Food-Potato, French Fried In Beef Tallow	1	Large	115.0	359	44	5	19	9	8
21137	Fast Food-Potato, French Fried In Beef Tallow and Veg Oil	1	Large	115.0	358	44	5	19	8	8
21138	Fast Food-Potato, French Fried In Vegetable Oil	1	Large	115.0	355	44	5	19	6	9
21139	Fast Food-Potato, Mashed	1/2	Cup	120.0	100	19	3	1	1	0
21026	Fast Food-Potatoes, Hashed Brown	1/2	Cup	72.0	151	16	2	9	4	4
21122	Fast Food-Roast Beef Sandwich w/ Cheese	1	Each	176.0	473	45	32	18	9	4
21121	Fast Food-Roast Beef Sandwich, Plain	1	Each	139.0	346	33	22	14	4	7
21052	Fast Food-Salad, w/o Dressing	1/2	Cup	69.3	11	2	1	0	0	0
21053	Fast Food-Salad, w/o Dressing, w/ Cheese and Egg	1/2	Cup	72.3	34	2	3	2	1	1
21054	Fast Food-Salad, w/o Dressing, w/ Chicken	1/2	Cup	72.7	35	1	6	1	0	0
21055	Fast Food-Salad, w/o Dressing, w/ Pasta and Seafood	1/2	Cup	139.0	126	11	5	7	1	2
21056	Fast Food-Salad, w/o Dressing, w/ Shrimp	1/2	Cup	78.7	35	2	5	1	0	0
21058	Fast Food-Scallops, Breaded and Fried	1	Each	24.0	64	6	3	3	1	2
21059	Fast Food-Shrimp, Breaded and Fried	1	Ounce	28.4	79	7	3	4	1	3
21123	Fast Food-Steak Sandwich	1	Each	140.0	315	36	21	10	3	4
21124	Fast Food-Submarine Sandwich w/ Coldcuts	1	Each	228.0	456	51	22	19	7	8
21125	Fast Food-Submarine Sandwich w/ Roast Beef	1	Each	216.0	410	44	29	13	7	2
21126	Fast Food-Submarine Sandwich w/ Tuna Salad	1	Each	256.0	584	55	30	28	5	13
21032	Fast Food-Sundae, Caramel	1	Each	155.0	304	49	7	9	5	3
21033	Fast Food-Sundae, Hot Fudge	1	Each	158.0	284	48	6	9	5	2
21034	Fast Food-Sundae, Strawberry	1	Each	153.0	268	45	6	8	4	3
21082	Fast Food-Taco	1	Large	263.0	568	41	32	32	17	10
21083	Fast Food-Taco Salad	1/2	Cup	66.0	93	8	4	5	2	2
21084	Fast Food-Taco Salad w/ Chili Con Carne	1/2	Cup	87.0	97	9	6	4	2	2
21088	Fast Food-Tostada w/ Guacamole	1	Ounce	28.4	39	3	1	3	1	1
21085	Fast Food-Tostada, w/ Beans and Cheese	1	Each	144.0	223	27	10	10	5	3
21086	Fast Food-Tostada, w/ Beans, Beef, and Cheese	1	Each	225.0	333	30	16	17	11	4
21087	Fast Food-Tostada, w/ Beef and Cheese	1	Each	163.0	315	23	19	16	10	3
40349	Hardee's-Big Cheese	1	Each	141.8	4950	280	300	300	–	–
40350	Hardee's-Big Deluxe	1	Each	248.1	6751	460	310	410	–	–
40356	Hardee's-Big Fish Sandwich	1	Each	191.4	514	49	20	26	–	–
40353	Hardee's-Big Roast Beef	1	Each	163.0	365	39	22	13	6	6
40351	Hardee's-Big Twin	1	Each	141.8	369	28	19	20	9	7
40358	Hardee's-Biscuit	1	Each	78.0	275	35	5	13	–	–
40348	Hardee's-Cheeseburger	1	Each	100.6	335	29	17	17	–	–
40357	Hardee's-Chicken Fillet	1	Each	191.4	510	42	27	26	–	–
40347	Hardee's-Hamburger	1	Each	100.1	305	29	17	13	–	–
40354	Hardee's-Hot Dog	1	Each	50.0	346	26	11	22	–	–
40355	Hardee's-Hot Ham & Cheese	1	Each	141.8	376	37	23	15	–	–
40352	Hardee's-Roast Beef Sandwich	1	Each	141.8	323	39	19	11	5	5
44118	Jack In The Box-Bacon Cheeseburger	1	Each	242.0	705	41	35	45	15	16
44101	Jack In The Box-Breakfast Jack	1	Each	126.0	313	29	19	14	5	5
44141	Jack In The Box-Cheesecake	1	Each	99.0	309	29	8	18	9	7
44115	Jack In The Box-Jumbo Jack	1	Each	222.0	497	41	25	26	10	11
44116	Jack In The Box-Jumbo Jack w/ Cheese	1	Each	242.0	559	40	28	31	13	11
44136	Jack In The Box-Regular French Fries	1	Each	109.0	351	45	4	17	4	7
44135	Jack In The Box-Small French Fries	1	Each	68.0	219	28	3	11	3	7
47265	K.F.C.-Colonel's Chicken Sandwich	1	Each	166.0	482	39	21	27	6	4
47261	K.F.C.-French Fries	1	Each	77.0	244	31	3	12	3	7
47260	K.F.C.-Mashed Potatoes and Gravy	1	Each	98.0	71	12	2	2	1	0
47239	K.F.C.-Original Recipe Center Breast	1	Each	103.0	261	9	25	15	4	4

Polyunsaturated fat (g)	Dietary Fiber (g)	Cholesterol (mg)	Folate (µg)	Vitamin A (RE)	Vitamin B-6 (mg)	Vitamin B-12 (µg)	Vitamin C (mg)	Vitamin E (mg)	Riboflavin (mg)	Thiamin (mg)	Calcium (mg)	Iron (mg)	Magnesium (mg)	Niacin (mg)	Phosphorus (mg)	Potassium (mg)	Sodium (mg)	Zinc (mg)
6	-	18	27	228	.7	.2	26	-	.2	.2	311	3	65	3.3	320	1166	382	1.9
5	-	30	30	173	.7	.3	29	-	.2	.3	308	3.1	69	4	347	1178	972	2.2
4	-	20	61	278	.8	.3	48	-	.3	.3	336	3.3	78	3.6	346	1441	485	2
1	-	32	51	174	.9	.2	32	-	.4	.3	411	6.1	111	4.2	498	1572	699	3.8
3	-	24	33	278	.8	.2	34	-	.2	.3	106	3.1	69	3.7	184	1383	181	.9
1	-	21	38	3	.3	.1	6	-	0	.2	18	1.6	38	2.6	153	819	187	.6
2	-	16	38	3	.3	.1	6	-	0	.2	18	1.6	38	2.6	153	819	187	.6
3	-	0	38	3	.3	.1	6	-	0	.2	18	1.6	38	2.6	153	819	187	.6
0	-	2	10	12	.3	.1	0	-	.1	.1	25	.6	22	1.4	66	353	272	.4
0	-	9	8	3	.2	0	5	.1	0	.1	7	.5	16	1.1	69	267	290	.2
4	-	77	40	46	.3	2.1	0	-	.5	.4	183	5.1	40	5.9	401	345	1633	5.4
2	-	51	40	21	.3	1.2	2	-	.3	.4	54	4.2	31	5.9	239	316	792	3.4
0	-	0	26	79	.1	0	16	-	0	0	9	.4	8	.4	27	119	18	.1
0	-	33	28	38	0	.1	3	-	.1	0	33	.2	8	.3	44	124	40	.3
0	-	24	23	32	.1	.1	6	-	0	0	12	.4	11	2	57	149	70	.3
3	-	17	33	213	.1	.6	13	-	.1	.1	24	1.1	17	1.2	68	200	524	.6
0	-	60	29	26	0	1.3	3	-	.1	0	20	.3	13	.4	53	135	163	.4
0	-	18	7	7	0	.1	0	-	.1	0	3	.3	5	0	49	49	153	.2
0	-	35	8	6	0	0	0	-	.2	0	14	.5	7	0	60	32	250	.2
2	-	50	62	31	.3	1.1	4	-	.3	.3	63	3.5	34	5	204	360	547	3.1
2	-	36	55	80	.1	1.1	12	-	.8	1	189	2.5	68	5.5	287	394	1651	2.6
3	-	73	45	50	.3	1.8	6	-	.4	.4	41	2.8	67	6	192	330	845	4.4
7	-	49	56	41	.2	1.6	4	-	.3	.5	74	2.6	79	11.3	220	335	1293	1.9
1	0	25	12	68	0	.6	3	.9	.3	.1	189	.2	28	.9	217	318	195	.8
1	0	21	9	57	.1	.6	2	.7	.3	.1	207	.6	33	1.1	228	395	182	.9
1	0	21	18	58	.1	.6	2	.8	.3	.1	161	.3	24	.9	155	271	92	.7
1	-	87	37	226	.4	1.6	3	-	.7	.2	339	3.7	108	4.9	313	729	1233	6
1	-	15	13	26	.1	.2	1	-	.1	0	64	.8	17	.8	48	139	254	.9
1	-	2	21	71	.2	.2	1	-	.2	.1	82	.9	17	.8	51	130	295	1.1
0	-	4	12	24	0	.1	0	-	.1	0	46	.2	8	.2	25	71	87	.4
1	-	30	75	85	.2	.7	1	-	.3	.1	210	1.9	59	1.3	117	403	543	1.9
	-	74	97	173	.2	1.1	4	-	.5	.1	189	2.5	68	2.9	173	491	871	3.2
1	-	41	15	96	.2	1.2	3	-	.6	.1	217	2.9	64	3.1	179	572	897	3.7
-	-	-	-	-	-	-	-	-	-	-	-	-	-	-	-	-	12510	-
-	-	-	-	-	-	-	-	-	-	-	-	-	-	-	-	-	10632	-
-	-	-	-	-	-	-	-	-	-	-	-	-	-	-	-	-	314	-
2	1	55	29	0	.3	3	0	.2	.4	.4	80	4.5	40	6.6	280	389	1071	7.4
4	1	45	28	14	.2	1.9	2	.7	.3	.2	66	3.3	29	5.5	161	229	475	3.8
-	-	-	-	-	-	-	-	-	-	-	-	-	-	-	-	-	650	-
-	-	-	-	-	-	-	2	-	.3	.5	-	-	-	5.5	-	-	789	-
-	-	-	-	-	-	-	-	-	-	-	-	-	-	-	-	-	360	-
-	-	-	-	-	-	-	2	-	.6	.6	-	-	-	6.4	-	-	682	-
-	-	-	-	-	-	-	-	-	-	-	-	-	-	-	-	-	744	-
-	-	-	-	-	-	-	-	-	-	-	-	-	-	-	-	-	1067	-
2	1	44	25	0	.3	2.6	0	.2	.4	.3	70	3.9	35	5.7	244	323	908	6.5
9	-	113	-	70	-	-	8	-	.5	.2	200	2.8	-	8.4	-	-	1240	-
3	-	190	-	138	.1	1.1	3	-	.5	.4	184	2.6	25	5.3	323	198	1080	1.9
2	-	63	-	-	-	-	-	-	.2	0	88	.3	-	1.9	-	-	208	-
2	-	72	-	67	.3	2.4	4	-	.3	.4	121	4.1	40	10.5	236	444	1023	3.8
2	-	98	-	196	.3	2.7	4	-	.3	.5	243	4.1	44	10.1	366	444	1482	4.3
-	-	0	-	-	-	-	26	-	0	.2	-	.7	-	3.6	-	-	194	-
-	-	0	-	-	-	-	16	-	-	.1	-	.4	-	2.3	-	-	121	-
9	1	47	29	14	.6	.3	0	2.3	.3	.4	100	3.1	41	10.6	261	297	1060	1.5
1	-	2	-	-	-	-	16	-	.1	.2	-	.3	-	1.9	-	-	139	-
0	-	-	-	-	-	-	-	-	0	-	16	.2	-	1.1	-	-	339	-
2	0	87	4	15	.6	4	0	5	1	1	16	1.2	31	11	238	265	600	1.1

Code	Name	Amount	Unit	Grams	Energy (kcal)	Carbohydrates (g)	Protein (g)	Fat (g)	Saturated fat (g)	Monounsaturated fat (g)
47240	K.F.C.-Original Recipe Drumstick	1	Each	57.0	169	5	12	12	2	3
47241	K.F.C.-Original Recipe Thigh	1	Each	95.0	324	11	16	24	6	6
47237	K.F.C.-Original Recipe Wing	1	Each	53.0	172	5	12	11	3	6
48215	McDonald's-Apple Danish	1	Each	115.0	390	51	6	17	4	11
48204	McDonald's-Bacon, Egg and Cheese Biscuit	1	Each	153.0	432	32	18	26	8	16
48174	McDonald's-Big Mac	1	Each	215.0	560	43	25	32	10	20
48205	McDonald's-Biscuit w/ Spread	1	Each	75.0	260	32	5	13	3	9
48170	McDonald's-Cheeseburger	1	Each	116.0	310	30	15	13	5	8
48187	McDonald's-Chef Salad	1	Each	265.0	215	7	20	12	6	6
48181	McDonald's-Chicken McNuggets	1	Each	18.5	45	3	3	3	1	2
48226	McDonald's-Chocolate Lowfat Milk Shake	1	Each	294.1	321	66	11	2	1	1
48189	McDonald's-Chunky Chicken Salad	1	Each	255.0	143	5	23	3	1	2
48217	McDonald's-Cinnamon Raisin Danish	1	Each	110.0	440	58	6	21	5	13
48198	McDonald's-Egg McMuffin	1	Each	135.0	284	27	18	11	4	6
48201	McDonald's-English Muffin w/ Spread	1	Each	58.0	170	26	5	4	2	2
48175	McDonald's-Filet O' Fish	1	Each	141.0	437	38	14	26	5	10
48188	McDonald's-Garden Salad	1	Each	189.0	50	6	4	2	1	1
48169	McDonald's-Hamburger	1	Each	102.0	255	30	12	9	3	5
48209	McDonald's-Hash Brown Potatoes	1	Each	53.0	130	15	1	7	1	4
48210	McDonald's-Hotcakes w/ Margarine and Syrup	1	Each	174.0	440	74	8	12	2	5
48216	McDonald's-Iced Cheese Danish	1	Each	110.0	390	42	7	21	6	13
48180	McDonald's-Large French Fries	1	Each	122.0	400	46	6	22	5	15
48176	McDonald's-McChicken	1	Each	187.0	415	39	19	20	4	9
48223	McDonald's-McDonaldland Cookies	1	Each	56.7	290	47	4	9	1	7
48172	McDonald's-McLean Deluxe	1	Each	206.0	320	35	22	10	4	5
48179	McDonald's-Medium French Fries	1	Each	97.0	320	36	4	17	4	12
48171	McDonald's-Quarter Pounder	1	Each	166.0	410	34	23	20	8	11
48218	McDonald's-Raspberry Danish	1	Each	117.0	410	62	6	16	3	11
48207	McDonald's-Sausage Biscuit	1	Each	118.0	420	32	12	28	8	17
48203	McDonald's-Sausage Biscuit w/ Egg	1	Each	175.0	505	33	19	33	10	20
48199	McDonald's-Sausage McMuffin	1	Each	135.0	345	27	15	20	7	11
48200	McDonald's-Sausage McMuffin w/ Egg	1	Each	159.0	430	27	21	25	8	14
48208	McDonald's-Scrambled Eggs	1	Each	100.0	140	1	12	10	3	5
48190	McDonald's-Side Salad	1	Each	106.0	30	4	2	1	0	1
48178	McDonald's-Small French Fries	1	Each	68.0	220	26	3	12	3	8
48227	McDonald's-Strawberry Lowfat Milk Shake	1	Each	294.1	320	67	11	1	1	1
48225	McDonald's-Vanilla Lowfat Milk Shake	1	Each	294.1	290	60	11	1	1	1
52366	Pizza Hut-Cheese Pizza, Hand Tossed	1	Slice	70.0	259	28	17	10	7	3
52359	Pizza Hut-Cheese Pizza, Pan	1	Slice	70.0	246	29	15	9	5	5
53322	Pizza Hut-Cheese Pizza, Thin'n Crispy	1	Slice	70.0	199	19	14	9	5	3
52363	Pizza Hut-Peperoni Pizza, Thin'n Crispy	1	Slice	70.0	207	18	13	10	5	5
52370	Pizza Hut-Pepperoni Personal Pan Pizza	1	Each	250.0	675	76	37	29	13	17
52367	Pizza Hut-Pepperoni Pizza, Hand Tossed	1	Slice	70.0	250	25	14	12	6	5
52360	Pizza Hut-Pepperoni Pizza, Pan	1	Slice	70.0	270	31	15	11	5	7
52365	Pizza Hut-Super Sprm Pizza, Thin'n Crispy	1	Slice	70.0	232	22	15	11	5	5
52362	Pizza Hut-Super Supreme Pizza, Pan	1	Slice	70.0	282	27	17	13	6	7
52369	Pizza Hut-Super Supreme, Hand Tossed	1	Slice	70.0	278	27	17	13	7	6
52371	Pizza Hut-Supreme Personal Pan Pizza	1	Each	250.0	647	76	33	28	11	17
52368	Pizza Hut-Supreme Pizza, Hand Tossed	1	Slice	70.0	270	25	16	13	6	7
52361	Pizza Hut-Supreme Pizza, Pan	1	Slice	70.0	295	27	16	15	7	8
52364	Pizza Hut-Supreme Pizza, Thin'n Crispy	1	Slice	70.0	230	21	14	11	6	6
54494	Red Lobster-Atlantic Ocean Perch, Lunch	1	Each	141.8	130	1	24	4	1	-
54506	Red Lobster-Calamari, Brded and Fried, Lunch	1	Each	141.8	360	30	13	21	6	-
54486	Red Lobster-Catfish, Lunch Portion	1	Each	141.8	170	0	20	10	3	-
54514	Red Lobster-Chicken Breast, Skinless, Lunch	1	Each	113.4	140	0	26	3	1	-
54487	Red Lobster-Cod, Atlantic, Lunch Portion	1	Each	141.8	100	0	23	1	0	-

Polyunsaturated fat (g)	Dietary Fiber (g)	Cholesterol (mg)	Folate (µg)	Vitamin A (RE)	Vitamin B-6 (mg)	Vitamin B-12 (µg)	Vitamin C (mg)	Vitamin E (mg)	Riboflavin (mg)	Thiamin (mg)	Calcium (mg)	Iron (mg)	Magnesium (mg)	Niacin (mg)	Phosphorus (mg)	Potassium (mg)	Sodium (mg)	Zinc (mg)
2	-	59	5	14	.2	.2	0	.4	.1	0	7	.7	13	3.4	99	130	268	1.7
3	0	103	8	28	.3	.3	0	.5	.2	.1	13	1.4	23	6.5	176	224	549	2.4
2	-	59	-	-	-	-	-	-	.1	0	24	.3	-	2.9	-	-	383	-
2	2	25	3	35	0	0	15	3.8	.2	.3	14	1.4	8	2.2	31	69	370	.2
2	1	248	18	157	.2	.6	0	1.5	.3	.4	181	2.6	30	2.5	442	232	1206	1.7
2	-	103	21	106	.3	1.8	2	-	.4	.5	256	4	38	6.8	314	237	950	4.7
1	1	1	6	0	0	.1	0	1.8	.1	.2	75	1.3	14	1.5	168	100	730	.7
1	-	50	18	118	.1	.9	2	.5	.2	.3	199	2.3	21	3.9	177	223	750	2.1
1	-	120	-	385	-	-	13	-	.3	.3	240	1.4	-	3.4	-	-	459	-
0	-	9	-	-	-	-	-	-	0	0	-	.1	-	1.3	-	-	97	-
0	-	10	-	92	-	-	0	-	.5	.1	333	.8	-	.4	-	-	241	-
1	1	80	28	373	.6	.6	20	11	.2	.2	35	1	38	8.7	262	445	235	3
2	-	34	-	33	-	-	4	-	.3	.3	32	1	-	2.9	-	-	430	-
1	1	221	43	147	.2	.8	1	1.8	.3	.5	250	2.7	32	3.6	312	208	724	1.8
1	2	9	51	37	.1	-	0	.1	.1	.3	151	1.6	12	2.5	60	74	285	.4
11	1	50	20	44	.1	.8	-	-	.1	.3	164	1.8	27	2.7	227	149	1023	.9
0	-	65	-	900	-	-	21	-	.1	.1	32	.8	-	.4	-	-	70	-
1	-	37	-	40	-	-	2	-	.2	.3	80	1.5	-	3.8	-	-	490	-
2	-	0	-	-	-	-	1	-	-	.1	-	-	-	.8	-	-	330	-
5	-	8	-	40	-	-	-	-	.3	.3	80	1	-	2.9	-	-	685	-
2	-	47	-	40	-	-	-	-	.3	.3	32	.8	-	1.9	-	-	420	-
2	-	0	-	-	-	-	15	-	-	.2	-	.6	-	2.9	-	-	20	-
7	-	50	-	20	-	-	2	-	.2	.9	120	1.5	-	8.6	-	-	830	-
1	-	0	-	-	-	-	-	-	.2	.2	-	1	-	1.9	-	-	300	-
1	-	60	-	100	-	-	6	-	.3	.4	120	2	-	6.7	-	-	670	-
2	-	0	-	-	-	-	12	-	-	.2	-	.4	-	2.9	-	-	150	-
1	-	85	-	40	-	-	4	-	.3	.4	120	2	-	6.7	-	-	645	-
2	-	26	-	-	-	-	4	-	.2	.3	-	.8	-	1.9	-	-	310	-
3	-	44	-	-	-	-	-	-	.2	.5	64	1	-	3.8	-	-	1040	-
3	-	260	-	60	-	-	-	-	.3	.5	80	2	-	3.8	-	-	1210	-
2	-	57	-	40	-	-	-	-	.3	.5	160	1.5	-	4.8	-	-	770	-
3	-	270	-	100	-	-	-	-	.4	.5	200	2	-	4.8	-	-	920	-
2	-	425	-	100	-	-	-	-	.3	.1	48	1	-	-	-	-	290	-
0	-	33	-	800	-	-	12	-	.1	.1	16	.4	-	-	-	-	35	-
1	-	0	-	-	-	-	9	-	-	.2	-	.2	-	1.9	-	-	110	-
0	-	10	-	60	-	-	-	-	.5	.1	280	-	-	.4	-	-	170	-
0	-	10	-	60	-	-	-	-	.5	.1	280	-	-	-	-	-	170	-
-	-	28	-	50	-	.3	5	-	.2	.2	300	1.5	32	2.6	220	198	638	2.3
-	-	17	-	45	-	.3	4	-	.3	.3	252	1.5	26	2.5	188	160	470	2
-	-	17	-	35	-	.3	2	-	.2	.2	264	.9	21	2.3	188	131	434	1.8
-	-	23	-	35	-	.3	3	-	.2	.2	180	.9	19	2.5	148	144	493	1.7
-	-	53	-	120	-	.4	10	-	.7	.6	584	3.2	53	7.8	360	408	1335	3.8
-	-	25	-	50	-	.3	4	-	.3	.3	176	1.4	28	2.7	156	208	634	1.9
-	-	21	-	50	-	.3	4	-	.2	.3	208	1.8	25	2.6	176	203	564	2.1
-	-	28	-	50	-	.4	4	-	.2	.3	184	1.4	26	2.6	168	232	668	2.3
-	-	28	-	60	-	.4	5	-	.3	.4	216	1.9	32	3	188	266	724	2.7
-	-	27	-	55	-	.4	6	-	.3	.4	176	1.9	33	3.5	168	258	824	2.4
-	-	49	-	120	-	.5	11	-	.7	.6	416	3.7	53	7.6	320	487	1313	3.8
-	-	28	-	55	-	.4	6	-	.3	.3	192	2.3	35	3.4	184	289	735	2.9
-	-	24	-	60	-	.4	5	-	.4	.4	200	1.4	33	2.9	184	290	832	2.8
-	-	21	-	50	-	.3	5	-	.2	.3	172	1.7	30	2.6	160	272	664	2.3
1	-	75	-	-	-	.3	-	-	.1	.1	-	-	21	1.5	160	-	190	.3
2	-	140	-	-	-	2	-	-	.1	.2	-	.6	21	1.5	360	-	1150	.9
2	-	85	-	-	-	0	-	-	.1	.3	-	-	21	1.9	160	-	50	.3
1	-	70	-	-	-	.1	-	-	.1	.1	-	.4	21	11.4	160	-	60	.9
1	-	70	-	-	-	.6	-	-	.1	0	-	-	28	.8	200	-	200	.3

Code	Name	Amount	Unit	Grams	Energy (kcal)	Carbohydrates (g)	Protein (g)	Fat (g)	Saturated fat (g)	Monounsaturated fat (g)
54510	Red Lobster-Deep Sea Scallops, Lnch Portion	1	Each	141.8	130	2	26	2	0	-
54488	Red Lobster-Flounder, Lunch Portion	1	Each	141.8	100	1	21	1	0	-
54489	Red Lobster-Grouper, Lunch Portion	1	Each	141.8	110	0	26	1	0	-
54490	Red Lobster-Haddock, Lunch Portion	1	Each	141.8	110	2	24	1	0	-
54491	Red Lobster-Halibut, Lunch Portion	1	Each	141.8	110	1	25	1	0	-
54513	Red Lobster-Hamburger, Lunch Portion	1	Each	151.2	410	0	37	28	11	-
54504	Red Lobster-King Crab Legs, Lunch Portion	1	Each	453.6	170	6	32	2	1	-
54507	Red Lobster-Langostino, Lunch Portion	1	Each	141.8	120	2	26	1	0	-
54500	Red Lobster-Lemon Sole, Lunch Portion	1	Each	141.8	120	1	27	1	0	-
54524	Red Lobster-Live Maine Lobster	1	Each	510.3	240	5	36	8	2	-
54492	Red Lobster-Mackerel, Lunch Portion	1	Each	141.8	190	1	20	12	4	-
54493	Red Lobster-Monkfish, Lunch Portion	1	Each	141.8	110	0	24	1	0	-
54498	Red Lobster-Norwegian Salmon, Lunch	1	Each	141.8	230	3	27	12	3	-
54495	Red Lobster-Pollock, Lunch Portion	1	Each	141.8	120	1	28	1	0	-
54502	Red Lobster-Rainbow Trout, Lunch Portion	1	Each	141.8	170	0	23	9	3	-
54496	Red Lobster-Red Rockfish, Lunch Portion	1	Each	141.8	90	0	21	1	0	-
54497	Red Lobster-Red Snapper, Lunch Portion	1	Each	141.8	110	0	25	1	0	-
54509	Red Lobster-Rock Lobster, Lunch Portion	1	Each	368.5	230	2	49	3	1	-
54511	Red Lobster-Shrimp, Lunch Portion	1	Each	198.5	120	0	25	2	1	-
54505	Red Lobster-Snow Crab Legs, Lunch Portion	1	Each	453.6	150	1	33	2	1	-
54499	Red Lobster-Sockeye Salmon, Lunch Portion	1	Each	141.8	160	3	28	4	1	-
54512	Red Lobster-Strip Steak, Lunch Portion	1	Each	255.1	560	0	47	40	17	-
54501	Red Lobster-Swordfish, Lunch Portion	1	Each	141.8	100	0	17	4	1	-
54503	Red Lobster-Yellow Fin Tuna, Lunch Portion	1	Each	141.8	180	6	32	2	1	-
62527	Subway-BMT, on Honey Wheat Bread	1	12 In.	220.0	1011	88	45	57	20	25
62559	Subway-BMT, on Italian Roll	1	12 In.	213.0	982	83	44	55	20	24
62560	Subway-Club Sandwich, on Honey Wheat Roll	1	12 In.	220.0	722	89	47	23	7	9
62561	Subway-Club Sandwich, on Italian Roll	1	12 In.	213.0	693	83	46	22	7	8
62562	Subway-Cold Cut Combo, on Italian Roll	1	12 In.	184.0	853	83	46	40	12	15
62563	Subway-Cold Cut Combo, on Wheat Roll	1	12 In.	184.0	853	88	48	41	12	15
62564	Subway-Ham and Cheese, on Italian Roll	1	12 In.	184.0	643	81	38	18	7	8
62526	Subway-Ham and Cheese, on Wheat	1	12 In.	194.0	673	86	39	22	7	8
62565	Subway-Meat Ball Sandwich, on Italian Roll	1	12 In.	215.0	918	96	42	44	17	17
62566	Subway-Meat Ball Sandwich, on Wheat Roll	1	12 In.	224.0	947	101	44	45	17	18
62567	Subway-Roast Beef, on Italian Roll	1	12 In.	184.0	689	84	42	23	8	9
62568	Subway-Roast Beef, on Wheat Roll	1	12 In.	189.0	717	89	41	24	8	9
62569	Subway-Seafood, on Italian Roll	1	12 In.	210.0	986	94	29	57	11	15
62570	Subway-Seafood, on Wheat Roll	1	12 In.	219.0	1015	100	31	58	11	16
62571	Subway-Spicy Italian, on Italian Roll	1	12 In.	213.0	1043	83	42	63	23	28
62572	Subway-Steak and Cheese, on Italian Roll	1	12 In.	213.0	765	83	43	32	12	12
62573	Subway-Turkey Breast, on Wheat Roll	1	12 In.	192.0	674	88	42	20	6	7
58318	Taco Bell-Bean Burrito	1	Each	206.0	387	63	15	14	4	-
58319	Taco Bell-Beef Burrito	1	Each	206.0	431	48	25	21	8	-
58321	Taco Bell-Burrito Supreme	1	Each	198.0	440	55	20	22	8	-
62585	Taco Bell-Light 7-Layer Burrito	1	Each	276.0	440	67	19	9	-	-
62583	Taco Bell-Light Bean Burrito	1	Each	198.0	330	55	14	6	-	-
62586	Taco Bell-Light Burrito Supreme	1	Each	248.0	350	50	20	8	-	-
62584	Taco Bell-Light Chicken Burrito	1	Each	170.0	290	45	12	6	-	-
62587	Taco Bell-Light Chicken Burrito Supreme	1	Each	248.0	410	62	18	10	-	-
62582	Taco Bell-Light Chicken Soft Taco	1	Each	120.0	180	26	9	5	-	-
62575	Taco Bell-Light Soft Taco	1	Each	99.0	180	19	13	5	4	-
62581	Taco Bell-Light Soft Taco Supreme	1	Each	128.0	200	23	14	5	-	-
62574	Taco Bell-Light Taco	1	Each	78.0	140	11	11	5	4	-
62588	Taco Bell-Light Taco Salad	1	Each	464.0	330	35	30	9	-	-
62580	Taco Bell-Light Taco Supreme	1	Each	106.0	160	23	14	5	-	-
58328	Taco Bell-Mexican Pizza	1	Each	223.0	575	40	21	37	11	-

Polyunsaturated fat (g)	Dietary Fiber (g)	Cholesterol (mg)	Folate (µg)	Vitamin A (RE)	Vitamin B-6 (mg)	Vitamin B-12 (µg)	Vitamin C (mg)	Vitamin E (mg)	Riboflavin (mg)	Thiamin (mg)	Calcium (mg)	Iron (mg)	Magnesium (mg)	Niacin (mg)	Phosphorus (mg)	Potassium (mg)	Sodium (mg)	Zinc (mg)
2	-	50	-	-	-	.4	-	-	.1	-	-	-	53	1.9	240	-	260	1.5
1	-	70	-	-	-	.3	-	-	-	0	16	-	21	1.5	48	-	95	.3
1	-	65	-	-	-	.1	-	-	0	.1	32	-	28	1.5	200	-	70	.3
1	-	85	-	-	-	.2	-	-	.1	0	-	-	21	2.9	160	-	180	.3
1	-	60	-	-	-	.3	-	-	-	.2	-	-	28	2.9	240	-	105	-
1	-	130	-	-	-	1.2	-	-	.3	.1	-	1.5	28	7.6	200	-	115	7.5
2	-	100	-	-	-	1.6	-	-	.2	.1	48	-	70	1.9	320	-	900	6
1	-	210	-	-	-	2	-	-	-	.1	16	.8	35	1.1	160	-	410	1.5
0	-	65	-	-	-	.4	-	-	.1	.1	-	-	21	.4	64	-	90	.3
4	-	310	-	-	-	2	-	-	.2	.2	320	.8	53	2.9	320	-	550	6.8
5	-	100	-	-	-	.8	-	-	.4	.2	16	.8	21	5.7	200	-	250	1.2
1	-	80	-	40	-	.2	-	-	.1	.1	-	1	14	.8	64	-	95	.3
5	-	80	-	-	-	.2	-	-	.1	.2	16	-	35	6.7	240	-	60	.3
1	-	90	-	-	-	1	-	-	.2	.1	-	-	28	.4	160	-	90	.3
4	-	90	-	-	-	1	-	-	.2	.1	80	-	21	2.9	200	-	90	.9
1	-	85	-	-	-	.6	-	-	.1	.1	-	-	21	.8	120	-	95	.3
1	-	70	-	-	-	.3	-	-	0	.1	-	-	21	4.8	120	-	140	.3
1	-	200	-	-	-	.5	-	-	.1	-	48	-	88	3.8	400	-	1090	6
1	-	230	-	-	-	.5	-	-	0	-	32	-	35	1.9	120	-	110	1.5
2	-	130	-	-	-	1.6	-	-	.1	0	80	.2	70	1.9	200	-	1630	6
2	-	50	-	-	-	2	-	-	.1	.4	-	-	35	7.6	280	-	60	.3
2	-	150	-	-	-	1.2	-	-	.3	.2	-	2	35	7.6	280	-	115	9
1	-	100	-	20	-	.3	-	-	.1	.1	-	-	28	3.8	80	-	140	.6
2	-	70	-	-	-	1.6	-	-	0	.1	-	.6	35	13.3	240	-	70	.3
7	6	133	-	-	-	-	-	-	-	-	-	-	-	-	-	1002	3199	-
7	5	133	63	67	.5	2.3	5	5.1	.3	.3	64000	4.3	66	5.1	308	917	3139	6.1
4	6	84	43	83	.5	.4	15	4.2	.4	.5	96000	3.2	40	9.3	247	1055	2777	1.4
4	5	84	47	74	.6	1	20	1.3	.3	.5	58000	3.1	66	12.5	384	971	2717	2.5
10	5	166	39	87	.2	1.2	17	.9	.3	.4	227000	2.9	28	3.8	315	876	2218	2.7
10	6	166	41	90	.2	1.3	18	.9	.4	.4	235000	3	29	3.9	327	1010	2278	2.8
4	5	73	45	174	.3	.8	17	3.8	.4	.5	304000	2.2	50	3.6	527	834	1710	2.8
4	6	73	-	-	-	-	-	-	-	-	-	-	-	-	-	918	2508	-
4	3	88	35	72	.4	3.2	19	1	.4	.3	78000	5	47	9.4	263	1210	2022	6.2
4	-	88	-	-	-	-	-	-	-	-	-	-	-	-	-	1498	2082	-
4	5	83	54	58	.4	2	5	4.4	.3	.2	55000	3.7	57	4.4	266	910	2288	5.3
4	6	75	56	59	.4	2.1	5	4.5	.3	.2	56000	3.8	59	4.5	273	994	2348	5.4
28	-	56	91	107	.3	6.5	5	2.5	.4	.5	230000	4.4	32	7	336	641	2027	5.3
28	3	56	-	-	-	-	-	-	-	-	-	-	-	-	-	557	1967	-
7	5	137	-	-	-	-	-	-	-	-	-	-	-	-	-	880	2282	-
4	6	82	36	119	.4	2.5	6	.8	.5	.3	231000	4.2	43	5.1	456	909	1556	6.8
7	7	67	-	-	-	-	-	-	-	-	-	-	-	-	-	605	2520	-
2	3	9	-	-	-	-	53	-	2	.4	190	4	-	2.8	-	495	1148	-
2	2	57	-	-	-	-	2	-	.3	.4	150	3	-	3.2	-	380	1311	-
2	3	33	-	-	-	-	26	-	2.1	.4	190	4	-	3.6	-	501	1181	-
-	-	5	-	350	-	-	5	-	-	-	300	2.5	-	-	-	-	1130	-
-	-	5	-	300	-	-	2	-	-	-	120	2	-	-	-	-	1340	-
-	-	25	-	600	-	-	9	-	-	-	96	1.5	-	-	-	-	1160	-
-	-	30	-	200	-	-	4	-	-	-	72	1.5	-	-	-	-	900	-
-	-	65	-	250	-	-	5	-	-	-	72	1.5	-	-	-	-	1190	-
-	-	30	-	150	-	-	5	-	-	-	48	.8	-	-	-	-	570	-
1	2	25	-	40	-	-	0	-	.2	.4	48	.6	-	2.8	-	196	554	-
-	-	25	-	100	-	-	2	-	-	-	48	.6	-	-	-	-	610	-
1	1	20	-	40	-	-	0	-	.1	.1	0	0	-	1.2	-	159	276	-
-	-	50	-	1200	-	-	27	-	-	-	120	1.5	-	-	-	-	1610	-
-	-	20	-	100	-	-	2	-	-	-	0	0	-	-	-	-	340	-
10	3	52					01	-	.0	.0	257	4	-	3	-	405	1031	-

Code	Name	Amount	Unit	Grams	Energy (kcal)	Carbohydrates (g)	Protein (g)	Fat (g)	Saturated fat (g)	Monounsaturated fat (g)
58325	Taco Bell-Nachos	1	Each	106.0	346	37	7	18	6	-
58323	Taco Bell-Nachos Bell Grande	1	Each	287.0	649	61	22	35	12	-
58329	Taco Bell-Pintos 'N Cheese	1	Each	128.0	190	19	9	9	4	-
58337	Taco Bell-Salsa	1	Each	10.0	18	4	1	0	0	-
58314	Taco Bell-Soft Taco	1	Each	92.0	225	18	12	12	5	-
58313	Taco Bell-Taco	1	Each	78.0	183	11	10	11	5	-
58332	Taco Bell-Taco Salad	1	Each	575.0	905	55	34	61	19	-
58333	Taco Bell-Taco Salad w/o Shell	1	Each	520.0	484	22	28	31	14	-
58316	Taco Bell-Tostada	1	Each	156.0	243	27	9	11	4	-
61273	Wendy's-Big Classic	1	Each	251.0	480	44	27	23	7	8
62322	Wendy's-Bkd Potato w/ Bacon and Cheese	1	Each	380.0	510	75	17	17	4	3
61287	Wendy's-Bkd Potato w/ Broccoli and Cheese	1	Each	411.0	450	77	9	14	2	3
62524	Wendy's-Bkd Potato w/ Cheese	1	Each	383.0	550	74	14	24	8	6
61281	Wendy's-Chicken Club Sandwich	1	Each	220.0	520	44	30	25	6	7
61292	Wendy's-Chili, Large	1	Each	340.0	290	31	28	9	4	2
61291	Wendy's-Chili, Small	1	Each	227.0	190	21	19	6	2	1
61285	Wendy's-French Fries, Biggie	1	Each	170.0	450	62	6	22	5	15
61284	Wendy's-French Fries, Medium	1	Each	136.0	360	50	5	17	4	12
61283	Wendy's-French Fries, Small	1	Each	91.0	240	33	3	12	2	8
61302	Wendy's-Frosty Dairy Dessert, Large	1	Each	402.2	570	95	15	17	9	4
61301	Wendy's-Frosty Dairy Dessert, Medium	1	Each	321.8	460	76	12	13	7	3
61300	Wendy's-Frosty Dairy Dessert, Small	1	Each	241.3	340	57	9	10	5	3
61271	Wendy's-Plain Single	1	Each	133.0	350	31	25	15	6	7
61272	Wendy's-Single w/ everything	1	Each	219.0	440	36	26	23	7	7
62477	White Castle-Cheeseburger Sandwich	1	Each	64.8	200	16	8	11	-	-
62481	White Castle-Chicken Sandwich	1	Each	63.8	186	20	8	7	-	-
62478	White Castle-Fish Sandwich, w/o Tartar	1	Each	59.3	155	21	6	5	-	-
62483	White Castle-French Fries	1	Each	96.9	301	38	2	15	-	-
62476	White Castle-Hamburger Sandwich	1	Each	58.5	161	15	6	8	-	-
62485	White Castle-Onion Chips	1	Each	92.1	329	39	4	17	-	-
62484	White Castle-Onion Rings	1	Each	60.2	245	27	3	13	-	-
62480	White Castle-Sausage Sandwich	1	Each	48.7	196	13	7	12	-	-
62479	White Castle-Sausage and Egg Sandwich	1	Each	96.3	322	16	13	22	-	-

Polyunsaturated fat (g)	Dietary Fiber (g)	Cholesterol (mg)	Folate (µg)	Vitamin A (RE)	Vitamin B-6 (mg)	Vitamin B-12 (µg)	Vitamin C (mg)	Vitamin E (mg)	Riboflavin (mg)	Thiamin (mg)	Calcium (mg)	Iron (mg)	Magnesium (mg)	Niacin (mg)	Phosphorus (mg)	Potassium (mg)	Sodium (mg)	Zinc (mg)
2	1	9	-	-	-	-	2	-	.2	-	191	1	-	.6	-	159	399	-
3	4	36	-	-	-	-	58	-	.3	.1	297	3	-	2.2	-	674	997	-
1	2	16	-	-	-	-	52	-	.2	.1	156	1	-	.4	-	384	642	-
0	0	0	-	-	-	-	-	-	.1	-	36	1	-	-	-	376	376	-
1	2	32	-	-	-	-	1	-	.2	.4	116	2	-	2.8	-	196	554	-
1	1	32	-	-	-	-	1	-	.1	.1	84	1	-	1.2	-	159	276	-
12	4	80	-	-	-	-	75	-	.6	.5	320	6	-	4.8	-	673	910	-
2	3	80	-	-	-	-	74	-	.4	.2	290	4	-	3.2	-	612	680	-
1	2	16	-	-	-	-	45	-	.2	.1	180	2	-	.6	-	401	596	-
7	-	75	-	60	-	-	12	-	.3	.5	120	3.5	-	6.7	-	500	850	-
8	-	15	-	100	-	-	36	-	.2	.5	80	2.5	-	6.7	-	1370	1170	-
7	-	0	-	200	-	-	60	-	.1	.3	80	2.5	-	4.8	-	1310	450	-
7	-	30	-	150	-	-	36	-	.2	.3	240	2	-	3.8	-	1210	640	-
9	-	75	-	20	-	-	9	-	.4	.6	80	8	-	15.2	-	470	980	-
1	-	60	-	150	-	-	12	-	.2	.2	80	4.5	-	2.9	-	660	1000	-
1	-	40	-	100	-	-	6	-	.1	.1	64	3	-	1.9	-	440	670	-
1	-	0	-	-	-	-	12	-	.1	.3	16	.8	-	3.8	-	950	280	-
1	-	0	-	-	-	-	9	-	0	.2	16	.6	-	2.9	-	760	220	-
1	-	0	-	-	-	-	6	-	0	.2	-	.4	-	1.9	-	510	150	-
1	-	70	-	100	-	-	-	-	1.4	.2	400	1	-	.8	-	1040	330	-
1	-	55	-	100	-	-	-	-	1	.2	320	.8	-	.8	-	830	260	-
-	-	40	-	80	-	-	-	-	.8	.1	240	.6	-	.4	-	630	200	-
2	-	70	-	-	-	-	-	-	.2	.4	80	3	-	5.7	-	280	510	-
7	-	75	-	60	-	-	9	-	.2	.4	80	3	-	6.7	-	430	850	-
-	3	-	-	-	-	-	-	-	-	-	-	-	-	-	-	-	361	-
-	2	-	-	-	-	-	-	-	-	-	-	-	-	-	-	-	497	-
-	1	-	-	-	-	-	-	-	-	-	-	-	-	-	-	-	201	-
-	5	-	-	-	-	-	-	-	-	-	-	-	-	-	-	-	193	-
-	2	-	-	-	-	-	-	-	-	-	-	-	-	-	-	-	266	-
-	4	-	-	-	-	-	-	-	-	-	-	-	-	-	-	-	823	-
-	3	-	-	-	-	-	-	-	-	-	-	-	-	-	-	-	566	-
-	2	-	-	-	-	-	-	-	-	-	-	-	-	-	-	-	488	-
-	3	-	-	-	-	-	-	-	-	-	-	-	-	-	-	-	698	-

Dietary Intake Assessment

Though it may seem overwhelming at first, it is actually very easy to track the foods you eat. One tip is to record foods and beverages consumed as soon as possible after the actual time of consumption.

I. Fill in the food record form that follows. A blank copy is supplied (see the completed example in Figure 12-4). Then, to estimate the nutrient values of the foods you are eating, consult food labels and the food composition table in Appendix A or use your Mosby's NutriTrac software package. If Appendix A does not use the serving size you need, adjust the value. If you drink $\frac{1}{2}$ cup of orange juice, for example, but the table has values only for 1 cup, halve all values before you record them. If you are using Mosby's NutriTrac, adjust the values by using the Amount Dialog. Then, consider pooling all the same food to save time; if you drink a cup of 1% milk three times throughout the day, enter your milk consumption only once as 3 cups. As you record your intake for use on the nutrient analysis form that follows, consider the following tips:

- Measure and record the amounts of foods eaten in portion sizes of cups, teaspoons,tablespoons, ounces, slices, or inches (or convert metric units to these units).
- Record brand names of all food products, such as "Quick Quaker Oats."
- Measure and record all those little extras, such as gravies, salad dressings, taco sauces, pickles, jelly, sugar, ketchup, and margarine.
- For beverages
  —List the type of milk, such as whole, skim, 2%, evaporated, chocolate, or reconstituted dry.
  —Indicate whether fruit juice is fresh, frozen, or canned.
  —Indicate type for other beverages, such as fruit drink, fruit-flavored drink, Kool-Aid, and hot chocolate made with water or milk.
- For fruits
  —Indicate whether fresh, frozen, dried, or canned.

  —If whole, record number eaten and size with approximate measurements (such as 1 apple—3 inches in diameter).
  —Indicate whether processed in water, light syrup, heavy syrup, or other medium.
- For vegetables
  —Indicate whether fresh, frozen, dried, or canned.
  —Record as portion of cup, teaspoon, or tablespoon or as pieces (such as 2 carrot sticks—4 inches long, $\frac{1}{2}$ inch thick).
  —Record preparation method.
- For cereals
  —Record cooked cereals in portions of tablespoon or cup (a level measurement after cooking).
  —Record dry cereal in level portions of tablespoon or cup.
  —If margarine, milk, sugar, fruit, or something else is added, then measure and record amount and type.
- For breads
  —Indicate whether whole wheat, rye, white, and so on.
  —Measure and record number and size of portion (biscuit—2 inches across, 1 inch thick; slice of homemade rye bread—3 inches by 4 inches, $\frac{1}{4}$ inch thick).
  —Sandwiches: list ALL ingredients (lettuce, mayonnaise, tomato, and so on) with amounts.
- For meat, fish, poultry, and cheese
  —Give size (length, width, thickness) in inches or weight in ounces after cooking for meat, fish, and poultry (such as cooked hamburger patty—3 inches across, $\frac{1}{2}$ inch thick).
  —Give size (length, width, thickness) in inches or weight in ounces for cheese.
  —Record measurements only for the cooked edible part—without bone or fat that is left on the plate.
  —Describe how meat was prepared.
- For eggs
  —Record as soft or hard cooked, fried, scrambled, poached, or omelet.

—If milk, butter, or drippings are used, specify kinds and amount.
- For desserts
  —List commercial brand or "homemade" or "bakery" under brand.

—Purchased candies, cookies, and cakes: specify kind and size.
—Measure and record portion size of cakes, pies, and cookies by specifying thickness, diameter, and width or length, depending on the item.

Food Record Form

Time	Minutes spent eating	M or S*	H† (0-3)	Activity while eating	Place of eating	Food and quantity	Others present	Reason for food choice

*M or S: Meal or snack
†Degree of hunger (0 = none; 3 = maximum).

II. Now, using your food record, complete the nutrient analysis form as shown in the sample below. A blank copy of this form follows for your use. Note that your NutriTrac software will create this table for you if you simply enter all food eaten.

Nutrient Analysis Form (Sample)

Name	Quantity	Energy (kcal)	Carbohydrates (g)	Protein (g)	Total fat (g)	Saturated fat (g)	Monounsaturated fat (g)	Polyunsaturated fat (g)	Dietary fiber (g)	Cholesterol (mg)	Folate (μg)	Vitamin A (RE)
Egg bagel, 3.5 inch diameter	1 ea.	180	34.7	7.4	1.0	0.1	0.2	0.4	0.7	44	16	7
Jelly	1 tbsp	49	12.7	—	—	—	—	—	—	—	2	—
Orange juice, prepared fresh or frozen	1½ cup	165	40.2	2.5	0.2	—	—	—	1.4	—	163	28
Cheeseburger, McDonald's	2 ea.	636	57.0	30.2	32.0	13.3	12.2	2.1	0.4	80	42	134
French fries, McDonald's	1 order	220	26.1	3.0	11.5	4.6	4.3	0.5	4.1	8	19	5
Cola beverage, regular	1½ cup	151	38.5	—	—	—	—	—	—	—	—	—
Pork loin chop, broiled, lean	4 oz.	261	—	36.2	11.9	4.1	5.3	1.4	—	112	6	3
Baked potato with skin	1 ea.	220	51.0	4.6	0.2	—	—	0.1	3.9	—	22	—
Peas, frozen, cooked	½ cup	63	11.4	4.1	0.2	—	—	0.1	3.6	—	46	53
Margarine, regular or soft, 80% fat	20 g	143	0.1	0.1	16.1	2.7	5.7	6.9	—	—	—	199
Iceberg lettuce, chopped	2 cup	14	2.3	1.1	0.2	—	—	0.1	1.6	—	62	37
French dressing	2 oz	300	3.6	0.3	32.0	4.9	14.2	12.4	0.4	—	—	—
2% low-fat milk	1 cup	121	11.7	8.1	4.7	2.9	1.3	0.1	—	22	12	140
Graham crackers	2 ea.	60	10.8	1.1	1.4	0.4	0.6	0.4	1.4	—	1	—
Totals		2584	300	99.0	112	33.4	44.1	24.8	17.9	266	395	607
RDA or minimal requirement*		2900		58					—		200	1000
% of RDA		89		170					—		198	61

*Values from inside cover. The values listed are for a male age 19 to 24 years. Note that number of calories is just a rough estimate. It is better to base energy needs on actual energy output.
g = gram
mg = milligram
μg = microgram
RE = retinol equivalent

Vitamin B-6 (mg)	Vitamin B-12 (µg)	Vitamin C (mg)	Vitamin E (mg)	Riboflavin (mg)	Thiamin (mg)	Calcium (mg)	Iron (mg)	Magnesium (mg)	Niacin (mg)	Phosphorus (mg)	Potassium (mg)	Sodium (mg)	Zinc (mg)
—	0.1	—	1.8	0.1	2.5	20	2.1	18	2.4	61	65	300	0.6
—	—	0.7	—	—	—	2	0.1	1	—	1	16	4	—
0.1	—	145	0.7	0.1	0.3	33	0.4	36	0.7	60	711	3	0.1
0.2	1.8	4.1	0.5	0.4	0.6	338	5.6	45	8.6	410	314	1460	5.2
0.2	—	12.5	0.2	—	0.1	9	0.6	26	2.2	101	564	109	0.3
—	—	—	—	—	—	9	0.1	3	—	46	4	15	0.1
0.5	0.8	0.4	0.4	0.3	1.3	5	1.0	34	6.2	277	476	88	2.5
0.7	—	26.1	0.1	0.1	0.2	20	2.7	55	3.3	115	844	16	0.6
0.1	—	7.9	0.4	0.1	0.2	19	1.2	23	1.1	72	134	70	0.7
—	—	—	2.1	—	—	5	—	—	—	4	7	216	—
—	—	4.3	0.1	—	0.1	21	0.5	10	0.2	22	177	10	0.2
—	—	—	15.9	—	—	7	0.2	5	—	3	7	666	—
0.1	0.8	2.3	—	0.4	0.1	297	0.1	33	0.2	232	377	122	0.9
—	—	—	—	—	—	6	0.3	6	0.6	20	36	86	0.1
2.1	3.65	204	22.5	1.79	5.5	792	15.4	298	25.9	1425	3732	3165	11.7
2	2	60	10	1.7	1.5	1200	10	350	19	1200	2000	500	15
107	180	340	225	105	368	66	154	85	132	118	187	633	78

Nutrient Analysis Form

Name	Quantity	Energy (kcal)	Carbohydrates (g)	Protein (g)	Total fat (g)	Saturated fat (g)	Monounsaturated fat (g)	Polyunsaturated fat (g)	Dietary fiber (g)	Cholesterol (mg)	Folate (μg)	Vitamin A (RE)
Totals												
RDA or minimal requirement*												
% of RDA												

*Values from inside cover. Note that number of kcal is just a rough estimate. It is better to base energy needs on actual energy output.

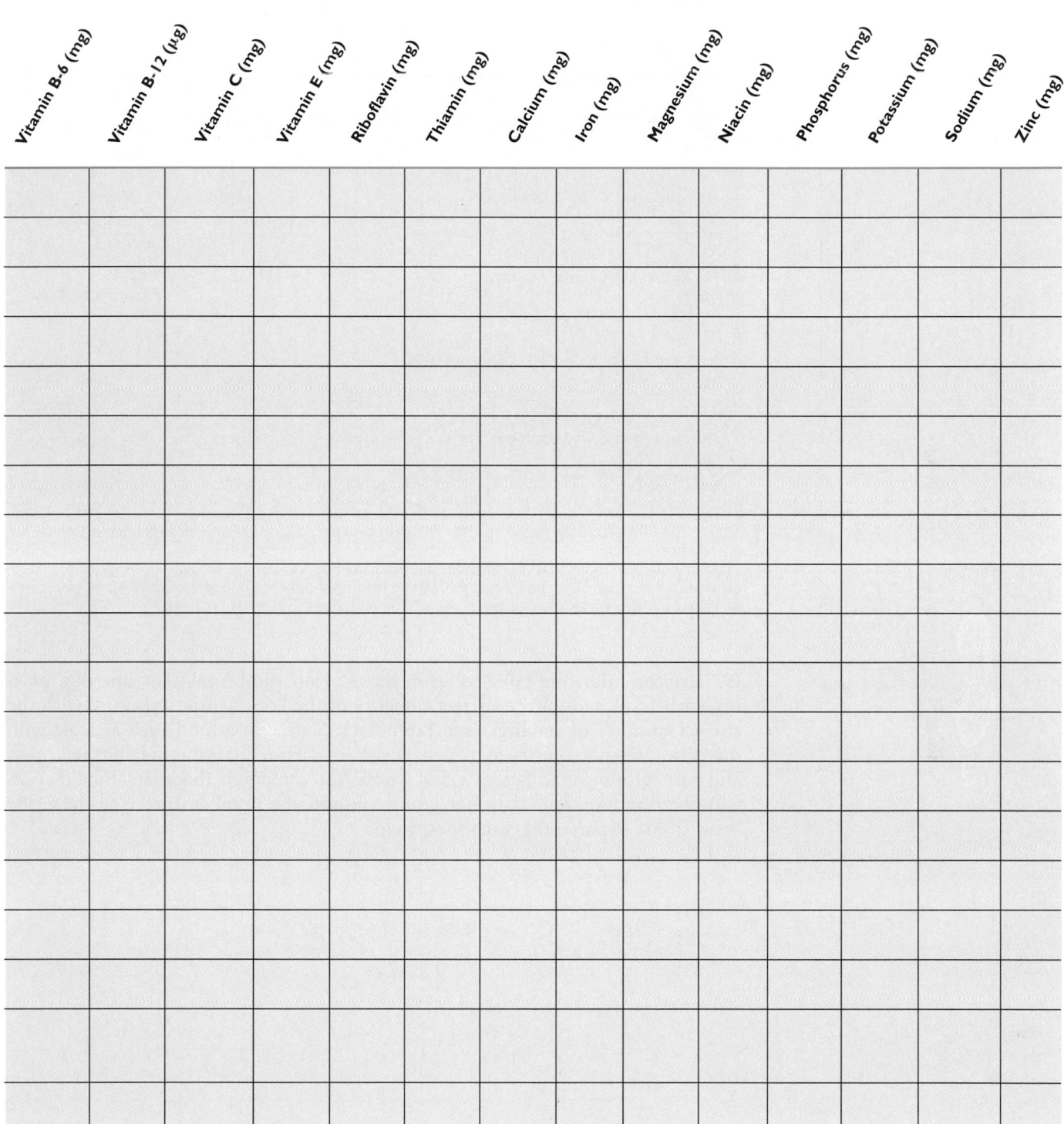

Vitamin B-6 (mg)	Vitamin B-12 (ug)	Vitamin C (mg)	Vitamin E (mg)	Riboflavin (mg)	Thiamin (mg)	Calcium (mg)	Iron (mg)	Magnesium (mg)	Niacin (mg)	Phosphorus (mg)	Potassium (mg)	Sodium (mg)	Zinc (mg)

III. Complete the following table as you summarize your dietary intake.

Percentage of kilocalories from protein, fat, carbohydrate, and alcohol

Intake

Protein (P):	_____ gram/day × 4 kcal/gram =	(P) _____ kcal/day
Fat (F):	_____ gram/day × 9 kcal/gram =	(F) _____ kcal/day
Carbohydrate (C):	_____ gram/day × 4 kcal/gram =	(C) _____ kcal/day
Alcohol (A)*:		(A) _____ kcal/day
	Total kcal (T)/day =	(T) _____ kcal/day

Percentage of kcal from protein:

$$\frac{(P)}{(T)} \times 100 = \underline{\hspace{1cm}} \% \text{ of total kcal}$$

Percentage of kcal from fat:

$$\frac{(F)}{(T)} \times 100 = \underline{\hspace{1cm}} \% \text{ of total kcal}$$

Percentage of kcal from carbohydrate:

$$\frac{(C)}{(T)} \times 100 = \underline{\hspace{1cm}} \% \text{ of total kcal}$$

Percentage of kcal from alcohol:

$$\frac{(A)}{(T)} \times 100 = \underline{\hspace{1cm}} \% \text{ of total kcal}$$

NOTE: The four percentages can total 99, 100, or 101, depending on the way in which figures were rounded off earlier.
*To calculate how many kcal in a beverage are from alcohol, look up the beverage in Appendix A. Determine how many kcal are from carbohydrate (multiply carbohydrate grams times 4), fat (fat grams times 9), and protein (protein grams times 4). The remaining kcal are from alcohol.

IV. Use the following table to again record your food intake for one day, placing each food item in the correct category of the Food Guide Pyramid, with the correct number of servings (see Table 2-1). Note that a food such as toast with margarine would contribute to two categories—namely, to the bread, cereal, rice, and pasta group and to fats, oils, and sweets. You can expect that many food choices will contribute to more than one group. Indicate the number of servings from the Food Guide Pyramid that each food yields.

Indicate the number of servings from the Food Guide Pyramid that each food yields							
Food or beverage	Amount eaten	Milk, yogurt, and cheese	Meat, poultry, fish, dry beans, eggs, and nuts	Fruits	Vegetables	Bread, cereal, rice, and pasta	Fats, oils, and sweets
Group totals							
Recommended servings							in moderation
Shortages in numbers of servings							

V.   **Evaluation.** Are there any weaknesses suggested in your nutrient intake that correspond to missing servings in the Food Guide Pyramid? Consider replacing the missing servings to improve your nutrient intake.

VI. **For the same day you keep your food record, also keep a 24-hour record of your activities.** Include sleeping, sitting, and walking, as well as the obvious forms of physical activity. Calculate your energy expenditure for these activities using Table 11-2 or Mosby's NutriTrac software. Try to substitute a similar activity if your particular activity is not listed. Calculate the total kcal you used for the day (total for column 3). Below is an example of an activity record. A blank form follows for your use. Ask your professor whether you are to turn in the form or the activity printout from the software.

WEIGHT (LB OR KG):

Energy Cost

Activity	Time (minutes); convert to hours	Column 1 kcal/hr (from App. K)	Column 2: time in hr	Column 3 (Column 1 × Column 2)
Example for a 150 lb man: Brisk walking	(30 min) 0.5 hr	299	0.5	150

WEIGHT (LB OR KG):

Energy Cost

Activity	Time (minutes); convert to hours	Column 1 kcal/hr (from App. K)	Column 2: time in hr	Column 3 (Column 1 × Column 2)
Total kcal expended (from adding all of column 3):				

This Appendix is now completed. See whether your professor wants you to complete more work before turning in this assignment.

APPENDIX C

RDIs, DRVs, and a Label-Reading Exercise

Daily Values (DVs) Established by FDA as Standards for Nutrient-Labeling Purposes are a Combination of RDIs and DRVs

Reference Daily Intakes (RDIs)*†§

Nutrient	Reference Amount
Vitamin A‖	5000 International Units (IU)
Vitamin C‖	60 mg
Thiamin	1.5 mg
Riboflavin	1.7 mg
Niacin	20 mg
Calcium‖	1 g
Iron‖	18 mg
Vitamin D	400 IU
Vitamin E	30 IU
Vitamin B-6	2 mg
Folic acid	0.4 mg
Vitamin B-12	6 µg
Phosphorus	1 g
Iodine	150 µg
Magnesium	400 mg
Zinc	15 mg
Copper	2 mg
Biotin	0.3 mg
Pantothenic acid	10 mg

Daily Reference Values (DRVs)†§

Nutrient	Basis for Calculating Daily Reference Value
Total fat	30% of kcal
Saturated fat	10% of kcal
Carbohydrate	60% of kcal
Dietary fiber	11.5 g of fiber per each 1000 kcal
Protein	10% of kcal for adults and children over 4 years

Nutrient	2000 Calories	2500 Calories
Total fat‖	<65 g	<80 g
Saturated fat‖	<20 g	<25 g
Cholesterol‖	<300 mg	<300 mg
Sodium‖	<2400 mg	<2400 mg
Total carbohydrate‖	300 g	375 g
Dietary fiber‖	25 g	30 g
Protein	50 g	65 g
Potassium	3500 mg	3500 mg

*Based on the National Academy of Sciences' 1968 Recommended Dietary Allowances (same as USRDA used until 1994). Values are highest RDAs except for pregnancy and breastfeeding.
†The DRV for protein does not apply to certain populations. An RDI for protein has been established for these groups: infants under 1 yr, 14 g; children 1-4 yr, 16 g; pregnant women, 50 g; and nursing mothers, 66 g.
‡Daily Value (DV) as used on label includes both RDIs for vitamins and minerals and DRVs for macronutrients and some minerals.
§Some DVs have been rounded to make label reading easier for consumers.
‖Percentages of DVs must be declared on label. Percentages of DV for other nutrients may be provided voluntarily. Note that the DVs for some nutrients (e.g., total fat) increase as energy intake increases.
g = gram
mg = milligram
µg = microgram

Label-Reading Exercise

Hone your label-reading skills by completing the following exercise. Choose a label on a cereal box. Be sure to show your calculations if this is to be turned in as part of your class assignments.

What is the weight in ounces of one serving?	_____ ounces
Convert the weight to grams	_____ grams
Does this serving size seem appropriate considering the nature of the food? Why/Why not?	

_____

Each serving contains how many grams of dietary fiber?	_____ grams
What percentage of the weight of one serving is dietary fiber?	_____ % weight

Next, refer to the carbohydrate information on the bottom of the label.

How many grams of complex carbohydrate are provided per serving?	_____ grams
How many kcal are provided by starch and related carbohydrates?	_____ kcal
How many kcal are provided by sugars?	_____ kcal
Approximately how many teaspoons of sugars is this (Hint: 5 grams = 1 teaspoon.)	_____ teaspoons
What percentage of the kcal in this cereal come from sugars?	_____ % kcal

Name the sugars provided by the fruit in this cereal.   _____ and _____

Name the sugar provided by milk.   _____

How would you classify the carbohydrates in this cereal?
   Circle one and explain:
      Mostly complex
      Mostly complex with simple sugars from fruit in the cereal
      Mostly simple sugars

Explain: _____

_____

_____

Refer to the top of the label where two columns, cereal and cereal plus milk, are listed:

What percentage of the kcal come from protein?	_____ % kcal
How many grams of protein are in ½ cup milk?	_____ grams
What type of milk was used for the label information?	_____

How much sodium is in a serving of this food?   _____

Is this cereal high in fat? (>5-7 grams per serving)   _____

What is the main ingredient in this cereal?   _____

Identify at least three vitamins added to the cereal.   _____

_____

_____

How is cholesterol identified on the food label? What is the maximum recommended intake?   _____

How much sodium is in a serving of this food?   _____

How much salt does this represent? (Hint: sodium × 2.5)   _____

What % of the Daily Value (DV) for sodium would one serving of this food contain?
   (Hint: mg ÷ DV for sodium)   _____

Would you buy or will you continue to eat this cereal based on your evaluation? Why/Why not?

_____

The Exchange System:
A Helpful Menu-Planning Tool

The Exchange System is a tool for quickly estimating the energy, protein, carbo-hydrate, and fat content of a food or meal. Although learning to use the Exchange System is a bit tedious, much like learning a foreign language, it greatly simplifies menu planning. The Exchange System organizes many details of the nutrient com-position of foods into a manageable framework. By using the Exchange System, you can plan daily menus without having to look up or memorize the nutrient values of numerous foods. So the time you spend now becoming familiar with the Exchange System will pay dividends in the future.

In the Exchange System, individual foods are placed into three broad groups: carbohydrate, meat and meat substitutes, and fat. Within these groups are lists that contain foods of similar macronutrient composition: various types of milk; fruit; vegetables; starch; other carbohydrates; various types of meat and meat substitutes; and fat. These lists are designed so that when the proper serving size is observed, each food on a list provides about the same amount of carbohydrate, protein, fat, and energy. This equality allows the exchange of foods on each list. Hence the term *Exchange System.*

The Exchange System was originally developed for planning diabetic diets. Diabetes is easier to control if the person's diet has about the same composition day after day. If a certain number of "exchanges" from each of the various lists is eaten each day, that regularity is easier to achieve. However, because the Exchange System provides a quick way to estimate the energy, carbohydrate, protein, and fat content in any food or meal, it is a valuable menu-planning tool.

Becoming Familiar with the Exchange System

To use the Exchange System, you must know which foods are on each list and the serving sizes for each food.

Table D-1 gives the serving sizes for foods on each exchange list, as well as the carbohydrate, protein, fat, and energy content per exchange. Note that the meat and milk lists are divided into subclasses that vary in fat content and hence in the num-ber of calories they provide. Foods on the meat and fat lists contain essentially no carbohydrate; those on the fruit and fat lists lack appreciable amounts of protein; and those on the vegetable, fruit, and other carbohydrates lists contain no fat. You need to study Table D-1 to become familiar with the sizes of the exchanges (i.e., serving sizes) on each list and the amounts of carbohydrate, protein, fat, and energy per exchange.

TABLE D-1

Nutrient Composition of Exchange System Lists (1995 Edition)

Groups/lists	Household measures*	Carbohydrate (grams)	Protein (grams)	Fat (grams)	Energy (kcal)
CARBOHYDRATE GROUP					
Starch	1 slice, ¾ cup raw, or ½ cup cooked	15	3	1 or less†	80
Fruit	1 small/medium piece	15	—	—	60
Milk	1 cup				
Skim/very low-fat		12	8	0–3†	90
Low-fat		12	8	5	120
Whole		12	8	8	150
Other carbohydrates	Varies	15	Varies	Varies	Varies
Vegetables	1 cup raw or ½ cup cooked	5	2	—	25
MEAT AND MEAT SUBSTITUTES GROUP	1 oz				
Very lean		—	7	0–1	35
Lean		—	7	3	55
Medium-fat		—	7	5	75
High-fat		—	7	8	100
FAT GROUP	1 tsp		—	5	45

The American Diabetes Association and American Dietetic Association: *Exchange lists for meal planning,* 1995.
*Just an estimate. See exchange lists for actual amounts.
†Calculated as 1 gram for purposes of energy contribution.

Before you can turn a group of exchanges into a daily meal plan, you must be aware of which foods are on each exchange list. The entire U.S. Exchange System is presented in Appendix E, which you should consult frequently while exploring the system to discover its various peculiarities. For example, the starch list includes not only bread, dry cereal, cooked cereal, rice, and pasta, but also baked beans, corn on the cob, and potatoes. These foods are not identical to those composing the bread, cereal, rice, and pasta group in the Food Guide Pyramid. The Exchange System is not concerned with the origin of a food, whether animal or vegetable. It is primarily concerned with the macronutrients carbohydrate, protein, and fat in each food on a specific list. For example, the carbohydrate composition of potatoes resembles that of bread more than that of broccoli, although potatoes are vegetables.

The very lean–meat list contains the white meat of chicken and turkey (without skin), water-packed tuna, shrimp, nonfat cottage cheese, and fat-free cheese. The lean-meat list contains round steak, lean ham, veal, the dark meat of chicken and turkey (without skin), fish, cottage cheese, and low-fat luncheon meat. The medium-fat meat list contains T-bone steak, pork loin roast, lamb rib roast, any fried fish, mozzarella cheese, and eggs. The high-fat meat list contains ribs, sausage, most luncheon meats (full fat), cheddar cheese, and peanut butter. Note that several foods on the meat and meat substitutes list are not meats, again demonstrating that origin is not important in classifying foods in the Exchange System.

The vegetable list contains most vegetables, but some starchy vegetables are on the starch list. Most vegetables, such as cabbage, celery, mushrooms, lettuce, and zucchini, can be considered "free foods"; their minimal energy contribution need not count in the calculations when they are eaten in moderation (1 to 2 servings per meal or snack). The fruit list contains fruits and fruit juices. The list of other carbohydrates includes jam, angelfood cake, fat-free frozen yogurt, and foods such as frosted cake that count as both other carbohydrate exchanges and fat exchanges.

The milk exchange list contains milk, plain yogurt, and buttermilk. The amount of fat in a product determines whether the serving is skim/very low fat, low fat, or whole.

The fat list contains margarine, mayonnaise, nuts and seeds, salad oils, olives, and full-fat sour cream and cream cheese. Bacon is listed as a fat, rather than as a high-fat meat.

Free foods, other than a moderate intake of most vegetables, include bouillon, diet soda, coffee, tea, dill pickles, and vinegar, as well as herbs and spices.

Using the Exchange System to Develop Daily Menus

Now let's use the Exchange System to plan a 1-day menu. We will target an energy content of 2000 kcal, with 55% coming from carbohydrates (1100 kcal), 15% from protein (300 kcal), and 30% from fat (600 kcal). This can be translated into 2 low-fat milk exchanges, 3 vegetable exchanges, 5 fruit exchanges, 11 starch exchanges, 4 lean meat exchanges, and 6 fat exchanges (Table D-2). Note that this is only one of many possible combinations; the Exchange System offers great flexibility.

Table D-3 arbitrarily separates these exchanges into breakfast, lunch, dinner, and a snack. Breakfast includes 1 low-fat milk exchange, 2 fruit exchanges, 2 starch exchanges, and 1 fat exchange. This total corresponds to $^3/_4$ cup of cold cereal, 1 cup of 2% milk, 1 slice of bread with 1 teaspoon margarine, and 1 cup of orange juice.

Lunch consists of 2 fat exchanges, 5 starch exchanges, 1 vegetable exchange, 1 low-fat milk exchange, and 2 fruit exchanges. This translates into 1 slice of bacon with 1 teaspoon mayonnaise on two slices of bread, with tomato. In other words, a bacon and tomato sandwich. You can also add lettuce to the sandwich. This can be considered a "free vegetable" choice. Add to this meal a 9-inch banana (1 exchange = 1 small banana), 1 cup of 2% milk, and 24 animal cookies.

TABLE D-2

Possible Exchange Patterns that Yield 55% of Energy as Carbohydrate; 30% as Fat; and 15% as Protein for Energy Intakes ≥2000 Kcal

Kcal/day	1200*	1600*	2000	2400	2800	3200	3600
EXCHANGE LIST							
Milk (low fat)	2	2	2	2	2	2	2
Vegetable	3	3	3	4	4	4	4
Fruit	3	4	5	6	8	9	9
Starch	5	8	11	13	15	18	21
Meat (lean)	4	4	4	5	6	7	8
Fat	2	4	6	8	10	11	13

This is just one set of options. More meat could be included if less milk is used, for example.
*Energy intakes of 1200 and 1600 kcal contain 19% of energy as protein and less carbohydrate to allow for greater flexibility in diet planning.

TABLE D-3

Sample 1-Day Menu Based on the Exchange System Plan*

BREAKFAST

1 low-fat milk exchange	1 cup 2% milk (put some on cereal)
2 fruit exchanges	1 cup orange juice
2 starch exchanges	3/4 cup cold cereal, 1 piece whole-wheat toast
1 fat exchange	1 tsp margarine on toast

LUNCH

5 starch exchanges	2 slices whole-wheat bread, 24 animal cookies
2 fat exchanges	1 slice bacon, 1 tsp mayonnaise
1 vegetable exchange	1 sliced tomato
2 fruit exchanges	1 banana (9 inches)
1 low-fat milk exchange	1 cup 2% milk

DINNER

4 lean meat exchanges	4 oz lean ham
2 starch exchanges	1 medium baked potato
1 fat exchange	1 tsp margarine
2 vegetable exchanges	1 cup broccoli
1 fruit exchange	1 kiwi fruit Coffee (if desired)

SNACK

2 starch exchanges	1 bagel
2 fat exchanges	2 tbsp regular cream cheese

*The target plan was a 2000 kcal energy intake, with 55% from carbohydrate, 15% from protein, and 30% from fat. Computer analysis indicated that this menu yielded 2050 kcal, with 55% from carbohydrate, 16% from protein, and 29% from fat—in close agreement with the targeted goals.

Dinner consists of 4 lean meat exchanges, 1 fruit exchange, 2 vegetable exchanges, 1 fat exchange, and 2 starch exchanges. This total corresponds to 4 ounces of lean ham, 1 medium baked potato (1 exchange = 1 small baked potato) with 1 teaspoon of margarine, 1 cup of broccoli, and 1 kiwi fruit. Coffee (if desired) is not counted because it contains no appreciable energy.

Finally, there is a snack containing 2 starch exchanges and 2 fat exchanges. This translates into 1 bagel with 2 tablespoons of regular cream cheese.

This 1-day menu is only one of many that are possible with the exchange lists we selected as an example. Apple juice could replace the orange juice; two apples could be exchanged for the banana. The lean ham could be 4 ounces of flank steak. The choices are endless. Notice that an exchange diet is much easier to plan if you use individual foods; however, the Exchange System tables list some combination foods to help you (see Appendix E). Using combination foods, such as pizza or lasagna, however, makes it more difficult to calculate the number of exchanges in a serving. For instance, lasagna typically has meat exchanges, vegetable exchanges, and starch exchanges. With experience, you will be able to tackle such complex foods. For now, using individual foods makes learning the Exchange System much easier. Finally, you might want to prove to yourself that our food choices really meet the exchange plan. This demonstration will give you practice turning exchanges into actual food servings.

Table D-2 gives you a head start in planning diets. Use this table and the following form to plan a day's diet for tomorrow. Then follow the diet you develop. Practicing this system makes it much easier to understand (Figure D-1).

Exchange List	Total Exchanges to be Consumed Daily	Exchanges Consumed at Each Meal		
		Breakfast	Lunch	Dinner
MILK				
VEGETABLE				
FRUIT				
STARCH				
MEAT AND SUBSTITUTES				
FAT				

Figure D-1 *Record the Exchange System pattern you have chosen in the left-hand column. Then distribute the exchanges throughout the day, noting the food to be used and the serving size.*

Exchange System Lists

Milk Exchange List

Skim and Very-Low-Fat Milk (12 g carbohydrate, 8 g protein, 0-3 g fat, 90 kcal)

1 cup	skim or nonfat milk (½% and 1%)
⅓ cup	powdered (nonfat dry, before adding liquid)
½ cup	canned, evaporated skim milk
1 cup	buttermilk made from nonfat or low-fat milk
¾ cup	yogurt made from nonfat milk (plain, unflavored)

Low-Fat Milk (12 g carbohydrate, 8 g protein, 5 g fat, 120 kcal)

1 cup	2% milk
¾ cup	plain nonfat yogurt (added milk solids)
1 cup	sweet acidophilus milk

Whole Milk (12 g carbohydrate, 8 g protein, 8 g fat, 150 kcal)

1 cup	whole milk
½ cup	evaporated whole milk
1 cup	goat's milk
1 cup	kefir

Vegetable Exchange List

(5 g carbohydrate, 2 g protein, 0 g fat, 25 kcal)
1 vegetable exchange equals:

½ cup cooked vegetables or vegetable juice
1 cup raw vegetables

artichoke	eggplant	peppers
artichoke hearts	green onions or scallions	radishes
asparagus	green pepper	salad greens
beans (green, wax, Italian)	greens (e.g., collard)	sauerkraut
bean sprouts	kohlrabi	spinach
beets	leeks	squash (summer)
broccoli	mixed vegetables (without corn, peas, or pasta)	tomato (fresh, canned, sauce)
brussels sprouts		tomato/vegetable juice
cabbage	mushrooms, cooked	turnips
carrots	okra	water chestnuts
cauliflower	onions	watercress
celery	pea pods	zucchini

Fruit Exchange List

Fruit (15 g carbohydrate, 0 g protein, 0 g fat, 60 kcal)

1 fruit exchange equals:

1	apple (small)
4 rings	apple, dried
½ cup	applesauce (unsweetened)
4	apricots, fresh
8 halves	apricots, dried
1	banana (small)
¾ cup	blackberries
¾ cup	blueberries
⅓ melon	cantaloupe (small)
1 cup cubes	cantaloupe
12	cherries (3 oz)
½ cup	cherries, canned
3	dates
2	figs, fresh (3½ oz)
1½	figs, dried
½ cup	fruit cocktail
½	grapefruit
¾ cup	grapefruit sections
17	grapes (small)
1 slice	honeydew melon (or 1 cup cubes)
1	kiwi
¾ cup	mandarin orange sections
½	mango (or ½ cup cubes)
1	nectarine (small)
1	orange (small)
½	papaya (or 1 cup cubes)
1	peach, fresh (medium)
½ cup	peaches, canned
½	pear, fresh
½ cup	pear, canned
¾ cup	pineapple, fresh
½ cup	pineapple, canned
2	plums (small)
½ cup	plums, canned
3	prunes, dried
2 tbsp	raisins
1 cup	raspberries
1¼ cup	strawberries (raw, whole)
2	tangerines
1 slice	watermelon (or 1¼ cups cubes)

Fruit Juice

½ cup	apple juice/cider
⅓ cup	cranberry juice cocktail
1 cup	cranberry juice cocktail, reduced-calorie
⅓ cup	fruit juice blends, 100% juice
⅓ cup	grape juice
½ cup	grapefruit juice
½ cup	orange juice
½ cup	pineapple juice
⅓ cup	prune juice

Starch Exchange List

(15 g carbohydrate, 3 g protein, 0-1 g fat, 80 kcal)
1 starch exchange equals:

Bread

½ (1 oz)	bagel
2 slices (1½ oz)	bread, reduced-calorie
1 slice (1 oz)	bread, white, whole-wheat, pumpernickel, or rye
2 (⅔ oz)	bread sticks, crisp, 4 in. long × ½ in.
½	English muffin
½ (1 oz)	hot dog or hamburger bun
½	pita, 6 in. across
1 (1 oz)	roll, plain (small)
1 slice (1 oz)	raisin bread, unfrosted
1	tortilla, corn, 6 in. across
1	tortilla, flour, 7-8 in. across
1	waffle, 4½ in. square, reduced-fat

Cereals and Grains

½ cup	bran cereal
½ cup	bulgur
½ cup	cereal
¾ cup	cereal, unsweetened, read-to-eat
3 tbsp	cornmeal (dry)
⅓ cup	couscous
3 tbsp	flour (dry)
¼ cup	granola, low-fat
¼ cup	Grape-Nuts
½ cup	grits
½ cup	kasha
¼ cup	millet
¼ cup	muesli
½ cup	oats
½ cup	pasta
1½ cup	puffed cereal
½ cup	rice milk
⅓ cup	rice, white or brown
½ cup	Shredded Wheat
½ cup	sugar-frosted cereal
3 tbsp	wheat germ

Starchy Vegetables

⅓ cup	baked beans
½ cup	corn
1 (5 oz)	corn on the cob (medium)
1 cup	mixed vegetables with corn, peas, or pasta
½ cup	peas, green
½ cup	plantain
1 (3 oz)	potato, baked or boiled (small)
½ cup	potato, mashed
1 cup	squash, winter (acorn, butternut)
½ cup	yam, sweet potato, plain

Crackers and Snacks

8	animal crackers
3	graham crackers, 2½ in. square
¾ oz	matzoh
4 slices	melba toast
24	oyster crackers
3 cups	popcorn (popped, no fat added or low-fat microwave)
¾ oz	pretzels
2	rice cakes, 4 in. across
6	saltine-type crackers
15-20 (¾ oz)	snack chips, fat-free (tortilla, potato)
2-5 (¾ oz)	whole-wheat crackers, no fat added

Dried Beans, Peas, and Lentils

(counts as 1 starch exchange plus 1 very-lean-meat exchange)

½ cup	beans and peas (garbanzo, pinto, kidney, white, split, black-eyed).
⅔ cup	lima beans
½ cup	lentils
3 tbsp	miso

Starchy Foods Prepared with Fat

(counts as 1 starch exchange plus 1 fat exchange)

1	biscuit, 2½ in. across
½ cup	chow mein noodles
1 (2 oz)	corn bread, 2 in. cube
6	crackers, round butter type
1 cup	croutons
16-25 (3 oz)	french-fried potatoes
¼ cup	granola
1 (1½ oz)	muffin (small)
2	pancakes, 4 in. across
3 cups	popcorn, microwave
3	sandwich crackers, cheese or peanut butter filling
⅓ cup	stuffing, bread (prepared)
2	taco shells, 6 in. across
1	waffle, 4½ in. square
4-6 (1 oz)	whole-wheat crackers, fat added

Other Carbohydrates Exchange List

One exchange equals 15 g carbohydrate, or 1 starch, or 1 fruit, or 1 milk

Exchanges per serving

¹⁄₁₂th cake	angelfood cake, unfrosted	2 carbohydrates
2 in. square	brownie, unfrosted (small)	1 carbohydrate, 1 fat
2 in. square	cake, unfrosted	1 carbohydrate, 1 fat
2 in. square	cake, frosted	2 carbohydrates, 1 fat
2	cookies, fat-free (small)	1 carbohydrate
2	cookies or sandwich cookies with creme filling (small)	1 carbohydrate, 1 fat
1	cupcake, frosted (small)	2 carbohydrates, 1 fat
¼ cup	cranberry sauce, jellied	1½ carbohydrates
1 (1½ oz)	doughnut, plain cake (medium)	1½ carbohydrates, 2 fats
3¾ in. across (2 oz)	doughnuts, glazed	2 carbohydrates, 2 fats
1 bar (3 oz)	fruit juice bars, frozen, 100% juice	1 carbohydrate
1 roll (¾ oz)	fruit snacks, chewy (puréed fruit concentrate)	1 carbohydrate

Other Carbohydrates Exchange List—cont'd

Exchanges per serving

1 tbsp	fruit spread, 100% fruit	1 carbohydrate
½ cup	gelatin, regular	1 carbohydrate
3	gingersnaps	1 carbohydrate
1 bar	granola bar	1 carbohydrate, 1 fat
1 bar	granola bar, fat-free	2 carbohydrates
⅓ cup	hummus	1 carbohydrate, 1 fat
½ cup	ice cream	1 carbohydrate, 2 fats
½ cup	ice cream, light	1 carbohydrate, 1 fat
½ cup	ice cream, fat-free, no sugar added	1 carbohydrate
1 tbsp	jam or jelly, regular	1 carbohydrate
1 cup	milk, chocolate, whole	2 carbohydrates, 1 fat
⅙ pie	pie, fruit, 2 crusts	3 carbohydrates, 2 fats
⅛ pie	pie, pumpkin or custard	1 carbohydrate, 2 fats
12-18 (1 oz)	potato chips	1 carbohydrate, 2 fats
½ cup	pudding, regular (made with low-fat milk)	2 carbohydrates
½ cup	pudding, sugar-free (made with low-fat milk)	1 carbohydrate
¼ cup	salad dressing, fat-free	1 carbohydrate
½ cup	sherbet, sorbet	2 carbohydrates
½ cup	spaghetti or pasta sauce, canned	1 carbohydrate, 1 fat
1 (2½ oz)	sweet roll or Danish	2½ carbohydrates, 2 fats
2 tbsp	syrup, light	1 carbohydrate
1 tbsp	syrup, regular	1 carbohydrate
6-12 (1 oz)	tortilla chips	1 carbohydrate, 2 fats
⅓ cup	yogurt, frozen, low-fat or fat-free	1 carbohydrate, 0-1 fat
½ cup	yogurt, frozen, fat-free, no sugar added	1 carbohydrate
1 cup	yogurt, low-fat, with fruit	3 carbohydrates, 0-1 fat
5	vanilla wafers	1 carbohydrate, 1 fat

Meat and Meat Substitutes Exchange List

Very-Lean-Meat and Substitutes List (0 g carbohydrate, 7 g protein, 0-1 g fat, and 35 kcal)

One very-lean-meat exchange equals:

Poultry:

1 oz	chicken or turkey (white meat, no skin), Cornish hen (no skin)

Fish:

1 oz	fresh or frozen cod, flounder, haddock, halibut, trout; tuna, fresh or canned in water

Shellfish:

1 oz	clams, crab, lobster, scallops, shrimp, imitation shellfish

Game:

1 oz	duck or pheasant (no skin), venison, buffalo, ostrich

Cheese with 1 g or less fat per ounce:

¼ cup	nonfat or low-fat cottage cheese
1 oz	fat-free cheese

Other:

1 oz	processed sandwich meats with 1 g or less fat per ounce, such as deli thin, shaved meats, chipped beef, turkey ham
2	egg whites
1/4 cup	egg substitute, plain
1 oz	hot dogs with 1 g or less fat per ounce
1 oz	Kidney (high in cholesterol)
1 oz	Sausage with 1 g or less fat per ounce

Counts as one very lean meat and one starch exchange:

1/2 cup	dried beans, peas, lentils (cooked)

Lean Meat and Substitutes List (0 g carbohydrate, 7 g protein, 3 g fat, and 55 kcal)

One lean meat exchange equals:

Beef:

1 oz	USDA Select or Choice grades of lean beef trimmed of fat, such as round, sirloin, and flank steak; tenderloin; roast (rib, chuck, rump); steak (T-bone, porterhouse, cubed), ground round

Pork:

1 oz	lean pork, such as fresh ham; canned, cured, or boiled ham; Canadian bacon; tenderloin, center loin chop

Lamb:

1 oz	roast, chop, leg

Veal:

1 oz	lean chop, roast

Poultry:

1 oz	chicken, turkey (dark meat, no skin), chicken white meat (with skin), domestic duck or goose (well-drained of fat, no skin)

Fish:

1 oz	herring (uncreamed or smoked)
6	oysters (medium)
1 oz	salmon (fresh or canned), catfish
2	sardines (canned) (medium)
1 oz	tuna (canned in oil, drained)

Game:

1 oz	goose (no skin), rabbit

Cheese:

1/4 cup	4.5%-fat cottage cheese
2 tbsp	grated Parmesan
1 oz	cheeses with 3 g or less fat per ounce

Other:

1 1/2 oz	hot dogs with 3 g or less fat per ounce
1 oz	processed sandwich meat with 3 g or less fat per ounce, such as turkey pastrami or kielbasa
1 oz	liver, heart (high in cholesterol)

Medium-Fat Meat and Substitutes List (0 g carbohydrate, 7 g protein, 5 g fat, and 75 kcal)

One medium-fat meat exchange equals:

Beef:

1 oz	Most beef products fall into this category (ground beef, meatloaf, corned beef, short ribs, prime grades of meat trimmed of fat, such as prime rib)

Pork:

1 oz	top loin, chop, Boston butt, cutlet

Lamb:

1 oz	rib roast, ground

Veal:

1 oz	cutlet (ground or cubed, unbreaded)

Poultry:

1 oz	chicken dark meat (with skin), ground turkey or ground chicken, fried chicken (with skin)

Fish:

1 oz	any fried fish product

Cheese (with 5 g or less fat per ounce):

1 oz	feta
1 oz	mozzarella
$\frac{1}{4}$ cup (2 oz)	ricotta

Other:

1	egg (high in cholesterol, limit to 3 per week)
1 oz	sausage with 5 g or less fat per ounce
1 cup	soy milk
$\frac{1}{4}$ cup	tempeh
4 oz or $\frac{1}{2}$ cup	tofu

High-Fat Meat and Substitutes List (0 g carbohydrate, 7 g protein, 8 g fat, and 100 kcal)

One high-fat meat exchange equals:

Pork:

1 oz	spareribs, ground pork, pork sausage

Cheese:

1 oz	all regular cheeses, such as American cheddar, Monterey Jack, Swiss

Other:

1 oz	processed sandwich meats with 8 g or less fat per ounce, such as bologna, pimento loaf, salami
1 oz	sausage, such as bratwurst, Italian, knockwurst, Polish, snoked
1 (10/lb)	hot dog (turkey or chicken)
3 slices (20 slices/lb)	bacon

Counts as one high-fat meat plus one fat exchange:

1 (10/lb)	hot dog (beef, pork, or combination)
2 tbsp	peanut butter (contains unsaturated fat)

Fat Exchange List
Monounsaturated Fats List (5 g fat and 45 kcal)

One exchange equals:

$\frac{1}{8}$ (1 oz)	avocado (medium)
1 tsp	oil (canola, olive, peanut)
	olives:
8	ripe, black (large)
10	green, stuffed (large)
6 nuts	almonds, cashews
6 nuts	mixed (50% peanuts)
10 nuts	peanuts
4 halves	pecans
2 tsp	peanut butter, smooth or crunchy
1 tbsp	sesame seeds
2 tsp	tahini paste

Polyunsaturated Fats List (5 g fat and 45 kcal)

One exchange equals:

	margarine:
1 tsp	stick, tub, or squeeze
1 tbsp	lower-fat (30% to 50% vegetable oil)
	mayonnaise:
1 tsp	regular
1 tbsp	reduced-fat
4 halves	nuts, walnuts, English
1 tsp	oil (corn, safflower, soybean)
	salad dressing:
1 tbsp	regular
2 tbsp	reduced-fat
	Miracle Whip Salad Dressing®:
2 tsp	regular
1 tbsp	reduced-fat
1 tbsp	seeds: pumpkin, sunflower

Saturated Fats List (5 g fat and 45 kcal)

One exchange equals:

1 slice (20 slices/lb)	bacon, cooked
1 tsp	bacon, grease
	butter:
1 tsp	stick
2 tsp	whipped
1 tbsp	reduced-fat
2 tbsp ($\frac{1}{2}$ oz)	chitterlings, boiled
2 tbsp	coconut, sweetened, shredded
2 tbsp	cream, half and half
	cream cheese:
1 tbsp ($\frac{1}{2}$ oz)	regular
2 tbsp (1 oz)	reduced-fat
	fatback or salt pork, see below†
1 tsp	shortening or lard
	sour cream:
2 tbsp	regular
3 tbsp	reduced-fat

†Use a piece 1 in. × 1 in. × 1/4 in. if you plan to eat the fatback cooked with vegetables. Use a piece 2 in. × 1 in. × 1/2 in. when eating only the vegetables with the fatback removed.

Free Foods List

A *free food* is any food or drink that contains less than 20 kcal or less than 5 g of carbohydrate per serving. Foods with a serving size listed should be limited to 3 servings per day. Foods listed without a serving size can be eaten as often as you like.

Fat-Free or Reduced-Fat Foods

1 tbsp	cream cheese, fat-free
1 tbsp	creamers, nondairy, liquid
2 tsp	creamers, nondairy, powdered
1 tbsp	mayonnaise, fat-free
1 tsp	mayonnaise, reduced-fat
4 tbsp	margarine, fat-free
1 tsp	margarine, reduced-fat
1 tbsp	Miracle Whip®, nonfat
1 tsp	Miracle Whip®, reduced-fat
	nonstick cooking spray
1 tbsp	salad dressing, fat-free
2 tbsp	salad dressing, fat-free, Italian
¼ cup	salsa
1 tbsp	sour cream, fat-free, reduced-fat
2 tbsp	whipped topping, regular or light

Sugar-Free or Low-Sugar Foods

1 candy	candy, hard, sugar-free
	gelatin dessert, sugar-free
	gelatin, unflavored
	gum, sugar-free
2 tsp	jam or jelly, low-sugar, or light
	sugar substitutes†
2 tbsp	syrup, sugar-free

†Sugar substitutes, alternatives, or replacements that are approved by the Food and Drug Administration (FDA) are safe to use. Common brand names include:
   Equal® (aspartame)
   Sprinkle Sweet® (saccharin)
   Sweet One® (acesulfame K)
   Sweet-10® (saccharin)
   Sugar Twin® (saccharin)
   Sweet `n Low® (saccharin)

Drinks

	bouillon, broth, consommé
	bouillon or broth, low-sodium
	carbonated or mineral water
1 tbsp	cocoa powder, unsweetened
	coffee
	club soda
	diet soft drinks, sugar-free
	drink mixes, sugar-free
	tea
	tonic water, sugar-free

Condiments

1 tbsp	catsup
	horseradish
	lemon juice
	lime juice
	mustard
1½	pickles, dill (large)
	soy sauce, regular or light
1 tbsp	taco sauce
	vinegar

Seasonings

flavoring extracts
garlic
herbs, fresh or dried
pimento
spices
Tabasco® or hot pepper sauce
wine, used in cooking
worcestershire sauce

Combination Foods List

	Entrées:	**Exchanges per serving:**
1 cup (8 oz)	tuna noodle casserole, lasagna, spaghetti with meatballs, chili with beans, macaroni and cheese	2 carbohydrates, 2 medium-fat meats
2 cups (16 oz)	chow mein (without noodles or rice)	1 carbohydrate, 2 lean meats
¼ of 10 in. (5 oz)	pizza, cheese, thin crust	2 carbohydrates, 2 medium-fat meats, 1 fat
¼ of 10 in. (5 oz)	pizza, meat topping, thin crust	2 carbohydrates, 2 medium-fat meats, 2 fats
1 (7 oz)	pot pie	2 carbohydrates, 1 medium-fat meat, 4 fats
	Frozen entrées:	
1 (11 oz)	salisbury steak with gravy, mashed potato	2 carbohydrates, 3 medium-fat meats, 3-4 fats
1 (11 oz)	turkey with gravy, mashed potato, dressing	2 carbohydrates, 2 medium-fat meats, 2 fats
1 (8 oz)	entrée with less than 300 kcal	2 carbohydrates, 3 lean meats
	Soups:	
1 cup	bean	1 carbohydrate, 1 very lean meat
1 cup (8 oz)	cream (made with water)	1 carbohydrate, 1 fat
½ cup (4 oz)	split pea (made with water)	1 carbohydrate
1 cup (8 oz)	tomato (made with water)	1 carbohydrate
1 cup (8 oz)	vegetable beef, chicken noodle, or other broth-type	1 carbohydrate

Fast (Quick-Service) Foods

		Exchanges per serving:
2	burritos with beef	4 carbohydrates, 2 medium-fat meats, 2 fats
6	chicken nuggets	1 carbohydrate, medium-fat meats, 1 fat
1 each	chicken breast and wing, breaded and fried	1 carbohydrate, 4 medium-fat meats, 2 fats
1	fish sandwich/tartar sauce	3 carbohydrates, 1 medium-fat meat, 3 fats
20-25	french fries, thin	2 carbohydrates, 2 fats
1	hamburger (regular)	2 carbohydrates, 2 medium-fat meats
1	hamburger (large)	2 carbohydrates, 3 medium-fat meats, 1 fat
1	hot dog with bun	1 carbohydrate, 1 high-fat meat, 1 fat
1	individual pan pizza	5 carbohydrates, 3 medium-fat meats, 3 fats
1	soft-serve cone (medium)	2 carbohydrates, 1 fat
1 sub (6 in.)	submarine sandwich	3 carbohydrates, 1 vegetable, 2 medium-fat meats, 1 fat
1 (6 oz)	taco, hard shell	2 carbohydrates, 2 medium-fat meats, 2 fats
1 (3 oz)	taco, soft shell	1 carbohydrate, 1 medium-fat meat, 1 fat

Summary of the Desired Characteristics of the Canadian Diet

1. **The Canadian diet should provide energy consistent with the maintenance of body weight within the recommended range.** Physical activity should be appropriate to circumstances and capabilities. While the importance of maintaining some activity throughout life can be stressed, it is not possible to specify a level of physical activity for the whole population. As a general guideline it is desirable that adults, for as long as possible, maintain an activity level that permits an energy intake of at least 1800 kcal while keeping weight within the recommended range.

2. **The Canadian diet should include essential nutrients in amounts recommended in this report.** While it is important that the diet provide the recommended amounts of nutrients, it should be understood that no evidence was found that intakes in excess of the RNI confer any health benefit. There is no general need for supplements except for vitamin D for infants and folate during pregnancy. Vitamin D supplementation might be required for elderly persons not exposed to the sun, and iron for pregnant women with low iron stores.

3. **The Canadian diet should include no more than 30% of energy as fat (33 grams per 1000 kcal) and no more than 10% as saturated fat (11 grams per 1000 kcal).** Dietary cholesterol, though not as influential in affecting blood cholesterol, is not without importance. A reduction in cholesterol intake normally will accompany a reduction in total fat and saturated fat. The recommendation to reduce total fat intake does not apply to children under the age of 2 years.

4. **The Canadian diet should provide 55% of energy as carbohydrate (138 grams per 1000 kcal) from a variety of sources.** Sources should be selected that provide complex carbohydrates, a variety of dietary fiber, and *beta-carotene.*

5. **The sodium content of the Canadian diet should be reduced.** The present food supply provides sodium in an amount greatly exceeding requirements.

While there is insufficient evidence to support a precise recommendation, potential benefit would be expected from a reduction in current sodium intake.

6. **The Canadian diet should include no more than 5% of total energy as alcohol, or two drinks daily, whichever is less.** The harmful influence of alcohol on blood pressure provides a more urgent reason for moderation. During pregnancy it is prudent to abstain from alcoholic beverages because a safe intake is not known with certainty.

7. **The Canadian diet should contain no more caffeine than the equivalent of four regular cups of coffee per day.** This is a prudent measure in view of the increased risk for cardiovascular disease associated with high intakes of caffeine.

8. **Community water supplies containing less fluoride than 1 milligram per liter should be fluoridated to that level.** Fluoridation of community water supplies has proven to be a safe, effective, and economical method of improving dental health.

In essence, suggested actions toward healthful eating as listed in Canada's *Guidelines for Healthy Eating* include the following:

- Enjoy a variety of foods.
- Emphasize cereals, breads, other grain products, vegetables, and fruits.
- Choose low-fat dairy products, lean meats, and foods prepared with little or no fat.
- Achieve and maintain a healthful body weight by enjoying regular physical activity and healthful eating.
- Limit salt, alcohol, and caffeine.

More details are available on RNI and diet recommendations in the 1990 publication *Nutrition Recommendations: The Report of the Scientific Review Committee.*

A separate Canadian food guide, illustrated on the following pages, provides a plan to meet these nutrient needs.

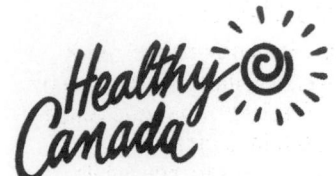

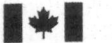 Health and Welfare
Canada

Santé et Bien-être social
Canada

CANADA'S
Food Guide
TO HEALTHY EATING

Enjoy a variety
of foods from each
group every day.

Choose lower-
fat foods
more often.

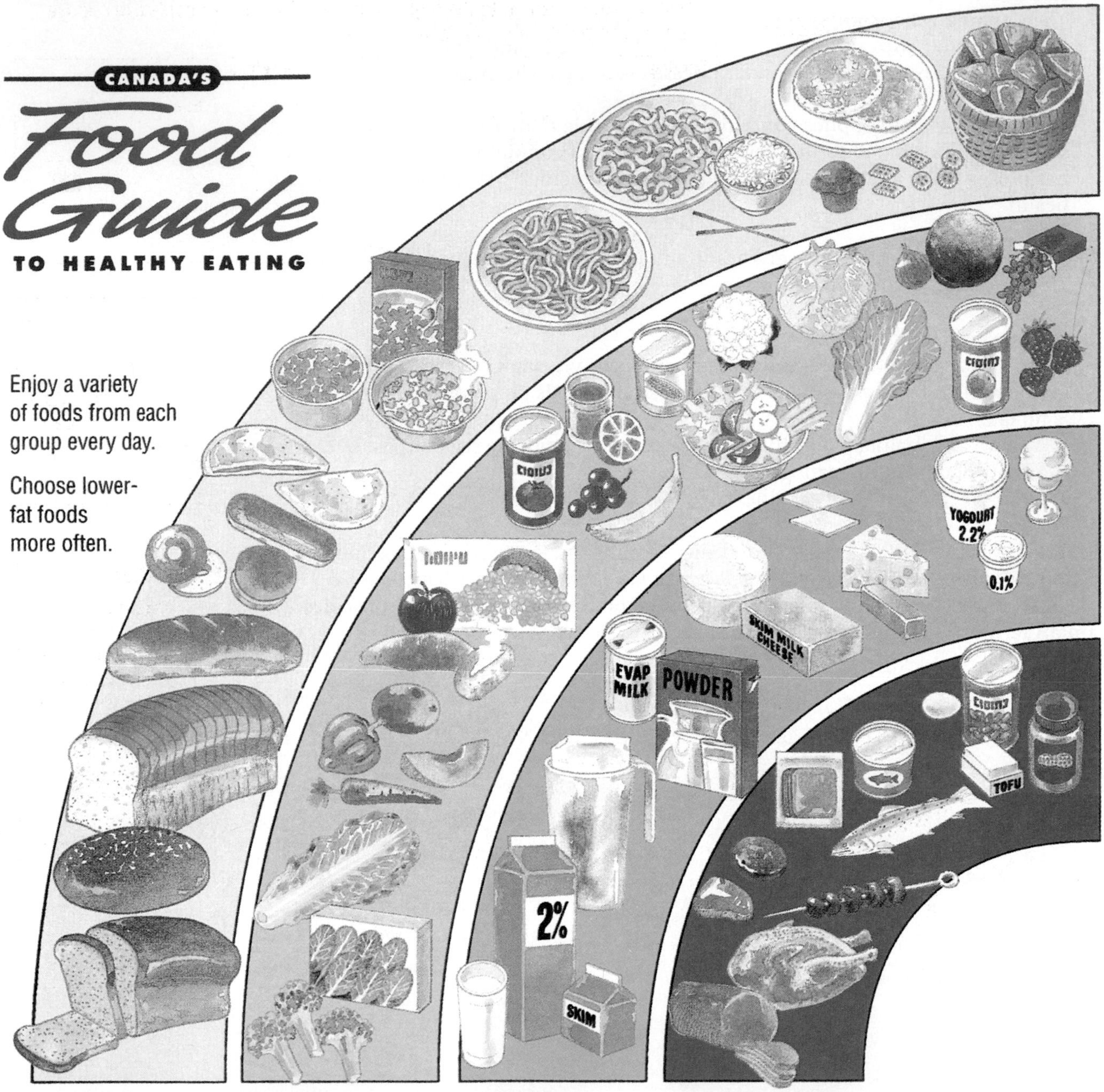

Grain Products
Choose whole grain
and enriched
products more
often.

Vegetables & Fruit
Choose dark green and
orange vegetables and
orange fruit more often.

Milk Products
Choose lower-fat
milk products more
often.

Meat & Alternatives
Choose leaner meats,
poultry and fish, as well
as dried peas, beans and
lentils more often.

Canada

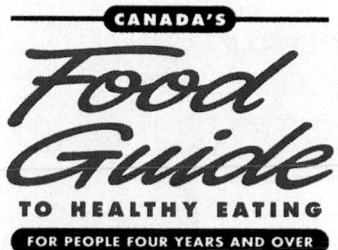

CANADA'S

Food Guide

TO HEALTHY EATING

FOR PEOPLE FOUR YEARS AND OVER

Different People Need Different Amounts of Food

The amount of food you need every day from the 4 food groups and other foods depends on your age, body size, activity level, whether you are male or female and if you are pregnant or breast-feeding. That's why the Food Guide gives a lower and higher number of servings for each food group. For example, young children can choose the lower number of servings, while male teenagers can go to the higher number. Most other people can choose servings somewhere in between.

Grain Products

5-12

SERVINGS PER DAY

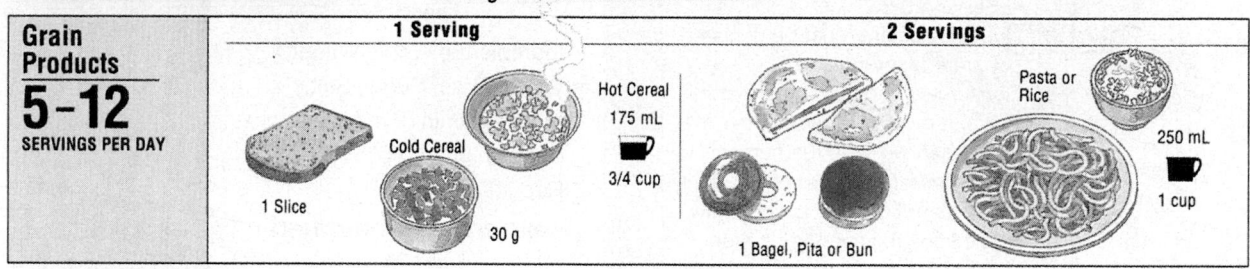

1 Serving

1 Slice

Cold Cereal

30 g

Hot Cereal
175 mL
3/4 cup

2 Servings

1 Bagel, Pita or Bun

Pasta or Rice
250 mL
1 cup

Vegetables & Fruit

5-10

SERVINGS PER DAY

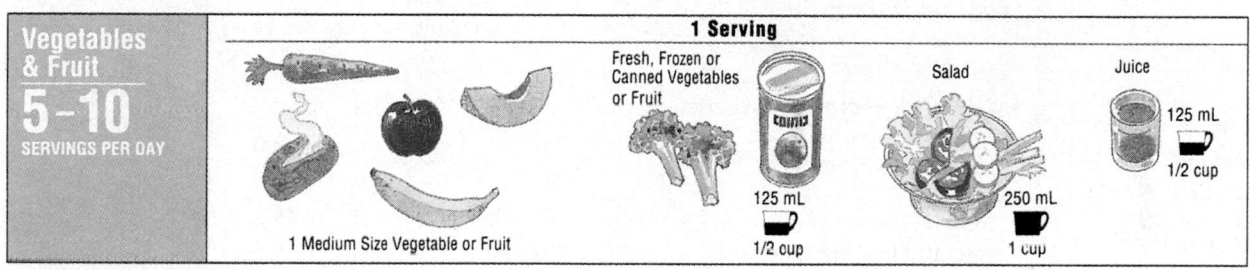

1 Serving

1 Medium Size Vegetable or Fruit

Fresh, Frozen or Canned Vegetables or Fruit
125 mL
1/2 cup

Salad
250 mL
1 cup

Juice
125 mL
1/2 cup

Milk Products

SERVINGS PER DAY

Children 4–9 years: 2–3
Youth 10–16 years: 3–4
Adults: 2–4
Pregnant & Breast-feeding Women: 3–4

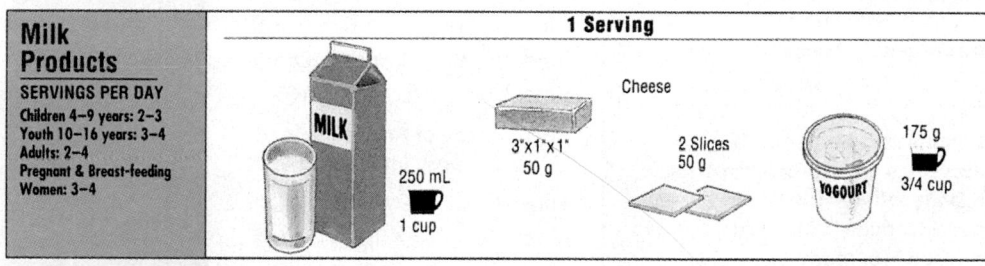

1 Serving

MILK
250 mL
1 cup

Cheese
3"x1"x1"
50 g

2 Slices
50 g

175 g
3/4 cup

Other Foods

Taste and enjoyment can also come from other foods and beverages that are not part of the 4 food groups. Some of these foods are higher in fat or Calories, so use these foods in moderation.

Meat & Alternatives

2-3

SERVINGS PER DAY

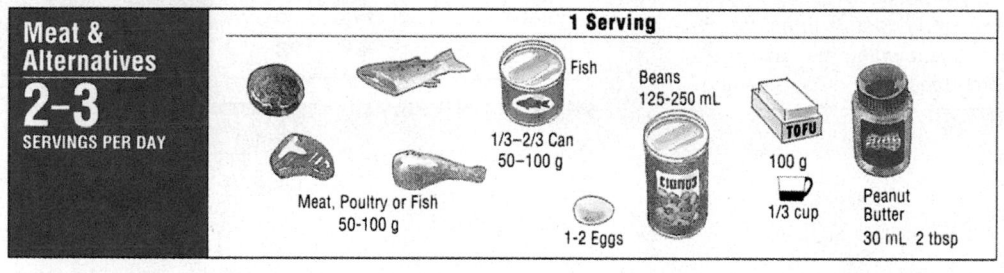

1 Serving

Meat, Poultry or Fish
50-100 g

1-2 Eggs

Fish
1/3–2/3 Can
50–100 g

Beans
125-250 mL
1/3 cup

TOFU
100 g

Peanut Butter
30 mL 2 tbsp

Enjoy eating well, being active and feeling good about yourself. That's VITALIT

© Minister of Supply and Services Canada 1992 Cat. No. H39-252/1992E No changes permitted. Reprint permission not required.
ISBN 0-662-19648-1

EXAMPLE OF THE FOOD LABEL FORMAT THAT IS CURRENTLY MANDATORY IN CANADA.

The nutrition label consists of:
- **A Heading**
- **Serving Size**

Nutrient content must be declared per *stated* serving size. Consumers should realize that if they eat more or less than the stated serving size, the nutrient values for fat, iron and other nutrients will change accordingly. Sometimes the serving size for the nutrition label differs from the Food Guide serving size.

- **Values for Energy, Protein, Fat and Carbohydrate**
  The nutrition label may also include:
- **Total fat broken down into Fatty Acids and Cholesterol**
- **Carbohydrate broken down into Sugars, Starch and Dietary Fibre**
- **Sodium and Potassium**

- **Vitamins and Minerals Expressed as a % of Recommended Daily Intake.** The RDI of a vitamin or mineral is a value developed for food labelling only. It is based on the highest Recommended Nutrient Intake (RNI), excluding the needs for pregnancy and breast-feeding.

CEREAL
Source of Fibre
Low in Fat

Ingredients: Whole Wheat, Wheat Bran, Sugar, Salt, Malt, Thiamin, Pyridoxine, hydrochloride, Folic Acid, Reduced Iron, BHT.

NUTRITION INFORMATION
per 30 g
Serving Cereal
(175 ml. 3/4 cup)

Energy	Cal	100
	KJ	420
Protein	g	3.0
Fat	g	0.6
Carbohydrate	g	24
Sugars	g	4.4
Starch	g	16.6
Dietary fibre	g	3.0
Sodium	mg	265
Potassium	mg	168

Percentage of Recommended Daily Intake

Thiamin	%	46
Niacin	%	6
Vitamin B$_6$	%	10
Folacin	%	8
Iron	%	28

From Guthrie HA, Picciano MF: *Human Nutrition*, St. Louis, 1995, Mosby.

Canada's Basic Labeling Requirements: under the Food and Drugs Act and the Consumer Packaging and Labeling Act

In general, prepackaged products must show the following basic label information:

1. THE COMMON NAME. This is either the name by which the food is generally known (e.g., orange drink, vanilla cookies, chocolate candies) or the name prescribed by a regulation (e.g., orange juice from concentrate, 60% whole wheat bread, milk chocolate, mayonnaise).

   When a prescribed common name is used, the product must conform to the compositional standard set forth in the regulations.

   The common name is to be shown on the principal display panel (i.e., main panel) in English and French in a minimum type height of 1.6 mm, based on the lower case letter "o."

2. A METRIC NET QUALITY declaration by volume (e.g., milliliters, liters), weight (e.g., grams, kilograms) or by count, as applicable. The net quantity declaration is to be shown on the principal display panel in English and French. The following symbols are considered to be bilingual:

   grams - g
   kilograms - k
   milliliters - ml or mL
   liters - l or L

   A minimum type height of 1.6 mm, based on the lower case letter "o", is required for all information in the net declaration except for the numbers which are to be shown in bold face type of not less than the following height:

   a) 1/16 inch (1.6 millimeters), where the principal display surface of the container is not more than 5 square inches (32 square centimeters);

   b) 1.8 inch (3.2 millimeters), where the principal display surface of the container is more than 5 square inches (32 centimeters) but not more than 40 square inches (258 square centimeters);

   c) 1/4 inch (6.4 millimeters), where the principal display surface of the container is more than 40 square inches (258 square centimeters) but not more than 100 square inches (645 square centimeters);

   d) 3/8 inch (9.5 milliliters), where the principal display surface of the container is more than 100 square inches (645 square centimeters) but not more than 400 square inches (25.8 square decimeters); and

   e) 1/2 inch (12.7 milliliters), where the principal display surface of the container is more than 400 square inches (25.8 square decimeters).

   Additional non-metric declarations (e.g., fluid ounces, pounds) are not required but may be shown grouped with the metric statement provided they are not false or misleading.

3. A LIST OF INGREDIENTS and their components (i.e., ingredients of ingredients) in descending order of proportion by weight. Spices, seasonings and herbs except salt, natural and artificial flavors, flavor enhancers, food additives, vitamin and mineral nutrients, may be shown at the end of the list in any order. Some components are completely exempt from a component declaration, while others are exempt depending on the amount used.

   Components of natural or artificial flavoring preparations, seasonings and spice or herb mixtures that are:

   a) flavor enhancers

   b) salt

   c) food additives which affect the finished product, and

   d) food additives listed in Table X of Division 16 of the Food and Drug Regulations must be shown in the ingredient list as if they were an ingredient of the finished food.

An ingredient or component must be shown in the list of ingredients by its common name.

The list of ingredients is to be shown in English and French on any label panel except the bottom. It is required to be displayed clearly and prominently and be readily discernible. A minimum type height of 1.6 mm based on the lower case letter "o" will usually satisfy this requirement.

4. THE NAME AND ADDRESS declaration of the responsible company. The company name must be the legal registered company name. The address should be complete enough for postal purposes and include the name of the country, if other than Canada or USA.

   This information is to be shown in either English or French on any label panel except the bottom, in a minimum type height of 1.6 mm based on the lower case letter "o."

   If only a Canadian company name and address is shown on an imported product that has been wholly manufactured outside of Canada, the Canadian declaration must be preceded by the appropriate terms "imported by/importé par" or "imported from/importé pour." Alternatively, the country of origin may be declared adjacent to the Canadian company name and address.

5. When a food has a DURABLE LIFE of 90 days or less, a "best before" date and storage instructions if they differ from normal room storage conditions must be declared. Additional information is available upon request.

6. When artificial flavors are used whether alone or with natural flavoring agents and a vignette on the label indicates a natural flavor source (e.g., picture of an apple) information that the added flavoring ingredient is imitation, artificial, or simulated must appear on or adjacent to the vignette in French and English in at least the same type height as required for the numbers in the net quantity.

7. Standard container sizes are specified for wine, glucose and refined sugar syrups, peanut butter, cookies, and biscuits. Specific information is available upon request.

Reprinted with permission of Consumer and Corporate Affairs CANADA.

The Human Cell—Primary Site for Metabolism

The cell is the basic unit of body structure, and it is where most metabolic reactions occur (Figure G-1). The cell is surrounded by a semipermeable membrane that controls the passage of nutrients and other substances in and out of it. Within the cell is fluid called the cytosol. Within the cytosol are small bodies called organelles that perform specific metabolic functions. The names and activities of the various cell parts are given below:

Nucleus: This spherical structure is bound by its own double membrane. Within the nucleus are chromosomes, which are long threads of DNA (also called chromatin) that contain hereditary information for directing cell protein synthesis and cell division. Although most cell types have only one nucleus, muscle cells contain many nuclei.

Mitochondria: These have their own outer membrane, as well as an inner membrane that is highly folded. The mitochondria are the major sites of energy production in the cell. Muscle cells contain many mitochondria.

Endoplasmic reticulum: This network of internal membranes seives as a communication network within the cell. Small granules called ribosomes are attached to parts of the outside of the endoplasmic reticulum, which is known as the rough endoplasmic reticulum. Ribosomes are the site for protein synthesis. Fat is synthesized in other areas of the endoplasmic reticulum where there are no ribosomes—namely, the smooth endoplasmic reticulum. In muscles, this organelle (called sarcoplasmic reticulum) plays a key role in muscle contraction.

Golgi complex: This consists of stacks of flattened structures that both package proteins for export from the cell and help form other cell organelles (Figure G-2).

Lysosomes: These small bodies contain digestive enzymes that break down worn-out cell parts and other cell debris. When a lysosome fuses with a particle that is to be digested, the digestive activity begins.

Storage forms of energy: These occur in the cell as glycogen granules and lipid droplets.

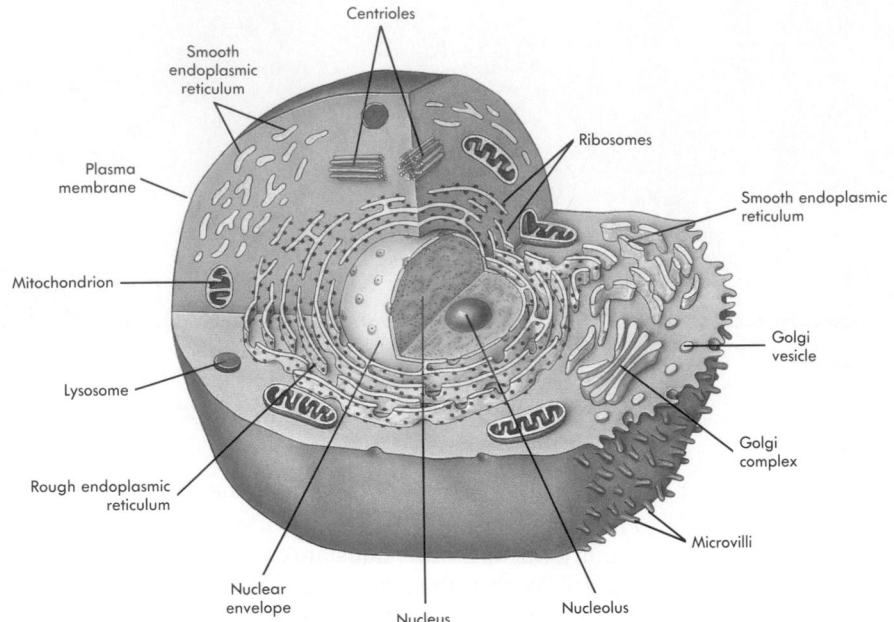

Figure G-1 *An animal cell.* Almost all human cells contain these various organelles.

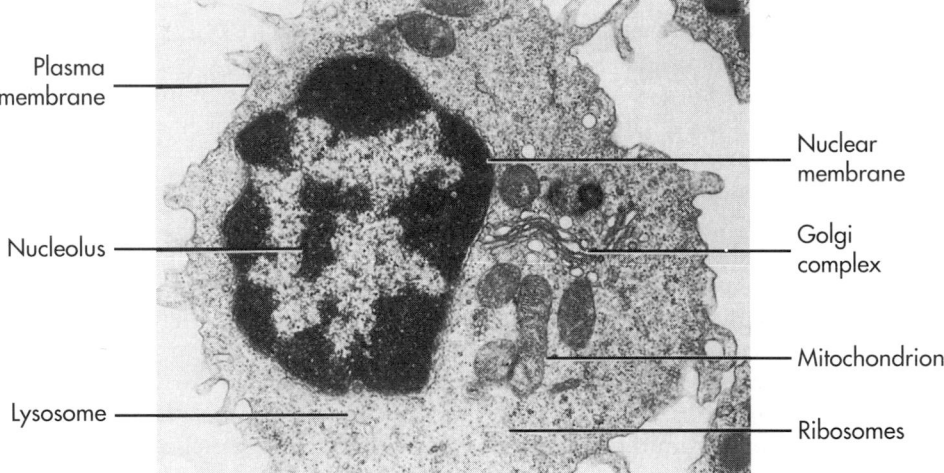

Figure G-2 *Electron micrograph of a cell, magnified 40,500 times. Our understanding of the structures in cells is based mainly on such pictures as this. (From Raven PH, Johnson GB: Biology, St. Louis, 1992, Mosby–Year Book.)*

Important Chemical Structures in Nutrition

Amino Acids

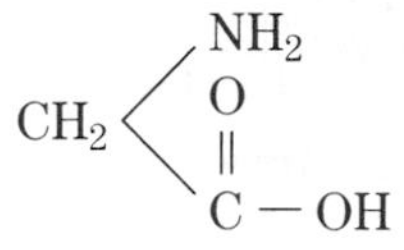

$$CH_2 \underset{C-OH}{\overset{NH_2}{\underset{\parallel}{\overset{O}{\big\langle}}}}$$

Glycine

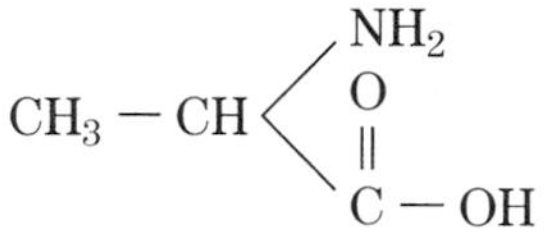

$$CH_3 - CH \underset{C-OH}{\overset{NH_2}{\underset{\parallel}{\overset{O}{\big\langle}}}}$$

Alanine

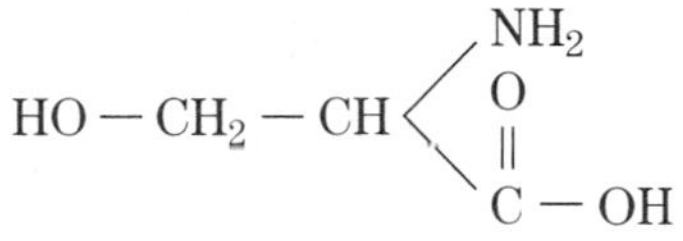

$$HO - CH_2 - CH \underset{C-OH}{\overset{NH_2}{\underset{\parallel}{\overset{O}{\big\langle}}}}$$

Serine

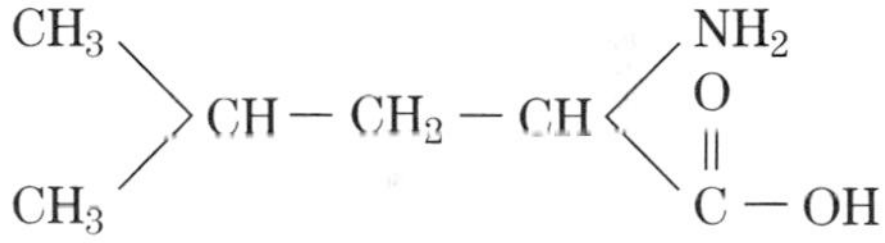

$$\underset{CH_3}{\overset{CH_3}{\big\rangle}} CH - CH_2 - CH \underset{C-OH}{\overset{NH_2}{\underset{\parallel}{\overset{O}{\big\langle}}}}$$

Leucine
(essential)

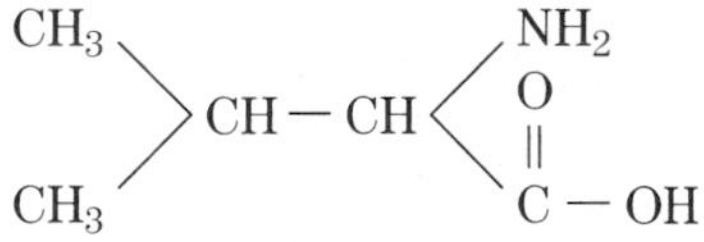

$$\underset{CH_3}{\overset{CH_3}{\big\rangle}} CH - CH \underset{C-OH}{\overset{NH_2}{\underset{\parallel}{\overset{O}{\big\langle}}}}$$

Valine
(essential)

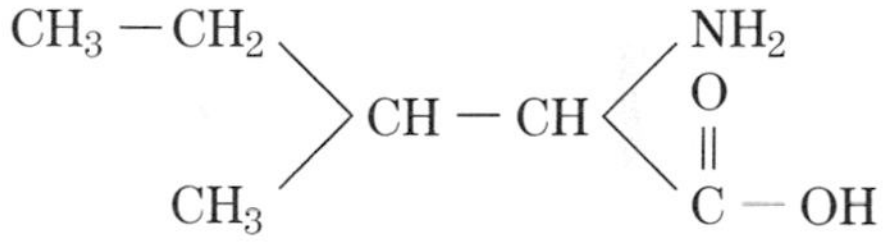

$$\underset{CH_3}{\overset{CH_3 - CH_2}{\big\rangle}} CH - CH \underset{C-OH}{\overset{NH_2}{\underset{\parallel}{\overset{O}{\big\langle}}}}$$

Isoleucine
(essential)

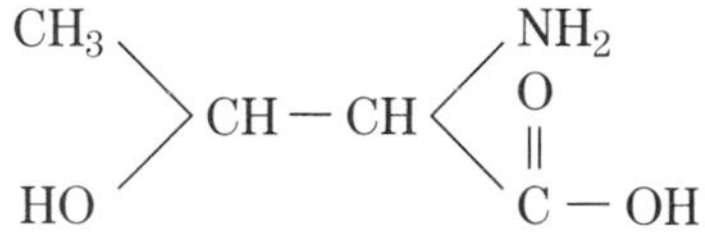

$$\underset{HO}{\overset{CH_3}{\big\rangle}} CH - CH \underset{C-OH}{\overset{NH_2}{\underset{\parallel}{\overset{O}{\big\langle}}}}$$

Threonine
(essential)

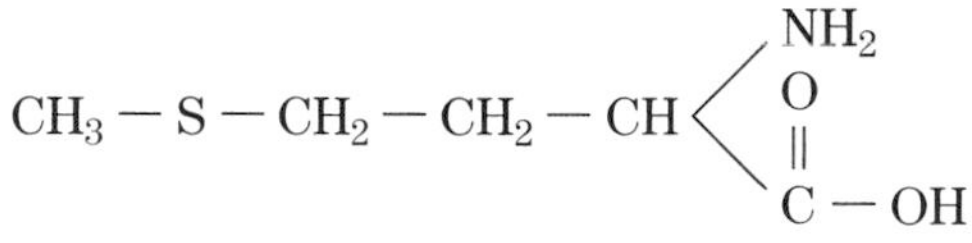

$$CH_3 - S - CH_2 - CH_2 - CH \underset{C-OH}{\overset{NH_2}{\underset{\parallel}{\overset{O}{\big\langle}}}}$$

Methionine
(essential)

$$HS - CH_2 - CH \underset{C-OH}{\overset{NH_2}{\underset{\parallel}{\overset{O}{\big\langle}}}}$$

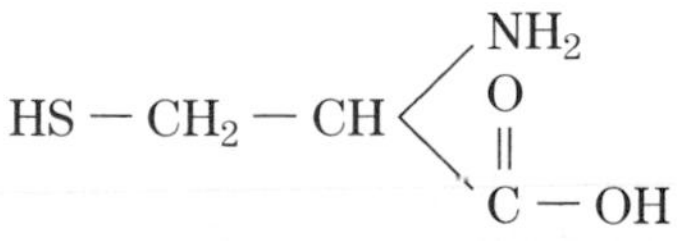

Cysteine

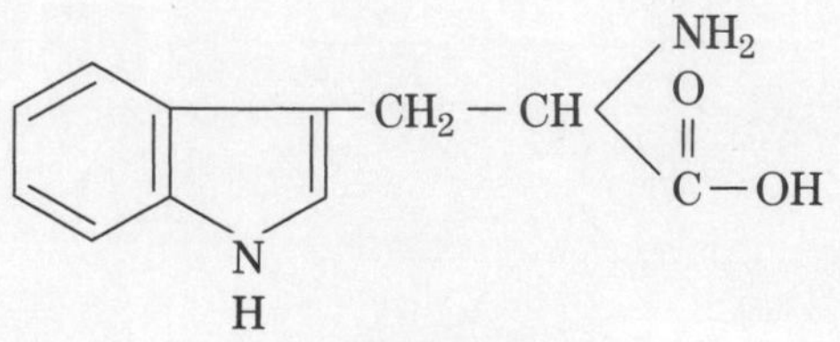

Tryptophan
(essential)

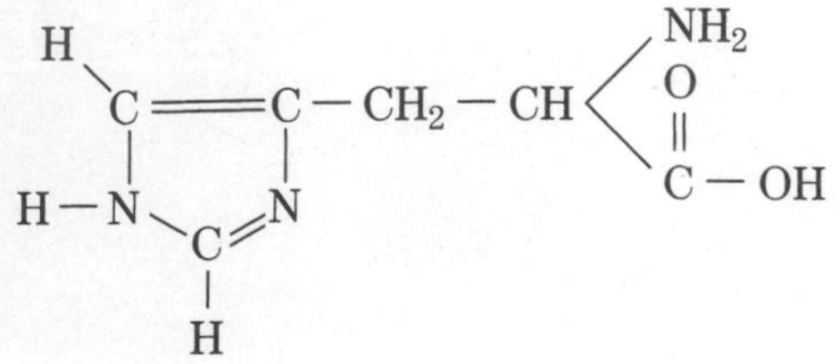

Histidine
(essential)

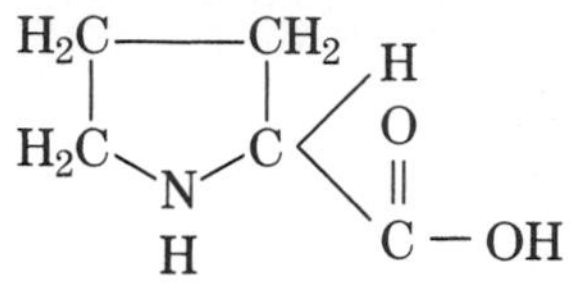

Proline

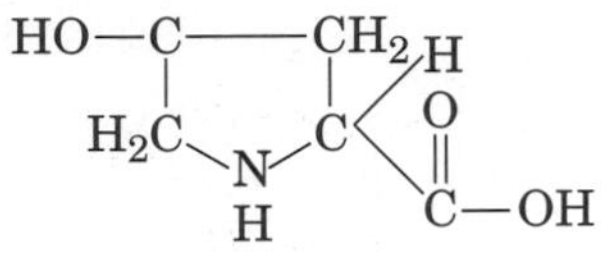

Hydroxyproline

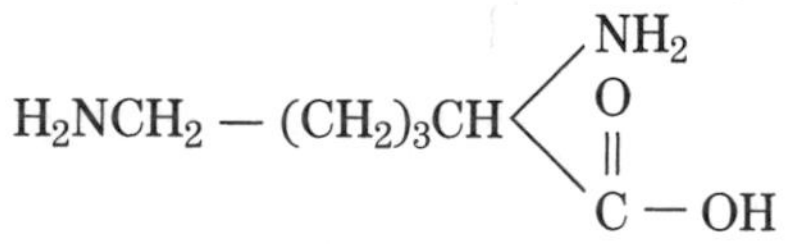

Lysine
(essential)

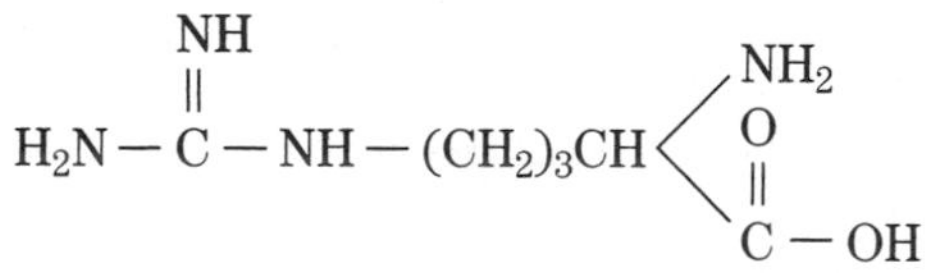

Arginine
(essential)

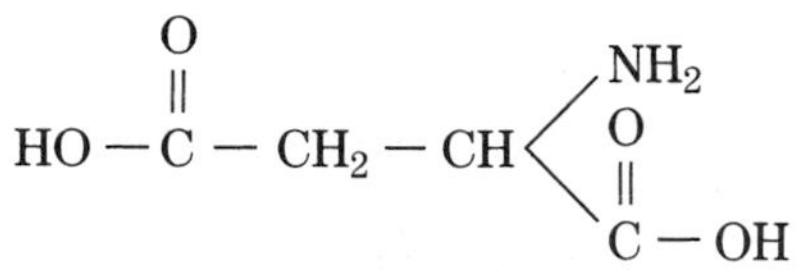

Aspartic Acid

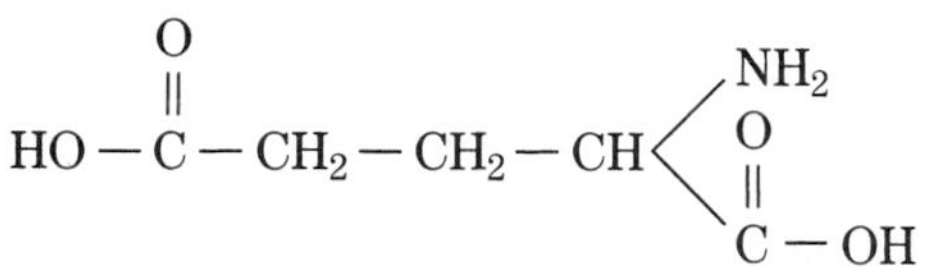

Glutamic acid

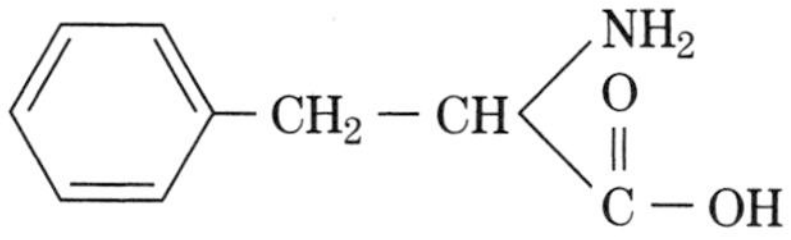

Phenylalanine
(essential)

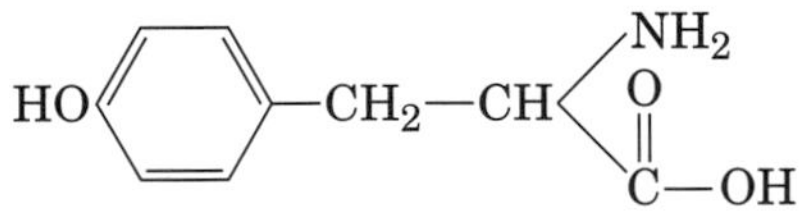

Tyrosine

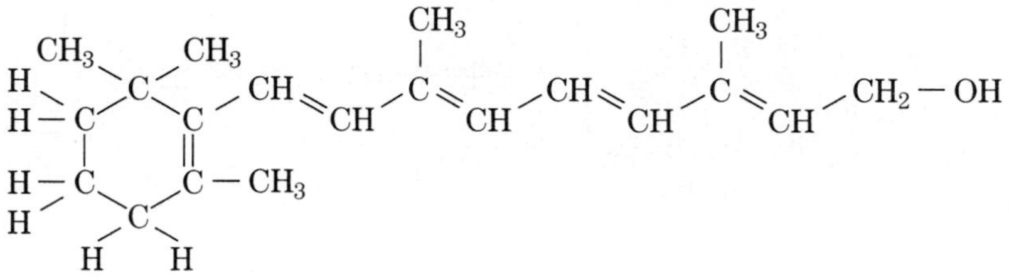

Vitamin A: retinol

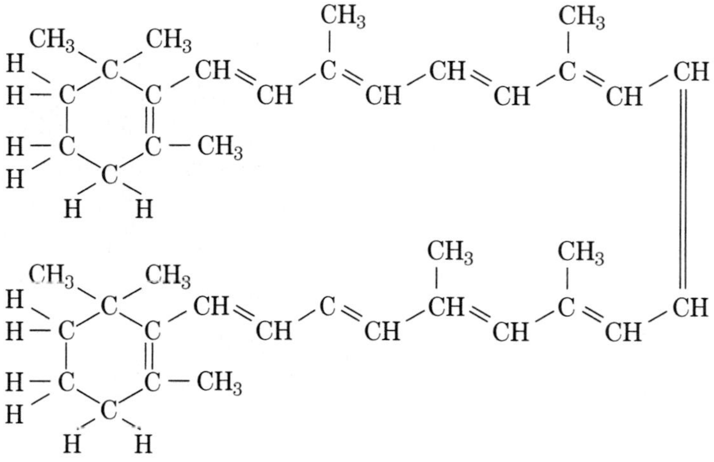

Beta-carotene

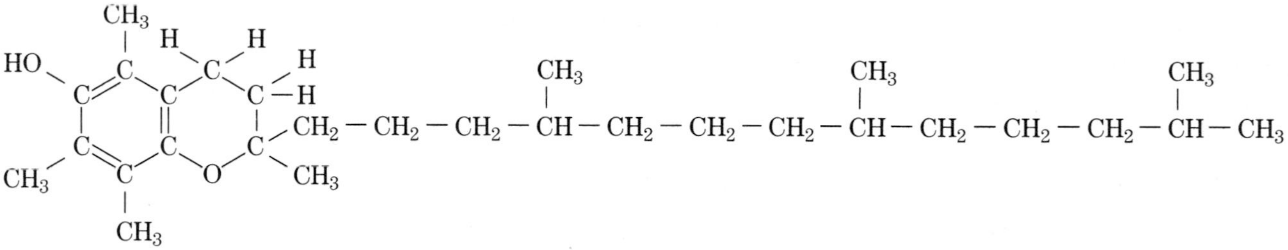

Vitamin E

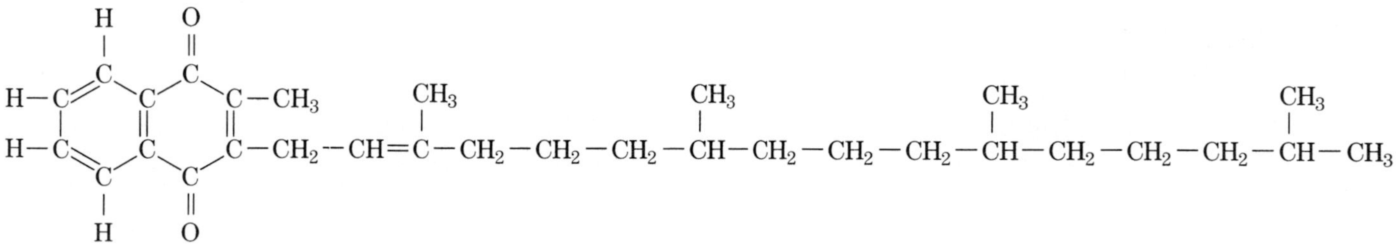

Vitamin K

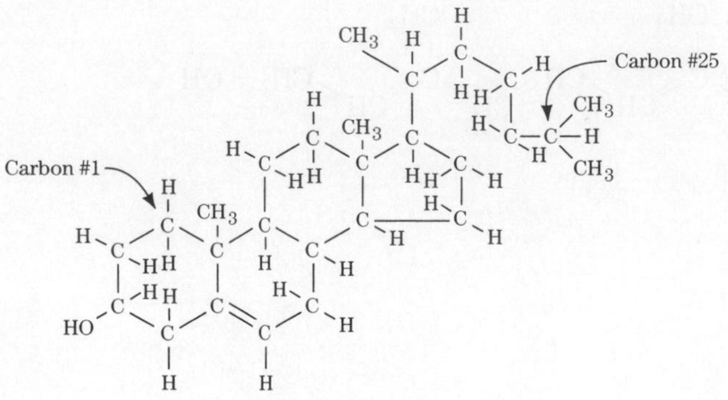

7-dehydrocholesterol

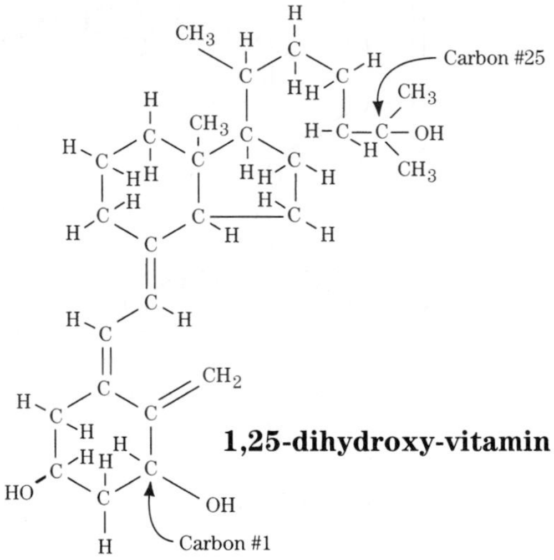

1,25-dihydroxy-vitamin D$_3$ (calcitriol)

Active vitamin D (calcitriol) and its precursor 7-dehydrocholesterol

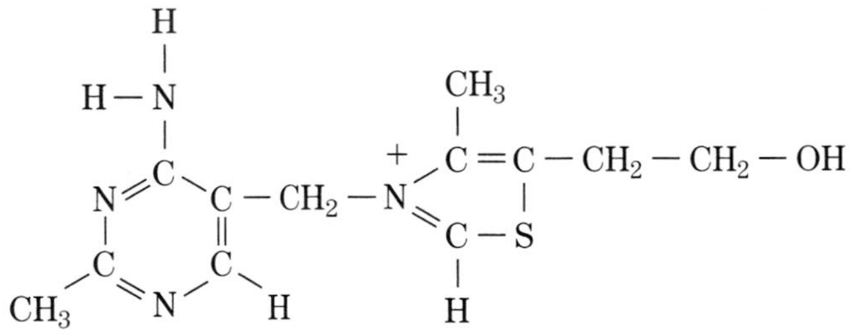

Thiamin

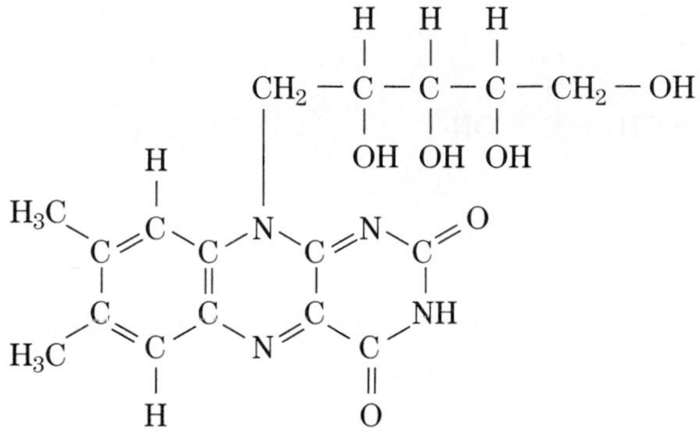

Riboflavin

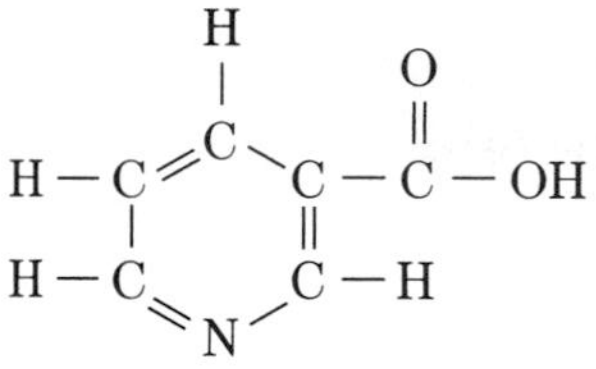

Nicotinic acid

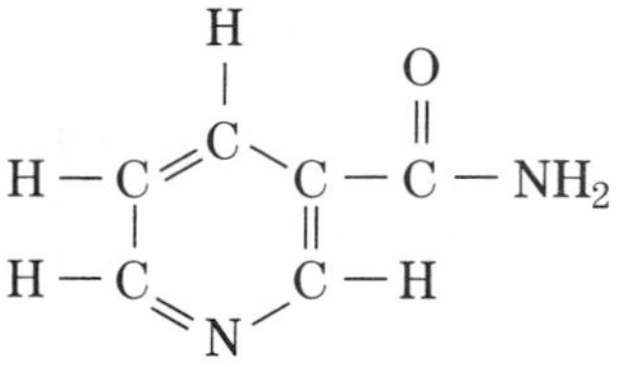

Nicotinamide

Niacin (nicotinic acid and nicotinamide)

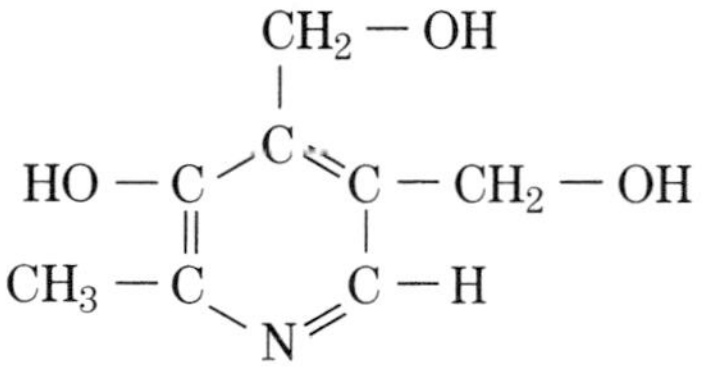

Pyridoxine

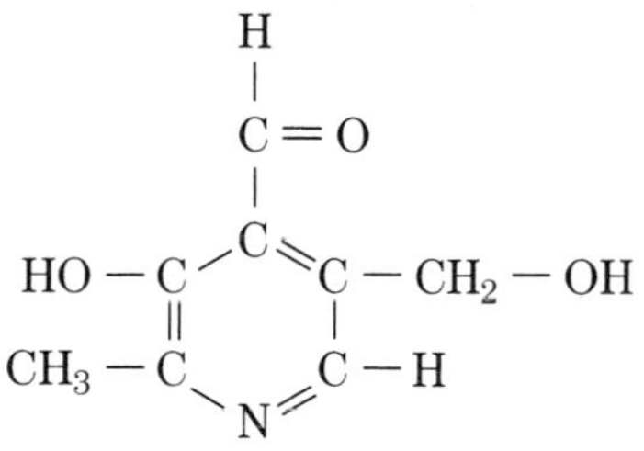

Pyridoxal

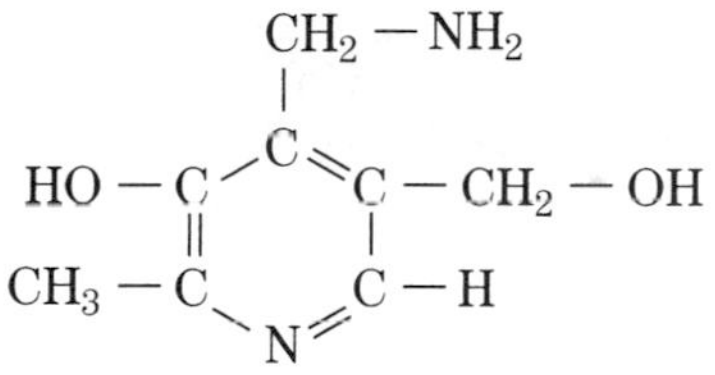

Pyridoxamine

Vitamin B-6 (a general name for three compounds—pyridoxine, pyridoxal, and pyridoxamine).

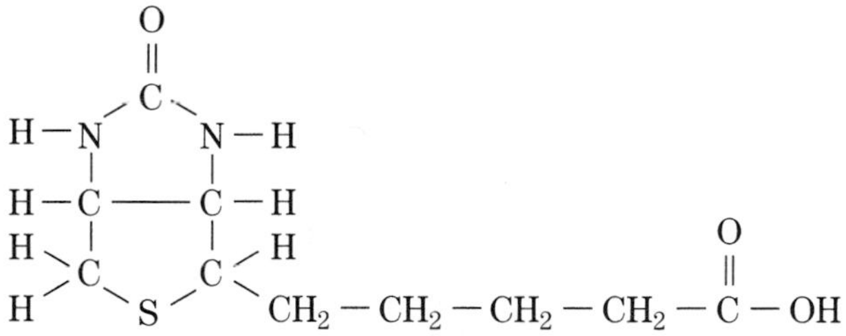

Biotin

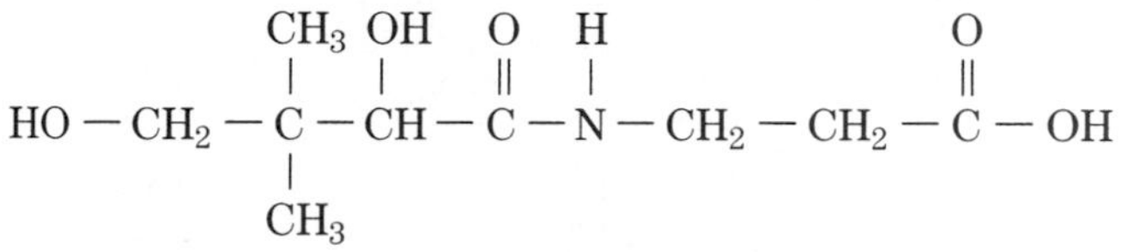

Pantothenic acid

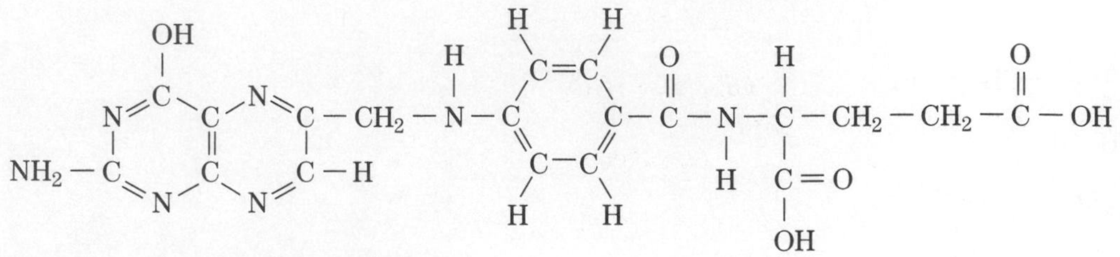

Folate (folacin or folic acid)

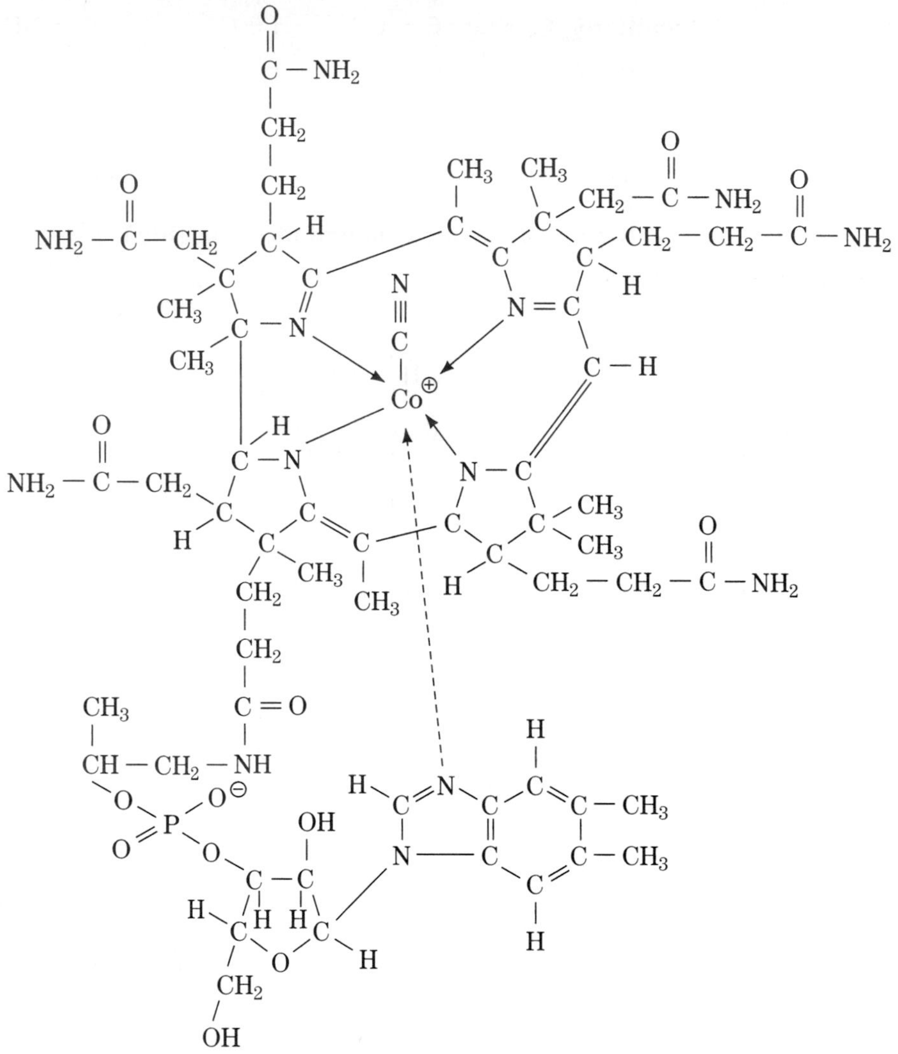

Vitamin B-12 (cyanocobalamin). The arrows in this diagram indicate that the spare electrons on the nitrogens attract them to the cobalt atom.

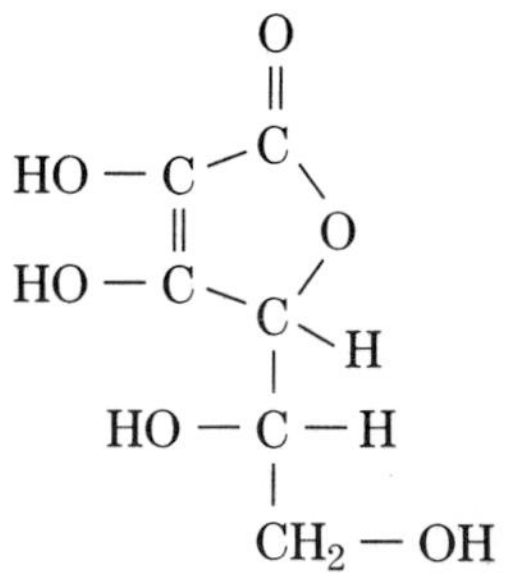

Vitamin C

Vitamin C (ascorbic acid)

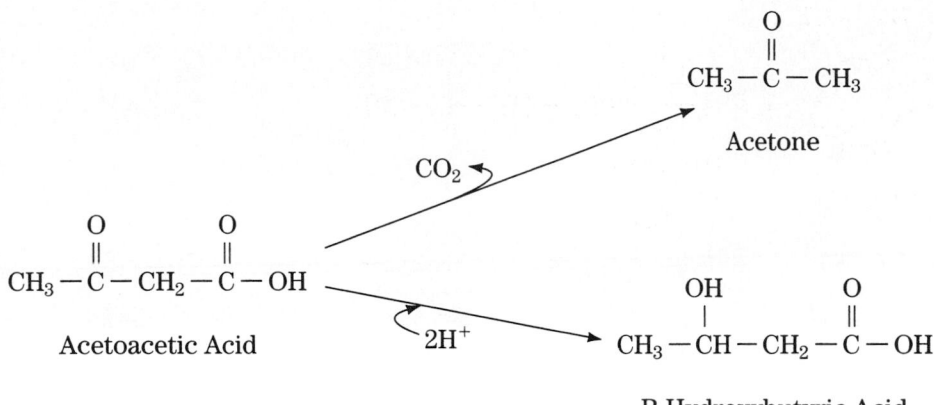

Acetoacetic Acid → Acetone (+ CO_2); Acetoacetic Acid → B-Hydroxybutyric Acid (+ $2H^+$)

OH
|
HO — P = O   Point of cleavage to yield
| ADP and energy release
O

Triphosphate   HO — P = O   Adenine
|
O

HO — P = O
|
O

Ribose   CH₂
(a sugar)

Determination of Frame Size

METHOD 1

Height is recorded without shoes.

Wrist circumference is measured just beyond the bony (styloid) process at the wrist joint on the right arm, using a tape measure.

The following formula is used:

$$r = \frac{\text{height (cm)}}{\text{wrist circumference (cm)}}$$

Frame size can be determined as follows:

Males	Females
r > 10.4 small	r > 11 small
r = 9.6–10.4 medium	r = 10.1–11 medium
r < 9.6 large	r < 10.1 large

From Grant JP: Handbook of Total Parenteral Nutrition, *Philadelphia, 1980, WB Saunders.*

METHOD 2

The patient's right arm is extended forward perpendicular to the body, with the arm bent so the angle at the elbow forms 90 degrees, with the fingers pointing up and the palm turned away from the body. The greatest breadth across the elbow joint is measured with a sliding caliper along the axis of the upper arm, on the two prominent bones on either side of the elbow. This is recorded as the elbow breadth. The following tables give elbow breadth measurements for medium-framed men and women of various heights. Measurements lower than those listed indicate a small frame size; higher measurements indicate a large frame size.

Men		Women	
HEIGHT IN 1" HEELS	ELBOW BREADTH	HEIGHT IN 1" HEELS	ELBOW BREADTH
5'2"–5'3"	2½–2⅞	4'10"–4'11"	2¼–2½
5'4"–5'7"	2⅝–2⅞	5'0"–5'3"	2¼–2½
5'8"–5'11"	2¾–3	5'4"–5'7"	2⅜–2⅝
6'0"–6'3"	2¾–3⅛	5'8"–5'11"	2⅜–2⅝
6'4" and over	2⅞–3¼	6'0" and over	2½–2¾

From Metropolitan Life Insurance Co., 1983.

Caffeine Content of Foods

BEVERAGES	mg
Carbonated beverages*	
Cherry Coke, Coca-Cola—12 fl oz (370 g)	46
cherry cola, Slice—12 fl oz (360 g)	48
Cherry RC—12 fl oz (360 g)	12
Coca-Cola—12 fl oz (370 g)	46
Coca-Cola Classic—12 fl oz (369 g)	46
Cola, RC—12 fl oz (360 g)	18
Mello Yello—12 fl oz (372 g)	52
Mr. Pibb—12 fl oz (369 g)	40
Mountain Dew—12 fl oz (360 g)	54
Dr. Pepper-type soda—12 fl oz (368 g)	41
Pepsi Cola—12 fl oz (360 g)	38
Carbonated beverages, low calorie*	
diet Cherry Coke, Coca-Cola—12 fl oz (354 g)	46
diet cherry cola, Slice—12 fl oz (360 g)	41
diet Coke, Coca-Cola—12 fl oz (354 g)	46
diet cola, aspartame-sweetened—12 fl oz (355 g)	50
diet Pepsi—12 fl oz (360 g)	36
diet RC—12 fl oz (360 g)	48
Pepsi Light—12 fl oz (360 g)	36
Tab—12 fl oz (354 g)	46
Coffee	
brewed—6 fl oz (177 g)	103
instant powder—1 tsp (1.8 g)	57
decaffeinated—1 rounded tsp (1.8 g)	2
with chicory—1 tsp (1.8 g)	37
prepared from instant powder—6 fl oz & 1 tsp powder (179 g)	57
amaretto, General Foods—6 fl oz & 11.5 g powder (189 g)	60
amaretto, sugar-free, General Foods—6 fl oz water & 7.7 g powder (185 g)	60

From Pennington JAT: *Bowes and Church's food values of portions commonly consumed*, ed 16, Philadelphia, 1994, JB Lippincott.
*Caffeine-free carbonated beverages and most noncola carbonated beverages contain no caffeine.

Continued.

Coffee—cont'd

decaffeinated—6 fl oz water & 1 tsp powder (179 g)	2
Francais, General Foods—6 fl oz water & 11.5 g powder (189 g)	53
Francais, sugar-free, General Foods—6 fl oz water & 7.7 g powder (185 g)	59
Irish creme, General Foods—6 fl oz water & 12.8 g powder (190 g)	53
Irish creme, sugar free, General Foods—6 fl oz water & 7.1 g powder (185 g)	48
Irish mocha mint, General Foods—6 fl oz water & 11.5 g powder (189 g)	27
Irish mocha mint, sugar-free, General Foods—6 fl oz water & 6.4 g powder (189 g)	25
orange cappuccino, General Foods—6 fl oz water & 14 g powder (191 g)	73
orange cappuccino, sugar-free, General Foods—6 fl oz water & 6.7 g powder (184 g)	71
Suisse mocha, General Foods—6 fl oz water & 11.5 g powder (189 g)	41
Suisse mocha, sugar-free, General Foods—6 fl oz water & 6.4 g powder (184 g)	40
Vienna, General Foods—6 fl oz water & 14 g powder (191 g)	56
Vienna, sugar-free, General Foods—6 fl oz water & 6.7 g powder (184 g)	55
with chicory—6 fl oz water & 1 tsp powder (179 g)	38

Tea, hot/iced

brewed 3 min—6 fl oz water (178 g)	36
instant powder—1 tsp (0.7 g)	31
with lemon flavor—1 rounded tsp (1.4 g)	25
with sugar & lemon flavor—3 tsp (23 g)	29
with sodium saccharin & lemon flavor—2 tsp (1.6 g)	36
prepared from instant powder	
1 tsp powder in 8 fl oz water (237 g)	31
Crystal Light—8 fl oz (238 g)	11
with lemon flavor—1 tsp powder in 8 fl oz water (238 g)	26
with sugar & lemon flavor—3 tsp powder in 8 fl oz water (259 g)	29
with sodium, saccharin & lemon flavor—2 tsp powder in 8 fl oz water (238 g)	36

CANDY

chocolate

German sweet, Bakers—1 oz square (28 g)	8
semi-sweet, Bakers—1 oz square (28 g)	13

chocolate chips

Bakers—1/4 cup (43 g)	12
German sweet, Bakers—1/4 cup (43 g)	15
semi-sweet, Bakers—1/4 cup (43 g)	14

DESSERTS
Frozen desserts

pudding pops, Jell-O

chocolate—1 pop (47 g)	2
chocolate caramel swirl—1 pop (47 g)	1
chocolate fudge—1 pop (47 g)	3

Frozen desserts—cont'd

    chocolate vanilla swirl—1 pop (47 g)   2

    chocolate with chocolate coating—1 pop (49 g)   3

    double chocolate swirl—1 pop (47 g)   2

    milk chocolate—1 pop (47 g)   2

Pies

chocolate mousse, from mix, Jell-O—$\frac{1}{8}$ pie (95 g)   6

Puddings, from instant mix

chocolate

    Jell-O—$\frac{1}{2}$ cup (150 g)   5

    sugar-free, D-Zerta—$\frac{1}{2}$ cup (130 g)   4

    sugar-free, Jell-O—$\frac{1}{2}$ cup (133 g)   4

chocolate fudge

    Jell-O—$\frac{1}{2}$ cup (150 g)   8

chocolate fudge mousse, Jell-O—$\frac{1}{2}$ cup (86 g)   12

chocolate mousse, Jell-O—$\frac{1}{2}$ cup (86 g)   9

chocolate tapioca, Jell-O—$\frac{1}{2}$ cup (147 g)   8

milk chocolate, Jell-O—$\frac{1}{2}$ cup (150 g)   5

MILK BEVERAGES

chocolate flavor mix in whole milk—2-3 tsp powder in 8 fl oz milk (266 g)   8

chocolate malted milk flavor powder

in whole milk—3 tsp powder in 8 fl oz milk (265 g)   8

with added nutrients in whole milk—4-5 tsp powder in 8 fl oz milk (265 g)   5

chocolate syrup in whole milk—2 tbsp syrup in 8 fl oz milk (282 g)   6

cocoa/hot chocolate, prepared with water from mix—3-4 tsp powder in 6 fl oz water (206 g)   4

MILK BEVERAGE MIXES

chocolate flavor mix, powder—2-3 tsp (22 g)   8

chocolate malted milk flavor mix, powder—3/4 oz (3 tsp) (21 g)   8

chocolate malted milk flavor mix with added nutrients, powder—3/4 oz (4-5 tsp) (21 g)   6

chocolate syrup—2 tbsp (1 fl oz) (38 g)   5

cocoa mix powder—1 oz pkt (3-4 tsp) (28 g)   5

MISCELLANEOUS

baking chocolate, unsweetened, Bakers—1 oz (28 g)   25

Common Food Additives

This list identifies the functions some of the more than 2800 additives allowed in the U.S. food supply

Additive	Function	Additive	Function
A		**D**	
Acetic acid	pH control‡	Dehydrated beets	color
Acetone peroxide	mat-bleach-condit§	Dextrose	sweetener
Apidic acid	pH control‡	Diglycerides	emulsifier
Ammonium alginate	stabil-thick-tex*	Dioctyl sodium sulfosuccinate	emulsifier
Annatto extract	color	Disodium guanylate	flavor enhancer
Arabinogalactan	stabil-thick-tex*	Disodium inosinate	flavor enhancer
Ascorbic acid	nutrient	Dried algae meal	color
	preservative		
	antioxidant	**E**	
Azodicarbonamide	mat-bleach-condit§	EDTA (ethylenediamine tetraacetic acid)	antioxidant
B			
Benzoic acid	preservative	**F**	
Benzoyl peroxide	mat-bleach-condit§	FD&C Colors:	
Beta-apo-89 carotenal	color	Blue No. 1	color
Beta carotene	nutrient	Red No. 3	color
	color	Red No. 40	color
BHA (butylated hydroxyanisole)	antioxidant	Yellow No. 5	color
BHT (butylated hydroxytoluene)	antioxidant	Fructose	sweetener
Butylparaben	preservative		
		G	
C		Gelatin	stabil-thick-tex*
Calcium alginate	stabil-thick-tex*	Glucose	sweetener
Calcium bromate	mat-bleach-condit§	Glycerine	humectant
Calcium lactate	preservative	Glycerol monostearate	humectant
Calcium phosphate	leavening†	Grape skin extract	color
Calcium silicate	anticaking‖	Guar gum	stabil-thick-tex*
Calcium sorbate	preservative	Gum arabic	stabil-thick-tex*
Canthaxanthin	color	Gum ghatti	stabil-thick-tex*
Caramel	color		
Carob bean gum	stabil-thick-tex*	**H**	
Carrageenan	emulsifier	Heptylparaben	preservative
	stabil-thick-tex*	Hydrogen peroxide	mat-bleach-condit§
Carrot oil	color		
Cellulose	stabil-thick-tex*	Hydrolyzed vegetable protein	flavor enhancer
Citric acid	preservative		
	antioxidant	**I**	
	pH control‡	Invert sugar	sweetener
Citrus Red No. 2	color	Iodine	nutrient
Cochineal extract	color	Iron	nutrient
Corn endosperm	color	Iron-ammonium citrate	anticaking‖
Corn syrup	sweetener	Iron oxide	color

From Lehmann P: More than you ever thought you would know about food additives, *FDA Consumer reprint, Health and Human Services Publication No. (FDA) 79-2115, 1979.*

Key to abbreviations: *stabil-thick-tex = stabilizers-thickeners-texturizers; †leavening = leavening agents; ‡pH control = pH control agents; §mat-bleach-condit = maturing and bleaching agents, dough conditioners; ‖anticaking = anticaking agents.

Additive	Function	Additive	Function
K		Sodium alginate	stabil-thick-tex*
Karaya gum	stabil-thick-tex*	Sodium aluminum sulfate	leavening†
		Sodium benzoate	preservative
L		Sodium bicarbonate	leavening†
Lactic acid	pH control‡	Sodium calcium alginate	stabil-thick-tex*
	preservative	Sodium citrate	pH control‡
Larch gum	stabil-thick-tex*	Sodium diacetate	preservative
Lecithin	emulsifier	Sodium erythrobate	preservative
Locust bean gum	stabil-thick-tex*	Sodium nitrate	preservative
		Sodium propionate	preservative
M		Sodium sorbate	preservative
Mannitol	sweetener	Sodium stearyl fumarate	mat-bleach-condit§
	anticakingi	Sorbic acid	preservative
	stabil-thick-tex*	Sorbitan monostearate	emulsifier
Methylparaben	preservative	Sorbital	humectant
Modified food starch	stabil-thick-tex*		sweetener
Monoglycerides	emulsifier	Spices	flavor
MSG (monosodium glutamate)	flavor enhancer	Sucrose (table sugar)	sweetener
N		**T**	
Niacinamide (niacin)	nutrient	Tagetes (Aztec Marigold)	color
		Tartaric acid	pH control‡
P		TBHQ (tertiary butyl hydro quinone)	antioxidant
Paprika (and oleoresin)	flavor		
	color	Thiamin	nutrient
Pectin	stabil-thick-tex*	Titanium dioxide	color
Phosphates	pH control‡	Toasted, partially defatted cooked cottonseed flour	color
Phosphoric acid	pH control‡		
Polysorbates	emulsifiers	Tocopherols (vitamin E)	nutrient
Potassium alginate	stabil-thick-tex*		antioxidant
Potassium bromate	mat-bleach-condit†	Tragacanth gum	stabil-thick-tex*
Potassium iodide	nutrient	Turmeric (oleoresin)	flavor
Potassium propionate	preservative		color
Potassium sorbate	preservative		
Propionic acid	preservative	**U**	
Propyl gallate	antioxidant	Ultramarine blue	color
Propylene glycol	stabil-thick-tex*		
	humectant	**V**	
Propylparaben	preservative	Vanilla, vanillin	flavor
		Vitamin A	nutrient
R		Vitamin C (ascorbic acid)	nutrient
Riboflavin	nutrient		preservative
	color		antioxidant
		Vitamin D (D-2, D-3)	nutrient
S		Vitamin E (tocopherols)	nutrient
Saccharin	sweetener		
Saffron	color	**Y**	
Silicon dioxide	anticakingi	Yeast-malt sprout extract	flavor enhancer
Sodium acetate	pH control‡	Yellow prussiate of soda	anticaking‖

Answers to Critical Thinking Questions

Chapter 1

1 Supplements purchased in a store can provide vitamins. Foods, on the other hand, supply not only vitamins but also carbohydrates, proteins, fats, and dietary fiber. The first three provide energy, and dietary fiber provides bulk for a healthy digestive system.
2 A diet consisting primarily of foods derived from animal sources contains mostly proteins and fats, with a high percentage of fats as saturated fats. Saturated fats reduce cholesterol clearance by the liver. High blood cholesterol is linked to increased risk of heart disease. A diet high in fat is also related to increased risk of colon, breast, and prostate cancer. Fruits and vegetables are rich in dietary fiber, which helps decrease blood cholesterol and increase the rate of peristalsis in the gastrointestinal tract. Fruits and vegetables, for the most part, contain low amounts of fats, if any, and are also low in energy, thus helping to maintain healthy body weight.

Chapter 2

1 Because the typical American diet consists of many foods high in fat and low in dietary fiber, Devan should assess his diet with respect to these components. He should list all of the foods he eats, preferably for a whole week, and estimate how much fat and dietary fiber he consumes. He then should change his eating habits to obtain recommended amounts of fat and dietary fiber. Most likely, Devan will need to decrease fat intake as well as increase dietary fiber in his diet.
2 A cup of skim milk provides 90 kcal, and a cup of whole milk provides 150 kcal. Both contain 8 grams of protein and about 290 milligrams of calcium. Skim milk delivers the same amount of protein and calcium as whole milk but with fewer calories. Thus skim milk is more nutrient dense with respect to protein and calcium than whole milk. The difference in the energy content of skim and whole milk results from varying fat contents: a cup of skim milk has only a trace of fat, whereas a cup of whole milk has 8 grams of fat.

Chapter 3

1 Early man lived only 30 years or so. Today our life expectancy is more than double that. History can give us clues to improve our diets, but only actual studies—such as double-blind research—can establish the actual advantages of any diet.
2 Many vitamins, such as the water-soluble ones, can be excreted when taken in excess; however, the fat-soluble vitamins are not as readily excreted. Vitamin A in particular can accumulate in large amounts, causing toxic effects. These effects can occur at just five or so times the Daily Values with regular usage of such excess quantities, especially in children, pregnant women, and the elderly. Large amounts of many water-soluble vitamins can also be toxic, but much higher doses are needed.

Chapter 4

1 Although taste receptors for sweet, salty, sour, and bitter flavors are located on the tongue, there are receptors associated with the nose that help us taste various flavors. These cells in the nose detect combinations of chemical molecules that, along with the taste receptors on the tongue, allow us to perceive the flavors in our foods. When you have a cold, the membranes in your nose secrete excess mucus, which prevents the molecules from exciting the receptors. Hence, your sense of taste is inhibited.
2 The small intestine is the most important absorption site in the digestive system because of its large surface area. Because much of the young girl's small intestine was removed, many of the nutrients she consumes are escaping absorption. Only a highly refined (liquid) diet or intravenous therapy is likely to succeed in keeping her adequately nourished.

Chapter 5

1 Diverticulosis is a condition in which tiny pouches form in the wall of the colon. When foods are eaten that are not easily digestible, like large pieces of nuts, these may become trapped in the pouches. Bacteria then metabolize these foodstuffs into acids and gases that irritate the diverticula, causing them to swell; this condition is called *diverticulitis*. The acids and gases in the swollen pouches cause cramping and abdominal pain.
2 Foods that remain in the mouth, usually caught between the teeth, are a source of food that bacterial can metabolize. As a by-product of this metabolism, bacterial produce acids that can decay tooth enamel, causing dental caries. Chewing gum after meals decreases the risk of caries because chewing stimulates the secretion of saliva, which helps to dislodge foods that remain in the mouth. Sugar-free gums also contain sugar substitutes, which bacteria can't metabolize. In addition, saliva helps to neutralize the acids produced by the bacteria.

Chapter 6

1 In addition to ensuring good health by supplying essential fatty acids, triglycerides in foods promote satiety (that is, a feeling of fullness). Triglycerides produce this effect by influencing certain hormonal responses, which in turn affect the rate of stomach emptying. After a nonfat meal the stomach empties rapidly, so one feels hungry in a short time. In contrast, after a meal containing some fat the rate of stomach emptying slows, so one feels satiated or satisfied for a longer period. If dieters with limited energy intakes would include a small amount of fat in their meals, they would not feel hungry as soon. (Increasing dietary fiber intake from fruits, vegetables, and whole grains provides the same benefit.) As a result, dieters would be less likely to give up their diets quickly and would have a better chance of long-term success.

2 The general term *fats* refers to lipids in foods without reference to their structure. Only dietary fats with a high proportion of saturated fatty acids have been associated with heart disease. In the body, fat (primarily in the form of tri-glycerides) has many beneficial functions. Triglycerides form the main energy stores in the body and can release fatty acids, which serve as fuel for many cells, such as those in muscles. Stored fat insulates the body and pro-tects vital organs. Absorption of fat-soluble vitamins from the small intestine is aided by their association with dietary fats. In addi-tion, the two essential fatty acids, linoleic acid and alpha-linolenic acid, are not synthe-sized by the body and must be in the diet to maintain health. Thus some fat is needed in the diet; moderation, not elimination, of intake is the goal.

Chapter 7

1 PKU is the abbreviation for the disease phenylketonuria. The liver of a person with phenylketonuria cannot readily convert phenylalanine, an essential amino acid, to tyrosine. This defect is caused by insufficient enzyme action. Because phenylalanine cannot be sufficiently degraded, tyrosine must be con-sidered an essential amino acid for people with PKU.

The inability to metabolize excess phenyl-alanine to tyrosine leads to the formation of abnormal products that arise from alternative metabolic pathways; these products can cause mental retardation. Thus determining which infants have PKU is vital, because the phenyl-alanine content in their diets must be moni-tored. However, because phenylalanine is an essential amino acid, some must be consumed.

2 Protein synthesis is a complex process by which a specific sequence and number of amino acids determine the structure of a protein. If enough of a given amino acid is not present during protein synthesis, produc-tion will stop. In other words, protein is an all-or-none product: all of the amino acids necessary to make the protein must be avail-able, or the protein will not be made at all. A mixed diet of plant products will contain enough of all 9 essential amino acids, so the all-or-none law won't typically be an issue in diet planning, even in vegetarianism.

Chapter 8

1 A possible explanation for the lack of clot dissolution in Tim's leg is that he has been consuming many foods rich in vitamin K. This vitamin assists in clot formation and is antagonistic to oral anticoagulant medications. If the vitamin K is not reduced in Tim's diet, the therapy won't be very effective.

2 Humans must obtain vitamin C from foods because the body cannot synthesize it.

An important function of this vitamin is to promote the formation of collagen, an important protein found in connective tissue. Collagen is an integral component of bone, skin, and blood vessels. Thus a low intake of vitamin C will impair wound healing. Defi-ciency can also lead to scurvy, the symptoms of which include bleeding gums and pinpoint hemorrhages on the skin.

Vitamin C is an antioxidant. It works with vitamin E against free radicals and helps "reactivate" vitamin E so that it can continue to function. Vitamin C also deters certain forms of cancer, modestly enhances iron absorption, assists in carnitine production, and synthesizes norepinephrine, a neurotransmitter. Finally, vitamin C is essential for immune system activity. However, vitamin C does not cure the common cold.

Chapter 9

1 When we do physical work, such as mowing the lawn, we perspire. The degree of perspi-ration varies among people and also depends on the time of day. Muscle strength and endurance decline significantly when there is a 3% loss of body weight. Symptoms such as thirst may indicate a 2% loss of body weight caused by dehydration. With greater water loss a headache and dizziness may develop. Even further water loss may induce a coma.

Anyone who anticipates loss of body water through perspiration would benefit from hydrating before the activity, such as in preparation for an athletic event. Doing so will minimize dehydration. Drinking fluids during exertion is also helpful.

2 Calcium is needed for normal bone growth and development. Bones serve as reservoirs of calcium for the bloodstream. Regulation of blood calcium may necessitate the breakup of bone mineral deposits for the release of calcium from bone. Bone mineralization is maximal before and during adolescence. Manuela is already an adult, but she can still consume calcium in amounts sufficient to decrease bone demineralization.

The best sources of calcium are milk and sardines, which Manuela, a vegan, will not eat. She should therefore acquaint herself with alternative sources—vegetables that contain calcium. She should also choose calcium-fortified foods, such as some brands of orange juice. However, if she cannot meet her calcium needs by modifying her diet, based on a nutrient analysis of her current intake, calcium supplements are advised.

3 The mineral selenium aids in the activity of the enzyme glutathione peroxidase. This enzyme participates in a system that metabo-lizes peroxides into less toxic alcohol deriva-tives and water. Peroxides tend to become free radicals, which in turn can attack and break down cell membranes, causing cell damage.

Selenium is considered important in protecting heart cells and other cells against oxidative damage through the action of glutathione peroxidase. In addition, because this enxyme reduces the amount of free-radical damage to cells, selenium may be important in protect-ing against cancer.

Chapter 10

1 Although Hal has seen a steady decrease in his weight for the duration of his diet thus far, his body has built-in mechanisms that tend to fight weight loss. One of those factors is the basal metabolic rate. The BMR tends to decrease to conserve energy as the number of calories in the diet decreases. Also, lipoprotein lipase activity increases in adipose cells, which increases lipid uptake into adipose (fat) cells. The increased activity of this enzyme allows the body to take up fats more efficiently from the blood after the dieting has stopped.

Thus, the body resists weight loss by phys-iological means; however, it may finally "surrender" to persistent dieting, and Hal will continue to lose weight as long as he continues to diet.

2 Low-carbohydrate diets, as well as "starvation diets," may lead to rapid reduction of body weight; however, they may also lead to problems. Weight lost in a short time generally results from loss of water and lean body tissue. Weight should be lost mostly from fat storage, not from muscle and other lean tissues. At the start of a diet, rapid weight loss may also be attributable to decreased salt intake and loss of glycogen from the liver and muscles. In addition, the liver is forced to undergo gluconeogenesis and ketogenesis to supply energy to "starving" cells. This type of diet, a quick-fix diet, yields only temporary results, with an eventual return to the higher weight.

Chapter 11

1 Marty has enhanced his cardiovascular fitness, a laudable goal. In addition, after a period of training, muscle cells worked on a regular basis will make more mitochondria. Because mitochondria are the sites of aerobic metabolism, more ATP can be generated. ATP is a necessary component for muscle contraction, so a greater amount of ATP production allows a greater amount of muscle contraction.

2 Many wrestlers and other athletes lose weight quickly by losing large amounts of water, usually by sweating. By doing so, an athlete can compete in a lower weight class and thus gain an advantage over an oppo-nent. However, losing weight this way can significantly impede performance. Over time, repeated dehydration episodes can lead to serious complications, such as kidney failure.

Athletes also risk becoming heat stressed during the event.

The loss of water before a competition is the quick way to lose weight. However, if an athlete is serious about his or her sport, a gradual change in diet to create the best possible weight/muscle composition should be the goal.

Chapter 12

1 The young woman would be advised to focus first on weight maintenance as she tries to organize the other aspects of her life. Then, possibly in six months or so, when she has time to focus on dieting, she can provide enough attention to this goal to make success more likely.

2 People may try to block success because they are jealous. Married people may fear that their spouse will become more attractive and therefore more desirable to others. Overall, change can threaten those around you, and this needs to be taken into account in any behavior change process.

Chapter 13

1 Signs that could indicate an eating disorder include the following:
(1) Compulsive behavior patterns
(2) Obsession with being and looking thin
(3) Obsession with counting calories
(4) Anxiety about eating with others (for example, refusing to go to a restaurant)
(5) Continual self-criticism and frequent comparisons of self with others, especially slender people
(6) Belief that one is fat

2 One of the most important topics Tom should discuss is proper nutrition. Using the concepts of variety, balance, and moderation, he can teach students about their diets. He should also present case studies of real people who have anorexia nervosa and bulimia nervosa so that his students can better understand the outcome of these diseases. Tom should also focus on increasing the self-esteem of young adults. The prepuberty and teenage years are a time of self-evaluation and criticism. It is important for Tom to help his students feel good about themselves by emphasizing the importance of self-worth—regardless of physical appearance. Finally, Tom can teach his students how to cope with difficult situations by showing them how to alleviate stress in positive and constructive ways.

Chapter 14

1 It is important to assess a woman's nutritional and health status before she begins trying to become pregnant. The dietary habits of the mother-to-be can affect the health of the newborn. Good nutrition is critical during a woman's childbearing years. Nutritional deficiencies have been shown to result in improper fetal development. An adequate vitamin and mineral intake in the months before conception and during the pregnancy can help prevent fetal defects, such as with the vitamin folate.

2 As the pregnancy advances, the uterus will continue to grow to accommodate the growing fetus. As the uterus enlarges, it presses against the stomach and intestines. Also, hormones produced in increased amounts during pregnancy relax muscles. This explains why heartburn may occur; the lower esophageal sphincter relaxes somewhat, allowing some foods and acid to regurgitate back into the esophagus causing heartburn. Ingesting smaller quantities of foods and not reclining after eating are recommended. High amounts of fats also decrease the rate of stomach emptying; therefore decreasing fat in the diet should also help. Because hormones relax muscles, the rate of peristalsis may also decrease and constipation may develop. Gradually increasing the amounts of dietary fiber and fluid in Sandy's diet to improve her digestive system's peristaltic activity would be wise.

Chapter 15

1 Human milk is low in iron. Although it provides the baby with many essential nutrients, it doesn't meet all of a baby's needs after about 6 months, because iron stores are depleted by this time. This iron deficiency can lead to anemia. Begin feeding infants iron-fortified cereal between 4 and 6 months of age to prevent iron-deficiency anemia. In addition, some pediatricians recommend giving iron supplements to breastfed infants, beginning shortly after birth.

2 Typical breakfast foods include cereal, eggs, toast, and pancakes, but any food can be a breakfast, lunch, or dinner food as long as it is nutrient dense. If Tim doesn't like the traditional breakfast foods but enjoys a sandwich, macaroni and cheese, or yogurt, his parents can offer these instead. These nutritious foods are no more beneficial at lunchtime than they are at 7 A.M. The depletion of carbohydrate stores that occurs during the night can cause children to be lethargic and inattentive in the morning. Eating early in the morning replenishes carbohydrate stores. Many experts believe that the nutrients consumed stimulate attention in children, allowing them to perform better in school.

Chapter 16

1 Science has established a considerable link between nutrition (diet) and health. For example, low-fat diets have been shown to reverse atherosclerosis and improve diabetes control in some people by reducing body fat. Although body cells will age no matter what health practices are followed, much of the risk for disease can be decreased through diet and lifestyle. A consistently healthful diet and a regimen of regular physical activity have proved effective in maintaining a healthy body: muscles are firmer, bone fractures are less likely, and the person looks and feels better. Overall, the secret to enjoying "youth" throughout life is to establish a healthy physical, mental, and social framework.

2 Many older people have experienced the death of a lifelong companion. Men and women who have lived with another person for twenty, thirty, and sometimes over fifty years find the loss of their loved one traumatic. If they have no means to cope with this overwhelming loss, they may become depressed. Depressed people often eat decreased amounts of food, show little interest in meals, and stop eating altogether. In addition, many older people depended on their loved ones for planning, buying, and preparing meals. The surviving partner may feel indifferent or overwhelmed by these tasks.

As the body ages, the senses lose their acuity. People lose some taste receptors in the tongue and some smell receptors in the nose. This loss of taste and smell contributes to apathy about eating (consider your appetite when you have a cold and can't smell or taste as well).

Chapter 17

1 USDA recommends cutting boards with unmarred surfaces made from nonporous materials. These include plexiglass, plastic, and marble, which are easy to clean. Grooves or cuts on surfaces provide a "home" where bacteria can thrive. If Jon wants to buy a wooden cutting board, he should plan to clean it using hot, soapy water every time he cuts something. He should also try not to use the same board for both meats and vegetables or fruits. If he must use it for everything, he should cut the vegetables first, wash the board in hot, soapy water, and then cut the meats. Jon should also sanitize any board once a week in a solution of two teaspoons chlorine bleach per quart of water to minimize any bacterial growth.

2 Bacteria thrive at room temperature, especially between 60° and 110° F. Some bacteria causes food-borne illness. Cooling by refrigeration slows down bacterial growth, but it does not stop it or destroy toxins already produced by the bacteria. Foods left at room temperature for 2 hours, or even 1 hour in hot weather, give microorganisms the opportunity to grow. Refrigeration after that time is too late. Diana is correct in wanting to discard the food.

Chapter 18

1 Undernourished children (and adults) often show short stature, apathy, muscular weakness, and decreased physical activity and work capability. Because undernutrition decreases resistance to disease, undernourished children are likely to have more frequent infections and recover more slowly from illness than well-fed children.

2 Where extreme food shortages exist, there is no choice but to supply hungry people with food—they are starving and dying. However, reliance on outside help is not a long-range solution. Rather, developing countries need to improve their economies and infrastructures so that people are able to produce or buy sufficient amounts of nutritious food to meet their needs. Appropriate development includes many aspects: education, availability of machinery and other agricultural tools, and alternative employment opportunities. Small farms and businesses should be encouraged. As the economy expands, more people will be able to afford nutritious food. Agricultural production should focus on basic food crops to be consumed by a country's own citizens, rather than on cash crops for export.

GLOSSARY

Medical Terminology to Aid in the Study of Nutrition

Term Meaning

a- Without, from
acyl A carbon chain
aden-, adeno- Gland
-algia Pain
aliment Food
-amine Containing nitrogen
andr-, andro- Man or male
apo-, ap- Detached
arteri-, arterio- Artery
arthr-, arthro- Joint
-ase Enzyme
-blast Immature form, embryonic
brady- Slow
buli- Ox
canc-, carcino- Malignancy
cardi-, cardio- Heart
centi- Divided into one hundred parts
chol-, chole-, cholo- Bile, gall
cholecyst- Gallbladder
chondr-, chondri-, chondro- Cartilage
chrom-, chromo- Color, colored
-clast Something that breaks
col-, coli-, colo- Colon
cyano-, cyan- Blue
cyt-, cyto- Cell
derm-, dermato- Skin
dextr-, dextro- Right, on or toward the right
duoden-, duodeno- Duodenum
dys- Difficult, painful
ect-, ecto- Without, outside, external
ectomy Excision of
-ein A protein
em- Blood
-emia In blood
encephal-, encephalo- Brain
endo-, ento-, end-, ent- Within
enter-, entero- Intestine
erythr-, erythro- Red
esophag-, esophago- Esophagus
eu- Well, easy, good
gastr-, gastro-, gastri- Stomach

gen- To become or produce
gloss-, glosso- Tongue
glyco-, glyc- Sugar
gynec-, gyn-, gyne- Woman or female (especially female reproductive organs)
hem-, hemat- Blood
hepat-, hepato- Liver
hexa-, hex- Six
histo- hist- Tissue
homeo-, homoeo-, homoio- Sameness, similarity
hydr-, hydro- Water
hyper- Excessive, above, beyond
hypo-, hyp- Under, beneath, deficient
hyster-, hystero- Uterus
idio- One's own, peculiar to, separate, distinct
ile-, ileo- Ileum
inter- Between, among
intra- Within, during, between layers of
-itis Inflammation of
jejun-, jejuno- Jejunum
kilo- One thousand
lact-, lacti-, lacto- Milk
leuc-, leuk- White, colorless
lev-, levo- Left, towards the left
lip-, lipo- Fat, lipid
litho-, lith- Stone
lymph-, lympho- Waterlike
lysis Destruction
mal- Bad, badly
malac-, malaco- Soft, a condition of abnormal softness
mega-, meg- Large, great
meta- After, later; change, exchange
metallo- Containing metal
micro- Divided into one million parts
milli- Divided into one thousand parts
mono- One
morph-, morpho- Form, shape
my-, myo- Muscle
myel-, myelo- Marrow, spinal cord
nas-, naso- Nose, nasal
necr-, necro- Dead

nephr-, nephro- Kidney
neur-, neuro- Nerve
-oid Formed like, resembling
-ol Alcohol
olig-, oligo- Few, scant
-oma Tumor
ophthalmo-, ophthalm- Eye, eyeball
-orex Mouth
-orexis Desire, appetite
-ose Sugar, carbohydrate
-osis Action, process, result, usually abnormal or diseased
ost-, osteo-, oste- Bone
ot- Ear
ovari-, ovario- Ovary
ovo-, ovi Eggs
pan- All
pancreat-, pancreato- Pancreas
para- Beside
parieto- Wall of a cavity, parietal bone
patho-, path- Disease
ped- Child, foot
-penia Without, lack of
-phobia Fear of
-plasm, -plasma Formative, formed, cell or tissue substance
pneum-, pneumo-, pneumono- Lung
-poiesis Production, format
poly- Many, much
post- After
pre- Before
prot-, proto- First
pseud-, pseudo- False
pulmo-, pulmon-, pulmono- Lung
pyel-, pyelo- Pelvis
pyr- Fever, fire
rect-, recto- Rectum
reni-, reno- Kidney
rhin-, rhino- Nose
-rrhagia Rupture, excessive fluid discharge
-rrhea Flow, discharge
sate To fill
scler-, sclero- Hard, hardness

G-1

-scopy Viewing
seb-, sebi-, sebo- Hard fat sebum, sebaceous glands
semi- Half
-soma, somat-, somato- Body
-stasia, -stasis Slowing or stopping of
stenosis Narrowing of
stomat-, stomato- Mouth, stoma

-stomy Surgical opening
sub- Under, below
super- Over, above
tachy- Swift, fast
thi-, thio- Containing sulfur
thromb-, thrombo- Blood clot
tox-, toxi-, toxo- Poison
trache-, tracheo- Trachea

-trophy Growth or mutation
ure-, urea-, ureo- Urine
uter-, utero- Uterus
vas-, vaso- Blood vessel
ven-, veni-, veno- Vein
vita- Life
xer-, xero- Dry

Glossary Terms

absorption The process by which substances are taken up by the GI tract and enter the bloodstream.

absorptive cells A class of cells, also called *enterocytes*, that line the villi; fingerlike projections in the small intestine that participate in nutrient absorption.

acesulfame (ay-see-SUL-fame) An alternate sweetener that yields no energy to the body; it is 200 times sweeter than sucrose.

achlorhydria (ay-clor-HIGH-dre-ah) A state of reduced acid production by the stomach, primarily resulting from loss of the acid-producing cells in the stomach, which is commonly associated with aging.

acid pH A pH less than 7. Lemon juice has an acid pH.

active absorption Absorption using a carrier and expending energy. In this way the absorptive cell absorbs nutrients, such as glucose, when a high concentration of the nutrient is already present in the absorptive cells.

adaptive thermogenesis Adaptive energy expended in heat production, such as when subjected to cold environmental conditions or overfeeding.

adenosine diphosphate (ADP) A breakdown product of ATP. ADP is synthesized into ATP using energy from foodstuffs and a phosphate group (abbreviated Pi).

adenosine triphosphate (ATP) (ah-DEN-o-sin try-FOS-fate) The main energy currency for cells. ATP energy is used to promote ion pumping, enzyme activity, and muscular contraction.

adipose (fat) tissue (ADD-ih-pos) A group of fat-storing cells.

ad libitum (ad-LIB-itum) At one's desire or pleasure.

adult-onset obesity Obesity that develops in adulthood; characterized by a normal number of adipose cells, but each cell is enlarged because of fat storage.

aerobic (air-ROW-bic) Requiring oxygen.

aerobic training In common usage this refers to activities that work the lungs and heart at a moderate to vigorous pace for a continuous period of time, such as brisk walking, jogging, swimming, or cycling. Duration is a key attribute of these types of activities.

alcohol Refers to ethyl alcohol or ethanol, CH_3CH_2OH.

alcohol dehydrogenase (dee-high-DRO-jen-ase) The enzyme used in alcohol (ethanol) breakdown; the major enzyme used in the liver when alcohol is present in low concentration.

aldosterone (al-DOS-ter-own) A powerful hormone produced by the adrenal glands that acts on the kidneys to cause sodium reabsorption and, in turn, water conservation.

alimentary canal (al-ih-MEN-tah-ree) Gastrointestinal tract.

alkaline (basic) pH A pH greater than 7. Baking soda in water yields an alkaline pH.

allergen A foreign protein, or antigen, that induces excess production of certain immune system antibodies; subsequent exposure to the same protein leads to allergic symptoms. While all allergens are antigens, not all antigens are allergens.

allergy A hypersensitive immune response that occurs when antibodies produced by the body react with a protein foreign to the body (antigen).

alpha glycosidic bond A type of glycosidic bond that can be broken by human intestinal enzymes in digestion.

alpha-linolenic acid (AL-fah-lin-oh-LE-nik) An essential acid with 18 carbon atoms and 3 double bonds (omega-3).

alveoli (al-VE-o-lye) Small air sacs of the lung.

amenorrhea (A-men-or-ee-a) The absence of three or more consecutive menstrual cycles; the absence of menses in a female.

amino acid (ah-MEE-noh) The building block for proteins containing a central carbon atom with a nitrogen atom and other atoms attached.

amniotic fluid (am-nee-OTT-ik) Fluid contained in a sac within the uterus. This fluid surrounds and protects the fetus during development.

amylase (AM-uh-lace) Starch-digesting enzyme from the salivary glands or pancreas.

amylose (AM-uh-los) A digestible straight-chain polysaccharide made of glucose units; primary component of starch in foods.

anabolic/anabolism (an-AH-bol-iz-um) Building compounds.

anaerobic (AN-ah-ROW-bic) Not requiring oxygen.

anaerobic training In common usage this refers to activities that consist of bursts of energy expenditure followed by a rest period, such as weightlifting or sprinting. Intense, short-term exertion is a key attribute of these types of activities.

anaphylactic shock (an-ah-fih-LAK-tic) A severe allergic response that results in lowered blood pressure and respiratory and gastrointestinal distress. This can be fatal.

androgen (AN-dro-jen) A general term for hormones that stimulate development in male sex organs; for example, testosterone.

android obesity (AN-droyd) Obesity in which fat storage is located primarily in the abdominal area; defined as a waist-to-hip circumference ratio greater than 1.0 in men and 0.8 in women. Android obesity is closely associated with a high risk of heart disease, high blood pressure, and diabetes.

anemia Generally refers to a decreased oxygen-carrying capacity of the blood. This can be caused by many factors.

anergy (AN-er-jee) Lack of an immune response to foreign compounds entering the body.

angiotensin I (an-jee-oh-TEN-sin) An intermediary compound produced during the body's attempt to conserve water and sodium; it is converted in the lungs to angiotensin II.

angiotensin II A compound produced from angiotensin I, which increases blood vessel constriction and triggers production of the hormone aldosterone.

animal model Study of disease in animals that duplicates human disease. This can be used to understand more about human disease.

anorexia nervosa (an-oh-REX-ee-uh ner-VOH-sah) An eating disorder involving a psychological loss of appetite and self-starvation, related in part from a distorted body image and to various social pressures; commonly associated with puberty.

anthropometry (an-throw-PO-meh-tree) The measurement of weight, lengths, circumferences, and thicknesses of parts of or the whole body.

antibody (AN-tih-bod-ee) Blood proteins that inactivate foreign proteins found in the body. This helps prevent and control infections.

antidiuretic hormone (ADH) (an-tie-dye-u-RET-ik) A hormone secreted by the pituitary gland that acts on the kidney to cause a decrease in water excretion.

antigen (AN-ti-jen) Any substance that induces a state of sensitivity and/or resistance to microbes or toxic substances after a lag period; substance that stimulates a specific aspect of the immune system.

antioxidant Generally a compound that prevents the oxidation of substances in food or the body, particularly lipids. Antioxidants are especially important in preventing the oxidation of polyunsaturated lipids in the membranes of cells. An antioxidant is able to donate electrons to electron-seeking compounds. This in turn reduces electron capture and thus breakdown of unsaturated fatty acids and other cell components by oxidizing agents. Vitamin E is one antioxidant cells use for protection. Some compounds have antioxidant capabilities (i.e., stop oxidation) but are not electron donors per se.

apoferritin (ape-oh-FERR-ih-tin) A protein in the intestinal cell that binds with the ferric form of iron (Fe^{3+}) to form ferritin.

apolipoproteins (APE-oh-lip-oh-PRO-teens) Proteins imbedded in the outer shell of lipoproteins. They help other enzymes function, act as lipid transfer proteins, or help bind to a receptor.

appetite The external (psychological) influences that encourage us to find and eat food, often in the absence of obvious hunger.

arachidonic acid (ar-a-kih-DON-ik) A fatty acid with 20 carbon atoms and four double bonds (omega-6).

areola (ah-REE-oh-lah) The circular dark area of skin at the center of the breast.

ariboflavinosis (ah-rih-bo-flay-vih-NOH-sis) A condition resulting from a lack of riboflavin. The a means "without," and the *osis* stands for "a condition of."

arithmetic progression A series of numbers in which the difference between each number is the same.

arthritis Inflammation at a point where bones join together. The disease has many possible causes.

aseptic processing (ah-SEP-tik) A method by which food and container are simultaneously sterilized; it allows manufacturers to produce boxes of milk that can be stored at room temperature. Variations of this process are also known as *ultra high temperature* (UHT) packaging.

aspartame (AH-spar-tame) An alternate sweetener made of two amino acids and methanol; it is about 200 times sweeter than sucrose.

atherosclerosis (ath-e-roh-scle-ROH-sis) A buildup of fatty material (plaque) in the arteries, including those surrounding the heart.

atom Smallest combining unit of an element.

autodigestion Literally, "self-digestion." The stomach limits autodigestion by covering itself with a thick layer of mucus and producing enzymes and acid only when needed for digestion of foodstuff.

autoimmune Immune reactions against normal body cells; self against self.

avidin (AV-ih-din) A protein found in raw egg whites that can bind biotin and inhibit its absorption. Avidin is destroyed by cooking.

bacteria A group of single-cell microorganisms, some of which produce poisonous substances called toxins that lead to ill health in humans. They contain only one chromosome and lack many organelles found in human cells. Bacteria produce enzymes that can digest substances around them. Some can live without oxygen and survive harsh conditions by means of spore formation.

baryophobia (bear-ee-oh-FO-bee-ah) A disorder of young children and young adults characterized by stunted growth resulting from underfeeding in an attempt to prevent development of obesity and heart disease.

basal metabolism (BAY-sal) The minimum energy the body requires to support itself when resting and awake. To have basal metabolic rate (BMR) measured, a person must not have eaten in the previous 12 hours and be maintained in a warm, quiet environment during the measurement. It amounts to roughly 1 kcal per minute or about 1400 kcal per day.

behavior contract A written agreement that outlines intended behavior changes, plans for reinforcement, and witnesses to monitor progress.

benign Noncancerous; tumors that do not spread.

beriberi (BEAR-ee-BEAR-ee) The thiamin deficiency disorder characterized by muscle weakness, loss of appetite, nerve degeneration, and sometimes edema.

beta glycosidic (BEY-tuh) bond A type of glycosidic bond that is not digested by human intestinal enzymes when it is part of a long chain of glucose monosaccharides.

BHA and BHT (Butylated hydroxyanisole and butylated hydroxytoluene) Two common synthetic antioxidants added to foods.

bile A substance made in the liver and stored in the gallbladder; it is released into the small intestine to aid fat absorption by emulsifying it into micelles.

bile acids Emulsifiers synthesized by the liver and released by the gallbladder during digestion to aid in fat digestion.

binge-eating disorder An eating disorder characterized by recurrent binge eating and feelings of loss of control over eating. Binge episodes can be triggered by frustration, anger, depression, anxiety, permission to eat forbidden foods, or excessive hunger.

bioavailability The degree to which the amount of an ingested nutrient is absorbed and so is available to the body.

biochemical deficiency symptoms Nutritional deficiency symptoms observed in the blood or urine, such as low concentrations of nutrient byproducts or low enzyme activities, indicating reduced body function.

bioelectrical impedance (im-PEE-dance) A method to estimate total body fat that uses a low-energy electrical current. The more fat storage a person has, the more impedance (resistance) to electrical flow will be exhibited.

biological value (BV) of a protein A measurement of the body's ability to retain protein absorbed from a food.

biotechnology A collection of processes that involve use of advanced scientific techniques to alter and, ideally, improve characteristics of animals, plants, and other forms of life.

bisphosphonates Compounds primarily composed of carbon and phosphorus that bind to bone mineral and in turn reduce bone breakdown.

blood doping A technique by which an athlete's red blood cell count is increased. Blood is taken from the athlete, and the red blood cells are concentrated and then later reinjected into the athlete.

body mass index Weight (in kilograms) divided by height squared (in meters). A value of 25 or greater indicates a higher risk for obesity-related health disorders.

bomb calorimeter (kal-oh-RIM-eh-ter) An instrument used to determine the energy content of a food.

bond A sharing of electrons, charges, or attractions linking two atoms.

bone mineral density Total mineral content of bone at a specific bone site divided by the width of the bone at that site, generally expressed as grams per cubic centimeter.

bone remodeling A process by which bone is first resorbed by osteoclast cells and then reformed by osteoblast cells. This process allows the body to form bone where needed, such as in areas of high mechanical stress.

bone-resorbing cells Specialized bone cells that remove bone material, also called *osteoclasts*.

brown adipose tissue (ADD-ih-pose) A specialized form of adipose tissue that produces large amounts of heat by metabolizing energy-yielding nutrients inefficiently. The energy released mostly just forms heat.

buffer Compounds that cause a solution to resist changes in acid-base balance.

bulimia nervosa (boo-LEEM-ee-uh) An eating disorder in which large quantities of food are eaten at one time (binge eating) and then purged from the body by vomiting, use of laxatives, or other means.

calcitriol (kal-sih-TRIH-ol) The active hormone form of vitamin D (1,25-dihydroxy-vitamin D). It contains a derivative of cholesterol as p.art of its structure.

cancer A condition characterized by uncontrolled growth of abnormal body cells.

cancer initiation The step in the process of cancer development that begins with alterations in DNA, the genetic material in a cell. This may cause the cell to no longer respond to normal physiological controls.

cancer progression The final stage in the cancer process in which the cancer cell grows to a sufficient mass so it will significantly affect body metabolism.

cancer promotion The step in the cancer process when cell division increases, in turn decreasing the time available for repair enzymes to act on altered DNA, and encouraging cells with altered DNA to develop and grow. Anything that increases the rate of cell division decreases the chance that the repair enzymes will find the altered part of the DNA in time to do their work.

capillary bed Minute vessels one cell thick that create a junction between arterial and venous circulation. It is here where gas and nutrient exchange occurs between body cells and the bloodstream.

carbohydrate (kar-bow-HIGH-drate) A compound containing carbon, hydrogen, and oxygen atoms; most are known as *sugars, starches,* and *dietary fibers.*

carbohydrate-loading A process in which a very high carbohydrate intake is consumed for 3 days before an athletic event while tapering exercise duration in an attempt to increase muscle glycogen stores.

carcinogens Compounds that have potential to cause cancer.

cardiac output (CARD-ee-ack) The amount of blood pumped by the heart.

cardiovascular Pertaining to the heart and blood vessels.

cariogenic (CARE-ee-oh-jen-ik) Literally "caries producing"; a substance, often carbohydrate-rich (such as caramel), that promotes dental caries.

carnitine (CAR-nih-teen) A compound used to shuttle fatty acids from the interior fluid of the cell into mitochondria.

carotenoids (kah-ROT-en-oyds) Plant pigments, some of which can yield vitamin A. Of the 600 or so carotenoids found in nature, about 50 yield vitamin A activity and thus are called provitamin A. Many have antioxidant properties as well. One example is beta-carotene.

carpal tunnel syndrome (CAR-pull) (SIN-drom) A disease in which nerves that travel to the wrist are pinched as they pass through a narrow opening in a bone in the wrist.

casein (KAY-seen) Protein found in milk that forms curds when exposed to acid and is difficult for infants to digest.

cash crop A crop grown by a country specifically for export, in order to gain the ability to purchase goods from other countries. Cultivation of cash crops diverts needed agricultural resources from production of crops needed to feed a country's own citizens. Examples are coffee, tea, cocoa, and bananas.

catabolic/catabolism (cat-ah-BOL-ik) Breaking down compounds.

catalyst (CAT-ul-ist) A compound that speeds reaction rates but is not altered by the reaction.

celiac disease (sea-lee-ak) Also known as *gluten-induced enteropathy.* It is caused by an allergy to protein found in wheat, rye, oats, and barley. If untreated, it causes severe flattening of the villi in the intestine, leading to severe malabsorption of nutrients.

cell A minute structure; the living basis of plant and animal organization. In animals it is bounded by a cell membrane. Cells contain both genetic material and systems for synthesizing energy-yielding compounds. Cells have the ability to take up compounds from and excrete compounds into their surroundings.

cellulose (SELL-you-los) A straight-chain polysaccharide of glucose mol-ecules that is undigestible; part of insol-uble fiber.

Celsius A centigrade measure of temperature. For conversion: (degrees in Fahrenheit − 32) × 5/9 = C°; (degrees in Celsius × 9/5) + 32 = F°.

cerebrovascular accident (CVA) (se-REE-bro-VAS-cue-lar) Death of part of the brain tissue due to a blood clot.

ceruloplasmin (se-RUE-low-PLAS-min) A blue, copper-containing protein component in the blood that can remove an electron from Fe^{2+} (the ferrous form) to yield Fe^{3+} (the ferric form). The Fe^{3+} form of iron can then bind with transport and storage proteins, such as transferrin.

chain-breaking Breaking the link between two or more actions that encourage problem behavior, such as snacking while watching television.

chelates (key-lates) Complexes formed between metal ions and substances with charged groups, such as proteins. The charged groups on the substance form two or more attachments with the metal ions, forming a ring structure. The metal ion is then firmly attached.

chemical reaction An interaction between two chemicals that changes both participants.

cholecystokinin (CCK) (ko-la-sis-toe-KY-nin) A hormone that stimulates enzyme release from the pancreas and bile release from the gallbladder.

cholesterol (ko-LES-te-rol) A waxy lipid; it has a structure containing multiple chemical rings (steroid structure).

chronic (KRON-ik) Long-standing, developing over time; slow to develop or resolve. When referring to disease, this indicates that the disease progress, once developed, is slow and tends to remain; a good example is heart disease.

chylomicrons (kye-lo-MY-krons) Lipoprotein made of dietary fat surrounded by a shell of cholesterol, phospholipids, and protein. These are made in the intestine after fat absorption and travel through the lymphatic system to the bloodstream.

chyme (KIME) A mixture of stomach secretions and partially digested food.

cirrhosis (see-ROH-sis) A loss of functioning liver cells, which are replaced by nonfunctioning connective tissue. Any substance that poisons liver cells can lead to cirrhosis. The most common cause is a chronic, excessive alcohol intake.

cis isomer (sis EYE-so-mer) An isomer form seen in compounds with double bonds, such as fatty acids, in which the hydrogens on both ends of the double bond lie on the same side of the plane of that bond.

citric acid cycle A pathway that breaks down acetyl-CoA, yielding carbon dioxide, $FADH_2$, NADH, and GTP. The pathway can also be used to synthesize compounds.

clinical Evidence of health or disease seen on physical examination.

clinical symptoms Generally, a change in health status noted by the individual (such as stomach pain) or noticed by a clinician during physical examination (the latter is technically called a clinical sign).

Clostridium botulinum (klo-STRID-ee-um BOT-you-LY-num) A bacterium that can cause a fatal type of food-borne illness.

coenzyme The active form of many vitamins; the coenzyme aids enzyme function.

cognitive restructuring Changing negative, self-defeating, or pessimistic thoughts that undermine weight control efforts to those that are positive, optimistic, and supportive of weight control. For one example, instead of using a difficult day as an excuse to overeat, substituting other pleasures for rewards, such as a relaxing walk with a friend could be done.

colic (KOL-ik) Periodic, inconsolable crying in a healthy young infant associated with sharp abdominal pain.

colostrum (ko-LAHS-trum) The first fluid secreted by the breast during late pregnancy and the first few days after birth. This thick fluid is rich in immune factors and protein.

complementarity of proteins Two food protein sources that make up for each other's insufficient contribution of specific essential amino acids, so that together they yield a high-quality (complete) protein diet.

complete proteins Proteins that contain ample amounts of all nine essential amino acids.

compound A group of different types of atoms bonded together in definite proportion (see molecule). Not all chemical compounds exist as molecules. Some compounds are made up of ions attracted to each other, such as Na^+Cl^- (table salt).

conceptus That produced as a result of conception; embryo.

conditioning The process through which an originally neutral stimulus repeatedly paired with a reinforcing agent elicits a predictable response.

congenital (con-JEN-i-tal) A term that means "present at birth." Thus a congenital abnormality is a defect that has been present since birth. These defects may be inherited from the parents, may occur as a result of damage or infection while in the uterus, or may occur at the time of birth.

conjugase (KON-ju-gase) Enzyme systems in the intestine that enhance folate absorption; they remove glutamate molecules from polyglutamate forms of folate.

connective tissue Protein tissue that holds different structures in the body together. Some structures are made up of connective tissue, notably tendons and cartilages. Connective tissue also forms part of bone and the nonmuscular structures of arteries and veins.

constipation A condition in which bowel movements are infrequent.

contingency management Forming a plan of action for responding to an environment in which overeating is likely, such as when snacks are within easy reach at a party.

control group Participants in an experiment whose habits or actions are not altered.

cortical bone (KORT-ih-kal) Dense, compact bone that comprises the outer surface and shafts of bone.

corticosteroid A steroid produced by the adrenal gland, an example of which is cortisol.

cortisol (KORT-ih-sol) A hormone made by the adrenal gland that, among other functions, stimulates the production of glucose from amino acids.

covalent bond (ko-VAY-lent) A union of two atoms formed by the sharing of electrons.

cretinism (KREET-in-ism) Stunting of body growth and poor mental development in the offspring that results from inadequate maternal intake of iodide during pregnancy.

Crohn's disease (Krown) A disease of unknown cause in which the small intestine becomes severely inflamed and its absorptive capacity limited.

crude fiber What remains of dietary fiber after extended acid and alkaline treatment. This consists primarily of cellulose and lignins.

cystic fibrosis (SIS-tik figh-BRO-sis) A disease that often leads to overproduction of mucus. Mucus can invade the pancreas, decreasing enzyme output. The lack of lipase enzyme then contributes to severe fat malabsorption.

cytochrome (SITE-o-krome) Electron-transfer agent that participates in the electron transport chain.

cytotoxic test (SITE-o-TOX-ik) An unreliable test to define food allergies that involves mixing whole blood with food proteins.

Daily Reference Values (DRV) Standards of intake for certain components of a diet (such as carbohydrate, fat, saturated fat, cholesterol, sodium, potassium, and dietary fiber) set by FDA for which no RDAs exist. These values are intended to be used for comparing intakes of these factors to desirable (or maximum) intakes. DRVs help consumers evaluate individual food choices and determine how they fit into a total diet as they form part of the Daily Values. The DRVs for cholesterol, sodium, and potassium are constant; those for other nutrients increase as energy intake increases. The DRVs constitute part of the Daily Values used in food labeling.

Daily Values A set of standard nutrient-intake values developed by the FDA and used as a reference for expressing nutrient content on nutrition labels. The

Daily Values include two types of standards—RDIs and DRVs.

dark adaptation A process by which the rhodopsin concentration in the eye increases in dark conditions, allowing improved vision in the dark.

deamination (dee-am-ih-NA-shun) The removal of an amino group from an amino acid.

Delaney Clause A clause to the 1958 Food Additives Amendment of the Pure Food and Drug Act in the United States that prevents the intentional (direct) addition to foods of a compound that has been shown to cause cancer in laboratory animals or man.

dementia (de-MEN-sha) General persistent loss or decrease in mental function.

denature (dee-NAY-ture) Alteration of the three dimensional structure of a protein, usually as a result of treatment by heat, acid, base, or agitation.

dental caries (KARE-ees) Erosions in the surface of a tooth caused by acids made by bacteria as they metabolize sugars.

deoxyribonucleic acid (DNA) The site of hereditary information in cells; DNA directs the synthesis of cell proteins.

dermatitis Inflammation of the skin.

dextrin Partial breakdown product of starch that contains few to many glucose molecules. These appear when starch is being digested into many units of maltose by salivary and pancreatic amylase.

diabetes (DYE-uh-BEET-eez) A disease characterized by high blood glucose (hyperglycemia), resulting from insufficient insulin action in the body (see **insulin-dependent diabetes** and **noninsulin-dependent diabetes**). Although this disease is commonly referred to as "diabetes," its technical name is *diabetes mellitus*.

diastolic blood pressure (dye-ah-STOL-ik) The pressure in the arterial blood vessels when the heart is between beats.

dietary fiber Substances in food (essentially from plants) that are not digested by the processes that take place in the stomach or small intestine. These add bulk to feces.

Dietary Goals Specific goals for nutrient intakes set in 1977 by a committee of the U.S. Senate.

Dietary Guidelines General goals for nutrient intake and diet composition set by government agencies—USDA and DHHS.

dietitian See **Registered Dietitian.**

digestibility (dye-JES-tih-bil-it-ee) The proportion of food substances eaten that can be broken down in the intestinal tract for absorption into the bloodstream.

digestion The process by which large ingested molecules are mechanically and chemically broken down to produce smaller forms that can be absorbed across the wall of the GI tract.

direct calorimetry (kal-oh-RIM-eh-tree) A method to determine energy use by the body by measuring heat that emanates from the body, usually using an insulated chamber.

disaccharides (dye-SACK-uh-rides) Class of sugars formed by the chemically linking of two monosaccharides.

diuretic (dye-u-RET-ik) A substance that, when ingested, increases the flow of urine.

diverticula (DYE-ver-TIK-you-luh) Pouches that protrude through the wall of the large intestine to the outside of the intestine.

diverticulitis (DYE-ver-tik-you-LITE-us) An inflammation of the diverticula caused by acids produced by bacterial metabolism inside the diverticula.

diverticulosis (DYE-ver-tik-you-LOH-sis) The condition of having many diverticula in the large intestine.

docosahexaenoic acid (DHA) (DOE-co-sa-hex-a-ee-no-ik) An omega-3 fatty acid with 22 carbons and six carbon-carbon double bonds. DHA is present in fish oils and is also synthesized from alpha-linolenic acid.

double-blind study An experiment in which the subjects and researchers are unaware of the subject's assignment (test or placebo) or the outcome of the study until it is completed. An independent third party holds the code and the data until the study is completed.

duodenum (doo-oh-DEE-num, or doo-ODD-num) The first 12 inches (30 centimeters) of the small intestine.

ecosystem A "community" in nature that includes plants and animals and the environment associated with them.

ectomorph (EK-tuh-morf) A body type associated with very long, thin bones and very long, thin fingers.

edema (uh-DEE-muh) The build-up of excess fluid in extracellular spaces.

eicosanoids (eye-KOH-san-oyds) Hormonelike compounds synthesized from polyunsaturated fatty acids. Within this class of compounds are prostaglandins, thromboxanes, and leukotrienes.

eicosapentaenoic acid (EPA) (eye-KOH-sah-pen-tah-ee-NO-ik) An omega-3 fatty acid with 20 carbon atoms and five double bonds; present in fish oils and is synthesized from alpha-linolenic acid.

electrolytes (ih-LEK-tro-lites) Substances that break down into ions in water and, in turn, are able to conduct an electrical current. These include sodium, chloride, and potassium.

electron A part of an atom that is negatively charged. Electrons orbit the nucleus.

electron transport chain A series of reactions using oxygen that help convert food energy into water and ATP energy.

elements Substances that cannot be broken down further by using ordinary chemical procedures.

elimination diet A restrictive diet that systematically tests foods that may cause an allergic response by first eliminating them for 1 to 2 weeks and then adding them back, one at a time.

embryo (EM-bree-oh) In humans, the developing human life form from about the third to eighth week after conception.

emulsifier (ee-MULL-sih-fire) A compound that can suspend fat in water by isolating individual fat drops using a shell of water molecules or other substances to prevent the fat from coalescing.

endocrine-onset obesity (EN-doh-krin) Obesity caused by rare hormonal abnormalities or rare genetic disorders. This is the cause of less than 10% of obesity cases in America.

endocytosis (phagocytosis/pinocytosis) Forms of active absorption in which the absorptive cell forms an indentation in its membrane and particles (phagocytosis) or fluids (pinocytosis) entering the indentation are then engulfed by the cell.

endometrium (en-doh-ME-tree-um) The membrane that lines the inside of the uterus. It increases in thickness during the menstrual cycle until ovulation occurs. The surface layers are shed during menstruation if conception does not take place.

endomorph (EN-doh-morf) A body type characterized by short, stubby bones, a short trunk, and short fingers.

endorphins (en-DOR-fins) Natural body tranquilizers that may be involved in the feeding response and function in pain reduction.

energy balance A state in which the energy intake, in the form of food or alcohol, matches the energy expended, primarily through basal metabolism and physical activity.

enriched A term generally meaning that the vitamins thiamin, niacin, and riboflavin and the mineral iron have been added to a grain product to improve nutritional quality.

enterohepatic circulation (EN-ter-oh-heh-PAT-ik) Recycling of compounds between the small intestine and the liver over and over again, as happens with bile acids.

enzyme (EN-zime) A compound that speeds the rate of a chemical process but is not altered by the chemical process. Almost all enzymes are proteins.

epidemiology (ep-uh-dee-me-OLL-uh-gee) The study of how disease patterns vary between different population groups, such as the cases of stomach cancer in Japan compared with that in Germany.

epigenetic carcinogens (promotors) (ep-ih-je-NET-ik car-SIN-oh-jens) Compounds that increase cell division and thereby increase the chance that a cell with altered DNA will develop into cancer.

epinephrine (ep-ih-NEF-rin) Also known as *adrenaline*. This hormone is released by the adrenal gland. A related form, norepinephrine, is released from various nerve endings in the body. Both hormones act to increase glycogen breakdown in the liver, among other functions.

epithelial cells (ep-ih-THEE-lee-ul) The surface cells that line the outside of the body and all external passages within it.

equilibrium (ee-kwih-LIB-ree-um) In nutrition, a state in which nutrient intake equals nutrient losses. Thus the body maintains a stable condition.

ergogenic (ur-go-JEN-ic) Work producing. An ergogenic acid is a physical, mechanical, nutritional, psychological, or pharmacological substance or treatment that is intended to directly improve exercise performance.

erythrocyte Mature red blood cell. This has no nucleus, and a lifespan of about 120 days; contains hemoglobin, which trans-ports oxygen and carbon dioxide.

erythropoietin (eh-REE-throw-POY-eh-tin) A hormone secreted mostly by the kidneys that enhances red blood cell synthesis and stimulates red blood cell release from bone marrow.

essential (indispensable) amino acids Amino acids not synthesized efficiently by humans. They therefore must be included in the diet. There are nine essential amino acids.

essential fatty acids Fatty acids that must be present in the diet to maintain health. These are linoleic acid and alpha-linolenic acid.

essential nutrient In nutritional terms, this represents a substance that, when left out of a diet, leads to signs of poor health. The body either can't produce these nutrients or can't produce them fast enough to meet its needs. Then, if added back to a diet before permanent damage occurs, the affected aspects of health are restored.

esterification (e-ster-ih-fih-KAY-shun) With regard to fats, the process of attaching fatty acids to a glycerol molecule, creating an ester bond and releasing water. Removing a fatty acid is called deesterification; reattaching a fatty acid is called reesterification.

estimated safe and adequate daily dietary intake (ESADDI) Nutrient intake recommendations made by the Food and Nutrition Board where a range for intake for some nutrients is given, because not enough information is available to set a more specific RDA.

eustachian tubes (you-STAY-shun) Thin tubes connected to the middle ear that open into the throat.

exchange The serving size of a food on a specific exchange list.

Exchange System A system for classifying foods into numerous lists based on their macronutrient composition and establishing serving sizes so that one serving of each food on a list contains the same amount of carbohydrate, protein, fat, and energy content.

experiment A test made to examine the validity of a hypothesis.

extracellular fluid Fluid present outside the cells; this includes intravascular and interstitial fluids.

extracellular space The space between cells.

facilitated absorption Absorption where a carrier is used to shuttle substances into the absorptive cells, but no energy input is needed. A concentration gradient higher in the intestinal contents than in the absorptive cell drives the absorption.

failure to thrive Inadequate gains in height and weight in infancy, often due to an inadequate food intake.

famine An extreme shortage of food that leads to massive starvation; often associated with crop failures, war, and political strife.

fasting hypoglycemia (HIGH-po-gligh-SEE-me-ah) Low blood glucose that follows about a day or so of fasting; generally caused by pancreatic cancer.

fat-soluble vitamins Vitamins that dissolve in such substances as ether and benzene, but not readily in water. These vitamins are A, D, E, and K.

fatty acids Acids found in lipids, composed of carbon atoms flanked by hydrogen atoms with an acid group

$$-\overset{\displaystyle O}{\overset{\|}{C}}-OH$$

$(-C-OH)$ at one end and a methyl group $(-CH_3)$ at the other.

feces (FEE-seas) Substances discharged from the bowel during defecation, consisting of the undigested residue of food, dead GI tract cells, mucus, bacteria, and other waste material. Another term for feces is *stool*.

feeding center A group of cells in the hypothalamus that, when stimulated, causes hunger.

female athlete triad A condition characterized by disordered eating, lack of menstrual periods, and low age-adjusted bone density.

fermentation The conversion, without use of oxygen, of carbohydrates to alcohols, acids, and carbon dioxide.

ferritin (FERR-ih-tin) A protein compound that serves as the storage form of iron in the blood and tissues.

fetal alcohol syndrome (FAS) (FEET-al) A group of physical and mental abnormalities in the infant that result from the mother consuming alcohol during pregnancy.

fetus (FEET-us) The developing life form from 8 weeks after conception until birth.

fluoroapatite (fleur-oh-APP-uh-tite) A tooth crystal containing fluoride ions. Presence of this crystal makes the tooth relatively acid resistant.

food-borne illness Sickness caused by ingestion of foods containing toxic substances produced by microorganisms.

food diary A written record of sequential food intake for a period of time. Details associated with the food intake are often recorded as well.

food intolerance An adverse reaction to food that does not involve an allergic reaction.

food sensitivity A mild reaction to a substance in a food that might be expressed as slight itching or redness of the skin.

fore milk The first breast milk delivered in the nursing session.

fortified A term generally meaning that vitamins, minerals, or both have been added to a food product in excess of what was originally found in the product.

fraternal twins Offspring that develop from two separate ova and sperm and therefore have separate genetic identities, although they develop simultaneously in the mother.

free radical Short-lived form of compounds that exist with an unpaired electron in the outer electron shell. This causes an electron-seeking nature, which can be very destructive to electron-dense areas of a cell, such as DNA and cell membranes.

free water The water not bound to the compounds in a food. This is available for microbial use.

fructose (FROOK-tose) A monosaccharide with six carbons that form a five-membered or six-membered ring with oxygen in the ring; found in fruits and honey.

fruitarian (froot-AIR-een-un) A person who eats primarily fruits, nuts, honey, and vegetable oils.

fungi Simple parasitic life forms including molds, mildews, yeasts, and mushrooms. They live on dead or decaying organic matter. Fungi can grow as single cells, like yeast, or as multicellular colonies, as seen with molds.

galactosemia (gah-LAK-toh-SEE-mee-ah) A rare, genetic disease characterized by the buildup of the single sugar galactose in the bloodstream resulting from the inability of the liver to metabolize it. If present at birth and left untreated, this disease causes severe mental and growth retardation in the infant.

gastric inhibitory peptide (GIP) (GAS-trik in-HIB-ih-tor-ee PEP-tide) A hormone that slows gastric motility and stimulates insulin release from the pancreas.

gastrin (GAS-trin) A hormone that stimulates enzyme and acid secretion in the stomach.

gastrointestinal (GI) tract The main sites in the body used for digestion and absorption of nutrients. It consists of the mouth, esophagus, stomach, small intestine, large intestine, rectum, and anus.

gastroplasty (GAS-troh-plas-tee) Surgery performed on the stomach to limit its volume to approximately 50 milliliters, the size of a shot glass.

gene (JEAN) The genetic material on chromosomes that makes up DNA. Genes provide the blueprint for the production of cell proteins.

generally recognized as safe (GRAS) A list of food additives that in 1958 were considered safe for consumption. Manufacturers were allowed to continue to use these additives, without special clearance, when needed for food products. FDA bears responsibility for proving they are not safe, but can remove unsafe products from the list.

genetic engineering Alteration of genetic material in plants or animals with the intent of improving growth, disease resistance, or other characteristics.

genotoxic carcinogen (initiator) (JEH-no-TOK-sik car-SIN-oh-jen) A compound that alters DNA in a cell, providing the potential for cancer to develop.

geometric progression A large group of numbers in which the division of each number by its immediate predecessor yields the same answer (e.g., 3, 9, 27, 81).

gestation (jes-TAY-shun) The period of the development of the offspring from conception to birth; this lasts about 40 weeks after the woman's last menstrual period.

gestational diabetes (jes-TAY-shun-al) Elevated blood glucose that develops during pregnancy but returns to normal after birth; one cause is placental production of hormones that antagonize blood glucose regulation.

glucagon (GLOO-kuh-gon) A hormone made by the pancreas that stimulates the breakdown of glycogen in the liver into glucose; this raises blood glucose. Glucagon also performs other functions.

gluconeogenesis (gloo-ko-nee-oh-JEN-uh-sis) The production of new glucose molecules by metabolic pathways in the cell. The source of the carbon atoms for these new glucose molecules is usually amino acids.

glucose (GLOO-kos) A six-carbon atom carbohydrate found in blood and in table sugar bound to fructose; also known as *dextrose,* it is one of the simple sugars.

glucose polymer A carbohydrate source used in some sports drinks that consists of a few glucose molecules bonded together.

glutathione peroxidase (gloo-tah-THIGH-own per-OX-ih-dase) A selenium-containing enzyme that can break down peroxides. It acts in conjunction with vitamin E to reduce free-radical damage to cells.

glycemic index (gligh-SEE-mik) A ratio used to measure the relative ability of a carbohydrate to raise blood glucose compared with the ability of white bread (or glucose) to raise blood glucose.

glycerol (GLISS-er-ol) A three-carbon alcohol containing three hydroxyl groups (—OH); used to help form the "backbone" of triglycerides.

glycocalyx (gly-co-KAY-licks) Hair-like projections that cover the microvilli of the absorptive cells.

glycogen (GLIGH-ko-jen) A carbohydrate made of multiple units of glucose; exhibits a highly branched structure; the storage form of carbohydrate for muscle and liver; sometimes known as *animal starch.*

glycolysis (gligh-COLL-ih-sis) The pathway that results in the breakdown of glucose into two three-carbon compounds.

glycosidic bond (gligh-coh-SID-ik) The bond present between two monosaccharides.

glycosylation The process by which glucose attaches to other compounds, such as proteins.

goiter (GOY-ter) An enlargement of the thyroid gland; this is often caused by insufficient iodide in the diet.

goitrogen (GOY-troh-jen) Substances in food that interfere with iodide absorption and metabolism, and so may cause goiter if consumed in large amounts.

gram Measure of weight in the metric system. One gram equals 1/28 of an ounce.

green revolution Increases in crop yields due to introduction of new agricultural technologies in less developed countries beginning in the 1960s. The key technologies were high-yielding, disease-resistant strains of rice, wheat, and corn; greater use of fertilizer; and improved cultivation practices.

growth hormone A pituitary hormone that causes body growth and the release of fat from storage, among other effects.

gum A dietary fiber containing chains of galactose, glucuronic acid, and other mono-saccharides; characteristically found in exudates from plant stems.

gynecoid obesity (GIGH-nih-coyd) Obesity in which fat storage is located primarily in the buttocks and thigh area.

H2 blockers Medications, such as cimetidine (Tagamet), that block the stimulation of stomach acid production caused by histamine.

Harris-Benedict equation An equation that predicts resting metabolic rate based on a person's weight, height, and age.

health fraud FDA defines health fraud as the promotion, advertisement, distribution, or sale of articles, intended for human or animal use, that are represented as being effective to diagnose, prevent, cure, treat, or mitigate disease (or other conditions), or provide a beneficial effect on health, but which have not been scientifically proven safe and effective for such purposes. Such practices may be deliberately deceptive, or done without adequate knowledge or understanding of the article.

heartburn A pain emanating from the esophagus, caused by stomach acid backing up into the esophagus and irritating the esophageal tissue.

heart attack Rapid fall in heart function caused by reduced blood flow through the heart's blood vessels. Often part of the heart dies in the process.

heart disease A disease usually caused by the deposition of fatty material in the blood vessels in the heart. This in turn reduces blood flow to the heart, thereby reducing heart function, which in turn can lead to death.

heat exhaustion Heat illness that occurs when heat stress causes depletion of blood volume from fluid loss by the body. This increases body temperature and can lead to headache, dizziness, muscle weakness, and visual disturbances, among other effects.

heat cramps Heat cramps are a frequent complication of heat exhaustion. They usually occur in individuals exercising for several hours in a hot climate who have experienced large sweat losses and have consumed a large volume of unsalted water. The cramps occur in skeletal muscles and consist of contractions for one to three minutes at a time.

heatstroke Heatstroke can occur when internal body temperature reaches 105° F. Sweating generally ceases if left untreated, blood circulation is greatly reduced. Nervous system damage may ensue and death is likely. Oftentimes individuals who suffer heatstroke, and their skin is hot and dry.

heat-labile (LAY-bile) A structure or activity that is changed by heating.

hematocrit (hee-MAT-oh-krit) The percentage of total blood volume made up of red blood cells.

heme iron (HEEM) Iron provided from animal tissues as hemoglobin and myoglobin. Approximately 40% of the iron in meat is heme iron; it is readily absorbed.

hemicellulose (hem-ih-SELL-you-los) A dietary fiber containing xylose, galactose, glucose, and other mono-saccharides bonded together.

hemochromatosis (heem-oh-krom-ah-TOE-sis) A disorder of iron metabolism characterized by increased iron absorption and deposition in the liver and heart tissue. This eventually poisons the cells in those organs.

hemoglobin (HEEM-oh-glow-bin) The iron-containing part of the red blood cell that carries oxygen to the cells and some carbon dioxide away from the cells. It is also responsible for the red color of blood.

hemolysis (hee-MOL-ih-sis) Destruction of red blood cells caused by the breakdown of the red blood cell membranes. This allows the cell contents to leak into the fluid portion of the blood.

hemorrhoid (HEM-or-oyd) A pronounced swelling in a large vein, particularly veins found in the anal region.

hemosiderin (heem-oh-SID-er-in) An insoluble iron-protein compound found in the liver. Hemosiderin stores iron when the amount of iron in the body exceeds the storage capacity of ferritin.

herbicide (ERB-ih-side) A compound that reduces the growth and reproduction of plants.

hexose (HEK-sos) A general term describing a carbohydrate containing six carbon atoms.

high-density lipoprotein (HDL) The lipoprotein synthesized primarily by the liver and intestine that picks up cholesterol from dying cells and other sources and transfers it to the other lipoproteins in the bloodstream, as well as directly to the liver. A low blood HDL value increases the risk for heart disease.

high-fructose corn syrup A corn syrup that has been manufactured to contain between 40% and 90% fructose.

high-quality (complete) proteins Dietary proteins that contain ample amounts of all nine essential amino acids.

hind milk (HYND) The milk secreted at the end of a nursing session; it is higher in fat than fore milk.

histamine (HISS-tuh-meen) A breakdown product of the amino acid histidine that stimulates acid secretion by the stomach and has other effects on the body, such as contraction of smooth muscles, increased nasal secretions, relaxation of blood vessels, and changes in relaxation of airways. It appears to decrease hunger and food intake.

homeostasis A series of adjustments that act to prevent change in the internal environment in the body.

hormone A compound secreted into the bloodstream that acts to control the function of distant target organ cells. Hormones can be either proteinlike or fatlike, such as insulin or estrogen.

hospice (HAHS-pis) A facility offering care that emphasizes comfort and dignity in death.

hunger The primary physiological drive to find and eat food, mostly regulated by internal cues to eating.

hydrogenation (high-dro-jen-AY-shun) The addition of hydrogen atoms to the double bonds of polyunsaturated and monounsaturated fatty acids to reduce the extent of unsaturation. This process turns liquid vegetable oils into solid fats and is used to make margarine and shortening. *Trans* fatty acids are a by-product of this process.

hydroxyapatite (high-drox-ee-APP-uh-tite) A compound, composed primarily of calcium and phosphate, that is deposited into the bone protein matrix to give bone strength and rigidity $(Ca_{10}[PO_4]_6OH_2)$.

hyperactivity A poorly defined term generally used to label inattention, irritability, and excessively active behavior in children.

hypercalcemia (high-per-kal-SEE-mee-ah) A high concentration of calcium in the bloodstream. This can lead to loss of appetite, calcium deposits in organs, and other health problems.

hypercarotenemia (high-per-car-oh-teh-NEEM-ee-ah) High concentration of carotene in the bloodstream, usually caused by a diet high in carrots or other yellow-orange vegetables.

hyperglycemia (HIGH-per-gligh-SEE-me-uh) High blood glucose, above 140 milligrams per 100 milliliters of blood.

hypergymnasia Exercising beyond the amount required for good physical fitness or maximum performance in a sport; excessive exercise.

hyperplasia (high-per-PLAY-zee-uh) An increase in cell number.

hypertension (high-per-TEN-shun) A condition in which blood pressure remains persistently elevated, especially when the heart is between beats; also called high blood pressure.

hypertrophy (high-PURR-tro-fee) An increase in cell size.

hypoglycemia (HIGH-po-gligh-SEE-mee-uh) Low blood glucose, below 40 to 50 milligrams per 100 milliliters of blood.

hypothalamus (high-po-THALL-uh-mus) A region at the base of the brain that contains cells that play a role in the regulation of hunger, respiration, body temperature, and other body functions.

hypothesis (high-POTH-eh-sis) An "educated guess" by a scientist to explain a phenomenon.

hysterectomy Surgical removal of the uterus.

identical twins Two offspring that develop from a single ovum and sperm and, consequently, have the same genetic makeup.

ileum (ILL-ee-um) Essentially, the area consisting of the last half of the small intestine.

incidental food additives Additives that appear in food products indirectly, from environmental contamination of food ingredients or during the manufacturing process.

incomplete (lower-quality) protein Food protein that lacks ample amount of one or more of the essential amino acids needed to support human protein needs.

indirect calorimetry (kal-oh-RIM-eh-tree) A method to measure the energy use by the body by measuring oxygen uptake. Formulas are then used to convert this gas exchange value into energy use.

infectious disease (in-FEK-shus) Any disease caused by an invasion of the body by microorganisms, such as bacteria, fungi, or viruses.

infrastructure The basic framework of a system or organization. For society, this includes roads, bridges, telephones, and other basic technologies.

inorganic Anything that is free of carbon atoms bonded to hydrogen atoms in the chemical structure.

insensible losses Fluid losses that are not perceptible to the senses, such as losses through lungs, feces, and skin (an exception is heavy perspiration).

insoluble fibers (in-SOL-you-bul) Fibers that, for the most part, do not dissolve in water nor are digested by bacteria in the large intestine. These include cellulose, some hemicelluloses, and lignins.

insulin (IN-suh-lin) A hormone produced by the beta cells of the pancreas. Insulin increases the synthesis of glycogen in the liver and the movement of glucose from the bloodstream into body cells, especially muscle and adipose cells, among other processes.

insulin-dependent diabetes A form of diabetes prone to ketosis and that requires insulin therapy.

intentional food additives Additives knowingly (directly) incorporated into food products by manufacturers.

international unit (IU) A crude measure of vitamin activity, often based on the growth rate of animals. Today these units have been replaced by more precise milligram and microgram quantities.

interstitial fluid (in-ter-STISH-ul) Fluid between cells.

intracellular fluid Fluid contained within a cell.

intrauterine Within the uterus.

intravascular fluid Fluid within the blood-stream (that is, in the arteries, veins, and capillaries).

intravenous (in-tra-VEEN-us) Introduced directly into the bloodstream.

intrinsic factor A proteinlike compound produced by the stomach that enhances vitamin B-12 absorption.

in utero (in YOU-ter-oh) "In the uterus" or, during pregnancy.

ion An atom with an unequal number of electrons and protons. Negative ions have more electrons than protons; positive ions have more protons than electrons.

ionic bond (eye-ON-ik) A union between two atoms formed by an attraction of a positive ion to a negative ion, as seen in table salt (Na^+Cl^-).

irradiation (ir-RAY-dee-AY-shun) A process whereby radiation energy is applied to foods, creating compounds (free radicals) within the food that destroy cell membranes, break down DNA, link proteins together, limit enzyme activity, and alter a variety of other proteins and cell functions that would otherwise lead to food spoilage. This process does not make the food radioactive.

isomers (EYE-so-mers) Different chemical structures for compounds that share the same chemical formula.

isotope (EYE-so-towp) An alternate form of a chemical element. It differs from other atoms of the same element in the number of neutrons in its nucleus.

jaundice (JAWN-diss) A yellow staining of the skin and sclera (white of the eye) resulting from a buildup of bile pigments in the bloodstream. Liver or gallbladder disease is often the cause.

jejunem (je-JOON-um) The first half of the small intestine (minus the first 12 inches, which is the duodenum).

juvenile-onset obesity Obesity that develops in childhood; often characterized by an excess number of adipose cells that are also very large because of abundant fat storage.

ketogenic A name often given to diets that lead to the abundant production of ketones by the liver. This can be caused by a low carbohydrate intake.

ketone (KEE-tone) Incomplete breakdown product of fat containing three or four carbons. An example is acetoacetic acid.

ketosis (kee-TOE-sis) The condition of having a high concentration of ketones in the bloodstream.

kidney nephrons (NEF-rons) Unit of kidney cells that filter wastes from the bloodstream and deposits them in the urine.

kilocalorie (kill-oh-KAL-oh-ree) (kcal) The heat needed to raise the temperature of 1000 grams (1 liter) of water 1 degree Celsius.

kilojoule (KIL-oh-jool) (kJ) A measure of work in which 1 kJ equals the work needed to move 1 kilogram a distance of 1 meter with the force of 1 newton. One kcal equals 4.18 kJ.

kwashiorkor (kwash-ee-OR-core) A disease occurring primarily in young children who have an existing disease and who consume a marginal amount of energy and considerably insufficient protein in the face of high needs. The child suffers from infections and exhibits edema, poor growth, weakness, and an increased susceptibility to further illness.

lactic acid (LAK-tik) A three-carbon acid; also called *lactate,* formed during anaerobic cell metabolism; a partial breakdown product of glucose.

lactobacillus bifidus factor (lak-toe-bah-SIL-us BIFF-id-us) A protective factor secreted in the colostrum that encourages growth of beneficial bacteria in the newborn's intestines.

lacto-ovo vegetarian A person who consumes only plant products, dairy products, and eggs.

lacto-ovo-peso vegetarian A person who consumes only plant products, dairy products, eggs, and fish.

lactose (LAK-tose) A sugar made up of glucose linked to galactose.

lactose intolerance (primary and secondary) Primary lactose intolerance occurs when lactase production declines for no apparent reason. Secondary lactose intolerance occurs when a specific cause, like long-standing diarrhea, results in a decline in lactase production.

lactovegetarian (lak-toe-vej-eh-TEAR-ree-an) A person who consumes only plant products and dairy products.

lanugo (lah-NEW-go) Downlike hair that appears on a person who has lost much body fat during semistarvation. The hair stands erect and traps air, which acts as insulation to the body, replacing the insulation properties usually supplied by body fat. Fetuses also have lanugo.

larva (LAR-va) An early developmental stage in the life history of some microorganisms, such as parasites.

laxative A medication or other substance that stimulates evacuation of the intestinal tract.

lean body mass The part of the human body that is free of all but essential body fat. About 2% of body weight as fat is essential. The rest of the fat in the body represents storage and so is not part of lean body mass. Lean body mass includes brain, muscle, bone, organs, connective tissue, skin, and other body parts, including body fluids such as blood.

lecithin (LESS-uh-thin) Any of several phospholipids containing two fatty acids, a phosphate group, and a choline molecule.

leptin A protein made by adipose cells that in turn influences food intake by communicating the degree of fat stores in the person (or laboratory animal).

"let-down reflex" A reflex stimulated by infant suckling that causes the release (ejection) of milk from milk ducts in the mother's breast.

life expectancy The average length of life for a given group of people born in a certain year, such as this year.

life span The potential oldest age to which a person can reach.

lignin (LIG-nin) An insoluble fiber made up of a multiringed alcohol (non-carbohydrate) structure.

limiting amino acid The essential amino acid in the lowest concentration in a food in proportion to body needs.

linoleic acid (lin-oh-LEE-ik) An essential fatty acid with 18 carbon atoms and two carbon-carbon double bonds; omega-6.

lipase (LYE-pase) Fat-digesting enzyme; gastric lipase is produced by the stomach and pancreatic lipase by the pancreas.

lipid (LIP-id) A compound containing much carbon and hydrogen, little oxygen, and sometimes other atoms. Lipids dissolve in ether or benzene and include fats, oils, and cholesterol.

lipid peroxidation Production of unstable lipids containing more than the normal amount of oxygen. In the formation of a fatty acid of this type first a carbon-carbon double bond is broken. The resulting breakdown products react with oxygen to form peroxides

$$(-\overset{\displaystyle H}{\underset{\displaystyle H}{C}}-\overset{\displaystyle H}{\underset{\displaystyle H}{C}}-O-O-H)$$

$$(-\overset{\displaystyle H}{\underset{\displaystyle H}{C}}-\overset{\displaystyle H}{\underset{\displaystyle H}{C}}-O-\overset{\bullet}{O}).\text{or free radicals}$$

lipofuscin (ceroid pigments) (lip-oh-FEW-shun) (SER-oyd) Lipid breakdown products in cells. These compounds have fluorescence, and in that way can be detected in aged cells, such as those in the eye, the heart, and the brain.

lipogenesis (lye-poh-JEN-eh-sis) The building of fatty acids using derivatives of acetyl-CoA molecules.

lipogenic (lye-poh-JEN-ik) Means creating lipid. The liver is the major organ with lipogenic potential in the human body.

lipolysis (lye-POL-ih-sis) The breakdown of triglycerides to glycerol and fatty acids.

lipoprotein (lye-poh-PRO-teen) A compound found in the bloodstream containing a core of lipids with a shell of protein, phospholipid, and cholesterol.

lipoprotein lipase (lye-poh-PRO-teen LYE-pase) An enzyme attached to the outside of some cells that line the bloodstream; it breaks down triglycerides into free fatty acids and glycerol.

liter (LEE-ter) (L) A measure of volume in the metric system. One liter equals 0.96 quarts.

lobules (LOB-you-els) Saclike structures in the breast that store milk.

long-chain fatty acids Fatty acids that contain 12 or more carbon atoms.

low birth weight (LBW) Infant weight at birth of less than 2.5 kilograms (5.5 pounds); usually caused by preterm birth; these infants are at higher risk for health problems.

low-density lipoprotein (LDL) The product of the VLDL containing primarily cholesterol; elevated LDL is strongly linked to heart disease risk.

low input sustainable agriculture (LISA) A form of farming that attempts to limit use of purchased materials, such as manufactured fertilizers and pesticides. Use of manure and crop rotation are typical substitutes.

lower-body obesity The type of obesity, also called gynoid, in which fat storage is primarily located in the buttocks and thigh area.

lower-quality (incomplete) proteins Dietary proteins that are low in or lack an ample amount of one or more of the amino acids essential for human protein needs.

lumen (LOO-men) The inside cavity of a tube, such as the GI tract.

lymphatic system (lim-FAT-ick) System of vessels that can accept fluid surrounding cells and large particles, such as products of fat absorption. This lymph fluid eventually passes into the bloodstream via the lymphatic system.

lymphocyte A class of white blood cells involved in the immune system, generally composing about 25% of all white blood cells. There are several types of lymphocytes with diverse functions, including antibody production, allergic reactions, graft rejections, tumor control, and regulation of the immune system.

lysosome (LYE-so-som) A cellular organelle that contains digestive enzymes for use inside the cell for turnover of cell parts.

lysozyme (LYE-so-zime) A set of enzyme substances produced by a variety of cells in the body that can destroy bacteria by rupturing their cell membranes.

macrocyte (MAC-row-site) A greatly enlarged mature red blood cell; it has a short life span.

macrophage Any large mononuclear, phagocytic cell that is able to engulf and digest cellular debris and invading bacteria.

major mineral A mineral vital to health that is required in the diet in amounts greater than 100 milligrams per day.

malignant Essentially to do anything malicious. In reference to a tumor, the property of locally spreading and spreading to distant sites.

malnutrition Failing health that results from a long-standing dietary intake that is insufficient to meet, or greatly exceeds, nutritional needs

maltose (MAWL-tose) Glucose bonded to glucose; a simple sugar.

marasmus (mah-RAZ-mus) A disease that results from consuming a grossly insufficient amount of protein and energy; usually seen in infancy. It is the equivalent of protein-energy malnutrition in adults. The person with marasmus has little or no fat stores and shows muscle wasting. Death from infections is common.

marginal Noticeable, but not severe.

mass movement A peristaltic wave that simultaneously coordinates contraction over a large area of the colon. Mass movements move material from one portion of the colon to another and from the colon into the rectum.

mast cells Cells that contain histamine and are responsible for some aspects of allergic and inflammatory reactions.

maximum volume of oxygen consumption (Vo_{2max}) The maximum oxygen consumption a person can achieve during exercise, such as when riding a bicycle or running on a treadmill.

meconium (mee-KOH-nee-um) The first thick, mucuslike stool passed after birth.

medium-chain fatty acids Fatty acids that contain 8 to 10 carbon atoms.

megadose Intake of nutrient in excess of 10 times human needs.

megaloblast (MEG-ah-low-blast) A large, immature red blood cell that results from the particular cell's inability for cell division at the appropriate time during red blood cell development.

menaquinones (men-AH-kwih-nones) Forms of vitamin K that come from animal food sources or bacterial synthesis.

menarche (men-AR-kee) The onset of menstruation. Menarche usually occurs around age 13, 2 or 3 years after the first signs of puberty start to appear.

menopause (MEN-oh-paws) The cessation of menses in women, usually beginning at about 50 years of age.

mesomorph (MEZ-oh-morf) A body type associated with average bone size, trunk size, and finger length.

metabolism (meh-TAB-oh-lizm) Chemical processes that occur in the body, enabling cells to release energy from foods, convert one substance into another, and prepare end products for excretion. In sum the processes allow for life.

metallothionein (meh-TAL-oh-THIGH-oh-neen) A protein that binds and regulates the release of zinc and copper in intestinal and liver cells.

metastasis Spread of cancerous cells from their site of origin to other areas of the body.

meter A measure of length in the metric system. One meter equals 39.4 inches.

micelle (MY-sell) An emulsification product in which individual emulsifiers organize with their fat-attracting parts to the center of the micelle and their water-attracting parts to the outside. Lipids are attracted to the center area, and water is attracted to the outside periphery.

microcytic (my-kro-SIT-ik) Literally means "small cell." Microcytic red blood cells are smaller than normal.

microcytic hypochromic anemia An anemia exhibiting small, pale red blood cells lacking sufficient hemoglobin (often caused by an iron deficiency); these red blood cells have reduced oxygen-carrying ability.

microfractures Small fractures, undetectable by x-rays or other bone scans, that may develop constantly in bones.

microsomal ethanol oxidizing system (my-kro-SO-mol) An alternative pathway for alcohol metabolism when alcohol is in high concentration in the liver; uses rather than yields energy for the body, in comparison to alcohol dehydrogenase activity.

minerals The basic chemical elements used in the body to help form body structures and regulate body processes. Examples are calcium and iron.

miscarriage Termination of pregnancy that occurs before the fetus can survive; also called *spontaneous abortion*.

mitochondria The main sites of energy production in a cell. Mitochondria also contain the pathway for burning fat for fuel, among other metabolic pathways.

modified food starch Starch molecules that have been chemically linked together to increase stability.

molecule A group of atoms chemically linked together; that is, tightly connected by attractive forces (see **compound**).

monoglyceride (mon-oh-GLIS-er-ide) A breakdown product of a triglyceride consisting of one fatty acid bonded to a glycerol backbone.

monosaccharide (mon-oh-SACK-uh-ride) A class of simple sugars, such as glucose, that is not broken down further during digestion.

monounsaturated fatty acid A fatty acid containing one carbon-carbon double bond.

mortality This represents a population's death rate. The term *morbidity* refers to the amount of sickness present.

mottling (MOT-ling) Discoloration or marking of the surface of teeth from fluorosis.

mucilage (MYOU-sih-laj) A dietary fiber consisting of chains of galactose, mannose, and other monosaccharides; characteristically found in seaweed.

mucopolysaccharide (MYOO-ko-POL-ee-SAK-ah-ride) Substance containing protein and carbohydrate parts; found in bone and other organs.

mucosa (MYOO-co-saw) Mucous membrane consisting of cells and supporting connective tissue. In the digestive tract there is also a layer of smooth muscle supporting the mucosa. Mucosa lines cavities that open to the outside of the body such as the stomach and intestine and generally contains glands that secrete mucus.

mucus (MYOO-cuss) A thick fluid secreted by glands throughout the body. It contains a compound that has both carbohydrate and protein parts. It acts as a lubricant and means of protection for cells.

mutation A permanent change in a cell's DNA; includes changes in sequence, alteration of gene position, gene loss or duplication, and insertion of foreign gene sequences.

mycotoxin (MY-ko-tok-sin) A group of toxic compounds produced by molds, such as aflatoxin B-1 found on moldy grains.

myocardial infarction (MY-oh-CARD-ee-ahl in-FARK-shun) Death of part of the heart muscle.

myoglobin (my-oh-GLOW-bin) Iron-containing compound that binds oxygen (O_2) in muscle.

negative balance The state in which nutrient losses from the body exceed intake, as in cases of starvation.

negative energy balance The state in which the energy intake is less than the energy expended. The result of this is a decrease in body weight.

neural tube defect A defect in the formation of the neural tube occurring during early fetal development. These are seen in about 2500 infants per year in the United States. The defect results in various nervous system disorders, such as spina bifida. Folate deficiency in the pregnant woman increases the risk of the fetus developing this disorder.

neuromuscular junction The junction between nerve and muscle.

neurotransmitter A compound made by a nerve cell that allows for communication between it and other cells.

neutron (NEW-tron) The part of an atom that has no charge.

night blindness A vitamin A deficiency condition in which the retina in the eye cannot adjust to low amounts of light.

nitrate A nitrogen-containing compound used to cure meats. Its use contributes a pink color to meats and confers some resistance to bacterial growth.

nitrosamines A carcinogen formed from nitrates and breakdown products of amino acids; can lead to stomach cancer.

nonessential (dispensable) amino acids Amino acids that can be readily made by the body in sufficient amounts. There are 11 nonessential amino acids.

nonheme iron Iron provided from plant sources and animal tissues other than hemoglobin and myoglobin. Nonheme iron is less efficiently absorbed than heme iron, as absorption is also more closely dependent on body needs.

non-insulin-dependent diabetes A form of diabetes in which ketosis is not commonly seen. Insulin therapy can be used, but often is not required; often associated with obesity.

nonpolar A neutral compound; no positive or negative poles present.

no observable effect level (NOEL) This corresponds to the highest dose of an additive that produces no deleterious health effects in animals.

nuclear receptor A site on the DNA in a cell where compounds (such as hormones) bind. Cells that contain DNA receptors for a specific compound are affected by that compound.

nucleus (NEW-klee-us) In chemistry, the core of an atom; it contains protons and neutrons.

nutrient density The ratio formed by dividing a food's contribution to the needs for a nutrient by its contribution to energy needs. When the contribution to nutrient needs exceeds that to energy needs, the food is considered to have a favorable nutrient density for that nutrient.

nutrient receptor Proposed site in the small intestine that is a mechanism to elicit a feeling of satiety.

nutrients Chemical substances in food that nourish the body by providing energy, building materials, and factors to regulate needed chemical reactions in the body.

nutrition The Council on Food and Nutrition of the American Medical Association defines nutrition as "the science of food; the nutrients and the substances therein; their action, interaction, and balance in relation to health and disease; and the process by which the organism (i.e., body) ingests, digests, absorbs, transports, utilizes, and excretes food substances."

nutrition label A label containing "Nutrition Facts" that must be included on most foods. It depicts nutrient content in comparison to the Daily Values set by FDA.

nutritional status The nutritional health of a person as determined by **a**nthropometric measures (height, weight, circumferences, and so on), **b**iochemical measures of nutrients or their by-products in blood and urine, a **c**linical (physical) examination, and a **d**ietary analysis (ABCD).

nutritionist A person who advises about nutrition and/or works in the field of food and nutrition. In many states in the United States a person does not need formal training to use this title. Some states reserve this title for Registered Dietitians.

obesity (oh-BEES-ih-tee) A condition characterized by excess body fat, often defined as 20% above healthy weight or a body mass index above 27-30.

oleic acid A fatty acid with 18 carbons and one carbon-carbon double bond; omega-9.

olfactory cells Cells in the nasal region that discriminate numerous chemical molecules and transmit that information to the brain. This information represents one of the components of what we describe as flavor.

oligosaccharides (ol-ih-go-SAK-ah-rides) Carbohydrates containing three to ten monosaccharide units.

omega-3 (ω-3) fatty acid An unsaturated fatty acid with its first double bond at the third carbon atom from the methyl end ($—CH_3$).

omega-6 (ω-6) fatty acid An unsaturated fatty acid with its first double bond at the sixth carbon atom from the methyl end ($—CH_3$).

omnivore (AHM-nih-voor) A person who consumes foods from both plant and animal sources.

oncogene (AHN-ko-jeen) Gene that codes for a protein that in turn leads to cellular growth and development.

oncotic force (ahn-KAH-tik) The osmotic potential exerted by blood proteins in the bloodstream.

opportunistic infection An infection that arises primarily in people who are already ill because of another disease.

organ A group of tissues designed to perform a specific function; for example, the heart. It contains muscle tissue, nerve tissue, and so on.

organic Anything that contains carbon atoms bonded to hydrogen atoms in the chemical structure.

organism A living thing. The human body is an organism consisting of many organs that act in a coordinated manner to support life.

osmosis Passive diffusion of a solution (water) through a semipermeable membrane from a less concentrated solution to a more concentrated compartment.

osmotic pressure The exerted pressure needed to keep particles in a solution from drawing liquid across a semipermeable membrane.

osteomalacia (OS-tee-oh-mal-AY-shuh) Adult form of rickets. This results from a vitamin D deficiency disease, leading to weak bones and increased fracture risk.

osteopenia (os-tee-oh-PEE-nee-ah) Decreased bone mass caused by cancer, hyperthyroidism, or other reasons.

osteoporosis (os-tee-oh-po-ROH-sis) Decreased bone mass where no outward causes can be found. Related to effects of aging, poor diet, and hormonal effects of menopause in women.

overnutrition A state in which nutritional intake exceeds the body's needs.

ovum An egg; female germ cell released from the ovary at ovulation.

oxalic acid (or oxalate) An organic acid found in spinach, rhubarb, and other leafy green vegetables that can depress the absorption of certain minerals, such as calcium.

oxidation Loss of an electron by an atom or molecule. In metabolism, often associated with a gain of oxygen or loss of hydrogen. Oxidation (loss of an electron) and reduction (gain of an electron) take place simultaneously in metabolism, because an electron that is lost by one atom is accepted by another.

oxidize (OX-ih-dize) To lose an electron or gain an oxygen atom.

oxidizing agent In one sense, a substance capable of capturing an electron from another compound. A compound is "oxidized" when it loses an electron.

p53 gene Tumor suppressor gene; it can be subject to mutations.

palatable (PAL-it-ah-bull) Pleasing to taste.

parathyroid hormone (PTH) A hormone made by the parathyroid glands that increases synthesis of the vitamin D hormone and aids calcium release from bone and calcium uptake by the kidneys, among other functions.

passive absorption Absorption that uses no energy. It requires permeability for the substance through the wall of the small intestine and a concentration gradient higher in the lumen of the intestine than in the absorptive cell. The higher concentration of the substance in the lumen of the intestine in comparison with that in the absorptive cells promotes the absorption of the nutrient.

pasteurization (pas-tur-ih-ZAY-shun) The process of heating food products to kill pathogenic microorganisms. One method heats milk at 161°F for at least 20 seconds.

pathway A metabolic progression of individual steps from starting materials to ending products, like $C_6H_{12}O_6$ (glucose) + O_2 yielding CO_2 + H_2O.

pectin (PEK-tin) A dietary fiber containing chains of galacturonic acid and other monosaccharides; characteristically found between plant cell walls.

peer-reviewed journal A journal that publishes research only after two or three scientists who were not part of the study agree it was well conducted and the results are fairly represented. Thus the research has been approved by peers of the research team.

pellagra (peh-LAHG-rah) A disease characterized by inflammation of the skin, diarrhea, and eventual mental incapacity; results from an insufficient amount of the vitamin niacin in the diet.

pepsin (PEP-sin) A protein-digesting enzyme produced by the stomach.

peptide bond A chemical bond formed to link amino acids in a protein.

peptide A few amino acids chemically bonded together; often two to four.

peptone A partial breakdown product of proteins.

percentile Classification of a measurement of a unit into divisions of 100 units.

peristalsis (per-ih-STALL-sis) A coordinated muscular contraction that is used to propel food down the gastrointestinal tract.

pernicious anemia (per-NISH-us ah-NEE-mee-ah) The anemia that results from a lack of vitamin B-12 absorption. It is pernicious (deadly) because of the associated nerve degeneration that can result in eventual paralysis and death.

pesticide A general term for an agent that can destroy bacteria, fungi, insects, rodents, or other pests.

pH A measure of the hydrogen ion concentration in a solution.

phagocytosis/pinocytosis (FAG-oh-sigh-TOW-sis/PIN-oh-sigh-TOW-sis) A form of active absorption in which the absorptive cell forms an indentation, and particles or fluids entering the indentation are then engulfed by the cell.

phenylalanine An essential (indispensable) amino acid.

phenylketonuria (PKU) (fen-ihl-kee-toh-NEW-ree-ah) A disease caused by a defect in the ability of the liver to metabolize the amino acid phenylalanine into the amino acid tyrosine. Toxic by-products of phenylalanine can then build up in the body and lead to mental retardation.

phenylpropanolamine (fen-ihl-pro-pan-OL-ah-meen) An over-the-counter decongestant that has a mild appetite- reducing effect.

phosphocreatine (PCr) (fos-fo-CREE-a-tin) A high-energy compound that can be used to reform adenosine triphosphate (ATP) from adenosine diphosphate (ADP).

phospholipid Any of a class of fat-related substances that contain phosphorus, fatty acids, and a nitrogen-containing base. The phospholipids are an essential part of every cell.

photosynthesis (foto-sin-tha-sis) The process by which plants use solar energy from the sun to produce energy-yielding compounds, such as glucose.

phylloquinone (fil-oh-KWIN-own) A form of vitamin K that comes from plants.

physiological anemia The normal increase in blood volume in pregnancy that dilutes the concentration of red blood cells, resulting in anemia; also called *hemodilution*.

phytic acid (phytate) (FY-tick, FY-tate) A constituent of plant fibers that binds positive ions to its multiple phosphate groups.

phytobezoar (fy-tow-BEE-zor) A pellet of fiber characteristically found in the stomach.

phytochemical A chemical found in plants. Some phytochemicals may contribute to a reduced risk of cancer or heart disease in people who consume them regularly.

pica (PIE-kah) The practice of eating nonfood items such as dirt, laundry starch, or clay.

placebo (plah-SEE-bo) A fake medicine used to disguise the roles of participants in an experiment; if fake surgery is performed, that is called a *sham operation*.

placenta (plah-SEN-tah) An organ formed in a woman only during pregnancy that secretes hormones to maintain the pregnant state and makes possible the transfer of oxygen and nutrients from the mother's blood to the fetus, as well as removal of fetal wastes.

plaque (PLACK) In terms of heart disease, a cholesterol-rich substance deposited in the blood vessels. It also contains various white blood cells and smooth muscle cells, cholesterol and other lipids, and eventually calcium. Sometimes called *atherosclerotic plaque* to distinguish it from bacterial plaque, which forms on teeth.

polar A compound with distinct positive and negative charges (poles) on it. These charges act like poles on a magnet.

polyglutamate form of folate (POL-ee-GLOO-tah-mate) Folate with more than one glutamate molecule attached.

polypeptide (POL-ee-PEP-tide) Fifty to 100 amino acids bonded together.

polysaccharide (POL-ee-SACK-uh-ride) Carbohydrate containing many glucose units, up to 3000 or more; also known as complex carbohydrates.

polyunsaturated fatty acid A fatty acid containing two or more carbon-carbon double bonds.

pool The amount of a nutrient stored within the body that can be easily mobilized when needed.

portal vein A large vein that distributes blood from the intestine to the liver through capillaries.

positive balance A state in which nutrient intake exceeds losses. This causes a net gain of the nutrient in the body, such as when tissue protein is gained during growth.

positive energy balance State in which energy intake is greater than energy expended, generally resulting in weight gain.

precursor A compound that comes before; to precede.

pregnancy-induced hypertension A serious disorder that can include high blood pressure, kidney failure, convulsion, and even death of the mother and the fetus. Although the exact cause is not known, good nutrition, especially calcium intake, and prenatal care may prevent or limit its severity. Mild cases are known as *preeclampsia;* more severe cases are called *eclampsia* (formally called *toxemia*).

premenstrual syndrome A disorder (also referred to as *PMS*) found in some women a few days before the onset of menses and characterized by depression, headache, bloating, and mood swings. Severe cases are currently termed premenstrual dysphoric disorder (PDD).

preservatives Compounds that extend the shelf life of foods by inhibiting microbial growth or minimizing the destructive effect of oxygen and metals.

preterm An infant born before 38 weeks of gestation; also known as premature.

prevalence The number of people at any one time that have a specific disease, such as obesity or cancer.

primary disease A disease process that is not simply caused by another disease process.

primary structure of a protein The order of amino acids in the protein molecule.

progestins (pro-JES-tins) Hormones, including progesterone, that are necessary for maintaining pregnancy and lactation.

prognosis (prog-NO-sis) A forecast of the course and end of a disease.

prohormone Precursor of a hormone.

prolactin (pro-LACK-tin) A hormone secreted by the mother that stimulates the synthesis of milk.

prostacyclin (prost-tah-SIGH-klin) A prostaglandin made by the blood vessel walls that is a potent inhibitor of blood clotting.

prostaglandin (pros-tah-GLAN-din) One of several potent hormonelike compounds made of polyunsaturated fatty acids that produce diverse effects in the body.

prostate gland A solid, chestnut-shaped organ surrounding the first part of the urethra in the male. The prostate gland is situated immediately under the bladder and in front of the rectum. The prostate gland secretes substances into the semen as the fluid passes through ducts leading from the seminal vesicles into the urethra.

protein Food components made of amino acids; contain carbon, hydrogen, oxygen, nitrogen, and sometimes other atoms, in a specific configuration. Proteins contain the form of nitrogen most easily used by the human body.

protein-energy malnutrition (PEM) A condition resulting from regularly consuming insufficient amounts of energy and protein. The deficiency eventually results in body wasting and an increased susceptibility to infection.

prothrombin (pro-THROM-bin) One of the numerous blood proteins needed for blood clotting that requires vitamin K for its synthesis.

proton (PRO-ton) The part of an atom that is positively charged.

proto-oncogene (PRO-tow-AHN-ko-jeen) Growth-promoting gene found naturally in human cells.

psyllium (SIL-ee-um) A mostly soluble type of dietary fiber found in the seeds of the plantain plant.

quack A person who does not have the medical skills or knowledge that he or she claims to have.

radiation Literally, energy that is emitted from a center in all directions. Various forms of radiation energy include x-rays and ultraviolet rays from the sun.

rancid (RAN-sid) Containing products of decomposed fatty acids; these yield off-flavors and odors.

rationalization The process of mentally distorting information and denying facts in an attempt to hold onto a certain opinion.

reactive hypoglycemia (HIGH-po-gligh-SEE-mee-uh) Low blood glu-

cose that may follow a meal high in simple sugars, with corresponding symptoms of irritability, headache, nervousness, and sweating. The actual number of cases of this disease in the population is low.

receptive framework for learning The process by which a person opens up to learning more about a problem; it usually involves seeking more information about the issue from books and people. In the case of seeking behavior changes, it involves examining background experiences to evaluate whether a behavior change is feasible.

receptor A site in a cell at which compounds (such as hormones) bind. Cells that contain receptors for a specific compound are partially controlled by that compound.

receptor pathway for cholesterol uptake A process by which LDL molecules (cholesterol-containing) are bound by cell receptors, with the incorporation of the LDL molecule into the cell.

Recommended Dietary Allowances (RDAs) Recommended intakes of nutrients that meet the needs of almost all healthy people of similar age and gender. These are established by the Food and Nutrition Board of the National Academy of Sciences.

Recommended Nutrient Intake (RNI) The Canadian version of RDA.

reduction In chemical terms the gain of an electron by an atom; takes place simultaneously with oxidation (loss of an electron by an atom) in metabolism because an electron that is lost by one atom is accepted by another. In metabolism reduction is often associated with the gain of hydrogen.

Reference Daily Intake (RDI) Standards established by FDA for expressing nutrient content on nutrition labels. RDIs are generally based on the maximum 1968 RDA values set for a nutrient that span a particular age range, such as children over 4 years through adults. *RDI* replaced the term *U.S. RDA*. The RDIs constitute part of the Daily Values used in food labeling.

Registered Dietitian (RD) (dye-eh-TISH-shun) A person who has completed a baccalaureate degree program approved by The American Dietetic Association, performed at least 900 hours of supervised professional practice, and passed a registration examination.

reinforcement A reaction by others in response to a person's behavior. Positive reinforcement entails encouragement; negative reinforcement entails criticism or penalty.

relapse prevention A set of strategies used by people to help prevent and cope with weight control lapses, such as recognizing high-risk situations and deciding beforehand on appropriate responses.

renin (REN-in) An enzyme formed in the kidney in response to low blood pressure; it acts on a blood protein to produce angiotensin I.

requirement The amount of a nutrient required by one person to maintain health. This varies between individuals. We do not know our individual requirements for each nutrient.

reserve capacity The extent to which an organ can preserve essentially normal function despite decreasing cell number or cell activity.

respiration The utilization of oxygen; in the human organism, the inhalation of oxygen and the exhalation of carbon dioxide; in cells, the oxidation (electron removal) of food molecules, particularly in the mitochondria, to obtain energy.

resting metabolic rate The amount of energy used during rest, without stringently controlling recent physical activity. Essentially the same as the basal metabolic rate, but the subject does not need to meet the strict conditions used for a basal metabolic rate determination. Today, both terms are often used interchangeably.

restraint A feeling that occurs as a result of restricted food intake, often associated with the belief that there are good and bad foods.

retinoids (RET-ih-noyds) Chemical forms of preformed vitamin A; one source is animal foods, like liver. Forms include retinol, retinal, and retinoic acid.

reverse transport of cholesterol The process by which cholesterol is picked up by HDL particles and transferred to the liver or to other lipoproteins that can dispose of it in the liver.

rhodopsin (row-DOP-sin) A protein involved in vision; it is made in the eye and incorporates a protein called *opsin* and a form of vitamin A; especially important in night vision.

ribose (RIGH-bos) A five-carbon sugar found in genetic material, specifically RNA.

rickets A disease characterized by softening of the bones because of poor calcium content. This deficiency disease arises in infancy and childhood from insufficient vitamin D activity in the body.

risk factor A characteristic or a behavior that contributes to the chances of developing an illness, such as smoking as a risk factor for developing lung cancer.

runner's anemia (ah-NEE-me-ah) A decrease in the blood's ability to carry oxygen, found in athletes, which may be caused by iron loss through perspiration and feces, red blood cell destruction due to the impact of exercise as the foot strikes the ground, or increased blood volume.

saccharin (SACK-ah-rin) An alternate sweetener that yields no energy to the body; it is 300 times sweeter than sucrose.

saliva (sah-LIGH-vah) A watery fluid produced by the salivary glands in the mouth that contains lubricants, enzymes, and other substances.

salt Generally refers to a compound of sodium and chloride in a 40:60 ratio.

satiety (suh-TIE-uh-tee) State in which there is no longer a desire to eat; a feeling of satisfaction.

saturated fatty acid A fatty acid containing no carbon-carbon double bonds.

scavenger pathway for cholesterol uptake A process by which LDL particles (cholesterol-containing) are taken up by scavenger cells embedded in the blood vessels.

scurvy (SKER-vee) The deficiency disease that results after a few weeks of consuming a diet that lacks vitamin C; pinpoint hemorrhages on the skin are an early sign.

sebaceous glands (seh-BAY-shus) Small glands surrounding hair follicles on the face, ears, chest, eyelid, back, and elsewhere. Blockage of a duct in a sebaceous gland by small particles can lead to an infection and local pressure, resulting in an acne lesion.

sebum (SEE-bum) Secretion of the sebaceous gland, consisting of waxes and various triglycerides.

secondary deficiency A deficiency caused not by lack of the nutrient in question, but by lack of a substance or process that is needed for that nutrient to function.

secondary disease A disease process that develops as a result of another disease.

secretin (SEE-kreh-tin) A hormone that causes bicarbonate ion release from the pancreas.

segmentation Contractions of the circular muscles in the intestines that lead to a dividing and mixing of the intestinal contents. This action aids digestion and absorption of nutrients.

self-monitoring A process of tracking foods eaten and conditions affecting eating; actions are usually recorded in a diary, along with location, time, and state of mind. This is a tool to help a person understand more about his or her eating habits.

self-talk The internal dialogue that each one of us carries on in our heads as we sort out beliefs, feelings, attitudes, and events happening in our lives.

semiessential amino acids Amino acids that, when consumed, spare the need to use an essential amino acid for their synthesis. Tyrosine in the diet, for example, spares the need to use phenylalanine for its synthesis.

sequesterants (see-KWES-ter-ants) Compound that binds free metal ions. By so doing, they reduce the ability of ions to cause rancidity in foods containing fat.

serotonin (ser-oh-TONE-in) A neurotransmitter synthesized from the amino acid tryptophan that appears to both decrease the desire to eat carbohydrates and induce sleep.

serum The portion of the blood fluid remaining after (1) the blood is allowed to clot and (2) the red and white blood cells are removed by centrifugation.

set point Often refers to the close regulation of body weight. It is not known what cells control this set point nor how it actually functions in weight regulation. There is evidence, however, that there are mechanisms that help regulate weight.

short-chain fatty acids Fatty acids that contain fewer than eight carbon atoms.

sickle cell anemia (ah-NEE-me-ah) An anemia that results from a malformation of the red blood cell because of an incorrect primary structure in part of its hemoglobin protein chains. The disease can lead to episodes of severe bone and joint pain, abdominal pain, headache, convulsions, paralysis, and even death.

sign A change in health status that is apparent on physical examination.

slough To shed or cast off.

small-for-gestational age (SGA) (jes-TAY-shun-al) Referring to infants who weigh less than the expected weight for their length of gestation. This corresponds to less than 2.5 kg (5.5 pounds) in a full-term newborn. A preterm infant who is also SGA will most likely develop some medical complications.

sodium bicarbonate An alkaline substance made basically of sodium and carbon dioxide ($NaHCO_3$).

soluble fibers (SOL-you-bull) Fibers that either dissolve or swell when put into water and are metabolized (fermented) by bacteria in the large intestine. These include pectins, gums, mucilages, and some hemicelluloses.

solvent A substance that other substances dissolve in.

sorbitol (SOR-bih-tol) An alcohol derivative of glucose that yields about 3 kcal per gram but is slowly absorbed from the small intestine. It is used in some sugarless gums and dietetic foods.

specific heat Heat required to raise the temperature of 1 g of a substance 1°C. Water has a high specific heat, meaning that a relatively large amount of heat is required to raise its temperature; therefore it tends to resist large temperature fluctuations.

sphincter (SFINK-ter) A muscular valve that controls flow of foodstuff in the GI tract.

spontaneous abortion Any cessation of pregnancy and expulsion of the embryo or nonviable fetus as the result of natural causes, such as a genetic defect or developmental problem; also called *miscarriage*.

spore A dormant reproductive cell capable of forming into an adult organism without the help of another cell. Various fungi and bacteria form spores.

starch A carbohydrate made of multiple units of glucose attached together in a form the body can digest; also known as *complex carbohydrate*.

steroids (STARE-oyds) A group of hormones and related compounds that are derivatives of cholesterol.

sterol A compound containing a multiring (steroid) structure and a hydroxyl group (—OH).

stimulus control Altering the environment to minimize the stimuli for eating; for example, removing foods from sight and storing them in kitchen cabinets.

stomach distention Expansion of the walls of the stomach (intestines as well) from the pressure caused by the presence of gases, food, drink, or other factors.

stress fracture A fracture that occurs from repeated jarring of a bone. Common sites include bones of the foot.

stroke Damage caused by part of the brain caused by interruption to its blood supply or leakage of blood outside vessel walls. Sensation, movement, or function controlled by the damaged area is impaired.

subclinical Not seen on a clinical (physical) examination.

subclinical disease Disease or disorder that is present but not severe enough to produce symptoms that can be detected or diagnosed.

subjects Participants in an experiment.

sucrose (SOO-kros) Fructose bonded to glucose; table sugar.

sugar Simple carbohydrate form with a chemical composition ratio of CH_2O.

superoxide dismutase (soo-per-OX-ide DISS-myoo-tase) An enzyme that can quench (deactivate) a superoxide negative free radical ($\cdot O_2{}^-$). This can contain the minerals manganese, copper, or zinc.

sympathetic nervous system Part of the nervous system that regulates involuntary vital functions, including the activity of the heart, smooth muscles, and adrenal glands. The sympathetic nervous system specifically accelerates heart rate, constricts blood vessels, and raises blood pressure. The parasympathetic nervous system slows heart rate, increases intestinal peristalsis and gland activity, and relaxes sphincters.

symptom A change in health status noted by the person with the problem, such as a stomach pain.

synapse (SIN-aps) Space between nerve cells. One nerve cell stimulates other nearby cells, including other nerve cells, by releasing chemicals that cross the synapse. These chemicals excite neighboring cells.

systolic blood pressure (sis-TOL-lik) The pressure in the arterial blood vessels associated with the pumping of blood from the heart.

teratogen (ter-A-toe-jen) An agent that causes physical defects in a developing fetus.

tertiary structure of a protein (TER-she-air-ee) The three-dimensional structure of a protein, formed by interactions of amino acids placed far apart in the primary structure.

tetany (TET-ah-nee) A state marked by sharp contraction of muscles with failure to relax afterward; usually caused by abnormal calcium metabolism.

theory An explanation for a phenomenon that has numerous lines of evidence to support it.

thermic effect of food The increase in metabolism that occurs during the digestion, absorption, and metabolism of energy-yielding nutrients. This represents about 5% to 10% of energy consumed.

"thrifty" metabolism A metabolism that characteristically uses less energy than normal, such that the risk of weight gain and obesity is enhanced.

thromboxane A stimulant of blood clotting made in the blood from polyunsaturated fatty acids.

thyroid-stimulating hormone A hormone that regulates the uptake of iodide by the thyroid gland and is secreted in response to a low concentration of circulating thyroxine.

tissue A group of cells designed to perform a specific function; muscle tissue is an example.

t-lymphocyte (tee-LYMF-oh-site) White blood cell processed by the thymus gland and responsible for recognition of foreign substances (such as viruses) in intracellular sites in the body.

tocopherol (tuh-KOFF-er-all) The chemical name for some forms of vitamin E. The alpha form is most potent.

tocotrienol (toe-co-TRY-en-ol) Compound related to tocopherol, but differs in the fatty acid side chain on the molecules, in that they contain more carbon-carbon double bonds.

toxic Poisonous; caused by a poison.

toxicity The capacity of a substance to produce injury or illness at some dosage.

toxin A poisonous compound that can cause disease. Some toxins are produced by organisms.

trabecular bone (trah-BEK-you-lar) The spongy, inner matrix of bone, found primarily in the spine, pelvis, and ends of bones.

trace mineral A mineral vital to health that is required in the diet in amounts less than 100 milligram per day.

transamination (trans-am-ih-NAY-shun) The transfer of an amino group from an amino acid to a carbon skeleton to form a new amino acid.

trans **fatty acids** A form of unsaturated fatty acids that, when found in food, is usually a monounsaturated fatty acid. In a *trans* fatty acid, the hydrogens of both carbons that form the double bond lie on opposite sides of the sides of that bond. A cis fatty acid has the hydrogens lying on the same side of the carbon-carbon double bond.

transferrin A blood protein that transports iron in the blood.

triglyceride (try-GLISS-uh-ride) The major form of lipid in the body and in food. It is composed of three fatty acids bonded to glycerol, an alcohol.

trimester The normal pregnancy of 38 to 42 weeks is divided into three 13- to 14-week periods called *trimesters*. Development of the embryo and fetus, however, is continuous throughout pregnancy with no specific physiological markers demarcating the transition from one trimester to the next.

trypsin (TRIP-sin) A protein-digesting enzyme secreted by the pancreas (in a zymo-gen form) that acts in the small intestine.

tumor Mass of cells; may be cancerous (malignant) or noncancerous (benign).

ulcer (UL-sir) Erosion of the tissue lining usually in the stomach (gastric ulcer) or the upper small intestine (duodenal ulcer). These are generally referred to as *peptic ulcers*.

umami A brothy, meaty, savory flavor in some foods. Monosodium glutamate enhances this flavor when added to foods.

undernutrition Failing health that results from a longstanding dietary intake that does not meet nutritional needs.

underwater weighing A method to estimate total body fat by weighing the individual first normally and then when submerged in water. The loss of weight when submerged in water is used to estimate total body fat.

underweight Body weight for height about 15% to 20% below healthy weight, or a body mass index below about 19. These cut-offs are less precise than for obesity because less study of this condition has been undertaken.

upper-body obesity The type of obesity, also called android, in which fat is stored primarily in the abdominal area; defined as a waist-to-hip circumference ratio of greater than 1.0 in men and 0.8 in women; closely associated with a high risk of heart disease, high blood pressure, and diabetes.

urea Nitrogen-containing waste product found in urine. Most nitrogen excreted from the body leaves in this form.

vagus nerves Nerves arising from the brain that branch off to other organs and are essential for control of speech, swallowing, and gastrointestinal function.

variability In a nutritional sense, the variation expected in nutrient requirements in a group of individuals.

vegan (VEE-gun) A person who eats only plant foods.

vegetarian A person who avoids eating animal products to a varying degree, ranging from consuming no animal products to simply not consuming four-footed animal products.

virus The smallest known type of infectious agent, many of which cause disease in humans. They do not metabolize, grow, or move by themselves. They reproduce by the aid of a living cellular host. Viruses are essentially a piece of genetic material surrounded by a coat of protein.

very-low-calorie diet (VLCD) Known also as *protein-sparing modified fast* PSMF), this diet allows a person 400 to 800 kcal per day, often in liquid form. Of this, 120 to 480 kcal is carbohydrate, while the rest is mostly high–biological value protein.

very-low-density lipoprotein (VLDL) The lipoprotein that initially leaves the liver. It carries both the cholesterol and lipid newly synthesized by the liver.

villi (VIL-eye) Fingerlike protrusions into the small intestine that participate in digestion and absorption of foodstuff.

visual cycle A chemical process in the eye that participates in vision. Forms of vitamin A participate in the process.

vitamins Compounds needed in very small amounts in the diet to help regulate and support chemical reactions in the body. Absence from the diet must result in a disease that timely replacement of the vitamin will cure.

water-soluble vitamins Vitamins that dissolve in water. These vitamins are the B vitamins and vitamin C.

whey (WAY) Proteins, such as lactalbumin, that are found in great amounts in human milk and are easy to digest.

white blood cells One of the formed elements of the circulating blood system; also called *leukocytes*. Five types of leukocytes are lymphocytes, monocytes, neutrophils, basophils, and eosinophils. White blood cells are able to squeeze through intracellular spaces and migrate. Leukocytes phagocytize bacteria, fungi, and viruses, as well as detoxify proteins that may result from allergic reactions, cellular injury, and other immune system cells.

whole grains Grains containing the entire seed of the plant, including the bran, germ, and endosperm (starchy interior). Examples are whole wheat and brown rice.

xanthine dehydrogenase (ZAN-thin de-HY-droj-eh-nase) An enzyme containing molybdenum and iron that functions in the formation of uric acid and the mobilization of iron from liver ferritin stores.

xenobiotic (ZEE-no-bye-OT-ic) Com-pound that is foreign to the body. The principal classes are drugs, chemical carcinogens, and environmental substances such as pesticides.

xerophthalmia (zer-of-THAL-mee-uh) Literally "dry eye." This is a cause of blindness that results from infection of the eye coupled with a vitamin A deficiency. The specific cause is linked to a lack of mucus production by the eye, which then leaves it more vulnerable to damage from surface dirt and bacteria.

xylitol (ZIGH-lih-tol) An alcohol derivative of the five-carbon monosaccharide, xylose.

yo-yo dieting The practice of losing weight and then regaining it, only to lose it and regain it again. This practice has been shown to lead to an increased risk for heart disease in some studies.

zymogen (zigh-MO-gin) An inactive form of an enzyme that requires the removal of some minor part of the chemical structure in order for it to work. The zymogen is converted into an active enzyme at the appropriate time, such as when released into the stomach or small intestine.

Credits

Chapter 14

Fig. 14-3. Wolff Communications.
P. 497. CLG Photographics.
P. 518. William Hubbell, Woodfin Camp and Associates.

Chapter 15

Fig. 15-4. CLG Photographics.
P. 542. CLG Photographics.
P. 552, top. Mark Kempf.
P. 552, left. Peter Beck/The Stock Market.
P. 554. Mike Clemmer/Picture Group.
P. 557. From Wong DL: Whaley & Wong's Nursing Care of Infants and Children, ed. 5, St. Louis, 1995, Mosby.

Chapter 16

P. 574. International Diabetes Center, Minneapolis, MN.
P. 589. John Lawlor/The Stock Market.
Fig. 16-6. Ron Chapple/ FPG International.
Fig. 16-7. Miro Vintoniv, The Picture Cube.
P. 607. Stewart Halperin.

Chapter 17

P. 614. Stewart Halperin.
P. 619. Wolff Communications.
Fig. 17-6. Stewart Halperin.
Fig. 17-8. Superstock/Four by Five.

Chapter 18

Fig. 18-1. AP/World Wide Photos.
P. 653. AP/World Wide Photos.
P. 659. AP/World Wide Photos.
Fig. 18-4. Larry Price/The Stock Market.
P. 672. Suzanne L. Murphy, FPG International.
P. 675. Stewart Halperin.
P. 681, left. Andrew Sacks/Tony Stone Images.
Fig. 18-7. Jay Freis/The Image Bank.

INDEX

Median Height and Weight and Recommended Energy Intake, 10th Edition RDAs

Category	Age (years) or condition	Weight (kg)	Weight (lb)	Height (cm)	Height (in)	REE* (kcal/day)	Multiples of REE	Average energy allowance (kcal) Per kg	Average energy allowance (kcal) Per day†
Infants	0-0.5	6	13	60	24	320		108	650
	0.5-1	9	20	71	28	500		98	850
Children	1-3	13	29	90	56	740		102	1300
	4-6	20	44	112	44	950		90	1800
	7-10	28	62	132	52	1130		70	2000
Men	11-14	45	99	157	62	1440	1.70	55	2500
	15-18	66	145	176	69	1760	1.67	45	3000
	19-24	72	160	177	70	1780	1.67	40	2900
	25-50	79	174	176	70	1800	1.60	37	2900
	51+	77	170	173	68	1530	1.50	30	2300
Women	11-14	46	101	157	62	1310	1.67	47	2200
	15-18	55	120	163	64	1370	1.60	40	2200
	19-24	58	128	164	65	1350	1.60	38	2200
	25-50	63	138	163	64	1380	1.55	36	2200
	51+	65	143	160	63	1280	1.50	30	1900
Pregnant	1st trimester								+0
	2nd trimester								+300
	3rd trimester								+300
Lactating	1st 6 months								+500
	2nd 6 months								+500

*Resting energy expenditure (REE); calculation based on FAO equations and then rounded. This is the same as RMR (resting metabolic rate).
†Figure is rounded.

1983 Metropolitan Life Insurance Company Height-Weight Table*†

Height Ft	Height In	WOMEN Frame* Small	WOMEN Frame* Medium	WOMEN Frame* Large	Height Ft	Height In	MEN Frame* Small	MEN Frame* Medium	MEN Frame* Large
4	10	102-111	109-121	118-131	5	2	128-134	131-141	138-150
4	11	103-113	111-123	120-134	5	3	130-136	133-143	140-153
5	0	104-115	113-126	122-137	5	4	132-138	135-145	142-156
5	1	106-118	115-129	125-140	5	5	134-140	137-148	144-160
5	2	108-121	118-132	128-143	5	6	136-142	139-151	146-164
5	3	111-124	121-135	131-147	5	7	138-145	142-154	149-168
5	4	114-127	124-138	134-151	5	8	140-148	145-157	152-172
5	5	117-130	127-141	137-155	5	9	142-151	148-160	155-176
5	6	120-133	130-144	140-159	5	10	144-154	151-163	158-180
5	7	113-136	133-147	143-163	5	11	146-157	154-166	161-184
5	8	126-139	136-150	146-167	6	0	149-160	157-170	164-188
5	9	129-142	139-153	149-170	6	1	152-164	160-174	168-192
5	10	132-145	142-156	152-173	6	2	155-168	164-178	172-197
5	11	135-148	146-159	155-176	6	3	158-172	167-182	176-202
6	0	138-151	148-162	158-179	6	4	162-176	171-187	181-207

*Based on a weight-height mortality study conducted by the Society of Actuaries and the Association of Life Insurance Medical Directors of America, Metropolitan Life Insurance Medical Directors of America, Metropolitan Life Insurance Company, revised 1983.
†Weights at ages 25 to 59 based on lowest mortality. Height includes 1-in heel. Weight for women includes 3 lb. for indoor clothing. Weight for men includes 5 lb. for indoor clothing. (See Chapter 10 for controversy surrounding the use and misuse of this table over the years and Appendix I for determination of frame size.)